Gynecology
Well-woman Care

Ronnie Lichtman, C.N.M., M.S., M.Phil.
Assistant Clinical Professor
Midwifery Program
Columbia University School of Nursing
New York, New York

Staff Midwife
Prevention of Prematurity Program
Harlem Hospital
New York, New York

Private Practice
New York, New York

Susan Papera, C.N.M., M.S.
Staff Midwife
North Central Bronx Hospital
Bronx, New York

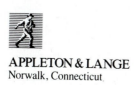

APPLETON & LANGE
Norwalk, Connecticut

0-8385-9682-7

92 93 94 / 10 9 8 7 6 5 4

Prentice Hall International (UK) Limited, *London*
Prentice Hall of Australia Pty. Limited, *Sydney*
Prentice Hall Canada, Inc., *Toronto*
Prentice Hall Hispanoamericana, S.A., *Mexico*
Prentice Hall of India Private Limited, *New Delhi*
Prentice Hall of Japan, Inc., *Tokyo*
Simon & Schuster Asia Pte. Ltd., *Singapore*
Editora Prentice Hall do Brasil Ltda., *Rio de Janeiro*
Prentice Hall, *Englewood Cliffs, New Jersey*

Library of Congress Cataloging-in-Publication Data

Gynecology: well-woman care / [edited by] Ronnie Lichtman, Susan
    Papera.
        p. cm.
    ISBN 0-8385-9682-7
    1. Gynecology. 2. Contraception. I. Lichtman, Ronnie.
    II. Papera, Susan. III. Title: Well-woman care.
    [DNLM: 1. Contraception—methods. 2. Gynecology. WP 100
G997153]
    RG101.G96 1990
    618.1—dc20
    DNLM/DLC
    for Library of Congress   89-17569
                                                                CIP

ISBN 0-8385-9682-7

9 780838 596821   90000

Acquisitions Editor: Marion K. Welch
Production Editor: Lauren Manjoney
Designer: M. Chandler Martylewski
Cover: Janice Barsevich

PRINTED IN THE UNITED STATES OF AMERICA

Contributors

Judith V. Becker, Ph.D.
Director
Sexual Behavior Clinic
New York State Psychiatric Institute
New York, New York

Associate Professor of Clinical Psychiatry
College of Physicians and Surgeons
Columbia University
New York, New York

Heather Clarke, C.N.M., M.S.
Midwife
Maternal-Infant Care/Family Planning Projects
New York, New York

Emily Coleman, M.A.
Coordinator
Sex Offender Program-Forensic Psychiatry Clinic
Bronx Lebanon Hospital
Bronx, New York

Maria Corsaro, C.N.M., M.S.
Staff Midwife
North Central Bronx Hospital
Bronx, New York

Private Practice
Ossining, New York

Cindy Dickinson, C.N.M., M.S., M.P.H.
Midwife
Comprehensive Perinatal Program
San Diego, California

†Therese Dondero, C.N.M., B.S.
Founder and Director
Midwifery Program
North Central Bronx Hospital
Bronx, New York

Founding Partner
Private Midwifery Practice
Hospital of the Albert Einstein College of Medicine
Bronx, New York

Marian E. Dunn, Ph.D.
Director
Center for Human Sexuality
Clinical Associate Professor of Psychiatry
State University of New York
Downstate Medical Center
Brooklyn, New York

Paula Duran, C.N.M., M.S.
Staff Midwife
Columbia Presbyterian Medical Center
New York, New York

Private Practice
Ossining, New York

Doreen C. Harper, R.N.C., A.N.P., Ph.D.
Associate Professor
Coordinator, Nurse Practitioner Programs
George Mason University
   School of Nursing
Fairfax, Virginia

Virginia Jackson, C.N.M., M.S.
Private Practice
Ossining, New York

Ronnie Lichtman, C.N.M., M.S., M.Phil.
Assistant Clinical Professor
Midwifery Program
Columbia University School of Nursing
New York, New York

Staff Midwife
Prevention of Prematurity Program
Harlem Hospital
New York, New York

Private Practice
New York, New York

Patricia Aikins Murphy, C.N.M., M.S.
Staff Midwife
Prevention of Prematurity Program
Harlem Hospital
New York, New York

---

†Deceased

Susan Papera, C.N.M., M.S.
Staff Midwife
North Central Bronx Hospital
Bronx, New York

Dayle Peck, C.N.M., M.S.
Supervisor
Midwifery Services
Jackson Memorial Hospital
Miami, Florida

Adjunct Faculty
University of Miami
Miami, Florida

Sarah G. Potter, M.S.N., C.A.N.P.
Adult Nurse Practitioner
Saint Francis Hospital and Medical Center
Hartford, Connecticut

Sharon Robinson, C.N.M., M.S.
National Executive Director
PUSH for Excellence
Washington, D.C.

Sr. M. Rose Carmel Scalone, R.S.M., C.N.M., M.P.H.
Staff Midwife
Maternity Center Association, Childbearing Center
New York, New York

Joanna Ferber Shulman, M.D.
Director of Obstetrics
North Central Bronx Hospital
Bronx, New York

Suzanne M. Smith, C.N.M., M.S., M.P.H.
Midwife in Private Practice
  with Privileges
Saint Vincent's Hospital
  and Medical Center
New York, New York

Clinical Instructor
New York Medical College
Valhalla, New York

Nancy Sullivan, C.N.M., M.S.
Instructor
Nurse-Midwifery/Women's Health Care
  Nurse-Practitioner Program
Oregon Health Sciences University
Portland, Oregon

Phyllis Turk, C.N.M., M.S.
Assistant Professor
School of Nursing
Radford University
Radford, Virginia

Contents

Preface

When Appleton & Lange approached us to write a textbook on gynecology, we were initially reluctant. A book loomed as a major undertaking in our already busy lives. But after gentle prodding from our editor, Marion Kalstein-Welch, we accepted the task; after all, we had been searching for a more appropriate reference for our gynecology practice and for a comprehensive textbook for our students. Marion agreed that sufficient time would be allotted for manuscript preparation; two years seemed reasonable.

That was five years ago. These have been tumultuous years. We have experienced upheavals in our professional and personal lives, as did many of our contributors—the challenge of career advancement, the deep sorrow of losing a parent and an admired colleague who was also a dear friend, and the indescribable joy and awesome responsibility of having children. Somehow through it all, we produced this book. The book evolved slowly, its content and format, scope and breadth always based on our own practice and teaching needs.

As we prepared each chapter we asked ourselves two questions: What do our students want and need to know? What do we, as experienced practitioners, want and need to know? We thus created a text that directly addresses our unique practice as nonmedical, independent managers of gynecologic care. Specifically, the book:

— provides a framework for clinical management while detailing the scientific background needed to make informed management decisions;
— discusses all components of patient care from teaching and counseling to self-help measures, from prescribing medication to referral for surgical intervention;

— covers in depth the problems that healthy women commonly face, such as vaginitis, premenstrual syndrome, and dysmenorrhea;
— suggests guidelines for consultation and referral for conditions requiring extensive diagnostic testing, medical or surgical management, or both;
— reviews current research findings on topics such as experimental methods of birth control and menopausal hormonal replacement;
— enables the practitioner to answer the increasingly sophisticated questions posed by women;
— offers students a single text that can replace the patchwork bibliography used in gynecology and midwifery courses.

The first section of *Gynecology:Well-woman Care* guides the student and practitioner in developing a general approach to all patients, taking the reader through female anatomy and physiology, and the basics of patient care—history taking, physical examination, and laboratory testing. Subsequent sections are organized according to the needs and problems with which women present for care. This format was chosen because of both its applicability to clinical practice and its usefulness in teaching.

Providing gynecologic care has rewarded us with tremendous satisfaction. It has given us the opportunity to interact with women of all backgrounds and to assist them with basic and often intimate needs—from choosing a contraceptive to adjusting to life changes from adolescence through menopause and beyond. We hope the joy we derive from our practice and the deep respect we have for our patients are communicated throughout this book.

Acknowledgments

A book is always a joint effort. For this one we have many to thank. First and foremost we wish to thank the patients we have seen during our careers as midwives. From them we have learned so much; through them our lives have been enriched. Our second most important teachers have been the midwifery students at Columbia University whom we have had the privilege to teach. They have stimulated our thinking, challenged our assumptions, and always returned to us far more than we ever gave. Of course, thanks are due to our own midwifery teachers at Columbia University, the faculty members of 1976 and 1977, and to the wonderful midwives we have had the honor to be associated with as faculty at Columbia from 1979 through the present. We owe gratitude for our professional growth to the midwives of North Central Bronx Hospital. Most appreciation is due the late Therese Dondero, C.N.M., B.S.; she was, for us both, a model of determination, conviction, and competence; a teacher of clinical excellence; a guide to the development of a clear and committed philosophy of midwifery care; and a dear friend whose passing has deeply saddened the entire midwifery community. We also have been influenced personally and professionally by our sisters involved in the women's movement. Their efforts have inspired our own struggle for women's rights as health care recipients and workers.

A number of physicians have been particularly supportive as consultants for our practice. Outstanding among them are Samuel Oberlander, Jack Maidman, and Steven Swersky.

Special thanks go to Barbara Decker, C.N.M., Ed.D., who recommended us for this book, and to Marion Kalstein-Welch, our editor at Appleton & Lange, whose unfailing enthusiasm and patience kept us going over several very difficult years. Lauren Manjoney, our production editor, is appreciated for her careful attention to the manuscript, her patience, and her good cheer. Our contributing authors must be acknowledged; without them there would be no book. The reviewers whose thoughtful critiques improved the text deserve recognition as well. Several people provided much needed assistance. We gratefully acknowledge Laura and Steven Lichtman, Delroy Williams, Janice Albert, Vernet Brown, Mei Chin, Deborah D'Amico-Samuels, and Julio Perez.

We wish to thank our families and friends, those who understood when we refused invitations because we had work to do, those whom we may have inadvertently neglected, but who never neglected us. They are too numerous to name but special love and appreciation is extended, in addition to those already mentioned, to Daisun Williams, Emanuel and Selma Lichtman, Allan and Kara Lichtman, Theresa Reubel, Vanessa Papera, and Bill Ewing. To Gillian Williams, there are apologies for any divided attention; the book should have been finished before your arrival.

The gestation of this book was marked by a number of births and deaths among its authors and their families. To the newborns, we offer a loving welcome and the hope for a future free from discrimination, poverty, and war. To the deceased, we offer the enduring memory of all they meant to us. We extend a particularly loving thank you to Gertrude Lichtman who generously relinquished time that should have been hers to allow us to work on this project, who offered encouragement and thoughtful suggestions, and who, to our great sorrow, missed the final product.

Introduction

As women have become more aware of their health needs and of the ways in which these needs are to be met, they are redefining the type of health services they seek. As a result, midwives, nurse-practitioners, and physician assistants have become increasingly sought-after providers of women's health care. Educated in a variety of ways, such practitioners represent simultaneously a new direction and a restoration of an age-old tradition of women as healers. In their care, women find an approach that differs from what has become today's conventional medical model, an approach characterized by a focus on health maintenance, rather than disease, by a recognition of each individual as a complete person, rather than a combination of body parts or systems, and by a commitment to return control of health and health care to the patient. It is in support of these concepts that this book has been written.

Because of the need for periodic gynecologic assessment and for reproductive control, many women use gynecologic caregivers as their main source of ongoing health care. We have therefore chosen to call these caregivers *primary women's health care practitioners* or *providers,* terms used interchangeably throughout this text.

This book fills many of the gaps in the literature currently available for women's health care practitioners. It offers a theoretical knowledge base geared toward a focus on health maintenance, using knowledge derived from a number of disciplines, including the self-help and women's movements. It provides a framework for the incorporation of this theory into clinical practice, based on the management process, defined briefly as follows:

1. Collection of data, including historic, physical examination, and laboratory data
2. Assessment of data, particularly with respect to the evaluation of normalcy
3. Development of a management plan
4. Implementation of the management plan. (This includes not only specific treatment, but teaching and counseling, self-help measures, and follow-up care. It may incorporate any or all of the three levels of management: primary management, consultation or co-management, or referral to other care providers or health team members.)
5. Evaluation of care

At the center of all management decisions is the woman who has come for care. Her input, her self-assessment, and her needs and priorities must always determine the services given. *She* is the leader of the health team. We call this a "woman-centered" approach. This can incorporate a family-centered approach, but only as the woman seeking care defines her family or support network and only to the extent that she desires its involvement.

We have chosen to use the term *patient* in referring to the woman seeking care, despite the fact that in most cases we are talking about healthy women. Other terms recently have come into vogue for healthy care seekers, including *consumer* and *client.* Proponents of these terms claim that the word patient connotes a sick person, helpless and dependent, unable to enter into an equal relationship with a health care provider, whereas the terms consumer and client connote a healthy, active participant. We recognize these connotations but we believe the solution lies in changing the reality, not the words.

Neither *consumer* nor *client* conveys the unique relationship that someone has with a health care provider. They merely cover up the sensitive issues involved in this relationship and obviate the attention needed to keep the relationship from becoming one of inequality. They also misrepresent the patient role. A patient is hardly comparable to someone purchasing a car or washing machine, for example. The term *consumer* also implies that power in health care relationships is, or should be, based on financial control, a concept we reject, particularly in our society where the privilege of buying health care is available unequally. Nor is a patient in the same relationship to a health care provider that she is to other professionals in relation to whom she is a client. In no other professional relationship is physical well-being at stake or is body integrity threatened.

We could use words like health care receiver or recipient, which have somewhat neutral connotations, but we wish not to deny the specialness of the health care encounter, nor to use words that, by definition, imply passivity. Instead, we retain the only word that relates specifically to this interaction. We hope our work contributes to the development of new connotations to the term "patient."

In referring to practitioners of well-woman gynecology, we have chosen to use the pronoun "she." This reflects the overwhelmingly female majority among nonphysician providers of well-woman gynecology.

We have chosen to call this text, *Gynecology: Well-woman Care.* To some, this may be a contradiction. Gynecology is, by definition (from *Taber's Cyclopedic Medical Dictionary,* 14th edition, 1981, F. A. Davis, Philadelphia) "The study of the diseases of the female reproductive organs, including the breasts" (p. G-50). How then can there be "well-woman" gynecology? We are not "gynecologists"; we are not specialists in "diseases" of the female reproductive system. We are specialists in its health maintenance and experts at screening for disease processes. There is no adequate terminology for this function as it relates to women in particular; there is no distinct name for this body of knowledge. In the past, midwifery programs have used life-cycle terminology and have called this phase of health care "interconceptional care." We object to this because it defines women by the process of conception. Many women are not "interconceptional"; they may be pre- or postconceptional or they may choose never to utilize their capability to conceive or be physiologically unable to do so. We refuse to use any terminology that defines women by their reproductive function. The term *gynecology* refers to the body system itself, not necessarily to its reproductive function.

Well-woman is not intended as an exclusionary term. A woman with a chronic illness, either in the reproductive tract, such as genital herpes, or outside the reproductive system, such as asthma, for which ongoing medical care has been obtained, may certainly choose nonphysician care for her gynecologic health maintenance. We believe that this type of care should be available to all women who seek it. Well-woman excludes only the independent management of serious medical or gynecologic conditions that require medical or surgical interventions for diagnosis or therapy.

Scope of Practice

The questions of how to define "serious medical or gynecologic conditions" and how to decide when consultation and/or referral is appropriate present many problems for nonphysician health care providers. This text does not resolve these issues. Research on what types of problems can be managed effectively by nonphysicians is lacking. The role and scope of practice of primary care women's health providers are defined differently in various educational programs, practice settings, and geographic regions. They are continually evolving. Throughout this book, in section introductions, specific chapters, and several appendices, implicit and explicit clarification of the nonphysician role in gynecologic health is provided. Undoubtedly, over time, components of this role will be refined.

Individual practitioners also have preferences for the degree of independence they wish to assume. Experience often dictates the degree of independence of which one is capable. In some states, specific functions are legislated or regulated; we urge each practitioner to become familiar with particular state laws, codes, and regulations governing her practice.

Organization of the Book

The organization of this book certainly attests to the broad scope of practice of nonphysician women's health care providers and its content speaks to the depth of our knowledge. We have chosen to organize *Gynecology: Well-woman Care* according to needs and problems that women present to gynecologic care providers. Section I, "Assessment," begins with a description of the anatomy and physiology of the female reproductive system, an understanding of which provides the basis for practice. This section then offers an overview of the first step in the management process: data collection, including history taking, physical examination, and laboratory testing. These areas together constitute the totality of health screening and the foundation from which all subsequent intervention is determined.

Section II, "Contraception," deals with a large component of practice in women's health: the provision of contraceptive services. Each chapter is devoted to a particular category of birth control method with the final chapter outlining what we can expect in the future. The introduction to Section II delineates issues in family planning and concepts that apply to all methods: utilization of birth control methods, contraceptive efficacy, informed consent, risk–benefit ratio, decision making, and self-assessment.

Section III, "Gynecologic Pathophysiology," discusses selected gynecologic diseases and disorders. This section is organized anatomically with a chapter devoted to sexually transmitted diseases (STDs). The introduction to this section concerns the role of the well-woman gynecologic practitioner in dealing with pathophysiology. It offers an evolving framework, developed empirically, for decision-making regarding the implementation of levels of management: primary, co-management or consultation, and referral. Using this framework, each practitioner can assess her own role in providing care and individualizing it to meet the needs of each patient.

Section IV, "Menstrual Issues," is devoted to problems relating to the menstrual cycle. Although some of these fall into the category of pathology, this is a separate section for several reasons. First, menstruation is a part of every woman's life whether it proceeds normally or not. It is crucial for women's health care practitioners to understand the great varieties of normalcy in menstruation and to promptly recognize abnormalities. Second, the most common problems related to menstruation may not be pathologic. The meaning of dysmenorrhea or premenstrual syndrome, for example, may vary among women faced with these conditions; most, however, do not consider themselves ill. Finally, because the physiology of menstruation is multisystem, disorders of menstruation do not easily lend themselves to the anatomic classification used for the section on pathology.

Section V, "Developmental Issues," singles out several developmental stages in the life-cycle that bear particular significance to women and to their health care providers: puberty and adolescence, the postpartum period, and the perimenopausal and aging years. All women face adolescence, menopause, and aging; most face pregnancy and the postpartum period. There are many other developmental issues that women confront such as marriage, divorce, becoming widowed, and career entry and change. Although an ability to relate to women during any potential developmental change or crisis is valuable for all health care practitioners, we have chosen to focus on those that have the most direct bearing on gynecologic health. While this book does not cover pregnancy, we do include the care of the postpartum woman in this section. In some hospitals or clinics, postpartum care is provided in gynecology or family planning setting. The practitioner working in these areas must be able to address the unique needs of the postpartum woman and family. Sometimes, ongoing postpartum care is needed beyond the routine examination at 4 or 6 weeks after delivery; this may not be provided by maternity practitioners, or a woman chooses to return to her former health care provider for these services. As the chapter on the postpartum period clearly demonstrates, postpartum adjustment is not necessarily limited to 6 weeks; women continue their emotional and physical adjustment to this tremendous change for many months. Prepregnancy screening and counseling is also an important issue for women's health care providers; this is discussed in Chapter 2, "The Well-woman Gynecologic Interview," and Chapter 4, "Laboratory Testing."

The final section of this book, "The Supportive Role," addresses topics which generally are not managed by the primary women's health care provider, although her input may be vital to patients facing problems and/or decision-making within these areas. The introduction to this section describes our reasons for choosing to place certain functions in this category and discusses the circumstances under which a practitioner may assume greater responsibility in these ares. The usual role of primary care practitioners in relation to sexuality, sexual abuse, infertility, abortion, and sterilization consists of screening, teaching and counseling, support, referral, and post-procedure care. We refer practitioners who wish to become more involved in the direct provision of care in any of these areas to gynecology or specialized textbooks for further information.

We also suggest that readers wishing to clarify or expand their practice roles refer to Appendices I and II. Appendix I, "American College of Nurse-midwives, Core Competencies," comprises two parts. Part A, "Nurse-midwivery, Management," delineates levels of management, and Part B, "Components of Nurse-midwifery Care, Family Planning/Gynecologic Care," outlines the *basic* knowledge in well-woman gynecology expected of a graduate of a midwifery educational program in the United States. Appendix II, "Guidelines for the Incorporation of New Procedures Into Nurse-midwifery Practice," also provided by the American College of Nurse-midwives, offers guidelines for expanding clinical practice. Other professional organizations may have similar standards and guidelines, and we encourage familiarity with those appropriate for each type of provider.

An additional appendix is included in the text. Appendix III presents a framework for the differential diagnosis of two common gynecologic problems: lower abdominal or pelvic pain and vaginal discharge. This appendix assists the practitioner in incorporating material contained in a number of chapters into the management process as utilized in clinical practice.

Literature Reviews

Many of the chapters in this text reflect extensive literature reviews from a variety of sciences. These include nursing, midwifery, medicine, epidemiology, psychology, sociology, anthropology, and feminism. In certain areas, we were struck by a relative dearth of nursing literature, particularly literature derived from research. We hope this text will offer encouragement to nurses to become increasingly involved in the development of the body of knowledge of well-woman gynecology.

In many chapters we have included in-depth discussions of current research on selected topics. These lengthy reviews have been provided to prepare the practitioner to discuss controversial areas with women and to provide guidance for informed patient decision-making. An example of such an area is hormonal replacement therapy, reviewed in Chapter 24, or treatment for premenstrual syndrome, a large focus of Chapter 19. While these may provide somewhat tedious reading at times, we strongly believe that practice and patient teaching must be based upon familiarity with research findings. Women today are highly aware of health issues and knowledgeable about them; the

practitioner must be able to address complex patient concerns. Information presented in this text, of course, must be supplemented by continual reading about new developments.

Philosophic Approaches in Gynecology Practice

Influence of the Women's Movement

In the mid- and late-1960s, women in the United States, and, indeed, throughout the world, began an organized struggle against sexist biases in society. Health care has been a major focus of this widely-supported movement with particular emphasis against patronizing attitudes of health care providers, unsafe but profitable practices, inequities of class and race, and the escalating emphasis on drugs and technology. This movement has inspired an increased awareness about health issues among many women and has encouraged large numbers of women to enter the health professions in a variety of capacities. It has influenced many aspects of health care and has fostered a long overdue recognition among health providers of the validity of issues raised both by individual women and by advocacy groups such as the National Women's Health Network.

The women's movement has taken two distinct, although complementary, directions. One thrust is the effort to create change within the health care system. The other is the self-help movement out of which has grown a sense of control over health among individuals and a network of alternative, women-directed institutions for health care delivery. Feminist health collectives and birthing centers are examples of these. We support both components of the feminist health movement; both have contributed to improving women's health and health care.

Self-help

Throughout the text, we refer to the concept of self-help. Self-help refers to particular practices, performed outside the professional encounter, whose purposes are the maintenance of health and the prevention or treatment of disease. For patients, self-help involves a continuum of attitudes and activities. Activities vary from minimal endeavors such as keeping written menstrual diaries, recording and reporting troublesome symptoms, or taking medications as prescribed to extensive involvements such as performing regular self speculum examinations, perhaps in the context of a support group. In between these ends of the spectrum lie such pursuits as practicing monthly self breast examination, correlating psychological, nutritional, stress, and other factors to premenstrual syndrome, developing and following nutritional programs, exercising regularly, making conscious efforts to improve communication within family or other support networks, and implementing stress reduction modalities. The extent to which an individual wishes to participate in self-help activities will vary according to interest, philosophy, past experience, the degree of troublesome symptoms, personal locus of control, age and maturity, cultural and educational background, current life circumstances, and the value given to self-help by significant others, including health practitioners.

We urge practitioners to incorporate discussions of self-help measures into all health care visits and to stress their value in the promotion and maintenance of health. Discussion should follow an assessment of the extent of a woman's involvement in self-help. It should then focus on assisting the woman to recognize her philosophies of health and to develop ways to increase or initiate self-help activities. Specific suggestions can be made and resources such as support groups and literature offered. The patient will accept or reject suggestions according to their compatibility with her abilities, life-style, and value system. She may choose self-help measures outside the realm of current scientifically-accepted health care. The practitioner can then review the practice, reinforce its potential benefits, and warn the patient about any possibly harmful effects. When the practitioner is unfamiliar with a given practice, it should be investigated. Alternative approaches can be offered. Each woman's decisions, however, must be respected.

Self-help measures do not replace practitioner-initiated health assessments and interventions. Self assessment for oral contraceptive danger signs, for example, is supplementary to, not instead of, practitioner assessment; self breast examination is not a substitute for regularly scheduled practitioner breast examination; knowledgeable patients continue to deserve careful teaching and counseling.

Holism

Although this book is limited to gynecologic health, we do not wish to imply that a woman consists only of her reproductive system or is defined or limited by its function. Throughout the text, we have borrowed many tenets from the holistic health care movement. These tenets hold that health or its lack in any body system is related to a vast number of influences including psychological, interpersonal cultural, and societal. A homeless person, for example, can't possibly follow advice to rest in bed; a woman with three small children may have difficulty reducing stress; a woman living without running water may find a diaphragm impossible to use safely. We believe that all such factors must be considered in assessing health and implementing interventions. For this reason, we have devoted entire chapters to the complete health history and physical examination and, in all chapters, have related social, psychological, family, and other issues to gynecologic practice.

This book does not separate the needs of women according to life-style, background, or degree of disability. We realize that these affect people, often profoundly. We realize, too, that no individual is bound by any of these conditions or circumstances. We have chosen not to emphasize differences among women, although we recognize their reality, because we believe that an understanding of the general health needs of women provides a strong base from which to adapt care for each individual. Flexibility and sensitivity are qualities that all health care providers must develop. We must be able to provide services without prejudice to women of all races, ethnicities, and cultural groups, socio-economic backgrounds and statuses. Whether a woman is single, married, separated, divorced, or widowed, heterosexual or lesbian, whether she lives alone, with a husband, a woman friend or friends, a male or female lover, or with a group, she must be seen as the unique person that she is. Whether she chooses to have children or not, how she chooses to do this, and how she defines her family are decisions mediated by society, culture, and technology, but ultimately made by the individual. Since many life-style decisions affect gynecologic health care, they should be discussed with patients, but never disrespected. An open approach to care and to people will enable the provider to serve a diverse group of women. For us, this is the challenge and the joy in being a women's health care provider.

Ronnie Lichtman, C.N.M., M.S., M.Phil.
Susan Papera, C.N.M., M.S.

SECTION I

Assessment

The Basis for Practice

An understanding of the body is the basis from which all health care derives. For this reason, we begin this book with a description of the female reproductive system, both anatomically and physiologically, for it is largely this system that makes women's health a distinct body of knowledge. Without this understanding, the practitioner's capability is limited.

Essential, too, for practice is the ability to collect data, to understand an individual woman's particular problems and needs. This section, therefore, devotes one chapter each to the three ways we learn about our patients—interview and history-taking, physical examination, and laboratory studies. From the data derived through these three modalities, the practitioner formulates the differential diagnosis and, ultimately, the diagnosis. Data collection must therefore be painstaking and thorough. The ability to collect a meaningful data base while maintaining sensitivity to the woman as a whole person is an essential clinical skill.

We have chosen to present a conventional medical description of the female reproductive system. We acknowledge, however, the work that various segments of the women's movement have done in extending our appreciation and understanding of women's bodies and in formulating "a new view of a woman's body."

An alternative interpretation of female anatomy has been proposed by a group of feminists involved in women's health care, the Federation of Feminist Women's Health Centers. They have expanded the traditional view of the clitoris to include additional external and internal structures. According to their analysis, the outer, visible portion of the clitoris includes the frenulum, the opening to the vagina, the hymen, the fourchette, the perineum, and the urethra. Several pelvic muscles and ligaments are seen as part of this organ: the anal sphincter, the transverse perineal, ischiocavernosus, and bulbocavernosus muscles, and the round and suspensory ligaments. In addition, these authors identify two types of internal erectile tissue as belonging to the clitoris. One is a soft tissue pad surrounding the urethra. They call this the *urethral sponge*. (It is possible that this pad corresponds to the G-spot; see Chapter 1, p. 5.) The other, comprising the lower border of the clitoris, lies between the anus and vagina and has been labeled the *perineal sponge*. For more discussion of this reinterpretation of women's anatomy and for drawings based upon it, see the illustrated guide, *A new view of a woman's body* (Federation of Feminist Women's Health Centers, published by Simon and Schuster, New York, 1981).

Although many health care providers may reject the analysis of the Federation of Women's Health Centers, we believe it behooves all practitioners to become aware of the philosophies and perspectives put forth by the women's health movement. Such an awareness expands our viewpoints and increases our sensitivity to patient concerns.

Whichever view one accepts of women's anatomy, it is important to recognize that the fundamentals for the provision of quality care come from learning fully about the system around which the care is based and from gaining proficiency in methods of data collection around which management is developed.

1

Anatomy and Physiology of the Female Reproductive System

Patricia Aikins Murphy

To present information useful to the practitioner, health care textbooks must divide the body into component parts. To fully appreciate each part, however, the practitioner must be able to conceptualize the whole; gynecologic practice requires an understanding of the anatomic relationships of the reproductive organs to each other, and the interactions between organs and systems that enable cohesive functioning.

This chapter reviews the anatomy of the female reproductive organs, including the external and internal genitalia and the breast. It discusses the functioning of the reproductive system, describing the neuroendocrine control of the menstrual cycle and detailing components of the ovarian and uterine cycles, and the effects of reproductive physiology on other body organs. Changes during the life cycle will be discussed briefly.

ANATOMY

The female reproductive organs are housed within the pelvis, a bony basin consisting of (1) the ilium, ischium, and pubis, which are fused into one structure surrounding the acetabulum; (2) the sacrum; and (3) the coccyx. These bones are linked by the symphysis pubis, the sacrococcygeal joint, and the sacroiliac joint (Fig. 1–1). Pelvic stability is maintained by sacroiliac, sacrospinous, and sacrotuberous ligaments.

External Genitalia

The term *vulva* refers to the structures that are visible externally in the perineal region (the area limited anteriorly by the symphysis pubis, posteriorly by the buttocks, and laterally by the thighs). The following structures are included (Figs. 1–2 and 1–3).

The *mons pubis* is a fatty tissue prominence overlying the symphysis. It is covered with coarse, curly pubic hair that forms the escutcheon which appears as a flattened inverted triangle over the symphysis. The appearance of this female escutcheon may vary in some women. The *labia majora* are two longitudinal folds of adipose tissue extending from the mons to enclose the *labia minora* and the structures in the vestibule (the area containing the urethral and vaginal openings). In nulliparous women, the *labia majora* are usually closely apposed; in multiparous women they may gape. The mons and the labia majora are well supplied with

sweat glands, blood and lymphatic vessels, and nerves. The outer surface of the labia is covered with pubic hair, which may extend out to the thighs in some women. The *labia minora* are thin firm folds of skin, inside and parallel to the majora. Anteriorly they form the clitoral hood (prepuce) and frenulum, then split to enclose the vestibule. The labia minora contain no hair follicles, are rich in sebaceous glands, and are well endowed with blood vessels and nerves, functioning as erectile tissue during sexual intercourse. In some women the minora are hidden by the labia majora; in others, they may protrude somewhat. Although they are paired structures, they may not be symmetric in appearance.

The *clitoris* is a small, cylindrical erectile organ. The internal structure consists of two crura covered by fibrous tissue and attached to the inferior pubic ramus. These crura converge to form the clitoral body, which contains the corpora cavernosa, that consists of two erectile structures. The body extends downward beneath the prepuce, ending in the glans. The glans, visible externally, lies between the prepuce and the frenulum. The clitoris is supplied by a branch of the pudendal nerve and is richly supplied with sensory nerve endings responsive to varying types of mechanical and psychoemotional stimuli.

The *vestibule* lies between the clitoris and the fourchette, which is a slightly raised ridge of tissue marking the posterior joining of the labia; the vestibule is bounded by the labia minora. Within the vestibule are the *urethral meatus*; the orifices of the *Skene's or paraurethral gland* on either side of the urethral opening; the orifices of the *Bartholin's glands* that are found at five and seven o'clock between the hymen and the labia minora; the *hymen*, a thin membranous fold of tissue over the vaginal opening; and the *vaginal opening* itself. In parous or sexually active women, the hymen may exist only as small tags of skin. The *fossa navicularis*, usually obliterated by childbirth, is found between the vaginal opening and the fourchette. Just beneath the vestibule are the *vestibular bulbs*, highly vascular tissue that becomes congested during sexual excitement.

Perineal Muscles

Superior to these external structures is the internal perineum, bounded by the symphysis pubis, the ischiopubic rami, the ischial tuberosities, the sacrum, and the coccyx (Fig. 1–4). The perineum is divided into an anterior urogenital diaphragm and a posterior anal triangle. The anterior

3

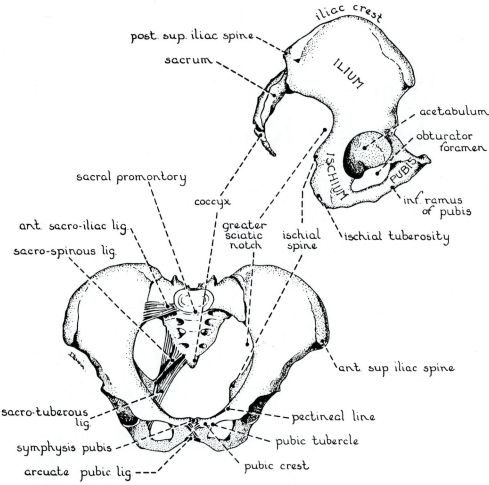

Figure 1–1. Bones and joints of the pelvis. *(From Oxorn, H., & Foote N. R. [1980].* Human Labor and Birth *[4th ed.]. New York: Appleton-Century-Crofts, p. 4.)*

muscles of the perineum include the *bulbocavernosus*, which surrounds the vagina and acts as a weak vaginal sphincter, reacting during sexual excitement by compressing the vestibular bulbs and the dorsal vein, promoting clitoral erection; the *ischiocavernosus*, which overlies the clitoral crura, compressing it when contracted to cause clitoral erection; and the *superficial and deep transverse perineal* muscles that blend with the *urethral sphincter*. The posterior muscles are the *external anal sphincter* and the *anococcygeal body*. The central point of the perineum is a fibrous structure formed by the common attachments of the bulbocavernosus, the superficial and deep transverse perineal muscles, the external anal sphincter muscles, and two levator ani muscles. (In obstetrics, this point is often referred to as the perineum.)

Pelvic Floor

Superior to the perineum are the structures of the pelvic floor or diaphragm, which separates the pelvic cavity from the perineal structures (Fig. 1–5). This diaphragm is a ''hammock'' of muscle extending from the pelvic brim to the sacrum and coccyx, and serves to support the pelvic organs. It is composed of the *levators ani* that consist of the *pubococcygeus* and *iliococcygeus* muscles, and the *ischiococcygeus* muscle. The pubococcygeus is further divided into the *pubovaginalis*, *puborectalis*, and *pubococcygeus proper*; these muscles are a dynamic and specialized part of the pelvic floor and may sustain damage in childbirth. The pubovaginalis is the actual vaginal sphincter, which acts as a sling for the vagina, and is the main muscular support of the pelvic organs. Damage to this muscle may result in cystocele, rectocele, or uterine prolapse. The puborectalis and pubococcygeus proper function to control the descent and passage of feces. Endopelvic fascia, connective tissue that forms a sheath for these muscles, also serves to support the pelvic organs. The iliococcygeus muscle functions primarily as a musculofascial layer, while the ischiococcygeus serves to supplement the levator ani.

Internal Organs

The *vagina* is a musculomembranous canal that connects the uterus to the external perineal area (Fig. 1–6). It is lined with mucous membrane of stratified squamous epithelium containing considerable amounts of glycogen. The normal bacterial flora of the vagina (lactobacilli) metabolize the glycogen, producing lactic acid and maintaining the vaginal pH in the acid range.

Normally reddish pink in color, vaginal tissue will take on a purplish hue with vasocongestion during sexual re-

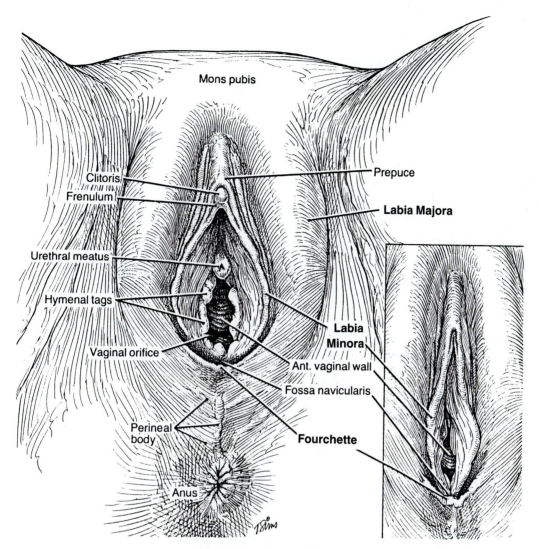

Figure 1-2. External organs of reproduction of women. The lower anterior vaginal wall is visible through the labia minora. In nulliparous women, the vaginal orifice is not so readily visible (inset) because of the close apposition of the labia minora. *(From Pritchard, J., Mac-Donald, P., & Gant, N. (1985). Williams Obstetrics [17th ed.]. East Norwalk, CT: Appleton-Century-Crofts, p. 8.)*

sponse or in pregnancy. Numerous ridges, or rugae, give the vaginal walls an almost corrugated appearance; these may fade gradually with repeated childbirth and after menopause.

The vagina is surrounded by the fascia and muscles of the pelvic diaphragm and perineum. Its collapsed length is 9 to 10 cm posteriorly and 6 to 7 cm anteriorly, inclining at about a 45° angle. The uterine cervix enters the upper vagina anteriorly, creating vaginal recesses around the cervix that are called *fornices.* The posterior fornix is separated from the rectum by a pouch called the *cul-de-sac.*

The vagina has great distensive capability during childbirth and sexual response, both lengthening and ballooning out, causing a loss of rugae. There are fewer nerve endings here than in other organs of sexual response; however, there are deep pressure receptors in the innermost vagina (Masters & Johnson, 1966). Some researchers also describe an area found about 2 inches inside the anterior vaginal wall that is extremely sensitive to pressure. This is known

as the *Gräfenberg spot* (G-spot). Stimulation of this area may lead to orgasm and ejaculation of a liquid through the urethra (Ladas, Whipple, & Perry, 1982). There is an extensive vascular supply, including a large venous plexus surrounding the vagina. Transudation from this plexus provides lubrication, especially during the excitement phase of sexual response.

The *uterus* (Figs. 1-7 and 1-8) is a pear-shaped, hollow muscular organ divided into the body and the cervix. The cervix, or lower neck of the uterus, is visible and palpable in the upper vagina; it is an oval structure, often pinker than the vaginal mucosa and firmer to touch because of the presence of more connective tissue. The cervical opening or os communicates to the inner uterus and is visible on the surface of the cervix as a small round opening in nulliparous women or as a slit-shaped, patulous or irregular opening in women who have borne children (Fig. 1-9). The outer cervix is composed of smooth, pink, stratified squamous epithelium of several layers: a thin basement mem-

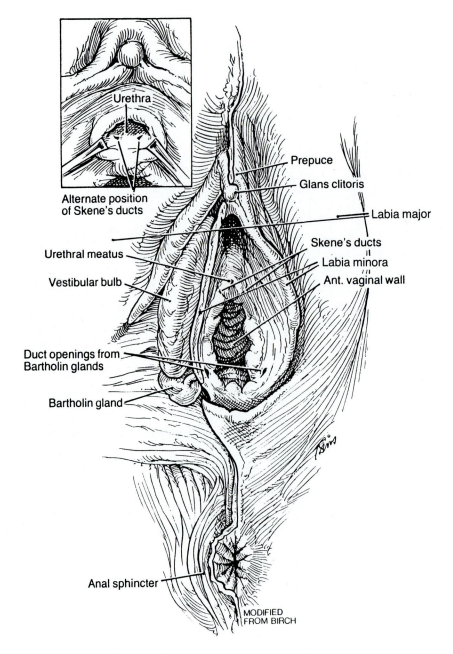

Urethra

Alternate position
of Skene's ducts

Prepuce

Glans clitoris

Labia major

Urethral meatus

Skene's ducts

Vestibular bulb

Labia minora

Ant. vaginal wall

Duct openings from
Bartholin glands

Bartholin gland

Anal sphincter

MODIFIED
FROM BIRCH

Figure 1–3. The external genitalia with the skin and subcutaneous tissue removed from the right side. *(From Pritchard, J., MacDonald, P., & Gant, N. [1985].* Williams Obstetrics *[17th ed.]. East Norwalk, CT: Appleton-Century-Crofts. p. 10.)*

brane, or basal layer, where mitosis occurs, and intermediate and superficial layers rich in glycogen. The superficial layer undergoes regular desquamation. Secretory endocervical glands produce mucus that changes in character under the influence of the menstrual cycle. Obstruction of these gland ducts produces Nabothian cysts on the surface of the cervix.

The endocervical canal connects the external os and the internal os that lies within the isthmus of the uterus. It is lined with tall, mucus-secreting columnar epithelium that appears as red "lumpy" tissue. This tissue may undergo squamous metaplasia if exposed to the acid pH of the va-

gina. The junction of squamous and columnar cells on the cervix is called the *squamocolumnar junction* and may be found within the endocervix or visible on the external cervix. The area of active squamous metaplasia in this junction is called the *transformation zone* and is thought to be particularly susceptible to neoplastic and carcinogenic changes (Martin, 1978).

The body of the uterus lies between the bladder and the rectum, usually at a right angle to the vagina. It may vary from 6 to 9 cm in length, 4 to 6 cm in width, and 2 to 4 cm in thickness; in parous women it may be slightly larger. Uterine position may be anteverted (inclined toward the

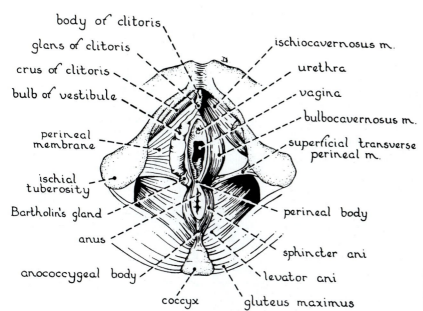

Figure 1–4. Perineal Muscles. *(From Oxorn, H., & Foote, N. R. [1980]. Human Labor and Birth [4th ed.]. East Norwalk, CT: Appleton-Century-Crofts. p. 11.)*

bladder), retroverted (inclined toward the rectum), or mid-position. Flexion refers to the relationship of the uterine body to the cervix: in anteflexion the anterior surface of the uterus inclines toward the cervix and in retroflexion the posterior surface is inclined toward the cervix. The uterus is commonly anteverted and slightly anteflexed.

The uterine body consists of the isthmus (just superior to the cervix), the corpus or main body, and the fundus (the portion across the top of the uterus between the insertion of the fallopian tubes). The thick-walled uterus is covered externally by peritoneum, composed of thick, myometrial muscle fibers, and lined by endometrium over stromal connective tissue. The endometrium is an inner mucous surface of high columnar cells that varies in composition under the influence of menstrual cycle changes. It is composed of three layers: the basalis, the spongiosa, and the compacta. Two groups of blood vessels supply the endometrium: straight basal arteries supply the basal third, and coiled, or spiral, arteries supply the middle spongiosa and superficial

compacta. These latter two layers are the most responsive to hormonal stimulation.

The uterus is not a fixed, but rather a mobile organ, and is supported, in part, by the muscles and fascia of the pelvic floor and perineum, and also by the cardinal, round, utero-sacral, and broad ligaments. Sensory nerve supply arises from the uterovaginal and hypogastric plexuses. Sensory nerves from the cervix arise from the sacral nerves.

The *fallopian tubes* are musculomembranous oviducts enclosed by the broad ligament and are responsible for the transport of ova from ovary to uterus. They attach in the upper uterus and run laterally for 10 to 12 cm to the ovaries. They consist of an interstitial portion within the uterine wall, a narrow isthmus, and a wider ampulla, and end in a funnel-shaped fimbriated structure partially projected around the ovary. The tubes are composed of inner and outer serous layers that surround layers of involuntary muscle. The inner tubes are lined with cilia that assist in ova transport.

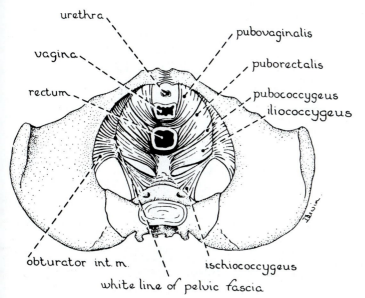

Figure 1–5. Pelvic floor. *(From Oxorn, H., & Foote, N. R. [1980]. Human Labor and Birth [4th ed.], New York: Appleton-Century-Crofts. p. 7).*

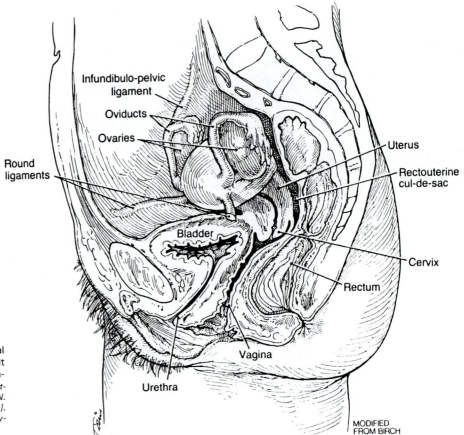

Infundibulo-pelvic
ligament

Oviducts

Ovaries

Round
ligaments

Bladder

Uterus

Rectouterine
cul-de-sac

Cervix

Rectum

Vagina

Urethra

MODIFIED
FROM BIRCH

Figure 1–6. Internal organs. Sagittal section of the pelvis of an adult woman that is illustrative of relations of the pelvic viscera. *(From Pritchard, J., MacDonald, P., & Gant, N. [1985]. Williams Obstetrics [17th ed.]. East Norwalk, CT: Appleton-Century-Crofts, p. 8.)*

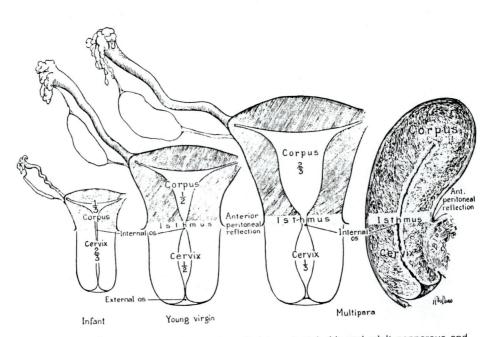

Corpus

Corpus
⅓
Corpus

Corpus
½

Corpus
⅔

Ant.
peritoneal
reflection

Isthmus

Internal os

Cervix
⅔

Anterior
peritoneal
reflection

Isthmus

Cervix
½

Isthmus

Internal
os

Cervix
⅓

Isthmus

Cervix

External os

Infant

Young virgin

Multipara

Figure 1–7. Comparison of the size of uteri of prepubertal girls and adult nonparous and parous women by frontal and sagittal sections. *(From Pritchard, J., MacDonald, P., & Gant, N. [1985]. Williams Obstetrics [17th ed.]. East Norwalk, CT: Appleton-Century-Crofts. p. 8.)*
(From Oxorn, H., & Foote, N. R. [1980].

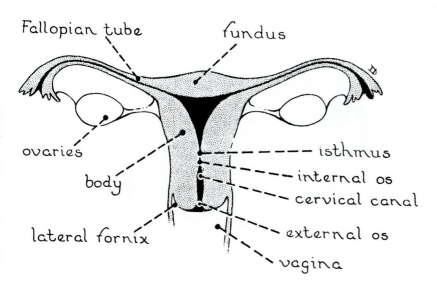

Figure 1–8. Uterus, cervix, vagina. *(From Oxorn, H., & Foote, N. R. [1980]. Human Labor and Birth [4th ed.]. New York: Appleton-Century-Crofts. p. 17.)*

The *ovaries* (Figs. 1-6, 1-8, and 1-14) are paired organs found near the fimbriated ends of the fallopian tubes. Measuring approximately 3 to 4 cm in length, 2 cm in width, and 1 to 2 cm thick, they are supported by the ovarian and suspensory (infundibulopelvic) ligaments. The inner ovary, or medulla, is composed of blood and lymphatic vessels, connective tissue, and nerve fibers. The outer ovary, or cortex, contains the ovarian follicles and is influenced by hormonal stimulation during the menstrual cycle.

Anatomy of the Breast

The breasts are modified sebaceous glands composed of glandular tissue, supporting connective tissue, and protective fatty tissue (Figs. 1-10, and 1-11). Each breast occupies a roughly circular space that is anterior to the pectoral muscles, extending from the second to the sixth ribs, and from the sternum to the midaxillary line. Glandular tissue may extend into the axilla. They are usually symmetric in size and shape, although it is not uncommon for one to be slightly larger than the other.

The mammary glands begin to develop in the early embryo, arising from a line of glandular tissue called the *mammary ridge* or "milk line," (see Fig. 10-4) that extends from the axilla to the groin. The breast and nipple buds will develop from one papilla along this line; other rudimentary papillae will generally atrophy later in embryonic life. In some women, vestiges of this ridge may be seen in the form of supernumerary nipples and breast tissue.

The size and shape of the breast varies greatly among women. Nonpregnant size may be influenced by heredity, nutrition, and cyclic fluctuations of the hormonal cycle.

Shape of the breast may vary during the life cycle, from conically protuberant in adolescents, to hemispheric in young and middle-aged women, to pendulous in older women.

The skin overlying the breast is similar to that of the abdomen, with some hair follicles around the central areola, which is a circular pigmented area surrounding the nipple. The nipple is a conical elevation containing milk ducts, sensory nerve endings, and smooth muscle fibers that contract with temperature, touch, or sexual stimulation. *Montgomery glands* are sebaceous glands opening into the areola; these may enlarge during pregnancy to look like nodules.

Each breast is composed of 15 to 20 lobes. Each lobe has a duct opening in the nipple; beneath the areola, these ducts dilate to form the lactiferous sinuses. Beyond the sinuses, the lobes branch to form 20 to 40 lobules; each lobule is subdivided into many secretory alveoli. The lobes are surrounded by, and embedded in, adipose tissue. Breast contour is largely due to the subcutaneous fat tissue. Fibrous connective tissue called *Cooper's ligaments* (Fig. 10-1), supports the mammary gland; affixing it to the overlying skin and retromammary fascia. The breast is further supported by muscles attaching to the ribs and clavicles.

Arterial and venous blood supply arises primarily from branches of the internal mammary, thoracic, and intercostal vessels, (Fig. 10-2). Lymphatic drainage, of concern in the metastasis of breast cancer, is abundant. The main flow is toward the axilla and anterior axillary nodes, but lymph drainage has been shown to pass in all directions from the breast; toward the opposite breast, the epigastric plexus, and the clavicular nodes (Fig. 1-12).

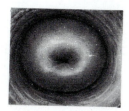

Cervical external os of a nonparous woman.

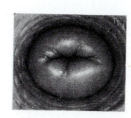

Cervical external os of a parous woman

Figure 1–9. External os of cervix. *(From Pritchard, J., MacDonald, P., & Gant, N. [1985]. Williams Obstetrics [17th ed.]. East Norwalk, CT: Appleton-Century-Crofts, p. 8.)*

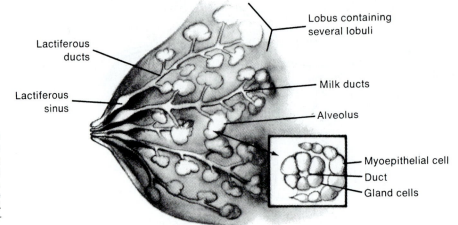

Figure 1–10. Simplified schematic drawing of duct system with cross section of myoepithelia around duct opening. Myoepithelia cells contract to eject milk. *(From Lawrence, R. [1980]. Breastfeeding: A Guide for the Medical Profession.* St. Louis, MO: C. V. Mosby. p. 21. Reprinted with permission.)

The nerve supply of the nipple and areola is extensive. Stimulation causes contraction of small muscles in the nipple, and, via a neuroreflex pathway to the hypothalamus, may promote the secretion of prolactin and oxytocin, and even lactation. Nipple erection and vasocongestion are produced by autonomic and tactile stimulation during sexual activity. The breast, itself, receives sensory innervation from the intercostal and supraclavicular nerves; thus, pain may be referred to the lateral chest, back, neck, and scapula.

THE MENSTRUAL CYCLE

To understand the menstrual cycle, one must understand the interactions of the hypothalamus, pituitary, and ovary. Hormonal secretions from these glands regulate physiologic responses in reproductive and other organs. The menstrual cycle is typically described as beginning on the first day of *menstruation,* followed by an ovarian *follicular/*uterine *proliferative* phase. The usual midpoint of the cycle is *ovulation,* followed by an ovarian *luteal/*uterine *secretory* phase, after which menstruation begins again.

Neuroendocrine Control

Within the hypothalamus of the brain are neurosecretory cells that share the characteristics of both neurons and endocrine gland cells. A neurohormone, gonadotropin releasing hormone (GnRH), originates in these cells and is responsible for control of the gonadotropin hormones, follicle-stimulating hormone (FSH), and luteinizing hormone (LH). These are secreted by the anterior pituitary in response to GnRH stimulation, and are essential for ovulation. Control of the reproductive cycle depends on the constant release of GnRH, which in turn is dependent on a complex interaction among GnRH, FHS, LH, and the ovarian steroid hormones, estrogen and progesterone. Other neurohormones (thyroid-stimulating hormone, growth hormone, and adrenocorticotropic hormone (ACTH) are also involved. Posi-

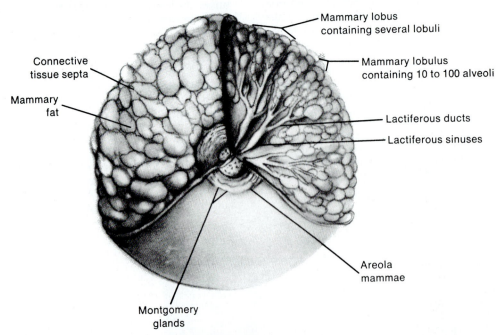

Figure 1–11. Morphology of mature breast with dissection to reveal mammary fat and duct system. *(From Lawrence. R. [1980]. Breastfeeding: A Guide for the Medical Profession.* St. Louis, MO: C. V. Mosby. p. 20. Reprinted with permission.)

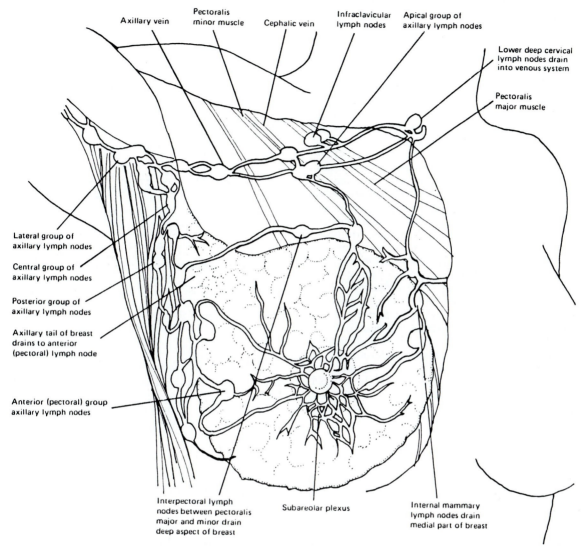

Figure 1–12. Lymphatic drainage of the breast. (From Martin, L. [1978]. *Health Care of Women* Philadelphia: J. B. Lippincott. Reprinted with permission.)

tive (stimulatory) and negative (inhibitory) feedback mechanisms govern these interactions.

The arcuate nucleus of the hypothalamus releases GnRH in a pulsatile fashion into the pituitary portal circulation (from the brain to the pituitary). Normal menstrual function depends on maintenance of this secretion in a critical range of frequency and concentration (Speroff, Glass, & Kase, 1983). GnRH production may be stimulated by norepinephrine and inhibited by dopamine (a prolactin-inhibiting factor) and serotonin; thus, both pharmacologic and psychologic factors may interfere with GnRH release. Endorphin (endogenous opiate) secretion may also affect GnRH release via direct inhibition of GnRH pulsatility or via dopamine inhibition, causing an increase in prolactin secretion. Prolactin has a well-known inverse relationship with gonadotropin secretion (Fritz & Speroff, 1983).

Although pulsatile GnRH is necessary for pituitary response, actual gonadotropin secretion from the pituitary is currently thought to be controlled by positive and negative feedback from the ovarian hormones on both the hypothalamus and the anterior pituitary cells (Speroff, et al., 1983; Fritz & Speroff, 1983). At the beginning of the menstrual

cycle, (Fig. 1–13), low levels of estrogen and progesterone stimulate secretion and release of GnRH and FSH, thus allowing follicular growth in the ovary. During the early follicular phase, levels of estradiol (an estrogen metabolite) begin to increase, causing increased synthesis and storage of gonadotropins. This results in the establishment of a pool of gonadotropins that is mobilized during the midcycle surge (Fritz & Speroff, 1983). Rising estradiol also inhibits pituitary response to GnRH and gonadotropin release, thus preventing premature release of this pool into the circulation. When estradiol reaches and maintains a critical level for a critical period (200 pg/mL), sustained for about 50 hours), this inhibitory effect becomes a stimulatory one, inducing a surge of LH secretion at midcycle and promoting a surge in FSH secretion as well (Fig. 1-13). These factors are responsible for the induction of ovulation.

After ovulation, there is a marked increase in secretion of progesterone (and a lesser increase in estrogen), causing profound inhibition of GnRH and gonadotropin release. In the latter part of the cycle, the production of ovarian hormones diminishes. FSH secretion is stimulated, menstruation occurs, and the cycle begins anew.

These neuroendocrine functions appear less abstract when considered in terms of ovarian function, uterine response, and the effects on other target organs.

The Ovarian Cycle

The ovarian cycle begins with the *follicular phase* (Fig. 1–15). Between 300,000 to 500,000 primordial follicles (oocytes arrested in a meiotic phase and surrounded by granulosa cells) are found in the ovary at puberty. Initial follicle growth is independent of gonadotropin stimulation; rather, it is a response to other physiologic circumstances (Speroff, et al., 1983). This growth is short-lived, however, and the majority of follicles (over 1,000 for every one that becomes a mature ovum) undergo only limited development followed by rapid atresia. At the beginning of each menstrual cycle, the rise in FSH levels saves a group of follicles for further development. The choice of follicle seems to be a combination of follicle "readiness" and FSH stimulation; the first follicle able to respond to the FSH apparently gains a developmental lead that it never loses (Fritz & Speroff, 1983).

This follicle then progresses to the *preantral* phase. The cell enlarges and the granulosa layer grows, forming an additional layer, called the *theca*. Under the influence of FSH, these cells both produce estrogen and convert androgen to estrogen, producing an optimal estrogenic environment. In conjunction with FSH, the estrogen works to produce and accumulate follicle fluid and to increase the number of FSH receptor cells as the granulosa proliferates. The follicular fluid provides an estrogen-rich environment for the follicle, now in the *antral* phase, and destined to ovulate (Fig. 1–14).

Estrogen production within the follicle has a stimulatory effect on maturation, whereas secretion of estrogen into the circulation (which occurs by day 5 of the cycle as levels in the follicle rise) acts to inhibit the release of FSH and LH from the pituitary. Another product of the granulosa cells, folliculostatin or inhibin, also acts to suppress FSH secretion as it is released by the growing follicle. The net result is to withdraw FSH support from the other follicles, limiting their own estrogen production and causing them to degenerate. Only the dominant follicle continues to develop; although it too remains dependent on FSH, its greater number of FSH receptor cells and the advanced de-

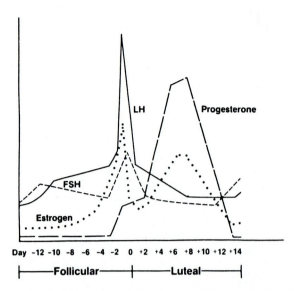

Figure 1–13. Serum hormone levels during the menstrual cycle. *(From Roberts, D., Van Sickle, M., & Kelly, R. [1983]. Role of sex steroid receptors. In Wynn, R. [Ed.],* Obstetrics and Gynecology Annual. *East Norwalk, CT: Appleton-Century-Crofts.*

velopment of the theca allow preferential delivery of FSH, thus maintaining FSH support despite declining FSH levels.

Primed by increasing levels of estrogen within the follicle, FSH begins to induce the development of LH receptors on the granulosa cells; these are crucial to later development of the corpus luteum. As estrogen levels rise higher in the circulation, the inhibition of LH is altered; with estradiol levels of 200 pg/mL sustained for 48 to 50 hours (Young & Jaffe, 1976), estrogen becomes capable of causing a stimulatory effect on LH release. In addition, these high levels of estrogen intensify the bioactivity of LH via modulation of the molecular structure (Marut, Williams, Cowan, et al., 1981). Thus, levels of a more bioactive LH rise in the late follicular phase, causing luteinization of the granulosa cell layer of the follicle, and resulting in the production of a small but crucial amount of progesterone.

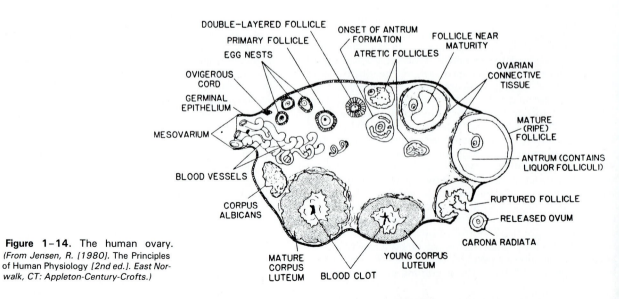

Figure 1–14. The human ovary. *(From Jensen, R. [1980].* The Principles of Human Physiology *[2nd ed.]. East Norwalk, CT: Appleton-Century-Crofts.)*

This *preovulatory* follicle continues to produce increasing amounts of estrogen, reaching peak levels 24 to 36 hours before ovulation. FSH drops to lower levels in response to the inhibitory effect of estrogen. LH increases and surges to a peak, causing an increase in progesterone secretion. Progesterone, in conjunction with the midcycle estrogen priming, facilitates the positive feedback mechanism and induces a surge in FSH secretion, ensuring a full complement of LH receptors in the granulosa cells (March, Goebelsmann, Nakamura, & Mishell, 1979; March, Marrs, Goebelsmann, & Mishell, 1981). There is also a concomitant rise in androgen levels at midcycle, derived from the atresia of unsuccessful follicles. As androgens are well known to influence libido, it is thought that this serves to stimulate the seeking of sexual activity at ovulation (Adams & Gold, 1978).

Ovulation occurs 10 to 12 hours after the LH peak, 24 to 36 hours after the estradiol peak, and 28 to 32 hours after the onset of the LH surge (Garcia, Jones, & Wright, 1981; WHO Task Force 1980). The wall of the follicle becomes more elastic due to progesterone influence. High prostaglandin concentrations in the follicular fluid, induced by the LH surge, promote follicular rupture, and the high levels of LH stimulate resumption of meiosis in the oocyte as it is released. The ovary now enters the *luteal phase*.

Within hours of the LH surge, there is a rapid drop in plasma estrogen as the high levels of LH suppress hormonal synthesis in the thecal tissue, and the midcycle rise in progesterone inhibits further granulosa cell multiplication (Speroff, et al., 1983). LH levels then fall abruptly with the loss of estrogen stimulation, the increasing production of progesterone in the luteinized cells of the follicle, and the inhibition of GnRH.

In the follicle, the granulosa cells continue to enlarge for 2 to 3 days, accumulating a yellow pigment (lutein). A capillary network develops within the follicle, reaching a peak of vascularization after 8 to 9 days. This is crucial in allowing the delivery of low-density lipoproteins (LDLs) to the corpus luteum; the ovarian hormone progesterone is manufactured from the cholesterol in the LDLs.

The *corpus luteum* develops at the site of the extruded ovum; its main function is the production of progesterone, which rises rapidly after ovulation, reaching a peak by day 8 of the luteal phase. Estrogen is also produced by the corpus luteum, with levels peaking at the same time as progesterone. These ovarian hormones serve to ready the uterus for implantation. Both estrogen and progesterone inhibit the secretion of gonadotropins by the pituitary, thus blocking new follicular growth.

After 9 to 11 days, if conception does not occur, the corpus luteum degenerates, probably as a result of the luteolytic action of the estrogen and altered prostaglandin levels. Estrogen and progesterone levels drop as the corpus luteum degenerates; when these hormone levels decline sufficiently, the secretion of GnRH and FSH is induced, allowing the cycle to begin again. If conception does occur, rapidly rising levels of human chorionic gonadotropin (hCG) will maintain the corpus luteum and its steroid production until the placenta is developed sufficiently to take over the role.

Uterine Response

The response of the uterine endometrium to hormonal stimulation is the most visible marker of neuroendocrine function. The upper two endometrial layers (compacta and spongiosa) and the coiled arteries supplying them undergo marked changes throughout the menstrual cycle (Fig. 1–15). The cycle begins with menstruation: the breakdown

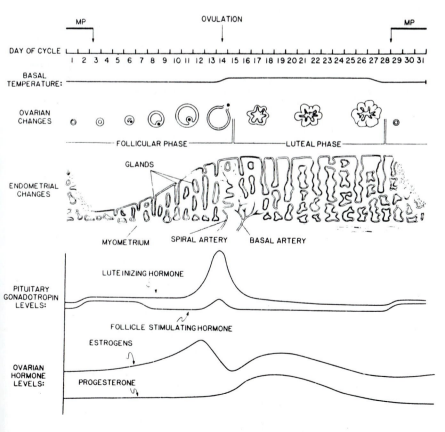

Figure 1–15. The menstrual cycle. *(From Jensen, R. [1980]. The Principles of Human Physiology [2nd ed.]. East Norwalk, CT: Appleton-Century-Crofts.)*

and sloughing of the endometrium. Immediately after menstruation, the endometrium is only 1 to 2 mm thick with cuboidal epithelium, narrow glands, and compact stroma. Under the influence of estrogen in the ovarian follicular phase, the endometrium enters its *proliferative* phase. It becomes taller, the epithelium more columnar, and the glands more tortuous. Mitotic activity is prominent. The endometrium grows to 3.5 to 5.0 mm in height as a result of estrogen-induced tissue growth as well as by "reinflation" of the stroma as it incorporates water, electrolytes, and amino acids (Speroff, et al., 1983). Spiral arteries extend into the endometrium forming a loose network.

After ovulation, under the influence of progesterone, *secretory* activity becomes more marked. The endometrium is edematous and vascular, measuring 5 to 7 mm in thickness. There is increased coiling of the spiral arteries. The endometrial glands assume a corkscrew pattern, the stroma becomes loose and edematous, and increasing amounts of glycogen are secreted, making the endometrium ripe for the implantation of a fertilized egg.

Degeneration of the endometrium begins well before menstrual bleeding with the decrease in ovarian hormone production and stimulation of prostaglandin effects in the endometrial tissue. Apparently, elevated progesterone levels in the luteal phase make the uterus resistant to prostaglandin stimulation; when progesterone levels fall, the uterus begins to respond to the prostaglandins normally found in secretory endometrium (Budoff, 1983; Csapo, 1980). Intense vasoconstriction of the coiled arterioles occurs several hours before the onset of bleeding, leading to endometrial ischemia and necrosis. Enzymes are liberated that further disrupt the endometrium, and the menstrual flow begins. The entire compacta and a large portion of the spongiosa are lost by the second day of the menses, although bleeding generally continues for a few more days. Endometrial tissue is regenerated by the unaffected basal layer, even as menstrual bleeding continues.

Dysmenorrhea, or painful menstruation, may be caused by increased levels of prostaglandins, causing stronger uterine contractions and thus more vasoconstriction and tissue anoxia. Endometriosis and pelvic inflammatory disease may also cause dysmenorrhea. (See Chapter 20 for more information on this phenomenon.)

Menstrual cycle length averages 28 to 30 days, but the range may extend from 21 to 35 days. Variation from one cycle to the next is common, and cycles are less regular at the extremes of reproductive years. The luteal, or secretory, phase is the most predictable in length, as the life span of the corpus luteum is relatively constant in women, lasting 14 +/- 2 days (Thorneycroft & Boyers, 1983). The follicular or proliferative phase is more variable and may last from 1 to 3 weeks (Pritchard, MacDonald, and Gant, 1985). The duration of menstrual flow is also variable, although generally similar from cycle to cycle for individual women, with a range of 2 to 8 days not being uncommon. Menstrual flow consists of the shed endometrium, blood, cervical and vaginal cells, and mucus. Clots may sometimes be present but menstrual blood is usually not coagulated. Thromboplastins in the endometrial tissue initiate clotting in the menstrual blood, but this is promptly counteracted by plasmin activators also present, causing clot lysis. Average menstrual blood loss ranges from 25 to 60 mL and represents an iron depletion of 150 to 400 mg each year (Pritchard, et al., 1985).

Effects on Other Organs

Effects of the hormonal cycles may be seen on other organs and systems. Effects on the reproductive system are outlined in Table 1–1.

In the vagina, estrogen stimulation in the first half of the cycle causes cornification of the vaginal cells. In the luteal phase, more basophils, leukocytes, and precornified cells are present.

There are marked changes in cervical mucus during the cycle. After menstruation, cervical secretions are sticky and viscid. With rising estrogen levels, the mucus becomes more watery and clear, resembling raw egg white, and can be stretched into a thread (*spinnbarkheit*). If spread on a slide and allowed to dry, it produces a fern pattern, as a result of the high sodium chloride content. This mucus pattern is associated with peak estrogen levels that precede ovulation and is thought to enhance sperm motility. In the luteal phase, the mucus again becomes viscid, cloudy, and tacky until menstruation.

The cervical os responds to estrogen by widening during the follicular phase until ovulation when it may be partially open or patulous. It returns to a closed state during the luteal phase.

The uterus increases in size because of the increased blood supply and thickness of the endometrium characteristic of the late proliferative and early secretory phases.

TABLE 1–1. ESTROGEN AND PROGESTERONE-MODULATED EFFECTS ON THE REPRODUCTIVE SYSTEM

Stage	Preovulation	Postovulation
Hormone Dominance	Estrogen	Estrogen and Progesterone

Effects	1. Oviducts
	   a. Increased motility
	   b. More dilute fluid secretion
	
	2. Cervix
	   a. Watery mucous secretion
	
	3. Uterus
	   a. Increased energy stores
	   b. Increased motility
	   c. Proliferated endometrium
		1. Oviducts
		   a. Lessened motility
		
		2. Cervix
		   a. Secretion of mucous plug
		
		3. Uterus
		   a. Quieted motility
		   b. Secretion of nourishing fluid
		   c. Augmented blood supply to endometrium

Purposes	1. Capture and retention of ovum 2. Facilitation of sperm entry and ascension to oviduct 3. Support of potential pregnancy	1. Conduct of ovum to uterus 2. Protection of potential pregnancy 3. Facilitation of fertilized ovum implantation

From Smith, E. (1982). Abortion: Health Care Perspectives. *East Norwalk, CT: Appleton-Century-Crofts.*

Rhythmic contractility of the uterus reaches a peak as estrogen levels rise, perhaps enhancing sperm motility toward the oviduct. The uterus becomes quiescent under the influence of progesterone, assisting the implantation process (Jones & Jones, 1982; Smith, 1982).

Estrogen dominance increases myocontractility of the oviduct to retain the ovum in the ampulla for fertilization; higher progesterone levels in the luteal phase inhibit contractility, allowing the ovum to travel back to the uterus for implantation (Smith, 1982).

Mittelschmerz, or intermenstrual pain, may occur at midcycle, lasting from a few hours to a day or so. It generally consists of crampy unilateral lower quadrant pain, sometimes radiating to the groin. The cause is unclear; current theories identify tubal peristalsis or increased peritoneal fluid as the source (Hann, Hall, Black, & Ferrucci, 1979; Hilgers, Daly, Prebil & Hilgers, 1981; Thorneycroft & Boyers, 1983).

Breast tissue responds to hormonal fluctuations with breast size, sensitivity, and nodularity peaking in the luteal phase. A few women also experience a midcycle increase in breast sensitivity (Hilgers, et al., 1981; Robinson & Short, 1977). Some researchers believe that this cyclic mastalgia is related to estrogen levels that stimulate the production of serotonin and prolactin (Labrum, 1981).

Basal body temperature (BBT) shows a characteristic biphasic pattern when recorded daily. During the first half of the cycle, BBT fluctuates around a mean of less than 98°F; in the luteal phase it shifts to fluctuate around a mean that exceeds the lower one by 0.4 to 1.0°F. The rise may be preceded by a slight decrease in temperature (Thorneycroft & Boyers, 1983).

Other body functions may be affected although the mechanisms are not always clear. The five senses (sight, hearing, smell, touch, and taste) are reported to reach a peak of sensitivity at ovulation (Barris, Dawson, & Theiss, 1980; Doty, Snyder, Huggins, & Lowry, 1981). There are reports of decreased appetite and food intake in the follicular and ovulatory phases (Dalvit, 1981). Other findings associated with the first half of the cycle include slower alpha waves on EEG, accompanied by an increase in psychological task score performance (Becker, Creutzfeldt, Schwibbe, & Wittke, 1982), and a general sense of alertness, well-being, pleasantness, and sexual arousal (Moos, Kopell, Melges, et al., 1969).

Elevated progesterone levels in the luteal phase promote renal excretion of salt. This leads to activation of renin, increased aldosterone production, and consequent retention of salt and water (London, Sundaram, Murphy, & Goldstein, 1983). Some studies of fluid retention and weight gain indicate a premenstrual increase, with a smaller increase sometimes noted at ovulation (Reeves, Garvin, & McElin, 1971), although other researchers dispute this (Reid & Yen, 1981). Faster alpha waves on EEG, impairment of short-term memory and attention, and the lowest level of performance on psychological performance scores are also associated with the late luteal phase (Becker, et al., 1982; Labrum, 1983).

A premenstrual increase in carbohydrate tolerance has been suggested to account for a frequently reported craving for sweets (Reid & Yen, 1981). Appetite and food intake increase in the latter half of the menstrual cycle, by about 500 cal/day (Dalvit, 1981). There is apparently an increased incidence of asthma, allergic reactions, and rhinitis premenstrually and at menstruation (Hanley, 1981; Reid & Yen, 1981). There are also reports of decreased sexual arousal and self-activation, accompanied by an increase in

drowsiness and fatigue during the luteal phase (Moos, et al., 1969) and reports of multiple physical and psychological symptoms (Beumont, Richards, & Gelder, 1975).

Depending on the source, differing numbers of women experience varying degrees of psychological and physical discomfort in the premenstrual period. These symptoms range from minor alterations (premenstrual molimina) to severe premenstrual tension syndrome (PMTS). A full discussion of theories relating to the etiology and preferred treatment of these symptoms is beyond the scope of this chapter; briefly, however, current theory indicates that there are several different groups of complaints that may have different physiologic bases. These groups are commonly referred to as PMTS—A (anxiety, irritability, and nervous tension), PMTS—B (water and salt retention, mastalgia, abdominal bloating, and weight gain), PMTS—C (premenstrual craving for sweets and increased appetite, sometimes accompanied by reactive hypoglycemia symptoms such as palpitations, fatigue, and dizziness), and PMTS—D (depression, withdrawal, insomnia, and confusion) (Abraham, 1983). (See Chapter 19 for a complete discussion of these problems.)

CHANGES DURING THE LIFE CYCLE

Puberty

Ovarian differentiation begins at about 10 weeks of fetal age. FSH and LH are found in fetal circulation, and ovarian germ cells develop, reaching a peak at about 20 weeks of gestation, declining thereafter. There is some gonadotropin secretion in infancy, but gonadotropin levels drop during childhood, a period characterized by low levels of gonadotropins, little pituitary response to GnRH, and maximal pituitary suppression (Speroff, et al., 1983).

The onset of puberty is characterized by several changes. The hypothalamus matures, becoming less inhibited by negative feedback mechanisms, and the pituitary becomes increasingly responsive to GnRH, resulting in increased gonadotropin secretion. This in turn promotes ovarian follicular development, increased sex steroid levels, and the development of secondary sex characteristics (Speroff, et al., 1983; Winter, Faiman, & Reyes, 1978). The age of onset of puberty is quite variable, influenced by heredity, nutrition, health, and other factors. It has been suggested that initiation of pubertal changes occurs at a particular body weight (48 kg) and percentage of body fat (17%), as estrogen release seems to depend on a mechanism requiring adequate body fat stores (Frisch & Revelle, 1971; Goldfarb, 1977); however, this is still debated by others who find that hard evidence is lacking (Garn, Lavelle & Pilkington , 1983; Scott & Johnston, 1982; Speroff, et al., 1983; Winter, et al., 1978). The critical factor seems to be a normal maturational process, especially of the central nervous system.

Pubertal development occurs over a period of 3 to 5 years, beginning around age 9 with a growth spurt and followed by budding of the nipples and breasts and the appearance of some pubic hair. Growth in the external and internal genitalia and breast tissue and increased axillary and pubic hair follow (Tables 1–2 and 1–3). Menarche usually occurs around age 13 in the United States, with a range of 10 to 16 years (Winter, et al., 1978; Zacharias, Rand, & Wurtman, 1976).

The decreased sensitivity of the hypothalamus to negative feedback mechanisms is crucial to pubertal develop-

TABLE 1-2. TANNER CLASSIFICATION OF FEMALE ADOLESCENT DEVELOPMENT

Stage	Breasts	Pubic Hair
I	Papillae elevated, preadolescent	None
II	Breasts and papillae, small mounds	Sparse, long, slightly pigmented
III	Breasts and areolae confluent, elevated	Darker, coarser, curly
IV	Areolae and papillae projected above breast	Adult type—pubis only
V	Papillae projected, mature	Lateral distribution

TABLE 1-3. MEAN ONSET OF FEMALE PUBERTAL CHANGES IN THE UNITED STATES

Age	Characteristic
9-10	Beginning of height spurt Growth of bony pelvis Female contour fat deposition Budding of nipples
10-11	Budding of breasts Appearance of pubic hair (may precede breast budding in 10%)
11-12	Appearance of vaginal secretions Growth of internal and external genitalia Increase in vaginal glycogen content; lowering of pH
12-13	Pigmentation of areolae Growth of breasts
13-14	Appearance of axillary hair Increase in amount of pubic hair Acne (in 75-90%) Menarche
15-16	Arrest of skeletal growth

From Goldfarb, A. (1977). Puberty and Menarche. Clinical Obstetrics and Gynecology 20(3), 629. Reprinted with permission.

ment, but the maturation of positive feedback response to estrogen does not occur until later. Lack of this positive estrogen feedback results in the absence of the LH surge and failure to ovulate (Altchek, 1977; Speroff, et al., 1983). The early menstrual cycles may be anovulatory and irregular until both negative and positive feedback mechanisms are fully developed. (See Chapter 22 for more discussion of adolescent changes.)

Menopause

The climacteric is a transitional period at the end of the reproductive years during which reproductive function diminishes until menopause, the cessation of menses. The average age of menopause in industrialized society is approximately 50, with the climacteric beginning as long as 8 years before this (Utian, 1980). Ovulation will begin to reduce in frequency by age 38 to 42 (Speroff, et al., 1983). The age of menopause has remained stable since medieval times, apparently independent of any physical or socioeconomic factors, except perhaps cigarette smoking (Edman, 1983).

The numbers of follicles and oocytes present in the ovary diminish with each menstrual cycle over the reproductive years, and it is thought that these residual follicles may also be less responsive to gonadotropin stimulation (Speroff, et al., 1983). The result is a gradual decrease in estrogen and folliculostatin production, resulting in an increase in FSH levels. FSH secretion produces rapid follicular development, initially shortening the cycles and further decreasing the number of follicles (Sherman, West, & Korenman, 1976). Estrogen levels continue to fall until they are too low to induce an adequate LH surge. Long, irregular cycles accompanied by a shortened luteal phase and anovulatory cycles accompanied by endometrial hyperplasia result. Estrogen-dependent tissues begin to atrophy. Soon, ovulation ceases entirely and the menopause occurs. (See Chapter 24 for further discussion of changes in this part of the life cycle.)

REFERENCES

Abraham, G. (1983, July). Nutritional factors in the etiology of premenstrual tension syndromes. *Journal of Reproductive Medicine,* 28(7):446-464.

Adams, D., & Gold, A. (1977, November 23). Rise in female initiated sexual activity at ovulation and its suppression by oral contraceptives. *New England Journal of Medicine,* 229(21):1145-1150.

Altchek, A. (1977, September). Dysfunctional uterine bleeding in adolescence. *Clinical Obstetrics and Gynecology,* 20(3):633-650.

Barris, M., Dawson, W., & Theiss, C. (1980, October 15). Visual sensitivity of women during the menstrual cycle. *Documenta Ophthalmologica,* 49(2):293-301.

Becker, D., Creutzfeldt, O., Schwibbe, M., & Wittke, W. (1982). Changes in physiological, EEG and psychological parameters in women during the spontaneous menstrual cycle and following oral contraceptives. *Psychoneuroendocrinology,* 7(1):75-90.

Beumont, P., Richards, D., & Gelder, M. (1975, May). Study of minor psychiatric and physical symptoms during the menstrual cycle. *British Journal of Psychiatry,* 126(594):431-434.

Budoff, P. (1983, July). Use of prostaglandin inhibitors for the premenstrual syndrome. *The Journal of Reproductive Medicine,* 28(7):469-478.

Csapo, A. (1980, October). Rationale for the treatment of dysmenorrhea. *Journal of Reproductive Medicine,* 25(supplement 4):213-221.

Dalvit, S. (1981, September). Effect of the menstrual cycle on patterns of food intake. *American Journal of Clinical Nutrition* 34(9):1811-1815.

Doty, R., Snyder, P., Huggins, G., & Lowry, L. (1981, February). Endocrine, cardiovascular and psychological correlates of olfactory sensitivity changes in the human menstrual cycle. *Journal of Comparative and Physiological Psychology,* 95(1):45-60.

Edman, C. (1983). The climacteric. In H. Buchsbaum (Ed.) *The menopause,* New York: Springer-Verlag.

Frisch, R., & Revelle, R. (1971, October). Height and weight at menarche and a hypothesis of menarche. *Archives of Disease in Childhood,* 46(249):695-701.

Fritz, M., & Speroff, L. (1983) Current concepts of the endocrine characteristics of normal menstrual function. *Clinical Obstetrics and Gynecology,* 26(3):647-689.

Garcia, J., Jones G., & Wright, G. (1981, September). Prediction of the time of ovulation. *Fertility and Sterility,* 36(3):308-315.

Garn, S., Lavelle, M., & Pilkington, J. (1983, August). Comparison of fatness in premenarcheal and postmenarcheal girls of the same age. *Journal of Pediatrics,* 103(2):328-331.

Goldfarb, A. (1977, September). Puberty and menarche. *Clinical Obstetrics and Gynecology,* 20(3):625-631.

Hanley, S. (1981, July). Asthma variation with menstruation. *British Journal of Diseases of the Chest,* 75(3):306-308.

Hann, L., Hall, D., Black, E., & Ferrucci, J. (1979, June). Mittelschmerz sonographic demonstration. *Journal of the American Medical Association,* 241(25):2731-2732.

Hilgers, T., Daly, D., Prebil, A., & Hilgers, S. (1981, August). Intermenstrual symptoms and estimated time of ovulation. *Obstetrics and Gynecology,* 58(2):152–155.

Jensen, R. (1980). *The principles of human physiology,* (2nd ed.) New York: Appleton-Century-Crofts.

Jones, H., & Jones, G. (1982). *Gynecology* (3rd ed.) Baltimore: Williams and Wilkins.

Labrum, A. (1983, July). Hypothalamic, pineal and pituitary factors in the premenstrual syndrome. *Journal of Reproductive Medicine* 28(7):438–445.

Ladas, A., Whipple, B., & Perry, J. (1982). *The G-spot and other recent discoveries about human sexuality.* New York: Holt, Rinehart & Winston.

Lawrence, R. (1985). *Breastfeeding: A guide for the medical profession* (2nd ed.) St. Louis: C. V. Mosby.

London, R., Sundaram, G., Murphy, L., & Goldstein, P. (1983, August). Evaluation and treatment of breast symptoms in patients with the premenstrual syndrome. *The Journal of Reproductive Medicine,* 28(8):503–508.

March, C., Goebelsmann, U., Nakamura, R., & Mishell, D. Jr. (1979, October). Roles of estradiol and progesterone in eliciting the midcycle LH and FSH surges. *Journal of Clinical Endocrinology and Metabolism,* 49(4):507–513.

March, C., Marrs, R., Goebelsmann, U., & Mishell, D. Jr. (1981, July). Feedback effects of estradiol and progesterone on gonadotrophin release. *Obstetrics and Gynecology,* 58(1):10–16.

Martin, L. (1978) *Health Care of Women.* Philadelphia: J.B. Lippincott.

Marut, E., Williams, R., & Cowan, B., et al. (1981), December). Pulsatile pituitary gonadotropin secretion: estrogen enhances the biological activity of LH. *Endocrinology* 109(6): 2270–2272.

Masters, W., & Johnson, V. (1966). *Human Sexual Response.* Boston: Little, Brown & Co.

Moos, R., Kopell, B., Melges, F., et al. (1969, March). Fluctuations in symptoms and moods during the menstrual cycle. *Journal of Psychosomatic Medicine,* 13(1):37–44.

Morehead, J. (1982, June). Anatomy and embryology of the breast. *Clinical Obstetrics and Gynecology* 25(2):353–357.

Oxorn, H., & Foote, N. R. (1980). *Human labor and birth* (4th ed.) New York: Appleton-Century-Crofts.

Pritchard, J., MacDonald, P., & Gant, N. (1985). *Williams Obstetrics* (17th ed.) East Norwalk: Appleton-Century-Crofts.

Reeves, B., Garvin, J., & McElin, T. (1971, April 1). Premenstrual tension symptoms and weight changes. *American Journal of Obstetrics and Gynecology* 109(7):1036–1041.

Reid, R., & Yen, S. (1981, January). Premenstrual syndrome. *American Journal of Obstetrics and Gynecology* 139(1):85–104.

Roberts, D., Van Sickle, M., & Kelly, R. (1983). Role of sex steroid receptors in obstetrics and gynecology. *Obstetrics and Gynecology Annual 1983* 12:61–78.

Robinson, J., & Short, R. (1977, May 7). Changes in breast sensitivity at puberty, during the menstrual cycle, and at parturition. *British Medical Journal* I(6070):1188–1191.

Scott, E., & Johnston, F. (1982, June). Critical fat, menarche and the maintenance of menstrual cycles. *Journal of Adolescent Health Care,* 2(4):249–260.

Sherman, B., West, J., & Korenman, S. (1976, April) The menopausal transition: analysis of LH, FSH, estradiol and progesterone concentrations during menstrual cycles of older women. *Journal of Clinical Endocrinology and Metabolism* 42(4):629–636.

Smith, E., (1982) *Abortion: Health Care Perspectives.* Norwalk: Appleton-Century-Crofts.

Speroff, L., Glass, R., & Kase, N. (1983). *Clinical Gynecologic Endocrinology and Infertility* (3rd ed.) Baltimore: Williams & Wilkins.

Thorneycroft, I., & Boyers, S. (1983). The human menstrual cycle: correlation of hormonal patterns and clinical signs and symptoms. *Obstetrics and Gynecology Annual 1983* 12:199–226.

Utian, W. (1980). *Menopause in modern perspective.* New York: Appleton-Century-Crofts.

Winter, J., Faiman, C., & Reyes, F. (1978, March). Normal and abnormal pubertal development. *Clinical Obstetrics and Gynecology,* 21(1):67–86.

World Health Organization Task Force (1980, October 15). Temporal relationships between ovulation and defined changes in the concentrations of plasma estradiol, LH, FSH, and progesterone. *American Journal of Obstetrics and Gynecology,* 138(4):383–390.

Young, J., & Jaffe, R. (1976, March). Strength and duration characteristics of estrogen effects on gonadotropin response to gonadotropin-releasing hormone in women. *Journal of Clinical Endocrinology and Metabolism,* 42(3):432–442.

Zacharias, L., Rand, W., & Wurtman, R. (1976, April). A prospective study of sexual development and growth in American girls: the statistics of menarche. *Obstetrical and Gynecological Survey,* 31(4):325–337.

2

The Well-woman Gynecologic Interview

Ronnie Lichtman

Communication between patients and providers is crucial to the provision of quality health care. Through communication, information is gathered from which problem lists, diagnoses, and plans can be developed. The communication process generally begins with the initial patient interview. With open communication, the interview is as significant to data collection as physical examination or laboratory testing. The interview has several additional purposes. It establishes a relationship between the care provider and the patient; it sets the tone for the entire visit and perhaps for subsequent visits as well.

This chapter discusses some theoretical and practical perspectives on the patient–practitioner relationship, outlines and describes the components of a complete health history, and suggest effective interview techniques. It concludes with a brief discussion of how to record the history and provides a sample writeup.

The chapter does not attempt to delineate or explore the various differential diagnoses relating to specific areas of the suggested history. Chapters that follow discuss the significance of historical data in relation to contraception, gynecologic problems, and clinical decision making. Appendix III on differential diagnosis outlines a diagnostic framework in which to place certain collected data. Bibliographic references can be referred to for more information on interviewing techniques.

THE PATIENT–PRACTITIONER RELATIONSHIP

The variety of possible relationships between patient and provider has concerned sociologists for many years. Their concern, however, has been largely restricted—in theoretical and empirical studies—to patient–*physician* relations. In early analyses, the patient and physician were each depicted in rigidly ascribed roles. Parsons, for example, characterized the physician's role as active and the patient's as dependent and passive. He saw them exclusively as a helping person and a person needing help. Later authors expanded Parsons's conception to encompass several types of possible interactions. Szasz and Hollander postulated three models: activity-passivity, guidance-cooperation, and mutual participation (Bloom & Wilson, 1979). Danziger (1978) assessed the input of the practitioner and the patient independently: a patient may be passive, active but dependent, or a potentially knowledgeable participant; a practitioner may act as an expert, a counselor, or a co-participant. In a study based on more than 100 observations of interactions between women and doctors, she found rapport to be dependent on the degree of compatibility between the two participants. Veatch (1972) has proposed an alternative formulation. He describes four interaction models—the "engineering," the "priestly," the "collegial," and the "contractual"—in which the health care provider acts respectively as a technician, a superior, an equal, or a party to a symbolic contract. Veatch calls the collegial model "a mere pipe dream," believing that "ethnic, class, economic, and value differences" make it impossible to implement. He describes the contractual model as "a true sharing of ethical authority and responsibility," avoiding, "the moral abdication on the part of the physician inherent in the engineering model . . . the moral abdication on the part of the patient in the priestly model . . . the false sense of equality in the collegial model" (p. 61).

Although we believe that there may be differences between patients and practitioners, they do not necessarily create inequalities. Veatch's conceptions are based on patient–*physician*—not patient–*practitioner* relationships. As Colombotos (1975) points out, there is less social distance between patients and nonphysician providers than there is between most people and physicians. In addition, the patient is less likely to *perceive* social distance, hence less inequality, in these relationships. This may be part of the reason that patients, particularly women, seek out such providers for their health care needs.

Promoting An Equal Partnership

In an equal partnership, each partner contributes expertise; the provider has knowledge about health and health care in general; the patient has knowledge about her own history and her own body. In assessing the role of the interview in primary care medicine, Barsky, Kazis, Freiden and associates (1980) suggest that it is a negotiation, or "consensus-seeking" encounter, and must therefore include the patient's perspective. When a practitioner expresses respect for what the patient brings to the encounter, the setting and implementation of common goals become possible. This patient-centered approach requires an ability to be nonjudgmental and accepting, authentic, and caring (Hein, 1980; Rogers, 1961, 1962). These attitudes necessitate self-awareness and consciousness of the communication process.

There are many behaviors that affect the quality of an

interaction. Some are clear; others may not be obvious. Some lead to the establishment of rapport; others work against it. A thoughtful care provider should try to become aware of behaviors that affect relationships with patients and make them conscious choices enhancing the desired effect. Bernstein and Bernstein (1980) call this "disciplined communication."

Both verbal and nonverbal behaviors provide emotional cues in communication. These begin with the introduction. If a nurse or receptionist calls the woman, it sets a tone for the practitioner–patient relationship that is less personal than if the practitioner goes to the waiting room to call the patient. This is especially true if the woman is asked to undress before the interview. Meeting a health care provider for the first time wearing only an examination gown does not promote feelings of equality on the patient's part.

Names are very important. How are patients addressed? How does the practitioner identify herself or himself? If practitioners use their own last names but call patients by their first names, a patronizing or disrespectful attitude may be communicated. Many practitioners establish relationships with patients on a first-name basis. This is both equal and personal. Other practitioners ask each woman to choose her preferred form of address. If a practitioner is most comfortable being called Ms., Mrs., Miss, Mr., or Dr., then the patient should be addressed in an equivalent manner.

Nonverbal behaviors include facial expressions, eye contact (or lack of it), posture and even touch (Long & Prophit, 1981). Smiling, when appropriate, conveys warmth and caring. A practitioner who continually looks down at the chart or stares off into space sets up social distance; a practitioner who maintains eye contact by frequently looking up from writing or waiting to write until the end of a conversation sends a message of interest. Slumping in one's seat creates an impression very different from the one created by sitting up or leaning toward the patient. Touching may or may not be appropriate; the important point is to be aware that it has meaning and to use it to instill trust rather than distrust. Handshaking, in our culture, is always a respectful form of physical contact.

The environment in which an interview is conducted may be conducive or nonconducive to trust. In private practice this is more within the control of the practitioner than it is in a clinic. Some practitioners choose not to sit behind desks, preferring round tables or couches and chairs which eliminate the authority emanating from the behind-the-desk posture. Where available furniture and seating arrangements are beyond the practitioner's control, the environment can still be positively manipulated. Doors should be closed, and curtains pulled. If this cannot be done, then at least "psychological privacy" (Bernstein & Bernstein, 1980; Zola, 1963) can be maintained. Voices can be soft; the practitioner can acknowledge awareness of the situation and give the patient complete attention. Interruptions can be avoided.

INFORMATION GATHERING

Of course, a primary purpose of the gynecologic interview is information gathering. For many women, visits to gynecologic care providers are their sole source of preventive health care, with the exception perhaps of dental or eye examinations. The purpose of these visits is, therefore, threefold: (1) detection, diagnosis, and treatment of gynecologic problems; (2) screening for other existing or potential health problems; and (3) general health maintenance and prevention of illness. To accomplish these purposes, an extensive history is necessary. The following categories are recommended:

- "Name tag" or identification
- Reason for visit
- Menstrual history
- Gynecologic history
- Obstetric history
- Contraceptive history
- Medical history/substance use
- Surgical history
- Family history
- Social/cultural history
- Occupational history
- Sexual history
- Nutritional history
- Exercise/activity history

The order in which this information is elicited may vary from practitioner to practitioner or from patient to patient, but all areas should be covered. Development of a systematic approach to history taking helps ensure completeness.

The order utilized in this chapter deviates somewhat from the traditional health history. This change reflects the special needs of a gynecologic visit. It emphasizes data most pertinent to problems presented in gynecologic practice and facilitates the interview process for women presenting for gynecologic care.

"Name Tag" or Identification

Full name, age, date and place of birth, address and phone number, workplace, and workplace address and phone number can be asked as part of the interview or obtained through a written form that the woman fills out while waiting. Often, this information is taken by a receptionist, nurse, or aide.

Reason for Visit

After introduction a good place to begin the interview is to find out why a woman has come for care, and what she expects from the visit. This is often referred to in the medical model as the "chief complaint" and charted as such. It may not, however, be a complaint. Health maintenance is a valid reason for a gynecologic assessment. A simple, open-ended question is "What brought you here today?" This allows the woman to speak to her primary concerns in her own terms and to give her input to the visit. It lets her know that you want to meet her needs and that she has control over her care. It also provides a direction for the rest of the interview; it focuses thinking and guides questioning to emphasize the areas most relevant to the patient's problem or concern.

It is wise, at this point, to explain to a woman how you intend to meet her needs and that as part of an overall assessment, you will be taking a complete health history. Explaining the purpose of such extensive questioning helps put a woman at ease and increases her willingness to provide complete data. Assurance that she can ask questions at any time is another method of increasing communication.

The order and format of the following parts of the history should be adjusted according to a particular woman's reason for seeking care. If she has a specific complaint, it is useful to mentally construct a differential diagnosis and ask questions to rule out each possible diagnosis. If her visit is for birth control provision, it may be best to start with contraceptive history. If she is seeing you for a general gynecologic screening, a variety of possibilities exists. Most important is the rational choice of an interview format so that thoroughness is never sacrificed.

Menstrual History

As the woman has contracted with you specifically for gynecologic care, this is often an appropriate place to start. She expects these questions. A menstrual history consists of the first day and duration of the last menstrual period (LMP), the age at menarche (often approximate), the usual menstrual interval, and the duration of menses. The last three can be written as 13 × 28–30 × 4.

Knowledge about the usual amount of flow and presence of clots, *mittelschmerz*, midcycle spotting, intermenstrual bleeding, premenstrual syndrome, and dysmenorrhea is integral to an understanding of a woman's experience of menstruation. The onset of and changes in these symptoms should be noted. The LMP should be investigated for its normalcy in relation to timing of onset, duration, amount, and character of flow, particularly if there is any possibility of pregnancy. Give the woman the opportunity during the interview to consult her calendar for retrieval of this information. If she does not keep a menstrual record, or has not brought it with her, provide her with a calendar to look at as this often will help her remember the start of the LMP. Always stress the value of menstrual record-keeping.

Specific menstrual symptoms should be fully explored (see Gynecologic History). Ascertain whether any of these are problematic for the woman and what, if any, remedies are used and their efficacy. Tampon use, including brand, strength, and frequency of changing tampons, should become part of all menstrual histories (see Chapter 18). Women over 40 should be queried about menopausal symptoms, such as changes in cycle intervals or duration, missed cycles, hot flushes, and decreased vaginal lubrication. If menstruation has ceased, the age of menopause should be noted along with details about any treatments currently or previously received (see Chapter 24).

Gynecologic History

Questions about past and current gynecologic problems are most pertinent to the care being sought. A gynecologic history focuses on genitourinary disorders and discomforts—vaginitis, sexually transmitted diseases, infertility, diseases of the female reproductive organs such as salpingitis or pelvic inflammatory disease, endometriosis, ovarian cysts, urinary tract infections, stress incontinence, and uterine and other structural abnormalities.

Often women do not know the specific names of previous disorders but remember their symptoms or how they were treated. They can be asked, for example, "Was the discharge thick or thin? Did it have an odor or was there itching? Were you treated with a vaginal cream or suppository, or with oral medication?" Any current symptomatology should be elicited—unusual discharge, itching, burning, dyspareunia, unusual bleeding between or with menses, dysuria or urinary frequency or urgency. Note also when the woman's last gynecologic checkup was and when she had her last Pap smear. Ask if she has had any abnormal Pap smears and if so what, if any, follow-up or treatment did she receive. Make a special note if this will be her first pelvic examination. Find out if she performs breast self-examinations.

Abdominal/Pelvic Pain and Vaginal Bleeding

Two symptoms are commonly experienced by women. Their differential diagnosis requires clear and precise information, and a number of questions should automatically be asked each time a patient reports either symptom. Because they are so basic to the gathering of complete data, these questions are explicitly delineated here:

Abdominal/Pelvic Pain

Onset/Related Factors: When did the pain first occur? When it first occurred, was it related to activity, exercise, eating (or not eating), specific food, medication, injury, trauma, sex, menses, urination, or bowel movements? Does its recurrence relate to any of these?

Character: What type of pain is it? (Examples can be given, such as sharp, dull, throbbing, burning, achy, cramplike, stabbing.)

Location: Exactly where is the pain? (Ask the patient to show you the area.) Is it internal or external? Deep or on the surface? Does it radiate? To where?

Frequency: Is it constant or intermittent? If intermittent, how often does the pain come?

Duration: How long does the pain last?

Intensity: Is the pain mild, moderate, or severe? Is it incapacitating? Can you [the patient] carry on normal activities while you have this pain? Are you bedridden?

Associated Symptoms: Do other symptoms occur before, during, or after the pain, such as constipation, diarrhea, nausea, vomiting, fever, anorexia, vaginal discharge or bleeding, urinary burning, frequency or urgency?

History/Relief Measures: Has it ever occurred before? Has it been getting worse or better, or has it changed in any way, since it first began or since its last occurrence? What do you do for it when it comes? Does this bring relief? To what degree? Have you ever seen a health care practitioner for this problem? What was the previous diagnosis and prognosis? Have you received treatment? What were the treatments and what were their effects?

Vaginal Bleeding

Onset/Related Factors:	(Ask the same questions as for onset of pain.)
Color:	Is it pink, bright red, dark red, brown, other?
Character:	Is it thin, thick, watery, mixed with mucus? Are there clots? If so, how large are the clots?
Amount:	Specify as best as you can how much bleeding you usually experience. (Give examples, such as drop(s); spots the size of a dime/ nickel/quarter/half-dollar; a cup or part of a cup.) Is the bleeding enough to wear a pad or tampon? What strength pad or tampon? How frequently is this changed? How saturated is the pad or tampon when it is changed?
Frequency:	How often do you have this bleeding? Is it related to your menstrual cycle? Does it occur after or before menses or midcycle?
Associated Symptoms:	Is it associated with pain with urination, urgency, frequency, diarrhea, constipation, rectal or vaginal itching or pain, midcycle pain, or pain with sex?
History/Relief Measures:	(Ask the same questions as for history/relief measures for pain.)
Contraceptive History:	What contraceptive do you use? When did the bleeding start in relation to the use of this contraceptive? What is the name and dosage (for oral contraceptives) and how are they taken? What is the type and size of an intrauterine device (IUD) (if one is in place)?

Obstetric History

"Have you ever been pregnant?" is a better question to ask than "Do you have any children?" as the interviewer wants to know about spontaneous and induced abortions and ectopic and molar pregnancies, as well as term and preterm births. A woman's parity and gravidy should be recorded. Parity is the total number of viable pregnancies; gravidy is the total number of pregnancies including a current one. Often, parity is written in a four- or five-digit code in which the numbers refer, in order, to full-term pregnancies, preterm births, abortions (spontaneous and induced), and number of children now living. In the five-digit code, a middle or final number is added, referring to multiple pregnancies. For example, G5, P3113 (or P31013 or P31130) means a woman has had five pregnancies of which three resulted in full-term deliveries, one in a premature birth, and another in an abortion. She has had no twin births and has three living children. The code does not indicate which of the four viable newborns is no longer alive, or when the death occurred. It is not possible to tell the number of stillbirths from this code or to differentiate spontaneous from induced abortions.

Births. Ask about the gestational age, place and type of delivery, weight, sex, and condition of the baby at birth, and complications or problems during the pregnancy, labor, delivery, or postpartum period. Treatments and sequelae of problems should be noted.

Abortions. It is important to know whether abortions were induced or spontaneous. Most women refer to the latter as "miscarriages," so questions about abortions must be carefully worded to be understood. The type of procedure undergone, if induced or incomplete, and sequelae, if any, are important data. Symptoms preceding and during the course of spontaneous abortions and the gestational age at the time of the abortion may also have significance, especially for women who have had more than one. The type of birth control used at the time of an unplanned pregnancy is another important piece of information to gather.

Ectopic and Molar Pregnancies. Ask about the type of surgery or other treatment, follow-up, and sequelae. Find out if an ectopic pregnancy was associated with IUD use.

Obstetric Plans. The interview should include questions regarding future obstetric plans. If a pregnancy is anticipated shortly, preconceptional screening should be implemented (see Chapter 4). Counseling on avoidance of drugs, medications, alcohol, cigarettes, x-rays, cat feces, raw meat and fish, and environmental pollutants should become a focus of the visit.

Contraceptive History

Ask about current and previously used contraceptives, including those that work and those that do not. It is important to know that somebody relies on withdrawal, for example, if that is all she does. Ask whether her partner uses condoms or if either of them has been sterilized. For each contraceptive, find out about onset, duration, and frequency of use, satisfaction, side effects and complications, and reasons for discontinuance of past methods. Be specific; find out the size and type of diaphragm or cervical cap, the name and dosage of oral contraceptive, the type and size of IUDs, and dates of usage. Sometimes a woman does not have all this information; pictures or actual devices can be shown to her so that she can identify which pill or type of diaphragm, cap, or IUD she has used. If a woman has been sterilized, find out the procedure used and if there have been any complications.

Questions about contraceptive planning should be included here. Does the patient want to continue with her present method or change it? Find out the reasons for any desired change.

Medical History

A complete medical history is an essential screening tool. Ask specific questions regarding kidney, liver, gastrointestinal, gallbladder, thyroid, lung and breast disease; blood and cardiovascular disorders, including hypertension, rheumatic heart disease or history of rheumatic fever, strokes, anemias, varicose veins, and phlebitis; diabetes cancer; epilepsy; infectious diseases, including tuberculosis and hepatitis; and asthma. Information about blood transfusions is especially important. If the patient has received any transfusions, find out whether this was after 1978 but before April, 1985, when screening of donated blood for human immunodeficiency virus (HIV) was begun (Centers for Disease Control, 1987; Friedland & Klein, 1987, p. 1126). Details regarding hospitalizations and treatments should be elicited. Childhood diseases, especially rubella, and immunization status should be noted.

Information about allergies is extremely important. All medication allergies should be highlighted in the history and on the front or inside of the chart folder.

Emotional and psychological problems and treatments should be discussed. Note the usage of psychoactive medications, past and current.

Substance use including tobacco, alcohol, and drug use is part of the medical history, although sometimes included in the social history or listed separately under the heading "Habits." Gather information regarding type, amount, onset, frequency or regularity, and duration of use. Be sure to include drugs obtained through prescription, over-the-counter, or in other ways. Ascertain whether the woman has self-administered intravenous drugs and if so, whether she has shared needles.

Record the woman's last complete medical checkup and optometric or ophthalmic and dental examinations. For a woman with current, chronic, or recurrent problems, ascertain whether she is currently under medical care and where this care is received. Note any medications or treatments she has received in the past or is currently using.

Surgical History

Record any surgeries; why, when, and where they were done; what procedure and anesthesia were used; and any subsequent complications. Ascertain whether blood transfusions were needed. When appropriate, ask about follow-up care.

Family History

A family history can be obtained by asking questions in two ways. If both are used, the chances of obtaining complete information is increased, especially with patients who need cues to stimulate memory. The diseases and disorders delineated in the section on medical history can be enumerated and the woman asked if anyone in her family has or has had them. Alternatively, specific family members can be mentioned, and the patient asked if they are alive and well or if they have any health problems. These include the woman's mother, father, maternal and paternal grandparents, siblings, and children. Aunts and uncles, related by blood, and cousins are less significant. You can ask if any relatives beyond the immediate family have any serious illnesses or whether there are any diseases that the patient knows run in her family. For immediate family members, record current ages and ages of onset of any illnesses. Include treatments that may indicate severity or etiology of the disorder, as in diabetes or hypertension. If any immediate relatives are deceased, find out their age at death and cause of death, if known.

Breast cancer, endometriosis, and osteoporosis are familial diseases of major concern in gynecologic practice. If a patient has a relative who has had breast cancer, ascertain whether it was pre- or post-menopausal and whether it involved one or both breasts. See chapters 10, 18, and 24 for more information on these entities. Another extremely important question to ask is whether the patient's mother took any medications when she was pregnant with her. Ask specifically about diethylstilbestrol (DES). If the patient is unaware of this, and was born between 1946 and 1971, it may help to ask if her mother had any problems with any of her pregnancies, such as bleeding, miscarriage or threatened abortion, toxemia, or diabetes, as women with such histories were most likely to have been given DES. See Chapter 18, Table 18-6, for a listing of names under which DES was marketed.

Social and Cultural History

Where and with whom a woman lives, what her support systems are, and their proximity to her may have profound effects on physical and psychological health and on health care needs. Knowing a woman's place of birth and cultural background helps a practitioner determine whether to screen for particular genetic disorders such as sickle cell anemia or thalessemia. Where she has lived—or recently traveled—provides clues to particular infectious agents, such as hepatitis virus or intestinal parasites, to which she may have been exposed. The Centers for Disease Control (1987) recommend counseling regarding testing for human immunodeficiency virus (HIV) for women of childbearing age born in countries or living in communities where there is a high prevalence of HIV among women.

Cultural and ethnic group identification may determine the meaning that a particular disease or health practice has for an individual (Harwood, 1981). Gynecologic practitioners, for example, may encounter cultural prohibitions against all or some forms of contraception. Cultures differ in attitudes toward bodily exposure and touch, in beliefs about blood and blood drawing, and in food habits. Medical anthropologists have made a distinction between "disease," which refers to biologic abnormalities, and "illness," which signifies the experience of sickness on a personal, interpersonal, and cultural level. Illness is influenced by perceptions, expectations, labeling, and values that are culturally determined. Both disease and illness must be treated for patient satisfaction and clinical effectiveness (Kleinman, Eisenberg, & Good, 1978). Members of any particular group, of course, may or may not subscribe to its predominant beliefs or follow all its customs. Although cultural sensitivity can enhance empathy, cultural stereotyping can be counterproductive to the establishment of rapport.

The following questions have been suggested by Kleinman and associates (1978) to identify cultural beliefs determining the patient's perception of illness:

1. What do you think has caused your problem?
2. Why do you think it started when it did?
3. What do you think your sickness does to you?
4. How severe is your sickness? Will it have a short or long course?
5. What kind of treatment do you think you should receive?

Culturally-determined treatments already sought or utilized should be discussed. Many cultural groups rely on folk healers and use a variety of herbal, spiritual, or naturalistic remedies.

Occupational History

Women's occupational hazards are an increasing subject of inquiry and include those involved in housework (Chavkin, 1984). Hazards to reproductive health, in particular, should be assessed in patients with fertility problems or in women who wish future childbearing (see Chapter 27). Occupational health specialists have urged that screening for occupational and environmental stresses and exposures be part of all routine health histories (Ginnetti & Greig, 1981; The Occupational and Environmental Health Committee, 1983). This can be done during the health interview, although a one-page written questionnaire can be utilized (Coye & Rosenstock, 1983). Areas to be covered are job title and industry, dates of employment, and specific hazards to which the worker is exposed. These include fumes and dust, chemicals, metals, solvents, heat or cold, noise, radiation, video display terminals (VDTs), heavy lifting or physical strain, shift work, and emotional stress. Safety conditions such as ventilation and available washing facilities should be assessed (Ginnetti & Greig, 1981). Family exposure should be elicited since toxicity can be brought home (Fletcher, Gowler, & Payne, 1980). Environmental as well as workplace pollutants should always be considered. Military service may also involve exposures that should not be ignored.

Sexual History

Sexuality is a highly charged issue in our society. Many practitioners refrain from asking questions about this area (Ende, Rockwell, & Glasgow, 1984). This may reflect their own discomfort with the subject matter or an unwillingness to tread on what is generally considered a private matter. Yet, women's health care cannot be complete without some knowledge of sexual functioning. Indeed, problems related to sexuality are frequent enough that they are discussed in this text in two chapters—one on sexual health (Chapter 25) and another on sexual abuse and its effects (Chapter 26).

In one study, 228 patients attending a general medical clinic were asked if they believed that a discussion of sexuality would be appropriate (Ende, et al. 1984). Ninety-one percent responded yes, although only 85 percent of the women patients answered yes. Among those whose physicians (in this study) actually discussed sexual functioning, 98 percent considered it appropriate.

At a minimum, the practitioner needs to know if a woman has sexual intercourse. Many practitioners ask "Are you sexually active?" This question can be misinterpreted; many women who have occasional sex may answer no and the practitioner may be misled. Be very precise in questioning. If a woman is not now having sexual relationships, find out if she has ever had relations. Do not make assumptions. Sex and intercourse do not necessarily mean the same thing. Relationships are not always heterosexual. Lesbian women have needs different from those of heterosexual women.

For sexually active women, find out the number of partners. This may be important if a woman wants to use the IUD for contraception or if her partner or partners require treatment for sexually transmitted diseases (see Chapters 8, 11, and 12). Frequency of intercourse may help determine an appropriate birth control method and may be important in infertility problems. A detailed sexual history is warranted if infertility is identified as a current problem (see Chapter 27).

Sexual risk factors for acquired immune deficiency syndrome (AIDS) should be evaluated. These include known exposure through sexual intercourse; having had sexual relations with an intravenous drug user, a bisexual male, a partner with hemophilia or who received blood products after 1978 but before April, 1985, or anyone whose drug or sexual behavior is unknown; or having engaged in prostitu-

tion (Centers for Disease Control, 1987). Questions about sexual practices that increase the risk of AIDS, as well as those that are protective, should be asked. Risk behaviors include anal intercourse and multiple partners, especially if they are casual encounters. Protective behaviors include monogamy and the use of condoms.

A woman should always be asked whether she has physical or emotional problems or areas of concern related to sexuality. If so, a more detailed history may be called for (see Chapter 25). An openness to her questions and need must be communicated. Conveying a nonjudgmental attitude and explaining reasons for the questions asked are particularly helpful in this part of the history taking.

Nutritional History

Good nutrition is basic to health; a good nutritional history is basic to health care. In addition to the overall benefit of eating well, certain dietary habits can specifically affect women's gynecologic or general health.

Chapters 7, 8, 10, 17, 19 to 24, and 27 all discuss known or suggested contributions of nutrition to health maintenance and disease prevention.

A comprehensive nutritional history takes time to obtain and this is often beyond the scope of a single office visit. It is certainly possible, however, to elicit an abbreviated version. To obtain a 24-hour recall of the previous day's intake or a description of a woman's usual eating habits is not too time consuming. Depending upon her method of birth control and the conditions for which she is at health risk, appropriate areas can be emphasized. Note any dietary restrictions; find out what, if any, nutritional supplements are used. Note the use of dietary stimulants such as caffeine, commonly found in coffee, tea, colas, and some other soft drinks. Ask about usual weight and any recent weight changes or frequent fluctuations. Discuss their possible causes.

Eating disorders such as anorexia and bulimia should be part of a nutritional history. These conditions are more common among young women and may have implications for gynecologic health (see Chapters 21 and 27). Birth control pills are not appropriate as a contraceptive for women with bulimia. Oral medication is problematic for these women. Habits such as fasting and pica should be identified in women planning pregnancy.

A 3-day written dietary history provides a more comprehensive nutritional account. Women identified as at risk nutritionally, or those contemplating pregnancies, for example, can bring a nutritional diary to a subsequent visit. It should consist of all food and fluid intake, time of ingestion, and associated activities. Suggest that it reflect 3 days of representative eating, not holiday or party "binges."

Exercise and Activity History

Activities of daily living and regular exercise have been increasingly related to health. Including these areas in the health history allows the practitioner to help patients structure their lives in ways that are most healthful for them. This might include, for example, routine exercise for all but especially for women with premenstrual syndrome or dysmenorrhea (see Chapters 19 and 20), a family history of cardiovascular disease (Ibrahim, 1983), those at risk for osteoporosis (see Chapter 24), or oral contraceptive users (see Chapter 7). Conversely, symptoms related to activity may be important clues to health problems. Find out specifically what types of activities the patient participates in and whether she experiences adverse effects after such activity ties. If so, have her specify the type and degree of activity related to the onset of the symptom or symptoms. This may alert you to the need for referral for further evaluation.

For women with physical disabilities, additional information about daily activities is important to assess each woman's degree of independence and manual skills, particularly in relation to potential contraception. The practitioner also will need to find out what assistance may be needed for the woman to get up to the examining table, to help prevent her from falling off the table, to dress and undress, and to manage her urinary drainage systems during the examination (Szasz, Miller, & Anderson, 1979, pp. 1354–1355).

INTERVIEW TECHNIQUES

Thoroughness in interviewing does not guarantee that the information obtained will be helpful. The approach to interviewing, the language used, and the type of questions asked all affect information gathering. Guidelines can be followed but often each of these areas must be adapted to individual women. The goal is to help a patient remember, identify, and verbalize—not always an easy task given the time constraints of an office visit and the variety of backgrounds of people in our society.

Language

Interview language must be understood clearly. Decisions need to be made regarding the degree of medical terminology to use. A patient's educational level, age, and ease with the English language give some clues as to how well technical words will be understood, but these can be misleading. A well-meaning practitioner who uses street terms with adolescents may be seen as patronizing and evoke embarrassment or hostility, particularly if the young woman senses discomfort with such terminology on the practitioner's part. On the other hand, an adolescent—or an adult—may be familiar with only the vernacular. Even a highly educated, articulate person may not understand much medical jargon. Sometimes it is best to use technical and nontechnical words in the same question. "Have you ever had hypertension, high blood pressure?" is an example of a question that should be understood by most patients.

A more difficult situation arises when the patient and practitioner do not speak the same language. If a patient's language ability is not obvious, Harwood (1981) recommends ascertaining the language she prefers. He also recommends using an interpreter rather than a phrase book if the interview is to be conducted in a language in which the practitioner is not able to ask for clarification or amplification of ideas. He advises the use of friends or relatives brought by patients as translators although he cautions against using non-adult children for this task because of the possible need to discuss subjects that are taboo between parents and children. Two guidelines to present to the interpreter are that the patient's own words be used whenever possible and clarification be requested whenever the patient or practitioner uses unfamiliar words or presents ideas that are unclear.

Questioning

Asking open-ended questions at the beginning of the interview, and at the beginning of each of its sections, is advisable. It gives the practitioner a chance to assess the language used by the patient and also reveals the concerns that are most salient to her. Linfors and Neelon (1981) assessed 55 outpatient visits and found that an open-ended interview best detected patient problems needing medical action. In a study that recorded and analyzed 74 office visits, questions that demanded only a yes or no answer were found to interrupt patients prematurely and to result in a loss of relevant information (Beckman & Frankel, 1984). Beginning the interview with such closed questions limited patient participation. A useful technique, therefore, is to start each category with an open-ended question, such as "Have you ever had any serious medical (gynecologic/obstetric, etc.) problems?" More pointed questions can then be asked specifying the conditions that are important for you to know about. Leading questions such as "You've never been hospitalized, have you?" are generally not advised. In asking questions about potentially sensitive areas, it is helpful to word questions in ways that communicate a nonjudgmental attitude. "How many partners will need to be treated for this infection?" may be better than "Do you have more than one partner who needs to be treated?" An alternative technique is to preface the question with information that implies acceptance: "Many young women today have problems with food. A common occurrence is forced vomiting after eating. Do you ever do this?"

How directive to be in an interview depends upon how responsive the patient is. Generally, at either extreme, direction is needed. The woman who answers questions briefly and incompletely needs much direction, often in the form of specific, fixed-choice questions that suggest appropriate answers to her. "What does that pain feel like?" may not bring forth as useful an answer as "I am going to give you some examples of words that describe pain. Tell me which one best fits the pain you have been having. Does it feel sharp like a knife, or is it a dull ache, or perhaps it feels like menstrual cramps?" Extremely verbal women may talk at length about areas that do not seem terribly relevant. It is generally rapport building and therapeutic to listen (Platt, 1981) and valuable information is gathered when the patient speaks freely. Some digressions, however, may need to be limited, especially if they indicate a need that you judge to be outside your scope of expertise or your time limitations. The practitioner can say something; "We can discuss that more later, or perhaps I can suggest someone who can help you with that. Right now, I have some more questions for you." However, Fletcher (1980, p. 931) cautions, "many interviewers . . . lost important clues by jumping in too soon with the next question. Interrupting to bring the patient back to the point may be needed to check irrelevance, but must be carefully done to avoid the risk of shutting the patient up."

Family Members or Friends

Some women have a family member or another person with them during the interview. If this is a mother or other close relative, she or he can be helpful in providing certain data. A parent usually knows the patient's childhood medical history. A sexual partner can sometimes add information about sexually transmitted diseases or birth control practices. Some women, however, are reluctant to speak in front of a third person. This may be true in the case of adolescents who are with their mothers. You may notice that the friend or relative answers most of the questions. It is valuable in these situations to speak to the woman alone, at least briefly. The history taking can extend into the examination part of the visit if no one else is present then. If the woman's support person stays with her for the physical, or if you have an assistant in the examination room, it may be wise to suggest that you would like to talk to the patient alone for a few minutes. At this time, she can be asked frankly if there is anything she would like to say to you privately.

Counseling

Another decision to be made is whether to combine history taking with counseling or whether to take a complete history and then counsel. The advantages of the first technique are that you avoid the problem of forgetting significant areas to cover in counseling and you need not inhibit a patient's queries that may arise as she is reporting historical data. The disadvantages are that this may become disorganized and inefficient. One area of counseling easily leads to another and the overall interview may suffer. Also, waiting to obtain additional data from the physical examination or from office laboratory tests will enhance teaching and counseling. Either way is acceptable, although most beginning practitioners find it easier to separate the two functions. In order not to omit important counseling needs, they jot down topics to be returned to.

The "Door-knob Syndrome"

A not infrequent occurrence in interviewing has been called the "door-knob syndrome" (Riegelman, 1981). This refers to the situation in which a patient suddenly remembers a problem or decides to give information previously avoided, just as the provider's or patient's hand is on the door-knob, signaling the visit's ostensible end. Discussion of problems brought up in this way should not be ignored, as they often are significant. In fact, they may indicate concerns so important or personal that the patient consciously or unconsciously suppressed them until she felt able to trust the practitioner.

Follow-up

It has been suggested that a complete history cannot be obtained at one session (Riegelman, 1981). It may be useful, for example, to counsel a patient on symptoms to look for and schedule a follow-up visit for further data collection. In gynecologic practice this might include the patient's keeping a bleeding history or a premenstrual symptom record. Specific characteristics of the problem or symptoms, its frequency, duration, timing relevant to the menstrual cycle, associated symptoms, or predisposing factors can be noted more accurately by the patient after careful discussion of relevant areas.

Directed Practice

Audio- or video-tapes can be utilized to increase the practitioner's consciousness of effective language and behaviors. These may be utilized in simulated (Lenkei & Bissonette, 1984; Shepherd & Hammond, 1984; Talento & Crockett-McKeever, 1983) or real patient encounters (Davis & Dans, 1981). Sometimes it can be difficult to listen to or watch oneself, but both can be invaluable in pointing out barriers to communication that most often can be eliminated with some effort. Of course, the patient's informed consent is needed for an interview to be taped, and in one study, 13 percent of patients refused when asked for permission to

allow a video camera in the consulting room (Martin & Martin, 1984). Patients with problems relating to the breast or reproductive system were found to be more likely to refuse consent. Among the consenting patients, 11 percent later expressed disapproval of the recording. To avoid jeopardizing rapport building with patients, it may be advisable to restrict video-taping to simulated encounters. Even without an audio- or video-recorder, simulation and role playing can improve the practitioner's interviewing effectiveness. These are often used in professional educational programs, but can be initiated in the work setting.

RECORDING THE INTERVIEW

Clarity and conciseness are two essential characteristics of the interview writeup. Both help practitioners organize their thoughts and sort out data that are relevant to the identification of problems and diagnoses. Clarity helps in planning for subsequent or follow-up care. This is especially important in a setting where the same provider may not be seen at each visit. Clarity also has a medicolegal function. The chart is a legal document, used in court as evidence should a malpractice or negligence suit arise. Vague or ambiguous statements can easily be misinterpreted.

Conciseness is essential if a chart is to be read by other practitioners. To be concise does *not* mean to be incomplete; it does mean avoiding verbosity. The best intentioned practitioner who records *everything* the patient says may actually be doing her a disservice: at future visits, vital information may be overlooked. An outline form, using widely accepted abbreviations with clear headings, is usually easier to follow than paragraphs written in whole sentences.

Recently, the computer has been advocated as an aid to record keeping. Among its benefits are decreased writing time (Farrell & Worth, 1982), facilitation of recall for return visits, and cost efficiency of maintaining backup records for weekend or night reference (Bradshaw-Smith, 1982). In addition, the sharing of records with patients can be eased through the use of computer printouts (Sheldon, 1982). Patient-held records have been suggested as a means of improving communication between health care agencies (Lakhani, Avery, Gordon, & Tait, 1984), increasing patient knowledge (Brophy, 1982), involving patients in their own health care, facilitating patient–practitioner communication (Snell, 1984), and sharing control and power with patients (Metcalfe, 1980). Problems of computer records include initial cost and disruption (Bradshaw-Smith, 1982), and the potential loss of patient privacy and confidentiality (Hiller, 1981; Hiller & Seidel, 1982). In a survey of 497 patients in two practices in England, one researcher found that nineteen percent of patients would be worried about the use of computers by their general practitioner. Twenty-seven percent felt that they would be unwilling to speak freely if their practitioner maintained computer records, and 7 percent stated that they would change practitioners rather than have their records kept in a computer file (Potter, 1981). Although a detailed discussion of the advantages and disadvantages of computer-kept records or of specific hardware or software is beyond the scope of this chapter, it is realistic to assume that this practice will become increasingly widespread in the near future. It should be mentioned that providing written health records to patients is not, however, dependent on computer technology. Photocopy machines work perfectly well for this purpose.

Sample Writeup

Patient	Anita Morales
Address	85 First Avenue, New York, NY 10003
Phone	(212)887-3426
Workplace	S&S, Inc.
Work Address	934 34th Street, New York, NY 10016
Date of Birth	5/24/60
Date	6/30/87
Reason for Visit:	27-year-old recently married, P0010, here for annual checkup and to discuss birth control methods. Uses diaphragm. Satisfied except slight discomfort in rear entry position and with deep thrusting.
Menstrual Hx:	LMP 6/12/85, 3 days, normal flow. 12 × 28–30 × 3-4. Heavy × 1 day, then light. Uses super Tampax × 1 day, then regular. Changes q ≈ 6–8 hr. ō dysmenorrhea or PMS.
Gyn Hx:	Last gyn checkup 2/84, Pap normal. Monilia × 1, 2 yr. ago. Rx'd c̄ vag. suppository. ? name. UTIs—recurrent 1979-1984, ≈2×/yr. No recurrence × 3 yr.
Obs Hx:	Ind. AB, 1980, 6 wk., vacuum, no problems. (Became pregnant using diaphragm, removed ā 6 hr.)
Contraceptive Hx:	Diaphragm × 7 yr., arcing spring, #70. IUD p̄ AB × several months → ↑'ed bleeding.
Medical Hx:	Last medical checkup for new job, 1984. Last dental exam, ≈ 6 mo. ago. Last eye exam, ≈2 yr. ago. Denies major illnesses. UCHD. Immunizations complete in childhood, including rubella. Boosters, last year. No smoking. Occ. alcohol: glass of wine, ≈1x/wk. Occ. marijuana: ≈1 joint/mo.
Family Hx:	M—A&W, age 55. No DES. F—CA of prostate, had surgery and radiation. Doing well. Age 58. Sibs—2 older sisters, A&W. MGf—A&W, age 89. MGm—died CA, intestinal, age 68. PGf—died pneumonia, age 75. PGm—A&W, age 70.
Social/Cultural Hx:	Born in Puerto Rico. In U.S. × 10 yr. Traveled to P.R. for 1 mo., 2/85. Lives with husband in 1-bedroom, 2-floor walkup apt.
Occupational Hx:	Secretary × 3 yr. Exposed to fluorescent lighting. Uses video display terminal ≈2hr/wk.
Sexual History:	1 partner × 3 yr. Several previous partners. Intercourse 3-4×/wk. No risk factors for AIDS. No problems except with diaphragm as noted above.
Nutritional Hx:	Generally 3 meals/day. Low-salt, low-fat, no red meat. Occ. sweets. 3 cups coffee/day, 1 cola. No supplementation. Usual wt: 135, no recent fluctuations.
Exercise/Activity Hx:	Aerobics 3 ×/wk. Walks 1-2 miles qd.

REFERENCES

Barsky, A. J., Kazis, L. E., & Freiden, R. B., et al. (1980, December). Evaluating the interview in primary care medicine. *Social Science and Medicine, 14A*(6):653–658.

Beckman, H. B., & Frankel, R. M. (1984, November). The effect of physician behavior on the collection of data. *Annals of Internal Medicine, 101*(5):692–696.

Bernstein, L., & Bernstein, R. S. (1980). *Interviewing: A guide for health professionals,* (3rd ed.), Norwalk, CT: Appleton-Century-Crofts.

Bloom, S. W., & Wilson, R. N. (1979). Patient–practitioner relationships. In H. Freeman, S. Levine, & Z. G. Reeder, (Eds.) *Handbook of medical sociology.* N.J.: Prentice-Hall.

Bradshaw-Smith, J. H. (1982, July). The role of the computer in general practice. *The Practitioner, 226*(1369):1211–1213.

Brophy, J. J. (1982, December 9 [letter]). Patients should be responsible for their own medical records. *The New England Journal of Medicine, 307*(24):1530.

Centers for Disease Control (CDC). (1987, August 14). Public health service guidelines for counseling and antibody testing to prevent HIV infection and AIDS. *Morbidity and Mortality Weekly Reports, 36*(31):509–515.

Chavkin, W., (Ed.) (1984). *Double exposure: Women's health hazards on the job and at home.* New York: Monthly Review Press.

Colombotos, J. (1975, Fall). The patient–physician relationship: Paper presented in the Program of General and Continuing Education in the Humanities, Professional and Humane Values, New York: Columbia University.

Coye, M. J., & Rosenstock, L. (1983, November). The occupational health history in a family practice setting. *American Family Physician, 28*(5):229–234.

Danzinger, S. K. (1978, September). Uses of expertise in doctor-patient encounters during pregnancy. *Social Science and Medicine, 12*(5A):359–367.

Davis, J. C., & Dans, P. E. (1981, October). The effects on instructor-student interaction of video replay to teach history-taking skills. *Journal of Medical Education, 56*(10):864–866.

Ende, J., Rockwell, S., & Glasgow, M. (1984, March). The sexual history in general medicine practice. *Archives of Internal Medicine, 144*(3):558–561.

Farrell, D. L., & Worth, R. M. (1982, March). Implementation of a computer-assisted medical record system in the family practice office. *Hawaii Medical Journal, 41*(3):89–92.

Fletcher, B. C., Gowler, D., & Payne, R. L. (1980, November 29). Transmitting occupational risks. *Lancet* II(8205):1193.

Fletcher, C. (1980, October 4). Listening and talking to patients, II: The clinical interview. *British Medical Journal, 281*(6245):931–932.

Friedland, G. H., & Klein, R. S. (1987, October 29). Transmission of the human immunodeficiency virus. *New England Journal of Medicine, 317*(18):1125–1135.

Ginnetti, J., & Greig, A. E. (1981, November–December). The occupational health history. *Nurse Practitioner, 6*(6):12–13.

Harwood, A. (1981). *Ethnicity and medical care.* Cambridge, Mass: Harvard University Press.

Hein, E. C. (1980). *Communication in nursing practice,* (2nd ed.). Boston: Little, Brown and Company.

Hiller, M. (1981, Fall). Computers, medical records, and the right to privacy. *Journal of Health Politics, Policy and Law, 6*(3):463–487.

Hiller, M. D., & Seidel, L. F. (1982, July–August). Patient care management systems, medical records, and privacy: A balancing act. *Public Health Reports, 97*(4):332–345.

Ibrahim, M. A. (1983, February). In support of jogging. *American Journal of Public Health, 73*(2):136–137.

Kleinman, A., Eisenberg, L., & Good, B. (1978, February). Clinical lessons from anthropologic and cross-cultural research. *Annals of Internal Medicine, 88*(2):251–258.

Lakhani, A. D., Avery, A., Gordon, A., & Tait, N. (1984, November). Evaluation of a home based health record booklet. *Archives of Disease in Childhood, 59*(11):1076–1081.

Lenkei, E., & Bissonette, R. (1984, November). Introduction to interviewing patients. *Journal of Medical Education, 59*(11):911–912.

Linfors, E. W., & Neelon, F. A. (1981, July). Interrogation and interview: Strategies for obtaining clinical data. *Journal of the Royal College of General Practitioners, 31*(228):426–428.

Long, L., & Prophit, P. Sr. (1981). *Understanding/responding: A communication manual for nurses.* Monterey, Calif.: Wadsworth Health Sciences Division.

Martin, E., & Martin, P. M. L. (1984, November). The reactions of patients to a video camera in the consulting room. *Journal of the Royal College of General Practitioners, 34*(268):607–610.

Metcalfe, D. H. H. (1980, July). Why not let patients keep their own records? *Journal of the Royal College of General Practitioners, 30*(216):420.

The Occupational and Environmental Health Committee of the American Lung Association of San Diego and Imperial Counties. (1983, November). Taking the occupational history. *Annals of Internal Medicine, 99*(5):641–651.

Platt, F. W. (1981, March). Research in medical interviewing. *Annals of Internal Medicine, 94*(3):405–407.

Potter, A. R. (1981, November). Computers in general practice: The patient's voice. *Journal of the Royal College of General Practitioners, 31*(232):683–685.

Riegelman, R. K. (1981, November). The hidden holes in the history. *Postgraduate Medicine, 70*(3):40–45.

Rogers, C. (1961). The characteristics of a helping relationship. In C. Rogers (Ed.). *On Becoming a Person*, Boston: Houghton Mifflin Company.

Rogers, C. (1962, Fall). The interpersonal relationship: The core of guidance. *Harvard Educational Review, 32*(4):415–429.

Sheldon, M.G. (1982, February). Giving patients a copy of their computer medical record. *Journal of the Royal College of General Practitioners, 32*(235):15–86.

Shepherd, D. & Hammond, P. (1984, March). Self-assessment of specific interpersonal skills of medical undergraduates using immediate feedback through closed-circuit television. *Medical Education, 18*(2):80–84.

Snell, P. (1984, December 15). Writing it down. *British Medical Journal, 298*(6459):1674–1678.

Szasz, G., Miller, S., & Anderson, L. (1979, June 9). Guidelines to birth control counselling of the physically handicapped. *Canadian Medical Association Journal, 120*(11):1353–1358.

Talento, B. & Crockett-McKeever, L. (1983, July/August). Improving interviewing. *Nursing Outlook, 31*(4):234–235.

Veatch, R. (1972, April). Updating the hippocratic oath. *Medical Opinion, 8*(4):56–61.

Zola, I. K. (1963, October). Problems of communication, diagnosis, and patient care: The interplay of patient, physician and clinic organization. *Journal of Medical Education, 38*(10):829–838.

3

The Physical and Pelvic Examinations

Susan Papera

The ability to perform physical examination is an essential skill of health care providers. In gynecologic practice, pelvic assessment can serve both screening and diagnostic purposes. The practitioner of well-woman gynecology must be equipped to perform a basic screening physical examination of the entire body and a complete and thorough pelvic examination.

This chapter provides the practitioner with a basic outline of specific procedures involved in performing a complete physical examination and with detailed information on the steps of a pelvic examination. Together with the information in Chapters 2 and 4, the skills needed for health assessment are covered completely.

Although the value of periodic health examinations is unquestioned, their timing and content are widely debated among clinicians, medical researchers and policy makers, epidemiologists, health educators, special interest groups such as the American Cancer Society, and recipients of such examinations. Introduced at the turn of the century, periodic screening examinations were adopted first by life insurance company physicians with the goal of increasing life expectancy, thereby reducing expenditures (Charap, 1981). Later, physical examinations became common in industry prior to employment and in the military prior to enlistment.

The basic premises underlying the screening physical are that (1) disease can exist in asymptomatic individuals; (2) disease can be detected by examination at an early stage; and (3) early discovery of disease can lead to arrest, reversal, or cure (Charap, 1981, p. 733). Early studies on health screening did not address the third premise, and, to this day, there remains little systematic research on the curative benefits of routine health examinations. As early as 1923, the value of routine annual health screening for all individuals was questioned (Council on Scientific Affairs, 1983). In more recent years, various researchers and groups have evaluated specific procedures used in health screening and have suggested guidelines for the incorporation of each of these into periodic examinations (American Cancer Society, 1980; Breslow & Somers, 1977; Canadian Task Force on the Periodic Health Examination, 1979; Frame & Carlson, 1975). Figure 3–1 summarizes the age-specific screening recommendations of four research groups. Each small blackened square within the larger square represents a procedure recommended by the group represented by that square. The key indicates the study group assigned to a given square.

The 1979 report of the Canadian Task Force on the Periodic Health Examination had a major impact on preventive health practices in many Western countries (Spitzer, 1984). This report provided age- and sex-specific recommendations for screening for numerous conditions. These recommendations were based on the effectiveness of the treatment or preventive measures employed after detection, and whether they would have greater effectiveness if begun in the asymptomatic stage rather than when symptoms developed; the "burden of suffering" of the disease; and the characteristics of the detection procedure, that is, its risks and benefits, the sensitivity and specificity of the maneuver or test (see Chapter 4), and the safety, simplicity, cost, and acceptability to the patient (Canadian Task Force on the Periodic Health Examination, 1979; Fletcher & Spitzer, 1980).

The Canadian Task Force report is updated annually; as the effectiveness of certain screening measures is revealed and better treatments are developed, the value of screening changes. The Task Force advised ongoing research to clarify the efficacy, effectiveness, and efficiency of various screening maneuvers and the most advantageous frequency of performance of each.

Among the most relevant recommendations for women's health are those relating to screening for cervical cancer, discussed more fully in Chapter 4, and those for breast cancer. In the 1985 update of its report, the Canadian Task Force (1986) recommended annual breast examination for women aged 40 and over, or 35 and over if risk factors exist (see Chapter 10). The American Cancer Society (1987) additionally advocates professional breast examinations every 3 years for women aged 20 to 40. Many gynecologists and women's health care practitioners continue to advise yearly physical examinations, including breast and pelvic assessments (Queenan, 1986); the American College of Obstetricians and Gynecologists (ACOG) (1980) recommends yearly screening for cervical cancer for all sexually active women, particularly in light of the high prevalence of risk for cervical cancer in the U.S. population today (see chapters 4 and 13).

In deciding how often to offer health screening and what to include, the practitioner should bear in mind that the recommendations of various groups are *minimal* standards (Canadian Task Force on the Periodic Health Examination, 1979, p. 1194). Risk factors should be assessed for each woman and frequency increased according to risk of the individual. Some conditions may need to be screened for at intervals more frequent than yearly. Symptomatic

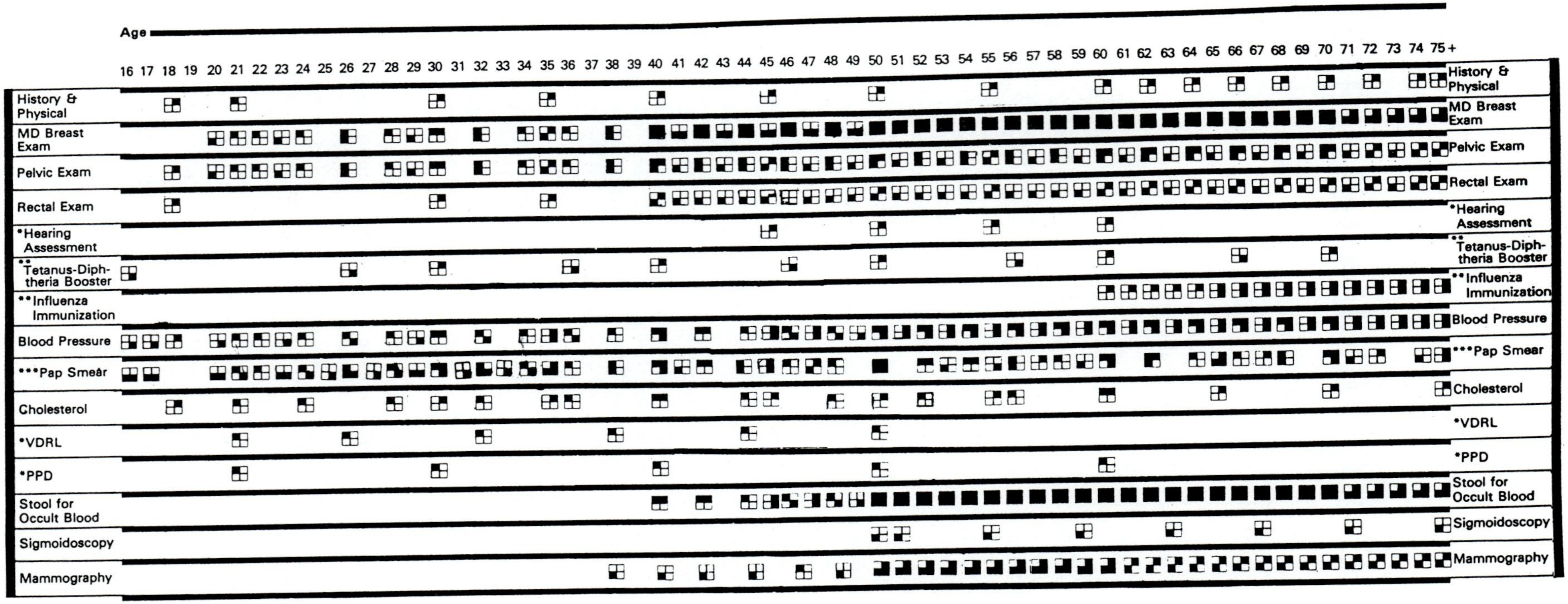

Age

16 17 18 19 20 21 22 23 24 25 26 27 28 29 30 31 32 33 34 35 36 37 38 39 40 41 42 43 44 45 46 47 48 49 50 51 52 53 54 55 56 57 58 59 60 61 62 63 64 65 66 67 68 69 70 71 72 73 74 75+

Row labels (left and right):
History & Physical
MD Breast Exam
Pelvic Exam
Rectal Exam
*Hearing Assessment
**Tetanus-Diphtheria Booster
**Influenza Immunization
Blood Pressure
***Pap Smear
Cholesterol
*VDRL
*PPD
Stool for Occult Blood
Sigmoidoscopy
Mammography

F	B&S
ACS	CTF

F   Frame and Carlson
B&S Breslow and Somers
ACS American Cancer Society
CTF Canadian Task Force on the Periodic Health Examination

A blackened square indicates that a study has considered the maneuver and recommended it. Squares left empty do not necessarily indicate that the study considered but did not recommend the maneuver.
* Canadian Task Force recommends that this be done on the basis of clinical judgment.
**At first visit physician should check past immunization history per Centers for Disease Control recommendations for rubella, mumps, poliomyelitis, diphtheria/tetanus toxoids, pertussis.
***If sexually active.

Figure 3–1. Summary of recommendations of the four major studies. *(Updated from Medical Practice Committee, American College of Physicians. [1981, December]. Annals of Internal Medicine, 95[6], 729–732. Reprinted with permission.)*

patients should be examined, regardless of the time interval from their last examination (Medical Practice Committee, 1981). Additional benefits of routine screening must also be considered: establishment of a trusting patient–practitioner relationship and continuing development of a data base. These enhance the relevancy and effectiveness of health teaching, counseling, and behavior modification (Council on Scientific Affairs, 1983; Fletcher & Spitzer, 1980).

No study has addressed the issue of prepregnancy health screening. We recommend a complete physical examination, comprehensive laboratory testing, outlined in Chapter 4, and health teaching for every woman planning a pregnancy within 3 to 6 months. This allows for detection and treatment of conditions that might negatively affect the pregnancy, birth, or neonate, such as syphilis, anemia, tuberculosis, or rubella susceptibility; implementation of treatments that should not be undertaken during pregnancy, such as radiation or chemotherapy; and initiation of health teaching, particularly on the avoidance of teratogenic exposures during the crucial first trimester.

Health care professionals should also consider the interests of patients in preventive health care. In a survey of 309 adults attending the Family Medical Center in Fayetteville, North Carolina, 91 percent expressed desire for an examination to prevent or detect disease; of these, 86 percent felt that such examinations were indicated every 6 months to 1 year. These patients wanted more extensive screening than performed by their physicians or recommended in published guidelines (Romm, 1984).

It is the responsibility of all practitioners to develop their own criteria for the timing and content of screening visits based on current recommendations and the needs of individual patients. A further responsibility inherent in well-woman care is providing adequate follow-up if a problem is identified that is not within the area of expertise of the practitioner.

As women's health care practitioners often are primary care providers (Queenan, 1986), gynecologic visits involve much more than pelvic organ assessment. A yearly complete physical examination with an accompanying interval history and laboratory testing as appropriate is advisable. A large part of the primary care visit is devoted to dialogue, education, and promotion of involvement of the woman in her own health. To accomplish these objectives, the woman must be viewed within the context of her entire life situation, with consideration of how her many roles and the stresses she experiences affect her attitudes and her ability to be healthy.

THE PHYSICAL EXAMINATION

The physical examination serves to detect abnormalities suggested by the history and/or unsuspected problems (Dignam, 1985, p. 5). The examination follows history taking and the establishment of a relationship that facilitates comfort. Specific information given during the history should guide the practitioner to areas of examination that may not be surveyed in a routine screening.

As baring the body for scrutiny by a relative stranger is anxiety provoking, the provider should develop or refine techniques to reduce this stress. Courtesy, respect, and sensitivity to each woman's feelings must be conveyed throughout the examination. Obvious stress-reduction measures include ensuring privacy, offering the woman a gown, explaining the procedures to be done and their rationale, exposing only the parts of the body being examined,

and keeping the examining room and instruments at a comfortable temperature.

Bates (1987, p. 128) suggests developing a consistent and logical order to the physical examination. This helps to ensure completeness and to decrease discomfort to the patient by lessening the number of times that she has to change positions.

The key maneuvers to be performed in physical assessment are inspection, palpation, percussion, and auscultation. This is the order in which they are generally carried out, although not all maneuvers are needed in the examination of a particular body system.

The following format is presented with an emphasis on the modalities utilized in a general health screening and their order. This is meant to be an adjunct to the more complete information contained in textbooks focusing entirely on physical examination. Further information on normal and abnormal findings is presented throughout the text in various chapters, particularly those in Section III, Gynecologic Pathophysiology.

Before beginning the examination process, and, indeed, during the interview, the practitioner should begin to form a general impression of the patient. Her overall appearance, gait, body posture, and speech patterns should be noted.

Height and Weight

Body weight in relation to height and body build can suggest nutritional or hormonal abnormalities.

With the patient sitting:

Blood Pressure and Pulse Rate. The Canadian Task Force recommends that every adult 25 years and older have a blood pressure measurement done on any visit to a physician. It is reasonable to interpret this to mean any visit to a health care provider. Obtain temperature as necessary.

Skin. Inspect the skin throughout the examination. Note its color, tone, presence of irregular pigmented lesions, scars, abnormal vasculature, bruising, and hirsutism.

(HEENT) Head, Eyes, Ears, Nose, and Throat

EYES. Inspect the eyes for obvious abnormalities such as discharge, inflammation, strabismus, opacity, and exophthalmos. Perform an ophthalmoscopic examination if hypertension is present or if warranted by historic data.

EARS. Perform an otoscopic examination if specific complaints are elicited.

MOUTH. Inspect the mouth for lesions and plaques. Inspect the tongue for position, lesions, moistness, and coatings. Inspect the teeth and gums for their general condition and the presence of caries, bleeding, and lesions.

THROAT. Inspect the pharynx, nose, and palate, and palpate the sinuses as warranted by information obtained in the history. Palpate the thyroid gland to determine size, configuration, consistency, and the presence of nodules or masses. Palpate the and palpate lymph nodes of the neck and supraclavicular areas.

Back. Palpate the spine for straightness and the presence of pain. Palpate the costovertebral angle to determine tenderness (CVAT) if an infection of the kidney is suspected.

Lungs. Inspect the chest for normal or abnormal movement. Percuss and auscultate the lungs posteriorly and laterally to determine the presence of abnormal sounds.

Breasts. Inspect the breasts. Use the breast examination to teach the woman all components of breast self-examination.

Good lighting is essential for adequate breast inspection. Inspect for symmetry, nipple alignment, nipple discharge, abnormal venous pattern, coloration, and skin appearance and changes including dimpling, puckering, and enlarged pores. Perform inspection with the patient in four positions: with her arms at her sides; with her arms raised above her head; with her hands on her hips with the pectoral muscles tightened; and with her arms extended forward and her face straight forward as she stands up and leans forward from the waist. When the woman is again seated, palpate the axillary area.

With the patient supine and the head and upper body elevated to a comfortable position:

Breasts. Palpate the breasts. Have the patient raise one arm over her head. If available, place a small pillow or rolled sheet under this shoulder. Palpate the entire breast on this side, gently pressing the breast tissue against the chest. A variety of techniques (see Fig. 10–10) can be used; the important consideration is to systematically palpate the entire breast. Possible techniques include palpating in a circular motion, working from the outside in to the areola or from the areola to the outer breast edge; dividing the breast into four quadrants and palpating from the outer to inner edge of each quadrant; or superimposing an imaginary wheel on the breast and palpating each of its spokes. Repeat the same procedure on the other side. It is not necessary or advisable to routinely attempt to express discharge from the nipple (Varney, 1987, p. 655).

The woman should repeat the examination under the practitioner's guidance. This demonstration increases the woman's familiarity with her breasts and provides her with a sense of what is normal. By observing her technique, the practitioner can correct any mistakes and encourage and reinforce effective techniques.

If an abnormality is found, repeat the palpation in both the sitting and the lateral recumbent positions (Dignam, 1985, p. 9). Ideally, the breasts should be examined after the menses, when the hormonal influence on the breast tissue is lowest. If normalcy of the breasts is unclear when the examination is done premenstrually, repeat the examination postmenses, especially if the woman has fibrocystic changes. Do not hesitate to consult with an appropriate physician, or refer the patient for a repeat examination, if an abnormality is present (see Chapter 10).

Heart. Note the rate, rhythm, and regularity of the heart with both the bell and the diaphragm of the stethoscope in four areas: the second right and left interspaces near the sternum; the lower sternal border; and the apex, the fifth or fourth left interspace medial to the midclavicular line (Bates, 1987, pp. 284–285). Determine the presence of murmurs or extra heart sounds and describe their location. Consult or refer as necessary.

Abdomen. Inspect the abdomen for contour, scars, obvious pulsations, and masses. Palpate first lightly, then deeply in each of the four quadrants. Percuss and palpate the liver, spleen, and the kidneys for enlargement and tenderness. If the woman has complained of abdominal pain, palpate that particular area last.

Inguinal Nodes. Palpate the left and right nodes for enlargement and tenderness.

Extremities. Inspect and palpate both extremities, noting varicosities, lesions, edema, erythema, warmth, and pain.

THE PELVIC EXAMINATION

It has been said that "the first pelvic examination is a rite of passage into American womanhood" (Hein, 1984, p. 47). The experience is one that is long remembered, affecting a woman's response to subsequent pelvic examinations and, indeed, general health care. To make this examination a positive experience, the provider needs to be cognizant not only of the proper techniques to be used but of the emotional, physical, and psychological input from the woman and her questions and concerns.

As the first gynecologic examination often occurs during adolescence, the particular concerns of teenagers regarding the event must be understood. Millstein, Adler, and Irwin (1984) found that fear of finding pathology and fear of pain were significant sources of stress among 84 young women seen in an adolescent clinic. Embarrassment and questions of personal cleanliness also were mentioned as creating anxiety. For a further discussion of the needs of this age group, see Chapter 22.

Adult women also approach the pelvic examination with varying degrees of anxiety. The procedure generally is seen as threatening, embarrassing, and uncomfortable (Willard, Heaberg, & Pack 1986). A woman's attitudes toward herself and her body, her comfort with her sexuality, and her past experiences all interact to increase or decrease her stress.

Involving the woman as an active participant in the pelvic examination is recommended to reduce examination anxiety. This can be accomplished by instructing the woman in the techniques used, explaining the sensations that she may feel, and using the opportunity of the examination to teach about the body and its functions. The woman is invited to visualize her external and internal genitalia by using a mirror, to voice concerns and raise questions, and to explore sexual and reproductive issues. This educational gynecologic examination has been found to have a positive impact on women exposed to it (Latta & Wiesmeier, 1982; Willard, et al., 1986). Use of a warm speculum and provider sensitivity to patient feelings also have been found to be important to women (Broadmore, Carr-Gregg, & Hutton, 1986).

Limiting discussion to *only* the mechanical aspects of the pelvic examination procedure, however, may be a source of anxiety. In a study of the experiences of 199 women with pelvic examinations, Broadmore et al., (1986) demonstrated the speculum beforehand to 36 women. Twenty-one of these women became less anxious; six, however, became more anxious. Unless information is included about associated feelings and sensations, anxiety may not be reduced (Thompson, 1981).

Before starting any explanation of the procedure, ascertain if it is to be a first pelvic examination. If not, find out what the woman's prior experiences have been. Assess her understanding of the procedures performed during a pelvic examination and their value. Find out whether the woman performs self-examinations; if so, ask how she does them and what she has noticed.

Techniques

The pelvic examination should follow other physical examination components, allowing the woman to become comfortable with the examiner. The same attitudes of respect and sensitivity should prevail. Privacy is paramount, although physical privacy may be difficult to achieve in some clinical settings. In these, and, indeed, all circumstances, the practitioner must guarantee emotional privacy by extreme and undivided attentiveness to each woman.

Whether or not to have a second professional person, assistant, or family member present during the examination depends on the specific requirements of the practice setting and the desires of the patient and practitioner. Broadmore and associates (1986) found that of 191 women surveyed, 146 (89 percent) preferred not to have a third person present; this was not significantly correlated with the sex of the examiner. In a study of adolescents (females and males) who were accompanied by a family member to a clinic, only 50 percent of 190 having a genital examination chose to have a family member present. This generally was viewed as beneficial by the physician performing the examination (Phillips, Bohannon, & Heald, 1986). In another investigation, Buchta (1986) found that most of 100 female adolescent patients in a private pediatric office preferred to be alone for pelvic examination; the sex of the physician influenced this preference only among adolescents aged 13 to 14. The younger adolescents preferred to have their mother present; the older adolescents chose a female nurse as the preferred chaperone.

The issue of draping also can be left to the woman, although the comfort of the examiner is a consideration. If a drape is used, it should be placed in such a way as not to impede eye contact between the patient and the practitioner (Fig. 3-2). A mirror should be offered to the woman.

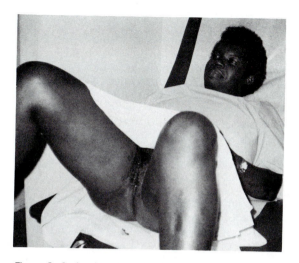

Figure 3-2. Correct draping in the semisitting position.

The patient assumes a supine or semisitting position (Fig. 3-2) with assistance, if necessary. Her head should be supported. Her feet should be placed in stirrups once all the necessary equipment is prepared. The stirrups should be at a comfortable length for the woman's height to prevent excessive abduction of the hips. The patient's hands should either be at her sides, over her chest, or holding the mirror at her knee or vulva (Fig. 3-3). These positions enhance abdominal muscle relaxation, whereas holding hands over the head tends to tighten these muscles. The semisitting position may be preferable to the supine as it is more comfortable for the patient, relaxes the rectus muscle, increases eye contact, and facilitates use of the mirror. Women in this position may feel less vulnerable and embarrassed, and verbal communication may be enhanced (Swartz, 1984).

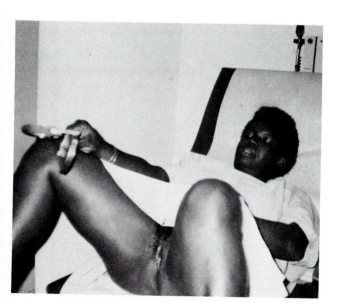

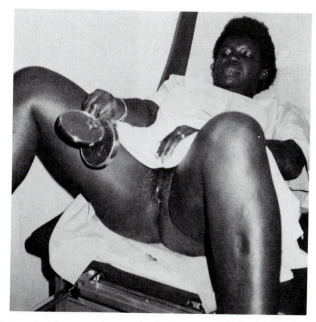

Figure 3-3. Use of the mirror.

Steps

The practitioner should wash her hands and glove both hands. Latex gloves are recommended. Avoid startling the patient by warning her that she will be touched and telling her where. Some practitioners begin by touching a less sensitive area such as the thigh (Primrose, 1984).

External Genitalia. Carefully inspect and palpate the external genitalia while explaining what each structure is, its location, and its function. Include the mons, labia majora, labia minora, prepuce, clitoris, urethra, perineum, and anal area. Note the hair pattern and any erythema, irritation, discharge, lesions, edema, infestation, or tenderness. Palpate Bartholin's and Skene's glands and the underside of the urethra for enlargement, pain, and discharge.

Vaginal Tone. With two fingers a short distance into the vagina, ask the woman to tighten her vaginal muscles or to squeeze the examining fingers. Then pronate the examining fingers in the vagina, spread them slightly and depress the posterior vaginal wall. Ask the woman to cough and then to bear down to assess for cystocele or rectocele and its degree. Explain Kegel exercises and the benefits of good vaginal tone (Table 3–1).

Speculum Examination. There are different types and sizes of specula. Both the width and depth of the blades vary. Specula are made in metal or plastic, and the manipulation of the blades differs between these two types. Metal specula are reusable after sterilization; plastic specula are disposable or can be given to patients for self-examination. The practitioner needs to be familiar with the instrument being used prior to inserting it to avoid undue discomfort to the woman.

Select a size of speculum that will be comfortable for the patient while allowing adequate visualization. Generally, a larger instrument is needed for a multiparous woman or woman with lax vaginal walls. Pediatric specula are available for adolescents or virginal women.

Warm water can be used to lubricate the speculum, but must be used sparingly because excess water can interfere with the accuracy of Pap smears. The speculum may be inserted after vaginal tone has been assessed, while the vagina still is depressed. This is advantageous to the patient because there is less manipulation, but the speculum must be warmed and lubricated beforehand. If the speculum was not inserted at that point, depress the perineum before insertion. Assist the woman to relax with breathing and visualization techniques. If she bears down with the pelvic musculature, as if having a bowel movement, insertion of the speculum is eased.

Insert the speculum at an oblique angle over the fingers in the vagina. When the speculum is in the vagina a short distance, remove your fingers and continue inserting the speculum into the posterior fornix. If the woman is extremely tense, hold the speculum just inside the introitus for a few moments, while the woman gets used to feeling it inside her vagina. Ask her to tell you when she is ready for you to advance it. Once the speculum has reached the posterior fornix, turn the blades to the horizontal position, withdraw slightly, and open the blades (Fig. 3–4). Inform the woman that she may feel increased pressure as the blades are opened.

The cervix should be visible; if not, ascertain where in the vagina the speculum is and adjust it accordingly. If the visible vaginal wall is rugated, the speculum is probably anterior to the cervix; if the visible tissue is smooth, the speculum is probably posterior to the cervix. The blades of the speculum should be closed before readjusting it. Once the cervix is in view, lock the speculum. If, after several attempts, the cervix cannot be located without undue discomfort to the woman, close the blades and withdraw the instrument. Find the cervix with the fingers and then reintroduce the speculum. Often, in this situation, the cervix will be extremely posterior or anterior or rotated to the left or right. Remember not to use lubricant on the fingers inserted into the vagina.

CERVICAL INSPECTION. Note the color of the cervix, any erythema, irregularities, lesions, ectropion, or friability, and the characteristics of any secretions. Also note the configuration of the os and if it appears to be dilated. Gently wipe away any excessive discharge. Obtain the Pap smear and any necessary cultures (see chapters 4, 12, and 13).

VAGINAL INSPECTION. Note the color, rugation, and presence of any abnormal tissue structures or discharge. Characterize any secretions according to color, consistency, amount, location, and odor. Obtain a specimen for a wet mount as necessary from the posterior vagina or lateral walls. Release the blades of the speculum and control them using the thumb lever. Inspect the vaginal walls by rotating the speculum blades from side to side. Gradually close the blades as the instrument is removed. The blades should be completely closed before the speculum is removed, to avoid pressure on the urethra.

Note the odor of any secretions on the speculum. Some

TABLE 3–1. KEGEL EXERCISES: INSTRUCTIONS TO PATIENTS

Kegel exercises, also called "pelvic floor exercises," are used to tone and strengthen the pubococcygeal muscle. This muscle is the major support for the urethra, bladder, vagina, uterus, and rectum. It is divided into the pubovaginalis, puborectalis, and pubococygeus proper muscles. Kegel exercises may be helpful in preventing or alleviating the problems of cystocele (weakened muscle between vagina and bladder), rectocele (weakened muscle between vagina and rectum), prolapsed ("falling") uterus, and urinary stress incontinence (loss of urine with sneezing, coughing, laughing, or other abdominal strain). The exercises can also enhance sexual pleasure. In the postpartum (after childbirth) period, the exercises promote healing of the perineum—the area stretched, and sometimes cut or torn, during childbirth.

To identify the pubococcygeal muscle, willfully stop and start the flow of urine or ask your care provider to identify this muscle during your next vaginal examination. The pressure you feel when stopping the flow of urine is caused by contraction of the pubococcygeal muscle. Once identified, you can exercise this muscle wherever and whenever convenient. Exercise consists of contracting the muscle, holding it, and releasing or relaxing it.

Kegel exercises can be done slowly, contracting the muscle for up to 10 seconds, or rapidly, releasing the muscle right after contraction. There is no limit on how frequently or how often the exercises should be done—the more the better.

Adapted from McKey and Dougherty (1986), Primrose (1984), and Varney (1987).

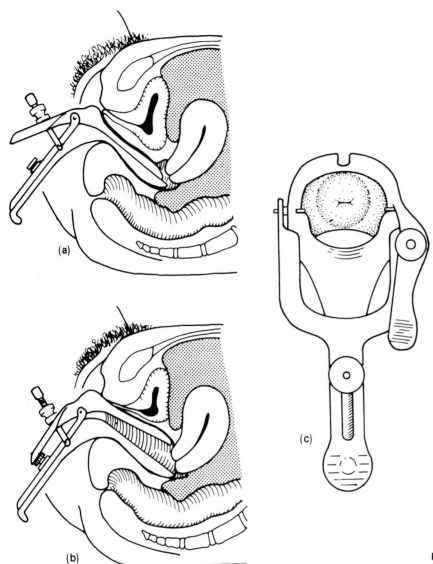

(a)

(b)

(c)

Figure 3–4. Placement of the speculum.

practitioners take a specimen of discharge from the speculum for the wet mount.

Bimanual Examination. Remove the glove from the nondominant hand. Discard it appropriately.

Relaxation of the abdominal muscles is essential for adequate palpation with minimal discomfort to the woman. Apply water-soluble lubricant to the index and middle fingers of the examining (dominant) hand. Warn the woman that the lubricant may feel cold. Insert these fingers into the vagina, in the vertical position. Place the fingers of the nondominant hand gently on the lower abdomen, palm down (Fig. 3–5).

VAGINA. Palpate the posterior and lateral aspects of the vagina for nodules or irregularities.

CERVIX. Locate the cervix, noting its position. Palpate the ectocervix, noting any irregularities. Feel the cervical consistency and whether there is dilation of the os. With one finger on each side of the cervix, note its length and inclination. Move it from side to side; assess its mobility and any associated pain.

UTERUS. Palpate the uterus to determine its position, size, shape, consistency, and degree of regularity. With the examining fingers still on either side of the cervix, apply upward pressure while applying downward pressure with the abdominal fingers. By following the inclination of the cervix either forward or backward, the position of the uterus can be determined as either anterior or posterior and then as either "verted" or "flexed" (Fig. 3–6). In any position, the uterus should be palpated with the vaginal fingers to the extent possible. Move the fingers of both hands laterally and up and down to outline the uterus.

It is often possible for a woman to feel her uterus through the abdominal wall if the examiner pushes it upward, particularly if the uterus is in the anterior position. If this is the case, ask the woman if she wishes to feel her

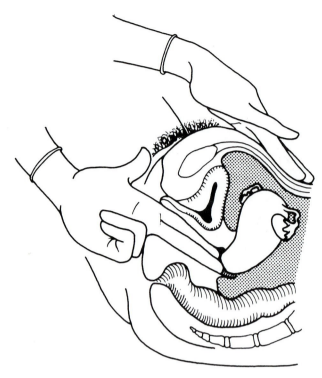

Figure 3–5. Bimanual palpation of the cervix and uterus.

uterus and help her place her fingers suprapubically to feel it.

If the uterus is retroverted or retroflexed, it is best evaluated during the rectovaginal examination.

ADNEXAE. Palpate the adnexae. Place the vaginal fingers into the right or left lateral fornix and move the abdominal hand laterally from above the uterine fundus (Fig. 3–7). Apply upward pressure with the vaginal fingers and downward pressure with the abdominal hand, and, moving the hands together, sweep the fingers toward the symphysis. If nothing is felt, move the fingers of both hands closer to the midline and repeat. This ensures adequate assessment of the entire adnexal area. Repeat the maneuver on the opposite side.

In palpating the adnexae, keep in mind that the normal anatomic relationship of the fallopian tubes and ovaries to the uterus is lateral and slightly posterior (see Chapter 1). This awareness will help guide the hands to the expected location and minimize discomfort to the woman.

Note any enlargements or irregularities of the ovaries and any thickening of the tubes. Normally, these structures are small and may not be palpable. The ovaries are sensitive when touched and some discomfort may be experienced. The woman should be warned of this to allay any anxiety that could arise if this pain is felt.

Rectovaginal Examination. After changing the glove of the examining hand, lubricate the middle finger of this hand. Visualize the rectal sphincter and place this finger, palm up, over the sphincter. Ask the woman to bear down. While she is straining, gently insert the lubricated finger into the rectum. Insert the index finger into the vagina and locate the cervix. Apply downward pressure with the abdominal hand and outline the uterus. Check the adnexal areas using both rectal and vaginal fingers. With the rectal

and vaginal fingers, palpate the sacral ligaments for consistency, smoothness, and tenderness and the rectovaginal septum for intactness. With the rectal finger, palpate the rectal walls and the tone of the anal sphincter. Note any masses, fistulas, fissures, or other lesions.

Depending on the woman's age, a test for stool guaiac may be warranted. The American Cancer Society advises annual rectal examinations from age 40 onward and annual stool guaiac examination after age 50 (American Cancer Society, 1987, p. 17). Some physicians, however, recommend testing the stool for guaiac every 2 years between ages 35 and the midforties (Queenan, 1986).

Occasionally, a woman will not be able to have the pelvic examination performed. If she is unable to tolerate two fingers in her vagina because of extreme anxiety, an intact hymen, or pain, the procedure should be attempted with one finger. If it is still intolerable, or the woman suffers from vaginismus, the examination should be stopped. The patient should be assisted to a sitting position and helped to explore the reasons for the difficulty. If a psychological or sexual problem is uncovered that the practitioner is not able to deal with, the woman should be referred for appropriate counseling. It may take more than one visit to accomplish the pelvic examination. If the cause of the woman's discomfort is physical, such as a tight hymenal ring, measures to alleviate the problem can be instituted. If she is willing, the patient can be taught techniques to manually dilate the vaginal opening. The woman should be instructed to assume a comfortable position at home and gently spread the hymen apart. She then should insert one finger deeply into the vagina on a daily basis, working up to inserting two fingers comfortably (Primrose, 1984). A follow-up appointment should be made to assess her progress and perform the pelvic examination if she is ready.

The woman with a physical or mental disability may have special needs. Depending on her particular disability, just getting to and from the examining table and into the necessary positions may be difficult. A woman with a spinal cord injury may need an assistant to hold her legs in the stirrups or to control leg spasms. To ensure complete care for disabled women, two or more visits may be necessary, the first to assess educational and physical needs, and the others to perform the examination with assistance (Szasy, Miller, & Anderson, 1979).

Sample Physical Examination Writeup

This follows the interview writeup (see Chapter 2).

Well-nourished, well-developed female in no apparent distress

Ht:	65″
Wt:	135 lb
BP:	110/74
Pulse:	84
Skin:	Clear, good tone, no lesions
HEENT:	Throat clear, good dentition, gums clear, thyroid nonpalpable, no lymphadenopathy
Back:	Spine straight, no CVAT
Lungs:	Clear to P&A[a]
Breasts:	Soft, nontender, no masses; nipples erect and intact
Heart:	RRR[b], no murmur
Abdomen:	Soft, nontender, no masses, no organomegaly
Inguinal nodes:	Nonpalpable, nontender
Extremities:	No varicosities, edema, or signs of phlebitis

[a]Percussion and auscultation
[b]Regular rate and rhythm

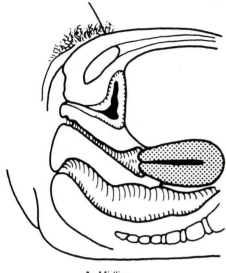

A. Midline

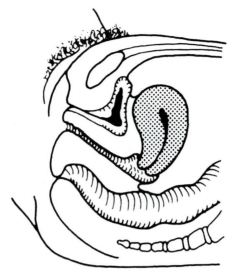

B. Anteverted

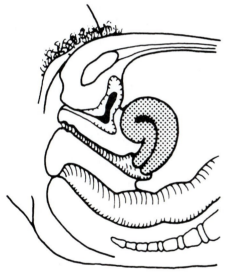

C. Anteflexed

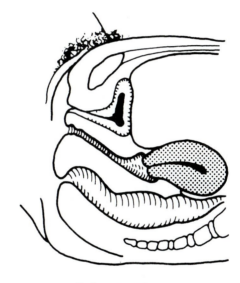

D. Retroverted

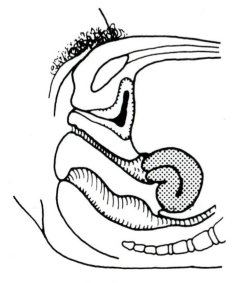

E. Retroflexed

Figure 3–6. Uterine positions.

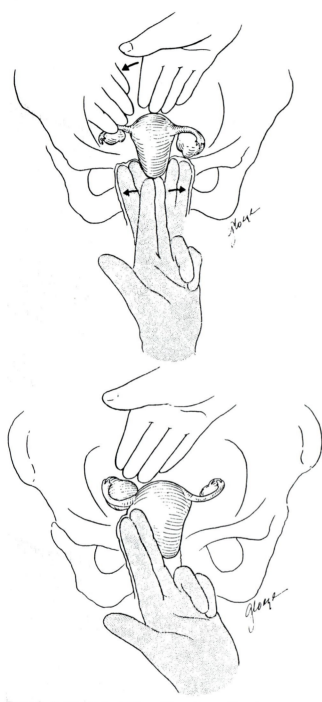

Figure 3-7. Bimanual palpation of the adnexae. *(From Dignam, W. J. [1985]. History and physical examination. In D. H. Nichols & J. R. Evrard [Eds.], Ambulatory gynecology. Philadelphia: Harper & Row. Reprinted with permission.)*

Pelvic:

External genitalia:	Normal female eschutcheon, vulva clear, BSU[c] s̄ discharge
Vagina:	Rugated; small amount of clear mucous discharge s odor; small cystocele, no rectocele; fair muscle tone
Cervix:	Midline, pink, clear, smooth, firm, mobile, nontender, os closed, no discharge
Uterus:	Retroverted, n1 size, smooth, firm, nontender

[c]Bartholin's, Skene's, and urethra

Adnexae:	Right: palpable, n1 size, no masses, nontender
	Left: nonpalpable, no masses, nontender
Rectovaginal:	No masses, fissures, or fistulas

REFERENCES

American Cancer Society. (1987). *Cancer facts and figures.* Washington, DC: American Cancer Society.

American Cancer Society. (1980, July/August). ACS Report on The Cancer Related Health Checkup. *Ca—A Cancer Journal for Clinicians, 30*(4), 194–240.

American College of Obstetricians and Gynecologists. (1980, June). *ACOG policy statement: Periodic cancer screening in women.*

Bates, B. (1987). *A guide to physical examination and history taking*(4th ed.). Philadelphia: J.B. Lippincott.

Breslow, L. & Somers, A.R. (1977, March). The lifetime health-monitoring program: A practical approach to preventive medicine. *The New England Journal of Medicine, 296*(11), 601–608.

Broadmore, J., Carr-Gregg, M. & Hutton, J.D. (1986, January 22). Vaginal Examinations: Women's experiences and preferences. *New Zealand Medical Journal, 99*(794), 8–10.

Buchta, R.M. (1986, November). Adolescent females' preferences regarding use of a chaperone during a pelvic examination: Observations from a private-practice setting. *Journal of Adolescent Health Care, 7*(6), 409–411.

Charap, M.H. (1981, December). The periodic health examination: Genesis of a myth. *Annals of Internal Medicine, 95*(6), 733–735.

Canadian Task Force on the Periodic Health Examination. (1979, November 3). The periodic health examination. *Canadian Medical Association Journal, 121*(9), 1193–1254.

Canadian Task Force on the Periodic Health Examination. (1986, April 1). The Periodic Health Examination. 2. 1985 update. *Canadian Medical Association Journal, 134*(7), 724–726.

Council on Scientific Affairs. (1983, March 25). Medical evaluation of healthy persons. *Journal of the American Medical Association, 249*(12), 1626–1633.

Dignam, W.J. (1985). History and physical examination. In D.H. Nichols & J.R. Evrard (Eds.), *Ambulatory gynecology.* Philadelphia: Harper & Row.

Fletcher, S.W. & Spitzer, W.O. (1980, February). Approach of the Canadian Task Force to the periodic health examination. *Annals of Internal Medicine, 92*(2, Part 1), 253–254.

Frame, P.S. & Carlson, S.J. (1975, February). A critical review of periodic health screening using specific screening criteria. *Journal of Family Practice, 2*(1), 29–36.

Hein, K. (1984, Summer/Fall). The first pelvic examination and common gynecologic problems in adolescent girls. *Women and Health, 9*(2/3), 47–63.

Latta, W. & Wiesmeier, E. (1982, July/August). Effects of an educational gynecological exam on women's attitudes. *Journal of Obstetric, Gynecologic and Neonatal Nursing, 11*(4), 242–245.

McKey, P.L. & Dougherty, M. (1986, September/October). The circum-vaginal musculature: Correlation between pressure and physical assessment. *Nursing Research, 35*(5), 307–309.

Medical Practice Committee, American College of Physicians. (1981, December). Periodic health examination: A guide for designing individualized preventive health care in the asymptomatic patient. *Annals of Internal Medicine, 95*(6), 729–732.

Millstein, S.G., Adler, N. & Irwin, C.E., Jr. (1984, April). Sources of anxiety about pelvic examinations among adolescent females. *Journal of Adolescent Health Care, 5*(2), 105–111.

Phillips, S., Bohannon, W. & Heald, F.P. (1986, July). Teenagers' choices regarding the presence of family members during the examination of the genitalia. *Journal of Adolescent Health Care, 7*(4), 245–249.

Primrose, R.B. (1984, January). Taking the tension out of pelvic exams. *American Journal of Nursing, 84*(1), 72–74.

Queenan, J. (Moderator). (1986, November). The periodic gyn exam: Establishing continuity of care [Symposium]. *Contemporary Ob/Gyn, 28*(5), 172–196.

Romm, F.J. (1984, August). Patient's expectations of periodic health examinations. *The Journal of Family Practice, 19*(2), 191–195.

Spitzer, W.O. (1984, May 15). The periodic health examination. 1. Introduction, *Canadian Medical Association Journal, 130*(10), 1276–1278.

Swartz, W.H. (1984, March 2). The semi-sitting position for pelvic examinations [Letter], *Journal of the American Medical Association, 251*(8), 1163.

Szasy, G., Miller, S. & Anderson, L. (1979, June). Guidelines to birth control counselling of the physically handicapped. *Canadian Medical Association Journal, 120*(11), 1353–1358.

Thompson, S.C. (1981, July). Will it hurt less if I can control it? A complex answer to a simple question. *Psychological Bulletin, 90*(1), 89–101.

Varney, H. (1987). *Nurse-midwifery* (2nd ed.). Boston: Blackwell Scientific.

Willard, M.D., Heaberg, G.L. & Pack, J.B. (1986, March/April). The educational pelvic examination: Women's responses to a new approach. *Journal of Obstetric, Gynecologic and Neonatal Nursing, 15*(2), 135–140.

4

Laboratory Testing

Patricia Aikins Murphy

Laboratory tests are used in a variety of situations in the well-woman gynecologic care setting. One very common use is in confirmation of a diagnosis suggested by history or physical findings; a pregnancy test or a wet smear falls into this category. Another use is in screening of asymptomatic women for certain conditions or illnesses: Pap smears and periodic tests for syphilis fall into this category. Tests may also be used to verify improvement in a patient's condition, assist in the selection of appropriate therapy, or document health or illness for insurance, disability, and employment purposes.

Laboratory tests are extremely useful in clinical practice, but they are meant to complement—not substitute for—the management process and to confirm information obtained by thorough history taking and physical examination. An isolated laboratory value is usually insufficient basis for making a diagnosis or a decision about the need for therapy. The practitioner must always review laboratory data wisely, bearing in mind that there are no perfect laboratory tests, only proper uses for and interpretation of them.

This chapter defines some concepts involved in the choice and interpretation of laboratory tests. A number of tests common to gynecologic practice are discussed: cytologic studies (Pap smears); tests for vaginitis and sexually transmitted diseases, including those that can be performed in office and those that are generally sent to the laboratory; and pregnancy tests and prepregnancy evaluations. Guidelines for the use of these tests and procedures for gathering specimens are outlined. Interpretation of tests and treatments to be initiated on the basis of test results are discussed in specific chapters that follow, particularly in Section III, "Gynecologic Pathophysiology." Laboratory tests specific to conditions that are less commonly seen in well-woman gynecologic practice, such as those evaluating infertility or bleeding disorders, are discussed in the appropriate chapters.

CONCEPTS INVOLVED

Results of laboratory tests usually fall into one of four categories:

1. True positive (TP): a positive result in a person who actually has the condition
2. True negative (TN): a negative result in a person who does not have the condition
3. False positive (FP): a positive result in a person who does *not* have the condition
4. False negative (FN): a negative result in a person who actually has the condition

Some test results are reported as falling within or outside a "reference range." For these tests, values obtained from a group of healthy people are used to develop a curve of test results. The upper and lower 2.5 percent are designated as the limits of the reference range. Results falling outside this reference range are often incorrectly interpreted as abnormal; actually, such a result indicates only that it is different from 95 percent of the population. Each laboratory sets its own reference ranges, based on differences in testing procedures and equipment.

Many factors affect the validity of test results. A Pap smear may be read as negative in a woman who has a cancerous lesion if she douched prior to the test, if the smear is inadequate for diagnosis, or if the slide is not prepared or read accurately. Tests for syphilis may be read as positive in patients who do not have syphilis as a result of the presence of certain other infections such as mononucleosis and influenza.

The sensitivity of a test refers to how well it identifies people who actually have the condition. Sensitivity is the percentage of positive test results obtained when testing only people with the disease. The lower the false-negative rate, the higher the sensitivity (see Table 4–1).

The specificity of a test refers to how well it eliminates those who do not have the disease. Specificity is the percentage of negative test results obtained when testing only people who do not have the disease. The lower the false-positive rate, the higher the specificity.

Tests that are highly sensitive are chosen when the purpose is to screen a population for a condition: a low rate of false negatives is desired to ensure detection of the disease. Tests that are highly specific for a certain condition should be chosen when a diagnosis must be made: a low rate of false positives is preferred when making decisions or initiating therapy based on a presumed diagnosis.

The results of any given test must also be viewed in relation to the prevalence of a given disease or condition in a certain population.* The positive predictive value (PPV)

The following discussion is based on an excellent chapter in The office laboratory *(Fischer, Addison, Curtis, & Mitchell, 1983).*

TABLE 4-1. CONCEPTS USED IN TEST RESULT INTERPRETATION

$$\text{Sensitivity} = \frac{\text{true positives}}{\text{total persons with disease}} = \frac{TP^a}{TP + FN} \times 100$$

$$\text{Specificity} = \frac{\text{true negatives}}{\text{total nondiseased persons}} = \frac{TN}{TN + FP} \times 100$$

$$\text{PPV} = \frac{\text{true positives}}{\text{total positives (true + false)}} = \frac{TP}{TP + FP} \times 100$$

$$\text{NPV} = \frac{\text{true negatives}}{\text{total negatives (true + false)}} = \frac{TN}{TN + FN} \times 100$$

[a]PPV, positive predictive value; NPV, negative predictive value; TP, true positive; TN, true negative; FN, false negative; FP, false positive.
Adapted from Fischer, P., Addison, L., Curtis, P., Mitchell, J. (1983). How good is the test? In The office laboratory. East Norwalk, CT: Appleton–Century–Crofts.

is the percentage of people with a positive test result who have the disease; the negative predictive value (NPV) is the percentage of people with negative test results who do not have the condition (Table 4–1). For example, suppose a test is developed that identifies condition X with 95 percent specificity (only 5 percent false positives) and 100 percent sensitivity (no false negatives). In a general population of 10,000 persons, condition X affects 1 in 1,000 people; if you screen all 10,000 persons, a total of 10 will have condition X. Because there is 100 percent sensitivity, all 10 will have a true positive test. Thus, 9,990 people in this group do not have the condition. Because the test is 95 percent specific, 5 percent, or approximately 500, of the healthy people will have false-positive tests. The PPV of the test (number of true positives divided by total number of positives) is 1.96 percent. In other words, less than 2 percent of those with positive results actually have condition X!

Suppose now that condition X usually coexists with a number of symptoms and physical findings that can be elicited during the history and physical examination of the person, and that 1 in every 10 persons with these findings has condition X. If the clinician limits screening to only 1,000 people who have these symptoms, 100 of those tested will have the condition. The PPV in this case is very different: dividing the true positives by the total positives results in a PPV of 67 percent, meaning that two thirds of those with positive results have condition X.

Proper selection of laboratory tests therefore depends on the purpose of the test and its sensitivity and specificity, as well as the prevalence of the condition for which the patient is being tested. Clinical knowledge and assessment skills enable the practitioner to choose properly and interpret wisely.

THE PAP SMEAR

The Papanicolaou (Pap) smear is an inexpensive screening test for cancer. Laboratory examination of cells obtained from the cervix can identify both cancerous and precancerous lesions, allowing timely intervention and treatment. The Pap smear has done "more to eradicate invasive cancer of the cervix and lower the death rate from cancer in women than any other scientific contribution to date" (Jordan, Linden, Friedman, et al., 1971, p. 180).

Obtaining a Pap smear is one of the major reasons a woman seeks gynecologic evaluation. Traditional recommendations have called for an annual Pap after initiation of sexual activity. Recently, these recommendations have been reevaluated and changed by certain medical groups,

generating considerable controversy over the timing and frequency of Pap smear screening.

A 1976 Canadian Task Force report on cervical cancer screening programs, the Walton report (Walton, 1976), questioned the cost-benefit/effectiveness of annual Pap smears in women not at "high risk" for cervical cancer, and changed recommendations for sexually active women in the low- or medium-risk category. The Walton report called for initiating Pap smears with the onset of sexual activity, and performing a second test within 1 year. If both were normal, Pap smears were recommended at 3-year intervals until age 35, then at 5-year intervals until age 60. After age 60, Pap smear screening could be stopped if all smears had been normal. Women at high risk for cervical cancer were still advised to seek annual Pap smears.

In April 1980, the American Cancer Society (1980) made new recommendations similar to those of the Walton report: women at low risk who had two negative Pap smears might prolong the screening interval to 3 years. A 1980 Consensus Development Summary report of the National Institutes of Health followed with the recommendation that after two negative Pap smears, the screening interval could be 1 to 2 years, depending on risk factors.

There was considerable disagreement in the medical community over these new recommendations, and other organizations reiterated the need for annual screening. The American College of Obstetricians and Gynecologists (1980) let its policy recommendations on periodic cancer screening stand at 1-year intervals for sexually active women, as did the Society of Gynecologic Oncology, the International Academy of Cytology, and the American Society of Cytologists (Eddy, 1981). In 1982, the Canadian Task Force revised its stand and changed recommendations to advise annual screening of sexually active women between 18 and 35 (American College of Obstetricians and Gynecologists, 1984).

Several considerations deserve emphasis in the debate over the appropriate interval for Pap smear screening. First, all groups stress the need for frequent (at least annual) screening of women at high risk for cervical cancer. The revised screening intervals of the Walton report and the American Cancer Society are aimed at low-risk women, generally defined as virgins or monogamous women with lifelong relationships, no history of venereal infection, and successive normal Pap smears (Fetherston, 1983). This fact was often overlooked in the publicity surrounding the issue. Categories of higher risk for cervical cancer are numerous and growing (Table 4–2), indicating that a large and increasing percentage of women are at risk for cervical cancer and should be screened at regular frequent intervals. It

TABLE 4–2. CHARACTERISTICS OF WOMEN AT RISK FOR CERVICAL CANCER

Early age at first coitus (<20)

Multiple sexual partners (three or more)

History of sexually transmitted disease (STD)

History of abnormal Pap smears

History of exposure to diethylstilbestrol (DES)

Promiscuity of male partner; history of STD in partner; history of penile or prostatic cancer in partner

Smoking[a]

[a]See Trevathan, Layde, Webster, et al. (1983, p. 499).

should be clarified that additional risk may also be conferred by "serial monogamy" or "multiple marital events" (i.e., one sexual partner at any given time but a number of different partners over the course of time). Medium-risk categories include women who initiated sexual activity after age 20 and have never had more than two partners. High-risk categories include those who initiated sexual activity before age 20 and have had three or more partners. Women who are initially monogamous but have several partners later in life (perhaps after divorce) are probably at higher risk as well (Richart & Barron, 1981).

A second consideration involves the actual rather than the theoretic frequency of obtaining Pap smears. Many practitioners express concern that in actual practice, "annual" Pap smears are sought at 18-month to 2-year intervals, thus implying a risk that recommendations of 3-year intervals might result in Pap smear screening only every 4 to 5 years (Richart & Barron, 1981).

A third concern involves the health maintenance screening that usually accompanies a gynecologic visit. Breast examination; screening for hypertension, gastrointestinal cancer, or other health problems, and identification of health concerns requiring treatment, surveillance, or counseling should be part of the annual exam; for many women, this is their only contact with a health care provider. Although recommended intervals vary for these procedures as well, any changes in recommendation for Pap smear screening should take into account the fact that additional health surveillance occurs at these visits.

A final consideration is the high rate of false-negative Pap smears described in the medical literature. Although many of these studies are open to some methodologic questions, there is general agreement that the usual estimate of 10 to 20 percent false-negative smears is low (Fetherston, 1983) and may in fact be closer to 33 percent (Richart, 1979; Richart & Barron, 1981). Diagnostic reliability is dependent on multiple factors: cooperation of the patient, method and quality of sample preparation, handling and staining techniques in the laboratory, proficiency of the technician and pathologist, and development of a quality assurance program in the laboratory (Wied, Bartels, Bibbo, & Keebler, 1981). The multitude of variables affecting reliability of results makes it difficult to control the false-negative rate. Recommendations for longer screening intervals may not be appropriate if as many as one third of women have false-negative cytology reports.

It seems reasonable in view of these considerations to continue to recommend annual Pap smear screening in sexually active women. In addition, individual practitioners should try to reduce the margin of error by using correct and appropriate sampling techniques when obtaining the Pap smear.

The woman should not be menstruating at the time of the Pap smear (blood makes proper evaluation of cells difficult). She should not have had intercourse, douched, or used any vaginal suppositories or products for 2 or 3 days prior to sampling. Douching or intravaginal products may remove or contaminate the cervical mucus and cells necessary for diagnosis. Coitus may cause trauma or uterine muscle contractions that could temporarily shrink the transformation zone (Singer, 1975). Pap smears can be obtained under these conditions if necessary, but reliability may be reduced.

The cervix should be inspected after insertion of an unlubricated speculum and before bimanual exam (lubricants and excessive water can produce distortion of the cytologic sample). Most practitioners agree that overt lesions should be referred for evaluation; the Pap smear is a *screening*—not a diagnostic—tool. In general, the cervix need not be cleansed before sampling; however, excessive exudate can be blotted or *gently* wiped away with a cotton ball.

Using a spatula, with the longer projection inserted into the cervical os, the practitioner should take a 360° scraping of the cervix, taking care to sample the squamocolumnar junction or transformation zone (T-zone). If the T-zone is not visible on the ectocervix, the scraping should still be done and an endocervical sample taken as described later. Spatulas with longer projections are available to allow scraping of the T-zone if it is located within the endocervix. The goal of the technique is to scrape exfoliated cells or those cells held loosely on the surface of the cervix. Vigorous scraping that abrades the cervix yields tissue that is virtually uninterpretable in the cytology smear (Richart, 1979). The value of wooden versus plastic spatulas has been studied, with some researchers claiming superiority of the plastic spatula, but this issue remains unclear (Rubio, 1977).

Scraping alone has a false-negative rate as high as 30 percent, even when the squamocolumnar junction is visualized on the ectocervix (Garite & Feldman, 1978; Richart, 1979). The lowest false-negative rates occur when both a scraping and an endocervical sample are obtained; appropriate technique thus necessitates that a sample be taken from the cervical canal. This is done in one of three ways: with an endocervical swab, a brush, or a pipette for endocervical aspiration. A fiber-tipped swab is introduced in the canal and rotated clockwise several times to obtain cells. A cotton-tipped swab should first be moistened with saline to prevent cells from adhering to the cotton; a synthetic fiber swab (such as Calgiswab) is nonabsorbent and can be used without moistening. Pap smears taken with an endocervical brush and spatula have been compared with those taken with a swab and spatula. Smears taken with a brush were found to have a greater likelihood of containing endocervical cells (Taylor, Andersen, Barber, et al., 1987). The brush is gently inserted into the endocervical canal, slowly rotated one-half to one full turn, and removed. The smear is prepared by rolling and twisting the brush onto a slide (International Cytobrush, undated). Alternately, the contents of the endocervix may be aspirated using a glass pipette placed at the external os. Many researchers believe that aspirated cells are better preserved and more abundant than those obtained by swabs; cells may be entrapped in cotton fibers or possibly damaged by rotation of the swab (Richart, 1979), but either technique is acceptable.

Although some practitioners use only the swab to obtain both endocervical and ectocervical specimens, studies have shown a high (60 percent) false-negative rate for this technique (Shen, Nalick, Schlaerth, & Morrow, 1984). Both scraping with a spatula and endocervical specimens are necessary for adequate sampling. If two endocervical specimens are needed (e.g., both a Pap smear and a gonorrhea smear), the Pap smear should be done first. Richart (personal communication, 1985) believes that the false-negative rate of the Pap may be increased by loss of the exfoliated endocervical cells in the gonorrhea specimen.

Once obtained, the specimen on the spatula should be spread uniformly over the surface of a glass slide labeled in pencil with the patient's name. Some researchers suggest that a counterclockwise circular or zig-zag motion makes the best and most uniform smear (Rubio, Kock, & Berglund, 1980). The swab or aspirated specimen is smeared on a second slide, taking care to rotate the swab in the direction opposite that from which the specimen was taken to release or ''unroll'' the mucus and cells. Practitioners should be sure that streaks of cervical mucus rather than just discharge are visible on the slide, as abnormal cervical cells are generally trapped within cervical mucus (Koss, 1982). A single slide may be used; if so, the endocervical specimen should be obtained first, placed on the slide, and then smeared together with the scraping specimen when that is obtained.

The specimen should be fixed immediately after spreading. Some laboratories accept air-dried specimens and attempt to reconstitute them; however, most researchers believe that air drying compromises cellular appearance and is not suitable for cytologic analysis (Richart, 1979). Spray fixatives are most commonly used; the slide should be held 12 in. from the container when fixing. If it is too close, the spray may ''blast'' cells off the slide; if it is too far, inadequate spray reaches the slide and drying distortion could result.

If desired, endocrine assessment (estrogen effect) is obtained by scraping the inner third of the lateral vaginal wall (see Chapter 24). Vaginal pool specimens are often recommended in perimenopausal women (sampling is done by scraping the posterior fornix with the other end of the spatula) for detection of endometrial cancer cells, but diagnostic accuracy is low; a 50 percent false-negative rate has been reported (Batzer, 1979).

TESTING FOR VAGINITIS AND SEXUALLY TRANSMITTED DISEASES

During the course of the gynecologic interview and the pelvic examination, the practitioner may decide that testing for vaginitis or a sexually transmitted disease (STD) would be appropriate.

Some clinics and practices establish policies of routine screening for certain asymptomatic infections that are capable of producing considerable morbidity (such as syphilis or gonorrhea); routine chlamydia screening in sexually active women has recently been suggested as well (Handsfield, 1985). Testing for other STDs is generally done if the practitioner obtains a history of symptoms in the patient or her partner, or if there is physical evidence of infection on examination; however, some studies suggest that only a minority of women have the classic signs and symptoms of vaginal infection (Fouts & Kraus, 1980), indicating a need to test more aggressively in women at risk.

Published recommendations for periodic health screening to detect venereal disease generally leave the frequency of testing to the discretion of the provider; one exception is syphilis, for which a serologic test has been recommended at least every few years in healthy adults (Frame & Carlson, 1975). Clinics and providers specializing in the care of sexually active women, however, see a need to screen aggres-

sively and frequently. Decisions about screening tests and intervals are best individualized to the patient, depending on her history of STD, sexual activity pattern, and risk for exposure. Women at risk should probably be screened annually or at each encounter. Several techniques and tests are available for testing for sexually transmitted diseases and vaginitis.

History and Clinical Findings

Although a full discussion of the signs and symptoms of the different vulvovaginal infections is beyond the scope of this chapter (see chapters 11 and 12), certain information must be sought before the practitioner can decide which tests are appropriate.

A patient's history provides little hard information for diagnosis. Women have different perceptions of symptomatology, and indeed the quality and degree of symptoms in each individual may vary over time. Physiologic discharge may be heavy at different times during the menstrual cycle, and may leave yellow-white stains on underwear. Lack of a history of vaginal discharge does not preclude the existence of a vaginal infection, nor does a report of heavy vaginal discharge always indicate an infectious origin.

Complaints of vulvar or vaginal irritation do suggest infection (usually trichomoniasis and candidiasis), and vaginal odor frequently accompanies bacterial vaginosis or trichomoniasis. (Bacterial vaginosis is the most current terminology for the condition that has been called *Gardnerella* and *Hemophilus*. See later text and chapter 11 for more discussion of the pathophysiology of this condition.) Dysuria may accompany herpes, moniliasis, or trichomoniasis (as the urine passes over inflamed vulvar tissue) or may be associated with either urinary tract infection or a urethral syndrome accompanying chlamydial or gonococcal cervicitis. Abdominal pain suggests pelvic infection, and generalized malaise or headache and fever may indicate primary herpes. Certain historic data (recent use of antibiotics or oral contraceptives, douching, sexual activity/partner) may also provide some clues for diagnosis. A history of recurrent STDs requires a careful evaluation for trichomoniasis. Some authorities believe that, because *Trichomonas* is a living parasite cell, it can itself become infected by organisms such as chlamydia, gonorrhea, and other bacteria. Within the cytoplasm of the trichomonad, these organisms can lie dormant and cause recurrences without reinfection; concurrent *Trichomonas* infection may play a significant role in the recurrence of STDs (Richart, Boon, Gupta, et al., 1984).

Physical findings are sometimes diagnostic, but usually require laboratory corroboration. There may be considerable overlap in the appearance of normal and pathologic discharge. The external genitalia should be normal if the discharge is physiologic. Erythema and fissures suggest *Candida*; edema of the vulva may accompany trichomoniasis or candidiasis. Copious discharge found on the surface and in the folds of vulvar tissue usually indicates trichomoniasis or bacterial vaginosis. Vesicles suggest herpes, and ulcerations should be investigated for herpes, chancroid, or syphilis. Condylomata or genital warts warrant screening for syphilis and a Pap smear. Flat cervical condylomata, a factor in the pathogenesis of cervical cancer, may not be visible to the naked eye but are present in 60 percent of women with vaginal warts (Kiviat, 1984).

Within the vagina, the discharge of a vaginal infection often adheres to the vaginal walls, as well as pooling in dependent areas where normal discharge is found. Bubbly or foamy discharge suggests trichomoniasis or bacterial vaginosis, as does discharge of low viscosity. Viscous discharge may be normal or associated with candidiasis (which may also present as a classic "cottage cheese" curdy discharge). Erythematous vaginal mucosa, although hard to quantify, is often described in candidiasis; punctate hemorrhages of the cervix or vagina may be seen with trichomoniasis. Yellow or green discharge is said to indicate trichomoniasis, but the color of the discharge can vary as with other infections. Discharge may in fact be minimal or absent in vaginitis. Vaginal odor indicates trichomoniasis or bacterial vaginosis. Other tests must therefore be utilized to distinguish between the two infections.

The cervix produces copious amounts of clear mucus during the immediate preovulatory phase of the menstrual cycle; purulent cervical discharge suggests gonococcal or chlamydial cervicitis (discharge and debris on the ectocervix must be wiped away with gauze or cotton before assessing this). Hypertrophic cervicitis (an erythematous friable columnar epithelium that may project above the plane of squamous epithelium) is highly suggestive of chlamydia (Eschenbach, 1980), erythema or inflammation around the cervical os may indicate gonorrhea. Ulcerative or necrotic lesions suggest herpes.

Office Laboratory Testing

Certain tests can be done and interpreted in the office to establish a diagnosis in cases of vaginal or urinary tract infection.

pH Tests. Applying a strip of pH indicator paper (such as Nitrazine Paper, Squibb & Sons) to the pool of discharge in the vagina or on the speculum blade can provide diagnostic clues. A pH of 4.5 or less indicates normal physiologic discharge or candidiasis; a pH of 4.5 or greater is consistent with trichomoniasis and bacterial vaginosis. Cervical mucus is alkaline, so care must be taken not to touch the paper to the cervix.

Swab Test. Mucopurulent secretion from the endocervix that appears yellow or green when viewed on a white cotton tip swab is a positive swab test. When found in conjunction with friable cervicitis and a large number of white blood cells in a cervical smear, it suggests chlamydial or gonococcal cervicitis (Centers for Disease Control, 1985a).

Amine or "Whiff" Test. In trichomonal vaginitis or bacterial vaginosis, diamines are present in the discharge that volatilize when in a highly alkaline environment, producing a "fishy" odor. A small amount of discharge should be mixed on a glass slide with a drop or two of potassium hydroxide (KOH) and "sniffed" immediately for the characteristic odor. In some women, this test is not necessary; a highly alkaline vaginal pH or recent sexual intercourse (semen is an alkaline fluid) may produce the "fishy" odor without special preparation. On the contrary, the amine test does not produce odor in the presence of concomitant candidiasis (Fleury, 1983). The amine test is considered by some to be 80 to 90 percent diagnostic of bacterial vaginosis (Erkkola, Jarvinen, Terho, & Meurman, 1983); other studies have found it present in trichomonal vaginitis as well, so further microscopic evaluation for clue cells or trichomonads should be done (Blackwell & Barlow, 1982). *Gardnerella* (an organism found in bacterial vaginosis) may be a normal inhabitant of the vagina and is thought to produce infection only in the presence of anaerobic bacteria; the KOH test confirms the presence of these anaerobes and should be part of the evaluation (Petersen & Pelz, 1983).

Wet Mount. The wet mount, a simple microscopic procedure, is the most useful technique available for the diagnosis of certain vaginal infections. A copious specimen of discharge from the vaginal vault is obtained with a cotton-tipped swab and placed in about 1 mL of warm normal saline (to separate the cells), mixed to produce a suspension, and placed on a glass slide for microscopic examination (Fig. 4–1 and Table 4–3).

Normal vaginal epithelial cells are flat with sharp clear edges (Fig. 4–2). Clue cells are epithelial cells covered with bacteria obscuring the edges of the cell and giving the cell a granular appearance (Fig. 4–3). The presence of clue cells strongly suggests bacterial vaginosis.

White blood cells are found in small numbers, one or two per high-power field (HPF), in normal vaginal discharge and should not exceed the number of epithelial cells (Eschenbach, 1983) (Fig. 4–3). Large numbers of leukocytes suggest infection of the cervix or vagina, but signifi-

TABLE 4–3. PREPARATION OF A WET SMEAR

Collect a copious amount of vaginal discharge with a cotton swab and place in a tube containing 1 mL of normal saline. Vigorously mix the swab in the saline.

Place a drop of the specimen mixture at each end of a clean glass slide or on two separate slides.

Add a drop of KOH (10%) to one specimen and sniff immediately for the characteristic "fishy" odor of bacterial vaginosis.

Cover both specimens with coverslips. Plan to view the plain saline specimen first to allow time for the KOH to lyse cells prior to looking for *Candida*.

With the 10× objective in place on the microscope, the light on low power, and the condenser in the lowest position, place the slide on the stage and lower the objective until it is as close to the slide as possible.

Adjust the eyepieces until a single round field is seen. Turn the coarse focus knob until the specimen is focused. Use the fine-focus knob to bring the specimen into sharp focus.

Be sure to use subdued light and a lowered condenser for a wet specimen. Try increasing the light and raising the condenser while viewing the specimen to see how the cells and bacteria disappear from view.

Move the slide until you have a general impression of the number of squamous cells. Switch to high power (40×); it may be necessary to increase the amount of light slightly.

Evaluate the slide for bacteria, white blood cells, clue cells, *Trichomonas*, and *Candida*. Even if one organism is identified, continue to scan the slide systematically to fully evaluate the specimen. Vaginitis may have multiple causes.

Move the KOH slide into position; switch back to low power to scan the slide for *Candida*. If hyphae are noted switch to high power to confirm the impression.

Be sure to wipe spilled fluid from the stage. If the objective becomes contaminated, use only special lens paper to clean it.

Adapted from Fischer, P., Addison, L., Curtis, P., and Mitchell, J. (1983). The office laboratory. East Norwalk, CT: Appleton–Century–Crofts.

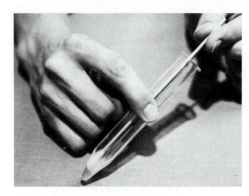

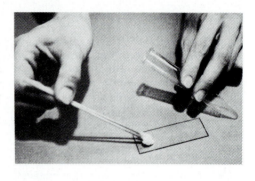

Figure 4–1. Preparation of a wet mount. **Top left.** Vaginal specimen swabs and saline in a plastic tube. **Top right.** Place the vaginal specimen on the microscope slide. **Bottom right.** Microscope slide with both a specimen saline and a KOH wet preparation. *(From Fischer, P., Addison, L., Curtis, P., & Mitchell, J. [1983]. The office laboratory. East Norwalk, CT: Appleton-Century-Crofts. Reprinted with permission.)*

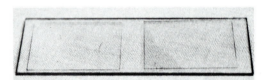

cant infection may exist without them. [Increased white blood cells are rare in bacterial vaginosis, for example, and if found should lead the practitioner to rethink the diagnosis (Blackwell & Barlow, 1982).] Trichomoniasis is often associated with excessive numbers of leucocytes, as is chlamydial or gonococcal cervicitis (Fischer, et al., 1983).

Normal vaginal bacteria, lactobacilli, are large rods and can be seen in the wet mount (Fig. 4–2). Lactobacilli are absent in bacterial vaginosis and are replaced by many small coccobacilli both in the fluid and adhering to the epithelial cells (Fischer, et al., 1983).

Trichomonads, ovoid flagellated organisms slightly larger than a leukocyte, are easily seen on wet mount, recognizable by their motility and undulating membrane (Fig. 4–4). Their motility is reduced when cold, and they assume a rounder shape when dry or drying, so it is important to keep the specimen warm and view it immediately for accurate diagnosis. Trichomonad motility is also hampered by large numbers of white blood cells; in this case, the practitioner must look under high power for the undulating membrane of the organism (Eschenbach, 1983).

Yeast structures may be seen on wet mount, but are

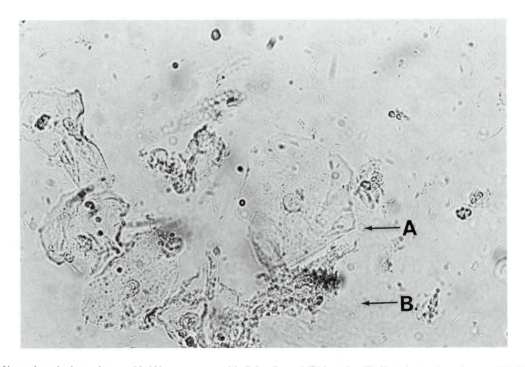

Figure 4–2. Normal vaginal specimen with (A) squamous epithelial cells and (B) lactobacilli. Note how clean these epithelial cells appear compared to those in Figure 4–3 (top and bottom) viewed under high dry objective. *(From Fischer, P., Addison, L., Curtis, P., & Mitchell, J. [1983]. The office laboratory. East Norwalk, CT: Appleton-Century-Crofts.*

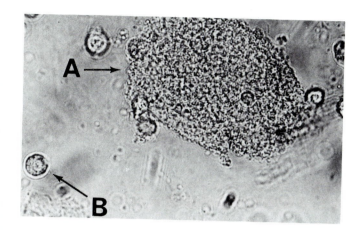

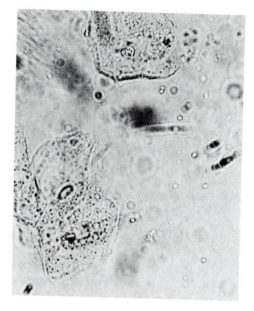

Figure 4–3. **Top.** (A) Clue Cell. (B) White blood cell in a vaginal wet preparation. Viewed under high dry objective. **Bottom.** Normal squamous epithelial cells with dark spots. These should not be confused with clue cells. Viewed under high dry objective. *(From Fischer, P., Addison, L., Curtis, P., & Mitchell, J. [1983]. The office laboratory. East Norwalk, CT: Appleton-Century-Crofts.)*

more easily discovered in a 10 percent KOH preparation. A generous specimen should be placed on a slide and mixed with a drop or two of KOH, which destroys leukocytes and bacteria and blanches the epithelial cells, leaving only the fungal organisms. It is important to wait a few minutes for this to occur; some advocate warming the slide briefly to enhance the lysing process. Candidal yeast forms are small ovoid structures, frequently seen budding, and may be normal flora in 25 to 50 percent of healthy women. Mycelia or hyphae are long tubular structures and are often seen in active fungal infections (Eschenbach, 1983) (Fig. 4–5).

The wet mount can have a high false-negative rate, probably related to poor specimen collection. A copious sample of vaginal discharge is crucial.

Urinalysis. Urinalysis may be done to confirm or rule out urinary tract infection in the evaluation of dysuria or other urinary tract complaints. Urine should be collected as a clean-catch midstream specimen: the woman should be instructed to wash her hands; then, while separating the labia with one hand, she should wipe the urethral–vaginal area two or three times, each time with a separate towelette containing a cleansing solution. She should then release a small amount of urine, stop the flow, place the specimen container, and continue urinating into the cup. If she has a heavy vaginal discharge, she should try to avoid contami-

nating the urine specimen by using a tampon or pad to absorb the vaginal secretions, in addition to meticulous cleansing.

The urine specimen should be tested or cultured within a few minutes of collection. If this is not possible, it should be tightly covered and refrigerated, and analysis should be performed within a few hours. Urine that is allowed to stand even one-half hour at room temperature begins to show bacterial overgrowth (Fischer et al., 1983).

Dipstick tests for protein, blood, glucose, ketones, pH, bilirubin, urobilinogen, and bacteria can be done in the office. Testing strips should be stored in a cool dry place and used before the expiration date to avoid deterioration. The test requires dipping the dipstick in a fresh urine specimen, and then comparing the color changes with the chart provided by the manufacturer. Timing must be accurate to ensure proper results. Many practitioners use dipsticks for nitrite as a screening test for occult bacteriuria. A first morning specimen is necessary, because the bacteria must have been in the bladder at least 4 hours for accuracy. Fischer and associates (1983) find this an insensitive screening test for asymptomatic women, however, and advise that anyone who is symptomatic should be carefully evaluated with a complete urinalysis and possibly a urine culture.

Microscopic urinalysis and Gram staining are best done

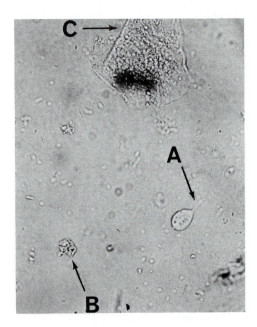

Figure 4–4. (A) *T. vaginalis.* The dark line is pointed at the flagellum which is very difficult to see. When viewed under the microscope, the flagellum would be moving. (B) White blood cell. (C) Squamous epithelial cell. Viewed under high dry objective. *(From Fischer, P., Addison, L., Curtis, P., & Mitchell, J., (1983). The office laboratory. East Norwalk, CT: Appleton-Century-Crofts.)*

red when properly decolorized and, if present, can be used as a check for proper procedure (Fischer, et al., 1983).

Gram-stained cervical smears can detect 38 to 60 percent of gonorrhea, but the test is insensitive and cultures are still needed for diagnosis (Riccardi & Felman, 1979). The finding of Gram-negative *intracellular* diplococci in a cervical smear may diagnose gonorrhea, but requires an experienced observer (Spence, 1983).

Finding more than ten white blood cells per oil immersion field (100×) in a Gram-stained smear of cervical secretions is highly indicative of chlamydial or gonococcal cervicitis (Centers for Disease Control, 1985a). Women with dysuria, frequency, and pyuria [more than ten white blood cells per high-power field (40×) in a specimen of urine sediment] in whom a Gram-stained smear of urine is negative for bacteria have the "acute urethral syndrome" often associated with chlamydia or gonorrhea (Centers for Disease Control, 1985a) (see Chapter 17).

Other Tests

Cytology. Pap smears detect some vaginal infections. Trichomoniasis may be identified in 60 to 70 percent of cases, but false positives are common (Eschenbach, 1983). Pap and other stained cytology smears such as Tzanck smears may identify the giant multinucleated cells characteristic of herpes and are highly specific, but sensitivity is thought to be only about 50 percent (Brown, Jaffee, Zaidi, et al., 1979; Mertz & Corey, 1984). Skin lesions are more likely to be positive than mucosal lesions. As a result of the rapid healing of recurrent lesions, one third to one half of suspected recurrent cases cannot be confirmed by laboratory tests; cervix, vagina, and labia should all be sampled to increase diagnostic accuracy as one area may be positive while other areas are not (Levin, 1984). These smears are difficult to obtain after the healing lesion is covered with membrane. Often, the center of the lesion has necrotic material; the active, diagnostically valuable part of the ulcer is at the margin, so this area should be scraped. Diagnostic accuracy can be as high as 90 percent in a margin-scraping specimen (Richart et al., 1984).

An experienced observer may detect chlamydial inclusions on a stained cytologic specimen, but sensitivity is usually low. Diagnostic accuracy of a cytologic specimen for chlamydia may be improved by taking a good pancervical scraping from high in the endocervical canal (Richart et al., 1984).

Immediate fixation is imperative for all cytologic specimens; the laboratory request should alert the cytologist to look for evidence of herpes or chlamydia.

on urine sediment (Fischer et al., 1983); unless the office is equipped with a centrifuge to spin down the urine specimen, the specimen should be sent to a laboratory for analysis.

Gram Stains. The Gram stain technique may be used in the office laboratory (Table 4–4). Many practitioners believe that the stain techniques have no real advantage over microscopic examination of the saline or KOH slides in the diagnosis of vaginitis. Normal vaginal flora may contain a variety of bacteria, so diagnosis is not necessarily aided by Gram stain. Others claim that the highlighting of cells and organisms during the staining process makes them easier to identify, thus facilitating diagnosis (Brucker, 1986; Mead, Thomason, Ledger, & Eschenbach, 1986).

In a properly stained specimen, Gram-negative organisms appear pink and Gram-positive organisms appear dark purple. Yeast cells stain purple, and bacteria are either pink or purple. Incorrect technique, especially when decolorizing, will cause false results. White blood cells appear

TABLE 4–4. GRAM STAINING

1. Spread a *thin* smear of the specimen on a glass slide. Air dry the slide completely, or dry it carefully high above a flame.
2. After the specimen is dry, fix it by passing it through a flame several times (with the specimen side away from the flame). Allow it to cool completely; otherwise, the reagents used in the staining process may precipitate on the slide.
3. Flood the slide with Gram crystal violet. Wait 10 seconds; then rinse with tap water.
4. Flood the slide with Gram iodine. Wait 10 seconds; then rinse with tap water.
5. Wash the slide with decolorizer until the fluid dripping from the slide changes from blue to colorless; then immediately rinse the slide with tap water. This step is crucial to ensure correct decolorizing.
6. Flood the slide with Gram safranin. Wait 10 seconds; then rinse the slide with tap water.
7. Allow the slide to air dry, or blot dry. Place the slide on the microscope stage and put a small drop of oil on the stained specimen. With the oil power objective in place, the condenser up, and the diaphragm open (for bright-field illumination), focus and examine several fields of the slide.
8. When finished, remove the oil from the lens with lens paper.

Adapted from Fischer, P., Addison, L., Curtis, P., and Mitchell, J. (1983). The office laboratory. East Norwalk, CT: Appleton–Century–Crofts.

Cultures. Media are available for culturing many bacterial and viral infections, but may not be accessible or economically available to individual practitioners or offices.

Gonorrhea is best diagnosed by direct inoculation of a swab from the endocervix onto a specified culture medium. The gonococcus invades the superficial epithelium of the endocervical glands, not the estrogen-stimulated vaginal tissue, so specimens must be taken from the endocervical canal (Smith & Lauver, 1984; Spence, 1983). Rectal and oropharyngeal samples are also appropriate if sexual exposure has occurred at these sites. No lubricant should be used during the examination, as it may be toxic to the gonococcus. Culture medium should be at room temperature before inoculation with the specimen. The cervix may be cleansed of excess exudate if necessary, and a swab inserted into the endocervical canal for 10 to 30 seconds to accumulate secretions, then rolled in a "Z" pattern onto the culture medium. Some authors recommend synthetic fiber-tipped swabs because of the possibility that the fatty acids in cotton may be toxic to the gonococcus (Fischer et al., 1983). Gonococci require a 2 to 10 percent carbon dioxide (CO_2) atmosphere for growth, so the culture medium should be placed in a CO_2-rich environment within 15 minutes of inoculation to ensure accurate results.

The most common medium used for gonorrhea testing is Thayer–Martin (TM) or modified TM. Inoculated plates may be placed in a candle jar; the candle must be lit and placed inside the jar each time it is opened to maintain an adequate CO_2 atmosphere. The plates should then be incubated within 1 to 2 hours for optimal results. Some systems use a carbon dioxide–generating tablet in a closed bag or container to create the necessary atmosphere.

Transgrow medium is a modification of TM medium, packaged in screw-type glass bottles that are charged with CO_2 at the time of manufacture. The CO_2 concentration can be lowered significantly if the bottle is not handled according to instructions, thus reducing accuracy of diagnosis.

Some large institutions culture specimens with nonnutritive Stuart's or Amies Transport medium, requiring reculture in the laboratory within a short period. This method has been found to be as sensitive as direct plating, as long as transport time is less than 3 hours (Ebright, Smith, Drexler, et al., 1982; Lue, Ellner, & Ellner, 1980). False-negative gonorrhea tests may result from prolonged time before incubation, incorrect incubation temperatures, inadequate CO_2 atmosphere after collection, antibiotic therapy, or poor specimen collection.

Gardnerella can be grown on standard culture medium; however, over 50 percent of women may be colonized with *Gardnerella* without signs or symptoms of vaginitis, so a culture is of little value. Many researchers believe that bacterial vaginosis results from combination of the *Gardnerella* organism with certain host–agent factors. Although not all of these are known, one is thought to be the presence of anaerobic bacteria; the amine test (see earlier) detects the presence of these bacteria (Embree, Caliando, & McCormack, 1984; Spiegel, Amsel, Eschenbach, et al., 1980).

Trichomonas can be cultured on Trichosel culture medium (this is not readily available in the United States but may sometimes be obtained from a parasitology lab). Twenty-four to forty-eight hours are required for diagnosis. Clinical and wet mount screening should be adequate for diagnosis in most cases.

Candida can be cultured on Nickerson's or Sabouraud's medium. Microstix-Candida is a plastic test strip of modified Nickerson's medium. These cultures are highly sensitive by 48 hours after inoculation. Isolation of the fungus does not prove disease, however, as *Candida* may be normal vaginal flora. Fungal cultures have been recommended in cases where the client is symptomatic but the KOH preparation is negative (Bergman, Berg, Schneeweiss, & Heidrich, 1984; Eschenbach, 1983).

Chlamydia cultures, if available, provide reliable diagnosis. *Chlamydia* is an intracellular parasite that attacks the cells of the transformation zone (Schachter, 1983). An endocervical specimen is necessary; the swab should be rotated in the cervical canal to increase recovery of the organism, and some abrasion of the surface is necessary for an optimal specimen. Some researchers recommend vigorously shaking the swab in the culture medium to release the organism, then discarding the swab; others find too many false-negative results with this technique (Mårdh, Weström, Colleen, & Wolner-Hanssen, 1981). Studies of various types of swabs suggest that synthetic fibers are better than cotton (Smith & Weed, 1983). Practitioners should follow the recommendations of the laboratory processing the specimen for appropriate equipment and technique.

Herpes is best diagnosed by culture. Ideally, the specimen should be collected 24 to 48 hours after the lesion appears, certainly within 4 to 5 days of illness onset, as viral shedding peaks during this time. Specimens from a vesicle punctured by a tuberculin needle provide the most sensitive results; if lesions are ulcerated, they should be scraped with a swab moistened with either saline or the fluid culture medium. Viral recovery is easier from primary lesions than recurrent ones. Specimens should be inoculated immediately on the medium, held at 4°C, and transported to a laboratory within 12 hours for optimal results (Oriel, 1983). Certain types of swabs may be toxic to the virus and should not be left in the medium (Schachter, 1983). Practitioners should follow the laboratory's guidelines regarding the best material and technique.

Some of these cultures may be expensive or not readily available to the practitioner; decisions about treating a suspected condition on clinical grounds must be made on an individual basis.

Serology. Certain serologic tests are available for the diagnosis of some sexually transmitted diseases.

Syphilis is best diagnosed by a dark-field microscopic examination of a specimen from a moist lesion, but an experienced microscopist and specialized equipment are required. Screening for syphilis is usually accomplished by a blood test for the amount of reagin (a substance believed to be a γ-globulin) present in the serum. Different tests are available: ART (automated reagin test), VDRL (Venereal Disease Research Laboratory), STS (serologic test for syphilis), and RPR (rapid plasma reagin). All test for the presence and titer of reagin, but the quantitative endpoints of each may differ so test results should not be cross-compared.

Positive screening tests are always followed by specific treponemal tests before making a diagnosis. Biologic false-positive reagin tests are common and may be caused by a variety of clinical entities, from bacterial or viral infection to immunization or autoimmune disease; diagnosis of syphilis must be based on a treponemal test. The most common is the fluorescent treponemal antibody absorption (FTA-ABS), which establishes the presence or absence of antibody to treponemes. It cannot distinguish between syphilis and other treponemal diseases. Once positive, the FTA-ABS will almost never become nonreactive. The Hemagglutination Treponemal Test for Syphilis (HATTS) is another specific test for the presence of syphilis. It is easier to perform than the FTA-ABS and compares favorably in sensitivity and specificity, except in cases of primary syphilis.

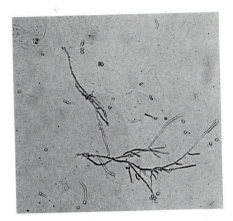

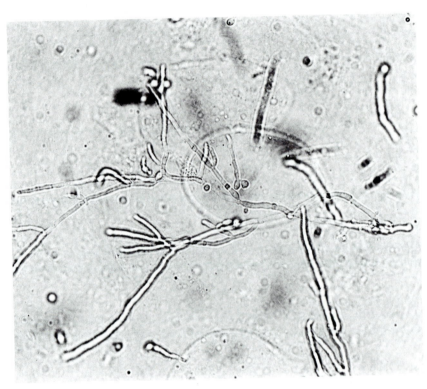

Figure 4–5. Top. *Candida* pseudohyphae in KOH preparation. Viewed under low power objective. **Bottom.** *Candida* pseudohyphae in KOH preparation. Same field as Figure 4–5 (top). Viewed under high dry objective. *(From Fischer, P., Addison, L., Curtis, P., & Mitchell, J., [1983]. The office laboratory. East Norwalk,, CT: Appleton-Century-Crofts.)*

The reagin tests are used to monitor the progress of the disease once the diagnosis is established. A fourfold or greater increase in two serologic specimens drawn 2 to 3 weeks apart indicates the presence of the disease; falling titers are used to monitor the effectiveness of therapy. The reagin test may become negative after successful treatment of the disease, or the titer may stabilize at a low level. Reinfection is indicated by rising titers.

Herpes may be diagnosed in primary cases by a four-fold increase of herpes antibody titer found in two samples of serum drawn 2 to 3 weeks apart. This is not valuable in recurrent herpes. Cultures are the most reliable diagnosis (Baker, 1983).

Gonorrhea, at least a past history of it, can be detected by a serologic test for antibody to the gonococcus. The test is not useful in the diagnosis of gonorrhea because of a lack of specificity (Spence, 1983). It may be of value in mass screening of large populations or detection of asymptomatic carriers (Toschach, Coull, Sigurdson, et al., 1979).

Monoclonal Antibody Tests. Monoclonal antibody tests have been developed for many uses in gynecologic care and offer a high degree of specificity and sensitivity. A monoclonal antibody is a hybrid cell usually derived by fusing a mouse plasma cell immunized against a specific antigen (such as *Chlamydia* or herpes) with a mouse myeloma cell that is capable of continuously reproducing (Nowinski, Tam, Goldstein, et al., 1983). Monoclonal antibodies thus ensure a uniform and continuous source of unique antibody.

Monoclonal antibody tests are based on detection of the antibody response to a specific antigen, thus reducing the problem of false results from cross-reactivity or past infections. False-negative results may still occur if there are several subtypes of an organism (as with *Chlamydia*); a monoclonal antibody may react with only one of these (Richart et al., 1984).

Some tests utilize fluorescein-labeled antibodies and require a fluorescent microscope for diagnosis. Others use enzyme-linked immunoabsorbent assay (ELISA) technology: if present, the antigen being tested for will bind to a monoclonal antibody that has been linked to an enzyme. Adding a reagent causes a marked color change in the mixture by provoking an enzyme reaction. Some of these tests must be read on a spectrometer in a laboratory; others are designed to be read by simple visual observation of the changes.

Monoclonal antibody tests are currently available for detection of *Chlamydia*, herpes, and gonorrhea. The sensitivity and specificity of these as compared with traditional diagnostic tests are still being evaluated. Continued research aimed at developing monoclonal antibody tests for other STDs, for certain gynecologic and breast cancer antigens, and for contraceptive and infertility applications will undoubtedly increase the uses of monoclonal antibody testing in years to come (Magil, 1985).

Hepatitis B Virus. Hepatitis B virus (HBV) can be a sexually transmitted disease; it can cause active infection or exist in asymptomatic carriers. People at risk include those of Asian descent or those from other endemic areas, people with acute or chronic liver disease, those with occupational exposure to blood (such as workers in dialysis units or other medical/surgical/dental situations), prostitutes, intravenous drug users, and those with intimate or household contact with HBV. Serologic tests are available to detect hepatitis B surface antigen (HBsAG), an early indicator of acute infection. HBsAG usually falls below detectable levels during convalescence, but some individuals remain HBsAG positive for life and can be chronic carriers. Two positive HBsAG titers taken at 6-month intervals indicate a carrier condition (Boehme, 1985). The presence of antibodies to HBsAG (anti-HBS) indicates immunity or a noninfectious state. Screening for and diagnosis of HBV infection should be done with the assistance of an expert consultant. Vaccines are available and recommended for people at risk.

Acquired Immune Deficiency Syndrome. AIDS is caused by the human T-lymphotropic virus type III/lymphadenopathy-associated virus (HTLV-III/LAV), now called human immunodeficiency virus (HIV). The virus is found in a number of body fluids; transmission currently is believed to occur through exchange of blood or semen via breaks in skin or mucous membranes. Transmission can occur during sexual intercourse or sharing of intravenous equipment. Infants can acquire HIV from their mothers during pregnancy, birth, or breastfeeding (Centers for Disease Control, 1985b). Women who are intravenous drug users, who are prostitutes, who received blood products between 1978 and April 1985 (Centers for Disease Control, 1987), or who have or have had sex partners who are at risk should be considered at risk for HIV infection. The Centers for Disease Control (CDC) recommend advising HIV testing for women in these high-risk categories. Because there is no currently available effective treatment for AIDS and because of the potential emotional and social consequences of a positive test result, practitioners must be able to explain the testing procedure and meaning of a positive test result to all patients considering being tested.

Current commercially available AIDS tests are serologic tests. A positive test detects antibody to HIV and indicates present or past infection with the virus; it does not necessarily diagnose AIDS or predict that AIDS will inevitably develop. Positive tests are presumed to indicate the ability to infect others.

The U.S. Public Health Service has set guidelines for considering an individual to have serologic evidence of HIV infection: (1) Two tests are performed: an enzyme immunoassay (EIA) screening test and a western blot (WB) or immunofluorescence assay; (2) the EIA test must be repeatedly reactive; (3) the WB test must validate the results. The WB test may be indeterminate; this may indicate very recent infection. When the WB test is indeterminate, a repeat test should be performed in 6 months. Only a repeat test showing clear reactivity is considered positive (Centers for Disease Control, 1987).

The EIA test has high sensitivity and specificity; tests licensed by the Food and Drug Administration show sensitivity and specificity greater than 99 percent (Centers for Disease Control, 1987); however, in populations with low prevalence of infection, even this high rate does not provide an acceptable predictive value. Repeating each reactive test reduces the number of false positives; subjecting each reactive test to a supplemental test that is highly specific (the WB test) further reduces the number of false positives. The false-positive rates achievable with this regimen have been shown to be as low as fewer than 1 in 100,000 tested individuals. Unlicensed tests may be highly accurate as well; this cannot be assured, however. Practitioners should therefore be aware of whether laboratories use licensed or unlicensed tests. The CDC further recommend that risk factors for AIDS be assessed whenever testing is implemented and that positive or indeterminate test results be interpreted in the context of historic, epidemiologic, clinical, and additional laboratory data. Complete assessment and referral to medical specialists familiar with AIDS patients must be part of the overall management for women testing positive for HIV. See Chapter 12 for more information about AIDS.

Knowledge about the significance of the HIV test is evolving; definitions of women at risk, recommendations for testing or screening, and interpretations of results change at frequent intervals. Current recommendations from CDC should be consulted when deciding to test a woman for HIV. The CDC maintains an AIDS hotline for up-to-date information: 1–800–342–AIDS. Complete informed consent must precede all HIV testing; see the Introduction to Section II for a full discussion of the components of informed consent.

PREGNANCY TESTING AND PREPREGNANCY EVALUATION

Pregnancy tests are used to rule out or confirm a diagnosis of pregnancy. Older biologic tests depended on the observation of ovulatory changes in animal reproductive tracts after injection with a pregnant woman's urine. These tests were clumsy and time consuming and are no longer used. Modern tests are based on the detection of human chorionic gonadotropin (hCG) in a woman's blood or urine. hCG is a hormone produced during pregnancy; it is present in low levels after fertilization and rises to detectable levels after implantation when the trophoblastic cells begin to proliferate rapidly. hCG levels in normal pregnancy rise predictably, doubling approximately every 1 to 2 days during the first 30 days of gestation. Peak levels occur 50 to 60 days after conception, after which levels drop and remain low for the remainder of pregnancy. It may take 7 to 10 days or longer for hCG to return to nonpregnant levels after a first-trimester abortion.

hCG contains an α subunit and a β subunit; α subunits are almost identical to LH, FSH, and TSH. Pregnancy tests that detect the α subunit can thus produce false-positive results in the presence of these hormones. The β subunit is specific for pregnancy; cross-reactivity is avoided in tests that detect only the β particle.

Immunologic tests are based on an antigen–antibody reaction. Urine tests require two reagents: one is a suspension of either latex particles bound to hCG or animal erythrocytes coated with hCG. The other reagent contains hCG antibody (anti-hCG). The patient's specimen is mixed with the anti-hCG solution. If she is pregnant, the hCG present in her urine will bind to the anti-HCG molecules in the reagent; if she is not pregnant, the anti-hCG will remain free and unbound. Next, the suspension containing hCG is added. If the woman is pregnant, the bound anti-hCG is not free to react with the new reagent, and there will be no visible reaction. If she is not pregnant, the free anti-hCG will bind to the hCG in the reagent and cause flocculation or agglutination: a visible precipitation of the reagents appearing as small white specks in the solution.

Most slide tests for pregnancy are rapid, 2-minute latex agglutination tests: a homogeneous solution with no visible agglutination indicates a positive pregnancy test; a solution that precipitates is a negative test. Some slide tests are designed with different endpoints, however; reading the instructions is imperative.

Tube tests for pregnancy (including some over-the-counter "at home" tests) are hemagglutination inhibition tests requiring 1 to 2 hours to perform. In the presence of sufficient hCG, the anti-hCG solution is neutralized and no agglutination occurs when hCG-coated particles are added. Different manufacturers have altered these tests to improve clarity and usefulness for the consumer; thus, the positive and negative endpoints of each of these tests must be interpreted according to the instructions.

Ultrasensitive immunoassays can be accurate within 14 days of conception; routine urine assays within 25 to 28 days. Both can cross-react with LH, but should be adequate for confirmation of normal pregnancy (Hatcher, Guest, Stewart, et al., 1984).

Monoclonal antibody/ELISA tests are being used more frequently for diagnosing pregnancy. These employ a monoclonal antibody specific for the β subunit of hCG, and an antigen–enzyme conjugate that can induce a simple color change reaction when β subunit of hCG is present. Results can be read on a spectrometer, or in some cases by simple visual observation. The newer home pregnancy tests are ELISA monoclonal antibody tests. Use of the β subunit–specific antibody allows for greater sensitivity and specificity. Sensitivity of each test depends on the amount of hCG it is designed to detect.

Radioimmunoassay (RIA) serum pregnancy tests utilize radiolabeled hCG in a fixed amount. The amount of this substance that can bind to the anti-hCG in a solution is reduced in proportion to the amount of hCG in the patient's serum, thus allowing quantitative measurement of hCG. These tests are specific for the β subunit; they can be accurate within 7 days of conception and are extremely useful in evaluating abnormal pregnancy (Hatcher, et al., 1984).

Radioreceptor assays (RRA) utilize hCG receptors (from the corpora lutea of animal tissue) and radiolabeled hCG. The amount of radiolabeled hCG that remains unbound to these specific receptor sites rises in proportion to the amount of hCG in the patient's specimen. Cross-reaction to LH can occur. These are accurate within 14 days of conception (Hatcher, et al., 1984).

Pregnancy tests vary in sensitivity and specificity. All tests must be interpreted according to the manufacturer's instructions. The endpoints of tests differ: some slide tests detect as little as 0.5 IU of hCG/mL; others turn positive only at a level of 1 to 2 IU/mL. Certain home tests are positive if a ring appears in the tube; others are negative.

False-negative pregnancy tests may result from an error in reading, dilute urine, incorrect procedure, performance of the test too early or too late in pregnancy, or a problem pregnancy (ectopic pregnancy or impending or missed abortion). Problems with urine tests can be minimized by collecting an early-morning specimen. This urine is the most concentrated and thus contains the highest level of hCG. If the urine has a specific gravity of at least 1.010, the risk of false-negative results is reduced. Urine should be tested within 12 hours if not refrigerated (Fischer et al., 1983).

False-positive tests can result from an error in reading, deterioration of the reagents, cross-reaction with LH, protein, or blood in the urine (urine specimens should be checked for these prior to testing), lipemia or turbidity of serum specimens, detergent residue in the test tube, drug interference (Aldomet, methadone, certain psychotropic drugs), and a variety of medical or gynecologic conditions (Hatcher et al., 1984).

Women seeking pregnancy may benefit from preconceptional examination and counseling. History and physical examination may reveal conditions that can be treated before pregnancy occurs. Nutritional status, including an anemia screen, can be judged and appropriate counseling initiated. Social habits that adversely affect the fetus can be identified (smoking, alcohol or drug use, occupational exposure to hazardous substances), allowing the woman time to reduce these risk factors before attempting pregnancy. Appropriate interval contraception can be discussed. Risk of genetic disease (such as sickle cell or Tay–Sachs) can be assessed and appropriate tests and counseling arranged. Rubella immunity can be determined and rubella vaccine offered (this vaccine should be offered to all rubella-susceptible women whether or not they are seeking pregnancy; in the absence of documented laboratory evidence of rubella immunity or without documentation of vaccination after the first birthday, serologic screening for rubella antibody should be offered). Tuberculin screening via skin testing can be done so that further workup, including x-ray, and treatment, when necessary, can be initiated before pregnancy.

A description of the normal menstrual cycle and useful concepts for identifying the most fertile period of the cycle can be discussed. Enzyme-linked monoclonal antibody tests to detect the LH surge have recently been developed for home use. As a single level of LH is less predictive than a rapidly increasing change in LH levels for assessing the time of ovulation, a woman needs to test her urine on successive days. Ovulation prediction test kits usually contain enough equipment for several test procedures.

PERIODIC HEALTH SCREENING

In addition to screening for cervical cancer and STDs, the gynecologic exam presents the opportunity to screen for the presence or risk of other health problems. Whether the provider of well-woman gynecologic services does the screening, ascertains that it has been done elsewhere, or refers the patient to another provider is less important than ensuring that the screening takes place.

The concept of periodic health screening or medical evaluation of healthy people has been the focus of considerable debate over the necessity, the benefit, and the cost effectiveness of routine physical and laboratory evaluations. Proponents argue that early detection of illness may lead to earlier and more successful treatment as well as reassurance of well individuals. Assessment of risk can alert patients to preventive measures and practitioners to the need for patient education and follow-up counseling.

The argument against periodic examination points to the inaccuracy of most screening tests: proper screening does not in fact occur if a test has a significant false-negative rate. The follow-up evaluation of healthy individuals with false-positive test results may be detrimental in both financial and psychological terms. In addition, the outcome of many conditions detected by periodic screening exams is not changed, thus creating a dubious benefit.

Recent analyses of the epidemiology of and current treatments for various conditions have led to a more specific or disease-oriented approach to screening. Criteria for effective screening tests are as follows (Rose, 1980):

1. The disease must result in significant morbidity or mortality.
2. There should be an effective treatment available for the disease.
3. The disease must have an asymptomatic period, and treatment begun in the asymptomatic period must give a better result or prognosis than treatment begun in the symptomatic period.
4. The screening test should be accurate, simple, and acceptable to the population.
5. The disease should have sufficient prevalence in the population to justify screening and follow-up costs.

Such selective screening tailored to groups at risk for specific conditions has been shown to be superior to general annual checkups of whole populations (Canadian Task Force, 1979).

Using these criteria, practitioners can make decisions about the appropriate periodic screening to be performed in practice. Hypertension, for example, meets most of these criteria, and the blood pressure reading used to detect it is simple and accurate, thus justifying regular screening. Anemia, on the other hand, may be prevalent in an asymptomatic phase, but does not usually result in significant harm; treatment before the symptomatic stage does not yield a therapeutic result superior to that obtained by treatment begun after symptoms develop. Thus, *routine* screening for anemia may be of dubious benefit (Rose, 1980). (This does not preclude screening in certain specific situations, such as prepregnancy counseling or during use of an intrauterine device for contraception.)

Further information, along with a summary of the recommendations for health screening of several research groups, is found in Chapter 3.

REFERENCES

American Cancer Society. (1980 July/August). Report on the cancer related health checkup. *Ca—A Journal for Clinicians, 30*(4), 194–240.

American College of Obstetricians and Gynecologists. (1984). Cervical cancer screening: How often? *ACOG Newsletter, 28,*4.

American College of Obstetricians and Gynecologists (1980, June). *Statement of policy 1980. Periodic cancer screening in women.*

Baker, D. (1983, March). Herpesvirus. *Clinical Obstetrics and Gynecology, 26*(1), 165–172.

Batzer, F. (1979). Laboratory procedures in gynecologic diagnosis. *Clinical Obstetrics and Gynecology, 22*(2), 463–474.

Bergman, J., Berg, A., Schneeweiss, R., & Heindrich, F. (1984, April). Clinical comparison of microscopic and culture techniques in the diagnosis of *Candida* vaginitis. *Journal of Family Practice, 18*(4), 549–552.

Blackwell, A, & Barlow, D. (1982, December). Clinical diagnosis of anaerobic vaginosis. *British Journal of Venereal Diseases, 58*(6) 387–393.

Boehme, T. (1985, March/April). Hepatitis B. *Journal of Nurse-Midwifery, 30*(2), 79–87.

Brown, S., Jaffe, H., Zaidi, A., et al. (1979, January–March). Sensitivity and specificity of diagnostic tests for genital infection with herpesvirus. *Sexually Transmitted Diseases, 6*(1), 10–13.

Brucker, M. (1986, May/June). Gram staining. *Journal of Nurse-Midwifery, 31*(3), 156–158.

Canadian Task Force on the Periodic Health Examination. (1979, November 3). Periodic health examination. *Canadian Medical Association Journal, 121*(9), 1193–1254.

Centers for Disease Control (1985a, October 8). 1985 STD treatment guidelines. *Morbidity and Mortality Weekly Report, 34*(4, Suppl.), 75s–108s.

Centers for Disease Control (1985b, December 6). Recommendations for assisting in the prevention of perinatal transmission of HTLV/LAV and AIDS. *Morbidity and Mortality Weekly Report, 34*(48), 721–732.

Centers for Disease Control (1987, August 14). Public health service guidelines for counseling and antibody testing to prevent HIV infection and AIDS. *Morbidity and Mortality Weekly Report, 36*(31), 509–515.

Ebright, J., Smith, K., & Drexler, L., et al. (1982, January–March). Evaluation of modified Stuart's medium in culturettes for transport of *N. gonorrheae*. *Sexually Transmitted Diseases, 9*(1), 45–47.

Eddy, D. (1981, October). Appropriateness of cervical cancer screening. *Gynecologic Oncology, 12*(2, Part 2), S169–S187.

Embree, J., Caliando, J., & McCormack, W. (1984, April–June). Nonspecific vaginitis among women in a STD clinic. *Sexually Transmitted Diseases, 11*(2), 81–84.

Erkkola, R., Jarvinen, H., Terho, P., & Meurman, O. (1983). Microbial flora in women showing symptoms of nonspecific vaginosis: Applicability of KOH test for diagnosis. *Scandinavian Journal of Infectious Diseases, 40*(Suppl.), 59–63.

Eschenbach, D. (1980, August). Recognizing chlamydial infection. *Contemporary Ob/Gyn 16*(2), 15–30.

Eschenbach, D. (1983, March). Vaginal infection. *Clinical Obstetrics and Gynecology, 26*(1), 186–202.

Fetherston, W. (1983, December). False-negative cytology in invasive cancer of the cervix. *Clinical Obstetrics and Gynecology, 26*(4), 929–937.

Fischer, P., Addison, L., Curtis, P., & Mitchell, J. (1983). *The office laboratory.* East Norwalk, CT: Appleton-Century-Crofts.

Fleury, F. (1983) Clinical signs and symptoms of *Gardnerella*-associated vaginosis. *Scandinavian Journal of Infectious Disease, 40* (Suppl.), 71–72.

Fouts, A., & Kraus, S. (1980, February). *Trichomonas vaginalis:* Re-evaluation of its clinical presentation and laboratory diagnosis. *Journal of Infectious Disease, 141*(2), 137–143.

Frame, P., & Carlson, S. (1975, June). A critical review of periodic health screening using specific screening criteria. Part 3. Selected diseases of the genitourinary system. *Journal of Family Practice, 2*(3), 189–194.

Frame, P., & Carlson, S. (1975d, August). A critical review of periodic health screening using specific screening criteria. Part 4. Selected miscellaneous diseases. *Journal of Family Practice, 2*(4), 283–289.

Garite, T., & Feldman, M., (1978, March/April). An evaluation of cytologic sampling techniques. *Acta Cytologica, 22*(2), 83–85.

Hansfield, H. (1985). Symposium: The volatile world of man and microbes. *News and Features from NIH, 85*(2), 4.

Hatcher, R., Guest, F., Stewart, F., et al. (1984). *Contraceptive technology 1984–1985* (12th rev. ed.). New York: Irvington.

International Cytobrush. (no date). *Product information . . . for Pap smear sampling.* Hollywood, FL: International Cytobrush.

Jordan, M., Linden, G., Friedman, E., et al. (1974, September 20). Has the survival rate from invasive carcinoma of the cervix been influenced by cytology screening? *Modern Medicine, 39*(19), 180–184, 188.

Kiviat, N. (1984). Cervical cytology. In B. Wentworth & F. Judson (Eds.), *Laboratory methods for the diagnosis of sexually transmitted diseases.* Washington, DC: American Public Health Association.

Koss, L. (1982). Cytologic evaluation of the uterine cervix. *Pathologist, 36*(8), 401–407.

Levin, M. (1984). Genital herpesvirus. In B. Wentworth & F. Judson (Eds.), *Laboratory methods for the diagnosis of sexually transmitted diseases.* Washington, DC: American Public Health Association.

Lue, Y., Ellner, P., & Ellner, D. (1980, October–December). Improved recovery of *N. gonorrheae* from clinical specimens by selective enrichment and detection by immunologic methods. *Sexually Transmitted Diseases, 7*(4), 165–167.

Magil, B. (1985, September). Monoclonals move into cancer surveillance. *Contemporary Ob/Gyn, 26*(9), 67–86.

Mårdh, P., Weström, L., Colleen, S., & Wolner-Hanssen, P. (1981, October–December). Sampling, specimen handling and isolation techniques in the diagnosis of chlamydial and other genital infections. *Sexually Transmitted Diseases, 8*(4), 280–285.

Mead, P., Thomason, J., Ledger, W., & Eschenbach, D. (1986, February). Symposium: Establishing bacterial vaginosis. *Contemporary Ob/Gyn, 27*(2), 186–203.

Mertz, G., & Corey, L. (1984, February). Genital herpes simplex infections in adults. *Urologic Clinics of North America, 11*(1), 103–119.

Nowinski, R., Tam, M., & Goldstein, L., et al. (1983, February 11). Monoclonal antibodies for the diagnosis of infectious disease in humans. *Science, 219*(4585), 637–643.

Oriel, J. (1983). Genital lesions. In W. McCormack (Ed.), *Diagnosis and treatment of sexually transmitted diseases*. Boston: John Wright-PSG.

Petersen, E., & Pelz, K. (1983). Diagnosis and therapy of nonspecific vaginitis. *Scandinavian Journal of Infectious Disease, 40*(Suppl.), 97–99.

Riccardi, N., & Felman, Y. (1979, December 14). Laboratory diagnosis in the problem of suspected gonococcal infection. *Journal of the American Medical Association, 242*(24), 2703–2705.

Richart, R. (1979, September). Screening techniques for cervical neoplasia. *Clinical Obstetrics and Gynecology, 22*(3), 701–712.

Richart, R., & Barron, B. (1981, March 1). Screening strategies for cervical cancer and cervical intraepithelial neoplasia. *Cancer, 47*(5, Suppl.), 1176–1181.

Richart, R., Boon, M., & Gupta, P., et al. (1984, October). Symposium: Stepping up the search for vaginal pathogens. *Contemporary Ob/Gyn, 24*(10), 194–215.

Rose, S. (1980, December). The periodic health examination. *Primary Care, 7*(4), 653–665.

Rubio, C. (1977, May). The false negative smear. II. The trapping effect of collecting instruments. *Obstetrics and Gynecology, 49*(5), 576–580.

Rubio, C., Kock, Y., & Berglund, K. (1980, January/February). Studies on the distribution of abnormal cells in cytologic preparation. *Acta Cytologica, 24*(1), 49–53.

Schachter, J. (1983). Laboratory support. In W. McCormack (Ed.), *Diagnosis and treatment of sexually transmitted diseases*. Boston: John Wright-PSG.

Shen, J., Nalick, R., Schlaerth, J., & Morrow, C. (1984, September/October). Efficacy of cotton-tipped applicators for obtaining cells from the uterine cervix for Papanicolaou smears. *Acta Cytologica, 28*(5), 541–545.

Singer, A. (1975, February). The uterine cervix from adolescence to menopause. *British Journal of Obstetrics and Gynaecology, 82*(2), 81–99.

Smith, L., & Lauver, D. (1984, June). Assessment and management of vaginitis and cervicitis. *Nurse Practitioner, 9*(6), 34–47, 67.

Smith, T., & Weed, L. (1983, August). Evaluation of calcium alginate-tipped aluminum swabs transported in culturettes containing ampules of 2-sucrose phosphate medium for recovery of *Chlamydia trachomatis*. *American Journal of Clinical Pathology, 80*(2), 213–215.

Spence, M. (1983, March). Gonorrhea. *Clinical Obstetrics and Gynecology, 26*(1), 111–124.

Spiegel, C., Amsel, R., & Eschenbach, D., et al. (1980, September 11). Anaerobic bacteria in nonspecific vaginitis. *New England Journal of Medicine, 303*(11), 601–607.

Taylor, P., Andersen, W., & Barber, S., et al. (1987, November). The screening Papanicolaou smear: Contribution of the endocervical brush. *Obstetrics and Gynecology, 70*(5), 734–738.

Toschach, S., Coull, L., & Sigurdson, S., et al. (1979, July–September). Evaluation of five serologic tests for antibody to *N. gonorrheae*. *Sexually Transmitted Diseases, 6*(3), 214–217.

Trevathan, E., Layde, P., & Webster, L., et al. (1983, July 22/29). Cigarette smoking and dysplasia and carcinoma in situ of the uterine cervix. *Journal of the American Medical Association, 250*(4), 499–502.

Walton, R. (1976, June 5). Cervical cancer screening program. *Canadian Medical Association Journal, 114*(11), 1003–1033.

Wied, G., Bartels, P., Bibbo, M., & Keebler, C. (1981, September–October). Frequency and reliability of diagnostic cytology of the female genital tract. *Acta Cytologica, 25*(5), 543–549.

SECTION II

Contraception

Issues and Concepts in Family Planning

Providing family planning services can be both satisfying and frustrating. This service meets a universal need of women: control over their reproductive function. It also provides healthy women an entree into the health care system and affords the practitioner an opportunity to provide an enormous amount of information. Not all women, however, will conclude the family planning encounter happily. For too many women, any available method of birth control represents a compromise of some sort. For some, these compromises are large; for others, less so. It challenges the health care provider to assist women to make choices, to determine, at any given stage of life, which method of birth control is appropriate. These choices sometimes involve medical questions, but they *always* involve questions of lifestyle, personal preference, and sexuality. It requires sensitivity, flexibility, openness, and self-awareness to be a guide and not a judge in providing contraceptive services.

The chapters in this section deal with the reversible methods of contraception. Together with the chapters on abortion, sterilization, and infertility, presented in Section VI, "The Supportive Role," they comprise the totality of family planning. The issues and concepts discussed in this introduction—utilization of birth control methods, effectiveness of methods, informed consent, risk-benefit ratio, decision-making, and self-awareness—can be applied to any family planning decision.

Utilization of Birth Control Methods. The National Center for Health Statistics, in its publication, *Use of Contraception in the United States*, 1982, by C. A. Bachrach and W. D. Mosher,* reported on utilization patterns among U.S. women aged 15 to 44 years old. They found that, in 1982, 54 percent of women in this age group were using some method of contraception. Among these, sterilization was the most popular method among ever-married women and oral contraceptives the most popular method among never-married women. Of sexually active women who were neither pregnant, postpartum, seeking pregnancy, nor involuntarily sterile, 12 percent were *not* using any contraceptive. In order, the most utilized methods of contraception in 1982 were:

- Male or female sterilization (18% of all women)
- Oral contraceptives (16%)
- Condoms (7%)
- Diaphragms (5%)
- IUDs (4%)
- Natural family planning methods (2%)
- Other (including withdrawal, douching, foam, and suppositories) (1%)

Contraceptive Effectiveness. Two types of analyses are mostly widely used to evaluate the effectiveness of a birth control method: life table analysis and the Pearl Index. Both methods attempt to assess the efficacy of the contraceptive in prevent-

---

*From Advance Data from Vital and Health Statistics, (1984, December 4). No. 103, DHHS Pub. No. (PHS) 85–1250. Public Health Service: Hyattsville, MD.

ing pregnancy by computing the number of pregnancies that can be expected in 100 women using the method for one year. To calculate a Pearl Index, the number of pregnancies seen are divided by the number of women in the study multiplied by the number of months the method is used by each. This is then multiplied by 1200, representing 100 women using the method for 12 months, or what is called 100 woman-years. This index has been criticized because it considers, without distinction, new method users and long-time method users. (See, for example, *Contraceptive Technology Update*, August 1986, pages 92–94). What makes this method potentially biased is that the latter have lower failure rates, since those who become pregnant early in their use of a given method generally do not continue to use the method. By considering only or mostly long-term users, a method can be made to look more effective than it really is. Rates of method continuation should be assessed, therefore, whenever the Pearl Index is reported. If a method is highly effective according to the Pearl Index, but has a low continuation rate, the reported effectiveness might reflect a bias. Life table analysis considers only women in their first year of use and is therefore subject to less bias than the Pearl Index.

Effectiveness of any birth control method must be evaluated according to theoretical and user rates. A theoretical effectiveness rate assumes that all users would use the method exactly as specified. It refers to the best rate possible. User effectiveness takes into consideration human error. For some methods of birth control, such as the IUD, which require minimal user input, these two rates are close.

For other methods, such as foam and condoms, these two rates may appear in some studies to be rather disparate since these methods require a lot of ongoing user participation. We caution practitioners in assessing user rates to remember that *their* input can strongly influence user rates. The time given to helping a woman or couple think about risks and benefits, to teaching and counseling, to ascertaining comfort with the method, to answering questions, to providing practice time in the provider's office, and to offering telephone and in-person follow-up all can considerably reduce user failures. Of course, in most cases, it is ultimately the patient who is the best judge of her willingness or ability to use a particular method correctly and consistently.

Informed Consent. Informed consent is a concept deriving from both law and ethics. Conscientiously following the guidelines of an informed consent will allow the practitioner to be legally protected for services offered and ethically secure in having provided all the information necessary to facilitate patient decision making. Informed consent is particularly important in the area of birth control because, unlike most medical treatments, family planning involves long- and short-term use of chemicals, hormones, and devices by perfectly healthy people.

The following discussion is adapted from the American Civil Liberties Handbook, *The Rights of Hospital Patients*, by George Annas, Avon Books, New York, 1975.

An overall guideline in informed consent is to provide all information in terms understandable to the patient. This may require vocabulary adjustments, oral, written, or sign-language translation, and the use of pictures in written communications. Without understanding, consent never can be informed. It is the practitioner's responsibility to assess the patient's understanding of information provided.

Informed consent for family planning encompasses the following:

- A description of the proposed method, how it works, what it does.
- The benefits of the proposed method, its effectiveness in preventing pregnancy, and other advantages.
- The disadvantages of the proposed method, including its risks.
- The cost of the proposed method, immediate and over time, including the need for provider follow-up and ongoing care.
- A full discussion of alternative methods, covering, for each method, a description, how it works, its benefits, effectiveness, advantages, disadvantages, risks, and cost. In family planning, alternative methods include all contraceptive choices, natural family planning, male or female sterilization, and abortion.
- A discussion of the benefits, advantages, effectiveness, disadvantages, risks, and costs of using no method of family planning.
- Assurance of the right to ask (and have answered) questions at any time.
- The right to withdraw consent at any time.
- Full disclosure of the experimental nature of any method when appropriate.

Each area of informed consent must be raised by the practitioner with each patient. For example, it is not enough to wait for the patient to ask questions; she must be told that she has the right to ask questions at any time and be given the opportunity to do so. She must be told explicitly that she can withdraw consent, or change her mind, even after she has signed a consent form.

Finally, all components of informed consent must be documented for legal verification. In some offices and clinics, this is done by having the patient sign a consent form; in others, it is up to the practitioner to include documentation as part of her note.

Risk-benefit Ratio.   There is no simple or universally applicable formula for calculating a risk-benefit ratio in family planning. What are considered to be risks and benefits and what are the relative importance of each differ among people and even differ at various stages in any individual. Practitioners need to be aware of the specific areas that should be considered by a woman in a self-evaluation of risks and benefits and how they must be put into priority. For example, a student may be willing to accept the medical risks inherent in the oral contraceptive because she wants the most effective reversible protection while she is in school. Later in her life, when her career is established and she is economically independent, she may choose a barrier method, preferring its slightly increased risk of pregnancy to the medical risks of hormonal use.

Obvious risk factors of contraceptives include medical risks and method-determined risks of pregnancy, both examined in the following chapters. Disadvantages of methods which may present risks to effectiveness for individual women may include "inconvenience" or "interference" with intercourse, high cost, or the need for frequent medical intervention, particularly where care is not readily accessible.

Benefits of methods include high effectiveness and lack of medical risk. Absence of a relationship to sex, low cost, availability without prescription or medical follow-up, and non-contraceptive medical benefits such as protection against sexually transmitted diseases (STDs), relief from dysmenorrhea, and reduced amount of vaginal discharge following intercourse may be additional advantages. Female control may be seen by some women as an advantage while others may prefer a method that requires male participation. Continuous protection or, conversely, the lack of continuous chemical exposure may be desirable.

Whether any of the above factors are risks or benefits depends upon a variety of considerations, which also influence the degree of importance of each identified risk and benefit. First, of course, are medical concerns. For example, with oral contraceptives, the risk of a cardiovascular problem, the most serious medical consequence of this method, is small for nonsmoking young women without a family history of such disease and who have no other risk factors for its development. This risk, however, is high for women over 40 who smoke.

Living situations and life-style characteristics are also major considerations. The degree of available privacy and accessibility to bathroom facilities and running water influence method choice. How likely a method is to be discovered by family members may be important; how awkward the method is to carry for a woman who has intercourse in more than one place may be equally significant. A woman in a monogamous relationship who has intercourse several times a week may assess her risk-benefit ratio very differently from someone who has occasional sex with a number of partners. These examples represent only two points on a varied spectrum of expressions of sexuality. And where a woman falls on this spectrum may change, often for some, rarely for others.

Sexual practices are important as well. Do a woman and her partner, for example, participate in oral-genital sex and therefore find creams and jellies distasteful? Does a woman often have repeated intercourse in a short time, making certain barrier methods unpleasant for her?

A woman's values figure into her decisions about birth control, as may those of her partner or significant others. Does she value the "natural," for example, and thus reject chemical methods of birth control? Does she have certain religious beliefs that make some methods more or less acceptable? Does the woman have convictions about the beginning of life that affect her attitude toward certain methods? Is she uncomfortable with a contraceptive whose mechanism of action is unclear? Does her cultural background proscribe certain methods or make their side effects, such as break-through bleeding, undesirable? Does the need to touch herself alter the acceptability of certain methods?

Future plans are relevant as well. Oral contraceptives, for example, may not be the method of choice for someone planning a family in the near future or for somebody contemplating immediate elective surgery. Plans for travel, inability to return for follow-up, or expected changes in living arrangements or sexual alliances may influence a woman's choice.

Finally, any degree of physical or mental disability of the patient may influence methods appropriate for her. When these might interfere with her ability to use a particular method, then that method is not appropriate for the woman, unless she has a partner or family member able to assume responsibility for its use. For methods with medical side effects, any risks that are increased secondary to a particular disability must be given special consideration.

As a practitioner, you will undoubtedly find other concerns raised by some of your patients. In addition, you may find that two women in ostensibly the same situation may make very different choices; while their risk-benefit ratios appear similar, the relative value of each parameter is assessed differently.

Decision-making. Although the decisions involved in family planning may seem awesome for some women, the thoughtful practitioner can provide concrete guidelines to make the decision manageable. The components of informed consent give the woman enough information so that decisions are based on knowledge; a discussion of risk-benefit ratio assists her in asking herself the appropriate questions for decision making. It allows her to decide what areas of her life are of concern in the family planning decision-making process and helps her to determine their relative importance.

In helping women to seek answers to questions about personal risks, it is useful to project interactions for patients to role play or at least consider. The woman who states, for example, that she has difficulty communicating with her partner but who chooses condoms as her birth control method may benefit from thinking about a variety of possibilities. How will she react, for example, if the man objects to wearing condoms? What will she do if they unexpectedly become involved in sexual foreplay and a condom is unavailable? Anticipation of specific scenarios can reinforce the reality of risk-benefit analysis and increase the efficacy of a chosen method for individuals. This technique may be particularly valuable in counseling young adolescents who may be most likely to find themselves in new, unplanned for situations.

One helpful bit of wisdom to share with patients is that decisions about family planning generally are not irreversible. Many women change contraceptive methods as their needs, lifestyles, relationships, health, and priorities change. At one time in a person's life, effectiveness may be the most crucial aspect in her decision making; at another time, minimizing health risks may become more important. For an adolescent, privacy, convenience, and separateness from sexuality may be the most important considerations in choosing a family planning method. As a young woman's sense of herself as a sexual being develops, she may change these priorities. A woman who has sex frequently (as she defines this) may have priorities different from somebody who needs more sporadic protection. These lifestyle choices themselves may be temporary. Reminding women of the possibility of change may make their decisions less threatening.

Self-assessment. We urge all health care practitioners to participate in self-assessment. This requires an honest appraisal of one's attitudes toward family planning. If you are a person who has had a need for family planning, your own decision making may inadvertently affect counseling and guidance given patients. Look at what methods you have chosen; examine why you chose them and review your experience with them. Use this information to identify your personal biases: did you have a negative experience with a method of birth control that makes you reluctant to offer it to patients? How does your previous experience compare to overall statistics? Is your negative attitude justified, based on objective data? Or conversely, do you favor a particular method because it has worked for you? Are the circumstances of your life that made it work for you universal? Definitely not. How might they differ for another woman? If you have not had personal experiences with birth control, think of friends or family members who have. Has their experience colored your perceptions? What other biases have affected you? Do you have cultural, philosophic, religious beliefs that influence your attitude toward contraception or toward any particular methods?

This type of self-assessment is essential to ensure that you as practitioner meet, not your own needs, but your patients' needs. Although we believe it is unrealistic to expect that any of us can provide totally objective care, we can minimize our biases by becoming aware of them and striving to balance them with an objective assessment of facts, just as we evaluate any reporting of data for its hidden biases. The facts presented in the following chapters should allow this analysis.

5

Natural Family Planning and Fertility Awareness

Sr. M. Rose Carmel Scalone

Despite the advances of modern contraceptive technology, in the last several decades there has been growing worldwide interest in methods of natural family planning/fertility awareness (NFP/FA). The reasons for this surge of interest range from the personal, moral, cultural, religious, and economic to dissatisfaction with contraceptive technology and concern about side effects and morbidity.

This chapter defines NFP/FA and describes each method of NFP/FA. The mechanism of action of NFP/FA and its effectiveness, advantages, disadvantages, and contraindications are discussed. The management of initial and follow-up visits for women and couples wishing to use these methods is outlined. Examples are provided of patient instructions for each method.

DEFINITION

Current methods of natural family planning are based on the concept of fertility awareness: the woman's ability to identify on a day-to-day basis certain physiologic changes that occur during her menstrual cycle. By applying a knowledge of fertile and infertile signs and sensations (Fig. 5-1), users of these methods are free to plan, to delay, or to avoid pregnancy. They learn to use the daily observations of these signals of the fertile and infertile phases of the menstrual cycle (Fig. 5-2) to determine the timing of intercourse or their use of birth control methods according to their desire to achieve or avoid pregnancy. For many women and couples, NFP/FA is a way of life involving periodic abstinence from sexual intercourse.

One major problem in the use of these methods by couples has been the unwillingness of one partner to agree to long periods of abstinence. Couples often solve this problem by combining techniques, that is, by using naturally occurring fertility signs to determine when some form of contraception (condom and foam or cervical cap or diaphragm with contraceptive cream or jelly) needs to be used. This is referred to as the fertility awareness method of family planning. The choice between use of abstinence or use of a barrier method of birth control during the fertile days is the major difference between natural family planning methods and fertility awareness methods. Most proponents of natural family planning believe that abstinence from intercourse and penile–vaginal contact during a woman's fertile time has a theoretical effectiveness rate of 100 percent. Use of an adjunct barrier method of contraception

during the woman's most fertile time decreases this effectiveness rate. Many proponents of NFP/FA encourage the use of noncoital means of sexual expression during fertile times and believe that this results in greater use effectiveness rates and increases the long-term use of these methods.

NFP/FA also includes the birth-spacing role of breastfeeding (see Chapter 23). Although not wholly reliable for any individual woman, Bonnar (1982) has documented that on a worldwide scale, lactation is responsible for more fertility control than all the contraceptive methods in current use. NFP/FA involves an educational and learning process in which primary care practitioners can play a major role. The continuity of care and formation of close relationships with patients enable them to provide psychosexual counseling and support in these chosen methods. NFP/FA can also be helpful in diagnosing certain gynecologic problems and may be used to help couples achieve pregnancy or to determine which couples need follow-up referral for infertility (see Chapter 27).

GENERAL CHARACTERISTICS

At present, there are three defined techniques for natural family planning:

1. The basal body temperature (BBT) method depends on identification of the elevation in body temperature characterizing the postovulatory phase of the menstrual cycle.
2. The ovulation method (OM), also called the cervical mucus method or Billings' method, depends on recognition of changes in the character of cervical mucus occurring prior to ovulation.
3. The sympto-thermal method (STM) uses both the BBT and the OM methods, as well as other symptoms, for establishing the fertile and infertile phases of each cycle.

At one time, the natural methods included the calculation or calendar method, also referred to as rhythm. This technique is now considered obsolete by many experts in NFP/FA, although some critics continue to single it out as proof that the natural methods are ineffective (Ross, 1977, p. 18).

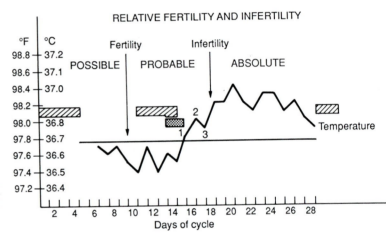

Figure 5–1. Top. Readily accessible NFP/FA parameters of the menstrual cycle. *(From Lanctot, C. [1979, April]. Natural family planning. Clinics in Obstetrics and Gynaecology, 6(1), 110. Reprinted with permission.)*

Figure 5–1. Bottom. Cyclic fertility of the menstrual cycle with observable signs and symptoms. *(From Lanctot, C. [1979, April]. Natural family planning, Clinics in Obstetrics and Gynaecology, 6(1), 110. Reprinted with permission.)*

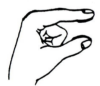 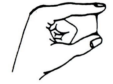 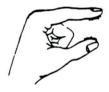

SOME CHARACTERISTICS OF FERTILITY MUCUS

1) Clear or slightly cloudy
2) Like raw egg white but may be stained pink, etc., from traces of blood
3) Thin, watery, "wet"
4) Dries leaving no residue
5) Slippery and lubricative
6) Stretchy and holds the stretch

SOME CHARACTERISTICS OF NON-FERTILE MUCUS

1) Opaque
2) Colored—white or yellow
3) Thick and sticky
4) Tacky and flakes when dry
5) Rubbery
6) "Gluppy"
7) Non-stretchy

OTHER NATURAL SIGNS AND SYMPTOMS OF FERTILITY (HIGHLY VARIABLE)

1) Abdominal pain
2) Inter-menstrual "bleeding" or "spotting"
3) Sustained temperature elevation
4) Changes in the cervix
5) Changes in sexual urge (perhaps)

Stress (physical or emotional) can inhibit or delay ovulation and change the mucus symptom in that particular cycle. In such a situation, watch **CLOSELY** for the possible return of fertility mucus after the designated peak.

Figure 5–2. Characteristics of cervical mucus.

Mechanism of Action

All NFP methods are based on the physiology of the menstrual cycle and the following basic assumptions:

1. Human ova are released only during the ovulatory phase of the menstrual cycle, which occurs only once per cycle. (If more than one egg is released during the same ovulation, it usually occurs within a few hours of the first ovulation.)
2. Human ova remain capable of being fertilized for about 24 hours.
3. Human sperm may remain alive in the female reproductive tract several days, but are capable of fertilizing the ovum probably no longer than 72 hours under ideal environmental conditions (Lanctot, 1979, pp. 109–110).
4. A menstrual cycle with ovulation occurs because of a delicately balanced relationship between the hormones secreted by the woman's pituitary gland and her ovaries. These cyclic hormonal patterns, that is, the rise in estrogen levels prior to ovulation and the rise in progesterone levels after ovulation, are accompanied by physiologic changes that can be observed by a woman throughout her cycle.

A review of the physiology of the menstrual cycle (see Chapter 1 and Figs. 5–1 and 5–2) indicates the major and readily accessible parameters that form the basis of NFP/FA methods.

Women, and ideally their partners when appropriate, are taught to keep a record of the days of their individual menstrual cycles and their monthly changes. They learn to recognize from these monthly observations when they are ovulating and thus when they are probably fertile. They use this information to decide when to avoid intercourse and penile–vaginal contact, or when to use a barrier method of birth control, if they do not want to get pregnant or when to have intercourse if they do want to get pregnant.

Effectiveness

The effectiveness of natural family planning methods varies widely in different studies. Pregnancy rates in published and unpublished studies range from a low of 0.4 pregnancy per 100 woman-years to a high of 39.7 pregnancies per 100 woman-years (Liskin, 1981). To meet the need for objective, scientifically rigorous, and internationally comparable data, the World Health Organization sponsored a prospective study of the ovulation method in three developing and two developed countries. According to the researchers, all study participants were highly motivated to use the method. All used NFP/FA with abstinence during fertile periods. The life-table pregnancy rate for the year after training was 20 percent (Liskin, 1981, p. I-44).

In almost every study to date, the low rate of effectiveness of natural family planning methods and thus the large majority of pregnancies have been attributed to couples' failure to abstain. This has prompted many family planning counselors and educators to recommend other forms of noncoital pleasuring and/or the use of barrier methods as an alternative to abstinence during the fertile period. In a U.S. study by Rogow, Rintoul, and Greenwood (1980, pp. 27–33), designed to measure the effectiveness of fertility awareness techniques, couples used either abstinence, barrier methods, or withdrawal during the fertile period. Eighty-six percent of the couples used barrier methods, withdrawal, or both. The life-table pregnancy rate for the group was 10.0 percent at 1 year. Offering women and couples an informed choice between abstinence and barrier methods, and discussing forms of noncoital sexual pleasuring during the fertile period, may correspond to the current practice of many, and thus help to make their family planning more effective.

Advantages and Disadvantages

The advantages and disadvantages of NFP/FA can be briefly summarized:

Advantages	Disadvantages
Self-awareness or self-knowledge promotes self-worth and self-esteem in women.	Interferes with sexual spontaneity—requiring periodic abstinence and/or modification of sexual behavior.
Safe; no hormones, medicines, or chemicals are administered or introduced into the woman's body; no physical side effects.	Requires high motivation for users to choose it initially and to stay with it.
Economical—free or relatively inexpensive; does not require medical follow-up.	Requires initial education and some ongoing counseling.
Acceptable to religious groups that oppose other contraceptive methods.	Records must be kept and charting must be done diligently to be accurate.
May be used for both planning and avoiding pregnancy.	Less effective in preventing pregnancy than most other methods.
Helps in recognition of the earliest signs of pregnancy.	Periodic abstinence may cause difficulties in relationships and stress; may be a source of tension and dissatisfaction.
Helps in recognition of abnormal cyclic patterns and/or gynecologic problems that may merit medical intervention.	The physiologic characteristics of some women—particularly if they are lactating, adolescent, premenopausal—may result in irregular cycles, and the fertile period may be difficult to detect.
Shared responsibility for family planning may lead to increased communication, cooperation, and other means of sexual expression for couples.	May be difficult to implement for women who see their partner infrequently or who have more than one partner.
May be esthetically more acceptable to some people than barrier methods.	

Contraindications

There are no contraindications to NFP/FA methods but there are certain gynecologic risk factors that decrease the methods' effectiveness. Practitioners need to be aware of these so that they may help their patients to decide whether or not NFP/FA is suitable for them. These are not rigid requirements, but rather are guidelines to consider before adoption of this method and are listed in the next section under Initial Visit. It must also be kept in mind that NFP/FA is not for everyone. Moderation is needed, and most advocates suggest that open communication and a warm, loving, stable, mutually supportive relationship are prerequisites for couples' use of any natural method.

MANAGEMENT OF THE VISITS

Today many practitioners are members of health care teams that offer NFP/FA methods within the full scope of family planning services. Practitioner responsibilities may include initial and follow-up physical examinations and/or education and counseling. Physical assessment and history taking are extremely important in helping patients decide whether or not NFP/FA methods are realistic choices for them. For practitioners whose responsibilities include education and counseling in NFP/FA methods, a special training course is highly recommended. These are offered by several centers throughout the world. (A listing of centers in the United States may be obtained by writing to The Human Life and Natural Family Planning Foundation.) An entire course includes information that is beyond the scope of this chapter and provides practice in interpreting NFP/FA in charts.

Initial Visit

Patients desiring NFP/FA should receive the information necessary to use the method in a structured program presented by an NFP/FA educator. It is important for the woman and her partner to share their personal views and the reasons they believe they are eligible for NFP/FA methods. By reviewing the specific charting techniques and interpretation of the signs of fertility with them, it is hoped that compliance with this method will be promoted. Abstinence should be recommended for the first cycle so that both the woman and her partner, when appropriate, have a chance to chart signs and symptoms and formulate questions or discuss problems at the next visit. Patients should also be warned that proficient use of NFP/FA methods may take up to 6 or 8 months. They must decide whether to continue abstinence, use barrier methods of contraception, or possibly increase the chances of a pregnancy until comfort with the method is achieved.

During the initial visit, determine whether the woman or couple wishes to space or limit family size or to achieve or plan a pregnancy. It is also important to determine what their past experience has been with periodic abstinence and their knowledge of and attitude toward other methods of family planning and past experience with them. Whether to use periodic abstinence, other means of sexual expression, and/or barrier methods during fertile times is entirely up to the couple. Professional understanding, support, and availability for follow-up discussions and problem solving are vitally important to the couple and their success with NFP/FA methods.

Certain medical and gynecologic problems, especially relevant to successful use of this method, should be ruled out during the history and physical examination.

The following are considered to be risk factors for pregnancy with the use of NFP/FA methods:

- Irregular menstrual cycles
- Menstrual cycles that are easily disrupted by stress, dietary changes, travel, season, and other factors
- History or presence of cervical erosion, cervicitis, or ectropion (see Chapter 13)
- History of frequent vaginal infection

Data Collection

HISTORY. Take a thorough history as outlined in Chapter 2.

PHYSICAL EXAMINATION. See Chapter 3. The physical examination is an excellent opportunity for the practitioner to help the woman to increase her body awareness and to reinforce learning. During the speculum examination, use a hand mirror to assist the woman in visualizing her cervix. Point out to her the configuration of the external os and the color, amount, and consistency of the cervical mucus in relation to the day of her menstrual cycle. After the bimanual examination, have the woman feel her cervix and describe how it feels in relation to her cycle.

LABORATORY TESTING. Perform routine screening tests (see Chapter 4). Include a wet mount regardless of the presence or absence of symptomatology. If any vaginal or cervical infections are found, the woman should be treated before she begins to learn the mucus-observing technique. If cervical mucus is present, smear a sample of it onto a slide, let it air dry, and check under the microscope for the "ferning pattern" characteristic of fertile mucus. Share the findings with the patient.

Intervention. Each woman or couple is encouraged to attend a minimum of two educational sessions taught by proficient, highly motivated instructors, ideally a male and female team, who will provide them with the necessary information about male and female anatomy and physiology, the menstrual cycle, periods of fertility and infertility with signs and symptoms, observation procedure, importance of recording observations, and psychosexual aspects. The care provider follows these educational sessions with individual sessions to review what was taught, answer questions, anticipate potential problems, and individualize instruction and counseling based on physical and psychosexual assessments.

Materials needed are workbooks or booklets explaining NFP/FA, a basal thermometer (Fig. 5–3), a supply of fertility awareness charts, and a folder or binder to hold the charts.

A new chart should be used for each menstrual cycle. On each chart, fill in the date, month, year, and method for taking the temperature (i.e., oral, rectal, or vaginal). The first day of menstrual flow is considered to be the start of the cycle, that is, day 1.

Certain symbols are used to record observations on the fertility awareness charts:

- Daily temperature recording
    - • = a period or a dot., (Connect the dots each day with a straight line.)
- Vaginal discharge
    - M   = menstruation
    - S   = spotting or scant bleeding
    - D   = dryness
    - W   = wetness or increased mucus
    - (W) = slippery, stretchable mucus or "PEAK" mucus
    - T   = thick or tacky mucus

BASAL THERMOMETER

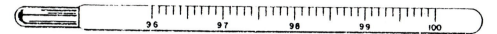

FEVER THERMOMETER

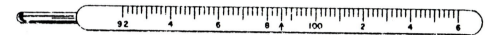

Figure 5–3. Each line on the basal thermometer is one tenth of a degree Fahrenheit and each line on the fever thermometer is two tenths of a degree Fahrenheit. *(From Gildenhorn, M. [1977]. Basal body temperature. Washington, DC: Natural Family Planning Federation of America, Inc. Reprinted with permission.)*

- Note other signs
  X = intercourse
  B = breast tenderness
  P = abdominal pain or cramps
- Disturbance of conditions
  Y = illness
  Z = later temperature or up late
  ? = abnormal vaginal discharge (e.g., itchy, greenish yellow, foul odor)

Teaching and Counseling. The following sections provide examples of patient instructions for each NFP/FP method. If used as written handouts, they may need to be revised for women or couples who do not read well enough to understand their content.

BASAL BODY TEMPERATURE METHOD. The term *basal body temperature* is by definition the lowest temperature reached by the body of a healthy person during waking hours. It is a resting temperature taken the same time daily, under the same conditions. A basal body shift is considered *ovulatory* when the temperature rise is at least 0.4° F above the average of at least the last six normal temperatures prior to the shift (Fig. 5–4).

Instructions

1. Using your basal thermometer, take your temperature about the same time each day. Before rising is the best time. Do this every morning even during menstruation. Be sure not to eat, drink, or smoke before taking your temperature. Keep the thermometer at your bedside.
2. Take your temperature either orally, vaginally, or rectally. Do not switch your method of temperature taking in the middle of a cycle. Take a reading after 5 full minutes. If you are too sleepy to read and chart your temperature before getting out of bed, or need glasses or contact lenses to see the mercury, you can read and chart later as long as the thermometer is not disturbed.
3. Record your temperature reading on your fertility awareness chart and connect the dots each day.
4. Your temperature does not have to be taken every day for the rest of your reproductive life. After you have established six or seven full charts and reviewed them with your NFP/FA counselor, you can cut the temperature taking to eight or nine times a

cycle, that is, 5 or 6 days before ovulation and 3 or 4 days after ovulation.
5. Any obvious reason for a temperature variation, such as a cold, infection, insomnia, and sleeping late, should be noted on your chart under the reading for that day.
6. Adequate charting and interpretation of the chart are very important. Your partner may help you to chart and interpret. Chart every day and do not rely on your memory of what the reading was yesterday or the day before.

Interpretation. The basal body temperature cannot tell you when ovulation will occur. It can tell you that ovulation has occurred. In one cycle, the basal body temperature goes through three phases:

Preovulation:	Low phase	Mostly fertile
Ovulation:	Rise	VERY FERTILE
Postovulation:	High phase	Mostly infertile

During the first part of your cycle (preovulation), the basal body temperature is in the low range. Postovulation, the temperature rises and remains elevated (high phase) until just before menstruation. The *third* consecutive day of high temperature is the start of the infertile time. The infertile time extends until the beginning of the next menstrual period.

For increased effectiveness of BBT interpretation, combine your awareness of other signs, such as cervical mucus secretions, intermenstrual pain or *mittleschmerz*, and intermenstrual spotting, to determine your most fertile time.

Easy Method for Determining the Temperature Shift: The Coverline

1. Do not take your temperature for the first 3 days of your menstrual cycle.
2. Begin taking your temperature on the fourth day of your cycle and take it for 6 consecutive days.
3. Take the highest of these six temperatures (there may be two or three that are equally the highest) and draw a line 0.1 of a degree (one square on your chart) above the highest of the first six temperatures. This is called a "coverline." Draw it across the chart. The coverline divides high and low temperatures; therefore, all temperatures below the coverline are

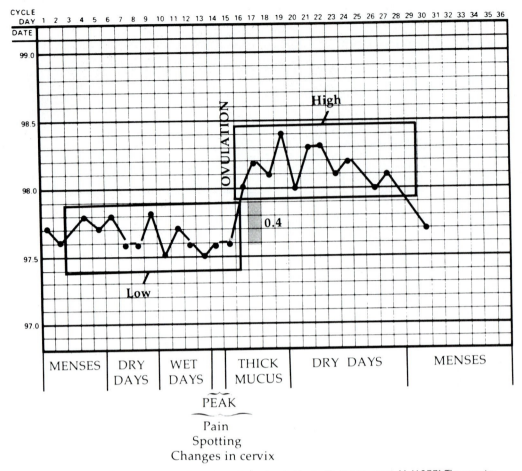

Figure 5–4. Signs of ovulation. *(From McCarthy, J., Martin, M., & Gildenhorn, M. [1977]. The sympto-thermal method. Alexandria, VA: The Human Life and Natural Family Planning Foundation. Reprinted with permission.)*

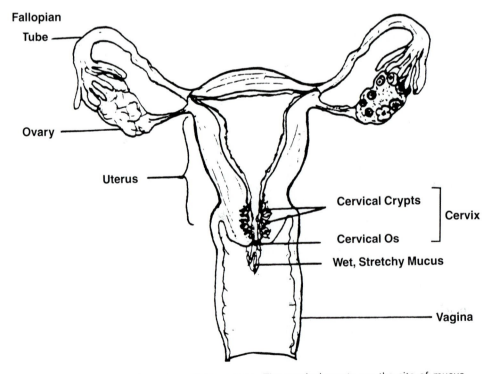

Figure 5–5. Estrogenic or preovulatory phase. The cervical crypts are the site of mucus production. Fertile mucus is wet, slippery, and lubricative.

A SUMMARY SHEET
THE OVULATION METHOD
OF NATURAL FAMILY PLANNING
Based on the Mucus Symptom

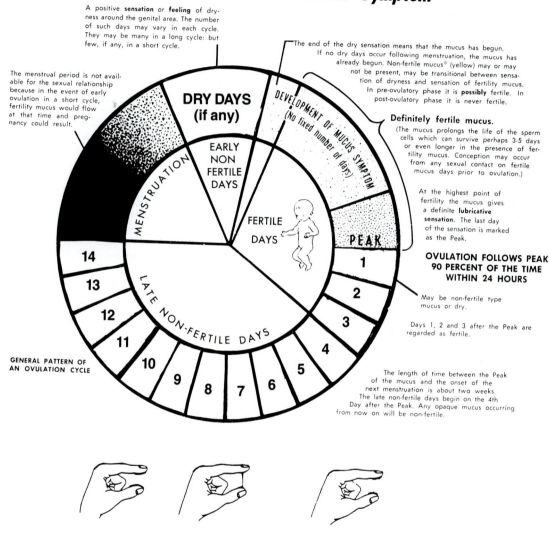

A positive **sensation** or **feeling** of dryness around the genital area. The number of such days may vary in each cycle. They may be many in a long cycle; but few, if any, in a short cycle.

The menstrual period is not available for the sexual relationship because in the event of early ovulation in a short cycle, fertility mucus would flow at that time and pregnancy could result.

DRY DAYS (if any)

DEVELOPMENT OF MUCUS SYMPTOM (No fixed number of days)

The end of the dry sensation means that the mucus has begun. If no dry days occur following menstruation, the mucus has already begun. Non-fertile mucus* (yellow) may or may not be present, may be transitional between sensation of dryness and sensation of fertility mucus. In pre-ovulatory phase it is **possibly** fertile. In post-ovulatory phase it is never fertile.

Definitely fertile mucus.
(The mucus prolongs the life of the sperm cells which can survive perhaps 3-5 days or even longer in the presence of fertility mucus. Conception may occur from any sexual contact on fertile mucus days prior to ovulation.)

At the highest point of fertility the mucus gives a definite **lubricative sensation.** The last day of the sensation is marked as the Peak.

EARLY NON FERTILE DAYS

MENSTRUATION

FERTILE DAYS

PEAK

OVULATION FOLLOWS PEAK 90 PERCENT OF THE TIME WITHIN 24 HOURS

May be non-fertile type mucus or dry.

Days 1, 2 and 3 after the Peak are regarded as fertile.

14 13 12 11 10 9 8 7 6 5 4 3 2 1

LATE NON-FERTILE DAYS

GENERAL PATTERN OF AN OVULATION CYCLE

The length of time between the Peak of the mucus and the onset of the next menstruation is about two weeks. The late non-fertile days begin on the 4th Day after the Peak. Any opaque mucus occurring from now on will be non-fertile.

SOME CHARACTERISTICS OF FERTILITY MUCUS
1) Clear or slightly cloudy
2) Like raw egg white but may be stained pink, etc., from traces of blood
3) Thin, watery, "wet"
4) Dries leaving no residue
5) Slippery and lubricative
6) Stretchy and holds the stretch

SOME CHARACTERISTICS OF *NON-FERTILE MUCUS
1) Opaque
2) Colored—white or yellow
3) Thick and sticky
4) Tacky and flakes when dry
5) Rubbery
6) "Gluppy"
7) Non-stretchy

OTHER NATURAL SIGNS AND SYMPTOMS OF FERTILITY (HIGHLY VARIABLE)
1) Abdominal pain
2) Inter-menstrual "bleeding" or "spotting"
3) Sustained temperature elevation
4) Changes in the cervix
5) Changes in sexual urge (perhaps)

Stress (physical or emotional) can inhibit or delay ovulation and change the mucus symptom in that particular cycle. In such a situation, watch **CLOSELY** for the possible return of fertility mucus after the designated peak.

Figure 5-6. A summary of the ovulation method. *(From Nofziger, M. [1979]. A cooperative method of natural birth control. Summertown, TN: The Book Publishing Co. Reprinted with permission.)*

in the low phase and all temperatures above it are in the high phase.

4. Continue taking your temperature and watch it with respect to the coverline. As soon as the temperature remains above the coverline for 3 consecutive days, the evening of the third day is safe to resume intercourse.

5. Temperatures falling on the coverline are neither high nor low and do not count. Also, occasionally something can throw off one of the first six temperatures and give you a false reading, for example, sickness, waking up later, and emotional upset. If one of the first six temperatures is abnormally high and you know why it is, disregard it in drawing the coverline. Go to the next highest temperature to draw the coverline.

6. If your pattern is not clear you cannot assume you are safe. Make an appointment with your NFP/FA counselor and take your charts with you.

OVULATION METHOD (OM) (MUCUS METHOD, BILLINGS' METHOD). It is the occurrence of ovulation that determines a woman's fertile days within her menstrual cycle. The ovulation method (OM) depends on the changes in the character and appearance of cervical mucus secretions and the cervix itself that occur just before ovulation (Figs. 5–5 and 5–6). Drs. John and Evelyn Billings of Australia pioneered the work in developing this monitoring system for human fertility and are responsible for making a significant contribution in the advancement of NFP programs throughout the world.

Cervical mucus secretions are a sign of the approach of ovulation, and there is evidence that the preservation of

sperm cells and their transport to the site of fertilization depends on the presence of a satisfactory cervical mucus. In addition, some women may experience other natural signs and symptoms of ovulation, such as a sudden sharp pain in the right or left side of the lower abdomen (*mittelschmerz* syndrome); intermenstrual bleeding; a softening of the cervix, a change in its position, and a slight dilation of the external os; mild breast tenderness; and changes in sexual urge. Young girls approaching puberty should be taught these signs and symptoms with other information about menstruation. Once a woman has been taught to recognize her bodily symptoms, she should keep a menstrual calendar or a record of the signs of ovulation on a fertility awareness chart.

Most proponents of the OM stress the value of periodic abstinence during the period of high fertility for women and couples who wish to avoid pregnancy (Fig. 5–7). With abstinence from intercourse and penile–vaginal contact during a woman's most fertile time, the OM has a 100 percent theoretic effectiveness rate. If barrier methods are used during the fertile time, their effectiveness rate must be assumed.

Instructions. Successful use of the OM is dependent on your recognition of the change in sensation of wetness in the vaginal area or, more precisely, at the opening of the vagina. Keep in mind that the quantity of mucus is not as important as the change in quality or characteristics of the mucus (Fig. 5–6). Become aware of the change in sensation.

All preovulatory mucus days are considered fertile. Clear, wet, stretchy, slippery, raw egg white–type, lubricative mucus indicates a very fertile time of the cycle. Sperm can survive in this mucus for relatively long periods.

OVULATION occurs on only **1 DAY** in each cycle	PREGNANCY can result from Contact of sexual organs on Fertile Mucus days Without Penetration or Ejaculation
EGG lives only 12–24 hours if not fertilized	
SPERM need **MUCUS** to survive	Intimate sexual contact on days of possible fertility may cause conception, even though contraceptive devices are employed
Sperm without Mucus Die within Hours Sperm with best Mucus may live 3–5 Days	When charting is commenced, COMPLETE ABSTINENCE for ONE CYCLE or ONE MONTH whichever is shorter, and until chart is reviewed by instructor
FERTILITY depends on OVULATION *AND* SATISFACTORY MUCUS	*SUCCESS* depends on: UNDERSTANDING ACCURATE OBSERVATION ACCURATE CHARTING MUTUAL MOTIVATION LOVING COOPERATION

Figure 5–7. Review of the ovulation method. *(From Marriage and Family Ministry, [undated]. Natural Family Planning Center, Akron, OH. Reprinted with permission.)*

1. Check your vaginal mucus each time you use the bathroom by observing after wiping with toilet tissue or by obtaining a mucus sample from the opening of the vagina prior to urinating and testing it between your thumb and forefinger for stretchability (Fig. 5–6).
2. If you are able to stretch your mucus 3 in. or more, consider yourself VERY FERTILE. This mucus gives a definite lubricative sensation and is considered "peak" fertility. As ovulation follows "peak" cervical mucus secretions within 12 to 48 hours and the egg survives up to 24 hours, fertilization is possible 3 days after "peak."
3. You may need to observe and record your mucus changes and other natural signs and symptoms for several cycles before you understand your own fertile period clearly enough to rely on this method of birth control. Your NFP/FA counselor will help you and your partner to interpret your fertility awareness records.
4. Chart daily. Late evening is the best time to fill in your chart because all of the signs and symptoms of the day will have been observed.
5. If your OM educator distributed colored stamps for you to use on your chart (McCarthy, Martin, & Gildenhorn, 1980) use them as follows:

Red stamp	Menstruation or bleeding during the cycle
Plain green stamp	Dry, infertile days
White stamp with a baby	Wet, stretchy, lubricative mucus
Circle around the white stamp with a baby	Peak day, that is, the last day of wet, stretchy, lubricative mucus (peak day can best be recognized as peak the next day)

A clear explanation of what to look for in the cervical mucus is provided in the Summary Sheet (Fig. 5–6). Descriptions of the mucus and the time that you have intercourse should be written on your charts.

6. If you do not use stamps, use written words or symbols (see earlier under Intervention) on your fertility awareness chart.
7. If pregnancy is to be avoided, abstain from vaginal intercourse and penile–genital contact or use a barrier method of birth control from the beginning of the mucus symptoms until the evening of the fourth day after peak.
8. Vaginal infections, semen, douching, contraceptive foam or jelly, lubricants, certain medications, and

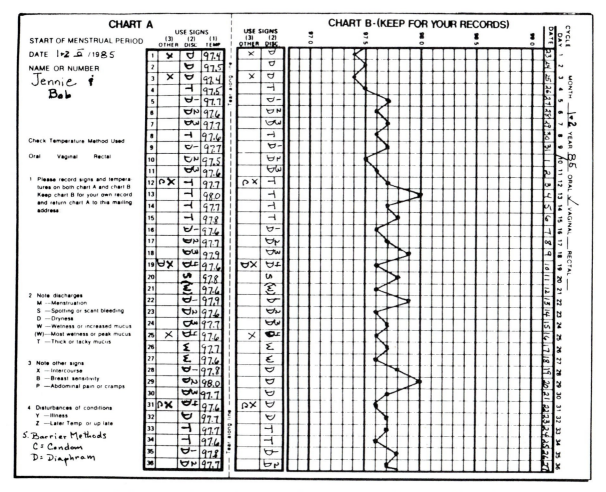

Figure 5–8. A chart of a partially breastfeeding woman. *(From McCarthy, J., Martin, M., & Gildenhorn, M. [1977]. The sympto-thermal method. Alexandria, VA: The Human Life and Natural Family Planning Foundation. Reprinted with permission.)*

even the normal lubrication of sexual arousal may interfere with your ability to notice your mucus changes. If your pattern is not clear, do not assume that you are safe.

9. Sometimes it is difficult to distinguish between seminal fluid and cervical mucus; therefore, during the dry days, intercourse and all genital contact are restricted to every other night, unless a condom is used. If avoiding pregnancy, remember the following rule: "Dry day, safe night, skip a day."

10. Avoid intercourse or use a barrier method during menstruation. All menstrual days are considered possibly fertile because menstruation may disguise the beginning of cervical mucus secretions.

11. Rules for avoiding pregnancy with use of the OM with abstinence are summarized as follows:

Early day rule for dry days	Intercourse at night on a dry day; abstain from intercourse and all genital contact on the next day and night.
Peak day rule	Abstain from intercourse and all genital contact until the fourth day after peak mucus (McCarthy et al., 1980, p. 43).

12. Combining the ovulation method with the basal body temperature method (see sympto-thermal method) is likely to improve effectiveness. Remember to take your fertility awareness charts with you whenever you visit your NFP/FA counselor.

Special Circumstances: Variations of the Normal Cycle. During puberty, after childbirth, after a spontaneous or voluntary abortion, after discontinuance of oral contraceptives, during and after breastfeeding (Fig. 5-8), when approaching menopause (Fig. 5-9), hormones are disturbed and the time of ovulation may vary. Most fertile women experience an occasional anovulatory cycle during their childbearing years. The following instructions are appropriate:

1. During these special circumstances, it is necessary to consider *all* mucus days as potentially fertile and adopt a "wait and see" attitude. It is important to heed the onset of the sensation of wetness even before any mucus is seen.

2. Use the "early day rule" on dry days only. If one or more days of thick, sticky, nonchanging mucus occur, avoid intercourse and all genital contact (or use a barrier method) until the evening of the fourth day after the last day of mucus.

3. If there are any days of bleeding or spotting, abstain

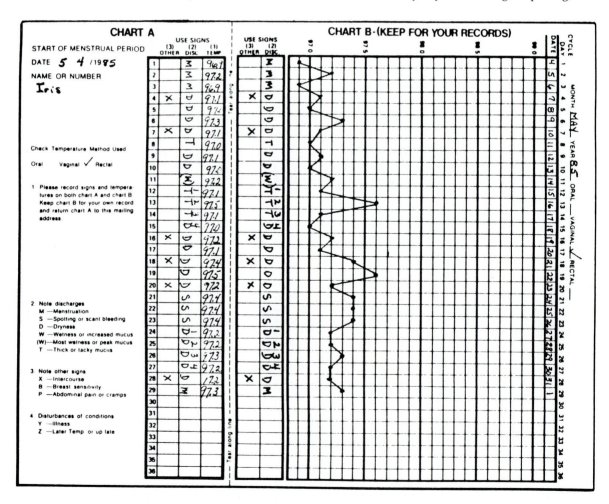

Figure 5-9. A chart of a premenopausal woman. *(From McCarthy, J., Martin, M., & Gildenhorn, M. [1977]. The sympto-thermal method. Alexandria, VA: The Human Life and Natural Family Planning Foundation. Reprinted with permission.)*

from intercourse and all genital contact or use a barrier method until the evening of the fourth dry day (McCarthy et al., 1980, pp. 46–49).

SYMPTO-THERMAL METHOD. The sympto-thermal method (STM) of family planning is a natural method that uses *both* the daily basal body temperature recordings and the ovulatory signs and symptoms (STM = BBT + OM) to recognize fertile and infertile phases of the woman's menstrual cycle. The basic instructions for patients would include those for BBT and OM. Daily charting produces an awareness of an individual woman's fertility pattern and the variation in her cycle lengths. (Fig. 5–10) By observation of the lengths of past cycles, the appropriate time of the start of the fertile phase in future cycles can be estimated. Once again, many advocates of the sympto-thermal method of natural family planning advise that the success of the method depends on abstinence from intercourse and all genital contact during the potentially fertile phases of the cycle, although many women and couples prefer to use barrier methods during these times.

Return Visits

At the end of the initial visit, review with the woman or couple the general structure of the NFP/FA program provided by your service and review with them the general sequence of follow-up visits:

1 month	Follow-up visit to review charting, answer questions, and reinforce learning
3 months	Follow-up visit to review charts, reinforce learning, answer questions, and help solve any problems
6 months	Follow-up by phone or visit to review all aspects of the method, answer any questions, and determine whether or not the woman or couple is happy with the method
Yearly visits	For well-woman gynecology checkups, to review any problematic charts and assess satisfaction with the method
Visits by appointments	When the woman or couple would like validation of their interpretation of their charting and use of the method or if physical or psychosexual problems arise

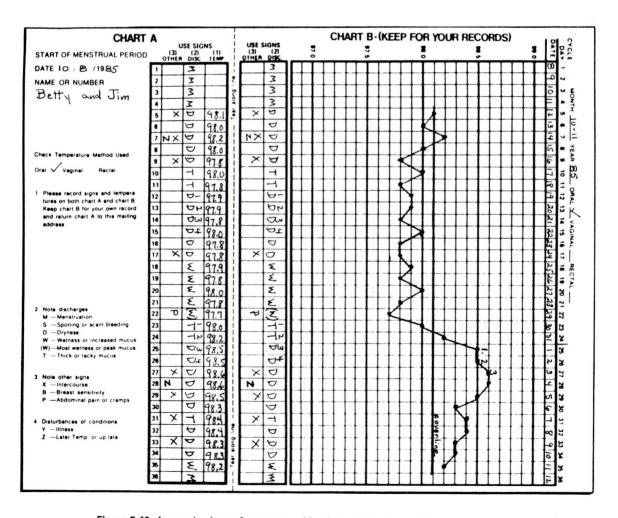

Figure 5-10. A sample chart of a woman with a long cycle. *(From McCarthy, J., Martin, M., & Gildenhorn, M. [1977]. The sympto-thermal method. Alexandria, VA: The Human Life and Natural Family Planning Foundation. Reprinted with permission.)*

If the health practitioner provides concise, accurate, and thorough NFP/FA instructions, a high percentage of the patients should be practicing the NFP/FA methods successfully within 6 to 8 months after initial instruction. Maintenance of accurate records should help the practitioner in diagnosing problems that need treatment, consultation, or referral, such as vaginitis, cervicitis, abnormal bleeding, and infertility.

SELF-HELP MEASURES

Many women and couples who have a positive experience with the NFP/FA method are available to help teach NFP/FA. Practitioners can recognize patients who are potential teachers and counselors. Do not hesitate to encourage their participation in NFP/FA programs. When problems with the method arise among patients, particularly with any of the disadvantages of the method, highly motivated and successful users of the method are often the best resource to help counsel and to share their experiences.

REFERENCES

Bonnar, J. (1982). Natural family planning including breastfeeding. In D. R. Mishell (Ed.), *Advances in fertility research*. New York: Raven Press.

Gildenhorn, M. (1977). *Basal body temperature*. Washington, DC: Natural Family Planning Federation of America, Inc.

Lanctot, C. (1979, April). Natural family planning. *Clinics in Obstetrics and Gynaecology, 6*(1), 109–110.

Liskin, L. (1981, September). Periodic abstinence: How well do new approaches work? *Population Reports, I*(3), I42–I43.

Marriage and Family Ministry. (undated). Akron, OH: Natural Family Planning Center.

McCarthy, J., Martin, M., & Gildenhorn, M. (1977). *The sympto-thermal method*. Alexandria, VA: The Human Life and Natural Family Planning Foundation.

McCarthy, J., Martin, M., & Gildenhorn, M. (1980). *The ovulation method—An instructional program with charts and text*. Washington, DC: The Human Life and Natural Family Planning Foundation.

Nofziger, M. (1979). *A cooperative method of natural birth control*. Summertown, TN: The Book Publishing Co.

Rogow, D., Rintoul, E. J., & Greenwood, S. (1980). A year's experience with a fertility awareness program: A report. *Advances in Planned Parenthood, 15*(1), 27–33.

Ross, C. (1977). *Natural family planning. 3. Introduction to the methods*. Washington, DC: The Human Life Foundation of America.

6

Barrier Methods

Maria Corsaro and Ronnie Lichtman

Barrier methods of birth control have existed since antiquity. Today, their appeal is based on a number of factors. Women see them as "natural," and appreciate their relative lack of medical side effects. These methods can be used intermittently and offer the user a large degree of control over her body. Increasingly, the protection they afford against sexually transmitted diseases (STDs) is considered a major advantage.

In initiating a barrier method, it is important to assess a woman's reason for using the method and her previous contraceptive history, with a particular focus on the method most recently used. Motivation for using a barrier method, and therefore its success, may vary according to the particular reason it has been chosen and past contraceptive experience. Counseling needs of the woman committed to the concept of barrier contraception may differ, for example, from those of the woman reluctantly switching from oral contraceptives or the intrauterine device (IUD) because of a medical contraindication. Women who previously depended on less user-intensive methods may need extra support to successfully adapt to barrier contraceptives, which require more involvement of the woman or couple.

Currently available barrier contraceptives are the diaphragm, foam and condoms, the cervical cap, the vaginal sponge, vaginal suppositories, and contraceptive film. This chapter describes each barrier method of contraception with discussion of effectiveness rates, advantages, disadvantages, and management issues. Distinctions are made between theoretical method effectiveness and use effectiveness. Because of the continual need for user input with barrier methods, these two rates can be widely divergent. Teaching guidelines are offered; these can be developed into handouts, modified as necessary to meet the particular needs, educational level, and language used by patients. In addition to instructions for each specific method, teaching must include all components of informed consent. These are outlined in the introduction to Section II, "Issues and Concepts in Family Planning."

Of the available barrier contraceptives, only the diaphragm and cervical cap require practitioner input for sizing and prescribing or dispensing. Women relying on other barrier methods, which are available over-the-counter, may not seek routine gynecologic care. Whenever possible, however, these women should be counseled on the value of regular health assessments. In addition, teaching and counseling provided by a practitioner can enhance the effective use of any barrier method. The understanding and caring practitioner can be highly influential in ensuring satisfaction with barrier contraceptives, as many disadvantages of these methods are based on subjective perceptions of the user. By carefully addressing patient concerns, many problems encountered with barrier methods can be overcome. This chapter therefore includes guidelines for method initiation and follow-up for each barrier contraceptive discussed. The provider should become comfortable handling all types of barrier methods and be familiar with variations among different brands of the same method.

Initial visits for all methods should include a complete history, physical examination, and appropriate laboratory testing. Section I, "Assessment," provides guidelines in each of these areas. Contraindications to the desired method must be evaluated. If a woman has not chosen a method, she should be assisted in making an informed choice. The Introduction to Section II, "Issues and Concepts in Family Planning," offers a framework for helping women evaluate their individual risk–benefit ratio for any contraceptive method.

THE DIAPHRAGM

Definition and Description

The diaphragm is a small cup of rubber with a rim stabilized by a rubber-covered steel spring. It ranges from 50 to 100 mm in diameter, with upper and lower limits dependent on the brand and type (Table 6–1). Sizes increase in 5-mm increments.

Diaphragms are classified according to the strength of their spring. This spring strength, combined with vaginal muscle tone and the anatomic shape of the pubic arch, is responsible for holding the diaphragm in place in the vagina. The three diaphragm types commonly available are the arcing spring, the coil spring, and the flat spring. The arcing spring is a double spring and is strong and firm. It is especially suited for the woman with fair to poor vaginal muscle tone, although all women can use this type. The arc shape, when folded (Fig. 6–1), facilitates insertion over the cervix. The coil spring diaphragm (Fig. 6–2) has an intermediate spring strength and is an appropriate diaphragm for women with average vaginal muscle tone. The flat spring diaphragm, which folds flat on insertion (Fig. 6–3), is a good choice for women with excellent vaginal tone, as it has a thin rim with gentle spring strength. It is particularly

TABLE 6-1. AVAILABLE DIAPHRAGMS BY SPRING TYPE AND MANUFACTURER

Spring Type (in descending order of strength)	Manufacturer			
	Ortho Pharmaceuticals	*Holland-Rantos*	*Schmid Products*	*Milex*
Arcing Spring	Allflex Sizes 55–95	Koroflex Sizes 60–95	Rames Bendex Sizes 65–95	Wide-seal Sizes 60–95
Coil Spring	Ortho Diaphragm Sizes 50–95	Koromex Sizes 50–95	Ramses Flexible Cushioned Sizes 50–95	Wide Seal Omiflex Sizes 60–95
Flat Spring	Ortho White Sizes 55–95			

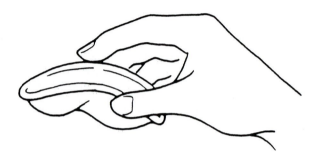

Figure 6-1. The arcing spring diaphragm.

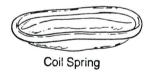

Coil Spring

Figure 6-2. The coil spring diaphragm. *(From Hatcher, R. A., Guest, F., Stewart, F., et al. [1986]. Contraceptive technology 1986–1987 [13th rev. ed.]. New York: Irvington Publishers. Reprinted with permission.)*

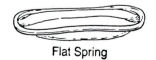

Flat Spring

Figure 6-3. The flat spring diaphragm. *(From Hatcher, R. A., Guest, F., Stewart, F., et al. [1986]. Contraceptive technology 1986–1987 [13th rev. ed.]. New York: Irvington Publishers. Reprinted with permission.)*

useful for the woman with a shallow pubic arch (Okrent, 1974). A woman using the coil or flat spring diaphragm needs to be quite comfortable feeling her cervix to ascertain proper coverage as these diaphragms do not fold into an arc and can be placed incorrectly above the cervix rather than over it. They can, however, be used with an introducer, which facilitates accurate placement.

The diaphragm is inserted into the vagina prior to intercourse, after contraceptive jelly or cream has been placed into the cup. Instructions on how much jelly or cream to use vary between a teaspoon and a tablespoon. The spermicide is placed in the center of the diaphragm. Many practitioners suggest spreading the cream or jelly thinly around the rim, but others have claimed that this may cause the diaphragm to be slippery and incorrectly placed (Craig & Hepburn, 1982). If spermicide is spread inside the inner rim only, the diaphragm is less slippery to insert than if the spermicide is placed on the outer part of the rim, yet the rim is still "sealed" with spermicide. A newly introduced diaphragm variation is the wide-seal rim, available with either an arcing or coil spring diaphragm. In this design, an inner rim added to the diaphragm theoretically holds the spermicide in place and seals the rim more effectively (Hatcher, Guest, Stewart, et al., 1986, p. 218).

In addition to differences in the type of spring among diaphragms, there are variations among brands in shades and texture of rubber and in the way the springs are folded. Some arcing spring diaphragms, such as the Koroflex (made by The Holland-Rantos Company) or the Ramses Bendex (made by the Schmid company), fold at only two points on the rim. Others, such as the Allflex (made by Ortho Pharmaceuticals), can be folded anywhere along the spring, as can all coil and flat spring types, except the new wide seal coil spring. Among the arcing spring diaphragms, the Koroflex and Ramses Bendex diaphragms may be easier to insert because they fold into a narrower shape than the Allflex (Hatcher et al., 1986, p. 218). Table 6-1 lists the currently available diaphragms.

The diaphragm has been properly placed when the anterior portion of its rim fits behind the symphysis pubis and the posterior rim is behind the cervix. The cervix should be covered by the cup part of the diaphragm.

Mechanism of Action

The contraceptive mechanism of action of the diaphragm is dual. First, it forms a barrier between the sperm and cervix. Second, it provides a holding receptacle for spermicide at close proximity to the cervix. There is controversy regarding which of these two actions is primary in contraceptive efficacy of the diaphragm. One research study found excellent results for the use of small (size 60 or 65) arcing spring diaphragms for all women without spermicide (Stim, cited by Tatum & Connell-Tatum, 1981, p. 4). Controlled, randomized clinical trials comparing the diaphragm's use as a barrier without spermicide to its use with cream or jelly have never been carried out, however. This question remains unresolved as does the question of whether additional spermicide is needed for repeated acts of intercourse (Craig & Hepburn, 1982).

Effectiveness

Method effectiveness of the diaphragm is 97 to 98.5 percent (Wortman, 1976). Use effectiveness rates, however, range from below 70 percent to over 90 percent, approaching theoretic effectiveness rates (Wortman, 1976).

Several large studies have shown excellent diaphragm effectiveness. One involved 2,168 young women at the Margaret Sanger Research Bureau in New York (Lane, Arceo, & Sobrero, 1976). Investigators followed women for 2 years and showed a use effectiveness rate of 97 to 98 per 100 users. Interestingly, lower failure rates were seen in women under 18 years old. The continuation rate for the method at the end of the first year was 8 in 10. The contraceptive success for the women in this study was felt to be due greatly to the initial fit of the diaphragm, the time spent with each woman in teaching correct use and practicing insertion and removal, and follow-up visits.

In another large study, Vessey and Wiggins (1974) found a failure rate of 2.4 per 100 woman-years. They found a decreasing failure rate with increasing age and duration of use.

In a 1-year prospective study of 721 diaphragm users, a pregnancy rate of 12.5 per 100 women was demonstrated (Edelman, McIntyre, & Harper, 1984). In this study, women less than age 25 showed a pregnancy rate of 16.8, whereas those over 25 showed a rate of 9.2. Increased failure rates were also correlated with single status, lower educational levels, and increased coital frequency.

Advantages/Benefits

When used correctly, the diaphragm is highly effective in pregnancy prevention with minimal side effects. In addition, there is some evidence that the spermicide *nonoxynol-9* may inhibit the growth of some bacteria and viruses associated with sexually transmitted diseases including syphilis, gonorrhea, herpes, and acquired immune deficiency syndrome (AIDS) (Asculai, Weis, Rancourt, & Kupferberg, 1978; Hicks, Martin, Getchell, et al., 1985; Postic, Singh, Squeglia, & Guevarra, 1978; Singh, Cutler, & Utidjian, 1972; Singh, Postic, & Cutler, 1976). The relationship of diaphragm use to cervical cancer has not been assessed although one large study hypothesized a protective effect (Melamed, Koss, Flehinger, et al., 1969).

Disadvantages and Risks

There are relatively few risks to diaphragm use compared with other methods. For some women, however, the method has a number of disadvantages. If there is desire to use the method, ways can be found to overcome many of these.

Disadvantages

DISCOMFORT. Female dyspareunia may result from a too large or too firmly rimmed diaphragm (Wortman, 1976 p. H-64). Occasionally the diaphragm can be felt by the partner. Sometimes this can be corrected with use of a different size or type of diaphragm.

PERCEIVED INTERFERENCE WITH SPONTANEITY OF LOVEMAKING. Interference with spontaneity is related mainly to the use of extra spermicide with each act of intercourse, although it may also be experienced if a woman does not insert the diaphragm prior to sexual foreplay. If the partner can learn to insert the diaphragm and/or the spermicide, insertion can become part of sexual interaction.

PERCEIVED MESSINESS. Messiness also relates to use of extra spermicide with each act of intercourse.

TASTE. Some men object to the taste of the spermicide used with the diaphragm. This may be reduced if the woman washes herself well after diaphragm insertion. Recently spermicides have been made with reduced taste and without perfumes. If these are still objectionable, the diaphragm can be inserted after oral sex, although this might be perceived to interfere with sexual spontaneity.

EXPENSE. Frequent use of spermicide can result in high costs.

NECESSITY OF TOUCHING THE GENITALS. Some women are uncomfortable touching their bodies for personal or cultural reasons. For some couples, this problem can be resolved by teaching the partner to insert and remove the diaphragm.

NEED FOR PRIVACY FOR INSERTION AND REMOVAL. A lack of privacy may be a particular problem for adolescent women and women or couples who share small living spaces with others.

Risks

ALLERGIC REACTIONS. Allergy to rubber or spermicide may occur in a woman or her partner. If allergy occurs with contraceptive cream, switching to jelly might resolve the problem, or vice versa. Changing brands may also alleviate allergic responses as the allergy may be to the inert ingredients, which vary among brands.

RECURRENT URINARY TRACT INFECTIONS. An association between diaphragm use and urinary tract infection, or cystitis, has been demonstrated in a number of research studies and in clinical practice (Fihn, Latham, & Roberts, et al., 1985a; Fihn, Running, Pinkstaff, et al., 1985b; Gillespie, 1984; Peddie, Gorrie, & Bailey, 1986; Percival-Smith, Bartlett, & Chow, 1983; Vessey, Doll, Peto, et al, 1976). Explanations for this association include urethral obstruction; alteration of the vaginal flora predisposing to colonization with Gram-negative organisms; and elevation of the bladder neck leading to increased residual urine, decreased rate of urinary flow, and increased intravesical pressure causing a susceptibility of the bladder mucosa to bacterial action (Gillespie, 1984, p. 29). Altering the diaphragm fit (see Initial Visit below) to allow increased space between the rim and pubic bone can alleviate this problem (Gillespie, 1984). A softer spring may also reduce the incidence of diaphragm-related urinary tract infections. Chapter 17 provides detailed discussion of the management of these infections.

TOXIC-SHOCK SYNDROME. A number of cases of toxic-shock syndrome (TSS) have been reported with diaphragm use. Use in the postpartum weeks, for more than 24 hours, and/ or during adolescence has been associated with this disease (Baehler, Dillon, Cumbo, & Lee, 1982; Jaffe, 1981; Lee, Dillon, & Baehler, 1982; Litt, 1983; Loomis & Feder, 1981; Wilson, 1983). See Chapter 18 for an in-depth discussion of TSS.

QUESTION OF BIRTH DEFECTS. In 1980, a retrospective study of karyotypes of spontaneously aborted fetuses conceived during the use of spermicidal agents showed an increase in postconception errors among such fetuses (Strobino, Kline, Stein, et al., 1980). In 1981, Jick and associates reported an increased incidence of birth defects among babies whose mothers had obtained a vaginal spermicide within the 600 days preceding delivery or abortion. These same researchers found an association between spermicide use and miscarriage (Jick, Shiota, Shephard, et al., 1982b). Another very small study corroborated the association between spermicide use and Down's syndrome (Rothman, 1982), and still another found a suggestion of a small adverse effect on the risk of congenital malformations (Huggins, Vessey, Flavel, et al, 1982).

These well-publicized findings led to much concern among diaphragm and other spermicide users, many of whom choose these methods for their relative lack of medical side effects. A number of subsequently published larger studies, however, did not support the conclusions of these reports (Louik, Mitchell, Werler, et al., 1987; Mills, Harley, Reed, & Berendes, 1982; Mills, Reed, Nugent, et al., 1985; Shapiro, Slone, Heinonen, et al., 1982; Warburton, Neugut, Lustenberger, et al., 1987), and the Jick report in particular has been widely criticized for weaknesses in its research design, methodology, and conclusions. The investigators made no attempt to ascertain whether women who had obtained vaginal spermicides had actually used them and, if so, when use had occurred. Using a cutoff of 600 days prior to delivery as the criterion for inclusion into the exposed group meant that some women had possibly used the product as long as 10 months prior to conception, if at all. In addition, several of the defects seen among supposed spermicide users were found to have an unusually low incidence in the study's control population, calling into question whether they actually did occur in greater numbers in the spermicide group. Finally, the lack of a clear syndrome among spermicide users makes any inference of causality impossible.

Most authorities agree at this time that if there is an association between spermicide use and fetal malformation, it is small. No causal relationship has been proven (Oakley, 1982). The author of a comprehensive review of the epidemiologic literature concluded that the evidence linking spermicides to either congenital malformations or spontaneous abortion is too weak to support any additional regulation of spermicides (Bracken, 1985). In December 1983, the Fertility and Maternal Health Drugs Advisory Committee to the Food and Drug Administration (FDA) determined that evidence does not warrant a warning on spermicide labels regarding use during pregnancy (Lemberg, 1984, p. 30).

Contraindications

The following preclude diaphragm use: allergy to rubber or all available spermicides; inability of the woman or her partner to insert or remove the diaphragm; inability to be properly fit with the diaphragm, as a result of uterine prolapse, severe cystocele, rectocele, or uterine retroversion.

A documented history of urinary tract infections may be a reason to discontinue diaphragm use, and their occurrence with previous use may preclude reinitiation, although a change in size or spring strength can be attempted to resolve this problem. A history of toxic-shock syndrome may be considered a contraindication. The method should not be used during the 6-week postpartum period.

Management of Visits

Initial Visit

METHOD INITIATION. Before diaphragm fitting, contraindications should be ruled out by history and pelvic examination. Specific assessment should be made of vaginal muscle tone, the presence of cystocele or rectocele, and uterine position.

To enhance correct diaphragm use, the woman should visualize and feel her cervix before practicing insertion and removal, especially if she has never seen or felt it before. This also gives her the opportunity to ask questions and to feel comfortable touching herself, and it allows the practitioner to provide information about normal anatomy and its variations. A mirror can be used during the speculum examination and the woman can be instructed to use one or two fingers to feel her cervix before the diaphragm is inserted by the practitioner for assessment of fit. The woman should also feel the pubic bone from inside the vagina so that she will be able to use this landmark to check her diaphragm placement.

Visual aids, such as a plastic pelvic model and charts, are helpful for teaching prior to patient practice. Proper diaphragm insertion can be demonstrated on the model and charts used to illustrate techniques and positions for method of insertion.

Each step of the diaphragm fitting procedure should be explained to the woman. The procedure is as follows:

First, insert two gloved fingers into the vagina to approximate the distance from the posterior cervix to the inner aspect of the symphysis pubis. When the middle finger has reached the posterior cervix, a finger from the other hand or the thumb of the same hand can be used to mark the place on the index finger of the examining hand where the symphysis pubis is felt. Match this length to the diameter of the fitting diaphragms to find the right size (Fig. 6-4). Diaphragms are preferable to rings for fitting because they can be assessed for buckling in the vagina, which may indicate too large a fit, and because they afford more realistic practice for the woman. Most diaphragm companies supply a set of fitting diaphragms if requested. These should be washed after each use and completely soaked for 20 minutes in a disinfecting solution: 70 percent alcohol (Hatcher et al., 1986; p. 219) or 10 percent bleach.

Insert the diaphragm so that the cervix is covered and the anterior rim is behind the pubic bone. In fitting, it is important to remember that during intercourse, the vagina expands 3 to 5 cm so that generally the largest size that will fit the vagina comfortably is recommended. For women with recurrent urinary tract infections, however, a smaller fit has been advised (Gillespie, 1984). Whether or not contraceptive efficacy is lost with a looser diaphragm fit is unknown. It is also important to remember that after the woman relaxes a bit, her vaginal muscle tone may also relax, which may necessitate a larger size. The initial estimate

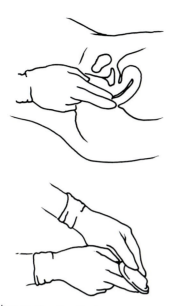

Figure 6-4. How to size the diaphragm. *(Courtesy of Ortho Pharmaceutical Company, Raritan, New Jersey 08069.)*

of size or type of diaphragm may change after the first attempt to fit. The diaphragm is the right size if: the cervix is covered completely; at least, but not more than, one finger fits between the anterior rim and the pubic bone; and the sides of the diaphragm do not buckle against the vaginal side walls, but are held firmly by the walls.

An additional check on diaphragm fit can be made if the woman coughs or bears down after it is in place. If it slips out from behind the pubic arch, it is most likely too large or too soft a rim. The woman should also walk around for a few moments with the diaphragm in place to make sure she cannot feel it. If feasible, exercising for 5 minutes can simulate vaginal wall expansion during intercourse. The fit can then be rechecked (Pyle, 1984).

Once fit has been established, the patient should feel the diaphragm in place, making sure that she feels the cervix through the rubber. She then can be instructed on insertion and removal. She can remove the diaphragm that the practitioner has placed or start with insertion. It is important to use for practice a diaphragm with the same type of rim that will be prescribed. It is also advisable to use the same brand; if this is not possible, the woman must be warned about the differences to expect, which were explained earlier under Definition and Description. For insertion, instruct the woman to follow these steps:

1. Assume a position of comfort (sitting; lying with knees or knees and hips bent; squatting; standing; placing one foot on a stool, chair, bed, or the toilet seat).
2. Squeeze between a teaspoon and tablespoon of contraceptive cream or jelly into the cup. Spread it thinly around the inside of the rim. Touch the spermicide only with the pinky of either hand so that the fingers that are used for diaphragm insertion do not become greasy.
3. Fold the diaphragm for easier insertion, with the dome facing downward, and hold it from above (Fig. 6-1). Remind the woman to hold the spring tightly; it can open and fly out of her hand when she is first learning. This happens especially with

the arcing spring as the firm spring strength makes it difficult to hold closed; the Koroflex and Ramses Bendex may be easier to hold closed than the Allflex.

4. Hold the diaphragm in the dominant hand. The other hand can be used to open the labia to facilitate insertion. Once part of the rim is in the vagina, the labia can be let go and the nondominant hand used to help push the diaphragm in further. The diaphragm should be inserted in a downward, backward direction.
5. Check to make sure that after the diaphragm is placed inside the vagina, the cervix is covered and the front portion of the rim is behind the pubic bone. The dome of the center of the diaphragm should be facing downward toward the floor of the vagina.

The practitioner must check to make sure that the woman's insertion and fit are correct. Some women have great difficulty with diaphragm insertion. A plastic inserter or introducer, designed to be used with a coil or flat spring diaphragm, is available for these women (Fig 6-6). It also facilitates proper placement when the cervix is very posterior. Instructions for use of the introducer are as follows:

1. Hold the diaphragm with the dome downward.
2. Hook the rim of the diaphragm onto the notch corresponding to its size. Hook the opposite side of the rim onto the front of the inserter.
3. Insert the introducer into the vagina as far posteriorly as it will go.
4. Twist the introducer 45° and withdraw it.
5. Check for proper diaphragm placement.

The following instructions are given for diaphragm removal:

1. Assume a position of comfort as in step 1 for insertion.
2. Insert the thumb or middle finger either between the front diaphragm rim and the pubic bone or on the rubber, a short distance behind the front rim, and push toward the rim.
3. Pull the diaphragm downward to release it from the bone, and then outward.
4. If the diaphragm is difficult to reach, bearing down with the vaginal muscles should bring the rim closer to the vaginal entrance.

During both insertion and removal, a woman may need encouragement and reassurance that learning to use the diaphragm may be a somewhat tedious and difficult process. She should not be rushed, but rather assured that eventually she will be able to insert and remove the device quickly. It is helpful to remind her of other skills she has learned and to emphasize that learning requires patience. All efforts should be praised. If the woman seems hesitant to touch herself in front of an onlooker, she can be given a few minutes of privacy to practice on her own, although sometimes observation reveals errors in technique that can be remedied with simple suggestions. After insertion and removal have been successfully accomplished, the woman should practice them one more time, or as many times as needed.

The diaphragm is dispensed only by prescription and must be prescribed by rim type and size. A woman may want a prescription for more than one diaphragm. If she has intercourse in more than one place, keeping a dia-

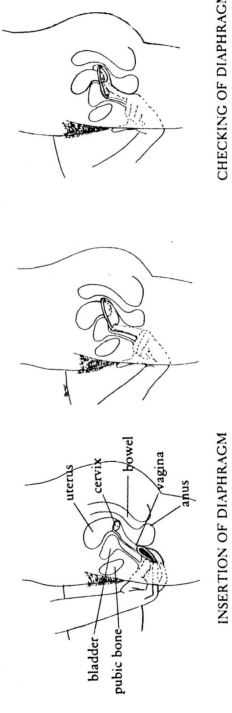

INSERTION OF DIAPHRAGM

uterus
cervix
bowel
vagina
anus
bladder
pubic bone

CHECKING OF DIAPHRAGM
Nina Reimer

Figure 6–5. Insertion and checking of diaphragm. (From The Boston Women's Health Book Collective [1984]. *The new our bodies, ourselves.* New York: Simon & Schuster, p. 227. Reprinted with permission.)

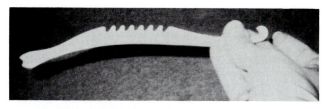

Figure 6-6. The diaphragm introducer.

phragm in each of these places may help her avoid being caught unprotected. Prescribing a refill will make it easier for her to replace the diaphragm, especially in an emergency situation.

TEACHING GUIDELINES. Several standard instructions for diaphragm use have been promulgated without research documentation. There is a lack of consensus on the length of time before intercourse that the diaphragm can be inserted. As the spermicide generally is considered active in vivo up to 6 hours, practitioners often consider 6 hours the upper limit, although many practitioners and manufacturers suggest 2 hours as the cutoff, or advise the addition of extra spermicide if more than 2 hours elapse from insertion to intercourse (Pyle, 1984). Diaphragm manufacturers and practitioners commonly advise adding additional cream or jelly externally to the diaphragm when repeated acts of intercourse occur within 6 to 8 hours. Studies proving or disproving whether this actually increases contraceptive efficacy are not available. Diaphragm users are told routinely to have the diaphragm refit for weight changes of at least 15 to 20 pounds. Although this recommendation has not been examined extensively, two small studies have considered it. A chart review of 80 diaphragm users found weight change greater than 10 pounds to be unrelated to the need

for change in diaphragm size (Fiscella, 1982). In another study, involving 125 women, adjustment in diaphragm size was found to be unnecessary with weight change up to about 25 pounds (Kugel & Verson, 1986).

The following instructions reflect current practice and pharmaceutical company advice. They have been adapted from Hatcher, Guest, Stewart, and associates (1984) and Connell and Tatum (1985a).

1. Before using the diaphragm for contraception, practice insertion and removal. Wear the diaphragm at least 8 hours to check your comfort. If you are at all uncertain about proper diaphragm placement, use a condom with the diaphragm if you have intercourse before you return for your diaphragm check.
2. Use the diaphragm with each act of vaginal intercourse.
3. Insert the diaphragm just prior to intercourse or up to 6 hours before.
4. If placed just prior to intercourse, your partner can insert the diaphragm.
5. Prior to insertion of the diaphragm, apply spermicidal jelly or cream (at least one teaspoon) in the dome and along the inner rim. Spermicides can be purchased at most pharmacies and some supermarkets and general stores. The choice between cream and jelly is one of personal preference or aesthetics. Make sure that whatever is chosen is specifically labeled to be used with the diaphragm. If an irritation occurs, switch from cream to jelly, or vice versa, or try a different brand. Many companies now manufacture clear spermicides, with reduced odor and taste, which may be preferable for some women or their partners.
6. After insertion, check placement of the diaphragm to make sure that the cervix is covered and the front rim is behind the pubic bone.
7. Remove the diaphragm no less than 6 hours after intercourse (the last act if it has been repeated) and no more than 24 hours after insertion.
8. With each act of intercourse, insert additional spermicide with either the finger or an applicator. An applicator can be purchased with spermicide in a "starter kit."
9. After use, clean the diaphragm with warm water and mild soap and dry well with a towel or by exposure to air.
10. Before storage, the diaphragm may be dusted with corn starch, which helps absorb excess moisture and odors. Do not use talc or perfumed powders, which may damage the rubber. Talc has also been linked to cervical cancer. Rinse the powder off before the next insertion.
11. Keep the diaphragm away from heat and petroleum jelly, which can deteriorate the rubber.
12. Check the diaphragm for holes, either before or after each use, by holding it up to the light or filling it with water to find leaks. Be especially careful to check around the rim where minute holes may be found. Check also for areas where the rubber appears to be wearing thin. Do not use a diaphragm with holes or thin areas; call your practitioner for a prescription or refill your previous one, if you do not have a spare.
13. With proper care, the diaphragm should last years.
14. You may need a new size or type diaphragm if you

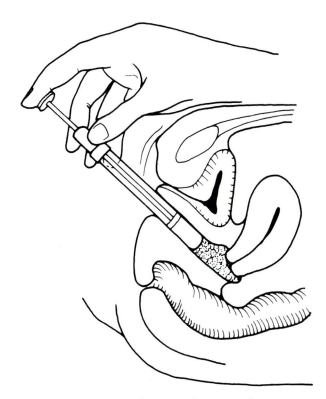

Figure 6-7. Insertion of contraceptive foam and its barrier action.

gain or lose 15 to 20 pounds; if you have discomfort with or without intercourse; after a pregnancy (birth, miscarriage, or abortion); after pelvic surgery; or if you have several urinary tract infections.

15. If at any time during diaphragm use you develop a high fever with vomiting or diarrhea, immediately call your practitioner or go to the nearest emergency room. These are the early symptoms of toxic-shock syndrome, a rare disease that on occasion is associated with the diaphragm.

Follow-up. At the end of the diaphragm fitting, the woman should be instructed to practice with it for 1 or 2 weeks and then return for a check. During this time, she should wear the diaphragm at least 8 hours whether or not she has intercourse so that comfort can be assessed when she returns. If she had difficulty practicing insertion, or is unsure of her ability to place the diaphragm properly, she should use condoms with the diaphragm until the check. She can come to the follow-up visit wearing the diaphragm or insert it at the visit. Of course, if a vaginal or cervical assessment needs to be made at the visit, the diaphragm should be inserted after the examination. Correct placement should be ascertained and satisfaction with the method reviewed. The woman must be given the opportunity to express concerns and ask questions.

The practitioner should always be available by phone to answer any questions and/or to see the woman, if needed. Time, education, patience, and encouragement are important to the success of the diaphragm as an effective contraceptive.

FOAM AND CONDOMS

Contraceptive foam and condoms can and are used alone, but because the contraceptive effectiveness is higher when both methods are used together, they will be presented here as a single method. It has been suggested, however, that since condoms are alone highly effective, it is not always wise to insist that spermicides be used with them because the overall effect may be to discourage their consistent use (Sherris, 1982, p. H-125). Foam can be used as an immediate back-up contraceptive should a condom break, leak, or fall off inside the woman (Craig & Hepburn, 1982) or it can be used only during the woman's most fertile times. Condoms also can be used to enhance the effectiveness of any other barrier contraceptive.

Definition and Description

Contraceptive foam consists of a spermicidal agent (usually nonylphenoxypoly polyethoxy ethanol or nonoxynol-9) in a foam medium. It comes in prefilled applicators or in cans with separate applicators whose sizes vary among brands. A condom is a sheath made of either latex or processed collagenous tissue (lambskin). Condoms can be lubricated or not, saturated with spermicide or not, and made with or without a reservoir tip to catch the sperm. They also come in a variety of colors, textures, and flavors.

Mechanism of Action

Foam works in two ways: First, through coital action and correct placement, it provides a barrier between sperm and the cervix (Fig. 6–7); second, its chemical action kills sperm. The condom creates a barrier between the cervix and sperm.

Effectiveness

Foam and Condoms. The theoretical effectiveness of foam and condoms used together is approximately 99 percent. This makes the combined method second only to oral contraceptives in theoretical effectiveness among the reversible methods of birth control.

Use effectiveness of foam and condoms together has not been widely investigated. It has been reported to be close to theoretical effectiveness (Hatcher, Stewart, Stewart, et al., 1980, pp. 86–87), although it can be as low as the use effectiveness of either method.

Foam. The theoretical effectiveness of foam is about 95 percent (Sherris, 1982, p. H-125). Use effectiveness is much lower, reported to be as low as 60 percent, although it can approach 95 percent (Bernstein, 1971, 1974; Tietze & Lewitt, 1967). Foam has not been as extensively studied as other birth control methods (Edelman, 1980, p. 341).

Condoms. Estimates of the theoretical effectiveness of the condom range from 98 to more than 99 percent (Sherris, 1982). Method failure results from breakage or leakage during use; statistics on how often this occurs are unavailable. Good-quality condoms are estimated to break no more often than once in every 1,000 condoms (Sherris, 1982, p. H-125). Since 1968, when rigorous guidelines were placed on condom manufacturers, the quality of condoms produced and marketed in this country has been excellent (Free & Alexander, 1976). In 1989, Consumers Union tested 40 condom varieties for defects and strength ("Can you rely on condoms?", 1989). Most models had a projected maximum failure rate of 1.5 percent. Six models had a projected maximum failure rate of 4 percent: Sheik Non-Lubricated Plain End, Ramses Sensitol Lubricated, Saxon Ribbed Lubricated, Ramses NuFORM, Mentor, and LifeStyles Nuda. Two models had a projected maximum failure rate of more than 10 percent: LifeStyles Extra Strength with Nonoxynol-9 and LifeStyles Nuda Plus. These are not recommended. Recently, condoms have been made with spermicidal lubrication, although more research is required to evaluate whether this addition improves contraceptive efficacy (Craig & Hepburn, 1982). It does, however, reduce the number of active sperm in the ejaculate in the condom (Hatcher et al., 1986, p. 236), and in one noncontrolled study the use of spermicidally lubricated condoms resulted in a failure rate of less than one per 100 woman-years (Potts & McDevitt, 1975).

Use effectiveness of condoms varies greatly. Use effectiveness rates have been reported as high as theoretical effectiveness and as low as 60 percent (Sherris, 1982, p. H-125). Differences may be related to age, family income, motivation to practice family planning, educational level, length of marriage, and experience with the method (Sherris, 1982). In one study in England, women over the age of 35 whose husbands had used condoms more than 4 years were found to have a pregnancy rate of just 0.7 per 100 couple-years of use. In this same study, women aged 24 to 35 whose husbands used condoms for the same period had a pregnancy rate of 3.6 per 100 couple-years (Sherris, 1982, p. H-125).

Advantages/Benefits

There are many advantages to foam and condoms, including a very small number of side effects and a high effectiveness rate with correct usage. Both foam and condoms are widely available without prescription. Condom use allows for the participation of men in the responsibilities of contraception.

A recently well-publicized advantage of condoms, and, to a lesser extent, of spermicides is protection against sexually transmitted organisms, including *Neisseria gonorrhoeae* (Jick, Hannan, Stergachis, et al., 1982a), *Treponema pallidum* (the syphilis spirochete) (Singh, et al., 1972), human immunodeficiency virus (HIV), and other viruses such as herpes and cytomegalovirus (Asculai et al., 1978; Conant, Hardy, Sernatinger, et al., 1986; Conant, Spicer, & Smith, 1984; De Gruttola, Moore, & Bennett, 1986; Liskin & Blackburn, 1986; Postic et al., 1978; Singh et al., 1976; Women's Health Update, 1987). Studies have found both latex and lambskin condoms to be protective, although whether the degree of protection differs is not known. Indeed, promotion of condom use is a major part of the public health response to the spread of AIDS.

A less widely known advantage of condoms is their protective effect against cervical dysplasia and their use in the treatment of dysplasia. Regression of dysplasia has been seen after initiation of condom use without other treatment (Richardson & Lyon, 1981). It is speculated that condoms prevent exposure to histones, which are proteins of the sperm head that may interact with cervical cells in a manner that promotes cancer (Baldwin & Goodwin, 1985, p. 330; Singer, Reid, & Coppleson, 1976). See chapters 12 and 13 for more discussion of these problems.

Disadvantages and Risks

There are a number of disadvantages, and a few risks, to the use of foam and condoms together or to each method separately. Many of these are amenable to change through counseling, particularly among women or couples who are motivated to use these methods.

Disadvantages

PERCEIVED INTERRUPTION OF LOVEMAKING. Because foam cannot be inserted more than 30 minutes before intercourse [although some authorities use 1 hour as the cutoff (Craig & Hepburn, 1982)], and because a condom can be placed only on an erect penis, many couples find that these methods interfere with spontaneity. They can be assisted in finding ways to incorporate use of the methods into their lovemaking; the woman, for example, can put the condom on her partner or the man can insert the foam into the woman.

PERCEIVED MESSINESS OF FOAM. If messiness presents so great a problem that the couple ends up using no protection, it is best to advise them just to use condoms with foam as a back-up should a condom break or slip off inside the woman.

TASTE OF FOAM. If a man objects to the taste of foam, couples can insert the foam after oral sex, prior to vaginal intercourse, should this prove to be a major deterrent to consistent contraceptive use.

PERCEIVED DECREASE IN SENSITIVITY OF PENIS DURING INTERCOURSE. Many brands and types of condoms are available today. Men can be advised to experiment with different types to find the most acceptable one. Often, condoms made of skin rather than rubber are thinner and perceived to interfere less with sensation.

Risks

ALLERGIC REACTIONS. Allergy to foam preparations or to condom material can occur in either partner. Relief may be ob-

tained by switching to a different brand of foam or another type of condom. Condoms made from natural animal skins may be less allergenic.

SPERMICIDES AND BIRTH DEFECTS. Although the issue has been raised, evidence linking spermicides to birth defects is not strong. See Question of Birth Defects, under The Diaphragm, for more discussion of this concern.

Contraindications

Contraindications to foam and condoms include allergy to foam or all condom materials; an inability to sustain an erection with condom use; and an inability to take responsibility for using this method consistently.

Management of Visits

Initial Visit

METHOD INITIATION. When initiating foam and condoms, it is useful to have samples of each available for demonstration. Different types of foam and condoms should be shown to women and, optimally, their partners. Models and illustrations can be helpful to show proper contraceptive placement. Condom placement also can be demonstrated on the index and middle fingers.

TEACHING GUIDELINES. The following instructions are adapted from those offered by Connell and Tatum (1985a, 1985b) and Hatcher and colleagues (1984) and from information in Free and Alexander (1976).

Foam

1. Foam can be purchased over-the-counter at most pharmacies and some supermarkets and general stores.
2. Shake the can of foam 20 times before using. This will ensure that there are a sufficient number of bubbles to act as a barrier.
3. Place the tip of the can into the applicator and fill the applicator with foam to where it is marked. Read the instructions provided by the manufacturer to see whether the applicator fills with pressure applied to the container tip or the applicator needs to be tilted.
4. Spread the lips of the vagina with one hand and insert the applicator into the vagina with the other as far as possible (Fig. 6–7); pull back one-half inch or so.
5. Push the plunger into the applicator and, without pulling back on it, remove the applicator from the vagina. Read the instructions that come with the particular brand of foam used, as some recommend two applicatorsful for contraceptive effectiveness. Generally, if the applicator holds at least 10 mL, one applicatorful is enough.
6. Insert foam no more than 30 minutes before intercourse because barrier effectiveness lessens after that time.
7. Use an additional applicatorful of foam with each act of intercourse.
8. As foam may have an unpleasant taste, you may want to insert it after oral sex.
9. If the foam is irritating to the vagina or external genitalia, or to your partner, try another brand.
10. To reduce messiness later, you can use a pad or tampon.

Condoms

1. Condoms can be purchased over-the-counter at pharmacies and some supermarkets and general stores.
2. The condom has to be placed on an erect penis by either the man or his partner. It must be placed before any penis-to-vagina contact.
3. Do not unroll the condom before placing it on the penis.
4. Place the condom on the tip of the penis and roll it down the length of the penis. If you are having difficulty rolling it down, try turning it inside out; you may have initially rolled it the wrong way.
5. Do not try to push the tip of the condom flush against the penis. You need a receptacle for semen that extends past the tip of the penis or the condom will break during ejaculation (Fig. 6–8). Many condoms have premade receptacle tips; if you purchase condoms without these tips; you must leave at least one-half inch of condom beyond the penis. Squeeze this area to let out the air.
6. After ejaculation, the penis should be removed from the vagina before it becomes soft. Prior to withdrawal of the penis from the vagina, it is important to hold the condom and penis together to prevent the condom from falling off and being left in the vagina.
7. Never use the same condom twice.
8. Never use petroleum jelly on condoms or keep them in warm places (such as seat pockets or wallets) as the rubber may deteriorate. Condoms packaged in sealed foil packages have a shelf life of up to 5 years.
9. Remember there are many different types, colors, textures, and sizes of condoms. It is worthwhile to find the type that is the most comfortable and enjoyable. Prelubricated condoms may increase sensitivity and have less of a chance of tearing. To lubricate the outside of the condom, use a water-soluble jelly like K-Y, contraceptive foam, or saliva. Many couples find condoms with a premade reservoir tip easier to put on properly.

Follow-up. Although foam and condoms do not require practitioner supervision, practitioner input may be helpful in successful method use. Whether the patient wishes or needs a visit to review contraceptive use depends on how well she (and her partner) are doing with this method. This can be determined by a phone call in 2 weeks or by advising the patient of your availability to answer questions or discuss concerns.

THE CERVICAL CAP

Definition and Description

The cervical cap is a small cuplike object made of rubber, Lucite, or polyurethane that fits over the cervix and is held in place by suction. Three types of cap are made—the vault or Dumas cap, the Vimule cap, and the Prentif cavity rim cap (Fig. 6–9). The most popular and widely available cap in the United States is the cavity rim (Fig. 6–9), which is made of rubber and resembles a thimble. It comes in four sizes measured according to diameter—22, 25, 28, and 31 mm—with the cap's depth increasing as the diameter increases. The Dumas cap is useful for women who cannot use a diaphragm because of poor vaginal muscle tone and cannot use a cavity rim cap because of a short cervix; the Vimule cap may be useful for women whose cervices are too short, too long, too large, or too irregular to wear the cavity rim cap (Bernstein, Kilzer, Coulson, et al., 1982; King, 1981, p. 2).

Some form of cervical cap has been described since antiquity. In its modern form, it was widely used in Europe in the late nineteenth and early twentieth centuries and remains popular in some European countries today. The cap was never used extensively in the United States, although it has become increasingly popular in recent years, largely as a result of advocacy efforts by women's health organizations (Fairbanks & Scharfman, 1980). In 1981, the Food and Drug Administration (FDA) made contraceptive cervical caps investigational devices. In 1988, the FDA approved the Prentif cavity rim cap as a contraceptive device while continuing study of the Dumas cap. Two components of the FDA approval were disappointing to some cap advocates: the stipulation that women fit for the cap must return in 3 months for a repeat Pap smear and that all users must be advised to restrict continuous wear of the cap to 48 hours. The FDA also stipulated that the cap must be fit by trained professionals, beginning with the physicians, midwives, nurses, and other providers who were approved for cap fitting during the FDA study period (Brown, 1988). It is expected that with approval, more practitioners will seek training to fit the cap. Caps have been available from Lamberts, Ltd., a London-based company, and are now available through their U.S. distributor, Cervical Cap (C&C) Ltd., P.O. Box 38003-292, Los Gatos, California 95031, 408–358–6264. Information regarding training for cap fitting is also available from C&C.

Cervical caps are made in a limited number of sizes and do not fit all women well. A custom-fitted cap with a one-way valve providing for the escape of mucus and menstrual fluid is currently being investigated in the People's Republic of China ("Valved Cervical Cap," 1987, p. 17), although two clinical trials of this cap in the United States have been discontinued because of unacceptable rates of displacement and pregnancy. The custom cap, designed by a dentist and a gynecologist, is made after a plaster mold is formed from an impression of the cervix, similar to the way dental molds are made. Theoretical advantages of this cap are that it would reduce dislodgement, could be worn continuously without spermicide, and would eliminate odors that occur when cervical mucus stagnates in spaces formed between the cap and cervix (Medical News, 1983).

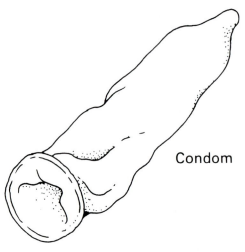

Condom

Figure 6–8. Unrolled condom with reservoir tip.

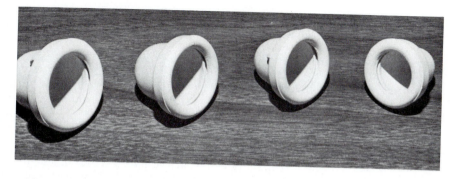

Figure 6–9. The Prentif cavity-rim cervical cap, in sizes. *(From Koch, J. [1982, February]. The Prentif contraceptive cervical cap: A contemporary study of its clinical safety and effectiveness, Contraception, 25[2], 137. Reprinted with permission.)*

Mechanism of Action

The cervical cap is a barrier method of contraception. Like the diaphragm, it prevents sperm from entering the cervical os. A small amount of spermicide is placed in the dome of the cap to aid its effectiveness, although studies have not been carried out to compare the cap's effectiveness with and without spermicide (King, 1981, p. 29).

Effectiveness

The effectiveness of the cervical cap varies widely in different studies although it can be said to approximate that of the diaphragm. Cap failure rates have been reported to be as low as 7.6 per 100 woman-years of use (Tietze, Lehfeldt, & Liebmann, 1953) and even lower when only consistent use is considered (Koch, 1982b). Overall failure rates have been reported as high as 16 to 17 (Johnson, 1984; King, 1981) and over 19 (Lehfeldt & Sivin, 1984) per 100 users. In one small study, failure rates were quite high, approaching 50 percent at the end of 2 years (Smith & Lee, 1984). The smallest-size Vimule cap was found to have the highest failure rate in this survey. Published studies are not consistent in the type of cap used or in the directions given for use, and this may contribute to the great divergence in reported effectiveness.

Dislodgement of the cap is thought to cause many cap failures. Therefore, cap fitters often encourage patients to use a condom as a backup method with the cap for a specified period after cap initiation and to check for proper cap placement after intercourse. Should the cap become dislodged during this test period, the woman must be refit or consider another method of birth control (Koch, 1982b, p. 140).

In one study, pregnancy rates were associated with increased wearing time after insertion (Powell, Mears, Deber, & Ferguson, 1986). This might be related to deterioration of the rubber; deterioration was noted after a year of cap use, particularly when the cap had been kept in for more than 3 days at a time.

Advantages/Benefits

There are many advantages to the cervical cap and most studies show high continuation rates. It provides effective contraception, separate from sexual intercourse. The cap has several advantages over the diaphragm. It can be fit even with lax vaginal muscle tone. It need not be refit after weight change. Less spermicide is used; additional spermicide need not be used with each act of intercourse. The cap is therefore less messy and less costly. Many women find the cap more convenient to use than the diaphragm because it can be left in place for a longer period, although the optimal time for both contraceptive efficacy and safety has not been determined. The cap is also less likely to cause pressure on the bladder and to be associated with urinary tract infections. There is some speculation that cervical caps may have a beneficial effect on cervical erosion (Koch, 1982b, p. 149).

Disadvantages and Risks

As with all barrier methods, many cap disadvantages can be overcome if motivation exists to use the method. Risks are few.

Disadvantages

LACK OF AVAILABILITY. The cap is not widely available at this time. It is not manufactured in this country and must currently be imported from England.

LIMITED SIZES AND RIGID SHAPE. Not all women can be fit with the cap, especially if the circumference of the cervix is very irregular in shape or if it points upward or downward.

DIFFICULTY IN INSERTION OR REMOVAL. Some women cannot reach their cervix, making cap insertion or removal, or both, difficult. Alternative positions, such as squatting, may make the cervix more accessible. Removal can be facilitated in a variety of ways. Bearing down during removal may bring the cap closer to the vaginal introitus. A diaphragm introducer can be used by hooking its end between the rim of the cap and the cervix so that the cap can be pulled off the cervix and into the vagina where it can be more easily removed. A string of unwaxed dental floss can be attached to the cap. The floss can be threaded through a needle and sewn into the extra piece of rubber found just beneath the cap's rim. Pulling on the string may help with removal. If insertion or removal remains impossible for the woman, the partner can be taught to insert and/or remove the cap.

PARTNER DISCOMFORT. If the cap is felt by the partner and not dislodged after intercourse, the woman can attempt to place it higher onto the cervix. If this continues to be a problem for the couple, another type of cap may work better, such as a Dumas cap. If the cap is felt secondary to dislodgement, a different size or type of cap should be tried. When the problem persists, another form of contraception should be considered.

ODOR. Odor is a frequently reported side effect with cap use that increases with duration of continuous use (Koch, 1982a). This problem can usually be resolved by soaking the cap for 15 to 30 minutes in water mixed with apple cider vinegar, lemon juice, baking soda, rubbing alcohol, bleach, or hydrogen peroxide, or putting a drop of chlorophyll into the dome before insertion (Chalker, 1987). Prolonged soaking should be avoided, however, as it may cause the cap to expand.

NEED FOR ALTERNATIVE METHOD DURING MENSES. The cap cannot be used during menstruation. Any other appropriate barrier method can be used during this time. This may present a problem for women or couples with objections to the other barrier contraceptives.

Risks

VAGINAL COMPLAINTS. Cap users have complained of vaginal or urinary discomfort, vaginal discharge, and itching (Koch, 1982a). The Vimule cap has been found to cause vaginal lacerations and has been removed from the FDA study. This side effect is seen most frequently among wearers of large-size Vimule caps and has been attributed to the flared, sharp edge of the cap and the rigidity and heaviness of the rim in the larger-sized caps (Bernstein et al., 1982).

CERVICAL CHANGES. Whether or not the cap causes adverse cervical changes is uncertain. In one study, cervical caps were not shown to be associated with adverse cervical changes; however, women were followed only for approximately 9 months (Koch, 1982b). In a study sponsored by the National Institutes of Health (NIH), cervical cap users were found to have Pap smear changes from class I to class III, described as inflammatory changes similar to those seen with papilloma virus infection. It is unknown whether these findings can be attributed to cap use ("Cervical Caps, Diaphragm," 1986, p. 32). This accounts for the FDA stipulation that the Pap smear be repeated 3 months after fitting; these changes are thought not to persist.

TOXIC-SHOCK SYNDROME. Although toxic-shock syndrome has not been reported with cap use, it is a theoretical possibility. The incidence of this disease is too low for an association to be seen considering the number of current cap users in this country. Some women choose to remove the cap 8 hours after intercourse to reduce the possibility of contracting toxic-shock syndrome.

Contraindications

The following conditions (adapted from King, 1981) preclude cap fitting: inability to be fit; allergy to rubber or all available spermicides; inability to insert and/or remove the cap if the partner is also unable to do this; cervical lacerations; malformations of the cervix; known or suspected gonorrhea or chlamydia; abnormal Pap smears; and cervical polyps, cysts, or warts.

A history of toxic-shock syndrome should be a signal for caution. Nabothian cysts are not necessarily contraindications unless they are large and positioned so that they interfere with cap suction. The cap should not be used during the 6-week postpartum period. Fitting in lactating women or women using oral contraceptives is problematic since the hormones affecting the cervix are altered in these women. Some practitioners advise women to discontinue oral contraceptives and wait until they have one or two

menstrual periods before cap fitting. If the cap is fit during lactation, the woman should use a backup method whenever the pattern of nursing changes to determine whether her fit has been affected.

Management of the Visits

Initial Visit. Before scheduling a woman for a cap fitting, it is advisable to explain the effectiveness of the cap, its advantages, and its disadvantages. The initial visit should be scheduled during ovulation so that the cap can be fit at the time it is most needed, because it sometimes fits differently at various stages in the menstrual cycle. This occurs secondary to cyclic cervical engorgement, dilation, and position changes.

A set of fitting caps can be ordered from C&C. They should be washed and soaked for about 20 minutes after each use. A 70 percent alcohol solution or 10 percent bleach solution can be used for sterilization.

METHOD INITIATION. After contraindications to cap use have been ruled out by history and speculum and bimanual examinations, and the woman has viewed her cervix, the cap can be fit. Visual aids, such as a plastic pelvic model and charts, are helpful for teaching prior to patient practice. Proper cap insertion can be demonstrated on the model and charts used to illustrate techniques and positions for method insertion. Explanations should be offered the woman during all steps of the following procedure:

First, perform a bimanual examination, noting the shape, length, and position of the cervix, and any irregularities in the shape of its circumference. Estimate the appropriate cervical cap size. Instruct and guide the woman to locate her cervix with one or two fingers. To do this, she may assume a squatting position, or lie with her legs bent up against her abdomen, or place one leg on a stool.

Squeeze the cap at the rim and insert it, dome outward, into the vagina. Place it on the cervix. Correct cervical cap fit, illustrated in Figure 6–10 is somewhat subjective. The fit can be considered good if the following criteria are met:

1. The cap covers the entire cervix; no portion of the cervix should be felt.
2. There is no space between the rim of the cap and the cervix. The entire circumference of the cap should be checked for this.
3. The suction is adequate and equal on all sides. Suction is checked by placing one finger on the rim and gently pulling the cap away from the cervix or by indenting the dome. The cap should not be pulled off easily; the indentation should remain at least 30 seconds (Koch, 1982b, pp. 138–139).
4. The dome of the cap is midline and faces the vaginal introitus. Thrusts of the penis thus will not hit the cap at an angle that might dislodge it (King, 1981, p. 43).

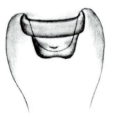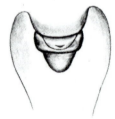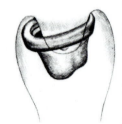

Figure 6–10. Correct and incorrect cervical cap placement. (From Chalker, R. [1987]. *The complete cervical cap guide.* New York: Harper & Row, p. 45. Copyright © 1987 by Rebecca Chalker. Illustrations copyright © by Suzann Gage. Reprinted with permission.)

Good fit   Too small   Too big

5. The cap is not close to the introitus, which would increase the likelihood of dislodgement or discomfort to either partner (Koch, 1982b, p. 139).

Whether or not the cap can be rotated on the cervix is not a significant criterion of fit. If it does rotate, check to ascertain that it does not tilt away from the cervix (Chalker, 1987).

Because of the subjective nature of cap fitting, it is advisable to confirm the fit by trying a cap one size larger and one size smaller than the cap chosen (King, 1981, p. 42). Sometimes it is necessary to go back and forth between sizes for better comparison. In some women, two sizes of cap fit equally well; the smallest size possible is advisable [Lamberts (Dalston) Limited, 1988].

After a good fit is verified, the woman should feel the cap in place. She should then be instructed on how to insert the cap, check its fit, and remove it. The cap is removed by inserting one or two fingers between the rim and the cervix and pulling the cap down and out of the vagina. Removal is easier if the woman can reach the posterior rim of the cap because the ball of her fingers face the cervix posteriorly. Many women cannot reach that far back, however, and can only remove the cap via the anterior rim. This is somewhat more awkward because the front of the fingers are facing the cervix.

The woman should insert and remove the cap as many times as she needs to feel comfortable with the technique. Whenever necessary, she should be afforded privacy to practice. If she is having difficulty, however, observation might reveal the problem. After the woman has inserted and removed the cap, the fitter should test her recognition of displacement by inserting the cap several times correctly and incorrectly without revealing where it will be placed. The woman should feel for the cap each time and report whether it is on the cervix or not (Koch, 1982b, p. 139).

If a woman continues to have difficulty with insertion or removal of the cap after several attempts, her frustration level may make further learning impossible. It may help for her to return for a second fitting session. If she is more relaxed and comfortable at that time, and in the interim has practiced feeling her cervix, she may be more successful. Alternatively, the partner can be taught insertion and/or removal.

TEACHING GUIDELINES. Patient instructions for cap use vary greatly. In a literature review, Leitch (1986) found, for example, that the recommended length of time for wearing the cap varied from 24 hours to 7 days, if it was specified. Table 6-2 summarizes the various instructions given. The FDA approval for cap use specifies a 48-hour maximum wearing time although many practitioners fitting the cap during the study period had been advising 72 hours (Brown, 1988).

The following are our recommendations on cap use, adapted from the literature and experience.

1. Before using the cap for contraception, practice insertion and removal. Wear the cap at least 8 hours and check the fit and your comfort after it has been on the cervix this length of time.
2. It is advisable to insert the cap at least one-half hour before intercourse. This helps increase the suction. Check to make sure the cervix is covered. You will know this because you will not be able to feel the cervix if the cap is correctly placed.
3. Prior to insertion, place spermicidal cream or jelly into one third of the cap's dome. Cream or jelly can be purchased over-the-counter at most pharmacies and some supermarkets and general stores; use the same spermicide that can be used with a diaphragm.
4. Use a condom along with the cap during the first month of its use, or, if you have intercourse fewer

TABLE 6-2. USE INSTRUCTIONS FOR THE CERVICAL CAP

Practitioner, Date	Wearing Time	Removal, Hours after Intercourse	Effectiveness
Boehm, 1983	Unspecified, insert > 1/2 hour before intercourse	8 hours	19.6/100 woman-years (100 wy) n = 47 (x̄ = 8.4 mos. use)
Denniston, 1981	5 days	unspecified	8.0/100w/6 mos. n = 110
Emma Goldman Clinic, 1983	2–3 days, insert >1/2 hour before intercourse	unspecified	15.6/100wy total 5.3/100wy method n = 429
Johnson, 1984	3 days	8 hours	16.9/100wy total 6.5/100wy method n = 56
Koch, 1982 (original instructions)	Up to 7 days (test for continued presence of spermicide on first use)	12 hours	8.4/100wy total 3/7/100wy method n = 371
Koch, 1983 (revised instructions)	5 days (same testing)	12 hours	~6% n ≅ 3000
Lehfeldt, 1984	7 days	8 hours	15.6–22/100wy 14/19 user, n = 130
Manufacturer's Instructions	24 hours	several hours	
Porterfield (Zodhiates)	7 days		30/100wy n = 60 (x = 4.8 mos.)
Smith, 1984	7 days	12 hours	6/15 cavity run 10/18 Vimule

From Leitch, W. S. (1986, October). Longevity of Gynol II and Ortho Creme in the Prentif cervical cap. Contraception, 34 (4), 365.

than eight times that month, then for at least eight acts of intercourse. During this "testing" period, check the cap after each intercourse and try to use different positions for intercourse. If the cap becomes dislodged more than once, you may need a different size or this may not be a good method for you. You may notice that the cap becomes dislodged only in a particular position of intercourse. You must then decide whether or not you want to continue using it.

5. With a new partner or in new positions, check the placement of the cap on the cervix. It is advisable to repeat the trial period explained in recommendation 4 with each new partner.
6. Wear the cap at least 8 hours after intercourse. If you have repeated intercourse, keep it on the cervix at least 8 hours after the last act. Do not leave it in longer than 2 days.
7. Wash the cap with mild soap and water. It should be inverted to make sure that neither cream or jelly nor cervical secretions build up in the inner fold. Dry the cap well with a towel or by exposure to air. You may powder it with corn starch before storing it. Do not use talc or perfumed powders.
8. Check for tears or holes in the cap by holding it up to the light or filling it with water to check for leaks. Do not use it if there are any holes.
9. Protect the cap from extreme heat, oils or petroleum jelly, as these may hasten the rubber's deterioration.
10. If you have had a vaginal infection, sterilize the cap by submerging it in rubbing alcohol for 20 minutes. This may help prevent reinfection.
11. If an unpleasant odor develops on the cap, you can either soak it in a solution of one teaspoon of apple cider vinegar to one quart of water, or put a drop of chlorophyll in the cap's dome prior to insertion. Chlorophyll can be purchased in most health food stores. Too frequent soaking, however, may cause the rubber to deteriorate.
12. Always bring the cap to an annual gynecologic examination so that the size can be rechecked.
13. Use a different method of birth control during your menstrual period if you have intercourse at that time.
14. The cap should be checked for fit after pregnancy (miscarriage, abortion, or full-term pregnancy). It should not be worn in the first 6 weeks after delivery. If at any time a cap that has been working properly becomes dislodged, it may be caused by deterioration of the rubber. The cap should be replaced and tested again with a backup method.
15. If at any time you or your partner experience burning or irritation, discontinue cap use and contact your health care provider. Do not, however, have unprotected intercourse if you do not wish to become pregnant.

Follow-up. Each woman should have the option of having the cap's fit and placement checked after 2 weeks to 1 month of use. The FDA currently mandates a 3-month follow-up Pap smear after cap initiation (Brown, 1988). After that, the woman should be seen within 1 year for visualization of the cervix, a Pap smear, and a complete gynecologic examination. Some practitioners and the FDA advise yearly replacement of all cervical caps (Powell et al., 1986). Certainly, dislodgement of the cap after a year or more of use may be a result of deterioration. A new cap should be purchased and put through a testing period with

a backup method. The practitioner must always be available to address patient concerns and problems.

If a woman cannot use the cap, she may need a lot of counseling to accept this. Because of the difficulty in obtaining a cap, she may have waited a long time to get one. Many women seeking this method see it as a last resort. Its failure can be viewed as devastating.

Ordering Caps

Caps can be ordered from C&C, Ltd. in any quantity. If it is expected that most patients will be nulliparas, it is advisable to order mostly sizes 22 and 25. If a practice or clinic serves mostly multiparas, then more size 28s are needed. Size 31 should be ordered in small quantities since it is used least often.

THE VAGINAL SPONGE

Definition and Description

The vaginal sponge (Fig. 6–11), known commercially as "Today," is a pliable round device, approximately 6 cm in diameter and 1.5 cm thick (Lemberg, 1984, p. 24). A loop to facilitate removal is attached. Made of polyurethane, the sponge contains 1 g of the spermicide nonoxynol-9 and small amounts of preservatives that maintain its pH at about 4 to 5 (Edelman et al., 1984, p. 70). The sponge is considered effective for 24 hours after insertion. It is available over-the-counter and costs about $1.00.

Mechanism of Action

The vaginal sponge works as a combination barrier and spermicidal contraceptive. It releases spermicide during intercourse while it absorbs semen and blocks the cervix.

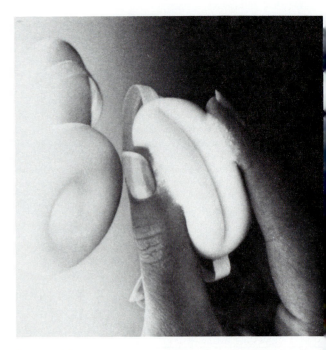

Figure 6–11. The vaginal sponge. *(Courtesy of the VLS Corporation.)*

Effectiveness

Original studies of the vaginal sponge showed it to be about 85 percent effective, although some studies have shown a failure rate as high as 27 percent. Its theoretic failure rate has been determined to be 9 to 11 per 100 women (Lemberg, 1984, p. 29). Effectiveness rates are lowest in the first 3 months of use, and a condom is useful as a backup during this time (Lemberg, 1984, p. 32). Further research is needed on the question of whether there are significantly higher failure rates among parous women; this finding was reported in a 1980 study comparing the sponge with the diaphragm, but was disputed by the sponge's manufacturer on the basis of criticisms of that study ("The Sponge," 1986, p. 81). Vaginal sponges can be used in conjunction with condoms, greatly enhancing effectiveness.

Advantages/Benefits

The sponge is easy to learn to use and convenient. It can be obtained without a prescription. It can be inserted well before intercourse; no additional user input is required at the time of intercourse. Preliminary findings of a study examining the sponge's effect on the transmission of STDs found a protective effect in vitro greater than the effect of an equivalent concentration of spermicide alone. Clinical studies have shown the relative risks for developing gonorrhea in sponge users and users of nonvaginal contraceptives to be 0.9 and 0.31; the risks for developing chlamydia have been reported to be 0.6 and 0.67 ("The Sponge," 1986; Rosenberg, Rojanapithayakorn, Feldblum, & Higgins, 1987). A firm assessment of the sponge's value in protecting against STDs is yet to be made ("The Sponge," 1986, p. 80).

Disadvantages and Risks

A number of disadvantages and risks are associated with sponge use, many of which can be overcome if there is commitment to using the method.

Disadvantages

PERCEIVED MESSINESS. Some women find vaginal sponges to be quite messy. The use of an absorbent sanitary pad may help with this problem.

ODOR/TASTE. Couples have complained of an odor and unpleasant taste with sponge use. The sponge can be inserted after oral sex if this proves to be a major problem, but this would negate the advantage it offers of being unrelated to intercourse. Spontaneity would be particularly interrupted because insertion requires the addition of water to the sponge.

DISCOMFORT. Discomfort with sponge use has been reported by both women and partners. Discomfort for women includes vaginal burning, stinging, soreness, dryness, itching, and a heat sensation. Male discomfort is related to feeling an obstruction (Edelman et al., 1984).

Risks

ALLERGIC REACTIONS. Allergic reactions to the sponge, in either a woman or her partner, may occur in response to the polyurethane or the spermicide.

VAGINAL IRRITATION/INFECTION. The sponge has been reported to cause vaginal irritation, especially in a woman with an infection (Lemberg, 1984 p. 30). In one clinical study, women using the sponge were found to have a rate of candidiasis vaginitis two and one-half times that of women using nonvaginal contraceptives (Rosenberg et al., 1987).

DISLODGEMENT. The sponge can be dislodged or expelled from the vagina. This may be especially true for women with uterine prolapse or poor pelvic muscle tone (Lemberg, 1984, p. 32). The risk associated with dislodgement or expulsion is, of course, pregnancy.

DIFFICULT REMOVAL/TOXIC-SHOCK SYNDROME. Difficult removal has been reported frequently with sponge use and may require practitioner assistance (North & Vorhauer, 1985). The sponge can fragment as it is being removed from the vagina. A number of sponge-related cases of toxic-shock syndrome have been documented. The estimated relative risk of developing this disease with sponge use compared with nonuse ranges from 7.8 to 40 (Faich, Pearson, Fleming, et al., 1986). This risk is highest with use during menstruation or the postpartum period; with difficult removal, particularly fragmentation; and with wearing time exceeding 30 hours.

QUESTION OF CARCINOGENICITY. When the sponge was originally marketed, there was concern among consumer groups and in the House of Representatives that both polyurethane and the spermicide nonoxynol-9 contained carcinogens: 2,4-TDA in the polyurethane as a by-product of its manufacturing process and dioxane and ethylene oxide in the spermicide (Lemberg, 1984, p. 30). The FDA addressed these issues and found that the type of polymer used in manufacturing the polyurethane in the sponge was not associated with 2,4-TDA. Analyses also failed to find the other two agents in the sponge.

QUESTION OF BIRTH DEFECTS. The question of teratogenicity has been raised with sponge use as it has with other spermicidal contraceptives. Evidence for an association is weak. (See Question of Birth Defects, under The Diaphragm.)

Contraindications

Contraindications to sponge use are known allergy to polyurethane and/or nonoxynol-9; history of toxic-shock syndrome; and inability of the woman and her partner to insert or remove the sponge.

The sponge should be used advisedly during menstruation, if at all. It should not be used in the postpartum period. Women with poor vaginal muscle tone may not be able to use the method.

Management of the Visits

Initial Visit

METHOD INITIATION. Samples of the sponge should be available for teaching. The device should be shown to the woman and an explanation given of how it works and how it is placed in the vagina. Visual aids, such as a plastic pelvic model and charts, are helpful for teaching prior to patient practice. Proper sponge insertion can be demonstrated on the model and charts used to illustrate techniques and positions for method of insertion.

The woman should visualize her cervix during the speculum examination and be taught how to feel it. After any explanation of sponge use, she should insert it into the vagina. Its placement should be checked by both practitioner and patient. The woman should remove the sponge.

TEACHING GUIDELINES. The following instructions are compiled from the Today sponge packet insert, prepared by the VLI Corporation, and from North and Vorhauer (1985) and Connell and Tatum (1985a).

1. The contraceptive sponge can be purchased over-the-counter at most pharmacies, some supermarkets, and other general stores.
2. The sponge can be placed at any time and left in the vagina up to 30 hours, but not necessarily that long. It is effective for 24 hours after insertion.
3. After the last act of vaginal intercourse, wait at least 6 hours before removal.
4. Do not use the sponge during menstruation. Another method of birth control is advised at this time.
5. For the first 3 months, it is recommended that another method of birth control be used as a backup. Condoms are excellent for this purpose and can be used with the sponge. This will enable you to become familiar with proper sponge usage. Most "sponge pregnancies" have occurred during the first 3 months of its use. Some couples continue to use condoms with the sponge at all times or during their most fertile periods (usually midcycle).
6. If redness, irritation, or discomfort is noted by either partner, discontinue sponge use, as this indicates a reaction to the sponge or spermicide.
7. Prior to placement of the sponge in the vagina, pour approximately two tablespoons of water into the dome of the sponge. This activates the spermicide and causes a sudsy appearance. Shake off the excess water, but do not remove the foam.
8. Fold the sponge and place it into the vagina. The loop of the sponge should be facing downward. To help insertion, separate the lips of the vagina with the fingers of the hand not holding the sponge. A sitting or squatting position may make insertion easier.
9. Slide the sponge deep into the vagina, making sure the loop is facing downward.
10. To check placement, insert one or two fingers into the vagina. The sponge should be high in the vagina. If it is not, gently push the sponge upward, closer to the cervix.
11. To remove the sponge, place one or two fingers into the vagina to find the loop. Hook your fingers around the loop and pull the sponge out gently.
12. Do not reuse the sponge.
13. A 24-hour toll-free telephone "talkline" has been established by VLI Corporation, makers of the Today sponge, for problems that seem to be related to sponge use: 800-223-2329.
14. If at any time during sponge use you develop a high fever with vomiting or diarrhea, call your practitioner immediately or go to the nearest emergency room. These are the early symptoms of toxic-shock syndrome, a rare disease that is on occasion associated with the sponge.

Follow-up. Return visits are indicated when there is difficulty using the vaginal sponge or if it appears that an allergic or inflammatory response has occurred. Practitioners should always be available to address the concerns of sponge users.

VAGINAL SUPPOSITORIES

Definition and Description

Vaginal suppositories consist of nonoxynol-9 spermicide in a semisolid suppository form. They are commercially marketed as Encare or the Encare Oval, Ortho-forms, Semicid, S'Positive, and Intercept (Tatum & Connell-Tatum, 1981, p. 8). Neo Sampoon is a foaming vaginal tablet manufactured in Japan and used internationally, but not yet approved for use in the United States. It contains the spermicide *menfegol*, which was approved by the FDA in 1980. Clinical trials of Neo Sampoon are underway (Borko, McIntyre, & Feldblum, 1985).

Mechanism of Action

When placed high in the vagina, a suppository reacts with the warmth and moisture of the vagina and produces an effervescence that occludes the cervical os and provides a barrier to sperm. In addition, suppositories have spermicidal properties.

Effectiveness

A wide range of effectiveness has been reported for vaginal suppositories—from about 60 to greater than 95 percent, depending on how they are used and how efficacy has been studied (Brehm & Hasse, 1975; Jackman, Berger, & Keith, 1981; Salomon & Hasse, 1977; Squire, Berger, & Keith, 1979). Data on effectiveness, however, are not extensive and studies suffer from methodologic weaknesses (Edelman, 1980, p. 341).

Advantages and Benefits

Suppositories can be obtained without a prescription. They are easy to use and can be combined with a condom to enhance their efficacy. They are small, relatively easy to insert into the vagina, and do not have to be removed.

Disadvantages and Risks

Vaginal suppositories have few disadvantages and risks, many of which can be overcome by motivated women and couples.

Disadvantages

PERCEIVED MESSINESS/INTERFERENCE WITH INTERCOURSE. Vaginal suppositories are considered by some women and couples to be messy or to interfere with intercourse, as the suppository must be placed within 1 hour of intercourse and an additional suppository is recommended if intercourse is repeated. After insertion, 10 to 15 minutes must elapse before intercourse.

TASTE. An unpleasant taste has been reported with suppository use. Suppositories can be inserted after oral sex, but couples must then remember to wait 10 to 15 minutes before vaginal intercourse.

SOFTENING OF SUPPOSITORIES. Heat causes suppositories to become soft in their package. This problem can be resolved by placing a wrapped suppository under cold water for a few minutes.

Risks. An allergic response to a suppository can occur in a woman or a man.

Contraindications

An allergy to nonoxynol-9 is a contraindication to suppository use. Otherwise, they can be used by most women.

Management of the Visits

Initial Visit

METHOD INITIATION. During pelvic examination, the woman should view her cervix and palpate it. If a pelvic model or illustration is available, it should be used to show her how the suppository is placed in the vagina. The woman should unwrap the suppository and its use should be reviewed.

TEACHING GUIDELINES. The following suggested instructions are adapted from Hatcher and associates (1984).

1. Vaginal suppositories can be purchased over-the-counter at pharmacies and many supermarkets and general stores.
2. Prior to intercourse, insert the unwrapped suppository as far into the vagina as it will go and wait 10 to 15 minutes or as long as the package instructions recommend. This is the time needed for effervescence to take place.
3. Intercourse should take place no more than 1 hour after insertion.
4. An additional suppository is required with each act of intercourse.
5. Do not douche for at least 6 hours after the last act of intercourse.
6. If redness, irritation, or other symptoms of discomfort are experienced by either partner, discontinue suppository use.
7. If, prior to insertion, the suppository is soft in its wrapper, place the wrapped suppository under cold water for a few minutes. This should harden the suppository.

Follow-up. The practitioner should be available by phone to answer questions. A woman should be seen if she is unhappy with the method or if an allergic response occurs as a new method of contraception needs to be considered and initiated.

CONTRACEPTIVE FILM

Contraceptive film is a relatively new method of birth control. It is made in England and has been marketed recently in the United States ("New Products Update," 1986, p. 25). The film is a 2-in., water-soluble, paper-thin product that contains nonoxynol-9, polyvinyl, alcohol, and glycerine. Its effectiveness has been reported as high as 93 percent and as low as 62 percent (Frankman, Raabe, & Ingemansson, 1975).

Contraceptive film is inserted no less than 5 minutes before intercourse and remains effective 2 hours after it has dissolved. A new film needs to be inserted with each act of intercourse. Its advantages over the suppository are that it takes less time to become effective after insertion and remains active twice as long. Its disadvantages are similar to those for the suppository and it is contraindicated in the presence of an allergy to the spermicide. Teaching guidelines for use of contraceptive film are similar to those for vaginal suppositories and can be adapted with changes reflecting the differences described.

REFERENCES

Asculai, S. S., Weis, M. T., Rancourt, M. W., & Kupferberg, A. B. (1978, April). Inactivation of herpes simplex viruses by nonionic surfactants. *Antimicrobial Agents and Chemotherapy, 13*(4), 686–690.

Baehler, E. A., Dillon, W. P., Cumbo, T. J., & Lee, R. V. (1982, August). Prolonged use of a diaphragm and toxic shock syndrome. *Fertility and Sterility, 38*(2), 248–250.

Baldwin, K. A., & Goodwin, K. (1985, November/December). The Papanicolaou smear. *Journal of Nurse-Midwifery, 30*(6), 327–332.

Bernstein, G. S. (1971, January). Clinical effectiveness of an aerosol contraceptive foam. *Contraception, 3*(1), 37–43.

Bernstein, G. S. (1974, March). Conventional methods of contraception: Condom, diaphragm, and vaginal foam. *Clinical Obstetrics and Gynecology, 17*(1), 21–33.

Bernstein, G. S., Kilzer, L. H., & Coulson, A. H., et al. (1982, November). Studies of cervical caps. I. Vaginal lesions associated with use of the Vimule cap. *Contraception, 26*(5), 443–456.

Boston Women's Health Collective. (1984). *The new our bodies ourselves.* New York: Simon & Schuster.

Borko, E., McIntyre, S. L., & Feldblum, P. J. (1985, April). A comparative clinical trial of the contraceptive sponge and Neo Sampoon tablets. *Obstetrics and Gynecology, 65*(4), 511–515.

Bracken, M. B. (1985, March). Spermicidal contraceptives and poor reproductive outcomes: The epidemiologic evidence against an association. *American Journal of Obstetrics and Gynecology, 151*(5), 552–556.

Brehm, H., & Hasse, W. (1975, September 5). The alternative to hormonal contraception? Importance and reliability of foam ovoid for vaginal contraception. *Medizinische Welt, 26*(36), 1610–1617.

Brown, L. (1988, May/June). The cervical cap—Here at last! *The Network News, 13*(3), 1,3.

"Can you rely on condoms"? (1989, March). *Consumer Reports,* 135–141.

Cervical caps, diaphragm provide equal protection from pregnancy. (1986, March). *Contraceptive Technology Update, 7*(3), 32.

Chalker, R. (1987). *The complete cervical cap guide.* New York: Harper & Row.

Conant, M., Hardy, D., & Sernatinger, J., et al. (1986, April 4). Condoms prevent transmission of AIDS-associated retrovirus. *Journal of the American Medical Association, 255*(13), 1706.

Conant, M. A., Spicer, D. W., & Smith, C. D. (1984, April–June). Herpes simplex virus transmission: Condom studies. *Sexually Transmitted Diseases, 11*(2), 94–95.

Connell, E. B., & Tatum, H. J. (1985a). *Barrier methods of contraception.* Durant, OK: Creative Infomatics, Inc.

Connell, E. B., & Tatum, H. J. (1985b). *Reproductive health care manual.* Durant, OK: Creative Infomatics, Inc.

Craig, S., & Hepburn, S. (1982, October). The effectiveness of barrier methods of contraception with and without spermicide. *Contraception, 26*(4), 347–359.

De Gruttola, V., Moore, K., & Bennett, W. (1986, March/April). AIDS: Has the problem been adequately assessed? *Reviews of Infectious Diseases, 8*(2), 298–305.

Edelman, D. A. (1980). Nonprescription vaginal contraception. *International Journal of Gynaecology and Obstetrics, 18*(5), 340–344.

Edelman, D. A., McIntyre, S. L., & Harper, J. (1984, December 1). A comparative trial of the Today contraceptive sponge and diaphragm. *American Journal of Obstetrics and Gynecology, 150*(7), 869–876.

Faich, G., Pearson, K., & Fleming, D., et al. (1986, January 10). Toxic shock syndrome and the vaginal contraceptive sponge. *Journal of the American Medical Association, 255*(2), 216–218.

Fairbanks, B., & Scharfman, B. (1980, Fall). The cervical cap: Past and current experience. *Women and Health, 5*(3), 61–80.

Fihn, S. D., Latham, R. H., Roberts, P., et al. (1985a, July 12). Association between diaphragm use and urinary tract infection. *Journal of the American Medical Association, 254*(2), 240–245.

Fihn, S. D., Running, K., & Pinkstaff, C., et al. (1985b). Diaphragms cause urinary obstruction in women with prior urinary tract infection. *Clinical Research, 33*(2), 720A.

Fiscella, K. (1982, July/August). Relationship of weight change to required size of vaginal diaphragm. *Nurse Practitioner, 7*(7), 21–22.

Frankman, O., Raabe, N., & Ingemansson, C. A. (1975). Clinical evaluation of C-Film, a vaginal contraceptive. *The Journal of International Medical Research, 3*(4), 292–296.

Free, M. J., & Alexander, N. J. (1976, September/October). Male contraception without prescription. *Public Health Reports, 91*(5), 437–445.

Gillespie, L. (1984, July). The diaphragm: An accomplice in recurrent urinary tract infections. *Urology, 24*(1), 25–30.

Hatcher, R. A., Guest, F., & Stewart, F., et al. (1984). *Contraceptive technology 1984-1985* (12th rev. ed.). New York: Irvington.

Hatcher, R. A., Guest, F., & Stewart, F., et al. (1986). *Contraceptive technology 1986-1987* (13th rev. ed.). New York: Irvington.

Hatcher, R. A., Stewart, G. K., & Stewart, F., et al. (1980). *Contraceptive technology 1980-1981* (10th rev. ed.). New York: Irvington.

Hicks, D. R., Martin, L. S., & Getchell, J. P., et al. (1985, December 21/28). Inactivation of HTLV-III/LAV infected cultures of normal human lymphocytes by nonoxynol-9 in vitro. *Lancet, 2*(8469/70), 1422.

Huggins, G., Vessey, M., Flavel, R., et al. (1982, March). Vaginal spermicides and outcome of pregnancy: Findings in a large cohort study. *Contraception, 25*(3), 219–229.

Jackman, M., Berger, G. S., & Keith, L. G. (1981). *Vaginal contraception.* Boston: G. K. Hall.

Jaffe, R. (1981, December 24). Toxic-shock syndrome associated with diaphragm use. *The New England Journal of Medicine, 305*(26), 1585–1586.

Jick, H., Hannan, M. T., & Stergachis, A., et al. (1982a, October 1). Vaginal spermicides and gonorrhea. *Journal of the American Medical Association, 248*(13) 1619–1621.

Jick, H., Shiota, K., Shephard, T. H., et al. (1982b). Vaginal spermicides and miscarriage seen primarily in the emergency room. *Teratogenesis, Carcinogenesis, and Mutagenesis, 2*(2), 105–210.

Jick, H., Waler, A. M., & Rothman, K. J., et al. (1981, April 3). Vaginal spermicides and congenital disorders. *Journal of the American Medical Association, 245*(13), 1329–1332.

Johnson, J. M. (1984, March 1). The cervical cap: A retrospective study of an alternative contraceptive technique. *American Journal of Obstetrics and Gynecology, 148*(5), 604–608.

King, L. (1981). *The cervical cap handbook.* Iowa City, Iowa: Emma Goldman Clinic for Women.

Koch, J. P. (1982a, February). The Prentif contraceptive cervical cap: Acceptability aspects and their implications for future cap design. *Contraception, 25*(2), 161–173.

Koch, J. P. (1982b, February). The Prentif contraceptive cervical cap: A contemporary study of its clinical safety and effectiveness. *Contraception, 25*(2), 135–159.

Kugel, C., & Verson, H. (1986, March/April). Relationship between weight change and diaphragm size change. *Journal of Obstetric, Gynecologic, and Neonatal Nursing, 15*(2), 123–129.

Lamberts (Dalston) Limited. (1988). *The Prentif® cavity-rim cervical cap for contraceptive use: Fitting instructions,* [Brochure]. London: Lamberts (Dalston) Limited.

Lane, M. E., Arceo, R., & Sobrero, A. J. (1976, March/April). Successful use of the diaphragm and jelly by a young population: Report of a clinical study. *Family Planning Perspectives, 8*(2), 81–86.

Lee, R. V., Dillon, W. P., & Baehler, E. (1982, January 23). Barrier contraceptives and toxic shock syndrome [Letter]. *Lancet, 1*(8265), 221–222.

Lehfeldt, H., & Sivin, I. (1984, October). The effectiveness of the Prentif cervical cap in private practice: a prospective study. *Contraception, 30*(4), 331–338.

Leitch, W. S. (1984, October). Longevity of Gynol II (R) and Ortho Creme (R) in the Prentif cervical cap. *Contraception, 34*(4), 363–379.

Lemberg, E. (1984, October). The vaginal contraceptive sponge: A new non-prescription barrier contraceptive. *Nurse Practitioner, 9*(10), 24–33.

Liskin, L., & Blackburn, R. (1986, July/August). AIDS—A public health crisis. *Population Reports,* Ser. L, No. 6, *14*(3).

Litt, I. F. (1983). Toxic shock syndrome. *Journal of Adolescent Health Care, 4*(4), 270–274.

Loomis, L., & Feder, H. M., Jr. (1981, December 24). Toxic-shock syndrome associated with diaphragm use. *The New England Journal of Medicine, 305*(26), 1585.

Louik, C., Mitchell, A. A., & Werler, M. M., et al. (1987, August 20). Maternal exposure to spermicides in relation to certain birth defects. *The New England Journal of Medicine, 317*(8), 474–478.

Medical News. (1983, October). Custom cervical cap reentering clinical trials. *Journal of the American Medical Association, 250*(15), 1946–1948.

Melamed, M., Koss, L. G., & Flehinger, B. J., et al. (1969, July 26). Prevalence rates of uterine cervical carcinoma in situ for women using the diaphragm or contraceptive oral steroids. *British Medical Journal, 3,* 195–200.

Mills, J., Harley, E. E., Reed, G. F., & Berendes, H. W. (1982, November 5). Are spermicides teratogenic? *Journal of the American Medical Association, 248*(17), 2148–2151.

Mills, J. L., Reed, G. F., & Nugent, R. P., et al. (1985, March). Are there adverse effects of periconceptional spermicide use? *Fertility and Sterility, 43*(3), 442–446.

New products update. (1986, March). *Contraceptive Technology Update, 7*(3), 25.

North, B. B., & Vorhauer, B. W. (1985). Use of the Today® contraceptive sponge in the United States. *International Journal of Fertility, 30*(1), 81–84.

Oakley, G. (1982, May 7). Spermicides and birth defects. *Journal of the American Medical Association, 247*(17), 2405.

Okrent, S. (1974). *A clinical guide to the intrauterine device and the vaginal diaphragm.* Wantagh, NY: author.

Peddie, B., Gorrie, S. I., & Bailey, R. R. (1986, April 4). Diaphragm use and urinary tract infection. *Journal of the American Medical Association, 255*(13), 1707.

Percival-Smith, R., Bartlett, K. H., & Chow, A. W. (1983, May). Vaginal colonization of *Escherichia coli* and its relation to contraceptive methods. *Contraception, 27*(5), 497–504.

Postic, B., Singh, B., Squeglia, N. L., & Guevarra, L. O. (1978, January–March). Inactivation of clinical isolates of herpesvirus hominis, types 1 and 2, by chemical contraceptives. *Sexually Transmitted Diseases, 5,* 22–24.

Potts, M., & McDevitt, J. (1975, June). A use–effectiveness trial of spermicidally lubricated condoms. *Contraception, 11*(6), 701–710.

Powell, M. G., Mears, B. J., Deber, R. B., & Ferguson, D. (1986, March). Contraception with the cervical cap: Effectiveness, safety, continuity of use, and user satisfaction. *Contraception, 33*(3), 215–232.

Pyle, C. J. (1984, March). Nursing protocol for diaphragm contraception. *Nurse Practitioner, 9*(3), 35–40.

Richardson, A. C., & Lyon, J. B. (1981, August 15). The effect of condom use on squamous cell cervical intraepithelial neoplasia. *American Journal of Obstetrics and Gynecology, 140*(8), 909–913.

Rosenberg, M. J., Rojanapithayakorn, W., Feldblum, P. J., & Higgins, J. E. (1987, May 1). Effect of the contraceptive sponge on chlamydial infection, gonorrhea, and candidiasis. *Journal of the American Medical Association, 257*(17), 2308–2312.

Rothman, K. J. (1982, April). Spermicide use and Down's syndrome. *American Journal of Public Health, 72*(4), 399–401.

Salomon, W., & Hasse, W. (1977). Intravaginal contraception: Results of a prospective long-term study of foam ovoid. *Sexualmedizin, 6*(1), 198–202.

Shapiro, S., Slone, D., & Heinonen, O. P., et al. (1982, May 7). Birth defects and vaginal spermicides. *Journal of the American Medical Association, 247*(17), 2381–2384.

Sherris, J. D. (1982, September/October). Update on condoms—

Products, protection, promotion. *Population Reports,* Ser. H, No. 6, *10*(5).

Singer, A., Reid, B. L., & Coppleson, M. (1976, September 1). A hypothesis: The role of a high-risk male in the etiology of cervical carcinoma. *American Journal of Obstetrics and Gynecology, 126*(1), 110–115.

Singh, B., Cutler, J. C., & Utidjian, H. M. D. (1972, February). Studies on the development of a vaginal preparation providing both prophylaxis against venereal disease and other genital infections and contraception. II. Effect in vitro of vaginal contraceptive and non-contraceptive preparations on *Treponema pallidum* and *Neisseria gonorrhoeae. British Journal of Venereal Diseases, 48*(1), 57–64.

Singh, B., Postic, B., & Cutler, J. C. (1976, October 15). Virucidal effect of certain chemical contraceptives on type 2 herpesvirus. *American Journal of Obstetrics and Gynecology, 126*(4), 422–425.

Smith, G. G., & Lee, R. J. (1984). The use of cervical caps at the University of California, Berkeley: A survey. *Contraception, 30*(2), 115–123.

The sponge at three years: Research studies new, rehashes old questions. (1986, July). *Contraceptive Technology Update, 7*(7), 80–82.

Squire, J. J., Berger, G. S., & Keith, L. (1979, June). A retrospective clinical study of a vaginal contraceptive suppository. *Journal of Reproductive Medicine, 22*(6), 319–323.

Strobino, B., Kline, J., & Stein, Z., et al. (1980). Exposure to contraceptive creams, jellies and douches and their effect on the zygote. *American Journal of Epidemiology, 112*(3), 434.

Tatum, H. J., & Connell-Tatum, E. B. (1981, July). Barrier contraception: A comprehensive overview. *Fertility and Sterility, 36*(1), 1–12.

Tietze, C., Lehfeldt, H., & Liebmann, H. G. (1953, October). The effectiveness of the cervical cap as a contraceptive method. *American Journal of Obstetrics and Gynecology, 66*(4), 904–908.

Tietze, C., & Lewitt, S. (1967). Comparison of three contraceptive methods: Diaphragm with jelly or cream, vaginal foam, and jelly/cream alone. *Journal of Sex Research, 3*(4), 295–311.

Valved cervical cap is focus of Chinese multicenter efficacy trial. (1987, February). *Contraceptive Technology Update, 8*(2), 17–18.

Vessey, M., Doll, R., & Peto, R., et al. (1976, October). A long-term follow-up study of women using different methods of contraception—An interim report. *Journal of Biosocial Science, 8*(4), 373–427.

Vessey, M., & Wiggins, P. (1974, January). Use–effectiveness of the diaphragm in a selected family planning clinic population in the United Kingdom. *Contraception, 9*(1), 15–21.

Warburton, D., Neugut, R. H., & Lustenberger, A., et al. (1987, August 20). Lack of association between spermicide use and trisomy. *The New England Journal of Medicine, 317*(8), 478–482.

Wilson, C. (1983, December). Toxic shock syndrome and diaphragm use. *Journal of Adolescent Health Care, 4*(4), 290–291.

Women's Health Update. (1987, January). Rely on condoms to protect your sexual health. *Contraceptive Technology Update's Patient Education Supplement,* S1–S2.

Wortman, J. (1976, January). The diaphragm and other intravaginal barriers—A review. *Population Reports,* Ser. H, No. 4.

7

Oral Contraceptives

Heather Clarke

Oral contraceptives, commonly known as ''the pill,'' have been widely used for birth control in the United States since their approval in 1960. Their introduction dramatically changed the nature of family planning. Women had available, for the first time, a reversible method of birth control that approached 100 percent effectiveness without directly interfering with sexual intercourse. This was hailed as a virtual revolution in contraception.

At the same time, however, the widespread use of oral contraceptives (OCs) meant that large numbers of healthy people were subjecting themselves to the almost-daily ingestion of highly potent systemic medication. As epidemiologic studies revealed the association of life-threatening complications with OC use, criticism of the pill grew. Individual women questioned whether they wanted to expose themselves to the many risks involved with hormonal contraception. Although OCs are still estimated to be the second most widely used method of reversible birth control in the world, surpassed only by the intrauterine device (IUD) in popularity (Hatcher, Guest, & Stewart, et al., 1984, p. 14), their use has shown a decreasing trend since 1977, both internationally and in the United States. Ten million American women used OCs in 1977 compared with 8.4 million in 1980.

In the last several years, however, adverse publicity regarding pill use appears to have diminished somewhat. This is due to several factors. The dosages of the two hormones present in most oral contraceptives have been decreased, and several noncontraceptive benefits have been documented.

When the Food and Drug Administration (FDA) first approved OC use, each pill contained 50 to 150 μg of estrogen and 1 to 10 mg of one of several progestins. Today, most of the commonly used combination brands contain 30 to 35 μg of estrogen and 1 mg or less of progestin in each pill. As the dosages decreased, manufacturers of OCs were faced with the problem of how to combine the steroids most appropriately to maintain a high level of efficacy *and* decrease the incidence of side effects such as breakthrough bleeding (BTB), spotting, and amenorrhea. These common problems among pill users are related primarily to an imbalance of estrogen relative to the progestin dosages and potency. By observing the normal menstrual cycle, manufacturers were able to develop brands in which the dosage of the steroids are adjusted to mimic the cyclic pattern, thereby controlling the incidence of these menstrual irregularities.

Ortho Pharmaceuticals was the first in 1982 to market Ortho 10/11. This biphasic pill provides 35 μg of ethinyl estradiol throughout the cycle, with only 0.5 mg of norethindrone for the first 10 days, increasing to 1 mg for the following 11 days. The progestin effect is similar to that of the normal menstrual cycle. During the first half of the pill cycle, the ratio of estrogen to progestin is high, stimulating endometrial development. In the second half, the dosage of progestin is increased to provide additional support. Although the biphasic pill did prove effective, its popularity was quickly overshadowed by the triphasic pill. This latest development in oral contraceptives has succeeded even further in mimicking the normal menstrual cycle. The ratio of estrogen to progestin is altered in three, rather than two, phases. Currently, three brands of triphasic pills are on the market, each with a different formulation: Ortho Novum 7/7/7 (Ortho), TriNorinyl (Syntex), and Triphasil or Tri-Levlen (Wyeth or Berlex/Wyeth) (see Table 7–1 for their compositions). Their use has been associated with a decreased incidence of menstrual irregularities, while at the same time they expose women to approximately 25 percent less progestin than do the regular 35 to 50 μg combination pills (Pasquale, 1984).

Minipills, approved for use in 1973, contain no estrogen and very small amounts of progestin. They have proven to be safe and effective for women with certain risk factors contraindicating the use of combination pills.

Despite new advances, OCs continue to engender controversy. The decision to use OCs as a method of birth control is one that must be made by each individual woman in conjunction with her health care provider. It must be based on a careful risk–benefit assessment, taking into consideration her unique needs, beliefs, and life-style. To offer informed choice to women, practitioners must be familiar with the components of OCs, their mechanisms of action, potency, benefits, recommended usage, and, most important, their complications and side effects and the risk factors for the development of each of these.

This chapter discusses each of these areas. It provides a framework for the management of OC use. It addresses the initiation of OC use and the ongoing care for women using this method of contraception. Combination pills, the progestin-only minipill, and postcoital pill use are covered.

MECHANISM OF ACTION

Synthetic estrogens and progestins in oral contraceptives have a combined synergistic effect on the female reproduc-

TABLE 7–1. ORAL CONTRACEPTIVES AVAILABLE IN THE UNITED STATES[a]

Drug (Brand Name and Company)	Estrogen	MCG	Progestin	MG	Endometrial Activity[b]
Ovulen (Searle)	Mestranol	100	Ethynodiol diacetate	1.0	7.7
Enovid-E (Searle)	Mestranol	100	Norethynodrel	2.5	10.9
Ortho-Novum, 2 mg (Ortho)	Mestranol	100	Norethindrone	2.0	6.1
Norinyl, 2 mg (Syntex)	Mestranol	100	Norethindrone	2.0	6.1
Ortho-Novum 1/80 (Ortho)	Mestranol	80	Norethindrone	1.0	4.8
Norinyl 1 + 80 (Syntex)	Mestranol	80	Norethindrone	1.0	4.8
Enovid, 5 mg (Searle)	Mestranol	75	Norethynodrel	5.0	7.4
Demulen (Searle)	Ethinyl estradiol	50	Ethynodiol diacetate	1.0	13.9
Ovral (Wyeth)	Ethinyl estradiol	50	Norgestrel	0.5	4.5
Norlestrin 2.5/50 (Parke Davis)[c]	Ethinyl estradiol	50	Norethindrone acetate	2.5	5.1
Norlestrin 1/50 (Parke Davis)[c]	Ethinyl estradiol	50	Norethindrone acetate	1.0	13.6
Ovcon-50 (Mead Johnson)	Ethinyl estradiol	50	Norethindrone	1.0	11.9
Norinyl 1 + 50 (Syntex)	Mestranol	50	Norethindrone	1.0	10.6
Ortho-Novum 1/50 (Ortho)	Mestranol	50	Norethindrone	1.0	10.6
Nelova[d] 1/50M (Warner Chilcott)	Mestranol	50	Norethindrone	1.0	10.6
Demulen 1/35 (Searle)	Ethinyl estradiol	35	Ethynodiol diacetate	1.0	37.4
Norinyl 1 + 35 (Syntex)	Ethinyl estradiol	35	Norethindrone	1.0	14.7
Ortho-Novum 1/35 (Ortho)	Ethinyl estradiol	35	Norethindrone	1.0	14.7
Nelova[d] 1/35 (Warner Chilcott)	Ethinyl estradiol	35	Norethindrone	1.0	14.7
Ortho-Novum 10/11 (Ortho), 10 days	Ethinyl estradiol	35	Norethindrone	0.5	19.6
Followed by 11 days	Ethinyl estradiol	35	Norethindrone	1.0	
Nelova[d] 10/11 (Warner Chilcott), 10 days	Ethinyl estradiol	35	Norethindrone	1.0	19.6
Followed by 11 days	Ethinyl estradiol	35	Norethindrone	0.5	
Brevicon (Syntex)	Ethinyl estradiol	35	Norethindrone	0.5	14.6
Modicon (Ortho)	Ethinyl estradiol	35	Norethindrone	0.5	14.6
Nelova[d] 0.5/35 (Warner Chilcott)	Ethinyl estradiol	35	Norethindrone	0.5	14.6
Ovcon-35 (Mead Johnson)	Ethinyl estradiol	35	Norethindrone	0.4	11.0
Tri-Norinyl (Syntex), 7 days	Ethinyl estradiol	35	Norethindrone	0.5	
Followed by 9 days	Ethinyl estradiol	35	Norethindrone	1.0	
Followed by 5 days	Ethinyl estradiol	35	Norethindrone	0.5	
Ortho-Novum 7/7/7, 7 days	Ethinyl estradiol	35	Norethindrone	0.5	
Followed by 7 days	Ethinyl estradiol	35	Norethindrone	0.75	
Followed by 7 days	Ethinyl estradiol	35	Norethindrone	1.0	
Triphasils 21 (Wyeth), 6 days	Ethinyl estradiol	30	Levonorgestrel	0.050	
Followed by 5 days	Ethinyl estradiol	40	Levonorgestrel	0.075	
Followed by 10 days	Ethinyl estradiol	30	Levonorgestrel	0.125	
Tri-Levlen (Berlex-Wyeth), 6 days	Ethinyl estradiol	30	Levonorgestrel	0.050	
Followed by 5 days	Ethinyl estradiol	40	Levonorgestrel	0.075	
Followed by 10 days	Ethinyl estradiol	30	Levonorgestrel	0.125	
Lo/Ovral (Wyeth)	Ethinyl estradiol	30	Norgestrel	0.3	9.6
Loestrin 1.5/30 (Parke Davis)	Ethinyl estradiol	30	Norethindrone acetate	1.5	25.6
Nordette (Wyeth)	Ethinyl estradiol	30	Levonorgestrel	0.15	
Levlen (Berlex/Wyeth)	Ethinyl estradiol	30	Levonorgestrel	0.15	
Loestrin 1/20 (Parke Davis)	Ethinyl estradiol	20	Norethindrone acetate	1.0	30.9
Ovrette (Wyeth)			Norgestrel	0.075	34.9
Nor-Q.D. (Syntex)			Norethindrone	0.35	42.3
Micronor (Ortho)			Norethindrone	0.35	42.3

[a]Some OCs are available in 21-day regimens or in 28-day regimens with seven placebo tablets.
[b]Percentage of spotting and bleeding in the third cycle of use.
[c]Available with seven iron tablets instead of seven placebo tablets.
[d]Generic OCs, available at lower cost than others, but with possibility of greater hormonal fluctuation.

tive system. The pseudomenstruation or withdrawal bleeding experienced by women on the pill is a result of hormonal withdrawal rather than the normal cyclic shedding of the endometrium in response to endogenous pituitary and ovarian hormones. In combination pills, the progestin effect is more powerful than that of estrogen (Speroff, Glass, & Kase, 1983). Progestin alone provides adequate contraceptive effects. Estrogen can be used alone as a luteal phase (postcoital) contraceptive. A number of theories explain the contraceptive action of the hormones in these various forms of oral contraceptives.

Ovulation

Women on combination oral contraceptives receive constant or varying levels of exogenous estrogen and progestin for 21 days. Low basal plasma levels of estrogen suppress secretions of follicle stimulating hormone–releasing factor (FSH-RF) within the hypothalamus. Subsequently, the anterior pituitary production of FSH and luteinizing hormone (LH) is inhibited. Midcycle surges of endogenous estrogen, FSH, and LH are eliminated. Ovulation is effectively suppressed in 95 to 98 percent of women. In a few instances, sufficient FSH is secreted to promote follicular development—more likely with the sub-50 μg preparations. In these cases, ovulation is still unlikely because the progestin component disturbs the normal positive feedback mechanism of estrogen and, subsequently, the LH surge (Fraser & Jansen, 1983).

Implantation

Estrogen, in high doses, may exert an antiprogestational effect within the uterus by interfering with the hypothalamic–pituitary–ovarian system (see Chapter 1). The normal secretory phase is altered and the endometrium becomes marked with areas of edema alternating with those of dense cellularity. These changes constitute a negative environment for implantation. Progestins produce atrophic endometrial glands, inhibiting implantation (Hatcher, Guest, Stewart, et al., 1986, p. 137; Speroff et al., 1983, p. 416).

Luteolysis

If ovulation does occur, high doses of estrogen may increase the rate of degeneration of the corpus luteum, inhibiting the production of endogenous progesterone and, subsequently, implantation and placental attachment (Hatcher et al., 1986, p. 137).

Ovum Transport

Progestins may decrease the rate of ovum transport by alterations in tubal secretion and peristalsis. This action may lead to an increase in ectopic implantations for women on certain progestin-only pills (Hatcher et al., 1986, p. 137).

Thick Cervical Mucus

Progestins promote scanty, thick, cellular cervical mucus that exhibits decreased ferning and spinnbarkeit, diminishing the ability of sperm to penetrate the cervix (Hatcher et al., 1986, p. 137; Speroff et al., 1983, p. 417).

Capacitation

Progestins may decrease capacitation—the action of hydrolytic spermatic enzymes which are responsible for alterations in the surface of spermatozoa—thus decreasing the sperm's ability to penetrate the ovum.

COMBINED ORAL CONTRACEPTIVES

Composition and Potency

A clear evaluation of the potency of oral contraceptives is difficult to make. Hormones in combination pills work both separately and together, and have synergistic and antagonistic effects. Each has effects on numerous organs and body functions and the potency of each of these effects is not necessarily the same. Studies in animals do not always apply to human beings, making the results of experimental studies difficult to interpret (Goldzieher, 1986).

Currently all combination pills available in the United States contain one of two estrogens—ethinyl estradiol or mestranol (Table 7–1). While it was believed previously that ethinyl estradiol may be 50 percent more potent than mestranol, recent studies have failed to find significant differences between the two (Goldzieher, Dozier, & de la Pena, 1980). Controversy still exists. Interestingly, all of the sub-50 μg formulations of OCs contain ethinyl estradiol.

There are a number of synthetic progestins in current use. Natural progestins cannot be utilized when taken orally. Unfortunately, synthetic progestins have androgenic effects, along with the estrogenic and antiestrogenic (progestational) effects expected of such compounds. Progestin potencies vary according to their type and dosage. Hatcher and associates (1984, p. 47) have assigned relative potencies to these three progestin properties in various birth control pills, although the reliability, validity, and clinical applicability of such estimates have been questioned (Goldzieher, 1986, p. 535).

Of progestins commonly used in OCs, *norgestrel* is considered the least estrogenic and the most androgenic; it is also highly antiestrogenic. *Norethynodrel* is the most estrogenic, and has no antiestrogenic or androgenic properties. *Norethindrone, norethindrone acetate* and *ethynodiol diacetate* are intermediate in estrogenic and androgenic effects, although norethindrone acetate is the most antiestrogenic of these progestins. See Table 7–1 for a listing of the pills that contain each of these progestins (Hatcher et al., 1984, p. 47).

Dickey (1984, p. 36) further classifies oral contraceptives according to endometrial activity, which is a result of the combined effects of three progestin activities and is related to the ratio of estrogen to progestin. Endometrial activity of a particular pill can be expressed in one of two ways: (1) the percentage of users who experience spotting or breakthrough bleeding (BTB) during their third cycle of use; (2) the percentage of users who fail to have withdrawal bleeding.

Unfortunately, OC manufacturers differ in their manner of reporting failure of menses. Practitioners can make more accurate comparisons among various brands by using the first measure. In general, the more potent progestins, norgestrel and norethindrone acetate, are associated with higher endometrial activity and less BTB or spotting than the weaker norethynodrel, ethynodiol diacetate, and, to a lesser degree, norethindrone. In trying to improve endometrial activity by manipulation of the progestin component, dosage, as well as potency, may be a factor.

Effectiveness

Oral contraceptives are not 100 percent effective. Effectiveness rates for typical users during the first year of use is reported at 98 percent, although the lowest observed failure rate is only 0.5 percent (Hatcher, et al, 1984, p. 3). Pasquale (1984) indicates that 30 to 35 μg of ethinyl estradiol is needed consistently to inhibit ovulation. In wide use, sub-50 μg preparations have proven effective. Their margin of error, however, is reduced: the risk of pregnancy is greater if pills are missed. As trends to decrease dose combinations continue, it is comforting to know that the newest effort—triphasics with significantly reduced progestin—appear not to have sacrificed effectiveness.

A number of factors may interfere with pill efficacy. During the first year, 40 to 60 percent of women discontinue use, primarily as a result of BTB or other non–life-threatening side effects. Failure to use another method after cessation of the pill can lead to pregnancy. Inconsistent or incorrect use of the pill will also reduce effectiveness, especially with 30 to 35 μg tablets, although formulations containing potent norgestrel may be associated with less breakthrough ovulation (BTO). BTO is more likely to occur if pills are missed early or late in the cycle, when FSH and LH are more sensitive to subtle hormonal changes (Fraser & Jansen, 1983). Switching from a more potent to a low-dose preparation may lead to BTO.

Gastrointestinal disturbances, such as severe diarrhea and vomiting, may result in decreased absorption of the hormones in OCs. Obese women also tend to have decreased rates of absorption and may require at least 50 μg of estrogen for fertility control (Fraser & Jansen, 1983). Caution must be utilized, however, as these women are at greater risk for cardiovascular disease. Long-term use of high-dose pills may further increase the risk of developing cardiovascular problems.

Low-dose OCs can interact with other systemic drugs, resulting in decreased contraceptive efficacy. This problem was first discovered when OC users taking rifampin became pregnant. It is now known that rifampin can induce hepatic enzymes that accelerate hormone metabolism, especially of progestin. Anticonvulsants and barbiturates increase enzymatic metabolism of estrogen. Antibiotics can interrupt the enterohepatic circulation of the pill. These medications deplete the colon of bacteria, leading to decreased steroid reabsorption, increased fecal excretion, and decreased plasma levels. The extent of interaction between OCs and other drugs varies greatly among users. Currently, no reliable method exists to identify women at risk. Practitioners should be suspicious of negative drug interaction when an established user presents with BTB and/or failure of withdrawal bleeding. BTB is more likely to occur if the drugs are introduced early or late in the cycle (Back, Breckenridge, Crawford, et al., 1981). See Table 7–2 for a listing of drug interactions and suggestions for management.

Risks of Combined Oral Contraceptive Use

Cardiovascular Disease. The most serious complications facing OC users are those associated with cardiovascular disease (CVD). It was previously believed that estrogen is responsible for the cardiovascular complications of oral contraceptives, but recent evidence implicates the progestin component as well; it is possible that venous complications are due to estrogen and those involving the arteries are due to both hormones (Bonnar & Sabra, 1986, p. 551; Kay, 1982).

The Royal College of General Practitioners in Great Britain (RCGP 1981) reported a 40 percent excess death rate among OC users. The majority of these deaths were related to CVD. OC users are four to eight times more likely to die from complications of CVD, thromboembolism, hypertension, stroke, and myocardial infarction than nonusers. Ory, Rosenfield, and Landman (1980) estimated that 3.7 deaths per 100,000 pill users in the United States will be attributed to CVD. In the same study, these investigators reported that of the approximately 8.4 million women who use oral contraceptives, 310 excess deaths per year occur. The great majority of complications related to CVD will occur in women 35 and older. Contraceptive Technology Update (CTU 1980–82), reporting from the RCGP (1981) and several other recent studies, suggested that it may be safer for a 15-year-old girl to use OCs for 20 years than for a 45-year-old woman to use them for one.

Smoking has a synergistic effect with age on the incidence of CVD (Goldbaum, Kendrick, Hogelin, & Gentry, 1987). Nicotine increases heart rate as well as systolic and diastolic blood pressure. The end result is a decrease in oxy-

TABLE 7–2. DRUGS THAT MAY REDUCE THE EFFICACY OF ORAL CONTRACEPTIVES

Class of Compound	Drug	Proposed Method of Action	Suggested Management
Anticonvulsant drugs	Barbiturates phenobarbital carbamazepin primidone ethosuximide phenytoin	Induces liver microsomal enzymes; Rapid metabolism of estrogen and increased binding of progestin and ethinyl estradiol to sex hormone–binding globulin.	Use another method, another drug, or higher-dose OCs (50 mg ethinyl estradiol).
Cholesterol-Lowering Agents	Clofibrate	Reduces elevated serum triglyceride and cholesterol; this reduces OC efficacy.	Use another method.
Antibiotics	Rifampin Isoniazid Penicillin Ampicillin Metronidazole Tetracycline Neomycin Chloramphenicol Sulfonamide Nitrofurantoin	Induces microsomal liver enzymes: see above. Enterohepatic circulation disturbed, intestinal hurry. Rifampin increases metabolism of progestins.	For short-course use of drug, use additional method or use another drug. For long course, use another method.
Sedatives and Hypnotics	Benzodiazepines Barbiturates Chloral hydrate Antimigraine preparations	Increases microsomal liver enzymes: see above.	For short-course use of drug, use additional method or another drug. For long course, use another method or higher-dose OCs.
Antacids	All	Decreases intestinal absorption of progestins.	Use additional method.

From Dickey, R. (1984). Managing contraceptive pill patients, (4th ed, pp. 116–117). Tulsa, OK: Creative Informatics, Inc. Reprinted with permission.

TABLE 7-3. EXCESS ANNUAL DEATHS AMONG 100,000 PILL USERS FROM CARDIOVASCULAR DISEASE IN GREAT BRITAIN

Age	Nonsmoker	Smoker
15-25	0	10.5
25-34	1.7	10.0
35-44	15.1	48.2
45+	40.9	178.8

From Royal College of General Practitioners. (1981). Further analysis of mortality in oral contraceptive users. Lancet, 541. Reprinted with permission.

gen consumption within the cardiovascular system. Prolonged and heavy smoking (defined as more than 15 cigarettes a day) impairs pulmonary function (Connell, 1984).

Current OC use is a more significant risk factor than former use. In an effort to balance the risk-benefit ratio, practitioners should note that the absolute risks involved with the use of OCs are less than those of pregnancy and childbirth in a healthy woman until age 35, even with the synergistic effect of smoking. After age 35, mortality significantly increases with the use of OCs, especially among smokers (Ory, 1983). (See Tables 7-3 and 7-4.)

Lipid Metabolism. There is sufficient evidence to suggest that elevated plasma levels of cholesterol and triglycerides are correlated with increased risk of CVD. Lipoproteins synthesized in the liver and intestines transport cholesterol and triglycerides in serum, and therefore play an important role in the control of lipid metabolism. Very-low-density lipoproteins (VLDLs) transport triglycerides to adipose tissue and low-density lipoproteins (LDLs) transport cholesterol into peripheral tissue. Increases in plasma levels of VLDLs, or LDLs, have positive correlations with increased risk of CVD. High-density lipoproteins (HDLs) transport cholesterol from peripheral tissue to the liver, resulting in a significant preventive effect on deposition of cholesterol in the arteries. HDL has two major components, HDL_2 and HDL_3. HDL_2 has a higher lipid content and is thought to provide protection against the development of CVD, while HDL_3 may not. Fotherby (1985) and other experts suggest that this protective effect exerted by HDL may be stronger than the atherogenic effect of LDL. Low plasma levels of HDL_2 may be more significant in predicting the increased risk of CVD than higher levels of LDL.

Both estrogen and progestin components of oral contraceptives are suspected of altering lipid metabolism. Estrogen may increase the hepatic secretion of LDL-cholesterol, whereas progestin may inhibit its uptake at the cell membrane level. Both actions thereby contribute to increases in plasma levels of LDLs, triglycerides, and cholesterol. Not all OC formulations have been found to affect lipid metabolism to the same extent. As the potency of progestins is more variable than that of estrogens in low-dose preparations, experts suspect that progestin has more significance in increasing plasma levels of LDLs. Brooks (1984) and Po-

well, Hedlin, Cerskus, and associates (1984) conducted two of the many studies associating the more potent progestins, norgestrel and norethindrone acetate, with higher levels of LDL. Similarly, HDL levels tend to be higher in women using more estrogenic preparations and lowest when the more potent progestin, norgestrel, is involved; however, pills with lower doses of norgestrel have, in several small studies that evaluated pill use of 6 to 12 months, been found to compare more favorably with the less potent progestins in their effect on HDLs (Briggs, 1983; Larsson-Cohn, Fahraeus, Wallentin, et al., 1981; WHO 1985). Recent reports suggest that the new triphasics—Ortho-Novum 7/7/7 and TriNorinyl—in which the norethindrone content is decreased, do not appear to alter HDL levels. Little change in lipid metabolism has been documented after 6 to 12 months of use of Triphasil, which contains norgestrel, leading to the conclusion that the total dose, rather than the type of progesterone, may be responsible for adverse changes in lipid metabolism (Roy, 1986, p. 547).

Other factors influence levels of lipoproteins in blood:

Genetic	Family history of hyperlipidemia may affect HDL-cholesterol (HDL-C) and LDL-cholesterol (LDL-C) levels, but not serum triglycerides.
Obesity	$HDL-C_2$ levels tend to be lower; triglyceride levels increase.
Exercise	Moderate strenuous exercise appears to offset the effects of OCs. $HDL-C_2$ levels increase while LDL levels are decreased (Gray, Harding, & Dale, 1983).
Dietary	Very high carbohydrate intake appears to decrease HDL-C concentrations while diets high in cholesterol tend to increase $HDL-C_3$ rather than HDL_2.
Alcohol	Consumption increases HDL_3 and triglyceride levels.
Smoking	Cigarette smoking increases triglycerides and decreases HDL-C levels.

TABLE 7-4. MORTALITY ATTRIBUTED TO PREGNANCY AND CHILDBIRTH, FIRST-TRIMESTER LEGAL ABORTION, AND USE OF VARIOUS METHODS OF BIRTH CONTROL BY AGE GROUP, BASED ON 100,000 USERS PER YEAR

Factors	15-19	20-24	25-29	30-34	35-39	40-49
Pregnancy and childbirth	12.9	12.0	15.3	26.5	53.9	89.1
Legal abortion	0.5	0.8	1.0	1.5	1.7	1.7
Oral contraceptives nonsmoker	0.3	0.5	0.9	1.9	13.8	31.6
Oral contraceptives smoker	0.2	3.4	6.6	13.5	51.1	117.2
IUD	0.8	0.8	1.0	1.0	1.4	1.4

From Ory, H. (1983). Mortality associated with fertility and fertility control. Family Planning Perspectives 15 (2), 52-63. Reprinted with permission.

Pathologic conditions   Diabetes mellitus and hyperthyroidism decrease, whereas hypothyroidism increases, HDL-C levels.

Carbohydrate Metabolism. Alterations in carbohydrate metabolism can accelerate atherosclerotic changes and increase the risk of CVD. It is known that high doses of estrogen decrease carbohydrate metabolism, whereas lower doses increase it. As the newer OC preparations maintain the estrogen component at a constant low dose, the more positive effect is probably achieved. Progestins are suspected of having a negative effect on carbohydrate metabolism, presumably interfering with the uptake of insulin at the cell membrane level. Potency is an important factor. Agents containing norgestrel are associated with the highest increase in serum glucose and plasma insulin levels (Spellacy, 1982). Women at risk for significant alterations in carbohydrate metabolism include those with a history of gestational diabetes or a history of a stillbirth or delivery of a macrosomic infant, those age 35 or older, the obese, and those with prior abnormal blood glucose tests or a first-degree relative with diabetes mellitus.

In light of current research on the effect of OCs on lipid and carbohydrate metabolism, and subsequently, on CVD, the following recommendations are made:

1. Use low-dose, sub-50 μg preparations containing less potent or intermediate progestins, that is, norethindrone 0.5 to 1 mg. (Medical Letter, 1983; Powell et al., 1984).
2. Institute strict screening for contraindications to identify women at risk for the development of complications (Hatcher et al., 1984).
3. Obtain baseline serum triglyceride and cholesterol levels before initiating OCs for women with risk factors, including a family history of myocardial infarction (MI) before age 50. To be accurately interpreted, these tests should be done after 12 hours of fasting. Additional testing is recommended 3 months after pill initiation and annually thereafter (Brooks, 1984). In women with elevated cholesterol and/or triglyceride levels, the risks of OC use must be carefully weighed against the benefits. Referral to or consultation with a physician is appropriate before initiation of OCs in the presence of these risk factors.
4. Institute additional screening for women at risk for alterations in carbohydrate metabolism, such as a fasting blood sugar (FBS) and a 2-hour glucose challenge test (GCT). Elevated values should be followed by a glucose tolerance test (GTT). The risk–benefit ratio should be carefully considered before initiation of OCs (Spellacy, 1982), and physician consultation and/or referral are appropriate in cases of elevated values.
5. Teach danger signs to all women on OCs (see "Teaching and Counseling").

Venous Thrombosis. The risk of superficial thrombosis of the leg increases in women using OCs by 50 percent from 2 per 1,000 to 3 per 1,000 annually (CTU, 1980–82). According to Ory, Rosenfield, and Landman (1980), the rate of deep-vein thrombosis is associated with a four- to sevenfold increase to a rate of 0.5 per 1,000 a year among women using low-dose OCs. For women using pills containing more than 50 μg, the increased risk may be tenfold compared with nonusers. Both progestins and estrogens may contribute to this risk. Progestin causes dilation of veins

and increases fibrinogen levels, and there is a strong relationship between estrogen and an increase in Factor VII levels. Hypercoaguability in the presence of dilated or obstructed veins can lead to clot formations.

An increased risk of thromboembolic disease is associated with current OC use only; it disappears when the pill is discontinued. Smoking significantly increases the risk. Women with Type A, B, or AB blood have three times greater risk than those with type O (Fraser & Jansen, 1983; Jick, Westerholm, Vessey, et al., 1969). Other risk factors include diabetes, increased age, obesity, full-term birth within the past 2 weeks and major surgery or immobilization. Moderate strenuous physical exercise 30 to 35 minutes a day, three times a week may decrease this risk. A possible explanation for this is that an increase of releasable plasminogen activator promotes an accelerated breakdown of clots (Williams, Logue, Lewis, et al., 1980). Clinical signs of venous thrombosis include pain to touch, localized to an extremity, swelling/warmth, and sometimes palpable cords.

Stroke (Cerebrovascular Accident). It is estimated that women on OCs have a five times greater risk of stroke than non-OC users. Cardiovascular accidents (CVAs) are responsible for 5 to 10 percent of deaths related to OC use, with mortality increasing with advancing age and the presence of hypertension (Connell, 1984). Although experts agree that the increased risk continues among former users and may be associated with length of use, there is a lack of documentation regarding the time involved (RCGP, 1981; Walnut Creek Contraceptive Drug Study, 1980).

There are two major types of stroke: (1) *thromboembolic stroke* results from blood clots and accounts for 85 to 90 percent of the total; (2) *common hemorrhagic stroke* is lethal; it results from bleeding from ruptured arteries and accounts for 10 to 15 percent. This type includes subarachnoid hemorrhage, the most common form of hemorrhagic stroke among women in the reproductive years.

Estrogen was originally blamed for the increased occurrence of stroke among OC users. Recent data, however, implicate progestins as well (Kannell, 1984). The incidence appears to be related to the dosages of both components. Women may complain of persistent unilateral headaches for weeks or months before a CVA occurs. Occasionally, hemiparesis is a warning sign. Practitioners should use caution in providing OCs to women with a history of migraine headaches, transient hemiparesis, or a close relative with a history of CVA. Smokers are also at increased risk (Goldbaum et al., 1987), particularly for the hemorrhagic type.

Myocardial Infarction. Women using OCs are three times more likely to be hospitalized for myocardial infarction (MI) than nonusers (Ory et al., 1980). The risk increases with age and smoking. Moderate use of cigarettes and OCs is associated with a two to five times greater possibility of experiencing an MI while the increased risk among heavy smokers is 7 to 34 times that of nonsmokers (Ory, Layde, & Schlesselman, 1982). Some data suggest that an increased risk persists for up to 10 years after discontinuation of OCs (RCGP, 1981), although other sources report less alarming data (Ory et al., 1982; Walnut Creek Contraceptive Drug Study, 1980). Generally, experts agree that arterial changes resulting from OC use do, theoretically, place current and previous users at greater risk of MI. Both estrogen and progestins are implicated, primarily as a result of their effect on lipid and carbohydrate metabolism (Fotherby, 1985). Women at risk for developing an MI while on OCs include smokers; women with hyperlipidemia, hypertension, diabetes, a history of preeclampsia in pregnancy; women age 35 and older; and women with a family history of MI before age 50. Clinical signs of MI include crushing chest pain, shortness of breath, and diaphoresis.

Liver Tumors. Hepatic adenoma is a benign tumor in the liver that can impair biliary secretion, causing an increase in hepatic blood flow. The danger lies in rupture of the tumor capsule, followed by extensive intraperitoneal hemorrhage, which can lead to death. Fortunately, such tumors are rare. The incidence among never users is 1.0 per million women. Among OC users up to age 31, the incidence is 1.3 per 100,000 users, increasing to 3 to 4 per 100,000 for older women (Rooks, Ory, Ishak, et al., 1979). Women who have used OCs 5 years or more appear to have 3.5 greater risk of developing a hepatic adenoma than nonusers. Age and hormonal potency have a positive correlation with the incidence of benign tumors. The estrogen component appears more responsible for tumor development. Genetic factors may also contribute to their development.

Some recent evidence suggests an increased risk of malignant tumors with pill use. In 1983, Forman, Doll, and Peto examined trends in mortality from liver cancer and found a small but consistent increase for young women over the preceding 24 years in the United Kingdom. This trend was not seen in four other developed countries, including the United States. Two case-control studies (Forman, Vincent, & Doll, 1986; Neuberger, Forman, Doll, & Williams, 1986) reported increased relative risks for developing liver malignancies in oral contraceptive users, particularly with use of 8 or more years. The absolute risk of this disease remains low, however; Forman and associates (1983, p. 352) estimate that no more than 10 deaths a year can be attributed to pill-induced hepatic cancer among 3.5 million users, assuming the data were conclusive. There also has been some concern that OCs may stimulate the rate of growth of preexisting tumors (Stubberfield, 1984).

A major clinical sign of liver tumors is acute abdominal pain. Such tumors are usually palpable and bruits may be present. Jaundice of the skin may be noticeable.

Hypertension. Women using OCs have up to six times increased likelihood of becoming hypertensive, defined as a blood pressure of 140/90 or greater (Connell, 1984). The risk is greater with increased age and duration of OC use. Both estrogen and progestins are implicated. Although the exact mechanism is unclear, the hormones in OCs are known to affect the renin–angiotensin–aldosterone system leading to increases in both systolic and diastolic readings. Women with preexisting hypertension should not be provided combined OCs since these steroids may worsen the condition, as well as interfere with the action of antihypertensive drugs.

The rise in blood pressure associated with OC use is generally minimal and tends to affect the systolic more than the diastolic reading. Fortunately, this negative effect on blood pressure appears to be associated only with current use. The majority of women return to normal pressure within a few months of discontinuation of the steroids (Connell, 1984). Those at risk include black women and women with a history of preeclampsia during pregnancy and/or a strong family history of hypertension. There is no evidence to suggest that the alterations in lipids and lipoproteins secondary to OCs further increase the risk of hypertension among users (Fotherby, 1985).

Gallbladder Disease. A study by the Boston Collaborative Drug Surveillance Program (1973) confirmed previous findings that OC users had a 50 percent greater chance of developing gallbladder disease than nonusers. A more recent study by the RCGP (1982) in Great Britain failed to find evidence to support such a claim. In fact, they suggested that the risk of gallbladder disease to OC users might be decreased. While the earlier study followed OC users up to 3 years, the study by RCGP followed women up to 10 years of use. Researchers in the latter study did witness an overall rise in the incidence of gallbladder disease during the first 4 years of OC use, followed by a subsequent gradual decrease over the next 6 years to rates below those of the controls. They suggest that the initial increased rates noted in both studies might reflect the long presymptomatic stage of gallbladder disease. It is possible then that the decreased incidence seen with long-term use provides a more accurate representation of the effects of OCs on gallbladder disease. Most experts agree that OCs do increase the incidence of gallbladder disease in susceptible women. Hatcher and associates (1984) include gallbladder disease as a contraindication to OC use. History of cholecystectomy is also listed among their possible relative contraindications because "the biochemical abnormality still exists following removal of the gallbladder and use of oral contraceptives could lead to stone formation in the common bile duct." Estrogen and, to a lesser degree, progestins, may be implicated in the development of gall stones because of their effect on LDL metabolism and on increasing serum cholesterol levels. Women with a history of severe liver damage, active mononucleosis, or infectious hepatitis are at risk for developing pill-related gallbladder disease. The primary clinical sign of gallbladder disease is severe abdominal pain.

Chlamydia Trachomatis. Genital infection with *Chlamydia trachomatis* occurs with greater frequency among OC users. Its overall incidence has increased in the past several years, and pelvic inflammatory disease (PID) related to *C. trachomatis* is now more common than PID related to *Neisseria gonorrhoeae* (Svensson, Mårdh, & Weström, 1983). *C. trachomatis* PID has a mild clinical course. Up to 70 percent of women are relatively asymptomatic. Women may get no treatment or receive oral antibiotic therapy, whereas women with *N. gonorrhoeae* PID often have to seek emergency room attention, and may require hospitalization for effective therapy. It appears, however, that the milder form of PID caused by *C. trachomatis* is associated with more tubal inflammation and subsequent adhesions.

Washington, Gove, Schachter, and Sweet (1985) postulate the following mechanisms to account for the increased occurrence of genital and pelvic infection with *C. trachomatis* among OC users:

1. Progesterone is known to suppress the growth of *N. gonorrhoeae*, however, recent studies in animals indicate that both estrogen and progesterone enhance the growth, survival, and ascension of genital *Chlamydia*. Synthetic hormones in OCs may have the same effects.

2. OC users have increased cervical ectropion, exposing more columnar epithelium. Theoretically, columnar cells are more susceptible to acquisition and growth of this intracellular organism.

Practitioners without the benefit of expensive *Chlamydia* cultures or monoclonal antibody tests (see Chapter 4) should become familiar with clinical diagnosis and appropriate antibiotic therapy for *Chlamydia* infections (see Chapter 12 for more information on *C. trachomatis*).

Additional Side Effects. The preceding discussion focused on the most serious complications of OC use, describing life-threatening conditions and changes that can lead to life-threatening events. The pill has been associated with numerous other effects. These are often referred to in the medical literature as "minor," although women's health advocates have criticized this designation. Many of the so-called minor side effects of the pill can be devastating to individual women and should, therefore, be taken seriously. Complaints should never be dismissed. One formulation may cause hormonal excess in one woman and hormonal deficiency in another; each woman responds differently based on her hormonal profile and other underlying physiologic factors. This explains the large variety of non–life-threatening, pill-related side effects. Once underlying pathology is ruled out, most of these side effects can be controlled by manipulation of the estrogenic, progestagenic, or androgenic activities of OCs to find a more suitable formulation.

Current literature does not support the practice of stopping OCs for a rest period to prevent the development of side effects. Many of the more common side effects disappear after the first 3 months of use. A practitioner's knowledge of the potency and combination of OC formulations

(Table 7–1), hormonal etiology of pill side effects (Table 7–5), and normal course and reversibility of most side effects (Table 7–5) will enable him or her to help each woman to successfully use OCs and avoid problems.

The Question of Breast Cancer. Although the characteristics of women at risk for breast cancer (e.g., nulliparity, childbearing delayed beyond age 30, history of early menarche, late menopause) suggest a hormonal etiology, most studies do not support the theory that OC users are at increased risk of developing breast cancer (Brooks, 1984). The Centers for Disease Control (CDC) study (1983a) indicates that OC users have a 0.96 relative risk of breast cancer compared to nonusers. The protective activity reflected in this reduced risk is more prevalent among nulliparous women. CDC failed to find an increased incidence of breast cancer among OC users at risk, including women with a history of benign breast disease or family history of breast cancer.

A number of studies, however, have questioned these findings, and suggest that there may be an association between pill use and breast cancer, particularly for certain

TABLE 7–5. PILL SIDE EFFECTS—HORMONE ETIOLOGY AND TIME FRAMEWORK*

Estrogen Excess	Progestin Excess	Androgen Excess	Estrogen Deficiency	Progestin Deficiency
1. Nausea, dizziness (1) 2. Edema and abdominal or leg pain with cyclic weight gain, bloating (1) 3. Leukorrhea 4. Increased leiomyoma size (3) 5. Chloasma (3,6) 6. Uterine cramps 7. Irritability, depression (2 or 4) 8. Increased fat deposition (2) 9. Cervical ectropion 10. Poor contact lens fit (1) 11. Telangiectasia 12. Vascular-type headache (+2 or +3) 13. Hypertension? (3,5) 14. Lactation suppression (1) 15. Headaches while taking pill (2) 16. Cystic breast changes (3) 17. Breast tenderness (1) 18. Increased breast size (ductal and fatty tissue and fluid retention) (1) 19. Thrombophlebitis (1,5) 20. Cerebrovascular accidents (2,6) 21. Myocardial infarction (3) 22. Hepatic adenoma (3,5,6) 23. Cyclic weight gain, edema (1)	1. Increased appetite & weight gain (non-cyclic) 2. Tiredness, fatigue, and weakness 3. Depression (2 or 4) 4. Decreased libido (2) 5. Oily scalp, acne (2) 6. Loss of hair (3 or 4) 7. Cholestatic jaundice (3) 8. Decreased length of menstrual flow (3) 9. Hypertension (3,5) 10. Headaches between Pill packages (3) 11. Monilial vaginitis/cervicitis (3) 12. Increased breast size (alveolar tissue) 13. Breast tenderness (1) 14. Decreased carbohydrate tolerance (1) 15. Dilated leg veins (1) 16. Pelvic congestion syndrome	1. Increased appetite and weight gain (non-cyclic) (3) 2. Hirsutism (3) 3. Acne (3 or 4) 4. Oily skin, rash 5. Increased libido 6. Cholestatic jaundice (3) 7. Pruritis	1. Irritability, nervousness 2. Hot flushes, vasomotor symptoms 3. Uterine prolapse, pelvic relaxation symptoms (3) 4. Early and midcycle spotting (1) 5. Decreased amount of menstrual flow (3) 6. No withdrawal bleeding (6) 7. Decreased libido (2) 8. Diminished breast size 9. Dry vaginal mucosa, atrophic vaginitis, and dyspareunia 10. Headaches (2 or 3) 11. Depression (3 or 4)	1. Late breakthrough bleeding and spotting (1) 2. Heavy menstrual flow and clots 3. Delayed onset of menses 4. Dysmenorrhea (1) 5. Weight loss

*Time framework is indicated by number in parenthesis where available: (1) Improves after 3 months; (2) Not time-related; (3) Worsens over prolonged use; (4) Worsens after discontinuation; (5) May or may not be reversible; (6) Consequences may be irreversible; + (2) During 3 weeks pills are taken; and + (3) During week pills are not taken.
Adapted from Hatcher, et al., Contraceptive Technology, 1984–85, (12th rev. ed.). and Dickey, R., (1984) Managing Contraceptive Pill Patients, (4th ed.).

groups of women. In a case-control study of several thousand women, Stadel, Lai, Schlesselman, and Murray (1988) found a 2-1/2 times increased risk of breast cancer among women who met 3 criteria: nulliparity, menarche before age 13, and pill use for 8 to 11 years. Women with the first 2 criteria who used pills for 12 or more years were found to have a rate of breast cancer 12 times higher than nonpill users. In another large study, the relative risk for breast cancer in women diagnosed between the ages of 30 and 34 was 3.3; it was 5.88 among women in that age group with 1 child at the time of diagnosis (Kay & Hannaford, 1988). It is possible that increased rates in young women represent increased surveillance secondary to pill use, rather than increased risk. In a study of 407 breast cancer patients and 424 women without cancer, the relative risk was 2.0 by age 45 for pill users and 4.1 for users of 10 or more years (Miller, Rosenberg, Kaufman, et al., 1989). These findings are suspect; they raise the question of why overall rates of breast cancer in young women have not increased dramatically in recent years.

Long-term prospective studies are warranted to clarify any association, delineate the risk groups, and demonstrate the findings of lifetime follow-up. Until this is accomplished, The National Women's Health Network (1989) recommends that young women should consider pill use for a maximum of 7 years and that all women, particularly long-term pill users, follow preventive and early detection measures for breast cancer, outlined in Chapter 10.

The Question of Teratogenesis.   An early study by Nora, Nora, Blu, and co-investigators (1978) raised much concern regarding life threatening birth defects resulting from the use of OCs. In this study, however, researchers failed to differentiate between women using OCs and those taking prescribed hormones to prevent spontaneous abortion. In 1980, when Janerich, Piper, and Glebatis evaluated the effects of OCs ingested during pregnancy, they found only a slight increase in the incidence of congenital defects among male offspring born to women over 30. Hypospadias and limb deformities constituted the defects. Children born to women who stopped OCs prior to conception were unaffected. More recently, Linn, Schoenbaum, Monson, and co-workers (1983) failed to find any association between the use of OCs during pregnancy and birth defects. Lammer and Cordero (1986) conducted a case control study of 1,091 infants with at least one of 12 major malformations, looking at the effects of first trimester exogenous sex hormone exposure. They found no statistically significant relationships between exposure to the hormones in oral contraceptives and any of the anomalies studied. Although these recent findings are reassuring, women who conceive while taking the pill and wish to carry to term should stop using the drug as soon as pregnancy is suspected; a backup method is advisable until pregnancy is confirmed.

Special Risks to Adolescents.   Of 29 million adolescents in the United States, 7 million males and 5 million females are sexually active (Tyrer, 1984a). Over one-third of females aged 15 to 18 are exposed to the relatively high mortality associated with pregnancy for this age group (see Table 7–4). Data on the use of various contraceptive methods by women aged 15 to 19 show the pill to be the first choice (1,539,000 users). No deaths related to serious cardiovascular complications have been reported for women under 18; however, the practitioner should be aware of some special considerations when prescribing OCs to teenage women in order to promote more efficient and safe fertility control.

POSTPILL AMENORRHEA.   Postpill amenorrhea and infertility resulting from the effects of OCs on the hypothalamic–pituitary–ovarian axis is a potential problem for adolescent pill users. Hatcher et al. (1984, p. 69) recommend waiting until the teenager has had 6 to 12 regular periods before providing her with OCs. They urge practitioners to be sensitive to the individual who is already sexually active with irregular and/or few menses. The risks of postpill amenorrhea and potential infertility associated with premature use of OCs must be weighed against the risks associated with adolescent pregnancy. The literature suggests that the risks of infertility after OC use are very small and probably temporary. Linn and associates (1982) found that it may take 24 months for 90 percent of former pill users to conceive while 90 percent of women using all other methods combined conceived within 13 months. Women with a history of irregular menses, which includes many adolescents, are likely to return to a similar pattern and take longer to conceive after discontinuing use of the pill.

GROWTH INHIBITION.   Another concern regarding adolescents and OC use is a possible inhibition of growth secondary to premature epiphyseal closure resulting from the pill's estrogen component. Tyrer (1984a) disputes this notion, noting that there is much documentation supporting the theory that epiphyseal closure is generally well under way in menstruating teens. It is highly unlikely that the use of popular low-dose OCs would adversely hasten the process.

USE FAILURES.   The incidence of improper use of OCs is higher among adolescents than nonadolescents; hence there are more pregnancies related to contraceptive use failure. Many of the reasons adolescents give for stopping the pill are related to side effects generally, for example exacerbation of acne and increased weight gain. Although not considered medically serious, both occurrences are very disturbing to young women concerned with body image. Nausea, chloasma, breakthrough bleeding, and development of stretch marks on thighs or breast can be equally disturbing. The practitioner should initiate low-dose, low-potency pills and provide anticipatory guidance with a discussion about relative risks of side effects versus pregnancy to all young women beginning OC use. The adolescent must be encouraged to take OCs correctly and not stop them without using another method.

NUTRITIONAL RISKS.   Adolescents typically have poor diets. They also fear weight gain from the use of OCs. They are usually at greater risk for nutritional deficiencies, especially of vitamin B_6. Good diet, counseling, and supplements are essential to their care.

Noncontraceptive Benefits

Despite the preceding discussion, it is important to remember that oral contraceptives offer women an extremely effective method of birth control, as well as a number of other benefits.

Benign Breast Disease.   Most data support a decreased incidence of benign breast disease with OC use. Up to 50 to 75 percent, or 20,000, surgical cases are prevented annually. Increased duration of use and low progestin potency appear to provide the greatest protection (Brooks, 1984).

Endometrial Cancer.   Endometrial cancer is the third leading cause of cancer deaths in women in the United States. Use of oral contraceptives decreases its incidence by 50 percent and averts 2,000 cases a year (Centers for Disease Control, 1983b; Rosenfield, 1983). The protective effect is greater with increased duration of use and nulliparity. The benefits are noted after 1 year of use and may, for former users, continue at least 10 years after cessation of use (Rosenfield, 1983).

Ovarian Cancer. The fourth leading cause of cancer mortality among women in the United States is ovarian cancer. OC use appears to decrease the incidence of ovarian cancer by one third. Nulliparous women enjoy the greatest protection (Rosenfield, 1983; Stubberfield, 1984). CDC (1983c) estimate that 1,700 deaths a year related to ovarian cancer are averted by the use of OCs. The rate of protection increases with duration of use and may continue up to 10 years in former users. Estrogen and progesterone are credited by their combined action with blocking incessant ovulation. The incidence of benign ovarian cysts is also decreased by the same mechanism.

Cervical Cancer. Data in this area are inconsistent. Some studies have shown an increased incidence of cervical dysplasia and carcinoma in situ with prolonged duration of OC use. They suggest that OCs may accelerate the degeneration of cervical dysplasia to more serious neoplastic lesions (Vessel, Lawless, McPherson, & Yeates, 1983). Other investigators, however, have failed to find positive correlation between the use of OCs and increased risk of cervical cancer (Stubberfield, 1984). Many extraneous variables complicate this area of investigation. Women using OCs have increased cervical erosion and more frequent Pap smears. Improved sampling with earlier detection of dysplasia may provide biased reporting. Furthermore, it is difficult to control the number of sexual partners—a major risk factor in the development of cervical cancer. Until more definitive investigations are complete, practitioners may take note of recent data indicating that folate, 10 mg daily, has a substantial beneficial effect on the cervical epithelium. Preliminary research data revealed several cases in which women with mild to moderate cervical intraepithelial neoplasia showed remarkable improvement with daily folate supplements compared to those women treated with a placebo. Notably, in many instances, the progression to dysplasia was averted (Medical News, 1980).

Rheumatoid Arthritis. The incidence of rheumatoid arthritis is decreased by 50 percent among OC users (Rosenfield, 1983; RCGP, 1978).

Pelvic Inflammatory Disease. There is evidence that the incidence of pelvic inflammatory disease (PID) in women on OCs is up to 50 percent less than in nonusers. The protective effect is noted after the first year of use and disappears after the pill is discontinued. It is estimated that hospitalizations for PID are reduced by 70 percent among OC users. The annual number of ectopic pregnancies secondary to PID is decreased. Because of widespread use of the pill, there are approximately 57,000 fewer cases of PID per year in the United States, 13,000 fewer hospitalizations, and 10,000 fewer ectopic pregnancies (CTU, 1980–82; Rosenfield, 1983). Several theories exist to explain this protective action:

- Decrease in menstrual blood, reducing the availability of this rich medium for incubation and growth of bacteria
- Hostile cervical mucus, deterring potential pathogens from entering the uterine cavity
- Decreased dilation of the cervical os at the time of menstruation and midcycle, inhibiting upward migration of pathogens
- Decreased strength of uterine contractions, reducing the possibility of infection spreading from the uterine cavity to the fallopian tubes

Recent investigations, however, document more cases of involuntary infertility secondary to a single episode of *C. trachomatis* than to *N. gonorrhoeae* (Svensson et al., 1983). In view of these findings, Washington et al. (1985) question the protective effect of OCs against PID and warn that users may have an increased risk of PID secondary to *C. trachomatis* exposure. *C. trachomatis*, as an intracellular organism, may be less dependent on quantities of menstrual blood. Washington and his associates urge practitioners to be cautious in providing OCs as a protective method for teenagers and women at risk for developing PID.

Other Benefits. Reduced menstrual flow and associated iron deficiency anemia, and lower incidence of acne, premenstrual syndrome, and dysmenorrhea have all been noticed among users of OCs (Rosenfield, 1983).

A Word About Nutrition

Metabolic actions of the contraceptive steroids can also affect vitamin and mineral metabolism. Decreased intestinal absorption is suspected to be the cause of many nutritional deficiencies among OC users. Notably, absorption of vitamins B_1, B_2, B_6, B_{12}, and C, and folic acid is affected.

Pyridoxine (B_6)	Estrogen appears to interfere with various steps in the conversion of vitamin B_6 to its coenzyme form, thus decreasing plasma levels of the vitamin (Smit Veninga, 1984).
Cobalamin (B_{12})	OCs may inhibit the production of glycoproteins necessary for its plasma transport.
Folacin (folic acid)	OCs may increase urinary excretion of folacin and, thereby, lower plasma levels.
Vitamin C	The decreased number of platelets and leukocytes noted in OC users suggest that steroids decrease absorption, alter normal tissue distribution, and decrease the levels of reducing compounds, including vitamin C.

Plasma levels of other nutrients appear to increase among OC users:

Vitamin A	OCs improve metabolism and redistribution.
Calcium	OCs increase absorption of dietary calcium without increased urinary excretion.
Iron	OCs decrease menstrual flow and increase absorption of iron from the gut.

Adolescents and poor women may have deficiencies in all areas, but especially of vitamin B_6, because of generally inadequate diets. Strict vegetarians may be deficient in B_{12} and zinc. Smokers tend to have a 30 to 50 percent lower level of plasma vitamin C than nonsmokers. Use of alcohol and illegal drugs can decrease appetite and increase the need for certain nutrients such as folacin.

Most experts believe that the alterations in vitamin and

mineral metabolism noted in OC users rarely lead to clinical levels of deficiency and toxicity. Routine supplementation of vitamins is generally not recommended, unless signs of deficiency occur (Tyrer, 1984b). Practitioners should be aware of signs of deficiency and include nutritional assessment and counseling as part of the routine health care for OC users (Table 7–6). Well-balanced, low-fat diets should be recommended although data on the extent to which diet affects adverse lipid changes secondary to OC use are not available.

Contraindications

The following list of contraindications is adapted from Hatcher et al. (1984). OCs should not be started in the presence of any absolute contraindication. Should such a contraindication develop during the use of OCs, they should be immediately discontinued. Strong relative contraindications are also often significant enough to warrant initiation of another method of birth control. For women with certain relative risk factors, such as diabetes and sickle cell disease, physician management or co-management of OC use may be appropriate. Consultations and referrals should be sought without hesitation whenever necessary.

It is important to always assist the individual woman in weighing the risks of oral contraceptives against their benefits for her particular life situation. The degree of acceptable risk varies among women, and for individual women at different times in the life cycle. In some situations, however, the practitioner may withhold a method based on her judgment of the limits of safety. In these instances, it is essential to assist the patient in accepting this necessity and to offer an alternative method of family planning.

Absolute Contraindications

1. Current or past thromboembolic disorder
2. Current or past cerebrovascular disease
3. Current or past artery disease
4. Known or suspected or past carcinoma of the breast
5. Known or suspected current or past estrogen-dependent neoplasia
6. Current pregnancy
7. Current or past benign or malignant liver tumor
8. Current impaired liver function

Strong Relative Contraindications

9. Severe headaches, particularly vascular and migraine
10. Hypertension with resting diastolic blood pressure of 90 or greater, or a resting systolic blood pressure of 140 or greater, on three or more separate visits, or an accurate measurement of 110 diastolic or more on a single occasion
11. Diabetes or prediabetes
12. Strong family history of diabetes
13. Active gallbladder disease
14. Previous cholestasis during pregnancy, congenital hyperbilirubinemia (Gilbert's disease)
15. Active mononucleosis

TABLE 7–6. VITAMIN AND MINERAL CHANGES ASSOCIATED WITH ORAL CONTRACEPTIVE USE

	RDA for Women	Serum Plasma or Blood Changes	Early Clinical Effects	Food Sources
Vitamin A	4,000–5,000 IU	Increased	Fissured skin, coarsening of hair, hepatomegaly	Liver, kidney, dairy products, eggs, dark leafy green and orange vegetables
Thiamine (B$_1$)	1.0 mg	Decreased	Anorexia, lethargy, depression, irritability (beriberi)	Pork, wheat germ, nuts, brown rice, organ meats, whole grains, beef, legumes, dry yeast
Riboflavin (B$_2$)	1.2 mg	Decreased	Glossitis, seborrhea, fissures at the corners of the mouth, conjunctival irritation	Milk, cheese, eggs, organ meats, green leafy vegetables
Pyridoxine (B$_6$)	2.0 mg	Decreased	Clinical depression, glucose intolerance	Yeast, wheat germ, meat, bananas, organ meats, fish, poultry, yams, legumes, whole grains, potatoes
Cobalamin (B$_{12}$)	3.0 mg	Decreased	Potentiation of pernicious anemia, folacin deficiency	Liver, kidney, fresh milk, poultry, seafoods, eggs (very small amounts)
Ascorbic acid (C)	45 mg	Decreased	Bleeding gums; swollen tender joints (scurvy)	Citrus fruit, raw leafy vegetables, tomatoes, cantaloupe
Folacin (folic acid)	0.4 mg	Decreased	Megaloblastic anemia, gastrointestinal disturbances	Liver, kidney beans, lima beans, green leafy vegetables, fish, nuts, asparagus, yeast, whole grains
Copper	2.0 mg	Increased	Pigment changes, Wilson's disease (hepatolenticular degeneration)	Liver, shellfish, whole grains, nuts, cherries, raisins, dried legumes
Iron	10 mg	Increased	None	Liver, meat, egg yolk, green leafy vegetables, clams, organ meats, dried peas and beans, dried fruit, nuts, oysters, molasses, whole grains, brewers yeast
Zinc	15 mg	Decreased	Delayed wound healing, alopecia, loss of taste	Meat, liver, eggs, seafood, milk, whole grains, peanuts, legumes

Adapted from Dickey, R., (1984). Managing Contraceptive Pill Patients, (4th ed.) Tulsa, OK: Creative Informatics, Inc. Reprinted with permission.

16. Sickle cell (SS) anemia or sickle cell–hemoglobin C (SC) disease
17. Undiagnosed, abnormal vaginal bleeding*
18. Surgery planned within the next 4 weeks or major surgery requiring immobilization
19. Long-leg casts or major lower-leg injury
20. Age 45 or older
21. Age 40 years or older, accompanied by a second risk factor for the development of cardiovascular disease
22. Age 30 years or older and currently a heavy smoker (15 or more cigarettes a day)
23. Impaired liver function within the past year

Other Possible Relative Contraindications. The following may contraindicate pill initiation.

24. Completion of term pregnancy within past 10 to 14 days
25. Weight gain of 10 or more pounds while previously on the pill
26. Failure to have established regular menstrual cycles
27. Patient with profile suggestive of anovulation and infertility problems such as late onset of menses or highly irregular painless menses
28. Current or past cardiac or renal disease
29. Conditions likely to make the woman unreliable in following pill instructions (mental retardation, major psychiatric problems, alcoholism or other drug abuse, or history of repeated incorrect use of oral contraceptives or other medication)
30. Gallbladder disease: postcholecystectomy
31. Lactation (see Chapter 23).

The following do not contraindicate pill initiation, but careful observation is required to determine whether the problem worsens or improves.

32. Depression
33. Hypertension with a resting diastolic blood pressure of 90 to 99 on a single visit
34. Chloasma or hair loss related to pregnancy (or history thereof)
35. Asthma
36. Epilepsy
37. Uterine fibromyomas
38. Acne
39. Varicose veins
40. History of hepatitis, but normal liver function tests for at least 1 year

Management Of Visits

The basic principle involved in providing oral contraceptives is use of a formulation with the least amount of hormones to decrease the risk of major side effects while achieving a high degree of contraceptive efficiency. After weighing the risks and benefits and ruling out absolute and strong relative contraindications, the practitioner is left to choose from a wide variety of agents. A correct choice enables a woman to avoid many side effects that may lead to discontinuation of the method and contraception failure.

Choosing the correct oral contraceptive may appear overwhelming. It is helpful to keep in mind the following points: Start everyone on a 30 to 35 μg pill, and avoid pills with potent or high doses of progestins. Become familiar with several low dose preparations and start women with these agents. Manipulate pill formulations first by increasing progestin potency, then raising the estrogen component to 50 μg. Rarely, if ever, should anyone be provided with more estrogen unless the use is temporary. If a woman is successfully using a 30 to 50 μg pill without problems, she should continue with that pill if at all possible.

Initial Visit

DATA COLLECTION

History. A complete history should be taken before initiating oral contraceptives (see Chapter 2). Certain areas are especially relevant to OC use: Why has the woman chosen OCs? What is her level of knowledge about them? What does she know about other methods of birth control? What is her age?

Family	Rule out premature MI, strong history of diabetes, breast cancer, hyperlipidemia, and hypertension.
Medical/ Surgical	Rule out all absolute and strong relative contraindications; determine other relative contraindications. Note current use of other medications, drugs, alcohol, tobacco.
Gynecologic	Rule out history of abnormal vaginal bleeding, PID, cervical dysplasia, chronic vaginitis or cervicitis, sexually transmitted diseases and treatments, and uterine fibroids.
Menstrual	Note menarche, last menstrual period (LMP), previous menstrual period (PMP), duration, frequency and flow, dysmenorrhea, irregular cycles or amenorrhea.
Obstetric	Note gravidy, parity, outcomes, timing of last delivery or abortion, history of gestational diabetes, macrosomic babies, stillbirths, cholestasis, hypertensive disorders during pregnancy, degree of nausea and vomiting.
Contraceptive	Inquire about methods used in the past, reason for discontinuing, side effects and complications, satisfaction of self and partner.
Sexual	Inquire about frequency, number of partners, satisfaction, problems.
Social	Determine ability to afford to come to clinic visits and to buy OCs and appropriateness of method to life-style.
Exercise	Determine if a prescribed exercise routine is followed.
Nutritional	Identify poor dietary habits that might induce deficiencies. Inquire about supplementation.

Physical Examination. Blood pressure, weight and height. Thyroid, heart, lungs, breast, abdomen, and extremities. Skin and hair distribution. Complete pelvic assessment (see Chapter 3).

---

*The American College of Obstetricians and Gynecologists (ACOG) and several clinicians recommend the inclusion of this in the list of absolute contraindications to OC use. Interpretation of the symptoms, however, is complex. It is important to determine an individual woman's bleeding pattern and ascertain whether or not a cause can be identified. Physician consultation should be obtained before providing OCs where there is any question of normalcy of the bleeding (Hatcher et al., 1984).

Routine Laboratory Tests. Pap smear, gonorrhea culture, serology, complete blood count (CBC) (Hgb/Hct may be sufficient), and wet smear. Routine chlamydial culture if available and whenever clinical signs or history warrant.

Other Laboratory Tests as Necessary. Fasting blood for serum triglycerides and total and HDL cholesterol, particularly in women with a family history of early-onset cardiovascular disease or risk factors such as hypertension (Mishkel, 1986, p. 569); SMA-12, fasting blood sugar, and glucose challenge test to screen and obtain a baseline for selected women at risk for diabetes.

ASSESSMENT. Determine whether there exist absolute or strong relative contraindications OR contraindications to the use of OCs.

INTERVENTION

Initiation. Choose an appropriate oral contraceptive agent. (See preceding discussion.) Provide a backup method if needed and teach the patient how to use it. Obtain additional laboratory data or arrange physician consultation depending on the severity of an identified contraindication and on institutional or practice protocols. Provide another method of birth control as necessary with appropriate counseling.

Practitioners must become familiar with specific recommendations of various manufacturers regarding the appropriate time for a woman to start her pills. Wyeth, for example, recommends starting Triphasils on day 1 of menses; others design their packs for initiation on day 5 or the first Sunday after menses begins. Recent data show the most reliable inhibition of ovulation when pills are started on the first day of the menstrual cycle (Killick, Eyong, & Elstein, 1987). This may be difficult to implement, however, because of packages that are designed for a Sunday start. Generally, the literature suggests the following options for initiation of OCs (Fraser & Jansen, 1983; Hatcher et al., 1984):

- *Days 1 or 2:* No backup method required.
- *Day 5 after menses:* Backup method suggested with low-dose formulations.
- *First Sunday after menses:* This may be a problem for women with history of 21-day cycles. Ovulation may occur on day 7. It takes OCs 48 hours to reach adequate blood hormone levels that effectively suppress ovulation. If the first Sunday falls on day 5 to 7, this may not be accomplished. Backup method is suggested for the first 1 to 3 months.
- *Anytime:* Initiation of OCs is recommended anytime, especially for women with history of irregular cycles. Pregnancy must be ruled out and no other contraindications apparent. Back-up method suggested.
- *Postdelivery:* Because of the increased risk of thromboembolism, experts recommend waiting at least 3 weeks before initiating OCs.
- *Lactating women:* Steroid hormones have been found in small amounts within breast milk of lactating women using OCs. Most data do not support negative effects to the newborn. Combined OCs are associated with decreased milk supply and subsequent slow weight gain of the infants involved. This is more apparent if the steroids are started before postpartum day 90 (Croxalto, Diaz, Peralta, et al., 1983; Peralta, Diaz, Juez, et al., 1983). Progestin-only pills (or minipills) do not appear to affect milk supply. Pedia-

tricians generally caution against the use of combined OCs by breastfeeding women and recommend use of minipills. Adverse effects in newborns have not been found with minipills, but data in this area are sparse and cannot be considered conclusive. If OCs are the only option, they should not be started before the 90th postpartum day, and close infant follow-up for adequate weight gain and neurologic development is recommended (American Academy of Pediatrics, 1981).
- *Postabortion:* After a first-trimester procedure, the risk of thromboembolism is low, whereas the possibility of ovulation within the first 14 days is high. OCs should be started immediately, or within 7 days of this procedure. If this is not done, they should be started with the first menses. Midtrimester abortions may carry the same risks as a full-term pregnancy. Therefore, OCs should not be started until 3 to 4 weeks later.

Teaching and Counseling. Time spent teaching and counseling will improve patient satisfaction and efficacy and safety of oral contraceptive use. Assessment of each woman's understanding of all that is taught is essential. The mechanism of action of oral contraceptives should be reviewed with all women who choose this method of birth control. The systemic nature of pill use and the many side effects associated with OCs should be discussed. The suppression of ovulation and menses should be described and an explanation of what monthly withdrawal bleeding entails should be provided.

Help each woman to choose an appropriate time to start her pills based on her particular situation and the specific pill involved. Encourage her to keep the pills out of the reach of children and animals. Review sequencing of pills with her so that confusion is eliminated regarding which pill to take; this is especially important with the new triphasics. The following instructions can be used or adapted for patient handouts regarding the specifics of pill use.

1. Take one pill by mouth each day at about the same time to maintain constant hormonal potency within the bloodstream. It may help to associate pill taking with another routine such as going to bed, brushing your teeth, or eating supper.
2. If you are using 21-day pills, you must stop taking the pills for 7 days between packs. Expect a "period" during this time. If it does not come and you have not missed any pills, begin your next pack on schedule.
3. If you are using 28-day pills, continue until the pack is completed and go directly to a new pack without missing a day. Expect your "period" during the last seven pills. If it does not come and you have not missed any pills, begin your next pack on schedule.
4. Use a backup method of birth control for the first 1 to 3 months if recommended. You should keep this method handy during this time and in case you miss pills.
5. If you miss one pill, take it as soon as you remember OR take two at your regular time. Pregnancy is unlikely, but breakthrough bleeding is possible. Keep a record of spotting and bleeding. Use a backup method for extra protection for the duration of the cycle.
6. If you miss two pills, take two as soon as you remember and then two the following day. For example, if you miss the Sunday and Monday night pills

and do not notice this until Tuesday, take two then and another two Wednesday night. Remember, doubling up is not as effective in preventing pregnancy. If you have sex around that time, you may become pregnant although this is unlikely. Use a backup method for the rest of the month and record any breakthrough bleeding.

7. If you miss three pills in a row, consider the following: ''Is this a good method for me?'' ''Is missing the pill a pattern of mine?'' ''Do I really want to be pregnant?'' Your chances of pregnancy are greater. It may be wiser for you to consider another method of birth control. If you want to continue the pills, you should do either of two things: (a) throw the pack away and use a backup method. Start a new pack with your next ''period,'' as before. You may have already started this bleeding when you realize that you have missed three pills. Continue a backup for the first 2 weeks. (b) ''double up'' for 3 days and use a backup method for the remainder of the cycle.

8. If you miss one period after missing one or more pills in a pack, you may be pregnant. Stop the pills or do not start a new pack of pills. Use an alternate method of birth control. Contact your care provider to have a pelvic exam and pregnancy test.

9. If you miss two periods in a row without missing any pills, you may be pregnant. Stop or do not restart a new pack. Use an alternative method of birth control and contact your care provider for a pelvic exam and pregnancy test. (It is important to inform women that the controversy still exists regarding possible teratogenic effects of OCs when taken during pregnancy.)

10. Notify any other health care providers that you are on the birth control pill. Several common drugs, such as antibiotics, may make the pill less effective. You may need to use a backup method or another method of birth control for the duration of other drug therapy.

11. If you have severe diarrhea or vomit 1 or 2 hours after taking the pill, you should take another pill. If the problem persists, use a backup method and contact your health care provider for advice.

12. Many women starting low-dose pills experience some light spotting or bleeding between periods for up to 3 months. This is normal. Your body is adjusting to the external hormones. It does not mean that your pills are ineffective. Do not stop the pills; continue to take them regularly. Use panty shields as necessary. Record amount, color, and duration of bleeding. Call for an appointment if it bothers you.

13. If you smoke, consider stopping! You are at increased risk of developing blood clots in your legs, a stroke, or a heart attack. Your risks further increase if you are over 30 years old.

14. If you want to become pregnant, you should stop the pill and use an alternative method for 3 to 6 months, or until you have at least three regular periods. Some women do not have a period immediately or soon after taking the pills. You can still become pregnant without seeing your period and it may be difficult to calculate your due date.

15. After using the pill, some women take longer to get pregnant than women who have not used the pill. If you are trying to become pregnant and have not conceived within 15 months of stopping the pill, contact your care provider for advice.

16. Be sure to eat a well-balanced diet while taking the pill.

17. It is advisable to do regular exercise such as aerobics, jogging, or swimming 30 to 35 minutes a day, at least three times a week.

18. Some women experience side effects such as nausea, weight gain, mild headaches, increased vaginal infections, and depression. Some of these go away after the first few months. Do not stop the pill! If these side effects bother you, call for an appointment.

19. Do not take other women's pills! The strength may be different. You could become pregnant or experience other side effects. Pills are usually prescribed for the individual woman.

20. If you plan major surgery requiring immobilization, call for an appointment. It is advisable to stop the pills four weeks before the surgery, and use an alternative method for two weeks after.

21. Call for your next appointment at the end of your next-to-last pack of pills so that you don't run out.

22. Know the pill's danger signs. If you develop any, stop the pills and come in to be seen immediately!

Danger Signs	Possible Problems
Severe or frequent headaches or headaches that persist after usual treatments (such as rest and/or over-the-counter pain medications)	Stroke, hypertension (increased blood pressure), migraine
Blurred vision, flashing lights, spots before eyes, temporary loss of vision	Stroke, hypertension
Severe chest pain and/or shortness of breath	Heart attack, pulmonary embolism (blood clot in the lungs)
Severe leg pain or redness, tenderness, warmth, or swelling of the leg	Thrombophlebitis (inflammation of the vein with a blood clot)
Severe abdominal pain	Gallbladder disease, liver tumor, pancreatitis, hepatic adenoma (benign liver tumor)
Temporary numbness or paralysis of any part of the body	Stroke, hypertension
Severe swelling of fingers, hands, ankles, or face	Stroke, hypertension, heart disease
Yellowing of skin	Liver tumor
Missed periods	Pregnancy
Severe depression	Vitamin B_6 deficiency

Return Visits. Timing of return visits after initiation of method varies among practitioners:

- 3 months, 3 months, 6 months, then annually
- 6 weeks, 3 months, every 6 months
- 3 months, then every 6 months

Some practitioners/clinics perform Pap smears every 6 months, however, annual smears are sufficient if the woman has a history of negative results and no additional risk factors (see Chapter 13).

Interval History	LMP, PMP
	Determine character and compare pattern prior to OC use. Note changes in family or personal medical surgical history, woman's/partner's satisfaction with method.
	History of use of OCs, and desire to continue/reason for discontinuing.

Physical Exam

Signs of complications and major side effects.

Assess patient's knowledge

Other side effects

Use of other medications, emergency room visits, etc.

Patient questions/concerns

Blood pressure, weight, breast, abdomen, lower extremities

Heart and lungs should be evaluated if patient complains of chest pain or shortness of breath

Complete pelvic assessment

(All physical exam components except blood pressure may be deferred at the first-interval visit if it is scheduled 6 weeks after pill initiation.)

Routine Laboratory Tests

Pap smear, wet smear as necessary, *C. trachomatis* culture or screening test if suspected. Complete physical exam and repeat of initial-visit labs and other more extensive lab work, as necessary, should be performed at annual visit.

MANAGEMENT OF SIDE EFFECTS AND COMPLICATIONS. If a woman presents with serious side effects or develops a disease that contraindicates OC use, stop the pill immediately and consult your physician backup as necessary for appropriate testing and followup. Provide an alternative method of birth control with instructions. For relatively minor side effects, determine their onset in relation to the length of OC use and timing in each cycle. Also note duration, intensity, and worsening. Try to determine the hormonal etiology of the problem (see Table 7–5). Nonpill-related differential diagnoses must be ruled out. It is also important to rule out other risk factors that might alter the course of the problem for a particular woman. If underlying pathology or other contributing factors are eliminated, the problem may be solved by switching to another pill formulation. In general, a switch to a higher potency drug may be made any time in the cycle, without need for backup. Assist women to switch packs without changing pill efficacy. It may be less confusing to switch at the start of a new cycle. In a change to a lower dose, the switch is best accomplished at the start of a new cycle, with a backup method provided for the first 2 weeks. If the change involves switching from a 28- to a 21-day regimen or vice versa, provide appropriate counseling (see previously). In some cases, the etiology of the specific problem may be difficult to determine, and intervention involves trial and error. The cause can sometimes be identified retrospectively, depending on whether pill manipulation was successful.

Differential Diagnosis and Interventions

Sign or Symptom	Possible Causes and Management (always take a careful history to determine)
Spotting/BTB	Normal adaptation to OCs, first 2 to 3 months: provide anticipatory guidance. Incorrect use of pill: provide patient teaching. Drug interaction: provide backup method, counseling (see Table 7–2). Other pathology, for example, fibroids, polyps: follow up appropriately. Estrogen deficiency, early bleeding, first 10 days: despite this etiology, most authors suggest first trying to increase progestin; if that does not work, increase estrogen to 50 μg; for example, if woman is using Ortho-Novum 7/7/7, first try Lo-Ovral 1/35 with stronger progestin or Ortho-

Novum 1/35 which has a consistent higher dosage of the same progestin; if that does not work, switch to Ortho-Novum 1/50.

Progestin deficiency, late bleeding, second 10 days: first increase progestin potency, then try increasing estrogen as above.

Amenorrhea	Suspected pregnancy: confirm by bimanual and pregnancy test; provide counseling and appropriate referral. Incorrect use of OC, that is, failure to stop 7 days on 21-day cycle: provide counseling. Drug interaction: see Table 7–2 for suggested management. Estrogen deficiency, especially in low-dose preparations: first try to increase endometrial activity (see Table 7–1); switch to a more potent progestin; if that does not work, increase estrogen to 50 μg.
Hypertension	Underlying pathology: provide referral and follow-up. OC induced, may be related to both estrogen and progestin: decrease estrogen component or switch to minipills and reevaluate 2 to 4 weeks later. If severe (diastolic greater than 100) or if other risk factors exist (smoking, obesity, headaches, or visual disturbances), stop OCs and provide another method. Consult as necessary.
Weight Gain	Suspected pregnancy: confirm by bimanual and pregnancy test. Provide counseling and appropriate referral. Anabolism as a result of progestin excess: decrease progestin potency. Increased subcutaneous tissue as a result of estrogen excess: decrease estrogen component. Cyclic weight gain worsening late in the cycle as a result of estrogen and fluid retention: decrease estrogen. Overeating: take history to assess other causes. Provide counseling and referral as necessary. Decrease progestin component.
Depression	Chronic depression: provide counseling and referral. Life causes, stress: provide counseling and appropriate referral. Estrogen or progestin excess: consider minipill. Estrogen deficiency: increase estrogen. Vitamin B$_6$, 25 mg daily, may improve the problem. If severe, stop OCs and observe; provide support and referral.
Headaches	Tension, unrelated to OC use, characterized by gradual increase in intensity without throbbing, usually bilateral in back of head and neck or temples: provide referral as necessary. Migraine—vascular spasms, usually unilateral and progressive in intensity, throbbing, nausea, dizziness; possibly numbness of leg and visual disturbances: stop OCs and provide another method; women may be predisposed to CVA. Reevaluate within 4 weeks. Fluid retention, estrogen excess associated with edema of leg, abdomen, breast tenderness and increased weight: consider use of minipill and reevaluate within 4 weeks.
Chloasma	Addison's disease: provide referral and follow-up. Pregnancy related: rule out pregnancy; provide appropriate referral. Estrogen excess: decrease estrogen component, consider minipill. Advise avoidance of direct sunlight. Counsel that it may be permanent.

TEACHING AND COUNSELING AT RETURN VISITS. Correct misinformation regarding use of method or side effects. Review danger signs. Provide sufficient cycles to cover length of next interval plus 1 month. Review use of backup method as necessary.

PROGESTIN ONLY MINIPILL

"Minipill" preparations eliminate estrogen and contain low quantities of progestin. Three minipills are currently available: Orvette, Nor Q.D., and Micronor.

Mechanism of Action

Minipills act by thickening cervical mucus, inhibiting capacitation, decreasing ovum transport, inhibiting implantation, and inhibiting ovulation.

Ovulation may occur in 40 percent of women on minipills; 21 percent have defective luteal function, while 39 percent are anovulatory. The other actions of progestins play a major role in preventing successful pregnancy (Graham & Fraser, 1982).

Effectiveness

Theoretically, minipills are less effective than the combined brands. Nor Q.D. and Micronor have a failure rate of 3.75 per 100 women, while Orvette has a slightly lower failure rate, 1.1 per 100 women. The 0.075 mg. of norgestrel in Orvette is more potent than the 0.35 mg of norethindrone in the other two brands.

Contraindications

Although the FDA recommends that the same absolute contraindications for combined OCs be followed for minipills, it remains unclear if there is actually an increased risk for development of hypertension and thromboembolic disease for women using minipills (Hatcher et al., 1984). Other strong relative contraindications include:

- Undiagnosed vaginal bleeding. If this occurs in older women particularly, it may be a sign of serious pathology. Minipills are frequently associated with irregular bleeding and may confuse the diagnosis.
- Acute mononucleosis
- History of irregular menses
- History of ectopic pregnancy

Complications

- Irregular menses, decreased duration and amount of menstrual flow, spotting, amenorrhea
- Headaches, less common than with combined OCs
- Hirsutism, edema
- Alteration in liver function tests—uncommon

Benefits

- decreased incidence of dysmenorrhea
- decreased total blood loss
- decreased PID related to *N. gonorrhoeae*

Management

Absolute and relative contraindications should be ruled out and, as with combined OCs, good history/physical exam and appropriate laboratory work obtained. Minipills may be beneficial to women desiring oral contraceptives who are 35 or older, and have a history of hypertension, severe varicosities, or migraine headaches, or who are lactating. Initiation is best on days 1 to 2 of the menstrual cycle, however, a woman can begin at any time.

Instructions to Women on Minipills

1. Be extra careful not to miss a day. Since your pills contain only small amounts of progestin, if you skip a pill you may ovulate and become pregnant.
2. If you miss one pill, double up the next day and use a backup method for the rest of the cycle. Return for a pelvic exam and pregnancy test if your period is late.
3. If you miss two pills in a row take one as soon as you remember, and also take your pill for that day. "Double up" the next day OR double up for 2 days to catch up. Be sure to use a backup method for the rest of the month, and return for a pelvic exam and pregnancy test if your period is late.
4. Most women experience spotting between periods and/or a decrease in the amount of menstrual flow. Wear panty liners as necessary. Your periods may become irregular. Some women do not have a period for 1 to 2 years while using this method. These side effects are normal and do not mean that the pills are not effective. If they bother you, call for an appointment. Keep a record of bleeding/spotting. If you do not have a period for 45 days, call to schedule a pelvic exam and pregnancy test. Remember to continue the pill. The likelihood of pregnancy is great if you stop. Do not stop pills without using a reliable alternative method of birth control.
5. Use a backup method of birth control for the first 2 to 3 months of minipill use.
6. Other side effects may include depression, irritability, and decreased sex drive. Call for an appointment; you may need a different pill.
7. Learn pill danger signs (these are the same as for combined OCs).
8. Return visits are conducted and timed similar to those for combined OCs.

POSTCOITAL ORAL CONTRACEPTION

The need for postcoital contraception will exist as long as people remain sexually active without reliable birth control. Adolescents, in particular, tend to have less knowledge and access to contraception and yet are sexually active in large numbers. Many women choose postcoital contraception in an attempt to avoid abortion. Diethylstilbestrol (DES) was a popular option for women desiring postcoital contraception, until its approval was withdrawn by the FDA because of possible teratogenic effects on infants after method failure. Dosages ranged from 25 to 50 mg of DES, the daily equivalent of 0.5 to 2.0 mg of ethinyl estradiol, for 5 days beginning within 72 hours of unprotected coitus.

Recent investigators (Van Santen & Hospels, 1985; Yuzpe, Smith, & Rademaker, 1982) have used Ovral for successful postcoital contraception. Two tablets are administered within 72 hours of a single act of unprotected coitus and repeated 24 hours later. Women receive a total of 200 mg of ethinyl estradiol and 2 mg of levonorgestrel. Reported failure rates vary from 0.16 to 1.6 percent. This compares favorably to those achieved with DES. The method appears particularly effective for women with a history of regular menses who are exposed to a single episode of unprotected coitus and take the first two tablets within 24 hours. According to studies, 98 percent of women bleed within 21 days of therapy. Mechanisms of action may include decreased motility of sperm and alterations in uterine contractions both inhibiting implantation; and subtle changes affecting either ovarian secretion of endogenous hormones or the endometrium directly (Ling, Wrixon, Acorn, et al., 1983).

Although the total dosage of hormones is less than with DES therapy or with one complete cycle of Ovral, there are some risks and side effects involved. At least one case of ectopic pregnancy has been reported, presumably related to decreased motility of sperm (Kubba, 1983). Nausea and vomiting occur in 37 and 39 percent of women, respectively; breast tenderness occurs in 12 to 14 percent of cases. Concurrent use of antiemetics may be initiated, however, this increases the incidence of breast tenderness (Van Santen & Hospels, 1985). Postpill amenorrhea is reported in three percent of women. There is no clear evidence of harm to offspring or women if this method fails. For years, many practitioners have informed women using Ovral regularly to double up for 2 days if two consecutive pills are missed. More research, however, remains to be done before FDA approval for routine use of Ovral as a postcoital method is obtained.

Instructions to Women

The following instructions must be covered before postcoital contraception is initiated.

1. Emergency nature of postcoital contraception, side effects, and potential risks to self and offspring if the method fails
2. Signs and symptoms of ectopic pregnancy
3. What to do if vomiting occurs within 1 to 2 hours after taking the pills (additional tablets may be needed; women should be encouraged to call for advice)
4. What to do if there is no period within 4 weeks (women should be advised to call for a pelvic exam and pregnancy test as this may indicate continued pregnancy)
5. Use of a backup method until menses
6. Contraceptive counseling with the provision of a more reliable and consistent method; excellent opportunity for positive intervention regarding family planning

SELF-HELP MEASURES

The following can be easily implemented by women and may help to avoid some side effects or pill dangers. These measures are advised for all OC users.

1. Participate in moderate aerobic exercise 30 to 35 minutes a day, 3 times per week.
2. Maintain a balanced diet.
3. Follow routine measures to avoid vaginitis, that is, wear cotton underwear, practice good hygiene, add yogurt to diet, avoid tight or wet clothing.
4. Become familiar with the danger signs and report them immediately to a care provider.
5. Keep a backup method of birth control available and be familiar with its use.
6. Report signs of pelvic discomfort or have partner(s) report urinary burning to his (their) care provider(s).

7. Discuss any minor problems with the care provider before stopping the pill.
8. Relax and enjoy the high degree of efficacy provided by use of the pills.

REFERENCES

American Academy of Pediatrics Committee On Drugs. (1981, July). Breast feeding and contraceptives. *Pediatrics, 68*(1), 138–140.

Back D., Breckenridge, A., Crawford, F., et al. (1981, January). Interindividual variation and drug interactions with hormonal steroid contraceptives. *Drugs, 21*(1), 46–61.

Bonnar, J., & Sabra, A. M. (1986, June). Oral contraceptives and blood coagulation. *Journal of Reproductive Medicine 31*(6, Suppl.), 551–556.

Boston Collaborative Drug Surveillance Program. (1973, June 23). Oral contraceptives and venous thromboembolic disease, surgically confirmed gallbladder disease and breast tumors. *Lancet I*(7817), 1399–1404.

Briggs, M. (1983, January). A randomized prospective study of the metabolic effects of four low-estrogen oral contraceptives. *The Journal of Reproductive Medicine 28*(1, Suppl.), 92–99.

Brooks, P. G. (1984, July). The relationship of estrogen and progesterone to breast disease. *Journal of Reproductive Medicine 29*(7, Suppl.), 530–538.

Centers for Disease Control (CDC) and Steroid Hormone Study. (1983a, March 25). Long-term oral contraceptive use and the risk of breast cancer. *Journal of the American Medical Association 249*(12), 1591–1595.

Centers for Disease Control (CDC) and Steroid Hormone Study. (1983b, March 25). Oral contraceptive use and the risk of endometrial cancer. *Journal of the American Medical Association 249*(12), 1600–1604.

Centers for Disease Control (CDC) and Steroid Hormone Study. (1983c, March 25). Oral contraceptive use and the risk of ovarian cancer. *Journal of the American Medical Association 249*(12), 1596–1599.

Connell, E. B. (1984, July). Oral contraceptives—the current risk benefits ratio. *The Journal of Reproductive Medicine 29*(7, Suppl.), 513–523.

Contraceptive Technology Update (CTU) (1980–1982). Choices, benefits and risks of oral contraceptives. Selected articles from *CTU Monthly Newsletter* D. Knowles, (ed.), with major contributions from R. Hatcher, M.D., M.P.H.

Croxalto, H. B., Diaz, S., & Peralta, O., et al. (1983, January). Fertility regulation in nursing women: IV. Long-term influence of a low dose combined oral contraceptive initiated at day 30 postpartum upon lactation and infant growth. *Contraception 27*(1), 13–25.

Dickey, R. (1984). *Managing contraceptive pill patients* (4th ed.) Oklahoma: Creative Infomatics, Inc.

Forman, D., Doll, R., & Peto, R. (1983, September). Trends in mortality from carcinoma of the liver and the use of oral contraceptives. *British Journal of Cancer 48*(3), 349–354.

Forman, D., Vincent, T. J., & Doll, R. (1986, May 24). Cancer of the liver and the use of oral contraceptives. *British Medical Journal 292*(6523), 1357–1361.

Fotherby, K. (1985, April). Oral contraceptives, lipids and cardiovascular disease. *Contraception 31*(4), 369–391.

Fraser, I., & Jansen, R. (1983, June). Mechanism of action of oral contraceptives. *Contraception 27*(6), 535–551.

Goldbaum, G. M., Kendrick, J. S., Hogelin, G. C., & Gentry, E. M. (1987, September 11). The relative impact of smoking and oral contraceptive use on women in the United States. *Journal of the American Medical Association 258*(10), 1339–1342.

Goldzieher, J. (1986, June). Use and misuse of the term potency with respect to oral contraceptives. *The Journal of Reproductive Medicine 31*(6, Suppl.), 535–551.

Goldzieher, J., Dozier, T., & de la Pena, A. (1980, January). Plasma levels and pharmacokinetics of ethinyl estrogens in various populations. II: Mestranol. *Contraception 21*(1), 17–27.

Graham, S., & Fraser, I. (1982, October). The progestogen only mini-pill. *Contraception 26*(4), 373–385.

Gray, P., Harding, E., & Dale, E. (1983, April). Effects of oral contraceptives on serum lipid profiles of women runners. *Fertility and Sterility 39*(4), 510–514.

Hatcher, R. A., Guest, F., & Stewart, F., et al. (1984). *Contraceptive Technology 1984–85* (12th rev. ed.), New York: Irvington Publishers, Inc.

Hatcher, R. A., Guest, F., & Stewart, F., et al. (1986). *Contraceptive Technology 1986–87* (13th rev. ed.), New York: Irvington Publishers, Inc.

Janerich, D., Piper, J., & Glebatis, D. (1980, July). Oral contraceptives and birth defects. *American Journal of Epidemiology 112*(1), 73–79.

Jick, H., Westerholm, B., & Vessey, M., et al. (1969, March 15). Venous thromboembolic disease and ABO blood type. *Lancet 1*(7594), 539–542.

Kannell, R. G. (1984, September). Oral contraceptives: the risks in perspective. *Nurse Practitioner 9*(9), 25–29, 62.

Kay, C. (1982, March 15). Progestogens and arterial disease-evidence from the Royal College of General Practitioners' study. *American Journal of Obstetrics and Gynecology 142*(6, Part 2), 762–765.

Kay, C. R., & Hannaford, P. C. (1988). Breast cancer and the pill—A further report from the Royal College of General Practitioners' oral contraception study. *British Journal of Cancer, 58,* 675–680.

Killick, S., Eyong, E., & Elstein, M. (1987, September). Ovarian follicular development in oral contraceptive cycles. *Fertility and Sterility 48*(3), 409–413.

Kubba, A. (1983, November 5). Case of ectopic pregnancy after postcoital contraception with ethinyl oestradiol–levongestrol. *British Medical Journal 287*(6402), 1343–1344.

Lammer, E. J., & Cordero, J. F. (1986, June 13). Exogenous sex hormone exposure and the risk for major malformations. *Journal of the American Medical Association 255*(22), 3128–3132.

Larsson-Cohn, U., Fahraeus, L., G. Wallentin, L., & Lador, G. (1981, February). Lipoprotein changes may be minimized by proper composition of a combined oral contraceptive. *Fertility and Sterility 35*(2), 172–178.

Ling, W., Wrixon, W., & Acorn, T., et al. (1983, November). Mode of action of d1-norgestrel and ethinyl estradiol combination in postcoital contraception. III: effect of pre-ovulatory administration following the luteinizing hormone surge on ovarian steroidogenesis. *Fertility and Sterility 40*(5), 631–635.

Linn, S., Schoenbaum, S. C., & Monson, R. R., et al. (1983, December). Lack of association between contraceptive usage and congenital malformations in offspring. *American Journal of Obstetrics and Gynecology 147*(8), 923–928.

Linn, S., Schoenbaum, S. C., & Monson, R. R., et al. (1982, February 5). Delay in contraception for former pill users. *Journal of the American Medical Association 247*(5), 629–632.

Medical Letter. (1983, July 22). Oral contraceptives and the risk of cardiovascular disease. *Medical Letter on Drugs and Therapy 25*(640), 69–70.

Medical News. (1980, August 15). Folate for oral contraceptive users may reduce cervical cancer risk. *Journal of the American Medical Association 244*(7), 633.

Miller, D. R., Rosenberg, L., & Kaufman, D. W., et al. (1989, February). Breast cancer before age 45 and oral contraceptive use: new findings. *American Journal of Epidemiology, 129*(2), 269–280.

Mishkel, M. (1986, June). Metabolic effects of oral contraceptives: a panel discussion. *Journal of Reproductive Medicine 31*(6), 569–572.

National Women's Health Network. (1989, February 23). Recommended guidelines on birth control pills. Washington, D.C.: National Women's Health Network.

Neuberger, J., Forman, D., Doll, R., & Williams, R. (1986, May 24). Oral contraceptives and hepatocellular carcinoma. *British Medical Journal 292*(6532), 1355–1357.

Nora, J., Nora, A., & Blu, J., et al. (1978, September 1). Exogenous progestins and estrogens implicated in birth defects. *Journal of the American Medical Association 240*(9), 837–843.

Ory, H. (1983). Mortality associated with fertility and fertility control. *Family Planning Perspectives 15*(2), 52–63.

Ory, H., Layde, P., & Schlesselman, J. (1982, March/April). The risk of myocardial infarction in former users of oral contraceptives. *Family Planning Perspectives 14*(2), 72–81.

Ory, H., Rosenfield, A., & Landman, L. (1980, November/December). The pill at 20: an assessment. *Family Planning Perspectives 12*(6), 278–283.

Pasquale, S. (1984). Sound rationale for a triphasic oral contraceptive. *The Journal of Reproductive Medicine 29*(7), 560–567.

Peralta, O., Diaz, S., & Juez, G. (1983, January). Fertility regulation in nursing women. V: long-term influence of low dose combined oral contraceptives initiated at day 90 postpartum upon lactation and infant growth. *Contraception 27*(1), 27–38.

Powell, M., Hedlin, A. M., & Cerskus, I., et al. (1984, June). Effects of oral contraceptives on lipoprotein lipids: a prospective study. *Obstetrics and Gynecology 63*(6), 764–770.

Rooks, J., Ory, H., & Ishak, K., et al. (1979, August). Epidemiology of hepatocellular adenoma—the role of oral contraceptive use. *Journal of the American Medical Association 242*(7), 644–648.

Rosenfield, A. (1983, October) The pill's many non–contraceptive benefits. *Contemporary Ob/Gyn 22*(4), 136–154.

Roy, S. (1986, June). Effects of oral contraceptives on cholesterol. *The Journal of Reproductive Medicine 31*(6), 546–548.

Royal College of General Practitioners' (RCGP) Oral Contraceptive Study. (1981, March 7). Further analysis of mortality in oral contraceptive users. *Lancet 1*(8219), 541.

Royal College of General Practitioners' (RCGP) Oral Contraceptive Study. (1982, October 30). Oral contraceptives and gallbladder disease. *Lancet II*(8305), 957–959.

Royal College of General Practitioners' (RCGP) Oral Contraceptive Study. (1978, March 18). Reduction in incidence of rheumatoid arthritis associated with oral contraceptives. *Lancet I*(8064), 569–571.

Smit Veninga, K. (1984, November/December). Effects of oral contraceptives on vitamins B_6, B_{12}, C and folacin. *Journal of Nurse-Midwifery 129*(6), 386–390.

Spellacy, W. (1982, March 15). Carbohydrate metabolism during treatment with estrogen, progestogen and low dose oral contraceptives. *American Journal of Obstetrics and Gynecology 142*(6, Part 2), 732–734.

Speroff, L., Glass, R. H., & Kase, N. G. (1983). *Clinical Gynecologic Endocrinology and Infertility* (3rd ed.). Baltimore: Williams & Wilkins Co.

Stadel, V. B., Lai, S., Schlesselman, J. J., & Murray, P. (1988, September). Oral contraceptives and premenopausal breast cancer in nulliparous women. *Contraception, 38*(3), 287–299.

Stubberfield, P. (1984, July). Oral contraceptives and neoplasia. *The Journal of Reproductive Medicine 29*(7, Suppl.), 524–527.

Svensson, L., Mårdh, P.-A., & Weström, L. (1983, September). Infertility after acute salpingitis with special reference to *Chlamydia trachomatis. Fertility and Sterility 40*(3), 322–329.

Tyrer, L. B. (1984a, July). Oral contraception for the adolescent. *The Journal of Reproductive Medicine 29*(7, Suppl.), 551–559.

Tyrer, L. B. (1984b, July). Nutrition and the pill. *The Journal of Reproductive Medicine 29*(7, Suppl.), 547–550.

Van Santen, M. R., & Hospels, A. A. (1985, March). Intercept II. Postcoital low dose estrogen and norgestrel combination in 633 women. *Contraception 31*(3), 275–293.

Vessel, M. P., Lawless, M., McPherson, K., & Yeates, D. (1983, October 22). Neoplasia of the cervix uteri and contraception: a possible adverse effect of the pill. *Lancet 2*(8356), 930–934.

Walnut Creek Contraceptive Drug Study. (1980, December). A prospective study of the side effects of oral contraceptives. *The Journal of Reproductive Medicine 25*(6, Suppl.), 245.

Washington, A. E., Gove, S., Schachter, J., & Sweet, R. L. (1985, April 19). Oral contraceptives, *Chlamydia trachomatis* infection, and pelvic inflammatory disease: a word of caution about protection. *Journal of the American Medical Association 253*(15), 2246–2250.

Williams, R. S., Logue, E., & Lewis, J., et al. (1980, May 1). Physical conditioning augments the fibrolytic response to venous occlusion in healthy adults. *New England Journal of Medicine 302*(18), 987–991.

World Health Organization (WHO). (1985, September). A randomized double-blind study of the effects of two low-dose combined oral contraceptives on biochemical aspects: report from a seven-centered study. *Contraception 32*(3), 223–236.

Yuzpe, A., Smith, R., & Rademaker, A. (1982, April). A multicenter clinic investigation employing ethinyl estradiol combined with D_1-norgestrel as a postcoital contraceptive agent. *Fertility and Sterility 37*(4), 508–513.

8

Intrauterine Devices

Heather Clarke

Intrauterine devices (IUDs) were introduced into the United States in the 1960s and rapidly gained popularity because they provided women with a highly effective and "carefree" method of birth control. There is no need for daily or consistent use as with oral contraceptives or coitus-related barrier methods. Furthermore, these devices are cost effective, requiring only annual medical visits for long-term use. In 1980, 60 million women around the world used IUDs compared with 55 million using the pill. IUDs are now the most widely used method of effective birth control in the world (Hatcher, Guest, Stewart, et al., 1984).

Despite these notable contraceptive advantages, the safety of IUDs has been a controversial issue since their introduction. The well-documented risks of uterine perforation, septic abortion, and pelvic inflammatory disease (PID or salpingitis) with the subsequent risk of infertility have led to criticisms of IUD use from medical and lay people alike. Devices that have been found to pose the greatest risks have been withdrawn from the market by the Food and Drug Administration (FDA). These include the Dalkon Shield, withdrawn in 1974 because of a high incidence of midtrimester septic abortion, leading to ten maternal deaths; the Hall-Stone ring and Brinberg Bow because of an increased incidence of uterine perforation and strangulated bowels; and the Majzlin Spring because of its tendency to embed within the uterine wall.

Negative publicity has led to a gradual decrease in the use of IUDs in the United States, especially among nulliparous women who face the risk of primary infertility secondary to PID (Cramer, Schiff, Schoenbaum, et al., 1985; Daling, Weiss, Metch, et al., 1985). Julius Schmid, Inc. ceased marketing the Saf-T-Coil in 1982 primarily for economic reasons. More recently, Ortho Pharmaceuticals, which has been manufacturing Lippes Loops since they were approved by the FDA in 1962, stopped marketing them in the fall of 1985. Ortho also cited falling profits as the prime reason for its decision. This action came after two national studies published in April 1985 (Cramer et al., 1985; Daling et al., 1985) reported a higher incidence of PID and subsequent tubal infertility with the Lippes Loop compared with copper-containing devices ("Ortho Stops," 1985). Subsequent to these studies, the FDA proposed a rule, published in the August 1985 *Federal Register*, that would require companies wishing to manufacture intrauterine devices to submit a premarketing approval application. The FDA has asked for a detailed discussion with supporting clinical studies addressing the following concerns:

pelvic actinomycosis; tubal infertility; length of time the IUD should remain in place; and the safety of leaving the IUD in place when contraception is no longer needed, that is, after menopause.

In early 1986, G. D. Searle withdrew its intrauterine devices—the Copper 7200 and the Tatum T (or Copper T)—from the U.S. market. These pharmaceutical company decisions are rather unfortunate for women in the United States, as Lippes Loops were the only remaining nonmedicated IUDs on the market, and the Copper 7's and Tatum T's were the only available copper-containing devices. They are used by thousands of women for long-term or terminal birth control. As of this writing, the only available IUDs in the United States are the Progestasert (Fig. 8-1), a progesterone-containing device, and the Copper T380A, a copper-containing device, newly introduced in 1988 by the Population Council, a nonprofit international family planning organization, and marketed by GynePharma, Inc. under the brand name ParaGard (Fig. 8-2).

This chapter describes the types of IUDs available; their mechanisms of action, effectiveness, side effects, risks, and benefits; contraindications to their use; and management of IUD patient visits. Saf-T-Coils, Lippes Loops, and Copper 7's and Tatum T's are discussed as they are still available in many offices and clinics and can be inserted safely until their expiration date. It is also possible that they will be remarketed if the demand exists. These recent marketing decisions—unlike that involving the Dalkon Shield—are *not* product recalls requiring discontinuance of the product ("Searle's Decision," 1986).

TYPES

The basic material of all recently used IUDs is inert plastic polyethylene with a monofilament nylon tail that protrudes from the cervix into the vagina. The tail serves to ease removal, allow the woman to check periodically for the presence of the device, and allow the practitioner to visualize for uterine retention.

IUDs may be classified as medicated and nonmedicated. Medicated devices are those to which copper or progesterone has been added. The Copper T200 (or Tatum T) and Copper 7200, initially marketed by the Population Council and G.D. Searle in 1972 and 1978, respectively, are both reinforced with 200 mm^2 of copper wire along their vertical arms to enhance contraceptive efficacy. The Copper

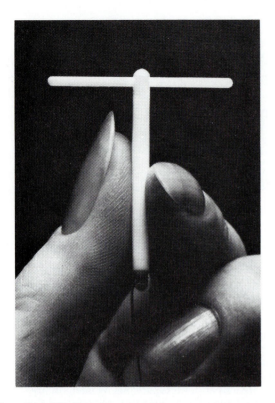

Figure 8–1. The Progestasert. *(Courtesy of the Alza Corporation.)*

T380A has a surface area of copper of 380 mm². The addition of copper has enabled the manufacturers to produce a smaller device that conforms better to uterine shape and configuration without significantly increasing the failure rate compared with other IUDs. In most clinical trials of women wearing the Copper T380A device, pregnancy rates were less than 1 percent after the first year of use (''Ortho Stops,'' 1985). This rate compares favorably with those for nonmedicated devices.

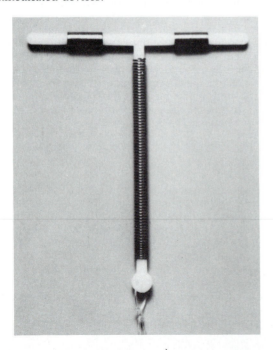

Figure 8–2. The Copper T380A. *(Courtesy of Gyne Pharma Inc.)*

Unfortunately, as the IUD's copper wire erodes over time, there is some question as to how long these devices can remain in place before their contraceptive efficiency decreases. Chantler, Scott, Filho, and associates (1984) found that although about one third of the IUD's copper is lost after 4 years of use, its rate of effectiveness did not appear altered. They still, however, recommend removal of the Copper T200 and Copper 7200 devices after 36 months of use because the rate of degradation of the copper wire increases thereafter. The Copper T380A has been approved by the FDA for 4 years (The Population Council, no date). Another Population Council device, the Copper T380AG is theoretically effective for many years because its copper wire contains a silver core that maintains the integrity of the copper over time. This device has not been approved in the United States. The Nova T, produced by G. D. Searle Company and readily available in other countries, also is highly effective and may prove to have longer-lasting effectiveness. The Nova T has barium sulfate added for radiopacity, and 200 mm² of copper on its vertical arm. Production of the reinforced copper devices was inhibited initially because of an apparent dispute regarding the patent rights between the two manufacturing companies (Copper T380A, 1985).

The Progestasert, marketed by Alza Corporation, has been available in the United States since 1976. The device is covered with a thin polymeric membrane that releases levonorgestrel into the endometrial cavity at the rate of 65 μg/24 hours. This addition of progesterone is thought to decrease the rates of failure, expulsion, and PID. The Progestasert, however, is the least studied of current devices. A major drawback to its widespread acceptance is that the levonorgestrel is significantly depleted after 12 months of use, necessitating annual removal and reinsertion.

MECHANISM OF ACTION

The exact mechanism of action of IUDs is unclear. Many experts agree that a number of factors contribute to IUD-induced infertility (Koch, 1980). Recent studies refute earlier findings indicating that the IUD acts mainly on the fertilized ovum or in prevention of implantation and suggest instead that the IUD prevents fertilization (Ortiz & Croxatto, 1987; Segal, Alvarez-Sanchez, Adejuwon, et al., 1985; Treiman & Liskin 1988; Videla-Rivero, Etchepareborda, & Kesseru, 1987). The following theories attempt to explain how contraception is achieved:

All IUDs

1. A prompt local inflammatory response is stimulated by the presence of a foreign body, with increased numbers of leukocytes, lymphocytes, plasma cells, and macrophages within the endometrial cavity (Moyer & Mishell, 1971; Sheppard, 1987). This may cause phagocytosis of sperm (Sağiroğlu, 1971).
2. Levels of prostaglandin (PG) in the endometrium and endometrial fluid are increased and, in turn, increase uterine contractibility, inhibiting implantation and/or disrupting the already implanted blastocyst (Tatum, 1977).
3. Mobility of the ovum in the fallopian tubes is increased.
4. Sperm transport is interfered with (Tredway, Umezaki, Mishell, & Settlage, 1975).

Additional Contraceptive Action of Copper-Releasing IUDs

5. The addition of copper significantly enhances the spermatocidal and spermatodepressive action of the IUD, immobilizing sperm as they pass through the uterine cavity.
6. Copper may inactivate enzymes, especially carbonic anhydrase and alkaline phosphatase, which are essential in reproductive physiology (Oster, 1972).
7. Copper may interfere with estrogen uptake within the endometrium, thereby inhibiting the intracellular changes necessary for implantation (Tatum, 1977).
8. Copper may cause precipitation of albumin leading to changes in the uterine wall unfavorable to implantation. The uterine secretions may also be affected in a manner that interferes with implantation (Oster, 1972).

Additional Contraceptive Action of Progesterone-Releasing IUDs

9. The progesterone released exerts a local effect within the endometrium. Ovarian function is not altered. Although many users of progesterone-releasing IUDs become amenorrheic, 75 percent continue to ovulate regularly even after 5 years of use (Nilsson, Lahteenmaki, & Luukkainen, 1984). It is theorized that the progesterone competes with estrogen receptors, thereby altering proliferative and secretory endometrial changes. Endometrial glands are poorly developed and atrophy. Stroma undergo diffuse predecidual changes and subsequent fibrosis. Implantation cannot take place in this negative environment. In addition, progesterone may also decrease the alkaline phosphatase activity of the sperm (Wan, Hsu, Ganguly, & Bigelow, 1977).

EFFECTIVENESS

Theoretical effectiveness of IUDs is between 97 and 99 percent; user effectiveness is about 90 to 96 percent (Hatcher et al., 1984). Because the IUD is a relatively carefree method, there is little room for human error. This is reflected in the closeness of these two rates. Most IUD failures probably result from partial expulsion, insertion into the lower uterine segment, or displacement of the device (Perlmutter, 1978). High fundal placement at the time of insertion is the most essential factor for high efficacy of an IUD. This depends greatly on the ability of the practitioner to accurately sound the uterus and select a device that will adapt most appropriately to the uterine shape and size. Copper- and progesterone-containing devices have slightly lower failure rates, particularly among nulliparous women. The addition of medication and the size and configuration of these devices, which facilitate high fundal placement, lead to greater contraceptive efficacy. User effective rates increase if women are encouraged to use a backup method for the first month following insertion [Hatcher and co-authors (1984, p. 103) strongly recommend the use of a backup for the first 3 months and at midcycle thereafter]; use self-help measures to tolerate the common initial side effects, and continue with the device; and feel for the string(s) periodically.

SIDE EFFECTS AND RISKS

As previously mentioned, a number of risks and side effects are associated with IUDs that decrease their attractiveness. Furthermore, many women have concerns about "having something inside of me." As health providers, it is important to understand the facts and present them to patients in a clear and nonjudgmental manner.

Bleeding and Anemia

The most frequent complaint among IUD users is heavier menstrual bleeding and/or spotting between periods. Incidence and severity are greatest immediately after insertion, and decrease after the first 3 months of use. Hatcher and associates (1984, p. 91) report that 15 percent of women who request removal of their IUDs do so because of this single side effect. Complaints include heavier and prolonged menstrual bleeding, spotting between menses, weakness, fatigue, and fainting. The primary cause of bleeding among IUD users is damage to the endometrium, resulting from abrasion or pressure exerted by the IUD. The amount of bleeding is less in the presence of the smaller copper devices. Local endometrial effects of the Progestasert further decrease the amount of menstrual bleeding experienced by users. According to Nilsson and associates (1984), many Progestasert users report longer menstrual cycles within 6 months of insertion with decreased blood flow, and 75 percent become amenorrheic after approximately 5 years of use.

Depletion of body iron stores and anemia can result from recurrent menstrual blood losses of 60 mL or greater (Goh, Hariharan, & Chan, 1984). Women using a copper device rarely experience anemia as heavy menstrual blood losses tend to taper off after the first year of use; anemia may be more commonly seen among those wearing a nonmedicated device, as heavy menstrual blood losses can continue through the duration of use. A recent study by Goh and associates (1984) confirms other findings that the Progestasert does not significantly decrease body iron stores. The Progestasert, therefore, may be an excellent choice for women who have a history of heavy menses and borderline anemia (hematocrit: 35 to 37 percent) and who desire an IUD. Unfortunately, this device is associated with a greater frequency of intermenstrual spotting. In their study involving 108 nulliparous and 84 parous women, Wan et al. (1977) reported that up to 56.5 percent of women wearing the Progestasert complained of spotting for the first 1 to 2 months after each insertion. The frequency of complaints decreases to 29.8 and 16.9 percent at 6 and 12 months, respectively. The spotting, which can last from 1 to 5 days, is the most common reason for discontinuation of the Progestasert.

Pain and Cramping

IUD users may complain of cramplike pain with discomfort in the lower abdomen and/or back. This is a frequent reason for removal of IUDs within the first year of use, secondary only to bleeding. Pain results from the contractions the uterus makes as it attempts to expel the foreign object. Cramping is usually strongest after insertion because of an immediate increase in local prostaglandin levels, which stimulate uterine contractions (Tatum, 1977). The frequency and intensity of cramps may decrease after 3 months as the uterus adapts, but often continue in a cyclic pattern with menses. Large, firm devices such as the Lippes Loop tend to cause more pain; smaller copper- or progesterone-containing IUDs adapt more readily to the uterine cavity, causing fewer contractions and less cramping.

Expulsion: Partial and Complete

If the uterus does not gradually adapt to the IUD, it may succeed in partially or completely expelling the foreign object. In a review of the literature, 5 to 20 percent of IUD users were reported to have expelled their devices within the first year of use (Hatcher et al., 1984). Losses are most likely to occur during the first 1 to 3 months of use, especially at the time of menses. Wan et al. (1977) found that among 192 Progestasert users, 77 percent of spontaneous expulsions occurred within the first month of use. Incomplete expulsions result in downward displacement of the IUD into the cervical canal. Clinical diagnosis of a partially expelled device is not difficult. The string lengthens into the vaginal vault, and, in many instances, the device itself can be visualized or palpated protruding from the os. Eventually, increased cervical stimulation results in strong expulsive forces from the entire uterus and complete expulsion commonly results. The diagnosis of complete expulsion can be made by ultrasound.

The rate of IUD expulsion is increased after postpartum insertion during which time the uterus is hypercontractible and involuting. It is therefore advisable to wait 6 to 8 weeks before attempting insertion. Some physicians, however, have found improved rates of postpartum retention with the insertion of a Copper T200 or Lippes Loop (Cole, McCann, Higgins, & Waszak, 1983; Cole, Edelman, Potts, et al., 1984; Stumpf & Lenker, 1984) that has been modified by adding two to three biodegradable sutures to the upper arms or loop of the devices, which are then called the Delta T and Delta Loop, respectively. This modification results in temporary embedding into the endometrium, enhancing retention. The sutures dissolve within 6 weeks. The devices are inserted as early as 10 minutes postpartum, but can be placed within 36 hours. Results are better if the devices are inserted high into the fundus by hand rather than forceps. The skill of the practitioner affects the efficacy of this technique.

Lactating women have a higher incidence of spontaneous IUD expulsions than those who bottle feed either following immediate postpartum insertion of a modified device or with insertion after 42 postpartum days (Cole et al., 1983, 1984). It is not until the sixth postpartum month that the differences in spontaneous expulsion between lactating and nonlactating women disappear.

Embedding

Continuous use of a nonmedicated IUD exceeding 5 years increases the risk of its embedding in the endometrium. Over time, as the device exerts pressure on the endometrial tissue, necrosis can result. With sustained pressure the device sinks deeper into the tissue. As the endometrium attempts to restore surface continuity it grows over the IUD. Usually this process is asymptomatic and may not be detected until removal of the device is attempted. With embedding, the risk of pregnancy is increased because the total surface area of the device is decreased. Removal is difficult and frequently accompanied by complaints of moderate to severe pain, as well as heavy bleeding (Tatum, 1977).

Perforations: Partial and Complete

An IUD may partially or completely perforate the uterine fundus or the cervix. Fundal perforations are most likely to occur at the time of insertion; cervical trauma can occur after downward displacement of a partially expelled device. Rates vary depending on the type of IUD, the technique of insertion, the skill of the practitioner, and uterine size, shape, consistency, and configuration. It is difficult to estimate the incidence rate because many perforations are not detected; however, rates in the literature range from 1 in 350 to 1 in 2,600 insertions (Heartwell & Schlesselman, 1983). According to Heartwell and Schlesselman, the relative risks (RR) for uterine perforation are not significantly different among various types of IUDs they studied, which included the Lippes Loop, Copper 7, and Copper T.

Perforations are more likely to be seen during the postpartum period, unless the device is inserted immediately or after 6 to 8 weeks. During the postpartum period, decreased serum estrogen leads to thinning of the endometrial walls, which, coupled with uterine hypercontractibility, increases the risk of uterine perforation after IUD insertion. In a study of 138 IUD users with a diagnosis of perforation requiring surgical removal, lactating women were found to have a tenfold increased risk for perforation over other IUD users. The higher rates were evident even if insertion took place after 8 weeks postpartum (Heartwell & Schlesselman, 1983).

Intrauterine embedding with subsequent difficult removal or pregnancy are among the major complications of partial perforation. With complete perforation, cases of IUDs trapped in the abdominal cavity with subsequent strangulation of an intestinal loop have been well documented.

String Problems

String complaints among IUD users include an inability to feel the string(s), lengthening or shortening of the string(s) and partner's being pinched by the string(s) during intercourse. Possible causes of the first two problems include partial or complete expulsion, pregnancy, upward movement of the device after the string was clipped too short, and fundal perforation. Many times, the string will be curled up within the cervical canal.

Hatcher and co-authors (1984, pp. 95–96) clearly point out some of the major problems with the string of the Copper 7. Its unique design places the string outside of the inserter barrel, where it poses the risk of upward bacterial invasion if contaminated during insertion. The string of the Copper 7 has also been shown to form a loop within the endometrial cavity at the time of insertion. If this loop slips down into the vagina, an incorrect diagnosis of partial expulsion may be made, and the device removed unnecessarily. On the other hand, if the device is partially expelled and the practitioner makes the assessment that the loop has slipped down and decides to leave the device in place, pregnancy and/or infection can result. Even if a correct diagnosis of the prolapsed loop of string is made, and the string is subsequently clipped, the loop can re-form within the uterine cavity, causing the string to shorten and disappear altogether. The practitioner is then faced with the problem of a lost string. Finally, if this loop becomes caught on the device, removal of the Copper 7 could be difficult.

Pregnancy

As IUDs do not prevent ovulation, pregnancy with an IUD in situ does occur. In a review of the literature Perlmutter (1978) found that IUD failure rates range from 0.0 to 5.6 per 100 woman-years, depending on the study and the device.

Copper-containing devices and the Progestasert have slightly lower failure rates than nonmedicated devices, probably because of their superior adaptation to the uterus. The risk of pregnancy increases if the device is inserted too low within the uterus, if it is inserted before the eighth postpartum week, if the uterus is too small (less than 6.5 cm) or too large (10 cm or greater), or if there has been partial or complete expulsion.

Women wearing nonmedicated devices have a higher incidence of pregnancy during the first 3 months after insertion; thereafter, the rate decreases with successive years. This decline in rate is absent with copper-containing devices. In fact, the majority of pregnancies reported in women using copper IUDs occur after 36 months of continuous use (Chantler et al., 1984). Efficacy of the Progestasert over a prolonged period has yet to be determined.

Pregnancy with an IUD in situ is one of the most serious complications for IUD users. The risk of spontaneous abortion is about 50 percent if the device is left in place and 25 percent if it is removed before 8 weeks of gestation. If history, pathologic findings, foul-smelling products of conception, and febrile morbidity are all considered signs of infection, then as many as 95 percent of spontaneous abortions with IUDs in situ may be accompanied by pelvic infection (Perlmutter, 1978). IUD users have up to a 50 times greater risk of developing sepsis than those who abort without an IUD. Ruptured membranes with foul-smelling odor are the usual presenting symptoms of septic abortion. The onset of sepsis usually begins with fever, chills, myalgia, and headaches. Pelvic or uterine symptoms may be absent. The course of the disease can be rapid, however. Some women who wore the Dalkon Shield died within 72 hours of onset of sepsis. Although the course is less rapid with other devices, maternal mortality is still possible.

Removal of the IUD as soon as possible is strongly advised if pregnancy occurs. Intrauterine pregnancy with an IUD in situ that continues to term is associated with higher rates of bleeding, amnionitis, premature labor, and stillbirth. There has been no increase in congenital anomalies documented among users of either copper or nonmedicated devices who have carried to term. Research regarding the Progestasert is more limited but so far no teratogenic effects have been reported. As this device releases progesterone, which is normally present at greater levels during pregnancy, rather than a synthetic progestin, it is theoretically unlikely that teratogenic damage would occur.

Another major complication of pregnancy with an IUD in situ is ectopic pregnancy. IUD users have a ten times greater risk over nonusers. The incidence of ectopic pregnancies among IUD users is 1 in 20 compared with 1 in 200 for nonusers (Perlmutter, 1978). Vessey, Yeates, and Flavel 1979) point out that the risk increases with duration of use. Most researchers support the theory that the increased incidence of ectopic pregnancies among IUD users reflects an actual *decrease* in the incidence of intrauterine pregnancies, rather than an increase in extrauterine gestations. A study by Vries, Shapiro, Degani, and co-workers (1983) confirmed that the IUD's most significant contraceptive effect occurs within the uterus, but that it is less effective in preventing conception within the fallopian tubes and virtually has no effect on the incidence of ovarian pregnancies. Therefore, the percentage of ectopic pregnancies among method failures automatically increases. Alteration in ovum or sperm movement through the tubes, however, does play an important role in increasing the rate of ectopic pregnancies among IUD users. If left undetected, a tubal or ovarian pregnancy eventually ruptures the confining space; the resulting hemorrhage and sepsis could be life threatening.

Pelvic Inflammatory Disease (PID)–Salpingitis and Infertility

PID (or salpingitis) currently accounts for the majority of IUD-related hospitalizations and deaths. Women wearing an IUD are nine times more likely to get PID than those not wearing one (Lee, Rubin, Ory, & Burkman, 1983). The risk varies according to the type of device. With the Dalkon Shield, the relative risk is 8.3 compared with nonusers. This risk is six and four times greater than those for users of copper-containing and Lippes Loop devices, respectively. Furthermore, the risk with the Dalkon Shield increases over time, but it decreases after the first 4 months with other devices (Lee et al., 1983).

Nulliparous women are at greater risk for developing PID and subsequent tubal infertility than are parous women. According to Weström, Bengtsson, and Mårdh (1976), nulliparous women who wear IUDs have a relative risk for developing PID of 6.8 compared with 1.7 among parous women who use IUDs. Among the factors increasing their risk are narrow cervical canals and smaller uteri, increasing the likelihood of trauma at the time of insertion and/or poor adaptation to the device. Therefore these women experience more partial expulsions and heavier menses—factors that may promote the development of PID.

Two large studies recently reported substantial evidence to link infertility with the use of IUDs. In a study of 159 nulliparous women with primary infertility, Daling and co-investigators (1985) found that 35 percent reported ever having used an IUD compared with 14 percent of fertile women chosen as matched controls. A history of smoking and, more significantly, multiple sexual partners were more prevalent among the infertile group. The relative risk of primary infertility among women with no prior history of PID [prior PID (PPID)] who ever used an intrauterine device was 2.6 compared with nonusers. Women who ever used a Dalkon Shield had the highest relative risk (6.8). Those who ever used a copper-containing device had the lowest (Table 8–1).

The other major study (Cramer et al., 1985) confirmed the findings suggesting that copper-containing devices held a significantly lower risk for both primary and secondary infertility associated with previous IUD use, regardless of age, number of sexual partners, duration of IUD use, or PPID (Table 8–2). In this study, parous women with secondary infertility who had ever used an inert device had a relative risk of 2.4 compared with a 1.6 relative risk among past users of copper devices. Women who discontinued their device within the first 3 months appeared to be at higher risk than women who wore them longer. Presumably, many of the reasons for removal shortly after insertion tended to be medical. Interestingly, among previous Lippes Loop users, the risk of tubal infertility decreased after the first 3 months of use, but gradually increased thereafter with each year of use. The single most important factor associated with increased risk of PID and subsequent tubal damage again found in this study is the number of sexual partners. This was true even among women with primary tubal infertility who never had used an IUD. Those with a history of multiple partners had a relative risk of 1.5 compared with IUD users with only one partner. Cramer and associates also found no significant difference in the risk between women who had PPID before using an IUD compared with women with negative histories for this condition.

The relationship of the Progestasert to PID is currently being studied. Soderstrom (1983) believes that it may de-

TABLE 8-1. RISK OF INFERTILITY BY IUD TYPE

IUD Type	Percentage That Used IUD		Adjusted Relative Risk
	Infertile Women (N = 159)	Fertile Women (N = 159)	
Ever used			
Any IUD	35.2	13.8	2.6
Dalkon Shield	14.5	2.5	6.8
Copper IUD	17.6	10.1	1.9
Lippes Loop/Saf-T-Coil	9.4	2.5	3.2
Only used			
Dalkon Shield	8.6	0.7	13.3
Copper IUD	12.1	8.6	1.3
Lippes Loop/Saf-T-Coil	7.1	0.7	4.5

(Adapted from Daling, J., Weiss, N. S., & Metch, B. J., et al. [1985]. Primary tubal infertility in relation to the use of an intrauterine device. New England Journal of Medicine, 312[15], 937–941. Reprinted with permission.)

crease the risk because of its quieting effect within the endometrium. Notably, menstrual blood loss and dysfunctional bleeding are decreased. Theoretically, the upward growth of bacteria is less likely. In support of this theory, Soderstrom found no microscopic evidence of endosalpingitis among 22 Progestasert users compared with a 49 percent incidence among 175 users of other devices, and a less than 1 percent incidence among 1,500 women who had never used an IUD. More research, however, is needed in this area.

Neisseria gonorrhoeae and *Chlamydia trachomatis* are two organisms commonly associated with the development of PID. Recently, *C. trachomatis* has been implicated as the most prevalent sexually transmitted disease (STD) and more likely to cause tubal damage than *N. gonorrhoeae*, because its mild clinical course is less frequently detected and treated. It appears that the use of an IUD and the presence of *C. trachomatis* have a synergistic effect leading to an increased risk of PID. As many as 76 percent of women with PPID and prior IUD use have evidence of *C. trachomatis* diagnosed on laparoscopy. The tubal damage tends to be bilateral (Gibson, Gump, Ashikaga, & Hall, 1984).

Colonization with *Actinomyces israelii*, a Gram-positive slow-growing bacteria, also occurs at a greater frequency in the presence of an IUD and is more likely to develop after 7 months of use. Keebler, Chatwani, and Schwartz (1983) reported incidences of 13.1 and 20.6 percent among Saf-T-Coil and Lippes Loop users compared with 2 percent among women using a copper-containing device. Presence of the ''Gupta bodies'' characteristic of the organism may be detected by Pap smear. Definitive diagnosis is made by endometrial or endocervical biopsy and direct immunofluorescence staining techniques (Yoonessi, Crickard, Cellino, et al., 1985). The clinical course of infection with *A. israelii* usually begins with endocervicitis, which can progress to endometritis and, less frequently, salpingitis or tubo-ovarian, abdominal, or pelvic abscess. *A. israelii*, however, is not a potent pathogen. Presence of a cervical infection does not necessarily result in PID, even with an IUD in situ. For this reason, a great deal of controversy exists regarding the management of asymptomatic women with Pap smears positive for *A. israelii*. There are four treatment options (Hatcher et al., 1984, pp. 101–102):

1. Provide treatment and remove the device.
2. Provide treatment and leave the IUD in place.
3. Do not provide treatment and leave the IUD in place.
4. Do not provide treatment and remove the device.

Most practitioners electing to treat prescribe a 7- to 10-day course of penicillin followed by a repeat Pap smear. It is advisable to treat each case individually. If the woman is well informed regarding danger signs and subsequent complications should PID develop, the device may be safely left in situ with or without treatment, should she desire continuing its use for contraception. In the woman willing to use another birth control method, it is probably wiser to recommend removal of the device, particularly if she may have difficulty recognizing or seeking treatment for the symptoms of PID.

Women with symptoms of PID, regardless of the etiol-

TABLE 8-2. RISK OF INFERTILITY BY DURATION OF USE AND IUD TYPE

	Percentage That Used IUD		Adjusted Relative Risk
	Infertile Women (N = 283)	Fertile Women (N = 3,833)	
Duration of IUD use			
Less than 3 mo	3.5	1.4	2.7
3–18 mo	8.1	5.2	1.7
18–36 mo	7.1	4.4	1.8
More than 36 mo	12.7	5.7	2.2
Device type			
Copper only	13.4	9.9	1.6
Noncopper	18.0	6.8	2.4
Loop/Saf-T-Coil	6.0	1.8	2.9
Dalkon Shield only	5.0	1.4	3.3

(Adapted from Cramer D., Schiff, I., & Schoenbaum, S. C., et al. [1985]. Tubal infertility and the intrauterine device. New England Journal of Medicine, 312 [15], 941–947. Reprinted with permission.)

ogy, should have the IUD immediately removed and begin a course of antibiotics to decrease the danger of tubal damage. (See Chapter 15 for a discussion of presenting symptomatology, diagnosis, and treatment of salpingitis.)

Other Complications

IUD users also have been reported to have a six times greater frequency of *Trichomonas* infections than nonusers (Blenkinsopp & Chapman, 1982). In this same study of 12,468 women, of whom 757 were using IUDs, there was a significant difference in the incidence of cervical intraepithelial neoplasia (CIN) among IUD users compared with nonusers, 1.0 percent compared with 0.3 percent. More research needs to be done in this area before a causal relationship can be claimed.

Women allergic to copper can develop a generalized urticaria in the presence of a copper-containing device. Lesions are small, intensely pruritic, with large erythematous halos. Complaints of headaches, palpitations and weakness may accompany this reaction. In a severe hypersensitive episode, the woman may develop large plaques of urticaria, angioedema, breathing difficulties, or even anaphylaxis. Time of onset is variable and can be influenced by exercise, emotional stress, or exposure to heat or cold. The exact mechanism is unknown, although copper is suspected as the antigen that triggers acetylcholine release within the autonomic nervous system. Removal of the IUD usually brings about prompt relief of symptoms (Shelley, Shelley, & Ho, 1983).

BENEFITS

Despite the preceding discussion, the IUD provides women with a highly effective method of birth control that requires little effort on their part. It is inexpensive to maintain and requires only annual medical visits. Unlike some barrier methods, use of an IUD does not interfere with foreplay or coitus, and women do not have to worry about forgetting to take pills or to insert a diaphragm, sponge, or cervical cap. There are no known systemic metabolic effects; thus, the IUD is an excellent choice for women who cannot use oral contraceptives.

Despite the problems noted with postpartum insertion, IUDs are more desirable for breastfeeding women than the pill. Heikkilä, Haukkamaa, and Luukkainen (1982) and Heikkilä and Luukkainen (1982) showed that even progesterone-containing devices do not alter the process of lactation. They found no significant changes in levels of progesterone in the serum of lactating women wearing the Progestasert. Furthermore, babies of mothers using this particular device were not significantly different from babies of nonusers with respect to growth and development.

According to Hatcher and co-authors (1984), some practitioners have found that insertion of an IUD can induce regular menstruation in women with postpill amenorrhea. The device may be beneficial in preventing adherence of endometrial walls in women with a history of Asherman's syndrome (see Chapter 14). Its insertion has been advocated during the healing process following a dilation and curettage for this syndrome to maintain an open uterine cavity (Nichols & McGoldrick, 1985, p. 441).

POSTCOITAL IUD INSERTION

Shortly after IUDs were introduced into the United States, they began to be used as an alternative to hormonal therapy for postcoital contraception. This was not a widely adopted practice, and little research has been done to document rates of effectiveness. As the copper device has been most extensively studied for postcoital use, it is generally recommended. This method has several benefits compared with hormonal postcoital contraception:

1. Women do not experience nausea.
2. The IUD can be retained as an ongoing contraceptive if desired.
3. Postcoital contraception with an IUD can be initiated within 5 days of unprotected intercourse. *The Family Planning Perspective News* ("Postcoital Copper IUD," 1979), reporting on a study by Tatum and associates, noted that of 300 women receiving postcoital IUD insertion, 2 percent received the device 6 to 7 days postcoitus and had subsequent menses, although it was suggested that a limit of 5 days would more likely ensure effectiveness.
4. If postcoital insertion fails, the woman may choose to continue the pregnancy without fear of birth defects if the device is removed early in the pregnancy.

Despite these benefits, the following risks of this method of postcoital contraception prevent its widespread use:

1. Insertion in a woman in whom implantation has taken place, as a result of an unreliable coital or menstrual history and/or incorrect uterine sizing, particularly if the woman has a retroverted uterus, resulting in disturbance of the pregnancy, could possibly endanger the woman's life. (This could be called an abortive procedure and expose the practitioner to medical–legal risk.)
2. Septic second-trimester spontaneous abortion if the method fails
3. Diagnosis of postinsertion bleeding as menses, leading to the unrecognized continuation of pregnancy

Should a patient and practitioner choose to use an IUD for postcoital contraception, close follow-up is essential. The decision to remove the device or seek a therapeutic abortion in the face of method failure should be made as soon as possible. The risks of pregnancy with an IUD in situ must be explained prior to insertion.

CONTRAINDICATIONS TO IUD INSERTION

The following list has been adapted from Varney (1987) and Hatcher and associates (1984). Practitioners should not insert IUDs in the presence of absolute or strong contraindications. The presence of some relative contraindications necessitates careful assessment of the risks and benefits to the individual woman. She should be well informed and provided with support to evaluate the risks involved and compare them with the benefits of an IUD at a given time of her life. Contraindications to IUD use may change throughout a woman's life cycle depending on her age, parity, history of PID, desire for future children, and, most significantly, number of sexual partners or number of sexual partners of her partner. Certain relative contraindications, such as acute cervicitis and anemia, may also require consultation with a physician and/or institutional protocols prior to deciding whether to insert a device.

Absolute Contraindications

1. Presence of PID
2. Known or suspected gonorrheal or chlamydial infection
3. Known or suspected pregnancy
4. Known genital actinomycosis

Strong Relative Contraindications

5. History of PID within the past 3 months, including postpartum endometritis or an infected abortion
6. History of chronic PID
7. History of an ectopic pregnancy, especially if future pregnancy is desired
8. Any episode of pelvic infection if the woman desires future pregnancy
9. Multiple sexual partners, or a partner with multiple sexual partners
10. Abnormal uterine bleeding
11. Uterus sounding to less than 4.5 cm
12. Unavailable or difficult-to-obtain emergency medical treatment
13. Impaired coagulation response or anticoagulant therapy
14. Valvular heart disease (IUD potentially increases the susceptibility to subacute bacterial endocarditis)
15. Abnormal Pap smear: suggestive of endometrial hyperplasia, cervical intraepithelial neoplasia, or cancer
16. Presence of myomas or other anomalies that distort the uterine cavity, for example, bicornuate uterus, endometrial polyps
17. History or presence of blood dyscrasia, including leukopenia, leukemia, sickle cell disease, and other hemoglobinopathies
18. Known or suspected allergy to copper (for copper-containing devices)
19. Diagnosed Wilson's disease (for copper-containing devices)
20. Impaired response to infection, for example, with diabetes, steroid treatment, chemotherapy, or acquired immune deficiency syndrome (AIDS)
21. Cervical stenosis
22. Endometriosis

Relative Contraindications

23. Anemia, that is, hemoglobin less than 10 g
24. Acute cervicitis
25. Uterus sounding between 4.5 and 6.5 cm, or 10 cm or greater
26. Past history of gonorrhea or chlamydia
27. Severe dysmenorrhea*
28. Severe menorrhagia*
29. Blood type incompatible with partner's
30. Impaired ability to recognize danger signals
31. Impaired ability to check for IUD string
32. Past history of vasovagal reaction or fainting in response to a previous attempt to insert an IUD
33. Nulligravidy—concern because of increased risk of PID resulting in infertility

---

*The Progestasert IUD may be therapeutic.

MANAGEMENT OF VISITS

Before deciding to insert an IUD, the practitioner should take a thorough history and perform a complete physical examination to screen for absolute and strong contraindications. Written informed consent should be obtained. A negative gonorrhea (GC) culture should be documented within the month preceding insertion. Those individuals who are quite nervous or who have a long distance to travel should be advised at the time the appointment is made to have someone accompany them when they come for insertion in case they experience immediate severe pain, bleeding, syncope, or nausea after insertion.

The Initial Visit

The initial visit may include IUD insertion if results of necessary cultures are available. Otherwise, a second visit is warranted for insertion and should be timed appropriately.

Data Collection

HISTORY. A complete history should be taken (see Chapter 2), focusing particularly on contraindications to IUD use. The patient's understanding of all birth control methods should be assessed as should her reasons for choosing the IUD and her knowledge level regarding this method. The patient's comfort or ability to touch her vagina and cervix should be a part of the sexual history.

The accessibility of emergency medical care is an additional piece of data to obtain. Screen for diets low in iron.

PHYSICAL EXAMINATION. The physical examination should be complete (see Chapter 3). Examination *must* include a careful assessment of the heart, the abdomen, and the pelvic organs. Specifically, pain with manipulation of the uterus or cervix, adnexal tenderness or masses, and uterine enlargement must be ruled out. Uterine shape, position, and presence of fibroids or unusual configurations need to be determined.

LABORATORY TESTING. Laboratory data should include a negative gonorrhea culture within the past month, a Pap smear, wet smear, chlamydia culture or screening on indication, and a complete blood count (see Chapter 4).

If contraindications are identified through historical, physical or laboratory data, additional laboratory data or physician consultation may then be appropriate, depending on the severity of the problem and institutional or practice-agreement protocols. When an absolute contraindication exists, provide another method of birth control if desired, with instructions on how to use it. If identified contraindications are not absolute, discuss the situation with the patient and together plan appropriate management. This may include, for example, nutritional counseling and iron supplementation with a return in 6 to 8 weeks for evaluation for possible insertion at that time. It may mean referral for colposcopy, with insertion dependent on the results of that test. Or it may consist of consultation with the physician managing the patient's diabetes or other medical problem(s). When necessary, interim birth control must be provided. Many times, the woman herself chooses another contraceptive method when faced with an IUD contraindication.

Intervention

Selection of the Appropriate IUD. In addition to availability, the choice of an IUD depends on several factors.

AVAILABILITY

WOMAN'S PREFERENCE. Continuation rate may be improved if a woman is fitted with the device of choice. Hatcher et al. (1984) caution never to use a device that the patient specifically does not want.

GOAL OF THE IUD—TERMINATION OF CHILDBEARING OR CHILD SPACING. If the woman desires no more children, then a nonmedicated device (if available) is desirable because it can be left in place indefinitely in the absence of complications. She is thus spared the trauma and increased risk of repeated insertions necessary with a copper- or progesterone-containing IUD. A copper-containing device may be preferable for a woman who desires to space her family because it is associated with a lower incidence of infertility.

SIZE OF THE UTERUS. If the uterus sounds to less than 4.5 cm, the IUDs currently available will probably not be tolerated. If it sounds to between 4.5 and 6.5 cm, a small Saf-T-Coil with a vertical length less than 3.0 cm will be best tolerated. Larger devices may increase the risk of perforation, heavy bleeding, or pregnancy. Most IUDs are acceptable for uteri that sound to between 6.5 and 9.5 cm. A large Saf-T-Coil, Size D Loop, Copper 7, Copper T, or Progestasert can be used when the uterus is sounded as 10 cm or greater. The device may not reach the fundus and expulsion is likely. Consider this a contraindication; strongly advise the use of a backup method at midcycle.

HISTORY OF PAINFUL OR HEAVY MENSES. The Progestasert may decrease both dysmenorrhea and menorrhagia. The Copper 7 or Copper T may be inserted in the presence of heavy menses because it is small and therefore adapts readily to the uterine cavity, resulting in less trauma.

OBSTETRIC HISTORY. Consider nulligravidity a contraindication unless the woman has one sexual partner who is also monogamous, definitely wants the device after being counseled about all other contraceptive methods, and is aware of the risk of infertility. If an IUD is to be inserted, consider a small Saf-T-Coil or Copper 7 or Copper T.

If the woman has had one or more abortions or preterm births, consider a small to medium Saf-T-Coil, Lippes Loop B, Copper 7, or Copper T.

For a woman who has had one or more full-term births, any IUD may be prescribed.

POSTABORTION OR POSTPARTUM. Immediately after a preterm birth or abortion, consider a small to medium Saf-T-Coil, Lippes Loop B, Copper 7, or Copper T. It should be noted, however, that the Lippes Loop decreases in effectiveness and increases in expulsion rate as size decreases. The pregnancy rate of the Lippes Loop D has been reported as 3.6 and its expulsion rate as 3.6, compared with rates of 8.0 and 6.5, respectively, for the Lippes Loop A (Hatcher et al., 1984, pp. 83–84).

After a full-term birth, a Delta T or Delta Loop may be inserted immediately after the placenta is delivered, or any IUD may be inserted 6 to 8 weeks postpartum.

POSTCESAREAN BIRTH. Most devices can be safely inserted 8 weeks after a cesarean. Consider a Copper 7, Copper T, or Progestasert, all of which can be inserted by withdrawal techniques.

HISTORY OF EXPULSION OF PREVIOUS IUDS. In the presence of a history of expulsion of previous IUDs, use a more rigid device, for example, the Lippes Loop. Consider a smaller device if one too large was used, or vice versa. Consider a Progestasert, which has a lower expulsion rate among multiparous women.

PRACTITIONERS' COMPETENCE AND FAMILIARITY WITH DIFFERENT IUDS. If no other circumstances exist, it is safer to insert a device that you are comfortable in handling.

Timing of Insertion. Most practitioners choose to insert IUDs during menses. At this time, the cervical canal is slightly dilated and, hence, the procedure is less traumatic. Most important, pregnancy is unlikely. Despite these two advantages, some practitioners do not limit their timing of insertion to menses. In fact, during this time, a woman may be more susceptible to the upward spread of infection, and the incidence of expulsion, presumably from increased uterine contractions, may be higher (Graham & Simock, 1982).

In addition to menses, an IUD may be safely inserted in the following situations:

1. When menses has started within the past 7 to 8 days with a history of 28-day cycles
2. On any day of the cycle if the woman is regularly using a reliable method of birth control or has not had sexual intercourse since her last normal period [Graham and Simock (1982) advocate midcycle insertions as the cervical os is also somewhat dilated at this time, and the risk of infections is less because of the presence of thick cervical mucus.]
3. At midcycle if the woman desires "morning-after" IUD insertion (The patient must understand clearly the risks of pregnancy with an IUD in situ and the effectiveness of this type of insertion, should sign an informed consent, and should be willing to return for close follow-up. The practitioner should carefully evaluate her feelings about postcoital IUD insertions.)
4. At 6 to 8 weeks postpartum if the woman has had no sexual contact since delivery
5. At 6 to 8 weeks postpartum if the woman has consistently used condoms and/or vaginal spermicides for each sexual contact (A pregnancy test is recommended prior to insertion.)
6. Immediately after an uncomplicated first-trimester abortion
7. Immediately after a delivery (Use a Delta T or Delta Loop.)

Procedure for Insertion. The following discussion has been adapted from Varney (1987). The technique of insertion of an IUD varies slightly depending on the particular device. Practitioners should study the instructions within the package insert prior to insertion. It is very important to move slowly throughout the procedure and not to use force. Certain general instructions should be followed.

1. Show the patient the device and explain the difference between the inserter barrel and the actual IUD.
2. Explain the procedure of insertion including speculum exam, Pap smear if necessary, and bimanual exam. Provide anticipatory guidance regarding expected discomfort.
3. Obtain written informed consent from the woman.
4. Perform a careful bimanual exam to rule out preg-

nancy and PID. It is important for the practitioner inserting the IUD to accurately determine the shape and position of the uterus.

5. Insert a metal speculum and adjust for maximum visualization and exposure of the cervix.

6. Change to sterile gloves and have an assistant open the IUD insertion kit. If an assistant is not available, open the kit before putting on sterile gloves.

7. Thoroughly wash the cervix with an antiseptic solution, for example, betadine or benzylonium if the woman is allergic to iodine. Wash from the os outward. The cervical canal can be washed with sterile cotton applicators soaked with antiseptic solution.

8. A paracervical block may be injected at this time (discussed later).

9. Apply a single-tooth tenaculum to the anterior cervical lip at 10 and 2 o'clock. Many practitioners apply the tenaculum to the posterior lip at 8 and 4 o'clock for posterior uteri. Be sure to firmly grasp the cervix 1.5 to 2.0 cm from the os to avoid tearing the cervix when tension is applied and to prevent obstruction of the cervical canal. Avoid placement at 9 and 3 o'clock. Major cervical blood vessels are located at those positions and heavy bleeding might result. An ''atraumatic'' tenaculum may be applied instead: with one side at 12 or 6 o'clock and the other just inside the os; the advantage is that it does not puncture the cervix. Some practitioners prefer to manipulate a tenaculum using two hands, one on each side of the instrument. Whether you use one hand or two, be sure to close the tenaculum *slowly*, but completely, one notch at a time. Forewarn the woman that she may feel a short sharp pinch. If this occurs, wait until it has subsided before proceeding with the next step. Rest the tenaculum gently on the speculum before reaching for the sound, allowing the woman time to relax.

10. Sound the uterus to confirm its position, to rule out obstructions within the canal and to measure the depth of the uterine cavity.

    a. Forewarn the woman that she may feel pulling and cramps as the sound passes through the cervical os. Encourage deep breathing for relaxation.

    b. Hold the sound between your thumb and first two fingers for sensitivity and control.

    c. Pull steadily and strongly on the tenaculum to straighten out the axis of the uterus (downward and outward for anteverted/anteflexed uteri or upward and outward for retroverted/retroflexed uteri). Using *gentle* pressure, insert the sound into the cervical os. DO NOT PUSH. Allow the sound to find its own way through the canal. At this point, one of three situations is possible:

       i. The sound passes easily through the internal os with little or no resistance.

       ii. The sound meets resistance at the internal os that is released by steady gentle pressure. Sometimes, gentle rotation redirecting the sound within the cervical canal or increased pressure on the tenaculum is effective in helping the sound to negotiate the internal os.

       iii. Spasms at the internal os resist the gentle pressure of the tip of the sound. This often occurs if the woman is tense. [A differential diagnosis of cervical stenosis should

be considered, especially in a woman with a history of induced abortion, dilation and curettage, or cervical surgery.] Patience here is usually the key to a successful insertion. Briefly provide explanation and reassurance to decrease the woman's anxiety. Encourage relaxation techniques. Alternatively, distracting conversation may be calming. Continue to apply steady and firm (but not forceful) pressure against the internal os. Make sure that sufficient pressure is applied to the tenaculum to straighten out the uterus. As the woman relaxes, you will feel the internal os relax and open, allowing the sound to slip into the uterine cavity. This may take several seconds to a few minutes, and you may need to repeat the process to pass the IUD inserter through the internal os. If, after a few minutes, release is not felt, or the woman requests that you stop or becomes more anxious, stop the procedure and remove all instruments.

11. Once the sound has passed the os, allow it to find its way into the uterine cavity. Do not push. The sound will confirm or refute your findings of uterine position and size.

12. Continue to gently push the sound until the tip taps the fundus.

13. Note the depth of the sound after its removal. It may be helpful to place a cotton-tipped applicator at the external os next to the sound, and remove both sound and applicator together. The depth is recorded by noting the position of the applicator next to the sound or the length of moisture on the instrument. If the uterus sounds to between 6.5 and 10 cm, proceed. Some IUDs, including the Copper T380A, are designed so that the portion of the inserter entering the uterus is set to equal the length of the uterine cavity determined by the sound.

14. Using sterile technique, load the IUD into the inserter. The Progestasert is loaded by pressing straight down on the inserter onto a sterile field. This causes the arms of the device to bend against the sides of the inserter. The arms of the Copper T380A should be inserted into the insertion tube only as far as necessary to ensure their retention in the tube. All devices should be inserted within a few minutes of being loaded so that they do not lose their shape.

15. Following manufacturer's instructions, proceed with insertion.

    a. Forewarn the woman that she will once again feel pulling and cramps as the device is inserted.

    b. Apply firm, steady pressure on the tenaculum (as in step 10c).

    c. Insert the IUD and inserter into the cervical canal and through the internal os. The inserter of the Progestasert can be bent slightly to conform to the shape of the uterus. Before insertion of this device, the thread-retaining plug should be checked to make sure it is secure in the inserter's end.

    d. Hold the cervical stop (or arm-cocker, in the case of a Progestasert) firmly at the external os.

    e. Use withdrawal or push technique to insert the device, depending on specific requirements. *Move slowly.* Undue force should never be used. If force seems required, stop and re-evaluate the condition of the cervix or uterus and/or the insertion technique. IUDs that require a push technique include all Lippes Loops and Saf-T-Coils. The Copper 7 may be inserted with a push or withdrawal technique; Copper T200, Tatum T, Copper T380A, and Progestaserts are inserted using withdrawal.

   f. Before inserting a Progestasert make sure the number on the shaft at the base of the arm-cocker is equal to the uterine depth measured on sounding.

16. Remove the inserter and plunger according to the specific instructions for the device. Alza Corporation suggests checking to make sure that no part of the Progestasert inserter is left in the uterus (Alza Corporation, 1986).

17. Cut IUD string(s) $2\frac{1}{2}$ in. (6 cm) from the os. This allows for subsequent palpation and visualization of the string(s) as the uterus resumes its shape or the IUD moves upward toward the fundus. The shorter string of the Progestasert, added to the depth of the uterus, should equal approximately 9 cm. This can be estimated as a check on the correct placement of this device.

18. Remove the tenaculum. Apply pressure to the puncture sites with a sponge stick and cotton ball or with several cotton applicators if bleeding is excessive. (Some bleeding is normal, and pressure from the vaginal walls may be sufficient to stop it.)

19. Remove the speculum.

20. Allow the woman to rest if necessary.

21. Give the woman the string clipping so that she will know what her string(s) feels like. All Lippes Loops and Saf-T-Coils have two strings as do the Copper T200, Tatum T, Progestasert, and Copper T380A. The Copper 7 has one string.

22. Teach the woman how to feel for her IUD string (see Teaching and Counseling).

23. Give the woman a perineal pad to wear.

24. Chart the procedure, including findings on bimanual exam, cleansing of the cervix, application of the tenaculum, depth of the sound, and type and size of device inserted. Note difficulties with insertion, amount of bleeding, patient's tolerance, length of string remaining in vagina, and teaching and counseling provided.

Immediate Postpartum IUD Insertion. Early postpartum IUD insertion is best accomplished immediately after delivery of the placenta. Insertion, however, may safely take place up to 36 hours postpartum (Cole et al., 1984). Whether or not this is a nonmedical function depends on your role in managing obstetric patients, institutional protocols, and your opportunity to learn this procedure with appropriate supervision.

1. Maintain sterile technique.

2. Tie three chromic catgut sutures to the upper arms of a Copper T200 or Lippes Loop. The tail on these devices must be a 10-in. (30-cm)-long monofilament nylon.

3. Stabilize the cervix with a ring forceps. (A tenaculum does not provide a good grip on the postpartum cervix. Furthermore, tearing would be likely with a tenaculum.)

4. Holding the IUD between the index and middle fingers, introduce it into the vagina, through the cervix, and high into the fundus. Be careful not to dislodge the device as the hand is removed and the IUD string(s) is directed toward the cervix.

Paracervical Block. IUD insertion can be very painful for some women, especially if they are anxious about the procedure. Nulliparous women or those with a history of vasovagal reactions are at risk for more difficult insertions. Paracervical anesthesia may be beneficial, particularly for insertion of an IUD in a woman in either of these two risk groups. It can be safely administered in the office if no more than 4 mL of 0.5 percent Lidocaine without epinephrine is used. The block is administered using sterile technique after the cervix has been thoroughly cleansed with betadine. It is important to rule out allergy to local anesthetic agents before beginning. Prior to using this type of anesthesia, nurse-practitioners are advised to ascertain whether it is legally permissible for them to administer paracervical blocks in their state. The following steps are adapted from Hatcher et al. (1984):

1. Draw up 4 mL of 0.5 percent Lidocaine into a sterile syringe using a 22-gauge needle.

2. Inform the woman that she should report any nausea, dizziness, or tingling of the lips after the procedure. These symptoms may be a normal reaction; however, should they occur, check the woman's vital signs to rule out toxicity.

3. Visualize the cervix completely and swab it with a Lidocaine-saturated cotton swab.

4. Insert the needle at 4 o'clock under the cervical mucosa. Aspirate lightly to avoid direct intravenous injection. If no blood is returned, inject 1 to 2 mL of 0.5 percent Lidocaine into the area. The vast amount of small blood vessels and capillaries in this region ensures rapid and adequate distribution of the drug.

5. Repeat step 4 at 8 o'clock.

6. Anesthesia should be achieved within 2 to 5 minutes.

7. Continue with IUD insertion (step 9).

Immediate Postinsertion Problems: Vasovagal Syncope. Syncope (fainting) may occur during or immediately after IUD insertion, especially in a nulliparous woman or one who is very nervous and fearful. The woman may complain of severe cramps, dizziness, visual disturbances, and lightheadedness. She may eventually faint. Her pulse can become weak and thready. Diaphoresis and decreased blood pressure may follow. The cause of this reaction is thought to be excessive pain; however, its occurrence is infrequent. Slow gentle manipulation of the instruments can reduce the risk, whereas abrupt or rushed movements may enhance it. It is important to continually talk to the woman during and after the insertion. Do not leave her alone until you are sure that she is not experiencing a syncopal reaction. Most reactions are transient and spontaneously subside if the practitioner is patient and temporarily stops the insertion procedure.

If the reaction continues, it may be necessary to place the woman in Trendelenberg position and offer spirits of ammonia. Recovery is usually prompt after removal of the device. If circulatory or respiratory depression continues, administer 0.4 to 0.5 mg of atropine sulfate intramuscularly. Continue to monitor vital signs and notify a backup physician. If the woman still desires an IUD, a repeat insertion attempt may be tried 1 month later. The use of paracervical block anesthesia and/or a smaller device is advisable (Hatcher et al., 1984).

Teaching and Counseling

Appropriate teaching and counseling at the time of IUD insertion provide a woman with information to deal with common side effects and recognize danger signs of IUD use, thereby increasing the safety and efficacy of this method. It is important to explain the theories regarding the mechanism of action of her device and its rate of effectiveness. The IUD user should also know the type and size of her particular device and the date it should be replaced, if necessary. Provide a card or literature with this information.

After the insertion procedure, the woman should be taught how to feel for the IUD string(s). If a mirror is available, it is helpful to show her the string(s) protruding from the os while the speculum is still in place. Have her feel the excess string from the insertion kit. Encourage her to wash her hands. Assist her to find a comfortable position, either squatting, lying down with her knees on her chest, standing with one leg on a chair or stool, or sitting on the toilet. Guide her to insert her longest finger into the vagina and direct it backward toward the cervix to locate the string at the os. Encourage her to note the length of the string(s) and the absence of the device itself at the os. She should be informed that, occasionally, the string(s) may curl up within the cervix. If this happens, she should gently probe the os with a finger to locate it. Caution her against tugging on the string(s).

The following important instructions, adapted from Hatcher and associates (1984) and Varney (1987), can be included in patient handouts and as part of verbal counseling regarding the specifics of IUD use. The language of written handouts may need to be adapted to the educational level of the patients receiving this literature.

1. a. Check for the IUD string routinely after each menstrual period.
   b. During the first month, the risk of expulsion is greater, so check for the string before intercourse.
   c. Examine sanitary napkins and tampons when you remove them, especially if you experience heavy menstrual bleeding and cramping.
2. Many women experience moderate to severe uterine cramps and heavier and more prolonged menstrual bleeding with or without clots for the first 1 to 3 months after insertion, until your body adapts to the IUD. You may also experience spotting between your periods, especially if you have been fitted with a Progestasert, although this particular device may *decrease* the amount of menstrual cramps and bleeding that you experience. You may find relief for cramps and increased bleeding from one or more of these self-help measures:
   a. Rest with a hot water bottle on the abdomen.
   b. Use analgesics, for example, aspirin, two tablets every 4 hours, or naprosyn (Naproxen) 250 mg, two tablets initially, followed by one tablet every 4 hours.
   c. Carry extra tampons and/or sanitary napkins and change frequently.
   d. Carry pantyliners for light-spotting days.
   e. Remember that you do not have to suffer with heavy bleeding and/or severe pain. You can return to your practitioner or clinic or go to an emergency room at any time to have the IUD removed.
   f. DO NOT TRY TO REMOVE THE DEVICE YOURSELF. If you or your partner attempt removal, you could hurt yourself.
3. Your IUD may be less effective during the first 1 to 3 months of use. Use a backup method such as foam or condoms during this time, and especially at midcycle. (Some practitioners recommend continued use of foam or condoms at midcycle. If you advise this practice, then teach the woman how to recognize midcycle.)
4. Avoid the use of tampons for the first 48 hours.
5. Avoid sexual intercourse for the first 24 hours.
6. You or your partner should *not* feel the string or device during intercourse. If either of you feel a "prick" by the string, it may be too long or too short. Return to your provider for evaluation and to have the string clipped shorter or the IUD changed.
7. If you miss a period or think that you might be pregnant, return to the office/clinic immediately. If you do become pregnant with an IUD in place, it is safer to have it removed immediately. Although you run a 25 percent risk of spontaneously aborting (miscarrying) after removal, the risk is 50 percent if you leave it in. Furthermore, a miscarriage is more likely to be infected with an IUD in place and this could seriously threaten your health. You should also seek immediate medical attention because you have a 5 percent increased risk of having an ectopic pregnancy (outside the uterus), which could rupture and cause pain and internal bleeding if not detected early.
8. If you are seen for any medical or surgical needs, notify the physician or health care provider that you have an IUD in place.
9. Maintain a diet high in iron or use iron supplements daily.
10. You may choose to avoid having more than one sexual partner and casual sexual contact because of the increased risk of pelvic infection and possible infertility.
11. Notify your care provider immediately if your partner has a discharge from his penis or burning on urination, or is treated for a sexually transmitted disease.
12. If you desire to become pregnant, wait about 3 months after the IUD is removed before trying. This may decrease the likelihood of an ectopic pregnancy.
13. If you have a Progestasert device, you may begin to skip periods after a while. As long as you have no signs of pregnancy and can still feel the string at the cervix, this is normal. You are probably not pregnant; however, call your practitioner for evaluation. This device should be replaced every year to maintain its effectiveness.
14. A copper-containing device should be replaced every 3 or 4 years. The Copper T380A can be worn 4 years; other copper devices must be changed every 3 years.
15. Know the IUD danger signs and seek medical care immediately.

Danger Signs	Possible Cause
Missed or late period	Pregnancy
Vague or severe lower abdominal, back, or pelvic pain	Pelvic Inflammatory Disease (PID), ectopic pregnancy

Fever and chills	PID
Foul-smelling vaginal discharge	Vaginitis; PID, pregnancy with miscarriage; partial expulsion of IUD
Severe menstrual cramping and/or heavy bleeding	Miscarriage; IUD expulsion; IUD adjustment or normal reaction to IUD
Breast tenderness or abdominal bloating, nausea, or vomiting	Pregnancy
String lengthens in vagina, or you feel the IUD with your fingers, or your partner feels it during intercourse	Lengthening of the string of the Copper 7; partial expulsion, perforation through the cervix
String missing	Complete expulsion, perforation through the uterus; pregnancy

Return Visits

The first return visit after an IUD insertion is scheduled for 4 to 6 weeks. During the interim, the woman should have had a period and possibly intercourse; therefore the practitioner can evaluate the retention of the device and specific problems experienced.

Data Collection

Interim History. For the last menstrual period, note the length, flow, pain, relief measures used, and compare with preinsertion menses; and for intermenstrual spotting/bleeding, the dates, amount, color, and pain.

Inquire of the patient the color, odor, consistency, and amount, of vaginal discharge and whether itching, dysuria, and associated pelvic discomfort were experienced.

Ask the woman how often she checks the string, when she last felt the string, and if the length has changed.

Question the patient with respect to sexual satisfaction (hers and partner's): Can her partner feel the string during intercourse? Does she consistently use a backup method? Does she experience pain with intercourse?

Is the patient taking any medications? Has she been seen by a doctor or in an emergency room since insertion? If so, when, why, and what treatment(s) did she receive?

Inquire about signs of pregnancy.

Ask about fever or chills and lower abdominal or back pain.

Physical Examination. Rule out lower abdominal tenderness.

If costovertebral angle tenderness (CVAT), rule out urinary tract infection (UTI) as a differential diagnosis if history indicates.

Perform a speculum examination to visualize the string at the os. Note length and trim if indicated. Note color of vaginal and cervical mucosa; presence of discharge (odor, color, etc.); obtain a wet smear if indicated. Perform a bimanual examination, noting pain with cervical or uterine manipulation, uterine and/or adnexal tenderness, uterine softening and/or enlargement, and adnexal masses.

Laboratory Tests. Obtain hemoglobin/hematocrit, urinalysis, and urine or other cultures if indicated; however, these are not routine at the 4- to 6-week revisit.

Assessment. If all findings are normal and the woman is satisfied with this method, she should continue with it. Review areas previously covered under Teaching and Counseling, especially danger signs. Answer questions. Make sure that she knows what type of device she has and the date that it should be replaced. Schedule her for an annual exam for an interim history and complete physical with Pap smear, gonorrhea culture, and other cultures and laboratory tests as indicated.

If complications have developed, treat and/or consult depending on the type and severity of the problem. The IUD may have to be removed.

Women who present for routine examinations with IUDs in place that you have not inserted require similar data collection. If the patient does not know what type of IUD she has, the device usually can be identified by the color and number of its strings. Lippes Loops have two strings; in sizes A and B, they are blue; in size C, yellow; and in size D, white. All Saf-T-Coils have two green strings. The Copper 7 and Copper T or Tatum T strings may both be light blue, or the Copper 7 string may be black. The Copper 7, however, has only one string. The Copper T380A has two white strings. The Progestasert has two clear strings. The Dalkon Shield, which should be removed unless the patient objects after a discussion of its life-threatening risks, has a multifilamentous string.

Management of Side Effects and Complications

Bleeding and Spotting

1. *Pregnancy (threatened spontaneous abortion or ectopic)*
   a. History: Sexual history; use of backup method; subjective signs of pregnancy; last menstrual period; pain.
   b. Physical: Uterine size and consistency; assessment of quality and quantity of bleeding.
   c. Lab: β subunit of human chorionic gonadotropin (hCG); complete blood count (CBC); blood type and Rh factor.
   d. Intervention: Remove IUD; consider ultrasound to rule out ectopic pregnancy; refer for dilation and curettage (D&C) or laparotomy as necessary.
2. *Endometritis*
   a. History: Fever, chills, foul discharge.
   b. Physical: Abdominal and pelvic exam; tenderness.
   c. Lab: CBC with differential; endocervical cultures.
   d. Intervention: Remove IUD; consult and treat according to protocols. Prescribe pelvic rest. Provide additional method of birth control at followup visit.
3. *Expulsion (partial or complete)*
   a. History: Pain or foul discharge; passage of clots; dysmenorrhea; intermenstrual bleeding; dyspareunia; postcoital spotting; feeling something hard at cervix; lengthening of string; inability to feel string or passage of the device; use of a backup method; signs and symptoms of pregnancy.
   b. Physical: Abdominal and pelvic to rule out pregnancy, PID; speculum exam to visualize partially expelled device or missing string.

c. Lab: β subunit of hCG as indicated.

d. Intervention: Remove partially expelled device; if device or string is not visible, probe cervix with alligator forceps and order ultrasound to diagnose expulsion. May insert another device if no contraindications (including possible pregnancy) exist and woman desires. Provide foam and condoms for back-up.

4. *Adjustment or normal reaction to IUD*

   a. History: Date of insertion (1 to 3 months ago); comparison of menstrual cycle before and after insertion.

   b. Physical: To rule out other diagnoses.

   d. Intervention: Provide anticipatory guidance and counseling with respect to diet, self-help, and danger signs. Remove IUD if woman desires; if she has a Lippes Loop, consider a copper-containing IUD or Progestasert or provide another method of birth control.

5. *Anemia* (not a cause of bleeding but an associated consequence)

   a. History: Signs and symptoms of anemia; diet history.

   b. Physical: Objective signs of anemia.

   c. Lab: CBC; further workup as necessary.

   d. Intervention: Offer dietary counseling and/or iron supplementation. Hatcher et al. (1984) suggest that the IUD be removed if the hematocrit is 30 to 32 percent or less. A Progestasert may reduce bleeding.

Pain and Cramping

1. *Postinsertion adjustment*

   a. History: Onset, frequency, intensity, and type of IUD and date of insertion.

   b. Physical: To rule out other diagnoses.

   c. Intervention: Provide anticipatory guidance. Prescribe hot water bottle or heating pad; aspirin 10 grains every 4 hours. A prostaglandin synthetase inhibitor—naprosyn—provides superior relief from dysmenorrhea and menorrhagia associated with IUD; Dosage: two tablets initially, then one tablet every 4 hours as needed (Othon & Nilsson, 1983).

2. *Device too large*

   a. History: Review of parity, depth of sound, type of device.

   b. Physical: Pelvic exam to rule out pregnancy and PID.

   c. Intervention: Remove and insert a smaller device; prescribe foam and condoms for 1 to 3 months as backup.

3. *Spontaneous abortion*
   See previous discussion.

4. *Ectopic pregnancy*
   See previous discussion.

5. *PID*
   Hatcher and co-authors (1984) strongly urge practitioners to consider immediately a diagnosis of PID when an IUD user presents with vague abdominal pain and/or foul vaginal discharge. The risk of subsequent infertility is increased if the possibility of chronic, mild, or acute PID is overlooked.

   a. History: Associated signs and symptoms—onset, character, and frequency of pain or discharge, previous PID; number of sexual partners and their symptoms and their numbers of partners.

   b. Physical: Bimanual pelvic exam for tenderness, mass, fixed uterus, and so forth.

   c. Lab: Endocervical cultures for gonorrhea, chlamydia, and anaerobes.

   d. Intervention: Remove IUD; consult and treat according to protocol (see Chapter 15). Counsel regarding pelvic rest. Partner may need to be referred for treatment. Arrange return visit to clinic in 1 to 2 weeks for evaluation, if not hospitalized. Provide another method of birth control at follow-up. Wait 3 months to 1 year before reinserting another device if desired. Consider one episode of PID a strong contraindication for reinsertion for women who are under 25, are of low parity, and/or desire more children.

6. *Fundal perforation at the time of insertion*

   a. Clinical presentation: Sharp pain with heavier bright red bleeding; often asymptomatic and undetected.

   b. Physical: Bimanual exam.

   c. Intervention: Stop procedure and remove the device; refer immediately if pain is severe. Advise pelvic rest or foam and condoms and a return for evaluation in 1 to 2 weeks if pain subsides.

7. *Subsequent fundal perforation (less common)*

   a. History: Shortening of string or inability to feel it; spotting or missed menses; signs and symptoms of pregnancy.

   b. Physical and lab: To rule out pregnancy.

   c. Intervention: Refer for hysteroscopy or laparoscopy if extrauterine location is suspected.

8. *Cervical perforation*

   a. History: Lengthening of string or ability to feel device itself; symptoms of pregnancy.

   b. Physical and lab: To rule out pregnancy.

   c. Intervention: Remove the device by exerting upward pressure on the dependent portion to dislodge the tip. Insert alligator forceps into the cervical canal; grasp and remove the device. Provide another method of birth control. Wait 3 months before reinsertion, if desired.

9. *Urinary tract infection/pyelonephritis*

   a. History: Dysuria, frequency, urgency, hematuria, lower back pain, previous UTIs.

   b. Physical: Suprapubic, bladder tenderness; CVAT.

   c. Lab: Clean-catch urine for urinalysis and culture and sensitivity (C&S).

   d. Intervention: Consult and treat according to protocols. May treat per symptoms and adjust based on C&S or wait for C&S. Counsel regarding self-help measures: fluids, hygiene, and sexual practices (see Chapter 17).

10. *Nonrelated gastrointestinal tract problem*

    a. History: To exclude other diagnoses; associated signs and symptoms (e.g., diarrhea, constipation, nausea, and vomiting).

    b. Physical: To exclude other diagnoses. Abdominal tenderness.

    c. Lab: To exclude other diagnoses.

    d. Intervention: Refer for diagnosis and possible treatment.

Lost IUD String

1. *Shortening of string*

   a. History: Type of IUD. When string was last felt. History of bleeding with clots, passage of the device, signs and symptoms of pregnancy.

b. Physical: To rule out pregnancy or PID.

c. Lab: To rule out pregnancy if indicated.

d. Intervention: Probe cervix with alligator forceps for string and remove device. May insert another if no contraindications exist.

2. *IUD in situ*

a. History, physical, and lab: See previous discussion.

b. Intervention: If string is not within the cervical canal, order an ultrasound for localization and rule out an intrauterine or ectopic pregnancy. Recent reports demonstrate that ultrasound can be safely used in wearers of copper IUDs. The risk of damage to the surrounding tissue is minimal because the copper poorly absorbs the sound waves (Grossman, 1978; Hatcher et al., 1984). If the IUD is visualized and pregnancy is ruled out, remove the device. Use sterile technique and follow the steps previously outlined for insertion. Sounding will direct you to the location of the device. Continue with traction on the tenaculum and slowly insert an alligator forceps into the cervical canal and into the uterine cavity. Grasp the IUD and slowly withdraw it from the uterus. Another device may be reinserted if indicated. Leave the string(s) long, and note their length.

3. *Partial or complete perforation*
See previous discussion.

Missed Period

1. *Intrauterine or Ectopic Pregnancy*

a. History: Last menstrual period, subjective signs and symptoms (see Chapter 15).

b. Physical: Abdominal and pelvic examinations.

c. Lab: β subunit of hCG and ultrasound as necessary.

d. Intervention: For an intrauterine pregnancy, counsel the woman regarding the risks of pregnancy with an IUD in situ (see Counseling and Teaching). Strongly advise removal of the device and do so immediately if the woman consents and the strings can be visualized. Do not attempt removal of the IUD with lost strings if a woman is pregnant. Refer for prenatal care or abortion as desired; some women may benefit from crisis-oriented counseling to help with decision making. For an ectopic pregnancy, refer the woman for immediate medical treatment. (See Chapter 15.)

Vaginal Discharge

1. *Vaginitis*

a. History: Color, consistency, odor of discharge; pruritis; relation to the menstrual cycle.

b. Physical: Speculum exam for clinical signs.

c. Lab: Wet smear; whiff test; cultures if necessary.

d. Intervention: Leave device in place. Treat vaginitis according to protocol. Refer partner for treatment or treat according to protocol as necessary. Suggest use of condoms if indicated. Arrange return in 1 to 2 weeks for evaluation. (See Chapters 11 and 12.)

2. *PID*
See previous discussion.

Partner Pinched By String

1. *String too long*

a. History: To rule out non–IUD-related problems. Complaints prior to IUD insertion. Other complaints of partner, for example, dysuria, penile discharge, lesions. History of sexually transmitted diseases.

b. Physical: Speculum exam to view string.

c. Intervention: Clip string and note new length on chart. Instruct woman to feel for string before she leaves office. Return for additional complaints.

2. *String too short*

a. History and physical: See previous discussion.

b. Intervention: Remove and replace IUD. If patient is midcycle and has had intercourse since menses without a backup method, have her return with menses for this.

3. *String type*

a. History: Type of IUD. (The Copper 7 which has a hard string, which many practitioners have found to be associated with pinching.)

b. Intervention: Change to another IUD, Tatum T or Copper T380A, if patient wishes copper device, or noncopper IUD if appropriate.

Difficult Removal: Embedding or Entanglement of String Within Device. This problem may not be suspected until an attempt at removal is made. Review the type of device and length of use. The following steps may help with a difficult removal.

- Continue to apply gentle steady traction to remove the device slowly.
- If the IUD fails to come out, insert a sound and slowly rotate it within the uterus; this may dislodge the device. Attempt removal by traction again.
- Paracervical block may be administered to decrease pain (see procedure).
- Cervical dilation using dilators can be done to increase the room for manipulation. Use small-size dilators and MOVE SLOWLY. Remember to inform the woman and talk to her to decrease her level of anxiety.
- Sound the uterus to locate the device.
- Use the alligator forceps to grasp the device and remove it from the uterine cavity.
- Consult with physician if the device does not come out.

Practitioners who are not skilled and confident in using cervical dilators or alligator-type forceps should refer the woman for removal by a physician or practitioner with experience in these techniques. If the preceding steps are unsuccessful, hospitalization for dilation and curettage may be required.

SELF-HELP MEASURES

The following measures may enable women to increase the effectiveness and safety of their IUDs. All IUD wearers have a right to information about these measures and their potential benefits. Some of these may involve life-style changes, and the extent to which an individual woman is willing to incorporate them into her life may vary. IUD wearers must understand the risks of not adhering to these measures and make decisions accordingly. Open discussion should be encouraged and a nonjudgmental attitude on the part of the practitioner adopted.

1. Limiting sexual partners to one at a time. Avoiding casual sexual contact. "Screening" potential partners for a history of sexually transmitted diseases and multiple sexual partners or contacts.
2. Using good vaginal hygiene. Changing tampons/sanitary napkins frequently. Wiping front to back (after a bowel movement). Avoiding vaginal contact after rectal contact.
3. Avoiding douching or limiting it to once a month after menses if it is important to the woman.
4. Developing body awareness, that is, knowing the normal amount and color of discharge and the signs of ovulation. Noting pelvic discomfort on cervical manipulation when checking for strings. Keeping a menstrual record for duration, date, interval length, and amount and character of flow, dysmenorrhea, premenstrual syndrome. Notifying a care provider of any changes.
5. Routinely checking for presence and length of IUD string(s). Notifying a care provider of any changes.
6. Knowing the type device used and when it should be replaced. Keeping all appointments.
7. Being familiar with IUD danger signs and reporting them immediately.

REFERENCES

Alza Corporation. (1986, July). Alza Product Information: Progestasert[R] Intrauterine Progesterone Contraceptive System. Palo Alto, CA: Alza Corporation.

Blenkinsopp, W., & Chapman, P. (1982, November). Prevalence of cervical neoplasia and infection in women using intrauterine contraceptive devices. *Journal of Reproductive Medicine,* 27(11), 709–713.

Chantler, E. N., Scott, K., & Filho, C. I., et al. (1984, February). Degradation of the copper-releasing intrauterine contraceptive device and its significance. *British Journal of Obstetrics and Gynaecology,* 91(2), 172–181.

Cole, L., Edelman, D., & Potts, D., et al. (1984, September). Postpartum insertion of modified intrauterine devices. *Journal of Reproductive Medicine,* 29(9), 677–782.

Cole, L., McCann, M., Higgins, J., & Waszak, C. (1983, April). Effects of breastfeeding on I.U.D. performance. *American Journal of Public Health,* 73(4), 384–388.

Copper T380A, Nova T IUDs not likely to be available in U.S. soon. (1985, October). *Contraceptive Technology Update,* 6(10), 144.

Cramer, D., Schiff, I., & Schoenbaum, S. C., et al. (1985, April). Tubal infertility and the intrauterine device. *New England Journal of Medicine,* 312(15), 941–947.

Daling, J., Weiss, N. S., & Metch, B. J., et al. (1985, April). Primary tubal infertility in relation to the use of an intrauterine device. *New England Journal of Medicine,* 312(15), 937–941.

Gibson, M., Gump, D., Ashikaga, T., & Hall, B. (1984, January). Patterns of adnexal inflammatory damage: Chlamydia, the intrauterine device, and a history of pelvic inflammatory disease. *Fertility and Sterility,* 41(1), 47–51.

Goh, T. H., Hariharan, M., & Chan, G. L. (1984, April). Anaemia and menstrual blood loss studies in women using Multiload Copper 250 and Progestasert IUDs, *Contraception,* 29(4), 359–366.

Graham, S., & Simock, B. (1982, October). A review of the use of intrauterine devices in nulliparous women. *Contraception,* 26(4), 323–341.

Grossman, M. (1978, July). Heating of metallic intrauterine contraceptive devices during ultrasound examination. *Obstetrics and Gynecology,* 53(1), 110–113.

Hatcher, R. A., Guest, F., & Stewart, F., et al. (1984). *Contraceptive technology 1984–1985* (12th rev. ed.). New York: Irvington.

Heartwell, S., & Schlesselman, S. (1983, January). Risk of uterine perforation among users of intrauterine devices. *Obstetrics and Gynecology,* 61(1), 31–36.

Heikkilä, M., Haukkamaa, M., & Luukkainen, T. (1982, January). Levonorgestrel in milk and plasma of breastfeeding women with a levonorgestrel-releasing IUD. *Contraception,* 25(1), 41–49.

Heikkilä, M., & Luukkainen, T. (1982, March). Duration of breastfeeding and development of children after insertion of levonorgestrel-releasing intrauterine contraceptive device. *Contraception,* 25(3), 279–292.

Keebler, M. D., Chatwani, A., & Schwartz, R. (1983, March). Actinomycosis infection associated with intrauterine contraceptive devices. *American Journal of Obstetrics and Gynecology,* 145(5), 596–599.

Koch, J. U. (1980, March). Sperm migration in the human female genital tract with and without intrauterine devices. *Acta Europaea Fertilitatis,* 11(1), 33–60.

Lee, N., Rubin, G., Ory, H., & Burkman, R. (1983, July). Type of intrauterine device and the risk of pelvic inflammatory disease. *Obstetrics and Gynecology,* 62(1), 1–6.

Moyer, D. L., & Mishell, D. R., Jr. (1971, September). Reactions of human endometrium to the intrauterine foreign body. II. Long-term effects on the endometrial histology and cytology. *American Journal of Obstetrics and Gynecology,* 111(1), 66–80.

Nichols, D. H., & McGoldrick, K. L. (1985). Minor and ambulatory surgery. In D. H. Nichols & I. R. Evrard (Eds.), *Ambulatory gynecology.* Philadelphia: Harper & Row.

Nilsson, C. G., Lahteenmaki, P., & Luukkainen, T. (1984, January). Ovarian function in amenorrheic and menstruating users of a levonorgestrel-releasing intrauterine device. *Fertility and Sterility,* 41(1), 52–55.

Ortho stops marketing loops: Cites economic factors. (1985, November). *Contraceptive Technology Update,* 6(4), 149.

Ortiz, M. E., & Croxatto, H. G. (1987, July). The mode of action of IUDs. *Contraception,* 36(1), 37–53.

Oster, G. K. (1972, January). Chemical reactions of the copper intrauterine device. *Fertility and Sterility,* 23(1), 18–23.

Othon, L., & Nilsson, B. (1983). Dysmenorrhea in women with intrauterine contraceptive device treatment with a prostaglandin synthetase inhibitor—Naproxen. *International Journal of Gynaecology and Obstetrics,* 21, 33–37.

Perlmutter, J. (1978, March). Pregnancy and the IUD. *The Journal of Reproductive Medicine,* 29(3), 133–137.

The Population Council. (no date). *The copper T380 IUD: A manual for clinicians.* New York: The Population Council, Program for the Introduction and Adaptation of Contraceptive Technology.

Postcoital copper IUD found to be effective in preventing pregnancy. (1979, May–June). *Family Planning Perspectives,* 11(3), 195.

Sağiroğlu, N. (1971, Jaunary–March). Phagocytosis of spermatozoa in the uterine cavity of woman using intrauterine device. *International Journal of Fertility,* 16(1), 1–14.

Searle's decision does not warrant arbitrary IUD removal. (1986, March). *Contraceptive Technology Update,* 7(3), 28.

Segal, S. J., Alvarez-Sanchez, F., & Adejuwon, C. A., et al. (1985, August). Absence of chorionic gonadotropin in sera of women who use intrauterine devices. *Fertility and Sterility,* 44(2), 214–218.

Shelley, W., Shelley, E. D., & Ho, A. K. S. (1983, April 16). Cholinergic urticaria acetylcholine receptor-dependent immediate-type hypersensitivity reaction to copper. *Lancet,* 1(8329), 843–846.

Sheppard, B. L. (1987, July). Endometrial morphological changes in IUD users: A review. *Contraception,* 36(1), 1–10.

Soderstrom, R. (1983, May). Will progesterone save the IUD? *Journal of Reproductive Medicine,* 28(5), 305–308.

Stumpf, P., & Lenker, R. (1984, October). Insertion technique not design affects expulsion rates of postpartum intrauterine devices. *Contraception,* 30(4), 327–330.

Tatum, H. (1977, January). Clinical aspects of intrauterine contraception: Circumspection 1976. *Fertility and Sterility,* 28(1), 3–78.

Tredway, D. R., Umezaki, C. U., Mishell, D. R., Jr., & Settlage, D. S. (1975, December). Effect of intrauterine devices on sperm transport in the human being: Preliminary report. *American Journal of Obstetrics and Gynecology,* 123(7), 734–735.

Treiman, K., & Liskin, L., (1988, March). IUDs—A new look. *Population Reports, 16*(1), 1–31.

Varney, H. (1987). *Nurse midwifery* (2nd ed.). Boston: Blackwell Scientific.

Vessey, M. P., Yeates, D., & Flavel, R. (1979, September 8). Risk of ectopic pregnancy and duration of use of an intrauterine device. *Lancet, 2*(8141), 501–502.

Videla-Rivero, L., Etchepareborda, J. J., & Kesseru, E. (1987, August). Early chorionic activity in women bearing inert IUD, copper IUD, and levonorgestrel-releasing IUD. *Contraception, 36*(2), 217–226.

Vries, K., Shapiro, I., & Degani, S., et al. (1983, February). Ovarian pregnancy in association with an intrauterine device. *International Journal of Gynaecology and Obstetrics, 21*(1–6), 65–70.

Wan, L. S., Hsu, Y., Ganguly, M., & Bigelow, B. (1977, October). Effects of the Progestasert on the menstrual pattern, ovarian steroids, and endometrium. *Contraception, 16*(4), 417–434.

Weström, L., Bengtsson, L. P., & Mårdh, P. (1976, July 31). The risk of pelvic inflammatory disease in women using intrauterine contraceptive devices as compared to non-users. *Lancet, 2*(7979), 221–224.

Yoonessi, M., Crickard, K., & Cellino, I. S., et al. (1985, January). Association of actinomycosis and intrauterine contraceptive devices. *Journal of Reproductive Medicine, 30*(1), 48–52.

9

Contraceptive Methods Under Investigation

Ronnie Lichtman

Perhaps one of the most frustrating experiences of a woman's health care provider is to be confronted with the woman who has exhausted all available birth control options. She has considered or tried all methods and each has proven to be unacceptable. Reasons for unacceptability among women include medical contraindications or fear of side effects, religious beliefs, aesthetic considerations, previous method failure, high cost, lifestyle or sexual incompatibility, and partner objections. None of these concerns is frivolous or trivial; not one of the available reversible contraceptives fully meets the criteria of infallibility, convenience, self-administration, low cost, and absence of side effects. Although these may be unattainable in any single method of birth control, the likelihood that any individual woman or couple will find a satisfactory contraceptive can only be increased through the widening of choices.

Various groups are involved in the quest for new and improved contraceptive methods. Major contraceptive research programs have been organized worldwide by government agencies, several nonprofit foundations, the United Nations, and a number of profit-making pharmaceutical companies (Atkinson, Schearer, Harkavy, & Lincoln, 1980). Much of the clinical research on contraceptives takes place in the Third World, where the need for improved birth control methods is said to be greater because of rapid population growth and where study protocols and standards for drug approval are not as stringent as they are in the United States. Critics of this practice cite the racism and paternalism involved in carrying out research in underdeveloped countries among poor and relatively uneducated women (Rosoff, 1984).

In the United States, the major source of public funding for contraceptive research is the Center for Population Research (CPR) of the National Institute for Child Health and Human Development (NICHD). In 1983, however, less than 10 percent of this agency's annual budget was allocated for the development of new contraceptive methods (Rosoff, 1984). This sum is less than 4 percent of the U.S. allocation recommended by a 1976 Ford Foundation report for "an adequate effort on a worldwide basis" (Rosoff, 1984, p. 29).

Given sufficient research efforts, the possibilities for new methods of birth control could encompass a number of areas including chemical and nonchemical methods either for men or women or for both sexes; however, analysis of U.S. public-sector funding for these various areas, summarized in Table 9–1, demonstrates that the over-whelming effort is concentrated on contraceptives for women, with the single largest expenditure going toward steroidal methods.

This chapter provides a brief overview of the research process involved in testing a new contraceptive and summarizes the following contraceptives currently being investigated or used in other parts of the world:

- Female methods
  Steroidal delivery systems: implants, vaginal rings and pills, injectables, intracervical devices, intranasal sprays
  Nonsteroidal antiovulatory chemicals
  Luteal phase (or postcoital or menses-inducing) contraceptives
  Antipregnancy immunization
  Chemical sterilization
  Techniques for ovulation detection/prediction
  Improvements of existing methods: diaphragm, cervical cap, vaginal spermicides, oral contraceptives, intrauterine device
- Male methods
  Steroidal agents
  Nonsteroidal agents
  Nonchemical methods
  Immunization
  Improvements of existing methods: condom

The discussion that follows is not intended to provide full clinical guidelines should any of these methods become available for use in the United States. It merely serves to acquaint the practitioner with what to anticipate in the future—near and not so near. Although technical improvements in surgical sterilization constitute an important component of ongoing research leading toward the development of simplified and reversible procedures, a discussion of surgical techniques is beyond the scope of this chapter.

EVALUATION OF A NEW CONTRACEPTIVE

Any new drug or medical device must be judged on at least three criteria: efficacy, safety, and utility (Borzelleca & Carmines, 1980, p. 32). Efficacy is the "ability to elicit a desired therapeutic effect"; for contraceptives, the desired effect is pregnancy prevention. Safety is the "absence of adverse

TABLE 9–1. PERCENTAGE DISTRIBUTION OF PUBLIC-SECTOR EXPENDITURES FOR DEVELOPMENT OF NEW CONTRACEPTIVE METHODS, 1978

Type of Method	Percentage
All female methods	**71.2**
Steroidal	37.2
Subdermal implants	(16.9)
Improved oral contraceptives	(9.9)
Injectables	(5.4)
Vaginal rings	(4.4)
Intranasal sprays	(0.5)
Vaccines against pregnancy[a]	10.1
Sterilization	2.0
Reversible	(0.4)
Nonsurgical	(1.6)
Antifertility and antiimplantation agents	8.3
Intracervical (ICD) and intrauterine (IUD) devices	6.9
ICDs	(1.6)
Postpartum IUDs	(1.6)
Other IUDs	(3.7)
Menses-inducing and abortifacient drugs	4.5
Barrier methods	2.2
All male methods	**6.1**
Systemic	5.5
Reversible sterilization and improved vasectomy techniques	0.6
Methods for couples and unclassified	**22.7**
Releasing factors[a]	5.1
Plant agents	3.9
Periodic abstinence	4.8
Other and unclassified	8.9
Total	100.0

[a]The percentage of total expenditures for releasing factors, derived from 1978 data, is almost certainly higher because of increased interest in this line of research, whereas the proportion devoted to steroidal male methods and to antipregnancy vaccines has probably decreased because of problems encountered with research on these methods.

From Atkinson, L., Schearer, B., Harkavy, O., and Lincoln, R. (1980). Prospects for improved contraception. Family Planning Perspectives, *12(4), 181. Reprinted with permission.*

effects at the therapeutic levels." Utility encompasses a number of characteristics including cost compared with other available drugs or devices, stability over time, and drug interactions.

To meet these criteria, drugs, including contraceptives, must be put through a number of phases of evaluation. The mechanism of action, degree of activity, and pharmacologic characteristics of the drug must be delineated and confirmed (Borzelleca & Carmines, 1980; Pasquale, 1980). In vitro studies to evaluate mutagenic effects must be performed. Before marketing, several phases of clinical trials are required: trials in animals to assess side effects, teratogenesis, tolerance, and safety of various doses and trials in humans to determine in vivo response, failure rates, and return to fertility. These stringent requirements explain the time and expense involved in the development of a new contraceptive.

FEMALE METHODS

Steroidal Delivery Systems

Alternative delivery systems for steroids are the most likely new contraceptives to become available in the near future. In fact, many of these methods, which include implants, vaginal rings and pills, injectables, intracervical devices,

and intranasal sprays, are already utilized in other parts of the world.

Implants. Subdermal implants for delivery of progestin have been in use for a number of years. NORPLANT is an implant consisting of six 2.4 mm × 3.4 cm Silastic (polydimethylsiloxane) capsules filled with progesterone (levonorgestrel). It was developed by the International Committee for Contraceptive Research of the Population Council, has been approved for marketing in seven countries including Finland and Sweden, is used in 31 countries, and is approved by the International Planned Parenthood Federation (IPPF) as a contraceptive available worldwide to IPPF-affiliated associations ("NORPLANT Gets Approval," 1986; The Population Council, 1987c). NORPLANT-2 is made of two covered rods containing levonorgestrel. It is easier to insert and has contraceptive effects comparable to those of the original NORPLANT (Diczfalusy, 1986b; Hingorani, Jalnawala, Kochhar, et al., 1986).

Implants are inserted subdermally via a trochar (Fig. 9–1) through a 3- to 5-mm incision into a woman's forearm or upper arm. Releasing a daily level of progestin comparable to the minipill, implants remain effective up to 5 years. Insertion can be accomplished under local anesthesia, without suturing, and can be as rapid as 3 minutes and rarely longer than 15 minutes (Sivin, Sanchez, Diaz, et al., 1983). Insertion takes place during menses. Some women experience tenderness, discoloration, bruising, and swelling at the insertion site for several days (The Population Council, 1987a). Except for the first few days, when the area of insertion should be protected, the implant needs no further care. Removal requires a 5-mm incision and takes approximately 10 to 20 minutes.

The contraceptive action of progestin-releasing implants is due to anovulation, endocrine abnormalities, inadequate luteal phase, changes in cervical function, and interference with oocyte maturation (Alvarez, Brache, Tejada, & Faundes, 1986; Brache, Faundes, Johansson, & Alvarez, 1985; Salah, Ahmed, Abo-Eloyoun, & Shaaban, 1987; Sivin, 1983). Studies show their failure rate to be less than one pregnancy per 100 woman-years of use (Holma, 1985; Sivin, 1983). Rare ectopic pregnancies have been reported with this method. Return to fertility was achieved in one 3-year trial within 1 year of termination in 77 percent of former users (Sivin, 1983). In another study, women discontinuing NORPLANT to become pregnant had all achieved pregnancy within 2 years, except for a few in whom male infertility was identified (Diaz, Pavez, Cardenas, & Croxatto, 1987).

The subdermal route with its constant low-level hormone release is considered more physiologic than the oral route (Johansson & Odlind, 1983). Hepatic effects are fewer and blood pressure changes have not been noted in studies of the implant. Although not extensively examined, changes in serum lipids in nonsmoking women using NORPLANT have been favorable (Shaaban, Elwan, Abdalla, & Darwish, 1984a), and effects on blood coagulation have been less pronounced than those seen with combination oral contraceptives (Shaaban, Elwan, El-Kabsh, et al., 1984b). Infants conceived during implant therapy have not manifested abnormalities, although their numbers are small (Diaz, Herreros, Johansson, & Croxatto, 1986).

Adverse effects do occur, however, with implant use. Most women experience menstrual irregularities with this method and these have been cited as major reasons for discontinuation; excessive bleeding often characterizes the first few months of use and is followed by diminished bleeding and possible amenorrhea with long-term use.

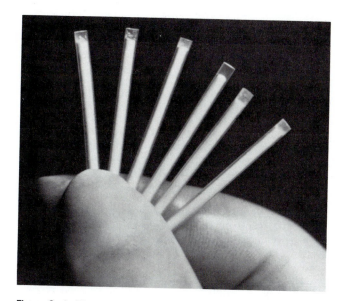

Figure 9-1. The six capsule NORPLANT method. *(Courtesy of the Population Council.)*

Overall long-term effects on hemoglobin status have been favorable, however, Other reported reasons for termination include mood changes, headaches, depression, loss of libido, nervousness, dizziness, and loss of sleep (Sivin, 1983). Skin problems such as acne or hirsutism have been noted. Changes in carbohydrate metabolism and plasma protein have been reported—both of unknown clinical significance (Johansson & Odlind, 1983; Sivin, 1983). Unacceptably high levels of levonorgestrel have been found in breastfed infants of mothers using NORPLANT (Shaaban, Odlind, Salem, et al., 1986). Implant effectiveness is reduced in women with epilepsy who take anticonvulsants, such as phenytoin, that induce metabolizing enzymes of the liver (Haukkamaa, 1986). In addition, the implants can be felt and sometimes seen, making them cosmetically unacceptable to some women (Connell, 1984, p. 54s), although the rods in NORPLANT-2 are less conspicuous.

Warning signs for women using NORPLANT include severe lower abdominal pain, heavy vaginal bleeding, arm pain, pus or bleeding at the insertion site, expulsion of an implant, migraine or repeated bad headaches, blurred vision, and delayed menses (The Population Council, 1987b).

An alternative type of subdermal contraception is the biodegradable implant. Its obvious advantage is elimination of the need for removal. A variety of such contraceptives are being studied (Gabelnick, 1983; Rivera, Gaita, Ortega, et al., 1984; Speidel, 1983).

Vaginal Rings and Pills

RINGS. Hormone-releasing contraceptive vaginal rings (CVRs) are based on the principle that the vagina is a dynamic site for absorption of a number of substances (Gallegos, 1980, p. 230). Available in several countries, most vaginal rings in use or under investigation release low-dose progestin or a progestin–estrogen combination. These rings are shaped like donuts with diameters of 50 to 75 mm and are inserted by the woman into the posterior vaginal fornix, around the cervix.

The advantages of a vaginal delivery system are that while rings can be kept in for prolonged periods, they deliver a minimal amount of steroid (Diczfalusy, 1986a) and can be removed at will (Nuttal, Elstein, & Spencer, 1985).

Progestin-releasing rings can be kept in place up to three to six cycles; estrogen-releasing rings remain in the vagina 3 weeks and are removed for 1 week each cycle (Diczfalusy, 1986a). This delivery system also exposes the liver to lower drug concentrations than the oral route (Nash & Jackanicz, 1982).

The contraceptive effect of progestin-containing rings results mainly from changes in cervical mucus, although endometrial changes have also been noted (Nuttal, et al., 1985). Rings containing estrogen have a greater effect on ovulation (Ahren, Victor, Lithell, et al., 1983; de Leede, Govers, & de Nijs, 1986; Schwan, Ahren, & Victor, 1983; Souka, Kamel, Einen, et al., 1985; Speidel, 1983).

Pregnancy rates with CVRs have been reported to be about 2 or slightly less than 2 pregnancies per 100 users (Nash & Jackanicz, 1982). Side effects include menstrual irregularities, such as breakthrough bleeding, spotting, and amenorrhea; vaginal irritation, erosion, discharge, or pain, especially with rigid rings (Nash & Jackanicz, 1982); occasional odor; and interference with coitus (Coutinho, da Silva, Carreira, et al., 1984; Hardy, Reyes, Gomez, et al., 1983). Some women have difficulty with insertion or removal of rings, and expulsions infrequently occur (Hardy et al., 1983; Nash & Jackanicz, 1982). Headaches, nausea, depression, nervousness, and dizziness have been seen less often than with oral contraceptives (Nash & Jackanicz, 1982).

PILLS. Daily vaginal administration of combination pills has been found to inhibit ovulation (Coutinho et al., 1984; Souka et al., 1985; Souka, El Sokkary, Kamel, & Hassa, 1986), while offering some of the same physiologic advantages as CVRs over oral contraceptives. Few vaginal side effects were reported in one trial of 124 women using these pills, and contraceptive effect over 6 to 20 months was excellent. Amenorrhea, breakthrough bleeding, and spotting occurred rarely (Coutinho et al., 1984).

Injectables. A method of birth control that is widely used in many countries, particularly underdeveloped countries, but engenders much controversy is the long-term injectable—the "shot." Full discussion of the arguments on both sides is beyond the scope of this chapter, but essentially the controversy revolves around potential side effects of this method and whether or not these effects have been adequately studied.

Two progestins — medroxyprogesterone acetate (DMPA or Depo-Provera) and norethisterone acetate (NET)—are most commonly used in injectable contraceptives. These provide protection against pregnancy for 90 and 60 days, respectively, inhibiting ovulation by acting on pituitary secretions, causing endometrial changes, and affecting the fallopian tubes and cervical mucus (Fraser & Halck, 1983). Reported pregnancy rates are less than one to slightly over one per 100 woman-years (Fraser & Halck, 1983; World Health Organization, 1982).

Menstrual irregularities are seen in most women after progestin injections, although clinical trials are in progress evaluating monthly injectables consisting of estrogen and progestin, which would decrease bleeding irregularities (Diaz-Sanchez, Garza-Flores, Jimenez-Thomas, & Rudel, 1987; Diczfalusy, 1986a). Abdominal bloating, headaches, mood changes, nervousness, fatigue, and weight gain have also been noted (Fraser & Halck, 1983). Possible serious side effects include teratogenicity, changes in carbohydrate and lipid metabolism (Liew, Ng, Yong, & Ratnam, 1985), prolonged infertility after discontinuation, and unknown long-term effects on infants breastfed by women receiving injections (World Health Organization, 1982). A suggested relationship between injectable progestins and the development of breast and endometrial cancer is particularly controversial, with debate focusing on the relevance to humans of studies in animals demonstrating carcinogenicity. Some critics of injectable contraceptives feel that despite widespread use, adequate follow-up of women using these contraceptives has not been carried out, especially as injections often are administered by paraprofessionals in traveling units; others (Minkin, 1980, 1981) believe that the evidence is sufficient to classify the progestins delivered by injection as unnecessarily dangerous.

An obvious disadvantage of the injectable contraceptive is that once injected, it cannot be removed from the system. Hormonal levels have been detected in the blood as much as 7.5 to 9 months after injection (Fraser & Halck, 1983). The United States Food and Drug Administration (FDA) has considered and denied approval of Depo-Provera as a contraceptive in this country. Considerable criticism has been leveled at groups that promote the use of any contraceptive in other countries, particularly in the Third World, that is banned from use for contraceptive purposes here (Levine, 1979).

Intracervical Devices. A progestin-releasing device that is inserted by a health care provider into the cervix after menses is under investigation. Advantages of intracervical devices (ICDs) over intrauterine devices (IUDs) are lack of mechanical irritation of the endometrium and, possibly, decreased risk of infection as a result of thickened cervical mucus (Kurunmaki, Toivonen, Lahteenmaki, & Luukkainen, 1984). Advantages over oral contraceptives are similar to those discussed for the vaginal ring (Kurunmaki et al., 1984). A distinct disadvantage of the ICD over vaginal delivery systems is the necessity for professional insertion with uterine sounding using a tenaculum (Moghissi, 1980). Discomfort, expulsion, spotting, and bleeding remain problems.

Intranasal Sprays. The possibility of administering the progestin norethisterone (NET) intranasally for contraception is currently under investigation. The advantage of this delivery system is increased bioavailability of the drug compared with oral administration, as gastric mucosa and hepatic degradation are bypassed. This allows lower doses to be effective, decreasing the body's overall drug load (Shah, Toddywala, Maskati, et al., 1985). Large-scale trials of intranasal sprays are planned.

Nonsteroidal Antiovulatory Chemicals

A group of chemicals used for treatment of infertility have been found, paradoxically, to have antifertility effects. Repeated doses of these peptide substances—analogs or agonists of gonadotropin-releasing hormone (GnRH) or luteinizing hormone–releasing hormone (LHRH)—apparently cause pituitary desensitization resulting in inhibition of follicular maturation and ovulation (Casper, Sheehan, Erickson, & Yen, 1980). Administered intranasally, these hormones work specifically on the hypothalamic–pituitary–ovarian system with fewer systemic effects than steroids (Bergquist, Nillius, & Wide, 1985). Short-term studies have shown good contraceptive results; side effects include bleeding irregularities and hot flashes. Slight nasal irritation and headaches early in usage have been reported (Bergquist et al., 1985; Nillius, Gudmundsson, & Bergquist, 1985). Further studies on metabolic effects are in progress (Gudmundsson, Nillius, & Bergquist, 1984). Interestingly,

these chemicals have antifertility effects for men as well and are discussed in the section on male contraception.

Luteal Phase or Postcoital Contraception

Contraceptives whose main effects are during the luteal phase of the menstrual cycle interfere with the process of fertilization, implantation, or continued pregnancy. Advantages are obvious: Contraception can be used only when intercourse takes place yet is not related to intercourse itself; contraception can be initiated after unprotected acts of intercourse. Short-term periodic administration could lead to fewer side effects and these would be localized rather than systemic (Hahn, McGuire, & Chang, 1980).

Luteal phase contraception—also called postcoital or menses-inducing contraception—takes a variety of forms and includes antiimplantive agents, morning-after pills, once-a-week pills, and interceptives and abortifacients (which interfere with pregnancy after implantation) (Hahn et al., 1980). A number of substances have been investigated as possible luteal phase contraceptives, including steroids, prostaglandins, LHRH and its agonists, antiprogesterones, and a number of products extracted from naturally occurring plants long used by traditional healers as abortifacients (Chatterton, Cheesman, Mehta, & Venton, 1980; Gallegos, 1985; Goldzieher & Quinones, 1980; Kabir, Bhattacharya, Pal, & Pakrashi, 1984; Pedron, Estrada, Ponce-Monter, et al., 1985).

Chapter 7 contains a discussion of "morning-after" pills: the use of a variety of oral contraceptive regimens for postcoital contraception within approximately 72 hours. Other agents, such as the antiprogestin mifepristone (RU 486), can potentially interrupt pregnancy for longer periods (van Santen & Haspels, 1987), up to 5 or more weeks after fertilization (Snyder & Schane, 1985).

Luteal phase contraception raises ethical and political questions for some opponents of abortion. Some consider any method that exerts its effect after fertilization to be an abortifacient. The introduction of luteal phase contraception may be met with attempts to block its use.

Antipregnancy Immunization

Another approach to luteal phase contraception is the antipregnancy vaccine, although vaccination could also be used to prevent penetration of the ovum by sperm (Talwar, 1982). Potential advantages of immunologic fertility control include long-term protection, ease of administration and use, and low cost (Stevens, 1983). Several problems arise, however, in the consideration of an antifertility vaccine: selection of an appropriate antigen (that would not cause reactions in nonreproductive tissues); achievement of immunity in at least 95 percent of the immunized; and reversal of immune effects. Antigen requirements include uniqueness to the reproductive tract (i.e., absence from other tissues) with a function that antibodies could inhibit or block (Anderson & Alexander, 1983). Possible antigens include reproductive hormones, particularly human chorionic gonadotropin (hCG), and substances found in the zona pellucida of the ovum, sperm, or embryonic, fetal, or placental tissue. Of these, hCG is the most widely studied.

One problem with hCG is that the *a* subunit is similar to many pituitary hormones and the *β* subunit is similar to LH. Concerns exist that development of nonspecific antibodies would cause immunologic damage in the pituitary or kidney (Anderson & Alexander, 1983, p. 560). One end of the *β* hCG chain, however, contains amino acids not found in LH; it is possible that a vaccine could target this area. Unfortunately, this portion of HCG has not been shown to be highly antigenic (Thanavals, 1981).

The ovum has two potential problems as an antigen: (1) Antibodies could cause undesirable reactions in the ovary and (2) women exhibit immunologic tolerance to natural antigens (Stevens, 1980, p. 396). Sperm enzymes hold greater potential as antigens. Indeed, some infertility is caused by naturally occurring sperm antibodies. An antisperm vaccine for women would make biologic sense because it would be to a foreign body rather than to an antigen found in the women's own bodies (Stevens, 1983). The placenta has a similar advantage; it is a "nonself" source; however, studies have shown severe side effects such as nephritis with this approach (Stevens, 1980).

The availability of monoclonal antibodies may enable the development of passive, short- or long-term, reversible immunization (Anderson & Alexander, 1983, p. 567). These substances hold great promise, but it is likely to be years before any antipregnancy vaccine becomes available.

Chemical Sterilization

The possibility of occluding the fallopian tubes with a variety of chemical agents has been studied in animals. To date, these agents have been found to carry a high degree of toxicity (Diczfalusy, 1986a) and are not reversible (Atkinson et al., 1980).

New Techniques for Detecting and Predicting Ovulation

Through assays of various urinary hormones or measurement of other cyclic changes such as electrical impulses transmitted via skin, it may become possible not only to detect ovulation with a high degree of accuracy, but to predict it in advance and to identify peak fertility periods (Baker, Holdsworth, & Coulson, 1984; Roy & Mishell, 1981; Schiphorst, Sallam, Adekunle, et al., 1984). Availability of self-administered predictive methods would greatly assist women using natural family planning.

Improvements on Existing Methods

A number of new developments could improve the efficacy, safety, or desirability of already existing contraceptives. In female methods, improvements have been suggested or are being investigated for the diaphragm, the cervical cap, vaginal spermicides and suppositories, and the IUD and oral contraceptives.

Diaphragm. Diaphragm improvements possible in the future include one-size-fits-all diaphragms, disposable diaphragms, and diaphragms impregnated with spermicide (*World Population,* 1982). Gillespie (1984) has proposed a U-shaped diaphragm (Fig. 9–2), which would decrease urethral and bladder neck pressure and eliminate the urinary tract problems that occur with diaphragm use. The literature, however, does not reflect research on this diaphragm modification.

Cervical Caps and Vaginal Spermicides. Individually molded cervical caps with one-way valves for increased wearing time have shown problems in clinical trials but are continuing to be investigated ("Contracap," 1983; "Valved Cervical Cap," 1987). Vaginal suppositories with increased doses of spermicides are being evaluated (Edelman & Thompson, 1982), and the spermicidal activity of a variety

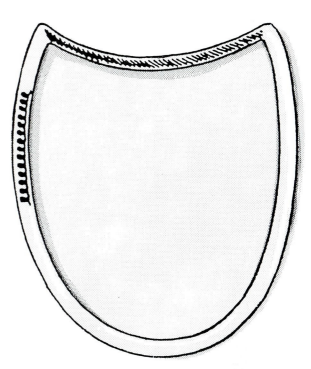

Figure 9–2. A proposed "U"-shaped diaphragm. *(From Gillespie, L. [1984, July]. The diaphragm: An accomplice in recurrent urinary tract infections.* Urology, 24[2], 25–30. Reprinted with permission.)*

of substances is being tested (Furuse, Ishizeki, & Iwahara, 1983; Mandal & Bhattacharyya, 1986; Waller, Zaneveld, & Fong, 1980). Surfactants, gossypol (see Male Methods, next section), and sperm enzyme inhibitors that would immobilize sperm or interfere with their ability to penetrate the ovum are among the proposed new vaginal spermicides. Propranolol, a β-blocking agent that also inhibits sperm motility and metabolism, has been suggested as an intravaginal spermicide (Patel, Warrington, & Pearson, 1983; Sherris, 1984; Zipper, Wheeler, Potts, & Rivera, 1983). Spermicide administration via a vaginal ring is under investigation; this would eliminate the need for precoital spermicide application (Burck & Zimmerman, 1984; World Health Organization, 1979).

Intrauterine Device. IUD improvements include extension of the period of release for steroids or copper (Ratsula, Haukkamaa, Wichman, & Luukkainen, 1983; Scommegna, 1980; Tso & Lee, 1982), addition of prostaglandins, hCG antibodies, or antiinflammatory compounds to the delivery system (Hurst & Peplow, 1985), and design of tailless devices, which have the potential to decrease the incidence of IUD-related pelvic inflammatory disease (Scommegna, 1980). Compounds that may aid in reducing the blood loss normally associated with IUD use are being investigated in the People's Republic of China (Diczfalusy, 1986b, p. 13).

Oral Contraceptives. Several types of oral contraceptives different from those used in the United States are available in China and may represent significant improvements (Chen & Kols, 1982, pp. J592–593). The "drip pill"—named after a step in its manufacturing process—is made from steroids in solution rather than from dusty powders. It enables the production of a much smaller pill and lowers exposure to steroids for workers involved in its production. The paper pill has the same advantages, and less expensive material is used in its production and packaging. The Chinese also rely more heavily than we do on a type of morning-after pill that is taken for 3 days after coitus and acts on the luteal phase of the menstrual cycle and on the endometrium. Its advantage is in less continuous use when intercourse is infrequent. A monthly oral contraceptive pill and an injectable contraceptive are also available in China.

MALE METHODS

Although the majority of contraceptive research funds is targeted to female methods, there is some support for methods for men. A number of steps in the male reproductive process could be amenable to intervention for contraception (Ritzen, 1983). These include the secretion of regulatory hormones (GnRH, LHRH, FSH, LH, and testosterone) and the processes of spermatogenesis, sperm maturation, and sperm transport. Organs involved in these processes include the hypothalamus, the pituitary gland, testes, seminiferous tubules, the epididymis, and the vas deferens.

A number of substances that interfere with one or more male reproductive functions have been identified and tested; the literature, however, reports varying degrees of side effects or practical problems with each of these and none has reached the stage of clinical trials in this country.

It has been pointed out that efforts at developing safe and effective male contraceptives are hampered by "a severe lack of information on male reproductive physiology; without more fundamental knowledge regarding the functions of the testis, epididymis, vas deferens, and accessory glands, it is unlikely that new methods for male contraception can be developed" (Patanelli, 1980, p. 194). Two questions remain: (1) Why is such minimal effort expended on decreasing these knowledge gaps? (2) Why are researchers apparently less tolerant of side effects for male methods than for female methods?

Steroidal Agents

Androgens, impeded androgens (which only partially stimulate organs), antiandrogens, progestins, and androgen-progestogen combinations have been evaluated as male contraceptives (Paulsen, Bremner, & Leonard, 1982). Estrogens have also been considered but have feminizing and other side effects including decreased libido and impotence and, therefore, are considered unacceptable for use in men (Bajaj & Madan, 1983; Smith, Rodriguez-Rigau, & Steinberger 1980).

Androgens: Testosterone. Exogenously administered testosterone has the potential for inhibiting spermatogenesis through a feedback mechanism on the hypothalamus and pituitary. Oral doses, however, have failed to achieve azoospermia (Smith et al., 1980). Injections that would lead to human contraception would have to be given on a daily or weekly basis, although longer-acting forms of testosterone have been tested in animals (Diczfalusy, 1986b). Subdermal delivery is possible but at present would require too large an implant for practical use (Bajaj & Madan, 1983). Testosterone injections can cause weight gain, acne, decreased testicular size, and possible cholestatic jaundice. The possibilities of increased susceptibility to atherosclerotic heart disease, hypertrophy or carcinoma of the prostate, and mutagenesis have been raised as well (Bajaj & Madan, 1983).

The future of testosterone as an acceptable male contraceptive depends on the results of long-term studies of side effects, especially on the cardiovascular system and prostate gland, and the development of longer-acting esters or derivatives that are active orally or can be practically implanted subcutaneously.

Progestins. Although progestins have the potential to cause oligospermia or azoospermia, doses sufficient to achieve sperm counts low enough for contraception also cause decreased libido and potency, gynecomastia, and nipple pain (Bajaj & Madan, 1983).

Progestin–Androgen Combinations. The addition of an androgen to a progestin theoretically should eliminate the problems of decreased libido and impotency. In trials conducted by the Population Council, however, such combinations did not consistently produce azoospermia. Side effects included weight gain, gynecomastia, decreased libido, night sweats, and, more seriously, increased serum transaminase (Bajaj & Madan, 1983; Smith et al., 1980). In one study, a combination of a form of testosterone and the progestin DMPA was found to cause decreased HDL cholesterol levels after withdrawal of the drugs (Friedl, Plymate, & Paulsen, 1985).

Antiandrogens. Antiandrogens inhibit the activity of androgen at target sites. Thus far, such agents have been found to reduce spermatogenesis but not to cause uniform azoospermia. In addition, they have possible affects on secondary sexual characteristics and other adverse side effects including negative protein and calcium balance (Bajaj & Madan, 1983).

Nonsteroidal Agents

Nonsteroidal agents effective for men exert contraceptive action in a variety of ways. Some of these inhibit spermatogenesis indirectly by affecting the hypothalamic–pituitary unit. A number of substances act directly either on spermatogenesis or on the sperm cells themselves. Some inhibit the capacity of sperm for fertilization; others modify sperm cells so that the resulting embryo is not viable; many have actions that as yet are not completely understood.

LHRH Analogs. A group of agents—LHRH analogs or agonists—that have potential for female contraception may also prove valuable in male reproductive control. Indeed, these neuropeptides have been referred to as the future "unisex" pill (Coutinho, 1974), although they are actually administered intranasally. Their contraceptive action in men has been hypothesized to result from (1) decreased gonadotropin secretion secondary to refractoriness at the pituitary level; (2) loss of testicular receptiveness as a result of increased release of gonadotropins; (3) negative feedback at the hypothalamic–pituitary level caused by high levels of gonadotropins and testicular steroid hormones; and/or (4) decreased spermatogenesis resulting from direct effects on the testes (Bajaj & Madan, 1983; Heber & Swerdloff, 1980).

Theoretically, antagonists of LHRH could also be used for male fertility control but these cause lowered LH and testosterone levels, thus interfering with libido and secondary sexual characteristics. LHRH analogs, however, may also reduce testosterone. A possible solution to this problem would be to administer testosterone with these agents.

Inhibin. Inhibin is a peptide hormone found in the gonads. Although current research on its effects is limited because it has not been isolated or purified, inhibin may prove to prevent sperm production by suppressing the release of pituitary FSH without interfering with LH. The advantage of this is that testosterone production would not be affected and some of the adverse side effects associated with decreased testosterone would thus be avoided (World Population, 1982). Although the role of FSH in male fertility is not entirely known, it is believed to be necessary for spermatogenesis (Bajaj & Madan, 1983). Currently, animal studies are underway to isolate inhibin as a first step toward eventual testing.

Other Agents With Effects on the Hypothalamic–Pituitary Unit. Substances that have been found to act on the hypothalamic–pituitary unit in men include a thiourate, ergot alkyloids, narcotics, such as morphine and methadone, and tranquilizers, such as the benzodiazepines. As Lobl, Bardin, and Chang (1980, p. 148) point out, it is not likely that these drugs could ever be used in contraception, but their "study may reveal novel actions which could be used to design new drugs." Other chemicals that affect spermatogenesis in known or unknown ways have been described by Lobl and associates (1980).

Naturally Occurring Plants

GOSSYPOL. Of the various drugs that have been considered for male contraception, gossypol has attracted the most attention. Gossypol is a compound present in the seed of the cotton plant. It was discovered in China in 1971 after an outbreak of illness and decreased fertility among Chinese farmers; this resulted when a change in processing techniques exposed them to raw cottonseed oil (Chen & Kols, 1982). Gossypol inhibits spermatogenesis and sperm motility (Donaldson, Sufi, & Jeffcoate, 1985).

Extensive clinical trials have been carried out in China confirming the consistent antifertility effects of gossypol but also revealing a number of toxic effects. These include fatigue, gastrointestinal symptoms, decreased libido, and hypokalemia. Hypokalemia can be severe in some cases but has been found primarily in men with diets low in potassium. It can be prevented by giving potassium salt to men who complain of fatigue and weakness or by increasing potassium in the diet (Shaozhen, Guangwei, Xiaoyun, et al., 1980). Gossypol also poses the problem of irreversibility after discontinuation, a problem that increases with increased duration of exposure (Prasad & Diczfalusy, 1983). It is possible that in the future a purified form or synthetic analog or derivative may retain antifertility properties with fewer side effects (Donaldson et al., 1985).

OTHER PLANTS. A number of other naturally occurring plants have sperm-inhibiting properties. Advantages to the use of plants in fertility regulation are their "folkloric history and established low toxicity potential" based on long-term use in indigenous medical systems, their familiarity to many people within such systems, and their low cost (Farnsworth & Waller, 1982). Disadvantages include the geographic limitations on availability of many such plants and the variability among plants. An extensive summary of plant products that inhibit sperm has been prepared by Farnsworth and Waller (1982).

Nonchemical Methods

An interesting attempt at inhibition of spermatogenesis has been described by Mieusset, Grandjean, Mansat, and Pontonnier (1985). They induced thermogenesis by pushing the testicles into the inguinal canal and keeping them there during waking hours by use of an adapted athletic supporter. During an experimental period of 6 to 12 months, sperm counts were lowered and sperm motility decreased after several months in all 14 volunteers. Normal sperm counts returned within 6 to 8 months. Whether this mechanical process could be used to induce infertility is unknown, however, because azoospermia was not achieved.

Immunization

Vaccination has been proposed for males as well as for females. A number of possible antigens have been identified in the male reproductive tract. Hormones produced by the hypothalamus, pituitary, or testes seem most amenable to the action of antibodies, as hormone antibodies are less likely to cause tissue damage than tissue antibodies (Wickings & Nieschlag, 1983). Further research is needed to assess the efficacy, side effects, and reversibility of male vaccines.

Improvements in Existing Male Contraceptives

Several recent innovations in condoms, such as lubrication with spermicides, have already been marketed. Another proposed improvement is the water-soluble condom. Its advantage is less reduction in sensation. A new male barrier contraceptive that would not interfere with sensation is a spermicidal film (similar to a film inserted intravaginally—see Chapter 6). This film would fit over the glans of the penis and dissolve at the cervix (Belsky, 1979).

THE FUTURE

New contraceptives require extensive and costly testing prior to widespread availability. Djerassi (1981) has suggested that the stringent FDA requirements for new contraceptives limit their development. Contraceptives, however, with high profit potential, such as the vaginal sponge, are more likely to be rapidly tested than those of low profit potential, such as the cervical cap. Although we do not favor lessening the requirements for contraceptive approval, we do favor increasing public funding for such research. National commitments to improving and developing new nonchemical methods, to supporting research on male contraceptives or those with shared responsibility, and to removing contraceptive research from the profit-making sector would be important toward bettering available methods and expanding choices.

REFERENCES

Ahren, T., Victor, A., & Lithell, H., et al. (1983, October). Ovarian function, bleeding control and serum lipoproteins in women using contraceptive vaginal rings releasing five different progestins. *Contraception, 28*(4), 315–327.

Alvarez, F., Brache, V., Tejada, A. S., & Faundes, A. (1986, February). Abnormal endocrine profile among women with confirmed or presumed ovulation during long-term NORPLANT use. *Contraception, 33*(2), 111–119.

Anderson, D. J., & Alexander, N. J. (1983, November). A new look at antifertility vaccines. *Fertility and Sterility, 40*(5), 557–571.

Atkinson, L., Schearer, B., Harkavy, O., & Lincoln, R. (1980, July/August). Prospects for improved contraception. *Family Planning Perspectives, 12*(4), 173–192.

Bajaj, J. S., & Madan, R. (1983). New approaches to male fertility regulation: LHRH analogs, steroidal contraception and inhibin. In G. Benagiano & E. Diczfalusy (Eds.) *Endocrine mechanism in fertility regulation.* New York: Raven Press.

Baker, T. S., Holdsworth, R. J., & Coulson, W. F. (1984). The dual analyte assay for the detection of the fertile period in women. In J. Bonnar, W. Thompson, & R. F. Harrison (Eds.), *Research in family planning.* Lancaster, England: MTP Press Limited.

Belsky, R. (1979). Water-soluble condom and vaginal contraceptive film insert. In G. I. Zatuchni, A. J. Sobrero, J. J. Speidel, & J. J. Sciarra (Eds.), *Vaginal contraception: New developments*, PARFR Series on Fertility Regulation. Hagerstown, MD: Harper & Row.

Bergquist, C., Nillius, S. J., & Wide, L. (1985, February). Peptide contraception in women. *Contraception, 31*(2), 111–118.

Borzelleca, J. F., & Carmines, E. L. (1980). New drug evaluation: Safety assessment. In G. I. Zatuchni, M. H. Labbok, & J. J. Sciarra (Eds.), *Research frontiers in fertility regulation.* Hagerstown, MD: Harper & Row.

Brache, V., Faundes, A., Johansson, E., & Alvarez, F. (1985, March). Anovulation, inadequate luteal phase and poor sperm penetration in cervical mucus during prolonged use of NOR-PLANT implants. *Contraception, 31*(3), 261–273.

Burck, P. J., & Zimmerman, R. E. (1984, February). An intravaginal contraceptive device for the delivery of an acrosin and hyaluronidase inhibitor. *Fertility and Sterility, 41*(2), 314–318.

Casper, R. F., Sheehan, K., Erickson, G., & Yen, S. S. C. (1980). Neuropeptides and fertility control in the female. In G. I. Zatuchni, M. H. Labbok, & J. J. Sciarra (Eds.), *Research frontiers in fertility regulation.* Hagerstown, MD: Harper & Row.

Chatterton, R. T., Cheesman, K. L., Mehta, R. R., & Venton, D. L. (1980). Postovulatory interception. In G. I. Zatuchni, M. H. Labbok, & J. J. Sciarra (Eds.), *Research frontiers in fertility regulation.* Hagerstown, MD: Harper & Row.

Chen, P., & Kols, A. (1982, January/February). Population and birth planning in the People's Republic of China. *Population Reports, 10*(1), J577–J618, Ser. J, No. 25.

Connell, E. B. (1984, March/April). Research on methods of fertility regulation. *Journal of Obstetric, Gynecologic, and Neonatal Nursing, 13* (2, Suppl.), 50s–56s.

Contracap makes crucial changes for expanded trials. (1983, October). *Contraceptive Technology Update, 4*(10), 114–115.

Coutinho, E. H. (1974, June). Male contraception and the "unisex" pill. *IPPF Medical Bulletin, 8*(3), 3–4.

Coutinho, E. M., da Silva, A. R., & Carreira, C., et al. (1984, September). Conception control by vaginal administration of pills containing ethinyl estradiol and *dl*-norgestrel. *Fertility and Sterility, 42*(3), 478–481.

de Leede, L. G. J., Govers, C. P. M., & de Nijs, H. (1986, December). A multi-compartment vaginal ring system for independently adjustable release of contraceptive steroids. *Contraception, 34*(6), 589–602.

Diaz, S., Herreros, C., Johansson, E. D. B., & Croxatto, H. B. (1986, April). Bleeding pattern, outcome of accidental pregnancies and levonorgestrel plasma levels associated with method failure in NORPLANT implants users. *Contraception, 33*(4), 347–356.

Diaz, S., Pavez, M., Cardenas, H., & Croxatto, H. B. (1987, June). Recovery of fertility and outcome of planned pregnancies after the removal of NORPLANT subdermal implants or Copper-T IUDs. *Contraception, 35*(6), 569–579.

Diaz-Sanchez, V., Garza-Flores, J., Jimenez-Thomas, S., & Rudel, H. W. (1987, January). Development of a low-dose monthly injectable contraceptive system. II. Pharmacokinetic and pharmacodynamic studies. *Contraception, 35*(1), 57–68.

Diczfalusy, E. (1986a, July). World Health Organization, Special Programme of Research, Development and Research Training in Human Reproduction: The first fifteen years: A review. *Contraception, 34*(1), 1–119.

Diczfalusy, E. (1986b, January). New developments in oral, injectable and implantable contraceptives, vaginal rings and intrauterine devices. *Contraception, 33*(1), 7–22.

Djerassi, C. (1981). *The politics of contraception: Birth control in the year 2001.* New York: Freeman.

Donaldson, A., Sufi, S. B., & Jeffcoate, S. L. (1985, February). Inhibition by gossypol of testosterone production by mouse Leydig cells in vitro. *Contraception, 31*(2), 165–170.

Edelman, D. A., & Thompson, S. (1982). Vaginal contraception—An update. *Contraceptive Delivery Systems, 3*(2), 75–81.

Farnsworth, N. R., & Waller, D. P. (1982, June). Current status of plant products reported to inhibit sperm. *Research Frontiers in Fertility Regulation, 2*(1), 1–16.

Fraser, J. S., & Halck, S. (1983). Depot medroxyprogesterone acetate. In D. R. Mishell, Jr. (Ed.), *Advances in human fertility and reproductive endocrinology. Vol. 2. Long-acting steroid contraception.* New York: Raven Press.

Friedl, K. E., Plymate, S. R., & Paulsen, C. A. (1985, April). Transient reduction in serum HDL-cholesterol following medroxyprogesterone acetate and testosterone cypionate administration to healthy men. *Contraception, 31*(4), 409–420.

Furuse, K., Ishizeki, C., & Iwahara, S. (1983, June). Studies on spermicidal activity of surfactants. I. Correlation between spermicidal effect and physicochemical properties of p-menthanylphenyl polyoxyethylene (8.8) ether and related surfactants. *Journal of Pharmacobio-Dynamics, 6*(6), 359–372.

Gabelnick, H. L. (1983). Biodegradable implants: Alternative approaches. In D. R. Mishell, Jr. (Ed.), *Advances in human fertility and reproductive endocrinology. Vol. 2. Long-acting steroid contraception.* New York: Raven Press.

Gallegos, A. J. (1980). Vaginal steroidal contraception. In G. I. Zatuchni, M. H. Labbok, & J. J. Sciarra (Eds.), *International workshop on research frontiers in fertility regulation*, PARFR Series on Fertility Regulation. Hagerstown, MD: Harper & Row.

Gallegos, A. J. (1985, May). The zoapatle. VI. Revisited. *Contraception, 31*(5), 487–497.

Gillespie, L. (1984, July). The diaphragm: An accomplice in recurrent urinary tract infections. *Urology. 24*(2), 25–30.

Goldzieher, J. W., & Quinones, R. G. (1980). Discussion: Luteal phase contraception. In G. I. Zatuchni, M. H. Labbok, & J. J. Sciarra (Eds.), *Research frontiers in fertility regulation.* Hagerstown, MD: Harper & Row.

Gudmundsson, J. A., Nillius, S. J., & Bergquist, C. (1984, August). Inhibition of ovulation by intranasal Nafarelin, a new superactive agonist of GnRH. *Contraception, 30*(2), 107–114.

Hahn, D. W., McGuire, J. L., & Chang, M. C. (1980). Contragestational agents. In G. I. Zatuchni, M. H. Labbok, & J. J. Sciarra (Eds.), *Research frontiers in fertility regulation.* Hagerstown, MD: Harper & Row.

Hardy, E. E., Reyes, Q., & Gomez, F., et al. (1983, November). User's perception of the contraceptive vaginal ring: A field study in Brazil and the Dominican Republic. *Studies in Family Planning, 14*(11), 284–290.

Haukkamaa, M. (1986, June). Contraception by NORPLANT subdermal capsules is not reliable in epileptic patients on anticonvulsant treatment. *Contraception, 33*(6), 559–565.

Heber, D., & Swerdloff, R. S. (1980). Brain peptides and fertility control in the male. In G. I. Zatuchni, M. H. Labbok, & J. J. Sciarra (Eds.), *Research frontiers in fertility regulation.* Hagerstown, MD: Harper & Row.

Hingorani, V., Jalnawala, S. F., & Kochhar, M., et al. (1986, March). Phase II randomized comparable clinical trial of NORPLANT® (six capsules) with Norplant -2 (two covered rods) subdermal implants for long-term contraception: Report of a 24-month study. *Contraception, 33*(3), 233–244.

Holma, P. (1985, March). Long-term experience with NORPLANT contraceptive implants in Finland. *Contraception 31*(3), 231–241.

Hurst, P. R., & Peplow, P. V. (1985, May). Suppression of leukocytosis by the intrauterine delivery of high doses of indomethacin in the rat. *Contraception, 31*(5), 445–451.

Johansson, E. D. B., & Odlind, V. (1983). NORPLANT: Biochemical effects. In D. R. Mishell, Jr. (Ed.) *Advances in human fertility and reproductive endocrinology. Vol. 2. Long-acting steroid contraception.* New York: Raven Press.

Kabir, S. N., Bhattacharya, K., Pal, A. K., & Pakrashi, A. (1984, April). Flowers of *Hibiscus rosa-sinensis*, a potential source of contragestative agent. I. Effect of benzene extract on implantation of mouse. *Contraception, 29*(4), 385–397.

Kurunmaki, H., Toivonen, J., Lahteenmaki, P. L. A. & Luukkainen, T. T. (1984, May). Intracervical release of ST-1435 for contraception. *Contraception, 29*(5), 411–421.

Levine, C. (1979, August). Depo-Provera and contraceptive risk: A case study of values in conflict. *Hastings Center Report, 9*(4), 8–11.

Liew, D. F. M., Ng, C. S. S., Yong, Y. M. & Ratnam, S. S. (1985, January). Long-term effects of Depo-Provera on carbohydrate and lipid metabolism. *Contraception, 31*(1), 51–64.

Lobl, T. J., Bardin, C. W., & Chang, C. C. (1980). Pharmacologic agents producing infertility by direct action on the male reproductive tract. In G. I. Zatuchni, M. H. Labbok, & J. J. Sciarra (Eds.), *Research frontiers in fertility regulation.* Hagerstown, MD: Harper & Row.

Mandal, A., & Bhattacharyya, A. K. (1986, January). Human seminal antiliquefying agents—A potential approach towards vaginal contraception. *Contraception, 33*(1), 31–38.

Mieusset, R., Grandjean, H., Mansat, A., & Pontonnier, F. (1985, April). Inhibiting effect of artificial cryptorchidism on spermatogenesis. *Fertility and Sterility, 43*(4), 589–594.

Minkin, S. (1980, Summer). Depo-Provera: A critical analysis. *Women and Health, 5*(2), 49–69.

Minkin, S. (1981, November). Nine Thai women had cancer . . . none of them took Depo-Provera, therefore, Depo-Provera is safe. This is science? *Mother Jones,* 34–54.

Moghissi, K. S. (1980). A progestogen-releasing intracervical contraceptive device: Fabrication and preliminary clinical evaluation. In G. I. Zatuchni, M. H. Labbok, & J. J. Sciarra (Eds.), *Research frontiers in fertility regulation.* Hagerstown, MD: Harper & Row.

Nash, H. A., & Jackanicz, T. M. (1982). Contraceptive vaginal rings. In D. R. Mishell, Jr. (Ed.), *Advances in human fertility and reproductive endocrinology. Vol. 1.* New York: Raven Press.

Nillius, S. J., Gudmundsson, J., & Bergquist, C. (1985, February). A new superagonist of GnRH for inhibition of ovulation in women. *Contraception, 31*(2), 119–122.

NORPLANT gets approval for IPPF contraceptive list. (1986, March). *Contraceptive Technology Update, 7*(3), 36.

Nuttal, I. D., Elstein, M., & Spencer, B. E. (1985, April). Progestogen-releasing vaginal rings—An update. *IPPF Medical Bulletin, 19*(2), 1–2.

Pasquale, S. A. (1980). Evaluation of new contraceptives: A study design. In G. I. Zatuchni, M. H. Labbok, & J. J. Sciarra (Eds.), *Research frontiers in fertility regulation.* Hagerstown, MD: Harper & Row.

Patanelli, D. J. (1980). Discussion: Pharmacologic and hormonal methods in male fertility control. In G. I. Zatuchni, M. H. Labbok, & J. J. Sciarra (Eds.), *Research frontiers in fertility regulation.* Hagerstown, MD: Harper & Row.

Patel, L. G., Warrington, S. J., & Pearson, R. M. (1983, October 29). Propranolol concentration in plasma after insertion into the vagina. *British Medical Journal, 287*(6401), 1247–1248.

Paulsen, C. A., Bremner, W. J., & Leonard, J. M. (1982). Male contraception: Clinical trials. In D. R. Mishell, Jr. (Ed.), *Advances in human fertility and reproductive endocrinology. Vol. 1.* New York: Raven Press.

Pedron, N., Estrada, A. V., & Ponce-Monter, H., et al. (1985, May). The zoapatle. VII. Antiimplantation effect in the rat of zoapatle aqueous crude extract (Zace) from *Montanoa tomentosa* and *Montanoa frutescens. Contraception, 31*(5), 499–507.

The Population Council. (1987a, August). NORPLANT Fact Sheet No. 2. *NORPLANT Worldwide, 8,* 2–3.

The Population Council. (1987b, November). NORPLANT Fact Sheet No. 3.

The Population Council. (1987c, April). The Norplant Tally: 31 countries and 44,000 women. *NORPLANT Worldwide, 7,* 4.

Prasad, M. R. N., & Diczfalusy, E. (1983). Gossypol. In G. Benagiano & E. Diczfalusy (Eds.), *Endocrine mechanisms in fertility regulation.* New York: Raven Press.

Ratsula, K., Haukkamaa, M., Wichmann, K., & Luukkainen, T. (1983, June). Vaginal contraception with gossypol: A clinical study. *Contraception, 27*(6), 571–576.

Ritzen, E. M. (1983). Steps in male reproductive endocrinology susceptible to regulation. In G. Benagiano & E. Diczfalusy (Eds.), *Endocrine mechanisms in fertility regulation.* New York: Raven Press.

Rivera, R., Gaita, J. R., & Ortega, M., et al. (1984, August). The use of biodegradable norethisterone implants as a 6-month contraceptive system. *Fertility and Sterility, 42*(2), 228–232.

Rosoff, J. (1984, January/February). Some organizational alternatives to increase support for reproductive and contraceptive research. *Family Planning Perspectives, 16*(1), 28–31.

Roy, S., & Mishell, D. R. (1981, December). Correlation of Ovutron readings and the basal body temperature (BBT) with serum sexhormone and luteinizing hormone levels. *Contraception, 24*(6), 635–646.

Salah, M., Ahmed, A. M., Abo-Eloyoun, M., & Shaaban, M. M. (1987, June). Five-year experience with NORPLANT implants in Assiut, Egypt. *Contraception, 35*(6), 543–550.

Schiphorst, L. E. M., Sallam, H. N., & Adekunle, A. O., et al. (1984). The optimization of an immunochemical test to locate the fertile period in women. In J. Bonnar, W. Thompson, & R. F. Harrison (Eds.), *Research in family planning.* Lancaster, England: MTP Press Limited.

Schwan, A., Ahren, T., & Victor, A. (1983, October). Effects of contraceptive vaginal ring treatment on vaginal bacteriology and cytology. *Contraception, 28*(4), 341–347.

Scommegna, A. (1980). Future IUD developments. In G. I. Zatuchni, M. H. Labbok, & J. J. Sciarra (Eds.), *Research frontiers in fertility regulation.* Hagerstown, MD: Harper & Row.

Shaaban, M. M., Elwan, S. I., Abdalla, S. A., & Darwish, H. A. (1984a, November). Effect of subdermal levonorgestrel contraceptive implants, Norplant, on serum lipids. *Contraception, 30*(5), 413–418.

Shaaban, M. M., Elwan, S. I., & El-Kabsh, M. Y., et al. (1984b, November). Effect of levonorgestrel contraceptive implants, Norplant, on blood coagulation. *Contraception, 30*(5), 421–430.

Shaaban, M. M., Odlind, V., Salem, H. T., et al. (1986, April). Levonorgestrel concentrations in maternal and infant serum during use of subdermal levonorgestrel contraceptive implants, NOR-PLANTS®, by nursing mothers. *Contraception, 33*(4), 357–363.

Shah, R. S., Toddywala, V., & Maskati, B. T., et al. (1985, August). Reproductive endocrine effects of intranasal administration of norethisterone (NET) to women. *Contraception, 32*(2), 135–147.

Shaozhen, Q., Guangwei, J., & Xiaoyun, W., et al. (1980, July). Gossypol related hypokalemia. *Chinese Medical Journal, 93*(7), 477–482.

Sherris, J. D. (1984, January/February). New developments in vaginal contraception. *Population Reports, 12*(1), H157–H190, Ser. H, No. 7.

Sivin, I. (1983). Clinical effects of NORPLANT subdermal implants for contraception. In D. R. Mishell, Jr. (Ed.), *Advances in human fertility and reproductive endocrinology. Vol. 2. Long-acting steroid contraception.* New York: Raven Press.

Sivin, I., Sanchez, F. A., & Diaz, S., et al. (1983, June). Three-year experience with NORPLANT subdermal contraception. *Fertility and Sterility, 39*(6), 799–808.

Smith, K. D., Rodriguez-Rigau, L. J., & Steinberger, E. (1980). Hormonal methods for male contraception. In G. I. Zatuchni, M. H. Labbok, & J. J. Sciarra (Eds.), *Research frontiers in fertility regulation.* Hagerstown, MD: Harper & Row.

Snyder, B. W., & Schane, H. P. (1985, May). Inhibition of luteal phase progesterone levels in the rhesus monkey by epostane. *Contraception, 31*(5), 479–485.

Souka, A. R., El Sokkary, H., Kamel, M., & Hassa, M. (1986, April). The effect of vaginal administration of low-dose oral contraceptive tablets on human ovulation. *Contraception, 33*(4), 365–371.

Souka, A. R., Kamel, M., & Einen, M. A., et al. (1985, June). Vaginal administration of a combined oral contraceptive containing norethisterone acetate. *Contraception, 31*(6), 571–581.

Speidel, J. J. (1983, November). Steroidal contraception in the '80s: The role of current and new products. *Journal of Reproductive Medicine, 28*(11), 759–769.

Stevens, V. C. (1980). Antipregnancy immunization. In G. I. Zatuchni, M. H. Labbok, & J. J. Sciarra (Eds.), *Research frontiers in fertility regulation.* Hagerstown, MD: Harper & Row.

Stevens, V. C. (1983). Potential methods for immunological fertility control in the female. In G. Benagiano & E. Diczfalusy (Eds.), *Endocrine mechanisms in fertility regulation.* New York: Raven Press.

Talwar, G. P. (1982). Contraceptive vaccines. In D. R. Mishell, Jr. (Ed.), *Advances in fertility research (Vol. I).* New York: Raven Press.

Thanavals, Y. (1981, June). Progress in immunological fertility control. IPPF *Medical Bulletin, 15*(3), 2–3.

Tso, W. W., & Lee, C.-S. (1982, February). Cottonseed oil as a vaginal contraceptive. *Archives of Andrology, 8*(1), 11–14.

Valved cervical cap is focus of Chinese multicenter efficacy trial. (1987, February). *Contraceptive Technology Update, 7*(3), 36.

van Santen, M. R., & Haspels, A. A. (1987, May). Interception, III. Postcoital luteal contragestion by an antiprogestin (mifepristone, RU 486) in 62 women. *Contraception, 35*(5), 423–431.

Waller, D. P., Zaneveld, L. J. D., & Fong, H. H. S. (1980, August). In vitro spermicidal activity of gossypol. *Contraception, 22*(2), 183–187.

Wickings, E. J., and Nieschlag, E. (1983). Immunological approach to male fertility control. In G. Benagiano & E. Diczfalusy (Eds.), *Endocrine mechanisms in fertility regulation.* New York: Raven Press.

World Health Organization. Special Programme of Research in Human Reproduction Task Force on Vaginal and Intracervical Devices for Fertility Regulation. (1979). Vaginal rings release spermicides. In G. I. Zatuchni, A. J. Sobrero, J. J. Speidel, & J. J. Sciarra (Eds.), *Vaginal contraception: New developments,* PARFR Series on Fertility Regulation. Hagerstown, MD: Harper & Row.

World Health Organization. (1982). *Injectable hormonal contraceptives: Technical and safety aspects.* Offset Publication No. 65. Geneva: WHO.

World population and fertility planning technologies: The next twenty years. (1982). Washington, DC: Congress of the United States, Office of Technology Assessment.

Zipper, J., Wheeler, R. G., Potts, D. M., & Rivera, M. (1983, October 29). Propranolol as a novel, effective spermicide: Preliminary findings. *British Medical Journal, 287*(6401), 1245–1246.

Gynecologic Pathophysiology

An Evolving Role

It is in the area of pathophysiology that primary health care practitioners most often ask the questions "What is my role?" "How far can I go in management?" "When do I need to consult?"

We do not attempt, in the following chapters, to give definitive answers to these questions. There is no guideline that can be established for all practitioners in all practice settings for all pathologic conditions. Little research has been done evaluating the effectiveness of nonphysician care in any individual disorder. All we can do is provide guidelines for an assessment, to be made by each practitioner or service, of the role of the primary care women's health practitioner when pathology presents. Some situations are clear; others are not. As each individual evolves and matures as a practitioner and as services grow and develop, decision making will change. Factors relating to the practitioner, the law, the institution, the patient, and the pathology itself must be considered in determining the role of the primary care women's health provider in gynecologic pathology.

Practitioner Considerations

EDUCATIONAL BACKGROUND. Primary care women's health practitioners are educated in a variety of ways. This education provides the basis of practice and sets limitations on one's capabilities. We refer you, for example, to Appendix I, Part A, for an outline of the minimum knowledge of well-woman gynecology acquired in midwifery educational programs. Consult, too, your own professional organization for its requirements and guidelines.

EXPERIENCE. A new graduate, of course, relies on physician consultation more frequently than someone with greater experience. This is quite appropriate; safety must always be the primary concern in providing patient care; one should not hesitate to consult when in doubt. This rule of thumb should be followed as well by experienced practitioners, particularly when confronted with something new or unfamiliar.

PERSONAL CONCERNS AND INTERESTS. Some practitioners may be more willing than others to seek in-depth knowledge about pathophysiology and may more readily accept the care of patients with complications. This is valid as long as patient safety remains the major consideration.

Legal Considerations.
States vary in the extent to which they legislate or regulate the practice of the health care provider. It is imperative that all practitioners become familiar with the legal basis of practice in their state and with the specific requirements, privileges, and restrictions afforded their practice. The professional organization is a resource for such information.

Institutional Considerations.
All nonphysician gynecologic care providers practice within the framework of an institution. This may be a freestanding clinic, a hospital clinic, a health maintenance organization, or a private practice. In the last, the provider may be an employee, a partner of a similar or different type of provider, or a solo practitioner. Whatever the circumstances, some type of agreement with a

physician generally exists. Protocols that are agreed on at the time of practice establishment or acceptance of employment must be followed. These may be quite specific and clearly outline the role of the primary care provider in any pathologic condition or may be vague, allowing for individual decision making. It is important that each provider become familiar with such protocols and be comfortable with them. Of course, such protocols can be changed as various considerations change.

Patient Considerations. Some patients may prefer the care of nonphysician providers and choose to be followed in a consultative arrangement, often seeing the nonphysician as an advocate or ombudsman. Others, at the onset of any pathologic change, prefer physician care. Patients have preferences, too, in the degree of specialization they choose for their care. Always, the patient's choice must be based on informed consent. In screening new patients, it is useful to assess whether they have pathologies that may be outside the provider's realm of expertise. The possibility of referral should be discussed so that the woman can choose to have her initial assessment with the person who will ultimately treat her pathology. For women already in your care, it may be beneficial to provide continuity and then referral.

Pathology Considerations. The type and degree of pathology, of course, play major roles in determining the extent of management involvement of the primary women's health care provider, with patient safety always the deciding factor.

Certain needs, problems, and minor pathologies clearly fall within the realm of practice of most primary care women's health providers. These include the provision of all methods of family planning, annual well-woman care, routine postpartum and postabortion care, including history taking, physical and pelvic examination, and laboratory screening. Standard routine laboratory testing includes Pap smears, pregnancy testing, screening for sexually transmitted diseases (STDs), complete blood counts, urinalyses, and stool for guaiac in women over 40. Common STDs and vaginal pathology generally can be managed by nonphysician health care providers, although legal considerations and/or practice or institutional policy may require physician consultation for the use of prescription medication. These disorders include trichomoniasis, bacterial vaginosis, candidiasis (monilia), herpes, chlamydia, gonorrhea, pediculosis, and primary syphilis. Dysmenorrhea generally can be managed by the nonphysician, except where an underlying pathology, such as endometriosis, is identified. Premenstrual syndrome not requiring experimental hormonal medication is also commonly managed by primary care providers.

Some conditions for which referrals are warranted are clear as well. Certainly, if the diagnosis of a pathology requires a technology with which the practitioner is unfamiliar or for which she has not been prepared, referral is in order. These include, for example, abnormal Pap smears requiring colposcopy, adnexal cysts greater than 6 cm, ectopic pregnancy, breast masses, and large or symptomatic fibroids. Any condition that does not respond to usual treatments also requires a consultation or referral. Examples include Bartholin's cysts not responsive to warm soaks or perineal condylomata acuminata that persist after a number of topical treatments.

Other conditions are not so clear; it is for these that each practitioner must consider legal, personal, institutional, and patient needs and circumstances for decision making. For example, does the primary care provider manage urinary tract infections? Does she follow women with in utero DES exposure? Does she follow women with small, asymptomatic fibroids or mild, asymptomatic endometriosis?

Although there are no pat answers to these questions, we suggest the following queries to aid in your decision making:

1. What is the patient's preference for treatment and follow-up? Does the patient understand the educational background and limitations of the nonphysician care provider as well as the advantages of this type of health care so that her choice is informed?
2. How often have you seen this pathology? How knowledgeable about it are you?
3. What is your relationship to your back up physician? Can a mutually agreeable co-management situation be arranged? An example of a condition often amenable to co-management is amenorrhea in a woman not desiring pregnancy; after a workup ruling out pathology (see Chapter 21), treatment can be provided with physician consultation and the patient co-managed if she responds appropriately.
4. Has the patient had a prior diagnostic workup, when applicable? If not, she can

be referred for initial diagnosis and treatment, and then sometimes returned for follow-up to the primary care provider. For example, a fibroid felt for the first time may require consultation and ultrasound for verification and then it is best followed by the same practitioner. This may be the nonphysician, particularly if the patient is more likely to return for care if she prefers this practitioner. If pathologic change or growth is detected, then the physician may once again be involved in this patient's care. In this case, a related issue is whether the primary care provider can order ultrasound without consultation in a given institution.

This question may apply as well to nongynecologic conditions that the practitioner uncovers or with which the patient presents. For example, if you hear a heart murmur in an asymptomatic patient who confirms that at a prior cardiac workup she was given the diagnosis of a functional murmur, then you may opt to continue her yearly screening without further referral. Sending for medical records may be useful in such situations. On the other hand, if you pick up a previously undetected murmur, then the patient deserves cardiac referral. The extent to which the practitioner can rule out serious pathology in nongynecologic conditions is another consideration. For example, mild or borderline anemia that one can attribute to IUD use or, on history taking and laboratory testing, to iron deficiency, and that is corrected with iron supplementation within a reasonable period may not require consultation. Severe or symptomatic anemia always does, as does anemia that fails to respond to therapy, has no clearly attributable causality, or is associated with pathology.

5. If the patient has a medical problem that affects gynecologic management, can the gynecologic component of her care be managed in collaboration with her medical provider? For example, if a woman chooses a nonphysician health care provider for her annual gynecologic checkups, but she has a metabolic disorder, such as diabetes, the practitioner may consult with the physician who manages the woman's medical condition to assess her eligibility for family planning methods and/or treatments.

6. If management requires a new skill, is the practitioner interested in learning it and is a supervised learning experience possible? Does the need exist for her to learn it? (This need may reflect patient desires or geographic or institutional factors.) Refer to Appendix II for guidelines on incorporating a new procedure into clinical practice.

For those practitioners who wish to participate in extended functions, such as colposcopy, we refer you to specialized texts and caution that competence in such practices requires formal, specialized education and continuing experience in their implementation.

Appendix I, Part A, defines levels of patient management. We refer all readers to this document for further elucidation of primary or independent management, co-management or consultation, and referral. We emphasize that co-management and referral in no way allow an abdication of responsibility for the patient. Appropriate follow-up should always be assured.

Before consultation or referral is implemented, we urge thorough data collection. Often, through history taking, physical examination, and/or laboratory testing, pathology can be ruled out. Assessment also can help determine the most appropriate consultant or source of referral. Time can be saved if test results can be obtained before another health provider is consulted or seen.

To facilitate co-management and referral, the practitioner must develop, within or outside of her institution, a network of collegial practitioners with whom she can consult and to whom she can refer. This includes, obviously, gynecologists, but also other physicians such as internists, radiologists, surgeons, oncologists, urologists, endocrinologists, dermatologists, pediatricians, psychiatrists, and general or family practitioners. Other nonphysician care providers must be part of a complete referral system. These include psychotherapists and sex therapists, who may be independently certified practitioners, social workers, or psychologists. Practitioners of alternative healing modalities such as chiropractic, massage, biofeedback, yoga, and other forms of stress management may be valuable sources of referral. Nutritionists and exercise physiologists are often helpful resources. Of course, the practitioner must be familiar with a provider's credentials and competence before making a referral. Self-help groups and organizations devoted to support for specific disorders, such as HELP for herpes sufferers, or Reach to Recovery, for victims of breast cancer, can be beneficial. Through the creative use of a variety of health team members, the best possible care can be offered to women.

10

The Breasts

Therese Dondero and Ronnie Lichtman

Every woman's health care practitioner undoubtedly will be faced with many patients who have concerns about their breasts or whose findings on routine breast examination lead to a suspicion of abnormality. The provider must be able to screen for breast pathology and determine when referral for confirmatory diagnosis and treatment is required. For all women, the practitioner must be able to assess for breast cancer risk and consistently provide teaching and counseling about risk factors, preventive measures, and breast self-examination and other screening modalities. The practitioner must be prepared to offer emotional support to women facing potential or diagnosed breast disease and to refer for intensive therapy when necessary.

Most complaints or concerns involving the breast are exaggerations of normal physiologic changes rather than pathologic abnormalities. Therefore, a thorough knowledge of the developmental and cyclic changes normally occurring in the breast is mandatory for any practitioner providing health care to women.

This chapter reviews the anatomy of the breast and breast development. Then, abnormalities—anatomic deviations from normal, benign breast conditions, and breast cancer—are discussed. The chapter provides the primary care provider with information necessary to perform each of the functions mentioned earlier.

ANATOMY

In essence the breast or mammary gland is a modified apocrine or sweat gland (Fig. 10–1). Located on the anterior chest wall, each breast is surrounded by fascia, separating it from the skin on one side and from the chest muscles on the other. These muscles, the pectoralis major and pectoralis minor, cover the ribs and help in arm movement. Each breast is composed of 15 to 20 lobes, which together form a circle with the tail of Spence extending from the outer quadrant into the axilla. The breast lobes are further divided into smaller lobules. Acinus cells (or alveoli), responsible for milk production, are found at the end of each lobule. Small ductules extend from each lobule and form into a larger duct. Before these ducts reach the nipple, each enlarges to form a lactiferous sinus, or ampulla. Each sinus has a tiny opening onto the nipple from which milk can be secreted. The breast nipple is surrounded by the more deeply pigmented areola, which contains the openings of underlying sebaceous glands called Montgomery's glands.

Connective tissue is found within and around the breast's lobes. Fibrous septa, called Cooper's ligaments, run from the breast's fascia around the lobes and fix the breast to its overlying skin while still permitting movement. A large part of the interlobule breast tissue is composed of fat, which varies in amount from person to person and at different life stages in the same woman.

Of particular importance in understanding the course of breast cancer is an appreciation of the breast's blood supply and its venous and lymphatic drainage. Three major arteries supply the breast. The internal mammary or thoracic artery, which enters the medial edge of the breast, brings the greatest amount of blood to the organ. The lateral thoracic artery is the second most important source of blood to the breast, entering it from the lateral edge. The pectoral branch of the thoracoacromial artery gives off branches to the posterior breast surface. The axillary artery has two branches to the breast. The breasts are well supplied with superficial subcutaneous veins, which drain mainly to the internal mammary vein whose route corresponds to the arterial blood supply—medially, laterally, to the axilla, and posteriorly (Fig. 10–2).

Many lymphatic vessels lie in the spaces between and around the breast lobes (Fig. 10–3). These vessels drain primarily into two clusters of lymph nodes: the axillary nodes found in the armpit and the internal mammary nodes found along the sternum. In addition, lymph fluid from the breast can drain into the supraclavicular nodes near the clavicle and the cervical nodes at the side of the neck. The lymphatic vessels of the two breasts also communicate with each other.

BREAST DEVELOPMENT

The breast undergoes many gross and microscopic changes at various times in the life cycle and during each menstrual cycle. The important stages of breast growth and regression are adolescence, pregnancy and lactation, and menopause. An interaction of a number of hormones appears to control breast changes (Wilson, 1986, p. 532).

The breast begins to grow at about the time of puberty. The first visible change is an elevation of the areola. Hypothalamic, pituitary, and eventually ovarian hormones stimulate breast growth. Insulin, thyroid hormone, growth hormone, and glucocorticoid are also necessary for breast development (McCarty, Glaubitz, Thienemann, & Rief-

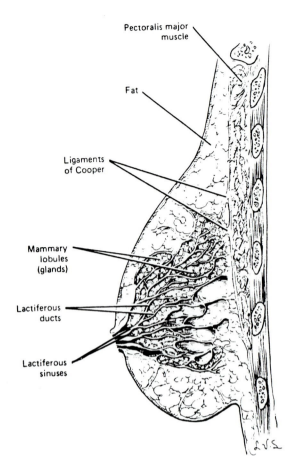

Figure 10–1. Sagittal section of the breast. *(From Lindner, H. H. [1989]. The breast. Clinical anatomy. Norwalk, CT: Appleton & Lange.)*

kohl, 1983, p. 2). The ductal system develops primarily under the influence of estrogen. This hormone also affects the breast's vascular supply and its connective and fat tissue. Lobules form under the influence of both estrogen and progesterone once ovulation occurs (Rush, 1984, p. 524; Townsend, 1980, p. 6).

During the menstrual cycle, the breasts undergo daily changes, although not uniformly in all lobules. There are premenstrual increases in vascularity and ductal and alveolar growth. It has been suggested that under repeated hormonal stimulation during the menstrual years, all breasts develop at least some degree of nodularity (Townsend, 1980, p. 6).

In pregnancy, the glandular tissue of the breast proliferates in response to placental stimulation. Estrogen, progesterone, placental lactogen, prolactin, and chorionic gonadotropin all have a role in breast development during pregnancy, as do growth hormone, adrenal corticosteroids, thyroid hormone, and insulin (McCarty et al., 1983, p. 7). With the withdrawal of estrogen and progesterone after delivery, prolactin, released from the anterior pituitary, becomes dominant and milk is actively synthesized in and secreted by the alveolar cells (Townsend, 1980, p. 8). At the end of lactation, there is a 3-month process of involution in which the lobules shrink in size, although not significantly in number. The breast, however, never returns entirely to its prelactation state.

With menopause, breast lobules slowly regress until all but a few small ones remain. Glandular tissue is replaced with fat.

ANATOMIC DEVIATIONS FROM NORMAL

Developmental deviations resulting from errors in the development of the ectoderm at the sixth week of embryonic life can cause anatomic deviations in the form of additional or absent breast tissue along the embryologic mammary ridge or "milk line," which extends from the axilla to the groin (Morehead, 1982, p. 356) (Fig. 10–4).

Polymastia is the presence of more than two breasts, usually along the milk line, with the axilla or abdomen as the most common site. This condition may not become apparent until pregnancy or lactation. If not large or causing emotional difficulties, the additional breasts should be left alone and the woman reassured that polymastia is a common finding.

Polythelia is the presence of supernumerary nipples, which may or may not be found along the mammary ridge. This condition is most frequently associated with normal breasts.

Amastia is a lack of development of one or both breasts. If it is unilateral, the breasts will be of unequal size.

Micromastia is a lack of breast development beyond the prepubertal state.

Macromastia is an extreme enlargement of the breasts in which their growth fails to cease after puberty. In some textbooks, this is termed *virginal hypertrophy*. The breasts can weigh up to 40 or 50 pounds in this condition.

Both micromastia and macromastia may present emotional difficulties relating to self-image. Macromastia also causes physical difficulties associated with pain on movement and shortness of breath when recumbent. Plastic surgery is available and should be reviewed with the woman as an option should you elicit concern on her part.

Inverted nipples are the result of the failure of the nipples to evert. This condition usually occurs a short time after birth and persists through adulthood. Inverted nipples occurring from birth can always be everted on physical examination. If eversion of the nipples is not possible, it may indicate an underlying malignancy and appropriate referral must be made. A recently occurring unilateral inversion or retraction must also be considered suspect (Wilson, 1986, p. 535).

Absence of one or both nipples is a quite rare physical finding. Absence of the underlying muscles may also occur rarely.

Asymmetry is unequal breast development. During adolescence, both breasts usually develop at the same pace; however, there are times when development is unequal and one breast becomes larger than the contralateral breast. Usually, the sizes become equal over time, and this information should be shared with the adolescent female. Occasionally, the breasts remain asymmetric. If the difference in size is striking and/or the woman is unhappy with her body image, plastic surgery is available to adjust the size difference. The expected results and risk–benefit ratio of the various surgical techniques are best reviewed with the surgical consultant.

All of the preceding anatomic deviations may cause varying degrees of emotional or physical distress, depending on the severity of the abnormality. The level of distress experienced by a woman should be elicited during an office visit and counseling or referral for correction of the more serious abnormalities offered. As most of the deviations described are minimal in their outward appearance, simple reassurance that the finding is a variation of "normal" and not uncommon in the general female population usually allays the concerns of being "different" (Morehead, 1982, pp. 353–357).

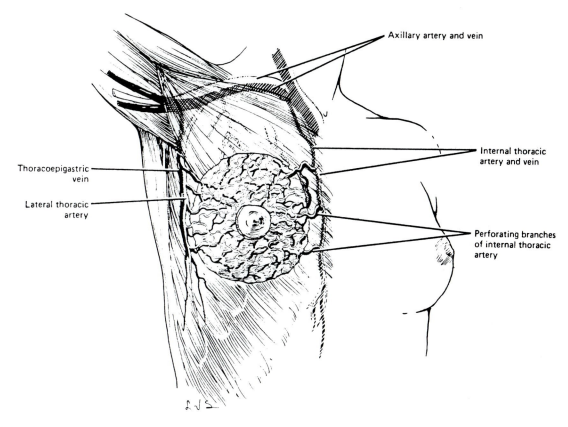

Figure 10-2. Blood supply to the breast. *(From Lindner, H. H. [1989]. The breast. Clinical anatomy.* Norwalk, CT: Appleton & Lange.)

Plastic surgery can reduce or enhance breast size or tighten the breast's support. Patients should be counseled that such procedures may have side effects and that results of these operations vary. Future lactation is theoretically possible with most reduction mammoplasty techniques; however, many women find that this is not possible after these procedures (Strombeck, 1986, p. 307). This surgery may also lead to infection, necrosis, hematomas, a large amount of scarring, and nipple retraction or malposition (Goldwyn, 1976, p. 150). Side effects of augmentation in-

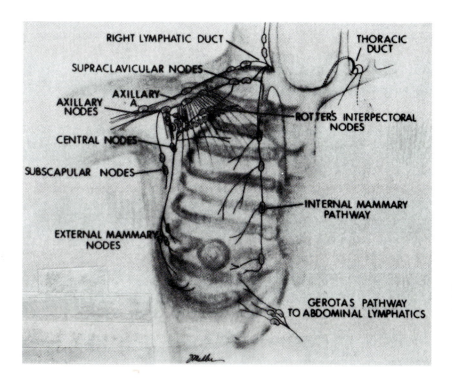

Figure 10-3. Lymphatic supply of the breast. *(From McCarty, K. S., Glaubitz, L. C., Thienemann, M., & Riefkohl, R., [1983]. The breast: Anatomy and physiology. In N. G. Georgiade, [Ed.]. Aesthetic breast surgery.* Baltimore: Williams & Wilkins. Reprinted with permission.)

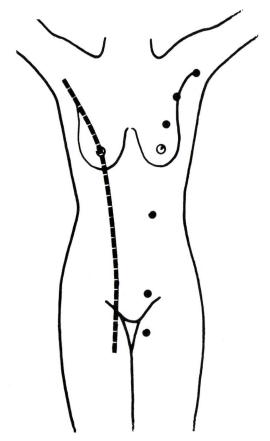

Figure 10–4. Embryologic ''milk line.'' *(From Morehead, J. R. [1982, June]. Anatomy and embryology of the breast.* Clinical Obstetrics and Gynecology, *25[2], 353–357. Reprinted with permission.)*

volving breast implants are similar to those discussed later under Breast Reconstruction. Augmentation procedures do not interfere with lactation ability (Lewis, 1983, p. 48).

Women considering breast surgery need to be counseled regarding realistic expectations of breast operations. They should be advised to thoroughly discuss expected results with the plastic surgeon before undergoing any procedure for aesthetic reasons. Although a changed body image may have positive effects, it can also create problems of adjustment and will not resolve deeper conflicts (Clifford, 1983; Goins, 1983).

BENIGN BREAST CONDITIONS

Most abnormal breast findings prove to be benign conditions related to the anatomic and physiologic development and changes of the normal breast. For many breast abnormalities, however, symptoms alone do not guarantee benign status, although age of the patient and type of symptom may strongly indicate a nonmalignant change. One of the main problems associated with benign breast conditions is diagnostic confusion with malignancies (Rush, 1984, p. 530). It is wise to consider abnormal findings as potentially cancerous until proven otherwise and to establish a safe referral system so that appropriate testing is performed to rule out malignancy.

Benign conditions of the breast, also called benign breast disease (BBD), include a variety of neoplasms and infectious disorders. Terminology used to classify the many

benign variations seen is not always consistent among authors and, in some instances, has changed over time. Schwartz (1982, p. 373), for example, points out that ''the constellation of symptoms characterized by excessive or irregular nodularity, engorgement, or increased density of the breasts related to the menstrual cycle is unfortunately given the misnomer of fibrocystic disease, when a better term is 'increased physiologic nodularity' or, when talking with patients, just 'lumpy breasts.' '' The following discussion is a synthesis of a number of sometimes conflicting sources.

Fibrocystic Breasts/Physiologic Nodularity

Definition. Fibrocystic or lumpy breasts can be defined as ''an exaggeration of the normal tissue response of the breast resulting from the ebb and flow of ovarian hormones'' (Greenblatt, Samaras, Vasquez, & Nezhat, 1982, p. 368). Fibrocystic breasts occur most commonly between the ages of 35 and 50.

On the basis of histologic findings, fibrocystic tissue may be classified in a number of ways. These include cystic glandular hyperplasia, which involves ductal tissue; adenosis or sclerosing adenosis, a more solid and fibrous variation occurring in younger women and most often confused with carcinoma; apocrine epithelium, which lines the lumen of the ducts and represents more primitive epithelial cells; ductal papillomatosis, a benign epithelial proliferation; and connective tissue hyperplasia. Lymphocytic infiltration is often, but not always, present. Cysts and fibroadenomas have also been designated as fibrocystic (Wilson, 1986, p. 539).

Clinical Presentation. Patients with fibrocystic breasts may complain of breast lumpiness or breast pain, usually increasing before menstruation. On palpation, fibrocystic breasts often feel symmetric. Masses may be generalized or localized. The most common areas of nodularity are the upper outer quadrants and the axillary tail. Such changes are least likely to be felt after the menstrual period.

Treatment. A variety of treatments for fibrocystic breasts has been suggested. The rationale underlying treatment of this condition includes relief from the pain that may accompany it and resolution of diagnostic dilemmas posed by the existence of nodularity. There is also speculation that treatment may reduce any increased risk of breast cancer related to fibrocystic changes (USDHHS, 1984, p. 16). (See Risk Factors under Breast Cancer for more discussion of this issue.)

The following treatments have been proposed (USDHHS, 1984, p. 16):

- Mild analgesics
- Warm compresses
- Nighttime supportive bra
- Low-salt diet
- Diuretics
- Restriction of methylxanthines, including caffeine, found in coffee, tea, cola, and chocolate
- Vitamin B_1
- Vitamin E
- Vitamin C
- Evening primrose oil, which contains essential fatty acids
- Thyroid hormone
- Sex hormones, including the androgen danazol, the

antiestrogen tamoxifen, the antiprolactin bromocriptine, and birth control pills

Prophylactic subcutaneous mastectomy or bilateral total mastectomy with breast reconstruction (see Prevention under Breast Cancer) is reserved for women with a history of multiple biopsies, intractable pain, or excessive fear of developing breast cancer.

Some of these treatments have been based on research studies; others have not. Table 10-1 provides a synopsis of findings regarding the efficacy of studied treatments in alleviating this condition or its symptoms. Research varies in the numbers of women studied and research methodologies utilized.

Treatments include the benign (e.g., warm compresses), the beneficial for overall health (e.g., restriction of caffeine), and the potentially dangerous (e.g., hormones and surgery). Their use must be considered carefully and the possible benefits measured against risks. Antiestrogen therapy, for example, can increase a woman's risk for the development of osteoporosis and may not be warranted when pain is not debilitating. Menopausal signs and symptoms may be seen with its use. Danazol is an extremely costly drug and has been reported to cause muscle cramps, acne, oily hair, menstrual disturbances or amenorrhea, weight gain, nervousness, hot flashes, hirsutism, changes in libido, and edema (Nezhat, Asch, & Greenblatt, 1980). Side effects have been reported with doses of vitamin E exceeding 800 daily units. These include thrombophlebitis, hypertension, fatigue, gynecomastia, breast tumors, vaginal bleeding, headache, dizziness, visual complaints, nausea, vomiting, cramps, muscle weakness, hypoglycemia, stomatitis, chapped lips, urticaria, and apparent aggravation of diabetes mellitus and angina pectoris (Roberts, 1981).

London, Sudaram, and Goldstein (1982, p. 522) advocate vitamin E 600 IU/day for up to six menstrual cycles for clinical relief of fibrocystic breast symptoms, once neoplasm is ruled out, followed by danazol therapy and finally tamoxifen or bromocriptine if both other treatments fail. Medications must be prescribed by a medical practitioner with experience in this area to ensure appropriate follow-up. There is no documented evidence, however, that any therapy for fibrocystic breast disease decreases the risks of breast cancer.

Benign Neoplasms

Cysts are benign fluid-filled sacs that vary greatly in size. They may be cyclic and either painful or not. Clinically, they are mobile, round, and soft or rubbery.

Diagnosis of a cyst can be aided by mammogram or ultrasound, which can differentiate fluid-filled from solid masses. Most often today, cysts are diagnosed by outpatient needle aspiration under local anesthesia. If the cyst collapses and disappears with aspiration, the diagnosis is confirmed; if no fluid can be withdrawn, if the lesion persists or recurs after aspiration, or if the aspirated fluid is bloody, then biopsy becomes necessary for diagnosis (USDHHS, 1984, p. 17).

Fibroadenomas are the most common benign breast tumors seen in women between the ages of 20 and 40. These may even be seen in adolescence (Schwartz, 1982, p. 374); a mass in a woman under the age of 25 is almost always a fibroadenoma.

A fibroadenoma presents as a painless mass that does not respond to cyclic changes. On palpation, it feels well circumscribed and mobile, usually round, but often lobulated or dumbbell-shaped. Its average size on detection is 2 to 2½ cm in diameter. Its consistency is rubbery and firm but not hard unless calcifications are present, as they sometimes are in older women (Schwartz, 1982, p. 375).

A fibroadenoma can be diagnosed only by biopsy and tissue examination. In any patient over the age of 20 this is recommended whenever a discrete mass is present (Schwartz, 1982, pp. 374–375). Fibroadenomas may be multiple. They have a 10 to 20 percent recurrence rate.

Surgical excision is the only treatment for a fibroadenoma and can be done on an outpatient basis under local anesthesia. Most often an incision around the areola can be used, providing a good cosmetic result (Schwartz, 1982, p. 376).

Cystosarcoma phyllodes is a type of fibroadenoma that exhibits rapid growth but is almost always benign (USDHHS, 1984, p. 17). Its presentation is similar to that of a fibroadenoma except that as it grows, it does not feel as smooth or uniform. Stretching of the skin overlying the tumor may occur to the point of ulceration. Diagnosis is made by biopsy. Excision is the recommended treatment, although if the tumor is large enough, a total mastectomy may be performed (Schwartz, 1982, pp. 376–377).

Intraductal papilloma is a lesion seen primarily in women in their forties. A papilloma is a small wartlike growth in the lining of the mammary duct, almost always occurring near the nipple (USDHHS, 1984, p. 17). Although not common, a papilloma is responsible for 75 percent of nipple discharge in women who are neither pregnant nor lactating. The associated discharge may be bloody or serous, may be intermittent or constant, and may occur spontaneously or only with manipulation. The differentiation of physiologic discharge from that associated with papilloma is in both its characteristics and how it can be elicited on palpation. A normal discharge is usually greenish black and sticky (Schwartz, 1982, p. 377). It is not secreted spontaneously but on palpation appears from many duct openings. The discharge occurring with papilloma is seen when a specific duct is palpated. Whenever a patient reports a bloody or serous discharge, around-the-clock palpation of the areola with pressure applied in the direction of the nipple is warranted to ascertain whether the discharge comes from a specific area. This locates the duct containing the papilloma. Sometimes the papilloma may be palpated as a small mass or the duct itself may be felt as a thin strand within the areola that disappears as fluid is discharged (Schwartz, 1982, pp. 377–378). Localized tenderness may be present.

Because these lesions continue to grow if not removed, surgical excision is recommended. When only one or a few ducts are removed, a woman can still nurse her children in the future although this issue is often moot as the lesion generally is seen around the perimenopause.

Multiple papilloma is a rare type of breast mass that is associated with an increased risk of invasive carcinoma. It is *not* the same as intraductal papilloma. It affects slightly younger women; 40 is the median age for this lesion. It must be diagnosed by biopsy. Excision or mastectomy is recommended, depending on the extent of the disease (Schwartz, 1982, p. 380).

Galactocele occurs after lactation is completed and involves the obstruction of a breast duct, usually beneath the areola in the ampulla. It may be tender and enlarged. Excision and drainage are recommended because the galactocele may become calcified and cause diagnostic confusion with malignancy (Wilson, 1986, p. 539).

Other benign breast neoplasms include any type of lesion that may appear in similar tissue elsewhere—lipoma, histiocytoma, leiomyoma, and granular cell tumors (often called myoblastomas).

TABLE 10-1. SELECTED RESEARCH FINDINGS ON TREATMENTS FOR FIBROCYSTIC BREASTS

Treatment	Study	Date	Number of Subjects	Study Design	Controlled	Parameter Studied	Findings
Antigonado-tropin Danazol: 200 or 400 mg/day	Mansel, Wisbey, & Hughes	1982	28	Prospective, double blind; random assignment	Y (crossover)	Pain and nodularity in cyclic mastalgia	400 mg/day: rapid relief 200 mg/day: slower relief, fewer side effects
Danazol: 100, 200, or 400 mg/day	Nezhat, Asch, & Greenblatt	1980	130	Prospective, nonrandom	N	BBD[a]: Pain, tenderness, and nodularity.	2/3: nodularity eliminated; 3 patients: not improved 1/3: some return of pain and tenderness 67 patients: side effects.
Danazol: 50, 100, or 200 mg/day	Baker & Snedecor	1979	25	Prospective, nonrandom	N	Severe fibrocystic breasts: pain, tenderness, and nodularity; mammogram after 6 months	100%: partial pain relief; part or complete regression of nodes; 13/16: reappearance after 12 months; 4: discontinued secondary to side effects
Danazol: 100–800 mg/day	Aksu, Tzingounis, & Greenblatt	1978	135	Prospective, nonrandom	N	BBD: pain, tenderness, and nodes	97%: overall pain relief 90.5%: relief of tenderness 73%: improved nodularity Recurrence: 6–10%
Danazol: 100–400 mg/day	Asch & Greenblatt	1977	58	Prospective, nonrandom	N	Lumpiness and tenderness	75.8%: total subjective and objective relief 50%: amenorrhea
Danazol: 800 mg/day	Greenblatt, Dmowski, Mehesh, & Scholer	1971	62 (8 voluntary controls)	Prospective, nonrandom	Y	Breast swelling, tenderness, and lump	60%: improved symptoms
Antiestrogen Tamoxifen: 20 mg/day	Fentiman, Caleffi, Brame, et al.	1986	60	Prospective, randomized with placebo group	Y	Severe mastalgia (pain)	71–75%: pain relief 33–38%: pain relief in controls 6 patients: discontinued secondary to side effects
Tamoxifen: 10 mg/day on days 5 to 24 of cycle	Shaabon, Movad, & Hassan	1980	31 (including 3 men)	Prospective; double blind; nonrandom	Y (crossover)	Fibrocystic mastopathy (pain), induration, and lumps	30: objective decrease of symptoms 9/27: decreased menses 3/27: hot flashes
Tamoxifen: days 5 to 25 of cycle	Ricciardi & Ianniruberto	1979	63	Prospective, experimental	Y	Clinical evidence of breast nodules, cystic changes, or severe subjective symptoms	71.43%: total remission 19%: improved

TABLE 10–1. SELECTED RESEARCH FINDINGS ON TREATMENTS FOR FIBROCYSTIC BREASTS (CONTINUED)

Treatment	Study	Date	Number of Subjects	Study Design	Controlled	Parameter Studied	Findings
Methylxanthine (caffeine) withdrawal							
	LaVecchia, Talamini, Decarli, et al.	1986		Case-control	Y	Breast cancer	No association between coffee consumption and malignancy
	Lubin, Ron, Wax, et al.	1985		Case-control dietary study	Y	Histologically confirmed BBD	No association
	Ernster, Mason, Goodson, et al.	1982	82	Prospective, random assignment; not blinded	Y	Clinically palpable breast findings; mammography	Decrease in breast findings; minimal change on x-ray
	Minton, Abou-Issa, Reiches, & Roseman	1981	85	Prospective, experimental	N	Clinical fibrocystic "disease," confirmed by mammogram	82.5%: total resolution 15%: improved
	Minton, Foecking, Webster, & Matthews	1979	20	Prospective, experimental	Y	Palpable breast nodules, pain, tenderness, and nipple discharge	65%: symptoms disappeared
Prolactin inhibitor Bromocriptine: 5 mg/day	Durning & Sellwood	1982	38	Prospective, double blind; placebo group	Y (crossover)	Severe cyclic breast pain with clinical assessment	Reduction in pain, tenderness, and nodes 21%: severe side effects
2-Br-α-Ergocriptine (CB-154)	Margin-Comin, Pujol-Amat, Cararach, et al.	1976	7	Prospective	N	Fibrocystic breast "disease"; nodules, pain, galactorrhea	5: improved 2: change or decrease in cyst size on mammogram
Thyroid hormone	Estes	1981	19	Prospective, nonrandom	N	Breast pain with nodularity	47%: total relief 73%: total or partial relief 11/18 with nodules: improved
	Daro, Gollin, & Samos	1964	286	Prospective	N	Nodular breasts with tenderness	Improved
Oral contraceptives Enovid (norethynodrel, mestranol)	Ariel	1973	110	Prospective, nonrandom	N	Fibrocystic breast "disease"; pain, tenderness, areas of firmness	76: objective remission 54: excellent response 1: thrombophlebitis
Vitamins α-Tocopherol acetate: 600 units/day	London, Sundaram, Schultz, et al.	1981	17 (6 controls)	Prospective; nonrandom	Y	Mammary dysplasia with cystic breast "disease"	88%: clinical improvement Controls: no change
α-Tocopherol: 600 mg/day	Sundaram, London, Manimekalai, et al.	1981	26 (5 controls)	Prospective; nonrandom	Y	Mammary dysplasia	85%: objective and subjective remission
Vitamin E: 200–400 mg/day	Abrams	1965	20	Prospective	N	Premenstrual pain, tenderness, and heaviness	16: moderate to complete relief 13: decrease or loss of cysts

[a]BBD, benign breast disease.

Breast Inflammation. *Fat necrosis* is a lesion that occurs in the breast after trauma, although the incident may have been so slight that it is not recalled. The pain, tenderness, and ecchymosis that are seen subsequent to the trauma, however, are usually remembered. On occasion, the precipitating trauma has been a previous breast biopsy. This lesion is usually felt superficially. Fibrosis generally follows hemorrhage and induration within the area of the mass, causing retraction and decreased mobility of the mass. As a result, cancer is often highly suspected. With a clear history, an experienced practitioner may watch this mass at biweekly intervals up to 6 weeks to determine if it decreases in size. Unless it disappears completely, biopsy is recommended (Schwartz, 1982). Treatment consists of excision.

Breast thrombophlebitis, also called *Mondor's disease*, presents with a cordlike, tender mass, showing retraction or dimpling with the arm raised. Because of these associated skin changes, it may be mistaken for a tumor and biopsy may be done, although it is not necessary to make this diagnosis. Mondor's disease may follow trauma. There is no treatment; it subsides within 3 to 4 weeks. Analgesics may be helpful.

Mammary duct ectasia is a dilation of subareolar ducts with fibrosis and inflammation. It has also been called plasma cell mastitis or comedomastitis. It usually occurs in perimenopausal women and presents with a nipple discharge of blood-stained sticky gray or greenish material. A mass may be present and produce retraction. Sometimes erythema, induration, and tenderness may be present above the mass. Regional nodes may be palpable. Biopsy is often necessary because of the difficulty in differentiating this lesion from cancer. Antibiotics may be ordered and warm compresses may be helpful. The duct may need to be removed should an abscess develop.

Subareolar abscesses may be recurrent, particularly in women with inverted nipples, and are usually caused by *Staphylococcus aureus* or anaerobic organisms. Antibiotics, drainage, or duct excision may be necessary.

Other infections of the nonlactating breast are rare but include protozoal infections, syphilis, and tuberculosis. Recently, an inflammatory lesion known as "granulomatous mastitis" has been identified (Schwartz, 1982, p. 385). This lesion involves the lobular areas rather than the breast ducts and is characterized by small, sterile abscesses with necrotic granulation tissue. Treatment is excision. Cancer may also present as an inflammatory lesion.

Lactational mastitis is the most common form of breast inflammation. It occurs in the postpartum period and is characterized by tenderness and erythema, followed by induration and breast edema. General malaise and fever may ensue. Three distinct entities causing lactational inflammation have been identified: mastitis resulting from milk stasis, noninfectious inflammation, and infectious mastitis. In a study of 213 women, milk stasis was found to be self-limiting, noninfectious mastitis responsive merely to breast emptying, and infectious mastitis responsive to breast emptying and antibiotics (Thomsen, Espersen, & Maigaard, 1984). Should infection progress to abscess, incision and drainage may be necessary to avoid necrosis. For more discussion of this disease process, see Chapter 23.

BREAST CANCER

Breast cancer is a major public health concern. One of every ten women in the United States develops this disease (American Cancer Society, 1987). The American Cancer So-

ciety (ACS) (1987, p. 8) has estimated an incidence of 130,000 new cases of invasive breast cancer among U.S. women in 1987. This greatly exceeds the rate of cancer of any other organ in either males or females. The estimated number of deaths for breast cancer in 1987 was 41,000, representing the second largest cancer killer of women. Indeed, until 1986, more women died of breast cancer than of any other form of cancer. In 1986 and 1987, only lung cancer replaced breast carcinoma as the leading cause of cancer death among U.S. females, although breast cancer continues to strike many more women.

The survival rate for localized breast cancer has improved from 78 percent in the 1940s to 90 percent today. Noninvasive cancer (in situ) has an almost 100 percent cure rate; metastatic breast cancer has only a 60 percent survival after 5 years (American Cancer Society, 1987, p. 10). The American Cancer Society reports that mortality for breast cancer has been stable for the past 50 years which it attributes to an increasing incidence balanced by longer survival. Relative 5-year survival rates for whites were reported as 63 percent in 1960–1963 and as 75 percent in 1977–1983. For blacks, the rates for these time periods were 46 and 62 percent, respectively (American Cancer Society, 1987, p. 17). Although these rates demonstrate increasing survival, an obvious gap remains between the races. In one analysis of this gap, poorer social class standing, not genetics, was found to be explanatory (Bassett & Krieger, 1986). Either decreased host resistance as a result of factors associated with poverty, such as malnutrition, or class differences in detection and/or treatment may be responsible.

Risk Factors

Although the cause or causes of breast cancer are unknown, many epidemiologic studies have examined factors associated with its development and a number of risk factors have been identified. These include certain demographic and geographic characteristics such as female sex, increased age, and urban residence; previous history of breast cancer; family history of premenopausal breast cancer; history of benign breast disease showing epithelial hyperplasia or proliferation; hormonal factors reflected in menstrual and reproductive history; diet; obesity; history of exogenous exposures including radiation and alcohol; history of certain other cancers; breast structure; and stress.

Although the pathogenesis of breast cancer remains elusive, it is helpful in understanding its development to appreciate the concepts of tumor "initiator" and tumor "promoter." Tumor initiators induce cell transformation during the process of cell division, thus causing development of a cancer; tumor promoters enhance cell proliferation (Thomas, 1983, p. 211). Only one definite breast cancer initiator has been identified to date: ionizing radiation. Most other known risk factors are thought to be tumor promoters, but the mechanisms by which they influence breast cancer have not been identified clearly.

Demography and Geography. Breast cancer is more than 100 times more common in women than in men. Its incidence rises steadily with age, although the rate of this increase declines after age 45 to 50 (Kelsey, 1979, p. 75). Whites have the highest rate among the races, although this gap has narrowed in recent years. Among ethnic groups, Jews have a high incidence. Social class differentials for this disease favor the lower classes. In the United States, breast cancer is seen more frequently in urban than rural areas and, for disease occurring in postmenopausal women, in the North rather than the South. Worldwide, it occurs most often in North America and Northern Europe.

Family History. Women with a first-degree relative (mother, sister, grandmother, or aunt) with breast cancer are at increased risk for developing the disease; the relative risk in most studies is estimated to be approximately 2 to 3 (Kelsey, 1979, p. 84; Moore, Moore, & Moore, 1983). Hereditary breast cancer has been postulated as a disease distinct from other forms of breast cancer (Lynch, Albano, Heieck, et al., 1984, p. 44). This type of breast cancer is characterized by an early age at onset (premenopausal), bilaterality, and an association with other cancers (e.g., of the bowel and endometrium). Several authors have theorized a genetic basis for familial breast cancer, identifying an autosomal dominant pattern in some families, passed to female offspring via the maternal or paternal line (Lynch et al., 1984, pp. 50–52). Others have suggested environmental or life-style factors (Moore et al., 1983, p. 197).

The attempt to find a genetic marker for breast cancer has thus far been unsuccessful. To date, the search for biologic markers—a particular body fluid elevated in cancer patients—has not yielded any that are sensitive and specific enough to be of clinical use in early detection. Plasma carcinoembryonic antigen (CEA) is elevated in 60 to 70 percent of patients with metastasis and may be helpful in determining patients most likely to develop recurrent disease. This requires further study (Waalkes, Enterline, Shaper, et al., 1984).

The Hormonal Link. The exact association between hormones and breast cancer is not understood. Hormonal factors have been hypothesized to be tumor promoters, although the evidence for their role is based on epidemiologic evidence of cancer patterns according to life events that affect a woman's hormonal milieu rather than on direct demonstration of specific pathogenic effects (Table 10–2).

Studies in rodents support the hypothesis that estrogen, and possibly prolactin, increases the risk of mammary cancer (Henderson, Ross, Pike, & Casagrande, 1982, p. 3233). The prolactin link, however, is confused by the fact that breastfeeding, a state when prolactin is notably increased, does not seem to increase breast cancer risk (Kelsey, 1979, p. 88). The relation of breastfeeding to breast cancer is indeterminate at this time (Moore et al., 1983, p. 205), although a recent case-control study suggests that it has a protective effect against breast cancer, particularly for premenopausal disease (McTiernan & Thomas, 1986).

Other hormones, including androgens and thyroid hormone, have been investigated (Kelsey, 1979), but more research about their relationship to breast cancer is needed to draw any firm conclusions. Progesterone deficiency has also been related to increased breast cancer risk (Cowan, Gordis, Tonascia, & Jones, 1981).

MENSTRUAL AND REPRODUCTIVE HISTORY. The clear association between menstrual and reproductive events and breast cancer lends strong support to the conclusion that hormonal factors are implicated in the development of the disease.

Early menarche and late menopause carry a small increase in relative risk for breast cancer development, implying that increased time exposure to endogenous sex hormones may play a role, although an alternative explanation is that a third factor, such as diet, influences both of these events and breast cancer.

Young age at first full-term birth affords protection against breast cancer; women whose first full-term delivery occurs before age 18 have been reported to have about one-third the risk of developing breast cancer of women whose first birth occurs after age 35 (Kelsey, 1979, p. 77). Although high parity has been cited as a protective factor, it is possible that this is more a result of a younger age at first birth among women of high parity than of the effects of births subsequent to the first.

Nulliparity increases breast cancer risk, although it does not result in as high an increased risk as bearing a first child after age 30. It has been suggested that perhaps an early full-term pregnancy prevents tumor initiation while a late first birth increases tumor promotion (MacMahon, Cole, & Brown, 1973, pp. 22–23). This may be related to a permanent decrease in circulating prolactin after the first birth. This theory was supported by a study showing higher prolactin levels among Catholic nuns than among their parous sisters but not among their nulliparous sisters (Moore et al., 1983, p. 209). The trend toward delayed childbearing may increase the incidence of breast cancer in the future (White, 1987). A recent case-control study found an increased risk among women who had an abortion prior to a first birth, although previous studies have been inconsistent regarding this factor (Hadjimichael, Boyle, & Meigs, 1986). Oophorectomy, particularly before age 35, is protective against breast cancer.

EXOGENOUS HORMONES. The relationship of exogenous sources of estrogen to breast cancer has been investigated.

TABLE 10–2. RISK FACTORS FOR BREAST CANCER: FACTORS IMPLICATING HORMONES AS TUMOR PROMOTERS

Factor	Influence on Risk	Remarks
Female sex	Increases risk	
Age	Increases risk	Effect of age diminishes after menopause
Age at menarche	Inversely related to risk	Influence diminishes with age
Age at menopause	Directly related to risk	Influence increases with age
Oophorectomy	Protection inversely related to age at oophorectomy	Influence increases with age
Nulliparity	Increases risk	
Age at first child	Directly related to risk (early birth protective)	Influence diminishes with age
Parity	Additional children may be weakly protective	
Lactation	Minimal	Unilateral nursing may influence laterality of tumor
Exogenous estrogens	Probably eliminates the protective effect of oophorectomy; risk in women with intact ovaries uncertain	Results of studies conducted to date are inconsistent

From Thomas, D. B. (1983). Factors that promote the development of human breast cancer. Environmental Health Perspectives, 50, *20. Reprinted with permission.*

Oral contraceptives, postmenopausal estrogen replacement, and diethylstilbestrol (DES) ingestion during pregnancy all have been examined, largely in case-control studies. A few such studies have shown some increased risk of breast cancer after oral contraceptive use, particularly in certain groups of women, for example, when used prior to a first pregnancy, by nulliparous women (Trapido, 1981), or by women with a family history of breast cancer (Black & Kwon, 1980). In a case-control study of several thousand women, Stadell, Lai, Schlesselman, and Murray (1988) found a $2\frac{1}{2}$ times increased risk of breast cancer among women who met 3 criteria: nulliparity, menarche before age 13, and pill use for 8 to 11 years. Women with the first 2 criteria who used pills for 12 or more years were found to have a rate of breast cancer 12 times higher than nonpill users. In another large study, the relative risk for breast cancer risk in pill users diagnosed between the ages of 30 and 34 was 3.3; it was 5.88 among women in that age group with 1 child at the time of diagnosis (Kay & Hannaford 1988). In a study of 407 breast cancer patients and 424 women without cancer, the relative risk was 2.0 for pill users and 4.1 for users of 10 or more years (Miller, Rosenberg, Kaufman, Stolley, Warshauer, & Shapiro, 1989). Yet, at least a dozen reports have found no association (Moore et al., 1983). Several of the studies whose results show an association have been criticized for methodologic weaknesses (see, for example, Rubin, Layde, & Peterson 1984; Stadel & Schlesselman, 1986; Vessey, McPherson, Yeates, & Doll, 1982); others, utilizing different methodology, have shown either no effect or a protective effect of oral contraceptives against breast cancer (Kelsey, Fischer, Holford, et al, 1981; Moore et al., 1983; Vessey et al., 1982). In 1983, the Centers for Disease Control reported on a large study (689 cases and 1,077 controls) that found no association between oral contraceptive use and breast cancer. The researchers included women in the study who had used oral contraceptives at least 15 years prior to the study and for a maximum of 11 years. Long-term prospective studies are needed to clarify the risk groups and to demonstrate the findings of lifetime follow-up.

Postmenopausal estrogens have been implicated in a few studies in increasing the risk of breast cancer. Ross, Paganini-Hill, Gerkins, et al. (1980) found increased risk in women with intact ovaries after a total dose exceeding 1500 mg. Jick, Walker, Watkins, et al. (1980) found an increased risk only for women experiencing natural menopause as opposed to those who had undergone surgically induced menopause. Other researchers, however, have not found this association (Gambrell 1982, pp. 467–469, 1984), and at this time the aggregate evidence does not seem to support such an association (see Chapter 24 for more discussion of this issue).

Studies examining whether DES ingestion during pregnancy increases breast cancer risk are conflicting; firm conclusions cannot be drawn at this time. The risk may be dose related (Beral & Colwell, 1980; Brian, Tilley, Labarthe, et al., 1980). Chapter 18 discusses this question in the section on DES exposure.

The Dietary Link. The association of breast cancer to dietary factors has never been demonstrated conclusively. Studies of diet and cancer are difficult to conduct; bias and contamination are unavoidable because intake can be neither strictly controlled nor monitored. Nevertheless, there exists a bulk of evidence linking diet to breast cancer. The aggregate data seem to support the possibility of a dietary component in the development of breast cancer, although

this finding has not been consistently upheld (Willett, Stampfer, Colditz, et al., 1987a).

High fat in the diet has emerged as a major dietary risk for breast cancer. Several explanations have been offered, including the production of estrogens from biliary steroids in the colon, which increases with a high-fat diet (Hill, Goddard, & Williams, 1971). This theory was supported by a study showing higher fecal steroid levels among women with breast cancer than among those without the disease (Papatestas, Panvelliwalla, Tartter, et al., 1982). Alternative explanations focus on the relationship of high fat consumption to obesity, which increases hormonal levels (Schindler, Ebert, & Friedrich, 1972; Siiteri, Schwartz, & MacDonald, 1974), and to diet's possible effect on age at menarche, another risk factor for breast cancer (Frisch & Revelle, 1971).

Several case-control studies have shown dietary differences between breast cancer patients and controls. Unfortunately, these studies have not been consistent in methodology or in the specific dietary factors examined. Increased overall intake of nutrients, total fat, beef, pork, butter, gravy, cheese, fat content of milk, and sweet desserts have each been implicated in increasing breast cancer risk (Hislop, Coldman, Elwood, et al., 1986; Le, Moulton, Hill, & Kramar, 1986; Lubin, Wax, & Modan 1986; Lubin, Burns, Blot, et al., 1981; Miller, Kelly, Choi, et al., 1978). Low intake of fish has been associated with increased risk (Hislop et al., 1986) and dietary fiber has been found to decrease breast cancer risk in women under age 50 (Lubin et al., 1986). In one study, carotene intake decreased risk in postmenopausal women (Hislop et al., 1986).

Other sources of data supporting the association of diet to breast cancer are less direct. It has been inferred from data in countries where statistics are available on cancer mortality and per capita consumption of animal protein or total fat (Armstrong & Doll, 1975) and from studies of migrants. The children of Japanese migrants to the United States have a rate of breast cancer greater than that of Japanese women living in Japan. This difference is thought to be related to change in dietary habits, leading to increased fat consumption after migration (Buell, 1973). Indeed, in Japan, breast cancer rates have increased as dietary fat intake has increased (Miller et al., 1978). In Iceland, this same increase has been seen as diets have become more Westernized (Bjarnason, Day, Snaedal, & Tulinius, 1974). Further circumstantial support for the theory that dietary intake of fats or animal products increases breast cancer risk comes from a study in which Armstrong, Brown, Clarke, and co-investigators (1981) found lower urinary levels of estriols and total estrogens, lower plasma prolactin levels, and higher sex hormone–binding globulin (SHBG) levels among vegetarian women than among nonvegetarian women, possibly explaining the lower breast cancer rates with low-fat diets. Soya protein has been found to have an antiestrogenic effect, possibly protective against breast cancer (Setchell, Borriello, Hulme, et al., 1984).

It has been suggested that diet early in life is more important in the pathogenesis of breast cancer than diet later in life (Moore et al., 1983, pp. 241–242), although not all researchers agree (Lubin et al., 1986). Further research is warranted before absolute dietary guidelines can be offered.

The National Cancer Institute (NCI) recently suspended a 10-year prevention trial, the Women's Health Trial (WHT), examining the link between dietary fat and breast cancer. In this study, women in the experimental groups were following a diet with fat intake limited to 20 percent of total calories (Foley, 1987). Twenty percent of fat is equal to 400 calories in a 2,000-calorie diet, or 44.4 g of fat per day (Rennie, Stallmeyer, & Orloff, no date). Although some researchers have called into question the reliability of following the diets of participants, this study had the potential for clarifying the role of diet in breast cancer prevention; its suspension is unfortunate.

Obesity. Body build has been shown to be moderately associated with breast cancer, particularly in postmenopausal women with the disease (Kelsey, 1979, pp. 92–93). In addition, obesity has been shown to have a negative effect on breast cancer prognosis (Wynder & Cohen, 1982, p. 196). There is disagreement in the literature over whether the effects of obesity on cancer risks are actually a result of the high-fat diets that lead to the obesity or the effects of dietary intake of fat are actually secondary to obesity (de Waard, 1983, p. 1675).

Exogenous Exposures. Radiation is the only known initiator of breast cancer. Evidence for its role comes from investigation in animals (Casarett, 1965); studies of atomic bomb victims of Hiroshima and Nagasaki (Jablon & Kato, 1972; McGregor, Land, Choi, et al., 1977; Tokunaga, Land, Yamamoto, et al., 1982; Wanebo, Johnson, Sato, & Thorslund, 1968); and studies of women who underwent x-ray treatment for postpartum mastitis in the 1940s and 1950s (Mettler, Hempelmann, Dutton, et al., 1969; Shore, Hempelmann, Kowaluk, et al., 1977) or fluoroscopy for tuberculosis from about the 1920s to mid-1950s (Boice & Monson, 1977; MacKenzie, 1965; Myrden & Hiltz, 1969).

Kelsey (1979, pp. 93–94) reports on several conclusions of interest that can be drawn from these studies. First, the greatest risk from radiation exposure occurs at ages 10 to 19, just before and during menarche and puberty. She suggests two possible reasons: rapid breast growth during this period and increased breast sensitivity to radiation before a first birth. It has been generally thought that women exposed to radiation before age 10 are not at increased risk for breast cancer, although at least one study (Tokunaga et al., 1982) provides evidence to contradict this finding. A second conclusion is that the cumulative effects of multiple radiation exposures may be equivalent to the effect of one large dose. Third, radiation effects are permanent. Last, the latent period between exposure and the development of cancer varies from 5 to 15 years, with a longer latent period in young women.

Two recent, large, prospective studies report a significant increase in breast cancer risk secondary to alcohol intake. These studies support the findings of a number of previous case-control investigations. The overall evidence for linking alcohol consumption to breast cancer risk is convincing (Graham, 1987). Schatzkin, Jones, Hoover, and associates (1987) found a 1.5 relative risk for developing breast cancer among women who reported any drinking compared to those who reported no drinking and a relative risk ranging from 1.4 to 1.6 for those drinking less than 1.3 g per day to those consuming at least 5 g per day (equivalent to three drinks per week). Willett, Stampfer, Colditz, and co-investigators (1987b) found age-adjusted relative risks of 1.3 for women drinking 5 to 14 g of alcohol a day (three to nine drinks per week) and 1.6 for those drinking 15 g or more per day.

Other exogenous exposures that have been studied include the antihypertensive drug, reserpine, hair dyes, and cigarette smoke. Smoking has been found to have no effect on breast cancer (Baron, Byers, Greenberg, et al., 1986;

Brinton, Schairer, Stanford, & Hoover, 1986). Evidence is lacking to link these other exposures to breast cancer, although further studies have been advocated (Kelsey, 1979, pp. 96–97; Moore et al., 1983, p. 219).

Benign Breast Disease (BBD). Women with BBD have long been thought to be at increased risk of developing breast cancer. In a critical review of the literature, Webber and Boyd (1986) found more evidence and better methodology in studies reporting an association between BBD and breast cancer than in those reporting no association. In one prospective study of 747 women with BBD, the age-adjusted rate of breast cancer was three times higher in the group with BBD than in the group of matched controls without the condition (Coombs, Lilienfeld, Bross, & Burnett, 1979). The investigators conducting this study believe that BBD is an indication of an abnormal hormonal milieu that results in both conditions, rather than a precancerous lesion. Women who have had breast biopsies have been found to account for a greater share of the increased risk from BBD than those who have not (USDHHS, 1984, p. 27). Nevertheless, relatively few women with BBD develop breast cancer. The risks for cancer are not necessarily the same as those for BBD (Ernster, 1981, p. 200). Research examining the particular benign lesions that appear to increase the risk of breast cancer has identified lobular or epithelial hyperplasia (Hutchinson, Thomas, Hamlin, et al., 1980; Page, Vander Zwaag, Rogers, et al., 1978).

The Viral Link. The possibility of a viral etiology for breast cancer has been investigated. Murine mammary tumor virus (MuMTV) has been identified in breast cancer in mice (Moore et al., 1983 p. 223); however, breast cancer in these rodents is unlike that in humans (USDHHS, 1984, p. 21). Particles similar to this virus have been found in the milk of breast cancer patients and their relatives, but have been found as well in women without the disease (USDHHS, 1984, p. 21). Moore et al. conclude (1983, p. 227) that ''there is at present no evidence for contagion or of transmission of a breast cancer virus via breast milk, although possible involvement of a MuMTV-related component in the etiology of some human breast cancer cannot be ruled out.''

Previous Breast Cancers. Breast cancer in one breast increases the risk of breast cancer in the other, or contralateral, breast. The increased risk has been reported to be up to 4- or 5-fold (Kelsey, 1979, p. 82) and has been called ''the best risk indicator available'' (Mansel, 1986, p. 364). Cancers of the endometrium (but not cervix), ovary, and colon and a tumor of the salivary gland also seem to increase the risk of developing breast cancer (Moore et al., 1983, p. 216; USDHHS, 1984, p. 28).

Breast Structure. The structure of the breast as seen on a mammogram may be associated with varying degree of breast cancer risk. Those breasts with dense parenchyma (glands and ducts) are considered at greater risk than those with less dense tissues (USDHHS, 1984, p. 28).

Stress. The relationship of a variety of personality and stress-related factors to the occurrence of breast and other cancers in both humans and animals has been investigated (Moore et al., 1983.) The ability to cope with stress has been cited as an important factor (Moore et al., 1983, p. 244). Nothing conclusive can be said about this risk at this time.

Role of the Immune System. It has been proposed that the immune system is linked to the etiology of breast cancer. A variety of immunologic agents have been studied in relation to risk for the disease or to its prognosis. No conclusions can be drawn currently, although this is a promising research frontier (Moore et al., 1983, p. 222).

Classification

Adenocarcinoma is the most common type of malignant breast tumor. A classification for breast cancer was proposed by Foote and Stewart and revised by the World Health Organization. This classification is based on the type of tumor, the breast structure in which it is located (nipple, lobule, or duct), and whether it can infiltrate tissues or remains localized. The following outline is adapted from Rush (1984, pp. 537–539) and Wilson (1986, p. 545) and descriptions summarized from these texts.

I. Paget's disease of the nipple
II. Carcinomas of mammary ducts
   A. Noninfiltrating
   B. Infiltrating
     1. Papillary carcinoma
     2. Comedocarcinoma
     3. Carcinoma with productive fibrosis
     4. Medullary carcinoma with lymphoid infiltrate
     5. Colloid carcinoma
     6. Tubular carcinoma
III. Carcinoma of mammary lobules
   A. Noninfiltrating
   B. Infiltrating
IV. Relatively rare carcinomas
V. Sarcoma of the breast

Paget's disease of the nipple accounts for only 1 percent of breast cancer. It is a primary carcinoma of the mammary ducts of the nipple that eventually invades the skin. This disease presents as a scaly lesion of the nipple, resembling eczema. Although Paget's disease has a slow natural history and skin manifestations may be the only evidence of neoplasm for many years, ultimately an underlying mass develops if it is left untreated. Biopsy is therefore indicated in any eczematoid lesion of the nipple that persists more than a few weeks in a postmenopausal woman. Patients with Paget's disease have a better prognosis than do other breast cancer patients. One third of women with this diagnosis show noninfiltrating carcinoma and their survival rate has been reported to be 100 percent at 5 years. The other two thirds are diagnosed with infiltrating carcinoma and their reported survival rate is 64 percent.

Noninfiltrating carcinomas of mammary ducts represent another 1 percent of breast cancers. Also called ductal carcinomas in situ, these lesions should be associated with a 5-year survival rate of 100 percent. These may be papillary cancers or comedocarcinomas.

Infiltrating papillary carcinoma, accounting for 5 percent of all breast cancers, evolves slowly and is associated with a better survival rate than the average breast carcinoma. It presents with a mass that is softer to palpation than most cancers and may reach a large size before metastasizing to the axilla.

Infiltrating comedocarcinoma refers to a histologic classification in which the cancer consists of collections of cancer cells showing extrusion of sebaceous-like material on cut section. This may be associated with inflammatory changes on breast examination. Tumors are usually large.

Infiltrating duct carcinoma with productive fibrosis is the most common form of breast cancer, responsible for about 75 percent of the disease. It has been called scirrhous carcinoma, fibrocarcinoma, and sclerosing carcinoma. This lesion presents as a very hard mass to palpation with uneven serrated edges.

Infiltrating medullary carcinoma has a favorable prognosis even in the presence of metastatic disease, with 5-year overall survival rates of 85 to 90 percent. Medullary cancer is the diagnosis in 5 percent of breast cancer cases. The tumor is soft, bulky, often large, and freely movable. If small, it may be mistaken for a cyst or fibroadenoma. Axillary metastasis occurs less frequently with this type of cancer than with the more common forms of the disease.

Infiltrating colloid carcinoma, seen in 1 percent of cancer patients, often involves only a single node. Clinically, this presents as a soft, cystic-type mass, possibly quite bulky before detection. Survival with this form of cancer is better than average.

Tubular carcinoma, also called "well-differentiated" or "orderly" cancer, occurs in 1.2 percent of cases and may be combined with other forms of breast cancer. If a breast cancer contains 90 percent or more of tubular lesions, the long-term survival nears 100 percent.

Noninfiltrating carcinoma of mammary lobules, also called lobular carcinoma in situ, involves the acini and terminal cells of breast lobules. In the in situ stage, it is a curable lesion. These cancers are multicentric and bilateral, and the contralateral breast is involved with in situ lesions in 35 to 59 percent of specimens.

Infiltrating carcinoma of mammary lobules is a rare lesion and may be indistinguishable from infiltrating duct carcinoma with productive fibrosis.

Relatively rare carcinomas include epidermoid carcinoma and adenoid cystic carcinoma of the breast. The latter rarely metastasizes, but the former is often advanced when identified. Breast cancer may also present as an inflammatory lesion. This form of the disease has a poorer-than-average prognosis.

Sarcoma of the breast is a very rare and predominantly benign lesion, and is actually a variant of fibroadenoma. Its malignant form is often called adenocarcinoma. The nonmalignant type occurs at an older age than other forms of adenocarcinoma. It produces a larger mass, typically averaging 5 to 10 cm, with a firm, rubbery consistency. The malignant form of breast sarcoma rarely metastasizes to the axilla.

In 1971, the concept of *minimal carcinoma of the breast* was defined to include carcinoma in situ and invasive masses measuring 5 mm or less in diameter, although later authors redefined this to include those with diameters less than or equal to 1 cm (Hartmann, 1984).

Diagnosis

In a practice that includes essentially healthy women who are coming for routine gynecologic care, the provider takes a general history, performs a basic breast examination, provides preventive teaching, and perhaps orders or advises laboratory testing. When, however, a woman presents with a chief complaint of a breast mass or abnormal breast symptoms, the provider's actions are quite different.

Some primary woman's health care practitioners may function in a clinic that only screens for abnormalities of the breast. This practice setting again requires a different approach and tends to more routinely involve invasive screening techniques such as mammography.

Data Collection

HISTORY. History taking for all patients presenting for annual or other well-woman examinations should include questions relating to breast disease and breast disease risk. Age, menstrual history, obstetric history, family history of breast disease, previous breast disease or work ups including biopsies and their results, contraceptive use, history of radiation exposure, medications including hormones such as oral contraceptives should all be part of routine history taking. A dietary history, assessing for fat and fiber intake, should be included.

For patients presenting with a complaint relating to the breast, more specific questions must be asked. Complaints may be pain, nipple discharge, or the finding of a lump or other abnormality, accidentally, through breast self-examination (BSE) or by the patient's partner.

When the complaint is pain, questions should include the type of pain, its onset and location, and its relationship to the menstrual cycle. In addition, history of trauma, remedies used to relieve the pain and their effect, and dietary intake of methylxanthines (or caffeine) found in coffee, tea, soda, and chocolate should be elicited. Haagensen (1986, p. 502) reports from his extensive experience that one type of pain may be suggestive of breast cancer, and causes him to assess the painful area with special care. This pain is intermittent, sharp, and localized with radiation outside the breast. It is described by patients as "sticking, stinging, stabbing, throbbing, or burning." Back pain, indicating vertebral metastasis, rarely may be a presenting symptom of breast cancer (Haagensen, 1986, p. 504).

Reported nipple discharges should be identified through history by color (clear, milky, greenish, blood tinged) and consistency (viscous, watery, bloody). Find out whether the discharge is unilateral or bilateral. Ask about amenorrhea or recent pregnancy, and about medication use, including oral contraceptives, phenothiazines, and reserpine, which may cause breast discharge. Amenorrhea coupled with discharge may indicate undiagnosed pregnancy or a pituitary tumor; serum prolactin levels may be useful to rule out the latter (see Chapter 21). If the discharge is milky, or thick and gray in a middle-aged woman, it may have been induced by the woman's repeated squeezing of the nipples; she should be advised against this practice (Haagensen, 1986, pp. 62–63). Nipple discharge may also be induced by sexual activity including breast manipulation and suckling. It may be seen in women who jog or run; friction between the nipples and clothing can stimulate prolactin production (O'Grady, 1986). Sexual and exercise histories are therefore warranted whenever nipple discharge is reported.

If the woman reports any other unusual finding, such as a lump, ask her when and how it was first noticed, how it has changed since then, whether it occurs or changes cyclically with the menstrual cycle, and whether pain or discharge is associated with it. Ask about other possibly associated symptoms such as bone, back, or joint pain, general malaise, weight loss, anorexia, fever, cough, hoarseness or chest pain, and changes in bowel habits or in menses.

These historic data can be correlated with signs and symptoms of the various benign breast conditions and of breast cancer to help develop a differential diagnosis.

PHYSICAL EXAMINATION. Examination of the breast involves inspection and palpation, as well as teaching of breast self-examination to the patient. As a screening technique, the American Cancer Society (1987, p. 10) recommends that breast examination be performed at 3-year intervals for women aged 20 to 40 and annually for women over age 40, although there is no reason not to perform this examination annually in all women who present for routine yearly checkups and to repeat it anytime a patient reports a breast change. It is only a screening examination and does not replace diagnostic procedures if there is any question regarding breast pathology. Its importance as a screening modality, however, cannot be overemphasized, as most breast cancers are asymptomatic. Although physical examination is less sensitive than mammography, it is more specific and has a greater predictive value (Rudolph & McDermott, 1987). Breast examination is best performed several days after menstruation when hormonal influences on nodularity are least significant.

Physical Examination Technique and Findings. The breasts can be inspected with the patient in the sitting or standing position. Good light and exposure, of course, are necessary. Symmetry of the two breasts is noted, although most often some degree of asymmetry in breast size is normal. Shape and contour of the breast and condition of the skin are observed. Dimpling, puckering, or retraction may indicate cancer, although these may be seen in Mondor's disease, fat necrosis, and duct ectasia. These changes occur when a tumor or its surrounding fibrosis involves and shortens Cooper's ligaments. Other changes of the skin, such as *peau d'orange*, in which open pores indicate lymph node involvement, are seen with more advanced disease (Marchant, 1982, pp. 360–361). The vascular pattern of the breast should be observed as should the condition of the nipple and areola. Paget's disease involves the nipple, often presenting with redness, thickening, erosion (Haagensen, 1986, p. 503), or scaly patches. A nipple pointing in an unusual direction or a difference in the direction of the two nipples may suggest a tumor (Townsend, 1980, p. 7). Flattening or retraction of the nipples, often noticed first by the patient, may indicate shortening of the duct system secondary to fibrosis developing around a carcinoma (Haagensen, 1986, p. 503). Bilateral venous engorgement may be seen with cystosarcoma phyllodes. Edema or redness may indicate blocked lymph nodes in advanced or inflammatory cancer.

Inspection of the breast should be performed first with the patient's arms at her sides, then with her arms held straight above her head, and next with her hands on her hips with the elbows brought toward the front of the body to contract the pectoralis major muscles. Finally, inspection should be done with the patient standing and leaning forward from the hips with her arms extended outward and her chin up (Haagensen, 1986, p. 542; Rush, 1984, p. 528). These positions may exaggerate breast changes, making them easier to see. With contraction of the pectoralis muscles, for example, a breast with cancer may rise more sharply than the normal breast or part of it may become abnormally elevated. This occurs secondary to a cancer's being fixed to the pectoral fascia (Haagensen, 1986, p. 534). See Figures 10–5 to 10–7 for examples of changes noted through inspection.

While this part of the examination is being performed, BSE can be introduced, with an explanation to the patient that as part of her self-exam, she should observe her breasts in front of a mirror in each of the positions assumed. What she is looking for should be reviewed.

Palpation of the breast must include both breasts and both axillae. Axillary examination affords assessment of breast tissue in the tail of Spence and of the axillary lymph nodes. Palpation should also include the supraclavicular

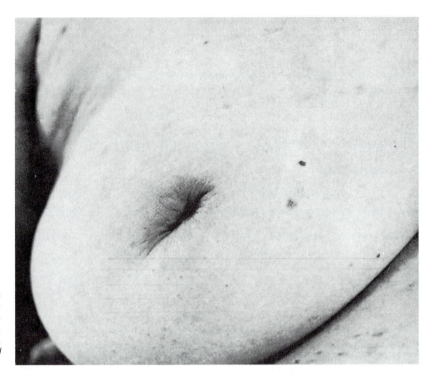

Figure 10-5. Example of breast changes seen on inspection. Simple inversion of the nipple—no disease of the breast. *(From Haagensen, C. D. [1986]. Diseases of the breast [3rd ed.]. Philadelphia: W. B. Saunders. Reprinted with permission.)*

lymph nodes as well as the internal mammary chain. Palpation is done with the balls or pads of the fingers, with firm but gentle pressure so as not to occlude any masses. To reduce friction between the hand and breast skin, powder can be used on the examining fingers (Haagensen, 1986, p. 522).

The axillary area is palpated with the patient erect (sitting or standing) and the arm held down and supported by the examiner so that the pectoralis muscles are not tensed (Fig. 10–8). The anterior portion of the axilla is palpated, where it lies under the clavicle, and the entire area is then felt to its base (Rush, 1984, p. 528).

The breast usually is palpated with the patient lying down with her arm on the side being examined raised above her head to flatten the breast on that side. A towel or wedge placed under the patient's shoulder on the same side helps elevate the breast and prevents it from falling to the side (Fig. 10–9).

A variety of methods can be used to ensure systematic examination of the entire breast. It can be palpated quadrant by quadrant, by dividing the breasts into spokes of a wheel and palpating from the lateral to medial aspect of each spoke, or in concentric circles, starting either around the outer edge of the breast or at the nipple and moving

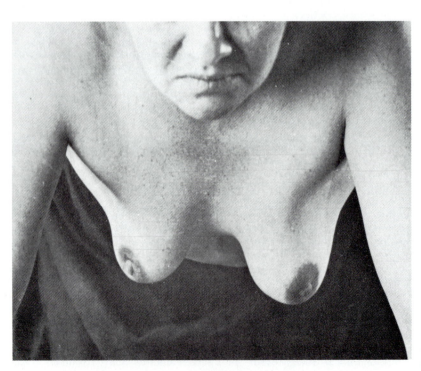

Figure 10-6. Example of breast changes seen on inspection. Right breast held up against chest wall, its areola and nipple deviated laterally, with patient in forward bending position—carcinoma of the upper central region of the right breast. *(From Haagensen, C. D. [1986]. Diseases of the breast [3rd ed.]. Philadelphia: W. B. Saunders. Reprinted with permission.)*

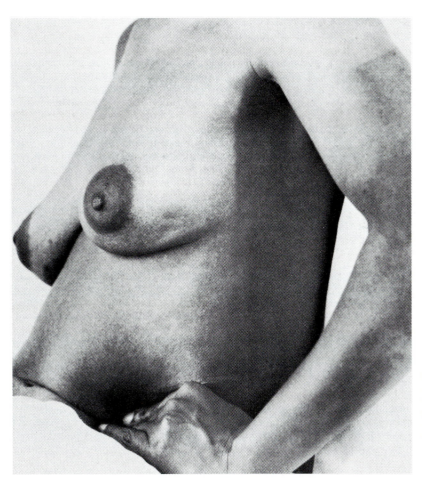

Figure 10-7. Example of breast changes seen on inspection. Pectoral contraction maneuver, arm pressed against the hip, bringing out small dimples in the skin over the carcinoma. *(From Haagensen, C. D. [1986]. Diseases of the breast [3rd ed.]. Philadelphia: W. B. Saunders. Reprinted with permission.)*

the fingers in a rotating fashion (Fig. 10–10). The entire circumference of the breast to the midaxillary line and the sternum should be covered. The areola and area under the nipple should be included. The examiner should not be confused by the inframammary ridge, a prominent bilateral

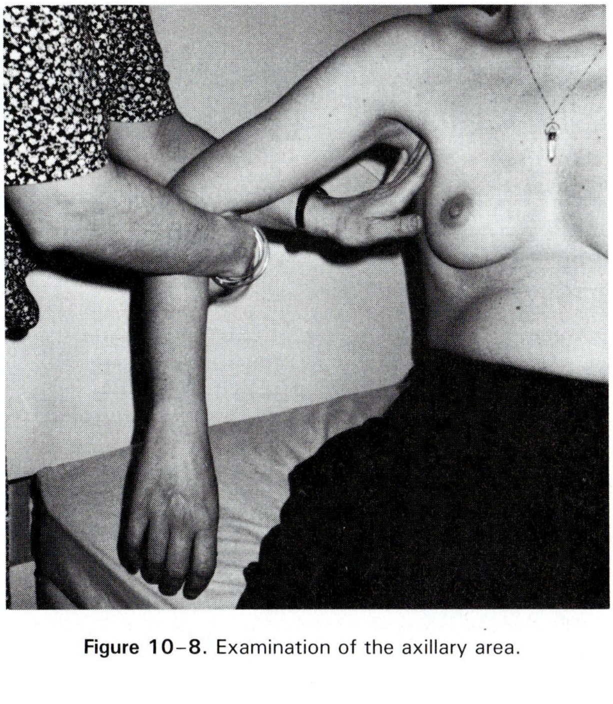

finding of dense nodular tissue at the lower edge of the breast felt in larger breasts, particularly in older women (Haagensen, 1986, pp. 523–524).

If the patient has complained of a nipple discharge, the areola should be stroked toward the nipple to see if discharge is elicited from a specific duct to identify papilloma. Discharge should be classified into one of the following types: milky, multicolored and sticky, purulent, watery, serous, serosanguineous, or bloody. This can usually be done by observation and palpation to feel stickiness. When the discharge is placed on white gauze, a reddish color with lighter shades of red extending to the periphery is noted if the discharge is bloody (Leis, 1977, p. 217).

The practitioner can use the examination time to explain the steps of BSE to the patient. Show the patient the

Figure 10-8. Examination of the axillary area.

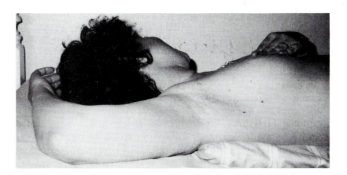

Figure 10-9. Position for breast palpation.

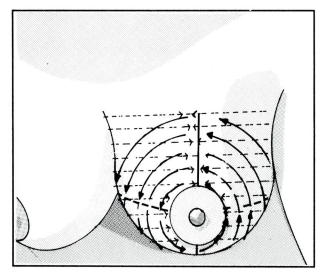

Figure 10–10 (Top). Systematic palpation of the breasts. Quadrant by quadrant *or* concentric circles.

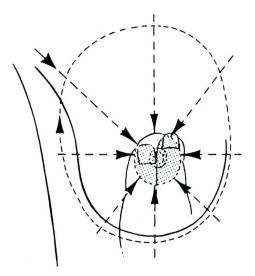

Figure 10–10 (Bottom). Wheel-spoke method. *(From Varney, H. [1987]. Nurse-midwifery [2nd ed.]. Boston: Blackwell Scientific. Reprinted with permission.)*

part of the fingers to use and caution her not to lift her fingers off the breast, but rather to use the rotating motion to slide them. One common mistake in BSE is not to make a wide enough circle around the entire breast circumference, particularly in the lateral areas. Patients can be instructed to use soap or powder (we recommend corn starch, which has no chemicals or perfumes) to help their fingers move more easily on their skin. Some women perform BSE in the shower as wet skin has the same effect.

It is advisable to watch the patient perform the examination to reinforce the learning process, correct errors in the technique, review findings in the various breast areas, and give positive feedback for her efforts. In at least one experimental study, teaching BSE with the opportunity to perform the examination and receive correction led to better lump detection than the passive methods of reading a

pamphlet or viewing a videotape (Assaf, Cummings, Graham, et al., 1985).

Breast examination findings should be recorded clearly, noting size of any lesions, their location, shape, regularity, mobility, consistency, and whether or not they can be easily outlined. Diagrams (Figs. 10–11 and 10–12) are helpful.

It is important to remember that the normal breast may feel nodular as a result of its lobular structure. This is especially prominent in the later part of the menstrual cycle (and during pregnancy and lactation). A typical cancerous lesion is solitary, unilateral, hard, with irregular or serrated edges, and poorly delimited. The edges of breast cancer tend to "fade out into the surrounding breast tissue" (Haagensen, 1986, p. 526). It is nonmobile and generally nontender. Its most common location is the upper outer quadrant (Leis, 1977, p. 213). Whenever there is even the smallest doubt, however, the practitioner must refer the patient for further evaluation. This may be as simple as an examination by a more experienced practitioner or as involved as mammogram and excisional biopsy.

LABORATORY TESTING.   X-ray of the breast or mammography is the standard laboratory test used either to screen women at risk for breast cancer or to help in the diagnosis of a palpated mass. Most experts agree that a mammogram, however, does not afford a final diagnosis (Kopans, 1985, p. 170). A mammogram suggesting nonmalignancy does not replace biopsy in the presence of a suspicious palpable mass. Conversely, in the absence of a palpable lesion, but with a suspicious mammogram, biopsy is indicated.

The basis for mammography as a screening examination for breast cancer is that it can detect smaller masses than can palpation, thus increasing survival rates and/or decreasing the need for extensive and debilitating surgical treatments (Homer, 1982, p. 398). Biologically, this is related to the way breast cancer grows. The lesion doubles at an approximate rate of every 100 days. At this rate of

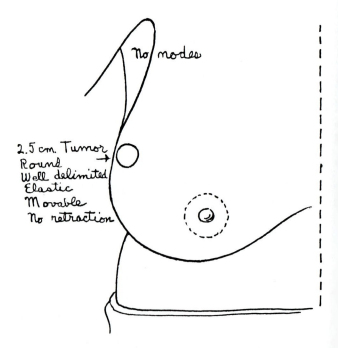

Figure 10–11. Example of diagram of breast finding. Sketch of the physical findings in a cyst of the breast. *(From Haagensen, C. D. [1986]. Diseases of the breast [3rd ed.]. Philadelphia: W. B. Saunders. Reprinted with permission.)*

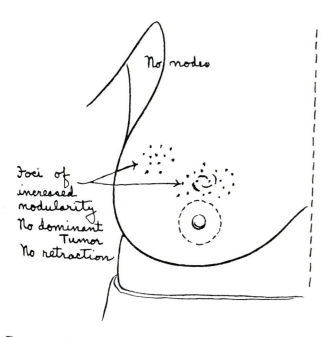

Figure 10–12. Example of diagram of breast finding. Sketch of the physical findings in a breast with increased nodularity. *(From Haagensen, C. D. [1986]. Diseases of the breast [3rd ed.]. Philadelphia: W. B. Saunders. Reprinted with permission.)*

growth, 8 years—or about 29 to 30 doublings—have elapsed before a tumor assumes a size of 1 cm, which is considered to be the minimum size at which it can be detected clinically (Speroff, 1985, p. 183).

Three techniques are currently available for mammog-

raphy: plain-film mammography, xeromammography, and electron radiography. In xeromammography, the image is reproduced on paper; in electron radiography, gas is used to form an electron image on clear plastic. Known as film-screen technique, this has the advantage of using the lowest dose of radiation of the three techniques, but is complex, associated with a lot of equipment breakdown, and not widely available. Xeromammography uses a higher dose of radiation than plain-film mammography but has several advantages including its ability to detect microcalcifications, which frequently indicate breast cancer. It is generally agreed that the best type of mammogram is dependent on equipment available and skill and experience of the radiologist performing the examination (Kopans, Meyer, & Sadowsky, 1984, p. 961; Speroff, 1985, p. 184; USDHHS, 1984, p. 37).

A mammogram takes a few minutes and involves two views of the breast, one from above and one from the side (Fig. 10–13). The woman undresses from the waist up and each breast is compressed in the mammography machine to get a more precise image. Some women find this painful.

The use of mammography for breast cancer screening has engendered controversy based on differing analyses of its usefulness and the possible risk it poses. In addition, criticisms have focused on its potential for increasing the number of biopsies performed and for leading to overaggressive surgical managmeent of carcinoma in situ, which does not lead to metastasis (Skrabanek, 1985, p. 317). (For more discussion of the prognosis and treatment of carcinoma in situ, see the section, Specific Therapies under Treatment.)

Few randomized controlled studies of mammography as a screening technique in breast cancer detection have been carried out. The first was conducted by the Health Insurance Plan of New York (HIP) from 1963 to 1968. This study, in which more than 60,000 women were assigned to

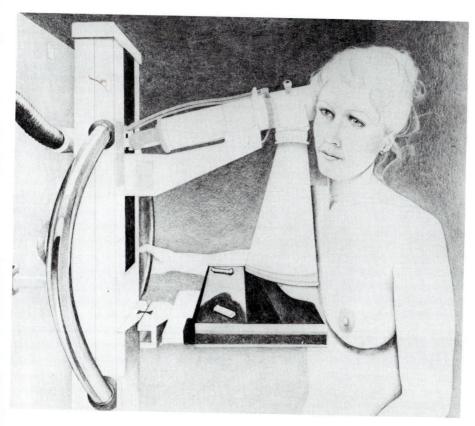

Figure 10–13. Mammography. *(From USDHHS [U. S. Department of Health and Human Services]. [1984]. The breast cancer digest [2nd ed.]. NIH Publication 84–1691, Bethesda, MD: National Cancer Institute, p. 37.)*

either an experimental or a control group, found a reduction in mortality of 33 percent in the experimental group. This group received annual mammograms and physical examinations for 5 years, whereas the control group received conventional medical care. Benefits have persisted to at least 14 years of follow-up (Strax, 1984). Most of the benefit in this study, however, was observed for women over the age of 50, for whom mortality was reduced more than 40 percent (Feig, 1984a, p. 14).

Mammography was enthusiastically accepted after this study and a large project offering mammographic screening was begun, sponsored jointly by the American Cancer Society and the National Cancer Institute. Known as the Breast Cancer Detection Demonstration Project (BCDDP), much of the current recommendations regarding use of mammography are based on data from this project, although it was not a clinical trial with random assignment to study and control groups. Early project data indicated that better technical quality resulting from improved equipment has increased mammographic efficacy for women under age 50 (Kopans, 1985, p. 172). Later reports also found increased survival for women in their forties, taking into consideration both lead-time and length-time biases. Lead-time bias refers to the time that screening would precede usual case finding; length-time bias refers to the possible early detection of a disproportionate number of slow-growing tumors (Seidman, Gelb, Silverberg, et al., 1987).

It is still agreed that the denseness of the normal breast tissue in women under age 35, as well as increased risk of radiation exposure in this age group, preclude routine use of mammography in these young women (Homer, 1982, p. 394). Some authors, however, advocate beginning screening mammography at age 30 for women with a mother or sister who had premenopausal breast cancer (Frankl, 1987).

Several recently reported studies from Europe confirm the findings of a substantial reduction in cancer mortality with mammographic screening. A randomized controlled study using single-view mammography every 24 to 33 months in 134,867 Swedish women aged 40 to 74 showed reductions of 31 percent in mortality and 25 percent in the rate of stage II or more advanced cancers. Differences in mortality were limited to women over age 49, although it is speculated that longer follow-up may demonstrate a benefit in the younger age group (Tabar, Fagerberg, Gad et al., 1985), as it has in the BCDDP study. Two case-control studies reported from The Netherlands also show benefits from mammography, with at least one of the studies showing beneficial results in women in all age groups over age 35 (Collette, Day, Rombach, & de Waard, 1984; Verbeek, Hendriks, Holland, et al., 1984).

The question of possible induction of breast cancer resulting from radiation exposure during mammography was raised in 1976 (Bailar, 1976). Since the original HIP study, the amount of radiation to which a woman is exposed during mammography has been reduced with newer machines, which expose a woman to approximately 0.025 to 0.5 rad (radiation *a*bsorbed *d*ose) to the midbreast for a two-view film of both breasts. Dose variation depends on equipment used, choice of plain-film mammography or xeroradiography, and size of the woman's breast (Homer, 1982, p. 394).

As risk of breast cancer from radiation exposure has been postulated from observations of women exposed to high doses, there is uncertainty over how to quantify risk from low doses. It is not clear whether the relationship between low- and high-dose risk is linear so that, for example, twice the exposure would double risk, or whether the risk increases geometrically with increased dose. By use of the linear extrapolation, which assumes the most risk from low radiation doses, it has been estimated that 7.5 breast cancer cases per year per rad per one million women might be expected after a 10-year latency period. For women exposed after the age of 35, the expected annual number of cases is 3.5 per million women per rad (Feig, 1984b, p. 6). With the average radiation dose currently received, it has been estimated that mammography carries a hypothetical risk of one excess cancer per year per one to two million women examined. With a 50 percent mortality rate, the hypothetical death rate would be one per two to four million women examined (Feig, 1984b, p. 8; Kopans et al., 1984, p. 961).

There remains a lack of consensus among experts on recommendations for mammographic screening. In 1977, the National Institutes of Health held a public Consensus Development Conference on breast cancer screening and recommended the following guidelines for mammographic screening (USDHHS, 1984, p. 34):

- Mammography should not be used to screen women under age 35.
- Mammographic screening of women aged 35 to 39 should be limited to women with a personal history of breast cancer.
- Annual mammography for women aged 40 to 49 is justified only for women with a personal history of breast cancer, or immediate relatives with a history of the disease.
- Mammographic examination can continue to be offered annually to women over age 50.

The American Cancer Society, the American College of Radiologists, and the American College of Obstetricians and Gynecologists promulgate their own recommendations as follows:

The American Cancer Society promotes "a baseline mammogram between the ages of 35 and 40, followed by annual or biennial mammograms from 40 to 49 and annual mammograms from 50 on" (USDHHS, 1984, p. 34).

The American College of Radiologists suggests that "for asymptomatic women, the first, or baseline, mammograms should be obtained by age 40. An earlier age is preferable when there is a personal history of breast cancer or a history of premenopausal breast cancer in the patient's mother and/or sisters. Subsequent mammographic examinations should be performed at one to two year intervals determined by the combined analysis of physical and mammographic findings and other risk factors, unless medically indicated sooner. Annual mammography and physical examination are recommended for all women over age 50" (USDHHS, 1984, p. 34).

The American College of Obstetricians and Gynecologists recommends "regular breast examinations including mammography at intervals to be determined by the physician," for women over the age of 50 and "for women between the ages of 35 and 50 . . . a 'baseline' mammogram be done in connection with a clinical physician examination." This organization states that the physician should determine the frequency of mammography based on "the results of this baseline evaluation and other examinations" (USDHHS, 1984, pp. 34–35).

Future data as well as technologic improvements are likely to lead to revisions in these guidelines.

Other Laboratory Techniques. Several techniques for breast cancer screening and/or diagnosis have been utilized in addition to mammography. These include ultrasound, thermography, computerized axial tomography (CT scanning), transillumination, digital radiography, magnetic resonance imaging, and the detection of biologic markers. Although no one technique is currently recommended for screening, some of these techniques have specific uses in the evaluation of symptoms. It is also possible that in the future, some of these techniques may be perfected and prove valuable in breast cancer screening.

Ultrasound utilizes high-frequency sound waves to form a computer image of the breast interior. Because it does not rely on ionizing radiation it has the potential to screen without increasing cancer risk. Currently, however, ultrasound is limited to the differentiation of cystic from solid masses, which may help avoid unnecessary surgeries, and to the examination of dense breasts, most often seen in younger women. A painless examination, ultrasound takes about 15 to 30 minutes to perform. The woman either lies on a table on her stomach with her breasts immersed in a tank of warm water or a water cushion is used (Kopans et al., 1984, p. 963; USDHHS, 1984, p. 39).

Thermography is a technique based on the fact that cancers may raise skin temperature. It is an attractive screening method because it is noninvasive, relatively simple, and inexpensive without concomitant risk; however, it results in excess false-positive and false-negative results. It is currently being evaluated for its use as an indicator of cancer risk but this is still experimental (Kopans et al., 1984, p. 964; USDHHS, 1984, p. 39).

Computerized axial tomography (*CT scanning*) is being investigated for use in detecting cancers in small dense breasts. Because it involves relatively large doses of radiation, it is not used routinely for screening, although it has been of help in diagnosis in selected cases (Kopans et al., 1984, pp. 964–965; USDHHS, 1984, p. 40).

Transillumination, also called *diaphanography* or *diaphanoscopy* or *light scanning*, involves shining a light through the breast, illuminating its interior. It does not, however, seem to illuminate small cancers detected by mammography. To determine its efficacy, clinical trials have been recommended and are being considered. It is possible that in the future, better technologies, involving, for example, lasers, may make this technique more useful in breast cancer screening (Kopans et al., 1984, p. 965; USDHHS, 1984, p. 40).

Digital radiography is not currently in use but offers the future potential for decreasing the radiation dose required for breast x-rays while enhancing their quality (Kopans et al., 1984, p. 965).

Magnetic resonance imaging (MRI), or *nuclear magnetic resonance (NMR)*, is an experimental technique that does not involve ionizing radiation. It may become most helpful in distinguishing benign from malignant lesions (Kopans et al., 1984, p. 966; USDHHS 1984, p. 40).

The detection of *biologic markers* in the serum or urine of women with breast cancer would provide an easy, noninvasive screening test with the potential for diagnosing cancer before the appearance of clinical signs. To date no such substance has been identified although several are currently being tested. These include oncologic proteins such as carcinoembryonic antigen (CEA) and α-fetoprotein (AFP), hormonal products such as human chorionic gonadotropin, enzymes, plasma proteins, and protein degradation products. Tests for particular antigens and responses to them are also being investigated. The use of monoclonal antibodies to evaluate such antigens may prove to be useful in detecting cancer sites and metastases (USDHHS, 1984, pp. 40–41).

Cytology has only limited value in breast cancer diagno-

sis. It can be performed on spontaneous nipple discharges, on fluid removed by needle biopsy from masses, or on breast fluid aspirated with a suction device. A negative result, however, cannot be relied on to rule out cancer, although a positive result strongly suggests its presence (USDHHS, 1984, p. 41).

Biopsy is currently the only definitive way to diagnose breast cancer, and most authors recommend its use whenever there is any doubt. In practice, if the primary care provider discovers a suspicious lesion, the patient should always be referred promptly to a physician—generally a gynecologist, surgeon, or oncologist—who will make the decision to biopsy.

Two types of biopsies are done, needle and surgical. Needle biopsies are performed with either a fine or a wide needle; surgical biopsies are either incisional or excisional, although excisional biopsy is currently replacing incisional biopsy (USDHHS, 1984, p. 41).

Fine-needle biopsy is used when a mass is most likely to be a fluid-filled cyst. In the case of a cyst, aspiration of breast fluid is both diagnostic and curative. When the mass disappears after withdrawal of fluid, it is clearly cystic and need just be followed closely to evaluate recurrence. If it recurs, or if, at the time of aspiration, it remains after fluid is withdrawn, or if no fluid can be withdrawn, then surgical biopsy is warranted (USDHHS, 1984, p. 41). Wide-needle biopsy involves use of a cutting needle to remove tissue for diagnosis. It can be done under local anesthesia as an outpatient procedure. As a negative finding does not rule out cancer, needle biopsy for solid masses has limited diagnostic value.

Surgical biopsies are used for most solid masses, although in 75 percent of cases, tumors turn out to be benign (USDHHS, 1984, p. 41). An excisional biopsy removes the entire lump and is therefore also called a "lumpectomy." This procedure can be done on an outpatient basis under local anesthetia for lumps less than 3 cm in diameter. When more extensive surgery is required, such as with a larger mass or with a nonpalpable lesion detected only by mammography, general anesthesia may be required and the procedure is done in hospital.

A *hormonal receptor assay* must be performed on all breast cancer biopsy specimens. This gives prognostic information and is helpful in choosing appropriate therapy, both for the original cancer and for later metastases. It is important that this test, which determines the tumor's response to estrogen and progesterone, can be performed by the laboratory to which the biopsy specimen is sent (USDHHS, 1984, p. 42).

One major change in the diagnostic practices for breast cancer is the use of a two-step procedure for diagnosis and treatment rather than a one-step procedure. This was recommended by a National Institutes of Health 1979 Consensus Panel at the urging of Rose Kushner, the consumer advocate to the panel (Kushner, 1984). In the past, it was thought that if a biopsy revealed cancer, delay and possibly the effect of the biopsy itself would adversely affect survival. Women were consequently routinely biopsied under general anesthesia after signing a consent for mastectomy. When cancer was determined by frozen section, a quick examination of a specimen, mastectomy was performed. In a National Cancer Institute survey conducted in 1979, 55 percent of women questioned about this procedure rejected it, preferring instead to have the time to seek a second medical opinion and explore treatment options. With the two-step procedure diagnosis can be based on permanent section, leading to more accuracy and less unnecessary surgery, and the extent of the disease can be determined prior to surgery. Evidence does not demonstrate adverse effects on survival of a short delay between diagnosis and treatment, and the two-step procedure is now widely advocated. As more therapeutic options become available, it makes even more sense, giving a woman time to make an informed decision about treatment and to emotionally accept the diagnosis while she is deciding (USDHHS, 1984, pp. 42–43).

In 1979, Massachusetts became the first state to pass a law requiring that all women with breast cancer be informed of every available treatment. Since then, this law has been passed in California and other states (Kushner, 1984, p. 186). Its adoption virtually mandates the separation of diagnosis from treatment.

Treatment

It is beyond the scope of this chapter to thoroughly explore breast cancer treatment and clearly beyond the scope of the primary care nonphysician to recommend a particular treatment modality. This is especially true because research on breast cancer and its therapies is continually evolving. Nevertheless, it behooves the practitioner to be familiar with the variety of treatment options available, to provide the patient with supportive counseling, and to develop a referral network that ensures her of informed choices.

Staging. Prior to the initiation of breast cancer therapy, the cancer should be "staged." Staging is based on the extent of the disease. It is determined by three factors—the characteristics of the tumor, the state of the regional lymph nodes, and the presence of metastases away from the original site—and is referred to as the *TNM* system (*t*umor, *n*odes, *m*etastases). Breast cancer stages range from I to IV (see Table 10–3). Prognosis is directly related to stage of disease and treatment is determined accordingly (USDHHS, 1984, pp. 46–47).

History, physical examination, and laboratory tests all contribute to breast cancer staging. Historic data include symptoms of possible metastasis including signs of impaired liver function such as anorexia or nausea, bone involvement such as back or joint pain, and neurologic effects. Physical exam involves a search for lymph nodes, liver enlargement, or disturbed neurologic signs. Blood tests such as liver function tests may help indicate metastases. X-rays of the chest, or scans of bones, liver, and brain may be indicated (USDHHS, 1984, p. 48).

Prognosis. The National Cancer Institute (USDHHS, 1984, pp. 48–49) reports the following factors as prognostic in breast cancer:

1. Lymph node involvement: Negative nodes on histopathologic exam or those showing only micrometastases (less than 0.2 cm) are associated with the most favorable prognosis.
2. Tumor size: Smaller tumors, especially those under 2 cm, are associated with increased survival rates.
3. Histologic characteristics of the tumors: Those composed of more mature and well-developed cells have a more favorable prognosis. Smooth and rounded tumors also carry a better prognosis than do those with irregularly shaped borders, which tend to infiltrate nearby tissues more readily.
4. Tumor type: The most common type—infiltrating ductal tumors—carries the poorest prognosis.
5. Tumor location: Tumors in the upper inner quadrant are thought to drain more readily into the in-

TABLE 10-3. BREAST CANCER STAGES

Stage I	Small tumor (< 2 cm) Negative lymph nodes No detectable metastases
Stage II	Tumor larger than 2 cm but smaller than 5 cm Lymph nodes negative <div align="center">OR</div>Tumor smaller than 5 cm Lymph nodes positive No detectable distant metastases
Stage III	Large tumor (> 5 cm) <div align="center">OR</div>Tumor of any size with invasion of skin or chest wall or "grave signs"[a] <div align="center">OR</div>Associated with positive lymph nodes in the collarbone area <div align="center">BUT</div>No detectable distant metastases
Stage IV	Tumor of any size Lymph nodes either positive or negative Distant metastases

[a]Edema, ulceration of the skin, "peau d'orange," or satellite skin nodules.
From the American Joint Committee TNM Staging of Breast Cancer. (1982). Also, from the U.S. Department of Health and Human Services. (1984). The Breast Cancer Digest (2nd ed.), NIH Publication 84-1691. Bethesda, MD: National Cancer Institute.

ternal mammary lymph nodes and, therefore, to be related to poorer outcome, although this is not universally agreed on.

6. Hormone receptor assays: Tumors revealing large numbers of estrogen receptors have a better prognosis than those considered estrogen receptor negative.
7. Results of tests examining the immune state of the patient: Positive results correlate with better prognoses. Such tests include white blood cell counts and skin tests that measure immune reactivity.
8. Age: Younger age tends to be associated with more aggressive cancers and poorer outcomes.
9. Body build: Obesity seems to be associated with cancers that recur more frequently.
10. Parity: Multiparity appears more likely to be associated with better prognosis than does nulliparity.

Specific Therapies. Until recently, the mainstay of breast cancer treatment was the radical mastectomy (often called the Halsted radical mastectomy after its developer, Dr. William S. Halsted). In this procedure, introduced in the late nineteenth century, the entire breast, skin, pectoral muscles, and axillary lymph nodes are removed, leaving the woman with a large scar and flattened or sunken chest. Some surgeons have even advocated an extended radical mastectomy, which adds the internal mammary nodes and usually a portion of the rib cage to the structures removed (USDHHS, 1984, p. 55). Lymphedema of the arm, shoulder stiffness, decreased muscle strength and possible lasting numbness in the arm on the operative side are common side effects of the radical mastectomy (USDHHS, 1984, pp. 54, 57).

The theory behind the use of radical mastectomy in breast cancer was that the disease is localized with spread through the adjacent lymph vessels. If the tumor and surrounding structures, including these lymph nodes, could be removed, the cancer's spread could be stopped.

Current theories regarding the natural course of breast cancer bring into question the basic premise of the radical mastectomy. Breast cancer is considered to be a systemic disease, spreading easily through both lymph and blood vessels. In this view of breast cancer, the breast's adjacent lymph nodes play less of a role in spread than does the body's entire immune system. Infiltration to the lymph nodes is considered prognostic and a "reflection of a host–tumor relationship that permits development of metastases, rather than an instigator of distant disease" (Fisher, 1981, p. 912). This perception of the disease, coupled with the fact that 76 percent of women with positive lymph nodes at the time of diagnosis and 25 percent of those with negative nodes experience cancer recurrences within 10 years, has led researchers to consider alternative forms of therapy for breast cancer, therapies that attack possible metastases with chemotherapeutic and hormonal agents while limiting surgery.

A number of surgical procedures have been studied and found to result in survival comparable to that after radical mastectomy, although there remains a lack of consensus on the optimal treatment for breast cancer. One of the problems in arriving at such a consensus is the fact that few women (less than 3 percent of patients with operable breast cancer) participate in clinical trials, which are prospective studies involving random assignment to various treatment and control groups and are considered the most scientific way of evaluating treatment (Fisher & Wickerham, 1986, p. 221). The relative effects of various treatment options thus take longer to investigate because of the difficulty of acquiring adequate numbers for study and because individual practitioners make decisions based on evidence acquired in nonscientific ways.

Surgical alternatives to radical mastectomy include the following (USDHHS, 1984, p. 55):

- *Total* (or *simple*) *mastectomy* with removal of the entire breast, leaving all or most of the axillary lymph nodes intact. A *total mastectomy with axillary dissection* adds removal of some or most of the axillary nodes. When the pectoralis minor muscle is also removed, this may be called a *modified radical mastectomy*.
- *Quadrantectomy* with removal of the quarter of the breast containing the tumor as well as the overlying skin, the fascia covering the pectoralis major muscle, and the pectoralis minor muscle. Axillary nodes in this procedure are excised either through the same or a separate incision, depending on the quadrant involved (Veronesi, Saccozzi, Del Vecchio, et al., 1981, p. 7).
- *Segmental mastectomy* (also called *partial mastectomy*) with removal of the tumor plus normal tissue around it to ensure tumor-free margins. This may or may not include fascia and some skin. Axillary dissection is usually performed with a separate incision.
- *Lumpectomy* or *tylectomy,* also called *local excision,* is similar to an excisional biopsy in that only the tumor is removed, possibly with a small amount of surrounding tissue. When axillary nodes are removed with this procedure, it is done through a separate incision.

Interestingly, research and clinical practice in Europe, including some randomized controlled studies, has suggested equivalent results for simple mastectomy or breast-sparing surgeries for stage I disease since the 1940s, 1950s, and 1960s (Bruce, 1971; Hayward, 1974; Kaae & Johansen, 1969; Rissanen, 1969). In the United States, clinical trials examining surgical options began in 1971 by the National Surgical Adjuvant Breast and Bowel Project (NSABP) and currently involve many institutions in this country and Canada. Ten-year survival rates have been evaluated for the first trial comparing radical mastectomy with total (or simple) mastectomy. They show clearly that for patients with primary operable breast cancer, radical mastectomy is no better than the lesser procedure with or without radiation (Fisher, Redmond, Fisher, et al., 1985b). A trial involving simple and segmental mastectomy has demonstrated that total mastectomy is no better than segmental mastectomy with or without radiation in terms of 5-year survival rates for patients with stage I and II cancers that are less than or equal to 4 cm in diameter and have margins free of tumor (Fisher, Bauer, Margolese, et al., 1985a). A firmer conclusion awaits 10-year survival rates. A similar study was reported on in 1981 (Veronesi et al.) comparing the results of quadrantectomy with axillary dissection and radiotherapy to those for radical mastectomy for tumors less than 2 cm. This research also found no benefit in the more extensive procedure.

Although clinical trials have demonstrated neither benefit nor detriment in removing lymph nodes, axillary dissection, involving removal of most or all nodes, or axillary sampling, involving removal of about ten nodes, is advisable as part of breast cancer staging (USDHHS, 1984, p. 56).

An additional treatment modality for localized breast tumors is radiation, used with breast-saving procedures to prevent local recurrences. In the NSABP trial of segmental mastectomy with and without radiation, those women who received radiation did in fact have a lower rate of recurrence in the same breast; overall 5-year survival rates were not affected, however. Another study, reported in 1982, did show benefit in 10-year survival rates with radiation after surgery (Tapley, Spanos, Fletcher, et al., 1982; USDHHS, 1984, p. 61). The NSABP researchers now recommend segmental mastectomy with axillary dissection followed by radiation as an effective alternative to total mastectomy (Fisher & Wickerham, 1986, p. 219), although some physicians prefer to wait until local recurrence occurs before using radiation (USDHHS, 1984, p. 61).

Breast irradiation is usually given as 5,000 rads over a 5-week period. Possible side effects include an erythematous skin reaction and increased pigmentation, which is often temporary. Telangiectasia may develop in the irradiated area. Thickening may also occur. A sore or dry throat or dry cough may occur because radiation is close to the throat and bronchi. Increased intake of fluids or sucking on hard candy may offer some relief (Eich, 1985). If the patient is also receiving chemotherapy, side effects may be increased. Whether radiation causes an increase in second primary tumors remains to be demonstrated (Fisher & Wickerham, 1986, p. 220).

Adequate rest, sufficient fluid intake, and good nutrition are essential to combat the effects of radiation. Women should keep the irradiated area dry and free from pressure, chafing, and exposure to heat or deodorants, lotions, ointments, and strong soap (Mast 1984). A bra may need to be avoided for about a week after treatment.

Other adjuvant breast cancer therapy is aimed primarily at systemic manifestations of the cancer. Such treatments include cytotoxic agents, hormones, and immune system stimulants.

The NSABP has conducted a number of clinical trials evaluating adjuvant therapy in the treatment of primary breast cancer with one or more histologically positive lymph nodes (Fisher & Wolmark, 1981, p. 1349). One major finding from these trials has been that all patients with positive nodes benefited from adjuvant therapy. A similar finding was reported by a group studying chemotherapeutic agents in Milan (Fisher & Wolmark, 1981, pp. 1355–1356). Currently, chemotherapy for women without positive nodes is not recommended, although its use is being studied because 20 to 30 percent of women in this group do develop systemic disease (Fisher & Wolmark, 1981, p. 1358). Chemotherapy has been shown to benefit primarily premenopausal breast cancer patients; its role in postmenopausal women is less clear. Current trials are underway to evaluate its use in this group of women (Fisher and Wickerham 1986, p. 221). A recent Consensus Development Conference held by the National Institutes of Health supported combination chemotherapy for women under age 50 with positive lymph nodes.

Several types of cytotoxic agents can be given orally, intramuscularly, or intravenously, for 6 months or longer after surgery and/or radiation as weekly, monthly, or daily regimens. The most beneficial length of time for therapy to continue is yet to be determined.

Of course, because of their toxic effects on cells, these drugs also affect noncancerous cells. Temporary side effects include nausea, vomiting, and diarrhea, decreased white blood cell production, hair loss, weight loss or gain, appetite changes, ulcerations of the mouth, nervousness, and irritability. Longer-term side effects include leukemia and cardiac disease. Such drugs are best administered by specialists familiar with their results. The appropriate combination to be used is determined on the basis of either the patient's condition or the clinical trial in which she is participating. Which are the best drug combinations for which patients remain to be determined (Fisher & Wolmark, 1981, p. 1357; USDHHS, 1984, p. 63).

Adequate hydration and a nutritious diet are essential for women receiving chemotherapy (Mast, 1984). Support is also an integral part of care for all cancer patients, particularly those receiving chemotherapy. This must be aimed at helping women cope with the disease, the physical and cosmetic side effects of treatment, family reactions, changes in values, and fears of complications and death (Warren, 1979). The need for information must be met. Individual and group teaching sessions can be effective (Reynolds, Sachs, Davis, & Hall, 1981).

Hormonal therapy has been effective in treating certain subgroups of breast cancer patients, particularly the postmenopausal group with estrogen-receptor–rich tumors. A variety of hormonal agents have been evaluated including antiestrogens (most commonly tamoxifen) and adrenal blockers (such as aminoglutethimide), which interfere with conversion of androstenedione to estrogen and progestins. Tamoxifen is currently recommended for initial hormonal therapy in postmenopausal women because of its high efficacy and low incidence of side effects. It is the standard against which new agents will be tested (Ingle, 1984, p. 775). Hot flushes, sweats, flushed face, and nausea are the most common side effects of tamoxifen; they usually subside within 1 week. A transient increase in the pain of metastasis may occur after 1 week of therapy. Hypercalcemia may occur; gastrointestinal complaints and neurologic symptoms alert the patient to this problem (Wissing, 1984).

Immunotherapy, which involves an effort to stimulate the body's own defenses against tumor cells, is highly experimental in breast cancer treatment. Interferon, an antiviral substance produced by the body's own cells, is an example of an immunotherapeutic agent. This area holds promise for the future (USDHHS 1984, p. 64).

The same therapies may be used to treat advanced cancers. Locally advanced cancer is a stage III tumor, a large mass that has invaded adjacent structures. A local recurrence is a tumor appearing in the area of the original mass and may indicate untreated cells or actually may be a metastasis. Metastatic cancer is the spread of cancer cells to another body part; in breast cancer, metastases are seen most often in bones, the lungs, the liver, and the brain (USDHHS 1984, p. 66).

Inflammatory cancer, because of its rapid progression and poor prognosis, demands treatment as advanced disease. Therapies include local radiation, chemotherapy, and immunotherapy, often followed by mastectomy (USDHHS, 1984, p. 65).

Noninvasive cancer, also called carcinoma in situ, poses a treatment dilemma. Although about 50 percent of women with in situ *ductal* carcinoma develop invasive cancer in the same breast, only about 25 to 33 percent of those with in situ *lobular* cancer later develop invasive disease. This may occur in the same or contralateral breast, and in more than one third of cases, is not evident for at least 20 years (Hutter, 1984, p. 798). Treatment for ductal carcinoma in situ usually involves mastectomy, although in a current trial, removal of the cancer coupled with careful follow-up is being evaluated for selected patients (USDHHS, 1984, p. 65). Treatments for lobular carcinoma in situ vary from careful follow-up to unilateral or even bilateral mastectomy, with or without a preceding biopsy of the contralateral breast. Recommended follow-up regimens for these women include monthly BSE after careful instruction, breast examination by an experienced clinician every 3 to 6 months, and mammography at regular intervals. Hutter (1984, p. 800) recommends mammography approximately every 6 months. The patient must receive informed consent to determine a treatment program that fits her idea of acceptable risk (Hutter, 1984, p. 799; Rosen, 1984, p. 96).

Referral to Clinical Trials. Although the treatment of breast cancer is outside the scope of the primary care practitioner, such providers can play a vital role in determining sources of referral for patients. It has been urged strongly by those involved in the NCI clinical trials of breast cancer treatment (Fisher & Wickerham, 1986) and by consumer advocate Rose Kushner, who is involved with the National Women's Health Network and has served as consumer representative to the NCI on breast cancer, that women be referred to institutions participating in NCI clinical trials for breast cancer treatment. The advantage to the individual patient is that it ensures that the physician involved treats large numbers of breast cancer patients, is familiar with recent therapies, and provides close follow-up. The advantage to the public is that widespread participation in clinical trials provides the *only* scientific way to evaluate treatments and develop the most efficacious regimens.

Today, NSABP clinical trials evaluating the role of adjuvant therapy in primary operable breast cancer and examining various chemotherapeutic or hormonal regimens are being conducted at more than 100 centers in the United States and Canada. Participation is available to patients in almost any geographic region of North America (Fisher & Wickerham, 1986, p. 217). A list of participating physicians and institutions can be obtained from the NSABP operations office at the University of Pittsburg (412-624-2671) and the Cancer Information Service at the NCI (1-800-4-CANCER).

In making decisions regarding treatment, Valanis and Rumpler (1985) have suggested that a woman needs information, appreciation of her own values, and time. To provide this, these authors advise discussing treatment options for breast cancer with all women before disease strikes. Although a woman's reactions may change once a diagnosis has been made, prior information enables her to think through her values and to weigh risks and benefits in the absence of the emotional upheaval created by a diagnosis of cancer. Of course, as treatment options are changing, this may not always be entirely possible.

Follow-up. The primary care provider can also help assess whether the breast cancer patient receives adequate follow-up after initial diagnosis and treatment. Such women are at high risk for recurrence and should never be followed in a haphazard manner (Horton, 1984). They are also at increased risk of developing cancer of the bowel, endometrium, and ovary. BSE should be stressed and yearly mammograms (or ultrasound for some young women) advised. Patients should be taught to recognize and report the following symptoms, indicating breast cancer recurrence or metastasis or the growth of a new cancer (Kushner, 1984, p. 336; Welch, 1980):

- Lump in the breast or any other breast changes
- Bone or joint pain
- Cough/hoarseness/dyspnea
- Persistent digestive problems such as nausea, vomiting, diarrhea, heartburn, and anorexia
- Unexplained weight changes
- Neurologic symptoms such as dizziness, blurred vision, frequent or severe headaches, numbing or tingling in the extremities, and difficulty with balance or gait
- Vaginal or rectal bleeding or changes in the menstrual cycle or bowel habits
- Incontinence

Breast Reconstruction. Another aspect of breast cancer treatment is breast reconstruction. After simple or total mastectomy, this can be accomplished with a silicone implant, leaving a scar across the reconstructed breast. In patients who have had radical mastectomy or in whom there is inadequate skin to cover an implant, such as may occur after radiation therapy (USDHHS, 1984, p. 86), additional skin and muscle are taken from either the latissimus dorsi or rectus abdominis muscles. The latter operation may allow for reconstruction without an implant, but may lead to abdominal weakness. The choice of location for the flap is dependent on both the surgeon's and the patient's preference and should be discussed prior to the procedure. Some patients prefer an abdominal scar, which can sometimes be hidden in the pubic hair, to an incision on the back.

Reconstruction of the nipple and areola can be achieved with skin grafts, although some women find that reconstruction of a breast mound is sufficient. Grafts can be taken from the other breast, the inner thigh, the vaginal lips, the buccal mucosa, the earlobe, or the area behind the ear. This procedure is often delayed for several weeks or months until the breast assumes its permanent shape and location (Dinner & Dowden, 1984, p. 811; Goldwyn, 1982, p. 445; Kincaid, 1984, pp. 443–444).

Breast reconstruction can be carried out at the time of mastectomy or postponed anywhere from 3 months onward. There are advantages and disadvantages in each decision. Simultaneous mastectomy and reconstruction eliminate the need for a second surgery and have been found to reduce psychiatric morbidity (Dean, Chetty, & Forrest, 1983), although some surgeons have suggested that women having immediate reconstruction may be less satisfied with

the results than those who have lived with their loss. In at least one study, however, in which 30 women were interviewed after the simultaneous procedures, a high level of satisfaction with few untoward effects was revealed (Noone, Frazier, Hayward, et al., 1982). Advantages of delaying the surgery until healing has taken place are to achieve a more cosmetic appearance, reduce the possibility of complications, and determine whether chemotherapy or radiation is indicated so that reconstruction can follow completion of such treatment (Goldwyn, 1982, p. 444; Kincaid, 1984, p. 437; USDHHS, 1984, pp. 90–91).

Complications of breast reconstruction include infection and hemorrhage, sometimes leading to skin necrosis with the need for replacement of the implant. A fibrous capsule of scar tissue can form around the implant and contract, giving the breast an unusual firmness and an unnatural shape and contour, and possibly leading to pain. Postoperative exercise and massage of the breast reduce the incidence of this complication as does placing the implant under the pectoralis muscle (Kincaid, 1984, p. 444; Riddle, 1986a, 1986b). Its occurrence may require surgical correction (USDHHS, 1984, pp. 93–94).

It is important for women to understand that a reconstructed breast will not look or feel exactly like the lost or remaining breast, although results of the surgery continue to improve (Kincaid, 1984). Many times, surgery to the contralateral breast is recommended to achieve symmetry. This may involve reduction, enlargement, or tightening (USDHHS, 1984, p. 90).

Today, breast reconstruction is considered an option for almost all women who have mastectomies, chosen at times even by those with advanced disease. Kincaid (1984, p. 438) cites inflammatory cancer and "very large aggressive tumors with questionable local eradication" as the only absolute contraindications to this procedure. It is not considered to affect the development or detection of a future cancer. In fact, placement of the implant under the muscle may facilitate the finding of a subsequent mass (USDHHS, 1984, p. 94).

It has been suggested that the availability of breast reconstruction may lead some women to earlier diagnosis and treatment for breast cancer (Goldwyn, 1982, p. 446; Rutledge, 1982). A major advantage for many women is that after reconstruction, they need not rely on external prostheses. This often makes participation in sports and other activities more comfortable. Recognizing the therapeutic role of breast reconstruction, a number of states, including California, New York, Illinois, and Connecticut, have mandated some type of reimbursement for it (USDHHS, 1984, p. 94).

Prevention

Analysis of the risk factors for breast cancer reveals difficulties inherent in its prevention. Hereditary factors, obviously, cannot be changed for women at risk for the familial type of cancer. Certain life-style decisions that affect breast cancer rates, such as delayed pregnancy, cannot be made solely on the basis of cancer prevention. There are, however, several primary, secondary, and tertiary prevention strategies that can be implemented.

Although the data on the role of diet in breast cancer promotion or prevention cannot yet be considered conclusive, there is no reason not to recommend low-fat, high-fiber diets, with high intake of vegetables, especially those containing carotene, for women at risk of developing this disease. Encouraging parents to adopt these diets for their children may be equally or more important.

Vitamins A, C, and E and some of the B-complex vitamins may have an effect in reducing breast cancer risk, and this too warrants further study. Hypervitamin therapy, however, may have side effects, and should not be advised routinely. Foods high in these vitamins can be suggested.

Women at risk of developing breast cancer should consider avoiding even moderate alcohol consumption. On the basis of current evidence, it is reasonable to advise that drinking for this group of women be limited to no more than three drinks per week.

Clearly, the most drastic suggestion for breast cancer prevention is prophylactic mastectomy. This has been recommended in the following high-risk groups (Snyderman, 1984):

1. Women with cancer of one breast, including carcinoma in situ
2. Women with strong family histories of breast cancer, especially the woman whose mother and sister had premenopausal, bilateral cancer
3. Women undergoing repeated breast biopsies showing atypia or hyperplasia

Opponents of prophylactic mastectomy point out that it results in large numbers of unnecessary surgeries. Prophylactic mastectomy removes the entire breast, including its tail, the nipple and areola, some skin, and the lower lymph nodes. A less extensive form of prophylactic surgery, the "subcutaneous mastectomy," used to be advocated. This removed as much tissue as possible through flaps made in the breast, leaving the nipple, areola, and outer skin intact. This operation is no longer considered acceptable for the purpose of prophylaxis because it leaves too much breast tissue in place (Snyderman, 1984, pp. 803–804).

Reconstruction can be done in women undergoing prophylactic mastectomy. Ultimately, the decision to undergo this procedure must be the patient's and must be based on informed consent.

Secondary prevention of breast cancer, that is, early detection, includes BSE, practitioner examination, and breast imaging. Recommendations and controversies regarding the timing of each of the latter two have been discussed previously. Although most authorities advocate monthly BSE, and it has been reported that more than 70 percent of palpable breast masses are found by women themselves (USDHHS, 1984, p. 110), a number of questions concerning the benefits of BSE have been raised.

Areas that have been looked at—although in relatively few research studies, each with methodologic limitations— include the efficacy of BSE as a screening technique and whether it has detrimental side effects. Those examining its efficacy have questioned whether cancer is actually diagnosed at an earlier stage in women who practice BSE and whether the practice of BSE is associated with increased survival time, unrelated to lead-time bias (meaning that longer survival reflects *only* earlier diagnosis) or length-time bias (meaning that the screening technique favors discovery of slow-growing tumors leading to increased survival secondary only to tumor characteristics) (Cole & Austin, 1981; Diem & Rose, 1985). Those looking at possible detrimental side effects of BSE have asked whether unnecessary anxiety is created by BSE when women falsely believe they have breast cancer after detecting a benign lump, whether unnecessary aspirational biopsies are done as a result of BSE, and whether breast examination by a health care practitioner is postponed by women who perform BSE.

In a review of the literature of BSE, Foster, Costanza, and Worden (1985, p. 481) found more positive than negative results of BSE and conclude that it "is efficacious in decreasing breast cancer mortality," although they concede "that assessment of the magnitude of the effect of BSE on survival has been limited." Based on the weight of evidence, they advise against randomized clinical trials of BSE. Cole and Austin (1981) suggest that the most beneficial effect of BSE is seen in women who do not or cannot avail themselves of other screening modalities. They emphasize, however, that BSE should not substitute for examination performed by a health care provider or for mammographic screening when appropriate.

Other concerns regarding BSE are how best to teach women the technique and how to motivate them to practice it consistently. In one study of 2,092 women with breast cancer (Huguley & Brown, 1981, p. 991), it was found that women who learned the technique from a physician or nurse were more likely to practice BSE once a month than those who learned it from any other source. These women were also more likely to perform it competently. Another study comparing three methods of teaching BSE found that demonstration with guided practice led to more frequent self-examination than either the provision of written information only or demonstration only (Marty, McDermott, & Gold, 1983). Other studies support the finding that teaching BSE can increase the performance of BSE among women; positive results have been found in both group and individual sessions, using demonstration and/or practice (Brailey, 1986; Edwards, 1980; Michalek, Walsh, Burns, & Mettlin, 1981). Confidence in examination skill also has been correlated with monthly performance (Keller, George, & Podell, 1980).

The following characteristics have been found to be associated with the practice of BSE: younger age, better educational background, and higher socioeconomic status (Massey, 1986; USDHHS, 1984, pp. 111–112). In a 1979 NCI survey, reasons for not practicing monthly BSE were given as not thinking about it or not being concerned. Ignorance of the importance of the examination, lack of knowledge about the method, and fear and anxiety, which were important reasons for not practicing regular BSE given in a NCI survey in 1973, were not found to be significant in 1979. Hallal (1982) found BSE to be correlated with three factors: (1) health beliefs, that is, perceived susceptibility and perceived benefits; (2) an internal health locus of control; and (3) high self-concept. Rutledge (1987) also found BSE to be related to its perceived benefits and to a high self-concept, as well as low perceived barriers to its practice.

These data certainly support the conclusions that hands-on teaching during routine health examinations is valuable in encouraging BSE and that women need positive reinforcement on their technique.

Tertiary prevention, or limitation of further disability, for breast cancer involves reducing recurrences and/or metastases. Recommendations for women with primary disease worthy of clinical trials include weight reduction and/or the reduction of dietary fats (de Waard, 1982; Wynder & Cohen, 1982) and alcohol, and the increase of dietary fiber and high vitamin A, C, E, and B-complex foods.

Emotional Aspects

Two issues must be addressed in a discussion of the emotional aspects of breast cancer: the impact of having a disease of the breast with the possibility of loss of that organ and the impact of facing a disease with an implicit threat to life. Response to each of these areas is individualized and influenced by many factors including age, marital status, social supports, knowledge, perception, self-image, employment, and general response to stress (Morris, 1983; USDHHS, 1984, p. 114).

The emotional impact of breast disease begins with the finding of a mass—by the patient or her partner, the health care provider, or mammography. Anxiety most often accompanies the period of awaiting diagnostic testing and results. It has been suggested that a woman's reaction at this time may predict her response to diagnosis and treatment (USDHHS, 1984, p. 114). Each subsequent phase requires additional adjustment—after diagnosis but before treatment, during treatment, after treatment, and possibly during recurrences and advanced disease stages. The primary care practitioner is most involved with the patient before diagnosis, although involvement may extend into any of the other periods.

A consistent research finding is that women often delay seeking medical advice from the time a symptom is detected. Denial and/or fear may be operable in these cases (Nichols, 1983, p. 163). By the time an appointment is made many misconceptions may be present. This initial visit, most often to a gynecologist, but possibly to a nonphysician or other primary woman's health care provider, is a crucial time for a woman to express her feelings and for the provider to correct misinformation. Many women want as much information as possible at this visit, including treatment options, even before diagnosis is confirmed. Some women find the time before biopsy to be the most stressful period in disease adaptation (Small, 1982, p. 450; USDHHS, 1984, pp. 114–115).

Interestingly, in one study, women who were reluctant to seek care were found to have not previously asked for medical advice about breast symptoms, nor to have received a breast examination from a health care provider or to have practiced BSE (Nichols, 1983, p. 164). The practitioner who routinely provides breast examinations, teaches BSE, raises the issue of breast symptoms with patients, and discusses treatment options may positively influence future care-seeking behavior.

After biopsy, the cancer patient must begin to cope with the reality of disease. She can use this period to seek a second medical opinion, to have tests to stage the disease, to choose appropriate treatment, and to prepare for hospitalization if necessary (USDHHS, 1984, p. 117). The patient's husband or partner should be involved in counseling and discussions as much as possible during each phase of diagnosis and treatment. This person is instrumental in the patient's eventual adjustment to the disease and may have his or her own set of fears and anxieties, which deserve attention (Northouse & Swain, 1987; Small, 1982, p. 450).

Small (1982, p. 450) reports the following myths that may need clarification to patients once diagnosis is made:

1. Cancer always recurs or kills.
2. Cancer is communicable and the patient may spread the disease.
3. The patient is responsible for the cancer because of past misdeed or because she has not taken proper care of herself.
4. The patient will no longer have sexual feelings or may be so changed that she will not be sexually acceptable.

Sexuality is a major concern for breast cancer patients, particularly after mastectomy or radiation, which may lead to physical changes. The NCI recommends facing this issue with patients shortly after primary treatment, with anticipatory guidance about the following expected reactions communicated to patients and partners: "fear of rejection manifested by withdrawal, temporary loss of sexual interest and self-confidence, fear of viewing the incision area, and concern about hurting it during sexual activity" (USDHHS, 1984, pp. 148–149).

Patients should be encouraged to resume sexual activity gradually, although touching and caressing can be encouraged as therapeutic at any time (USDHHS, 1984, pp. 149, 151). For patients without current partners, the issue of future sexual relationships needs to be raised. Discussion of sexual issues should be done by a practitioner with experience and comfort in this area. Oncology nurses are often good counselors and Reach to Recovery volunteers can be helpful in sharing their own experiences. If any provider feels that the patient's adjustment problems are severe, she should be referred for intensive counseling.

Some premenopausal women with breast cancer are concerned with the effect of the disease on their ability to become pregnant in the future and of the effect of pregnancy on the disease. Except for some chemotherapeutic agents, which may cause sterility, neither the disease nor its treatment precludes subsequent childbearing. Studies do not show effects on disease-free interval or overall survival from pregnancy (Donegan, 1979; Harvey, Rosen, Ashikiar, et al., 1981). It is recommended that women delay pregnancy at least 2 years after initial diagnosis because this is when disease is most likely to recur, especially for women with positive nodes (Donegan, 1979).

Women with breast cancer can be referred to a variety of support groups. Referral for social, psychological, or financial assistance may be necessary as well. A team approach is imperative. Funch and Mettlin (1982) found social, professional, and financial support related to psychological and physical recovery in 151 breast cancer patients in the 3 to 12 months after surgery. Support groups have been found to be particularly useful for patients with recurrent or advanced disease whose problems become increasingly similar to those of other cancer patients (Morris, 1983, p. 1729). Table 10-4 lists resources for breast cancer support and education. Several mail-order suppliers for postmastectomy clothing are also included (Feather & Lanigan, 1987).

Educational materials can be obtained by contacting a local chapter of the American Cancer Society or by writing to the organization at 90 Park Avenue, New York, NY 10016. The NCI, at Building 31, Room 10A18, Bethesda, MD 20205, provides pamphlets on topics such as BSE, breast lumps, breast biopsy, breast cancer treatment, breast reconstruction, and recurring breast cancer. *The Breast Cancer Digest*, a guide for health professionals from which much of this chapter is adapted, is available from the NCI as well.

Several books can be suggested to patients. *Alternatives: New developments in the war on breast cancer* by Rose Kushner (New York: Warner Books, 1984) is the consumer's "everything you always wanted and needed to know about breast cancer and more," as well as a personal account of the author's struggle against the disease. Another stirring book by a cancer patient is *The cancer journals* by Audre Lorde (Argyle, NY: Spinster, Ink., 1980). Its author is a poet, feminist, and lesbian who offers a strong and unconventional approach to confronting mastectomy. Each work documents a courageous woman's emotional triumph over the disease and each offers its own inspiration and hope.

TABLE 10-4. BREAST CANCER SUPPORT AND EDUCATION GROUPS[a]

Name of Group	Services Offered	Address	Phone
American Cancer Society (ACS)	Literature, films, exhibits, special programs, and support services for cancer patients	National Headquarters: 777 Third Avenue New York, NY 10017	212–371–2900
ACS Programs: Reach for Recovery	American Cancer Society patient volunteer support and education service for breast cancer patients and families	Local ACS chapters	See local listings.
CanSurmount	Cancer patient volunteer meets with cancer patients and families on physician referral	Local ACS chapters	See local listings.
I Can Cope	Series of eight classes for patients and families	Local ACS chapters	See local listings.
Memorial Sloan–Kettering Cancer Center	Rehabilitative support services for patients and families	Box 166 1275 York Avenue New York, NY 10021	New York City Cancer Information Service: 212–794–7982
Postmastectomy Project	Psychotherapy for women and husbands	Stanford University 735 Mayfield Avenue Stanford, CA 94305	415–857–0857
RENU (Reconstruction Education for National Understanding)	Educational services for women considering breast reconstruction		Philadelphia: 215–635–1499 Washington, DC: 202–483–2600 Cleveland: 216–356–2683
ENCORE (Encouragement, Normalcy, Counseling, Opportunity, Reaching Out, Energies revived)	YWCA exercise program for postoperative breast cancer patients	Local YWCA branches	See local listings.
The St. Francis Center Counseling Program	Individual and group therapy for patients and families	1768 Church Street, NW Washington, DC 20036	202–234–5613
Hospice in America, The National Hospice Organization (NHO)	Information on hospice locations and services	1901 North Fort Meyer Drive Arlington, VA 22205	703–243–5900
Make Today Count	Discussion groups for patients, families, and health professionals; local chapters around the country	P.O. Box 383 Burlington, IA 52601	319–753–6521
Cancer Information Service (CIS)	Latest information on cancer for patients, families, and health providers		800–4–CANCER
American College of Surgeons	Information on certified, hospital-based cancer programs throughout the country.	55 East Erie Street Chicago, IL 60611	
Y-ME	Counseling and support for cancer patients; 24-hour volunteer patient hotline	P.O. Box 483 18220 Harwood Avenue Homewood, IL 60430	312–799–8228
Cancer Care, Inc. and the National Cancer Foundation	Counseling and support for patients with advanced disease	One Park Avenue New York, NY 10016	212–679–5700
Lumpectomy/Radiation Therapy Information Service, The West Coast Cancer Foundation	Volunteer hotline for women with early-stage breast cancer considering this treatment	50 Francisco Street San Francisco, CA 94133	415–981–4590
The Cancer Consultative Service	Multidisciplinary, multiinstitutional recommendations on breast cancer treatment provided on physician referral	Building 1805 14th Avenue and Lake Street San Francisco, CA 94129	415–221–2132
Lifeline	Small-group counseling for patients and families prior to treatment.	915 South Limestone Street Lexington, KY 40536	606–233–6541
Metropolitan Mastectomy Association of Denver	Meetings four times a year for all women who have had mastectomies	1809 East 18th Avenue Denver, CO 80218	303–321–2464
Cancer Risk Counseling Service	Counseling on cancer risk	824 Cragmont Avenue Berkeley, CA 94708	415–527–8938
Information Hotline	Information on screening, diagnosis, staging, and treatment for breast cancer, community resources, and counseling and emotional supports; various workshops	Health Care Division Palo Alto Medical Foundation 300 Home Avenue Palo Alto, CA 94301	415–321–4121

TABLE 10-4. BREAST CANCER SUPPORT AND EDUCATION GROUPS[a] **(CONTINUED)**

Name of Group	Services Offered	Address	Phone
Mail-order catalogs for postmastectomy clothing		Regenesis, Inc. 18 East 53rd Street New York, NY 10022	
		Airway (Truman) 3960 Rosslyn Drive Cincinnati, OH 45209	
		Camp International, Inc. P.O. Box 89 Jackson, MI 49204	
		Sear's and Penney's catalogs	

[a]Information is taken from USDHHS (1984, pp. 187–197). See this reference for additional cancer resource listings, including those concerned with financial aid and legal assistance for cancer patients.

REFERENCES

Abrams, A. A. (1965, May 20). Correspondence: Use of vitamin E in chronic cystic mastitis. *New England Journal of Medicine, 272*(20), 1080.

Aksu, M. F., Tzingounis, V. A., & Greenblatt, R. B. (1978, September). Treatment of benign breast disease with danazol: A follow-up report. *Journal of Reproductive Medicine, 31*(3), 181–184.

Ariel, I. M. (1973, October 15). Enovid therapy (norethynodrel with mestranol) for fibrocystic disease. *American Journal of Obstetrics and Gynecology, 117*(4), 453–459.

Armstrong, B.K., Brown, J. B., & Clarke, H. T., et al. (1981, October). Diet and reproductive hormones: A study of vegetarian and nonvegetarian postmenopausal women. *Journal of the National Cancer Institute, 67*(4), 761–767.

Armstrong, B., & Doll, R. (1975, April 15). Environmental factors and cancer incidence and mortality in different countries, with special reference to dietary practices. *International Journal of Cancer, 15*(4), 617–631.

Asch, R. H., & Greenblatt, R. B. (1977, January 15). The use of an impeded androgen—danazol—in the management of benign breast disorders. *American Journal of Obstetrics and Gynecology, 127*(2), 130–134.

Assaf, A. R., Cummings, K. M., & Graham, S., et al. (1985, Fall). Comparison of three methods of teaching women how to perform breast self-examination. *Health Education Quarterly, 12*(3), 259–272.

Bailar, J. C., III. (1976, January). Mammography: A contrary view. *Annals of Internal Medicine, 84*(1), 77–84.

Baker, H. W., & Snedecor, P. A. (1979, November). Clinical trial of danazol for benign breast disease. *American Surgeon, 45*(11), 727–729.

Baron, J. A., Byers, T., & Greenberg, E. R., et al. (1986, September). Cigarette smoking in women with cancers of the breast and reproductive organs. *Journal of the National Cancer Institute, 77*(3), 677–680.

Bassett, M. T., & Krieger, N. (1986, December). Social class and black–white differences in breast cancer survival. *American Journal of Public Health, 76*(12), 1400–1403.

Beral, V., & Colwell, L. (1980, October 25). Randomised trial of high doses of stilbestrol and ethisterone in pregnancy: Long-term follow-up of mothers. *British Medical Journal, 281*(6248), 1098–1101.

Bjarnason, O., Day, N., Snaedal, G., & Tulinius, H. (1974, May 15). The effect of year of birth on the breast cancer age—Incidence curve in Iceland. *International Journal of Cancer. 13*, 689–696.

Black, M. M., & Kwon, S. (1980). Precancerous mastopathie: Structural and biological considerations. *Pathology, Research and Practice, 166*(4), 491–514.

Boice, J. D., & Monson, R. R. (1977, September). Breast cancer in women after repeated fluoroscopic examinations of the chest. *Journal of the National Cancer Institute, 59*(3), 823–832.

Brailey, L. J. (1986, September). Effects of health teaching in the workplace on women's knowledge, beliefs, and practices regarding breast self-examination. *Research in Nursing and Health, 9*(3), 223–231.

Brian, D. D., Tilley, B. C., & Labarthe, D. R., et al. (1980, February). Breast cancer in DES-exposed mothers: Absence of association. *Mayo Clinic Proceedings, 55*(2), 81–93.

Brinton, L. A., Schairer, C., Stanford, J. L., & Hoover, R. N. (1986, April). Cigarette smoking and breast cancer. *American Journal of Epidemiology, 123*(4), 614–622.

Bruce, J. (1971, December). Operable cancer of the breast: A controlled clinical trial. *Cancer, 28*(6), 1443–1452.

Buell, P. (1973, November). Changing incidence of breast cancer in Japanese-American women. *Journal of the National Cancer Institute, 51*(5), 1479–1483.

Casarett, G. W. (1965). Experimental radiation carcinogenesis. *Progress in Experimental Tumor Research, 7*, 49–82.

Centers for Disease Control and Steroid Hormone Study. (1983, March 25). Long-term contraceptive use and the risk of breast cancer. *Journal of the American Medical Association, 249*(12), 1591–1595.

Clifford, E. (1983). Augmentation, reduction, and reconstruction: Psychological contributions to understanding breast surgery. In N. G. Georgiade, (Ed.), *Aesthetic breast surgery.* Baltimore: Williams & Wilkins.

Cole, P. & Austin, H. (1981, June). Breast self-examination: An adjuvant to early cancer detection (Editorial). *American Journal of Public Health, 71*(6): 572–574.

Collette, H. J., Day, N. E., Rombach, J. J., & de Waard, F. (1984, June 2). Evaluation of screening for breast cancer in a non-randomised study (The DOM Project) by means of a case-control study. *Lancet, 1*(8388), 1224–1226.

Coombs, L. J., Lilienfeld, A. M., Bross, I. D. J., & Burnett, W. S. (1979). A prospective study of the relationship between benign breast diseases and breast carcinoma. *Preventive Medicine, 8*, 40–52.

Cowan, L. D., Gordis, L., Tonascia, J. A., & Jones, G. S. (1981). Breast cancer incidence in women with a history of progesterone deficiency. *American Journal of Epidemiology, 114*(2), 209–217.

Daro, A. F., Gollin, H. A., & Samos, F. H. (1964, January). The effect of thyroid on cystic mastitis. *Journal of the International College of Surgeons, 41*(1), 58–59.

Dean, C., Chetty, U., & Forrest, A. P. M. (1983, February 26). Effects of immediate breast reconstruction on psychosocial morbidity after mastectomy. *Lancet, 1*(8322), 459–462.

de Waard, F. (1982). Nutritional etiology of breast cancer: Where are we now, and where are we going? *Nutrition and Cancer, 4*(2), 85–89.

de Waard, F. (1983, December). Epidemiology of breast cancer: A review. *European Journal of Cancer and Clinical Oncology, 19*(12), 1671–1676.

Diem, G., & Rose, D. P. (1985, August). Has breast self-examination had a fair trial? *New York State Journal of Medicine, 85*(8), 479–480.

Dinner, M., & Dowden, R. V. (1984, February 1). Breast reconstruction. State of the art. *Cancer, 53*(3, Suppl.), 809–814.

Donegan, W. L. (1979). Mammary carcinoma and pregnancy. In W. L. Donegan & J. S. Spratt (Eds.), *Cancer of the breast* (2nd ed.). Philadelphia: W. B. Saunders.

Durning, P., & Sellwood, R. A. (1982, May). Bromocriptine in severe cyclical breast pain. *British Journal of Surgery, 69*(5), 248–249.

Edwards, V. (1980, September–October). Changing breast self-examination behavior. *Nursing Research, 29*(5), 301–306.

Eich, S. J. (1985, February). Promising early breast cancer treatment—Without mastectomy. *Cancer Nursing, 8*(7), 51–58.

Ernster, V. L. (1981). The epidemiology of benign breast disease. *Epidemiologic Reviews, 3,* 184–202.

Ernster, V. L., Mason, L., & Goodson, W. H., et al. (1982, March). Effects of caffeine-free diet on benign breast disease: A randomized trial. *Surgery, 91*(3), 263–267.

Estes, N. C. (1981, December). Mastodynia due to fibrocystic disease of the breast controlled with thyroid hormones. *The American Journal of Surgery, 142*(6), 764–766.

Feather, B. L., & Lanigan, C. (1987, August). Looking good after your mastectomy. *American Journal of Nursing, 87*(8), 1048–1049.

Feig, S. A. (1984a). Benefits and risks of mammography. *Recent Results in Cancer Research, 90,* 11–27.

Feig, S. A. (1984b). Hypothetical breast cancer risk from mammography. *Recent Results in Cancer Reserch, 90,* 1–10.

Fentiman, I. S., Caleffi, M., & Brame, K., et al. (1986, February 8). Double-blind controlled trial of tamoxifen therapy for mastalgia. *Lancet, 1*(8476), 287–288.

Fisher, B. (1981, September–October). New concepts in the treatment of breast cancer. *Israel Journal of Medical Science, 17*(9), 911–915.

Fisher, B., Bauer, M., & Margolese, R., et al. (1985a, March 14). Five-year results of a randomized clinical trial comparing total mastectomy and segmental mastectomy with or without radiation in the treatment of breast cancer. *New England Journal of Medicine, 312*(11), 666–673.

Fisher, B., Redmond, C., & Fisher, E., et al. (1985b, March). Ten-year results of a randomized clinical trial comparing radical mastectomy and total mastectomy with or without radiation. *New England Journal of Medicine, 312*(11), 674–681.

Fisher, B., & Wickerham, L. (1986, April). Answers to questions about breast cancer. *American Family Physician, 33*(4), 214–222.

Fisher, B., & Wolmark, N. (1981, December). The current status of systemic adjuvant therapy in the management of primary breast cancer. *Surgical Clinics of North America, 61*(6), 1347–1360.

Foley, M. J., (1987, November/December). Breast cancer update: The women's health trial: Down for the count? *The Network News, 12*(6), 1, 3.

Foster, R. S., Costanza, M. C., & Worden, J. K. (1985, August). The current status of research in breast self-examination. *New York State Journal of Medicine, 85*(8), 480–482.

Frankl, G. (1987, October 15). The use of screening mammography. *Cancer, 60*(8, Suppl.), 1979–1983.

Frisch, R.E., & Revelle, R. (1971, February). The height and weight of girls and boys at the time of initiation of the adolescent growth spurt in height and weight and the relationship to menarche. *Human Biology, 43,* 149–159.

Funch, D. P., & Mettlin, C. (1982). The role of support in relation to recovery from breast cancer. *Social Science and Medicine, 16*(1), 91–98.

Gambrell, R. D. (1982, April). The menopause: Benefits and risks of estrogen–progestogen replacement therapy. *Fertility and Sterility, 37*(4), 457–473.

Gambrell, R. D. (1984, September 15). Proposal to decrease the risk and improve the prognosis of breast cancer. *American Journal of Obstetrics and Gynecology, 150*(2), 119–132.

Goins, M. K. (1983). Psychological aspects of aesthetic surgery of the breast. In N. G. Georgiade (Ed.), *Aesthetic breast surgery.* Baltimore: Williams & Wilkins.

Goldwyn, R. M. (1976). Remarks on reduction mammaplasty. In R. Goldwyn (Ed.), *Plastic and reconstructive surgery of the breast.* Boston: Little, Brown.

Goldwyn, R. M. (1982, June). Breast reconstruction. *Clinical Obstetrics and Gynecology, 25*(2), 443–446.

Graham, S. (1987, May 7). Alcohol and breast cancer. *New England Journal of Medicine, 316*(19), 1211–1212.

Greenblatt, R. B., Dmowski, W. P., Mehesh, V. B., & Scholer, H. F. L. (1971, February). Clinical studies with an antigonadotropin—danazol. *Fertility and Sterility, 22*(2), 102–112.

Greenblatt, R. B., Samaras, C., Vasquez, J. M., & Nezhat, C. (1982, June). Fibrocystic disease of the breast. *Clinical Obstetrics and Gynecology, 25*(2), 365–371.

Haagensen, C. D. (1986). *Diseases of the breast* (3rd ed.). Philadelphia: W. B. Saunders.

Hadjimichael, O. C., Boyle, C. A., & Meigs, J. W. (1986, February). Abortion before first livebirth and risk of breast cancer. *British Journal of Cancer, 53*(2), 281–284.

Hallal, J. C. (1982, May/June). The relationship of health beliefs, health locus of control, and self-concept to the practice of breast self-examination in adult women. *Nursing Research, 31*(3), 137–142.

Hartmann, W. H. (1984, February 1). Minimal breast cancer: An update. *Cancer, 53*(3, Suppl.), 681–684.

Harvey, J. C., Rosen, P. P., & Ashikiar, R., et al. (1981, November). The effect of pregnancy on the prognosis of carcinoma of the breast following radical mastectomy. *Surgery, Gynecology and Obstetrics, 153*(5), 723–725.

Hayward, J. (1974, February). Conservative surgery in the treatment of early breast cancer. *Cancer, 33*(2), 593–599.

Henderson, B. E., Ross, R. K., Pike, M. C., & Casagrande, J. T. (1982, August). Endogenous hormones as a major factor in human cancer. *Cancer Research, 42*(8), 3232–3239.

Hill, M. J., Goddard, P., & Williams, R. E. (1971, August 28). Gut bacteria and aetiology of cancer of the breast. *Lancet, 2*(7722), 472–473.

Hislop, T. G., Coldman, A. J., & Elwood, J. M., et al. (1986). Childhood and recent eating patterns and risk of breast cancer. *Cancer Detection and Prevention, 9*(1/2), 47–48.

Homer, M. J. (1982, June). Mammographic detection of breast cancer. *Clinical Obstetrics and Gynecology, 25*(2), 393–400.

Horton, J. (1984, February 1). Follow-up of breast cancer patients. *Cancer, 53*(3, Suppl.), 790–797.

Huguley, C. M., & Brown, R. L. (1981, March 1). The value of breast self-examination. *Cancer, 47*(5), 989–995.

Hutchinson, W. B., Thomas, D. B., & Hamlin, W. B., et al. (1980, July). Risk of breast cancer in women with benign breast disease. *Journal of the National Cancer Institute, 65*(1), 13–20.

Hutter, R. V. P. (1984, February 1). The management of patients with lobular carcinoma in situ of the breast. *Cancer, 53*(3, Suppl.), 798–802.

Ingle, J. N. (1984, February 1). Additive hormonal therapy in women with advanced breast cancer. *Cancer, 53*(3, Suppl.), 766–777.

Jablon, S., & Kato, H. (1972, June). Studies of the mortality of A-bomb survivors. 5. Radiation dose and mortality, 1950–1970. *Radiation Research, 50*(3), 649–698.

Jick, H., Walker, A. M., & Watkins, R. N., et al. (1980, November). Replacement estrogens and breast cancer. *American Journal of Epidemiology, 112*(5), 586–594.

Kaae, S., & Johansen, H. (1969, December). Simple mastectomy plus postoperative irradiation by the method of McWhirter for mammary carcinoma. *Annals of Surgery, 170*(6), 895–899.

Kay, C. R., & Hannaford, P. C. (1988). Breast cancer and the pill-A further report from the Royal College of General Practitioners' oral contraception study. *British Journal of Cancer, 58,* 675–680.

Keller, K., George, E., & Podell, R. N. (1980). Clinical breast examination and breast self-examination experience in a family practice population. *The Journal of Family Practice, 11*(6), 887–893.

Kelsey, J. L. (1979). A review of the epidemiology of human breast cancer. *Epidemiologic Review, 1,* 74–109.

Kelsey, J. L., Fischer, D. B., & Holford, T. R., et al. (1981, August). Exogenous estrogens and other factors in the epidemiology of breast cancer. *Journal of the National Cancer Institute, 67*(2), 327–333.

Kincaid, S. B. (1984, May). Breast reconstruction: A review. *Annals of Plastic Surgery, 12*(5), 431–447.

Kopans, D. B. (1985, September). Use mammography to detect cancer earlier. *Contemporary Ob/Gyn, 26*(3), 170–179.

Kopans, D. B., Meyer, J. E., & Sadowsky, N. (1984, April 12). Breast imaging. *New England Journal of Medicine, 310*(15), 960–967.

Kushner, R. (1984). *Alternatives: New developments in the war on breast cancer.* New York: Warner Books.

La Vecchia, C., Talamini, R., & Decarli, A., et al. (1986, September). Coffee consumption and the risk of breast cancer. *Surgery, 100*(3), 477–481.

Le, M. G., Moulton, L. H., Hill, C., & Kramar, A. (1986, September). Consumption of dairy produce and alcohol in a case-control study of breast cancer. *Journal of the National Cancer Institute, 77*(3), 633–636.

Leis, H. P., Jr. (1977, July–August). The diagnosis of breast cancer. *Ca—A Cancer Journal for Clinicians, 27*(4), 209–232.

Lewis, J. R. (1983). Augmentation mammoplasty. In N. G. Georgiade, (Ed.), *Aesthetic breast surgery.* Baltimore: Williams & Wilkins.

Lindner, H. H. (1989). *The breast. Clinical anatomy.* East Norwalk, CT: Appleton & Lange.

London, R. S., Sundaram, G. S., & Goldstein, P. J. (1982, April). Medical management of mammary dysplasia. *Obstetrics and Gynecology, 59*(4), 519–523.

London, R., Sundaram, G. S., & Schultz, M., et al. (1981, September). Endocrine parameters and alpha-tocopherol therapy of patients with mammary dysplasia. *Cancer Research, 41*(9, Part 2), 3811–3813.

Lorde, A. (1980). *The cancer journals.* Argyle, NY: Spinsters, Ink.

Lubin, F., Ron, E., & Wax, Y., et al. (1985, April 26). A case-control study of caffeine and methylxanthines in benign breast disease. *Journal of the American Medical Association, 253*(16), 2388–2392.

Lubin, F., Wax, Y, & Modan, B. (1986, September). Role of fat, animal protein, and dietary fiber in breast cancer etiology: A case-control study. *Journal of the National Cancer Institute, 77*(3), 605–612.

Lubin, J. H., Burns, P. E., & Blot, W. J., et al. (1981, December). Dietary factors and breast cancer risk. *International Journal of Cancer, 28*(6), 685–689.

Lynch, H. T., Albano, W. A., & Heieck, J. J., et al. (1984, September). Genetics, Biomarkers, and Control of breast cancer: A review. *Cancer Genetics and Cytogenetics, 13*(1), 43–92.

MacKenzie, I. (1965). Breast cancer following multiple fluoroscopies. *British Journal of Cancer, 19*(1), 1–8.

MacMahon, B., Cole, P., & Brown, J. (1973, January). Etiology of human breast cancer: A review. *Journal of the National Cancer Institute, 50*(1), 21–42.

Mansel, R. E. (1986, June 30). Benign breast disease and cancer risk: New perspectives. *Annals of the New York Academy of Sciences, 464*, 364–366.

Mansel, R. E., Wisbey, J. R., & Hughes, L. E. (1982, April 24). Controlled trial of the antigonadotropin danazol in painful nodular benign breast disease. *Lancet, 1*(8278), 928–930.

Marchant, D. J. (1982, June). History, physical examination, and breast self-examination. *Clinical Obstetrics and Gynecology, 25*(2), 359–363.

Margin-Comin, J., Pujol-Amat, P., & Cararach, V., et al. (1976, December). Treatment of fibrocystic disease of the breast with a prolactin inhibitor: 2-Br-alpha ergocryptine (CB-154). *Obstetrics and Gynecology, 48*(6), 703–706.

Marty, P. J., McDermott, R. J., & Gold, R. S. (1983). An assessment of three alternative formats for promoting breast self-examination. *Cancer Nursing, 6*(3), 207–211.

Massey, V. (1986, May/June). Perceived susceptibility to breast cancer and practice of breast self-examination. *Nursing Research, 35*(3), 183–185.

Mast, M. (1984, February). Primary care of the mastectomy patient. *Nurse Practitioner, 9*(2), 27–34, 78.

McCarty, K. S., Glaubitz, L. C., Thienemann, M., & Riefkohl, R. (1983). The breast: Anatomy and physiology. In N. G. Georgiade, (Ed.), *Aesthetic breast surgery.* Baltimore: Williams & Wilkins.

McGregor, D. H., Land, C. E., & Choi, K., et al. (1977, September). Breast cancer incidence among atomic bomb survivors, Hiroshima and Nagasaki, 1950–69. *Journal of the National Cancer Institute, 59*(3), 799–811.

McTiernan, A., & Thomas, D. B. (1986, September). Evidence for a protective effect of lactation on risk of breast cancer in young women. *American Journal of Epidemiology, 124*(3), 353–358.

Mettler, F. A., Hempelmann, L. H., & Dutton, A. M., et al. (1969, October). Breast neoplasms in women treated with X rays for acute postpartum mastitis. A pilot study. *Journal of the National Cancer Institute, 43*(4), 803–811.

Michalek, A. M., Walsh, D., Burns, P., & Mettlin, C. (1981, October). Report on a BSE educational program for lay audiences conducted by nurse health educators. *Cancer Nursing, 4*(5), 385–388.

Miller, A. B., Kelly, A., & Choi, N. W., el al. (1978, June). A study of diet and breast cancer. *American Journal of Epidemiology, 107*(6), 499–509.

Miller, D. R., Rosenberg, L., & Kaufman, D. W., et al. (1989, February). Breast cancer before age 45 and oral contraceptive use: New findings. *American Journal of Epidemiology, 129*(2), 269–280.

Minton, J. P., Abou-Issa, H., Reiches, N., & Roseman, J. M. (1981, August). Clinical and biochemical studies on methylxanthine-related fibrocystic breast disease. *Surgery, 90*(2), 299–304.

Minton, J. P., Foecking, M. K., Webster, D. J. T., & Matthews, R. H. (1979, September 1). Response of fibrocystic disease to caffeine withdrawal and correlation of cyclic nucleotides with breast disease. *American Journal of Obstetrics and Gynecology, 135*(1), 157–158.

Moore, D. H., Moore, D. H., II, & Moore, C. T. (1983). Breast carcinoma etiological factors. *Advances in Cancer Research, 40*, 189–253.

Morehead, J. R. (1982, June). Anatomy and embryology of the breast. *Clinical Obstetrics and Gynecology, 25*(2), 353–357.

Morris, T. (1983, December). Psychosocial aspects of breast cancer: A review. *European Journal of Cancer and Clinical Oncology, 19*(12), 1725–1733.

Myrden, J. A., & Hiltz, J. E. (1969, June 14). Breast cancer following multiple fluoroscopies during artificial pneumothorax treatment of pulmonary tuberculosis. *Canadian Medical Association Journal, 100*(22), 1032–1034.

Nezhat, C., Asch, R. H., & Greenblatt, R. B. (1980, July 1). Danazol for benign breast disease. *American Journal of Obstetrics and Gynecology, 137*(5), 604–607.

Nichols, S. (1983, March). Reluctance to seek medical advice about breast symptoms. *Journal of the Royal College of General Practitioners, 33*(248), 163–166.

Noone, R. B., Frazier T. G., & Hayward, C. Z., et al. (1982, April). Patient acceptance of immediate reconstruction following mastectomy. *Plastic and Reconstructive Surgery, 69*(4), 632–638.

Northouse, L. L., & Swain, M. A. (1987, July/August). Adjustment of patients and husbands to the initial impact of breast cancer. *Nursing Research, 36*(4), 221–225.

O'Grady, L. (1986). Breast. In C. Havens, N. D. Sullivan, & P. Tilton (Eds.), *Manual of outpatient gynecology,* Boston: Little, Brown.

Page, D. L., Vander Zwaag, R., & Rogers, L. W., et al. (1978, October). Relation between component parts of fibrocystic disease complex and breast cancer. *Journal of the National Cancer Institute, 61*(4), 1055–1062.

Papatestas, A. E., Panvelliwalla, D., & Tartter, P. I., et al. (1982, March 15). Fecal steroid metabolites and breast cancer risk. *Cancer, 49*(6):1201–1205.

Rennie, S., Stallmeyer, J., & Orloff, T. (no date). *The diet your doctor won't give you.* Washington, DC: The National Women's Health Network. [pamphlet].

Reynolds, S. A., Sachs, S. H., Davis, J. M., & Hall, P. (1981, June). Meeting the information needs of patients on clinical trials: A new approach. *Cancer Nursing, 4*(3), 227–230.

Ricciardi, I., & Ianniruberto, A. (1979, July). Tamoxifen-induced regression of benign breast lesions. *Obstetrics and Gynecology, 54*(1), 80–84.

Riddle, L. B. (1986a, March). Augmentation mammaplasty. *Nurse Practitioner, 11*(3), 30–40.

Riddle, L. B. (1986b, December). Expansion exercises: Modifying contracture of the augmented breast. *Research in Nursing and Health, 9*(4), 341–345.

Rissanen, P. M. (1969, June). A comparison of conservative and radical surgery combined with radiotherapy in the treatment of stage I carcinoma of the breast. *British Journal of Radiology, 42*(498), 423–426.

Roberts, H. J. (1981, July 10). Perspective on vitamin E as therapy. *Journal of the American Medical Association, 246*(2), 129–131.

Rosen, P. P. (1984). Lobular carcinoma in situ and intraductal carcinoma of the breast. *Monographs of Pathology, 25,* 59–105.

Ross, R K., Paganini-Hill, A., & Gerkins, V. R., et al. (1980, April 25). A case-control study of menopausal estrogen therapy and breast cancer. *Journal of the American Medical Association, 243*(16), 1635–1639.

Rubin, G., Layde, P. M., & Peterson, H. B. (1984, July). Is this study valid? A closer look at the OC–breast Ca data. *Contemporary Ob/Gyn. 24*(1), 171–176.

Rudolph, A., & McDermott, R. J.(1987, April). The breast physical examination. *Cancer Nursing, 10*(2), 100–106.

Rush, B. F. (1984). Breast. In S. I. Schwartz, (Ed.), *Principles of surgery* (4th ed.). New York: McGraw–Hill.

Rutledge, D. N. (1982, December). Nurses' knowledge of breast reconstruction: A catalyst for earlier treatment of breast cancer? *Cancer Nursing, 5*(6), 469–474.

Rutledge, D. N. (1987, March/April). Factors related to women's practice of breast self-examination. *Nursing Research, 36*(2), 117–121.

Schatzkin, A., Jones, D. Y., & Hoover, R. N., et al. (1987, May 7). Alcohol consumption and breast cancer in the epidemiologic follow-up study of the First National Health and Nutrition Examination Survey. *New England Journal of Medicine, 316*(19), 1169–1173.

Schindler, A. E., Ebert, A., & Friedrich, E. (1972, October). Conversion of androstenedione to estrone by human fat tissue. *Journal of Clinical Endocrinology and Metabolism, 35*(4), 627–630.

Schwartz, G. F. (1982, June). Benign neoplasms and "Inflammations" of the Breast. *Clinical Obstetrics and Gynecology, 25*(2), 373–385.

Seidman, H., Gelb, S. K., & Silverberg, E., et al. (1987, September). Survival experience in The Breast Cancer Detection Demonstration Project. *Ca—A Cancer Journal for Clinicians, 37*(5), 258–290.

Setchell, K. D. R., Borriello, S. P., & Hulme, P., et al. (1984, September). Nonsteroidal estrogens of dietary origin: Possible roles in hormone-dependent disease. *The American Journal of Clinical Nutrition, 40*(3), 569–578.

Shaabon, M. M., Movad, F., & Hassan, A. R. (1980). Treatment of fibrocystic mastopathy by an antiestrogen, Tamoxifen. *International Journal of Gynaecology and Obstetrics. 18*(5), 348–350.

Shore, R. E. Hempelmann, L. H., & Kowaluk, E., et al. (1977, September). Breast neoplasms in women treated with x-rays for acute postpartum mastitis. *Journal of the National Cancer Institute, 59*(3), 813–822.

Siiteri, P. K., Schwartz, B. E., & MacDonald, P. C. (1974, August). Estrogen receptors and the estrone hypothesis in relation to endometrial and breast cancer. *Gynecologic Oncology, 2*(2/3), 228–238.

Skrabanek, P. (1985, August 10). False premises and false promises of breast cancer screening. *Lancet, 2*(8450), 316–320.

Small, E. C. (1982, June). Psychosocial issues in breast disease. *Clinical Obstetrics and Gynecology, 25*(2), 447–454.

Snyderman, R. K. (1984, February 1). Prophylactic mastectomy: Pros and cons. *Cancer, 53*(3, Suppl.), 803–808.

Speroff, L. (1985, September). Why mammography is effective. *Contemporary Ob/Gyn, 26*(3), 183–190.

Stadel, V. B., Lai, S., Schlesselman, J. J., & Murray, P. (1988, September). Oral contraceptives and premenopausal breast cancer in nulliparous women. *Contraception, 38*(3), 287–299.

Stadel, B. V., & Schlesselman, J. L. (1986, March). Oral contraceptive use and the risk of breast cancer in women with "prior" history of benign breast disease. *American Journal of Epidemiology, 123*(13), 373–382.

Strax, P. (1984, February 1). Mass screening for control of breast cancer. *Cancer, 53*(3, Suppl.), 665–670.

Strombeck, J. O. (1986). Reduction mammaplasty. In J. O. Strombeck & F. E. Rosato (Eds.), *Surgery of the breast.* New York: Georg Thieme.

Sundaram, G. S., London, R., & Manimekalai, S., et al. (1981, April). Alpha-tocopherol and serum lipoproteins. *Lipids, 16*(4), 223–227.

Tabár, L., Fagerberg C. J. G., & Gad, A. et al. (1985, April 13). Reduction in mortality from breast cancer after mass screening with mammography. *Lancet, 1*(8433), 829–832.

Tapley, N. D., Spanos, W. J., Jr., & Fletcher, G. H., et al. (1982, March 15). Results in patients with breast cancer treated by radical mastectomy and postoperative irradiation with no adjuvant chemotherapy. *Cancer, 49*(6), 1316–1319.

Thomas, D. B. (1983, April). Factors that promote the development of human breast cancer. *Environmental Health Perspectives, 50,* 209–218.

Thomsen, A. C., Espersen, T., & Maigaard, S. (1984, July 1). Course and treatment of milk stasis, noninfectious inflammation of the breast, and infectious mastitis in nursing women. *American Journal of Obstetrics and Gynecology, 149*(5), 492–495.

Tokunaga, M., Land, C. E., & Yamamoto, T., et al. (1982, October 23). Breast cancer in Japanese A-bomb survivors [Letter]. *Lancet, 2*(8304), 924.

Townsend, C. M. (1980). Breast lumps. *Clinical Symposia, 32*(2),

Trapido, E. J. (1981, November). A prospective cohort study of oral contraceptives and breast cancer. *Journal of the National Cancer Institute, 67*(5), 1011–1015.

USDHHS (U.S. Department of Health and Human Services). (1984, April). *The breast cancer digest* (2nd ed.), NIH Publication 84-1691, Bethesda, MD: National Cancer Institute.

Valanis, B. G., & Rumpler, C. H. (1985, June). Helping women to choose breast cancer treatment alternatives. *Cancer Nursing, 8*(3), 167–175.

Varney, H. (1987). *Nurse-midwifery* (2nd ed.). Boston: Blackwell Scientific.

Verbeek, A. L. M., Hendriks, J. H. C. L., & Holland, R., et al. (1984, June 2). Reduction of breast cancer mortality through mass screening with modern mammography. *Lancet, 1*(8388), 1222–1224.

Veronesi, U., Saccozzi, R., & Del Vecchio, M., et al. (1981, July 2). Comparing radical mastectomy with quadrantectomy, axillary dissection, and radiotherapy in patients with small cancers of the breast. *New England Journal of Medicine, 305*(1), 6–11.

Vessey, M. P., McPherson, K., Yeates, D., & Doll, R. (1982, March). Oral contraceptive use and abortion before first term pregnancy in relation to breast cancer risk. *British Journal of Cancer, 45*(3), 327–331.

Waalkes, T. P., Enterline, J. H., & Shaper, J. H., et al. (1984, February). Biological markers for breast carcinoma. *Cancer, 53*(3, Suppl.), 644–651.

Wanebo, C. K., Johnson, K. G., Sato, K, & Thorslund, T. W. (1968, September 26). Breast cancer after exposure to the atomic bombings of Hiroshima and Nagasaki. *New England Journal of Medicine, 279*(13), 667–671.

Warren, B. (1979, February). Adjuvant chemotherapy for breast disease: The nurse's role. *Cancer Nursing, 2*(1), 32–37.

Webber, W., & Boyd, N. (1986, August). A critique of the methodology of studies of benign breast disease and breast cancer risk. *Journal of the National Cancer Institute, 77*(2), 397–404.

Welch, D. A. (1980, July-August). Spinal metastases from carcinoma of the breast. *Nurse Practitioner, 5*(4), 8–10.

White, E. (1987, April). Projected changes in breast cancer incidence due to the trend toward delayed childbearing. *American Journal of Public Health, 77*(4), 495–497.

Willett, W. C., Stampfer, M. J., & Colditz, G. A., et al. (1987a, January 1). Dietary fat and the risk of breast cancer. *New England Journal of Medicine, 316*(1), 22–28.

Willett, W. C., Stampfer, M. J., & Colditz, G. A., et al. (1987b, May 7). Moderate alcohol consumption and the risk of breast cancer. *New England Journal of Medicine, 316*(19), 1174–1180.

Wilson, R. E. (1986). The breast. In D. C. Sabiston, Jr. (Ed.), *Davis-Christopher textbook of surgery* (13th ed., Vol. I). Philadelphia: W. B. Saunders.

Wissing, V. S. (1984, September). Breast cancer. The hormone factor. *American Journal of Nursing, 84*(9), 1117–1119.

Wynder, E., & Cohen, L. A. (1982). A rationale for dietary intervention in the treatment of postmenopausal breast cancer patients. *Nutrition and Cancer, 3*(4), 195–199.

11

The Vulva and Vagina

Ronnie Lichtman and Paula Duran

Problems associated with the lower genital tract—the vulva and the vagina—are a large focus of well-woman gynecologic practice. Such disorders range from mild skin or mucous membrane lesions or vaginitis to serious diseases. Clinical manifestations range from local discomfort to systemic involvement and sequelae. The practitioner of well-woman gynecology must be familiar with the variety of illnesses presenting as lower genital tract lesions and develop the clinical expertise to diagnose these conditions accurately, assess the need for treatment, consultation, or referral, and provide complete teaching and counseling regarding both primary and secondary prevention.

This chapter describes and discusses the management of selected vulvar and vaginal diseases. These include some sexually transmitted diseases (STDs); however, the discussion in this chapter is limited to those disorders that tend to affect only the vulva and the vagina. Many sexually transmitted organisms, although they enter the body through the vagina, may manifest themselves as cervical, uterine, tubal, multiorgan, and systemic disorders. These are covered in Chapter 12 or in the appropriate chapter.

The chapter begins with a discussion of the general approach to the diagnosis of vulvar and vaginal disorders and the role of the primary care provider. Because of the multitude of problems that may exist in the lower genital tract, this approach must be kept in mind throughout all subsequent sections.

FRAMEWORK FOR MANAGEMENT OF VULVAR AND VAGINAL PROBLEMS

The discussion of vulvar and vaginal pathology that follows is based on each distinct diagnostic entity. Women, however, do not present with diagnoses; they present with a symptom or symptoms, a physical finding or findings on examination, or a history of exposure to an organism, defined or undefined. From the historical and clinical picture presented, the practitioner must be able to construct a differential diagnosis, complete the historic database, perform appropriate parts of a physical assessment, and obtain or order diagnostic laboratory tests. She must also determine her ability to make a final diagnosis and, if necessary, treat the presenting disorder. She must be able to provide appropriate referrals when diagnosis is beyond her expertise or treatment requires techniques or the provision of medications outside her legal or ethical scope of practice.

Data Collection

Historic Data. Vulvar and vaginal disorders commonly present with vaginal discharge; pruritis; odor, pain or discomfort including local burning, stinging, pressure, cramping, dysuria, or dyspareunia; or spotting. A woman may complain of a blister, bump, lump, or lesion on the external genitalia. The practitioner must be familiar with the wide range of possible causes of each symptom and be able to correlate symptoms with diagnoses. We refer readers to Appendix III, Parts A and B, for an outline of diagnoses that present with vaginal discharge or pelvic pain. Chapter 2 provides a series of questions that ensure establishment of a complete database when patients present with pain or bleeding. Chapter 2 also reviews the components of a complete history; elements of the menstrual, gynecologic, sexual, contraceptive, obstetric, medical, and family histories provide clues to the appropriate diagnosis. The history often narrows the diagnostic possibilities and, in many cases, focuses on the specific disorder.

Physical Examination. Until the physical examination is complete, the practitioner should maintain openness to diagnostic possibilities. What sounds, from history, like one disorder may, on inspection, appear to be something quite different. Careful visualization, including a speculum examination, thorough palpation of the inguinal area and all pelvic organs, milking of the urethra for secretions, and assessment of odor of vaginal secretions, is essential to the diagnostic workup. Chapter 3 describes techniques of assessment. Inspection of other body parts also may provide clues to diagnosis. The vulva is part of the skin; both dermatologic and systemic diseases may manifest themselves there. Lesions occurring elsewhere on the body may lead the practitioner to suspect a nongynecologic diagnosis and clarify the need for medical referral.

Laboratory Testing. Although history and physical examination often point to a diagnosis, this must be confirmed by laboratory testing. Not all disorders present at all times with classic signs and symptoms. Or, more than one infectious agent may be present; this could easily be missed by relying only on historic and physical examination data. The practitioner must know when to use and how to obtain and interpret a Pap smear, vaginal pH testing, a wet mount, the whiff test, serologic or antibody testing, urinalysis, and vaginal, rectal, urine, and oral cultures and sensitivities.

Chapter 4 provides a detailed discussion of these various tests including instructions on their performance.

Intervention

Treatment and Consultation. Whenever doubt exists regarding diagnosis or whenever treatment lies outside the realm of expertise of the primary care practitioner, consultation or referral should be implemented without hesitation. Consultants or sources of referral must include not only gynecologists but dermatologists, infectious disease specialists, venereal disease (VD) or sexually transmitted disease (STD) clinics, as well as support groups, therapists, and counselors who can help women cope with the psychological consequences of certain disorders.

The necessity for consultation depends on a number of factors including clinic or practice protocols providing for standing orders for nonphysician's prescribing or dispensing of medications; state law governing prescription-writing privileges and the formulary of medications included in such privileges; experience of the practitioner; the seriousness or associated complications of the presenting condition; and whether the condition is recurrent or persistent. Practitioners must consult individual state statutes or regulations and protocols within their practice setting for clarification of their rights regarding treatment.

The following sections outline standard treatments, relying, where available, on recommendations of the Centers for Disease Control (CDC). They also outline, whenever possible, self-help preventive and curative measures. In some cases, scientific evidence for these remedies is lacking. As long as the measures are not deemed to be harmful, however, they may be implemented; many women find them useful and more acceptable than medical therapies.

Medication regimens recommended in this chapter generally apply to nonpregnant, nonnursing women. For medication regimens acceptable in pregnancy and during lactation, consult an obstetrics or other specialized text.

Teaching and Counseling. Teaching and counseling must be specific to the disorder presented; however, certain overall guidelines apply in most situations. All teaching and counseling must be provided in a sensitive manner, with recognition that problems involving the vulva and vagina often have emotional consequences. They affect body image and sexuality; they affect important, intimate relationships. Diagnoses or diagnostic possibilities must be fully shared with each woman; she must understand the cause or possible causes of her problem and participate in decision making regarding treatment.

Complete and careful instructions about medication usage must be provided, in writing if necessary, and every effort made to ensure and assess each woman's understanding of prescribed medication regimens. Side effects, risks, and benefits of the treatment must be supplied. Advantages and disadvantages of treatment itself must be discussed, particularly with asymptomatic disease. Women must understand that once a treatment regimen is initiated, it should be completed as prescribed, even if symptoms abate. Follow-up for a test of cure should be offered, especially in the case of asymptomatic infections, and a thorough explanation of symptoms that indicate persistence or recurrence should be given. Treatment of possible resistant or recurrent conditions should not, however, be provided without seeing the woman and completely reevaluating her problem. What appears to be treatment failure or reinfection may actually be an untreated coexisting problem or a reaction to the medication used.

THE VULVA

The vulva is composed of skin of ectodermal origin. It is also a sexual organ. It is, therefore, subject to skin diseases and to STDs.

In this section a number of vulvar disorders are discussed. These discussions are not intended to provide the primary care practitioner with the ability to diagnose or treat these disorders. Their intent is rather to acquaint the provider with the great variety of inflammatory, noninflammatory, traumatic, neoplastic, and systemic lesions of the vulva and alert her to the need for consultation whenever diagnosis is in doubt or the presenting condition has serious potential. For detailed information on these disorders, the reader is referred to a more specialized textbook such as that by Gardner and Kaufman (1981).

Developmental Abnormalities of the Vulva and External Genitalia

Developmental abnormalities of the vulva and external genitalia are rare. They include *clitoral hypoplasia* or *hypertrophy, vulvar hypoplasia, labial fusion,* and *hypertrophy of the labia minora.* Chromosomal abnormalities including *true hermaphroditism* and *pseudohermaphroditism, androgen insensitivity syndrome,* and *gonadal dysgenesis* can also lead to abnormalities of vulvar structures. Abnormalities of the urinary system may be noted and include *ectopic urethral orifices, episadias, ectopic anus,* and a *high rectovaginal fistula* (Malinak & Franklin, 1981). The primary care practitioner should be aware of these deviations even though they are encountered rarely. Referral for genetic workup and possible medical or surgical treatment is warranted.

Vulvitis

Vulvitis is an inflammation of the vulva. Vulvitis may result from sexually transmitted organisms, discussed in Chapter 12, or other infectious organisms. The vulva may also be subject to a number of noninfectious conditions. These include *contact dermatitis, intertrigo* and *seborrheic dermatitis, psoriasis, vulvodynia,* and *focal vulvitis.* Inflammation may also be secondary to systemic disease with vulvar manifestation.

Contact Dermatitis. Contact dermatitis (Figure 11–1) is a common benign disorder of the external genitalia. Formerly called eczema, the name *contact dermatitis* reflects the causality of this disorder: local irritants (Woodruff, 1986). Such irritants include tight, nonabsorbent underwear or the detergents or bleach in which they are washed, aerosol sprays, bath oils and bubble bath, toilet paper dye, perfumed soaps and powders, and vulvar deodorants.

Contact dermatitis presents with pruritis and a rash. The rash may be vesicular or blisterlike.

Contact dermatitis must be differentiated from other vulvar lesions, described in this section, from various types of vulvovaginitis discussed later in the chapter, and from sexually transmitted diseases with vulvar manifestations, discussed in Chapter 12.

A thorough history can often reveal possible irritants. A recent change in habits in vulvar hygiene often precedes the appearance of dermatitis and helps identify the cause.

Through physical examination, the practitioner can locate the extent of the lesion, describe its appearance, and assess associated signs that may exclude this diagnosis.

Laboratory testing is done to exclude specific organ-

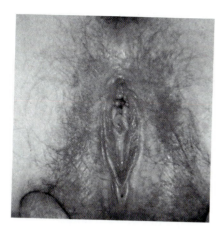

Figure 11–1. Acute dermatitis: Erythema of the external genitalia. *(From Woodruff, J. D. [1985]. Noninfectious diseases of the vulva. In D. H. Nichols & J. R. Evrard [Eds.], Ambulatory gynecology. Philadelphia: Harper & Row. Reprinted with permission.)*

isms. A patch test may help determine whether a woman is sensitive or allergic to a particular agent. The agent can be applied to the skin surface—usually the back or forearm—and an adhesive bandage placed over it for 48 to 72 hours (Gardner, 1981b); however, a positive reaction may not be seen on skin as it is not damp like the vulva.

Diagnosis involves an attempt to pinpoint the offending irritant. This is done by exclusion, through history, physical examination, and laboratory tests, of other vulvar or vulvovaginal lesions. The woman herself must eliminate possible irritants one by one until she is free of the dermatitis. Consultation with a dermatologist or allergist may be necessary for diagnosis. This should be undertaken when all gynecologic diagnoses have been ruled out.

The best treatment for contact dermatitis is elimination of the offending organism. Local hydrocortisone ointments can be used for symptomatic relief. These should be used sparingly and in low strengths, 0.1 to 0.25 percent. Such ointments can be purchased over-the-counter at most pharmacies. Women should be advised against prolonged usage, which can cause systemic reaction or local fibrosis (Woodruff, 1986).

Avoiding the use of soap on the vulva may bring some relief. Women should be warned against using vulvar or vaginal deodorants and perfumes. Extra rinsing of clothing may help in removing perfumes and fabric softeners used in detergents (Pincus & Stadecker, 1987, p. 19). Cotton underwear washed in mild detergent without bleaching is least likely to cause problems.

Intertrigo and Seborrheic Dermatitis. Intertrigo or seborrheic dermatitis is dandruff of the vulva. In its extreme form, it manifests as thickening and cracking of the crural and intralabial skin folds (Woodruff, 1985). It is commonly seen in diabetic women. Diagnosis consists of identification of this risk factor and the elimination of other causes for the lesion. Treatment is local and includes dusting with cornstarch to absorb moisture and topical application of low-strength hydrocortisone cream for pruritis (Woodruff, 1986).

Psoriasis. Although psoriasis classically is characterized by silver scabs and redness with excoriation of the skin, vulvar psoriasis is not a scaly lesion. It appears as an erythematous patch. Diagnosis is made by examination of the

rest of the body, revealing classic lesions of psoriasis, and exclusion of other vulvar diagnoses. A family history may be a clue, as this disorder tends to be familial (Pincus & Stadecker, 1987, p. 20). Treatment is best managed by a dermatologist.

Vulvodynia/Burning Vulva Syndrome. The term *vulvodynia* was proposed at a 1983 Congress of the International Society for the Study of Vulvar Disease to refer to chronic vulvar discomfort, especially of a burning (or stinging, irritating, or raw) nature. It may have a number of causes. The *burning vulva syndrome* (BVS) was defined at that Congress as vulvodynia that has no known physical cause and is resistant to usual treatments (McKay, 1985).

Vulvodynia and BVS present with a subjective complaint, most often without physical findings, except, at times, sensitivity of the vulva to touch. Findings differ from those in chronic pruritus with no known cause because excoriation, erythema, and edema are absent. Organisms responsible for vulvovaginitis are not present.

Diagnosis of these conditions must be made by exclusion. Treatment consists of reassurance and counseling on vulvar hygiene, including wiping from front to back and avoiding strong soaps or vigorous scrubbing of the area. Local anesthetics may be helpful; compresses of cool milk, Crisco shortening, or oil may help with dry skin. Topical low-dose hydrocortisone cream can be applied. Biofeedback has shown some success in alleviating symptoms. With time, the symptoms often subside (McKay, 1985). Dermatologic consultation may be appropriate once gynecologic pathology is ruled out and before a final diagnosis is made.

Focal Vulvitis. Focal vulvitis is a syndrome of unknown etiology characterized by superficial dyspareunia with one or more tiny, tender areas of inflammation or ulceration of the mucosa of the vestibule (Peckham, Maki, Patterson, & Hafez, 1986). Most lesions in this syndrome appear around Bartholin's ducts or between them posteriorly. Onset can be gradual or sudden during sexual intercourse. Diagnosis is made by exclusion of other causes for the disorder, including vaginitis and identifiable dermatologic conditions.

Approximately one half of women with these lesions undergo spontaneous remission. Local treatment with lidocaine (Xylocaine) ointment applied directly to the lesions by the woman using a mirror or by her partner can afford temporary relief, allowing for comfortable sexual intercourse. Peckham and associates (1986, p. 864) report relief with surgical excision of the hymenal ring and contiguous mucosa of the vestibule. They reserve surgery, however, for women with "unremitting dyspareunia of unknown cause associated with the characteristic focal inflammatory lesions for at least six months." Because of the relationship of focal vulvitis to sexual intercourse and because treatment is often palliative, not curative, women with this disorder require much caring support.

Other Inflammatory Vulvar Lesions. Other inflammatory lesions of the vulva may be caused by staphylococci, hemolytic streptococci, and anaerobic bacteria. Infections can occur in hair follicles, apocrine glands, or the epiclitoral regions. Pyogenic ulcers such as impetigo can occur, and tissue glands can become infected as in erysipelas and cellulitis (Kaufman & Faro, 1987, pp. 280–281).

Risk factors for infection of the vulva include obesity, sweating, malnutrition, diabetes, seborrhea, scabies, and pediculosis (see Chapter 12).

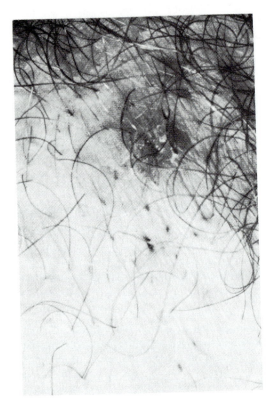

Figure 11–2. Folliculitis: Single, erythematous, raised lesion. *(From Gardner, H. L., [1981]. Pyodermas of the vulva. In H. L. Gardner & R. H. Kaufman [Eds.], Benign diseases of the vulva and vagina [2nd ed.]. Boston: G. K. Hall Medical Publishers. Reprinted with permission.)*

Folliculitis is caused by staphylococcal invasion of the sebaceous ducts and hair follicles (Figure 11–2). A *furuncle* occurs when the infection spreads and causes localized cellulitis (Figure 11–3). Furuncles are often referred to as "boils" (Kaufman & Faro, 1987, p. 282). A *carbuncle* results when several follicles in close association are infected (Figure 11–4). Symptoms include pain, tenderness, and lymphadenitis. Spontaneous healing usually occurs.

Periclitoral abscesses have no known cause. Their onset is acute with severe pain, edema, and inguinal adenopathy. After several days, the abscess points (Kaufman & Faro, 1987, p. 283).

Infection of apocrine glands is called *hidradenitis suppurativa* (Figure 11–5). Initially, this appears as multiple nodules in the skin. Staphylococci or streptococci are often involved in this infection. The lesions form abscesses that rupture with purulent and foul-smelling discharge. Infection may become widespread, involving the entire vulva (Kaufman & Faro, 1987, pp. 283–284). Spontaneous resolution may lead to scarring and induration.

Impetigo contagiosum, a contagious disorder seen mostly in children, is caused by bacterial invasion of the skin secondary to mosquito bites and scratching. It presents initially as a superficial vesicle and then becomes a pustule. Spontaneous rupture leaves a crusted over superficial ulcer (Kaufman & Faro, 1987, p. 285).

Erysipelas results from trauma and spreads rapidly in the lymph system. It presents with a well-defined, erythematous, tender lesion and chills, fever, and malaise. Systemic antibiotic therapy is required.

Cellulitis of the vulva occurs secondary to surgical procedures. It presents with swelling, tenderness, and erythema around the wound. Pain and low-grade fever are usually present. Spontaneous drainage may occur (Kaufman & Faro, 1987, p. 286).

Candida may be noted on the vulva, although it is usually associated with vaginal infection. (See The Vagina.)

Tinea cruris (Figure 11–6), a fungal infection, is usually associated with lesions on other parts of the body, including the adjacent skin surfaces. These lesions are slightly elevated and sharply marginated. Diagnosis is made by examining scrapings of the lesions under the microscope, showing hyphae characteristic of fungi. Clotrimazole (Lotrimin), miconazole nitrate (Monistat), and tolnaftate (Tinactin) are effective as local treatment (see Candidiasis).

Other Dermatologic Diseases. Dermatologic disorders occurring anywhere on the body may at times affect the vulva. Such disorders include *bullous pemphigoid, pemphigus, dermatitis herpetiformis,* and *erythema multiforme.* These diseases generally present with blisters, although vulvar blisters often rupture and instead leave an excoriated area. They may be confused with herpes genitalis. Physical

Figure 11–3. A draining furuncle. *(From Gardner, H. L. [1981]. Pyodermas of the vulva. In H. L. Gardner & R. H. Kaufman [Eds.], Benign diseases of the vulva and vagina [2nd ed.]. Boston: G. K. Hall Medical Publishers. Reprinted with permission.)*

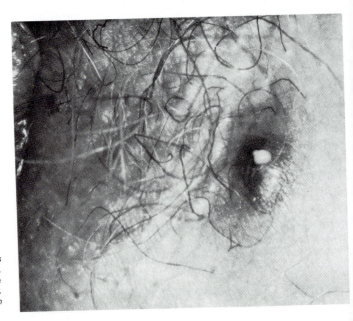

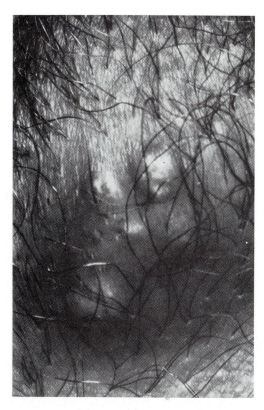

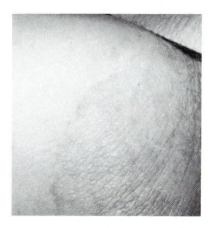

Figure 11–6. Tinea cruris. *(From Woodruff, J. D. [1985]. Noninfectious diseases of the vulva. In D. H. Nichols & J. R. Evrard [Eds.], Ambulatory gynecology. Philadelphia: Harper & Row. Reprinted with permission.)*

Systemic Disease with Vulvar Manifestations. Woodruff (1985) estimates that 25 percent of women with *Crohn's disease* have perineal involvement. Usual manifestations include fistulas or draining sinuses in the perineum or vaginal outlet or linear excoriations in these areas with lymphedema. An autoimmune disease, *Behçet's disease*, may lead to vulvar and perineal ulcerations with similar ulcers on the oral mucous membranes. *Iritis*, which can become a total neurologic disease, may also manifest itself with vulvar ulcerations. The practitioner must appreciate the fact that whenever persistent lesions of the vulva cannot be diagnosed as a common gynecologic disease or STD, referral for further medical workup is required.

Nonneoplastic White Lesions of the Vulva

Leukoplakia, a commonly known term for white patches on the vulva, is generally not used today and has been replaced by the term *dystrophy*. Dystrophic lesions fall into two categories: *hyperplastic dystrophy*, also known as *hyperkeratosis*, and *lichen sclerosus*.

The characteristics of dystrophic lesions are "a keratin layer of varying thickness (accounting for the white or grayish-white color), an abnormal thinning or thickening of the epithelial layer, an underlying chronic inflammatory infiltrate, and varying degrees of change in the subepithelial connective tissue" (Woodruff, 1986, p. 1018).

Hyperkeratosis (also called hyperplastic dystrophy) is the increased deposition of keratin, often occurring with inflammation or irritation. The deposition of keratin occurs as a protective response to the original irritative lesion. It appears as a white or grayish-white area. Excoriation and fissures may be seen secondary to scratching. Local corticosteroid therapy is usually prescribed for this lesion.

Lichen sclerosus (Figure 11–7) is a patchy white change in the labia. It is often called *lichen sclerosus et atrophicus*. Although lichen sclerosus can appear at any age, it is most common in midlife. Asymptomatic in its early stage, in the postmenopausal woman lichen sclerosus may cause severe pruritus and even lead to malignancy. The cause of the disorder is unknown but a hereditary component may be involved (Friedrich & MacLaren, 1984). Trauma from the friction of clothing may contribute to disease onset (Friedrich, 1985b). Typical lesions are "flat, ivory, lightly erythematous, depressed, polygonal papules," with varying degrees of scaling (Pincus & Stadecker, 1987, p. 12). As disease advances, the papules may be less apparent and scratching

Figure 11–4. A carbuncle: Multiple lesions in close association. *(From Gardner, H. L., [1981]. Pyodermas of the vulva. In H. L. Gardner & R. H. Kaufman [Eds.], Benign diseases of the vulva and vagina [2nd ed.]. Boston: G. K. Hall Medical Publishers. Reprinted with permission.)*

examination reveals lesions on other parts of the body. Referral to a dermatologist for diagnosis (usually by biopsy) and treatment (usually with corticosteroids) is warranted (Stage, Humeniuk, & Easley, 1984).

Vulvar Parasites. Vulvar parasites are discussed in Chapter 12.

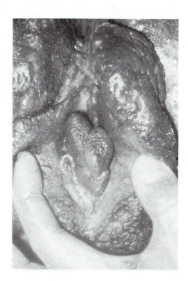

Figure 11–5. Hidradenitis supporativa: Infection of apocrine glands and distortion of the vulva. Draining sinuses identified by irregular and prominent gland swellings. *(From Woodruff, J. D. [1985]. Noninfectious diseases of the vulva. In D. H. Nichols & J. R. Evrard [Eds.], Ambulatory gynecology. Philadelphia: Harper & Row. Reprinted with permission.)*

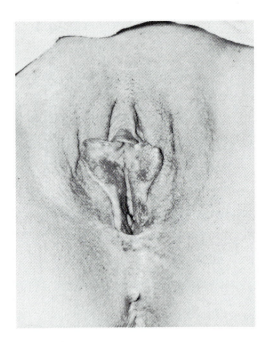

Figure 11–7. *Lichen sclerosus*: Whitish alterations on labia minora and at fourchette. *(From Woodruff, J. D. [1986]. Lesions of the vulva and vagina. In D. N. Danforth & J. R. Scott [Eds.], Obstetrics and gynecology (5th ed.). Philadelphia: J.B. Lippincott Company. Reprinted with permission.)*

may produce purpura or petechiae. Local edema may occur with induration, thickening, and firmness. Eventually, tissue atrophies and loss of the labia occurs. Diagnosis by biopsy and hormonal treatment with progesterone cream have been advocated (Pincus & Stadecker, 1987).

Leukoderma or *vitiligo* (Figure 11–8) is loss of vulvar pigmentation, often seen at puberty and associated with a similar loss of pigmentation on other parts of the body. The lesions are not significant and often transitory. Leukoderma may be associated with inflammation.

White lesions warrant referral for diagnosis by colposcopy and/or biopsy to rule out cellular atypia (Townsend, 1984; Woodruff, 1986, p. 1020).

Traumatic Vulvar Lesions

Traumatic lesions of the vulva and/or vagina include hematomas and lacerations. They may result from injury from a rigid structure such as a bicycle bar, foreign bodies inserted into the vagina, or sexual abuse. In addition to medical and possibly surgical treatment, evidence of sexual abuse requires reporting in the case of minors and referral for psychological assessment and treatment (see Chapter 26).

Vulvar Neoplasms

Vulvar neoplasms include solid and cystic lesions, malignant and nonmalignant.

Benign Solid Tumors. Solid tumors of the vulva include granular cell myoblastoma, lipoma, fibroma, hemangioma ("strawberry mark"), varicocele or other vascular lesions, hidradenoma, nevus, fibroepithelial polyp, endometrioma (associated with endometriosis), and granuloma.

The most common benign skin lesion of the vulva is the *hidradenoma* (Figure 11–9). This tumor occurs postmenarche and is superficial, well circumscribed, and movable. It may appear solid or cystic. It is most often solitary but may be multiple and is usually less than 2 cm in diameter. Generally appearing on the labia majora, the tumor may also involve the labia minora, skin around the labia, or perineum. Most are asymptomatic although they may be pruritic or ulcerate and bleed.

The *fibroepithelial polyp* is commonly referred to as a "skin tag" (Figure 11–10). It is a soft, skin-colored, wrinkled structure without hair, varying in size from a few millimeters to more than a centimeter (Kaufman, 1981b). It may become swollen, ecchymotic, or ulcerated.

Usually women with tumors present with a lump or bump. History taking should include the duration the pa-

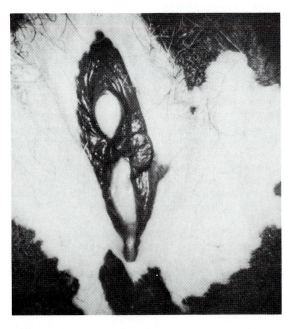

Figure 11–8. Vitiligo. *From Woodruff, J. D. [1986]. Lesions of the vulva and vagina. In D. N. Danforth & J. R. Scott [Eds.], Obstetrics and gynecology [5th ed.]. Philadelphia: J. B. Lippincott Company.*

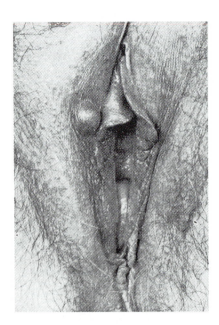

Figure 11–9. Hidradenoma. *From Woodruff, J. D. [1986]. Lesions of the vulva and vagina. In D. N. Danforth & J. R. Scott [Eds.], Obstetrics and gynecology [5th ed.]. Philadelphia, J. B. Lippincott Company.*

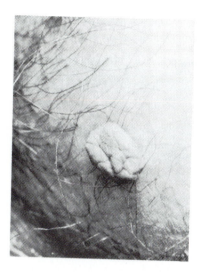

Figure 11–10. Skin tag. *(From Kaufman, R. H. [1981]. Cystic tumors. In H. L. Gardner & R. H. Kaufman [Eds.], Benign diseases of the vulva and vagina [2nd ed.]. Boston: G. K. Hall Medical Publishers. Reprinted with permission.)*

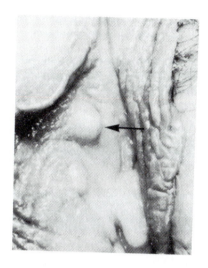

Figure 11–12. Mucous cyst. *(From Kaufman, R. H. [1981]. Cystic tumors. In H. L. Gardner & R. H. Kaufman [Eds.], Benign diseases of the vulva and vagina. [2nd ed.]. Boston: G. K. Hall Medical Publishers. Reprinted with permission.)*

tient has had the lump, any changes it has undergone, and associated symptoms such as pain. Any firm, noncystic lesion requires referral for biopsy for appropriate diagnosis. Some authors advocate colposcopic examination of lesions such as nevi or any neoplasm (Townsend, 1984). The pigmented nevus may develop into malignant melanoma (Kaufman, 1981b).

Cystic Lesions. Cystic lesions are commonly seen. These include inclusion cysts, mucous cysts, hydroceles or cysts of the canal of Nuck, and Bartholin's duct cysts or abscesses. These often need no treatment other than reassurance or local therapy and may be managed by the knowledgeable primary care provider.

EPIDERMAL INCLUSION CYSTS. Epidermal inclusion cysts (Figure 11–11) were previously called sebaceous cysts, because pressure on the cyst often produces discharge of an oillike material. This exudate actually consists of desquamated epithelial cells. Inclusion cysts commonly appear as multiple subcutaneous nodules on the vulva. They may be related to trauma, most commonly repair of a vaginal laceration or episiotomy, secondary to entrapment of fragments of mucosa at the repair site (Kaufman, 1981a). Inclusion cysts

need to be excised or drained if they are infected or irritating but ordinarily require no treatment.

MUCOUS CYSTS. Mucous cysts are seen on the inner surfaces of the labia minora at the introitus or in the vagina behind the hymenal ring (Figure 11–12). They are usually blocked minor glands of the vestibule. The cysts are typically single but may occasionally be multiple, and are generally small but range from 2 to 30 mm in diameter. They may be pedunculated and may be painful (Michael & Roth, 1987). Treatment, if necessary, consists of excision.

HYDROCELES/CYSTS OF THE CANAL OF NUCK. Hydroceles or cysts of the canal of Nuck (Figure 11–13) appear in the labia majora near the inguinal area or midvulva. They may be 1 cm or larger and rarely are symptomatic (Kaufman, 1981a). These must be differentiated from a hernia, which involves the bowel. If they are cosmetically unacceptable to the woman or cause discomfort, they can be removed surgically.

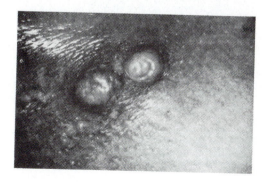

Figure 11–11. Epidermal inclusion cysts. *(From Woodruff, J. D. [1985]. Noninfectious diseases of the vulva. In D. H. Nichols & J. R. Evrard [Eds.], Ambulatory gynecology. Philadelphia: Harper & Row. Reprinted with permission.)*

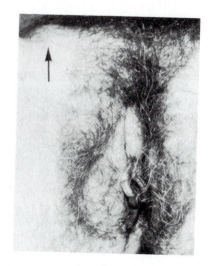

Figure 11–13. Cyst of the canal of Nuck (hydrocele) in right inguinal region. *(From Kaufman, R. H. [1981]. Cystic tumors. In H. L. Gardner & R. H. Kaufman [Eds.], Benign diseases of the vulva and vagina. [2nd ed.]. Boston: G. K. Hall Medical Publishers. Reprinted with permission.)*

BARTHOLIN'S GLAND CYST/BARTHOLIN'S GLAND ABSCESS. Bartholin's glands are duplicate structures located on either side of the vaginal orifice and slightly posterior to it. Cysts of these glands are the most common vulvar cysts (Michael & Roth, 1987). These glands grow rapidly at puberty and involute at menopause; cysts are usually found in women during the menstruating years. Bartholin's cysts (Figure 11–14) may be asymptomatic and present only as a mass. In this case, treatment is unnecessary.

Recurrent cysts may be treated with a surgical procedure known as marsupialization (Figure 11–15), which maintains the patency of Bartholin's duct and the function of the gland. The procedure is associated with minimal morbidity. It involves making an incision in the mucous membrane overlying the cyst, just outside the hymenal ring, draining the cyst cavity, excising a portion of the cyst lining, and forming a stoma, which eventually shrinks. The edges of the cyst wall are everted and sutured to the surrounding skin and mucous membranes (Tancer, Rosenberg & Fernandez, 1956).

An abscess of Bartholin's gland may result from secondary infection of a cyst or from a primary infection that causes edema and inflammation that occludes the duct (Michael & Roth, 1987). The woman may present with localized pain and systemic manifestations including fever, chills, and malaise.

Neisseria gonorrhoeae, Escherichia coli, Proteus mirabilis, and mixed bacterial flora have been cultured from Bartholin's gland abscesses. A sexual history and history of exposure to gonorrhea is important, therefore, when a woman presents with this problem; gonorrhea cultures are appropriate (see Chapter 12). A discussion of perineal hygiene should be undertaken.

If conservative treatment, consisting of warm vaginal baths and soaks, fails to cause drainage of an abscess, or if systemic symptoms are present, consultation and/or referral is indicated for antibiotic therapy and/or incision and drainage of the abscess.

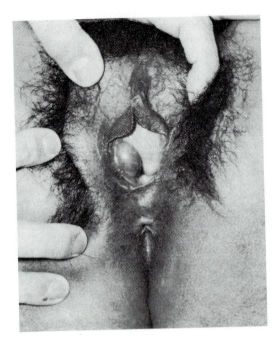

Figure 11–14. Bartholin duct cyst. *(From Woodruff, J. D. [1986]. Lesions of the vulva and vagina. In D. N. Danforth & J. R. Scott [Eds.], Obstetrics and gynecology [5th ed.]. Philadelphia: J. B. Lippincott Company.)*

Cancer of the Vulva. Cancers of the vulva include carcinoma in situ, Paget's disease, invasive cancer, and melanomas, as well as secondary malignancies and other less common types of cancers (Woodruff, 1986). Rarely, carcinoma may be found in Bartholin's gland (Copeland, Sneige, Gershenson, et al., 1986). Vulvar cancer accounts for less than 5 percent of gynecologic cancers among women in North America (American Cancer Society, 1987).

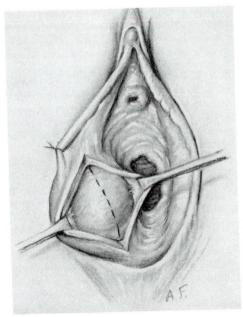
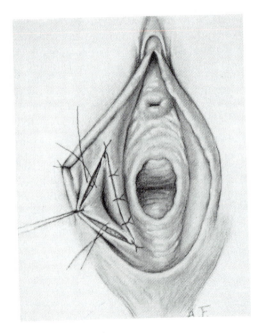

Figure 11–15. Left, Incision for marsupialization of Bartholin's duct cyst. **Right,** Suturing the marsupialization. *(From Tancer, M. L., Rosenberg, M., & Fernandez, D. [1956, June]. Cysts of the vulvovaginal [Bartholin's] gland. Obstetrics and gynecology. 7[6]:608–610. Reprinted with permission.)*

CARCINOMA IN SITU. Carcinoma in situ of the vulva appears in any age group although it is most commonly seen in women in the third and fourth decades of life. Its incidence is increasing, particularly in younger age groups (Woodruff, 1985, p. 390). Its association with STDs has been suggested as a reason for this increase (Jones & McLean, 1986; Wolcott & Gallup, 1984), although increased use of biopsy for suspicious lesions has been cited as a confounding factor. Human papillomavirus (HPV), particularly HPV types 6 and 11 has been found to be associated with vulvar carcinoma (Sutton, Stehman, Ehrlich, & Roman, 1987) (see Chapter 12).

Carcinoma in situ of the vulva may be asymptomatic or present as a lump or with pruritus. Cancerous lesions of the vulva may be scaly or white, red, or irregularly pigmented. Figures 11–16 to 11–23 represent varying presentations of vulvar carcinoma in situ.

Referral for diagnosis in cases of any suspicious lesions of the vulva is mandatory. Diagnosis is made by biopsy. Colposcopy may reveal the extent of lesions and has been advocated as a means of choosing therapy with the least chance of recurrence (Townsend, 1984).

A number of treatments have been advocated for carcinoma in situ of the vulva, including simple and radical surgery, laser surgery, and topical treatment with chemotherapeutic or immunologic agents. Vulvectomy has not been shown to prevent invasive cancer more than local excision, as this disease rarely progresses to invasive cancer (Morley, 1981; Wolcott & Gallup, 1984), particularly among women in their twenties (Woodruff, 1985, p. 391). Local incision avoids the disfigurement and sexual dysfunction that occurs with even simple vulvectomy (Kaplan, 1985). Laser therapy has been advocated for localized lesions (Gomez-Carrion, Kaufman, & Richart, 1988). Follow-up is always essential, however, because of the possibility of recurrence (Jones & McLean, 1986).

PAGET'S DISEASE OF THE VULVA. Paget's disease affects apocrine gland areas of the body. It occurs largely in women in their fifties and sixties. The disease presents with burning and pruritis. Lesions are multiple and bright red with white patches. Paget's disease may also involve the perianal area and breast. Invasive disease is rare. Diagnosis is made by biopsy. Vulvectomy has been advocated as treatment for Paget's disease (Woodruff, 1985, p. 393). Because recurrences are common, careful follow-up is essential.

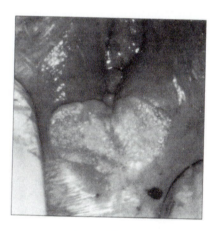

Figure 11–16.

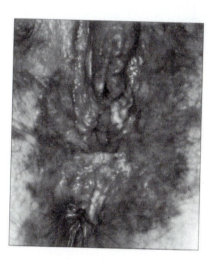

Figure 11–17.

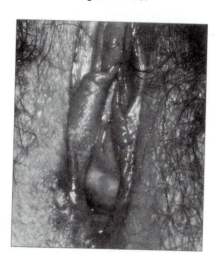

Figure 11–18.

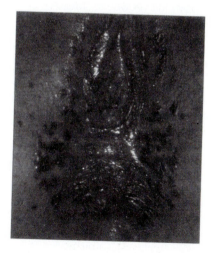

Figure 11–19.

Vulvar cancer in situ.

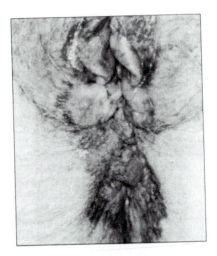

Figure 11-20.

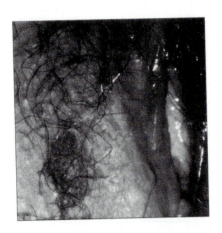

Figure 11-21.

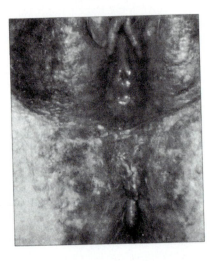

Figure 11-22.

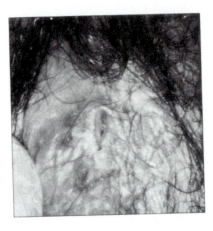

Figures 11-23. Vulvar cancer in situ. *(From Richart, R. M., Gomez-Carrion, Y. & Kaufman, R. H. [1988, February]. Treatment priorities for vulvar neoplasia. Contemporary Ob/Gyn. 31 [21]: 79-80, 82-83, 81-88, 91, 94. Reprinted with permission.)*

Vulvar cancer in situ.

INVASIVE CARCINOMA OF THE VULVA. Invasive cancer of the vulva rarely occurs before age 40. Diseases associated with cancer of the vulva include hypertension, cardiovascular disease, obesity, STDs, and, most commonly, diabetes. Breast, endometrial, and cervical cancers are associated malignancies (Perez, DiSaia, Knapp, & Young, 1985).

Cancer of the vulva is found most commonly in the labia, particularly the labia majora. The clitoris and Bartholin's gland may be involved. Cancer may be asymptomatic or present with a mass or growth, pruritus, bleeding, or pain.

Invasive cancer of the vulva may spread to adjacent organs or through the lymphatic system (Figge, Tamini, & Greer, 1985). The lymphatics of the vulva are extensive and diffuse. Blood vessels are not usually a source of spread except in advanced disease (Perez et al., 1985).

Diagnosis must be made by biopsy and the disease staged. Conventional staging has depended on the size of the tumor, involvement of lymph nodes, and spread to other structures.

Treatment for cancer of the vulva is generally surgical; extent of the surgery depends on the disease stage, with individualization of therapy recommended (Iversen, 1985).

Surgical techniques are not completely agreed on; techniques advocated include wide local excision for early disease (DiSaia, 1987), bilateral lymph node dissection of the groin, vulvectomy, and, in advanced cancer, pelvic exenteration. Radiation therapy has been suggested as a component of treatment (Fairey, MacKay, Benedet, et al., 1985).

VULVAR MALIGNANT MELANOMA. Malignant melanoma is an increasingly common lesion. Although malignant melanoma of the vulva is rare, it accounts for about 10 percent of malignant neoplasms of the vulva (Pierson, 1987, pp. 170-171). It usually occurs in the postmenopausal woman and presents with a mass, pruritus, and bleeding. Cure rates for malignant melanoma range from 30 to 50 percent. Surgical removal remains the treatment of choice. In malignant melanoma of the vulva, surgery consists of radical vulvectomy with bilateral groin dissection.

THE VAGINA

The vagina is an opening extending from the external genitalia to the cervix of the uterus. It consists of an anterior, a posterior, and two lateral walls that are made up of smooth muscle and lined with stratified squamous epithelium. The walls of the vagina are in contact with each other except where the cervix protrudes into the vagina. Before the initiation of sexual intercourse, the opening to the vagina is usually covered by folds of mucous membrane called the *hymen*. The spaces created by the cervix and vaginal walls are called *fornices*. Several glands, providing lubrication, line the walls of the vagina (Crafts, 1986).

Disorders of the vagina include congenital anomalies, muscular weaknesses, neoplasms, and infectious processes, which may be sexually transmitted.

Congenital Anomalies of the Vagina

Imperforate Hymen. With an imperforate hymen, a young woman undergoes puberty, but, at menarche, has no bleeding. After about 6 months, pain ensues. On examination, bulging and thinning of the hymen are noted and the distended vagina can be felt on rectal examination (Altchek, 1985, p. 57). Hymenectomy can be performed to correct this problem.

Rigid Hymen. A rigid, inelastic hymen is a problem if intercourse is not possible. A young woman with this problem can be taught gradual dilation with her fingers or dilators. This is best accomplished while tub bathing (Nichols & McGoldrick, 1985). If dilation is unsuccessful, a woman can be referred for hymenectomy. A rigid vaginal introitus has also been described and referral for possible surgical correction advised (Nichols & McGoldrick, 1985).

Septate Vagina. A septate vagina may occur with or without other müllerian abnormalities; associated anomalies include uterine didelphys, septate uterus, and, less commonly, a bicornuate uterus (Buttram, 1983), fully described in Chapter 14. A vaginal septum may be partial or complete and may run longitudinally or transversely. These defects can be corrected through dilation, displacement, or surgical division (Pritchard, MacDonald, & Gant, 1985, p. 495).

Double Vagina. A double vagina differs from a septate vagina in that it has a double introitus and each passage ends in a separate cervix. Sometimes, however, one vagina ends blindly.

Vaginal Effects from Diethylstilbestrol. The effects of diethylstilbestrol (DES) on vaginal development are covered completely in Chapter 18.

Congenital Absence of the Vagina. Congenital absence of the vagina is an anomaly of müllerian development. It usually occurs with congenital absence or abnormality of the cervix and/or uterus (see Chapters 13 and 14). Absence of the uterus and vagina is known as *Mayer–Rokitansky–Kuster–Hauser syndrome*, or *müllerian agenesis*. It has been reported in one in 2,500 to one in 5,000 births but is found in 18 percent of women with primary amenorrhea (Altchek, 1985; Buttram, 1983). In this condition, the ovaries are normal and the vulva appears normal on gross inspection. There is no vaginal opening, however, and the uterus is found to be absent on rectal examination. Sonogram is considered less reliable for diagnosis than physical examination; laparoscopy can confirm the diagnosis. Treatment, usually accomplished in late adolescence, consists of developing a neovagina, which can be done with manual dilation or surgery.

In about 5 percent of women with absent vagina, there is a functioning uterus. This results in retrograde menstruation and requires surgery to create an exit for menstrual blood as soon as the condition is discovered.

Noninfectious Disorders of the Vagina

Cystocele and Rectocele. Cystocele and rectocele occur when the support between the vagina and bladder or vagina and rectum, respectively, is weakened. These problems usually occur secondary to trauma associated with childbearing. Small cystoceles and rectoceles may be asymptomatic and require no treatment. Symptoms associated with cystocele include pressure and poor bladder emptying. Rectocele may lead to discomfort and difficulty emptying the bowel. Cystocele and rectocele can be identified on vaginal examination (see Chapter 3).

Pelvic floor exercises ("Kegels") are recommended to restore vaginal muscle tone. These should be done daily in sets repeated at frequent intervals. The exercises are described in Chapter 3 (Table 3–1) and Chapter 17. Surgical treatment for severely symptomatic cystocele and/or rectocele consists of anterior and/or posterior colporrhaphy, respectively. Surgery is usually deferred until the woman no longer desires childbearing. High-fiber diets, regular bowel habits, and possibly stool softeners have been advised for women with rectocele to avoid constipation and straining (Neeson & Stockdale, 1981).

Enterocele. Herniation of the fascia of the posterior vagina above the rectovaginal septum and below the cervix is called an enterocele. This condition may be asymptomatic or cause a dragging sensation, low backache, and rarely deep pelvic pain (Tovell & Danforth, 1986). A large enterocele may protrude through the vagina. A symptomatic enterocele requires surgical correction. Unfortunately, the condition is sometimes mistaken for a rectocele, and surgery is therefore not successful. Referral must be made to a specialist in vaginal repairs.

Vaginal Prolapse. Vaginal prolapse is a rare complication of hysterectomy or an occasional result of obesity, old age, or chronic malnutrition. It is often associated with enterocele and cystocele (Tovell & Danforth, 1986). Referral for surgical correction is necessary.

Foreign Bodies in the Vagina. The insertion of a foreign body into the vagina can lead to discomfort, trauma, discharge, and odor. A woman may present with an inability to remove the object, or she may forget about the object, and present with any of these symptoms. Most often, the object is a tampon. Retained tampons create a typical picture: onset of symptoms shortly after menses, possibly bloody or serosanguineous discharge, and, most noticeable, a strong odor. Odor may be noted by the partner during sexual relations. The puritis and discharge typical of vaginitis are absent. The object may be lodged in the posterior fornix and may be missed on speculum examination, but felt during bimanual palpation.

Treatment consists of removal of the foreign body. Associated trauma may require medical or surgical consultation or referral. Sexual abuse should be ruled out, especially in the case of a minor. After removal of a tampon, the examining room may need to be aired out or deodorized before the next patient is seen. Embarrassment often follows this problem and the provider needs to show sensitivity and provide reassurance.

Vaginal Neoplasms

BENIGN LESIONS.   Although very rare, blue *nevi* have been reported in the vagina. Usually they involve adjacent organs. These lesions must be biopsied to rule out malignant melanoma, which is more common.

Gartner's duct is a remnant of the wolffian or mesonephric duct found along the anterior part of the vaginal sidewall. *Gartner's duct cysts* (Figure 11-24) may be multiple or single. Usually these cysts are a few millimeters in size, but occasionally they achieve a large size. Large cysts may cause discomfort or difficulty with intercourse and may need to be excised (Green, 1977, p. 237). Gartner's duct cysts may be palpated on vaginal examination or may protrude through the introitus and be confused with a cystocele. Diagnosis can be made by determining whether the cyst originates in the anterior vaginal wall or the sidewall.

VAGINAL CANCER.   Most malignant tumors of the vagina are metastases from other sites (Hilborne & Fu, 1987, p. 181). Vaginal cancer is infrequent; among gynecologic cancers, only cancer of the fallopian tube is less common. Vaginal cancer accounts for less than 2 percent of all gynecologic cancers (Perez et al., 1985).

Like cervical cancer (see Chapter 13), vaginal cancer shows a progression from vaginal intraepithelial neoplasm (VAIN) to invasive cancer (Lenehan, Meffe, & Lickrish, 1986). Unlike cervical cancer, however, rates of carcinoma in situ are lower than those of invasive cancer. The lesion occurs most commonly in postmenopausal women with an average age of 58 to 65 years—approximately 10 years older than women with cervical cancer (Hilborne & Fu, 1987, p. 181).

A history of cancer of the cervix or vulva is the biggest risk factor for the development of vaginal cancer because of the similarity of tissues. The upper part of the vagina is of müllerian origin, comparable to the cervix; the lower part arises from the urogenital sinus, as does the vulva. Prior ionizing radiation to the vagina may also be a risk factor (Hilborne & Fu, 1987). Exposure to DES in utero is a risk for vaginal clear cell adenocarcinoma. This is discussed fully in Chapter 18.

Vaginal dysplasia and VAIN are usually asymptomatic

and are diagnosed by cytology. Symptoms, when present, may include dyspareunia, spotting after intercourse, burning, and leukorrhea. Lesions of vaginal cancer generally are white and granular, with sharp borders and sometimes a reddened or pinkish area. The majority of lesions appear in the upper vagina and on the posterior vaginal wall (Perez et al., 1985, p. 1058).

Women with invasive cancer of the vagina present most commonly with abnormal vaginal bleeding. Other common symptoms are vaginal discharge, a visible or palpable mass, pelvic pain, and urinary symptoms. Invasive cancer may, however, be asymptomatic (Al-Kurdi & Monaghan, 1981; Davis & Franklin, 1975; Johnston, Klotz, & Boutselis, 1983; Pride, Schultz, Chuprevich, & Buchler, 1979).

One type of vaginal cancer—*verrucous carcinoma*—presents as a cauliflower-like lesion that may be confused with condylomata acuminata (see Chapter 12). It tends to ulcerate and become infected and usually appears as a single large lesion, whereas condylomata acuminata are smaller and multiple (Hilborne & Fu, 1987, pp. 196–197).

Although rare, pigmented lesions of the vagina do appear and are most often malignant melanoma. Most women with malignant melanoma of the vagina present with vaginal bleeding or a vaginal mass (Liu, Hou, & Li, 1987).

Diagnosis involves complete and careful inspection of the vagina with a speculum, rotating it to fully expose all areas of the vagina. Palpation should follow. Specimens taken for cytology using a cotton swab moistened with saline or a wooden spatula are warranted if a cancer is suspected. The entire vaginal canal should be sampled. Referral for colposcopy and biopsy of suspicious lesions is mandatory. Biopsy must be made of any undiagnosed pigmented lesion.

Prognosis for women with vaginal cancer depends on the stage of disease, which is based on disease extent. The overall disease-free rate at 5 years is 45 percent; it ranges from 50 to 85 percent for stage I to 0 to 25 percent for stage IV (Benedet, Murphy, Fairey, & Boyes, 1983). Malignant melanoma is often fatal within 5 years (Liu et al., 1987).

Treatment of vaginal cancer must be individualized according to type of cancer, stage of disease, age, general health of the woman, and previous therapy (Benedet et al., 1983; Hilborne & Fu, 1987). Treatments for VAIN and precancerous lesions including carcinoma in situ are local excision, cryosurgery, laser therapy, partial or total vaginectomy, topical chemotherapy, and radiation. Invasive cancer is treated by radiation and/or radical pelvic surgery. Some authors advise radiation therapy as the preferred treatment, because it leads to fewer side effects and less dysfunction (Perez et al., 1985). Conservative surgery consisting of partial or total vaginectomy has been advocated for microinvasive carcinoma of the vagina (Peters, Kumar, & Morley, 1985).

As for any person with cancer, psychosocial support is essential for women with vaginal cancer. In this case, not only does the woman face a potentially life-threatening disease, but a disease of an organ intrinsically related to sexuality. Radical pelvic surgery has been shown to result in difficulties of adjustment related to body image, self-concept, and sexuality (Fisher, 1979, p. 223). The woman's family and supportive others must be included in the pre- and postdiagnostic and pre- and posttreatment phases of care. Lamb and Woods (1981) suggest several ways of promoting sexual health. These include initiating and encouraging open communication about sexuality; providing anticipatory guidance regarding what to expect; validating

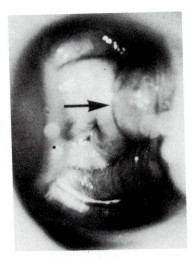

Figure 11-24. Gardner's duct cyst. *(From Kaufman, R. H. [1981]. Cystic tumors. In H. L. Gardner & R. H. Kaufman [Eds.], Benign diseases of the vulva and vagina. [2nd ed.]. Boston: G. K. Hall Medical Publishers. Reprinted with permission.)*

normalcy of sexual behaviors as well as sexual thoughts, desires, and dreams; and educating patients about sexuality including alternate ways of expressing physical love. These functions may require consultation with other care providers. Referral for individual, family, or group therapy may be appropriate.

Vaginal Infections

To recognize an infectious process of the vagina, the practitioner must be aware of the normal vaginal environment, particularly its secretions.

Vaginal Secretions. Normal vaginal secretions are influenced by hormonal changes. Throughout the menstrual years, every woman secretes discharge through the vagina in response to the fluctuation of estrogen and progesterone during the menstrual cycle (Horos, 1975).

Vaginal discharge begins in the cells of the cervix. Normal discharge is clear to cloudy in appearance, slightly slimy, and nonirritating. It has a mild unoffensive odor and may turn yellow after drying (Monif, 1982). Through the force of gravity, this cervical mucus travels into the vagina where a small amount of additional liquid is added by the vagina itself. Although the vagina has no major glands, the epithelium of the vaginal walls is usually moist. Bartholin's glands secretions also make up a portion of the vaginal fluid (Wagner & Levin, 1978).

Vaginal mucus helps to carry away some of the sloughed-off squamous epithelial cells of the vagina. These cells have a high content of glycogen, which is metabolized in the vagina by healthful vaginal flora called *lactobacilli* or *Döderlein's bacilli*. The metabolic by-product is lactic acid, which sets up the naturally acidic environment of the vagina (Horos, 1975).

The acid nature of vaginal secretions helps promote vaginal health as most common bacteria and infectious organisms prefer to grow in a more alkaline medium. The normal pH range of vaginal secretions is 3.8 to 4.2 (Monif, 1982). Cohen (1969) examined a group of women with active vaginal infections and found the mean (range) vaginal pH values in women with infections to be 5.2 (4.2–7.5) for gonorrhea; 5.2 (4.0–7.0) for trichomoniasis; and 4.8 (4.0–5.5) for candidiasis. Any interference with the delicate balance of vaginal secretions sets up an environment conducive to infection.

Amount of vaginal discharge is not in and of itself an indication of infection. Vaginal secretions increase normally at the time of ovulation, just before menstruation, during pregnancy, and with sexual arousal (Horos, 1975). Any other change in vaginal discharge may indicate a problem. Malodorous, irritating, abnormally colored, and unusually heavy discharge needs to be carefully assessed. Whenever a woman perceives a change in vaginal discharge, her observation deserves investigation.

Prevention of Vaginal Infections. The frequency and severity of vaginal infections can be diminished by careful explanation of preventive measures for all women. Providing an explanation of the normalcy of vaginal secretions and giving each woman an opportunity to view her genitalia and her normally occurring secretions, to ask questions, to discuss cultural beliefs, and to air her feelings about her vagina may go a long way toward promoting vaginal health. Although research on behavioral factors and vaginitis is lacking (Ervin, Komaroff, Baranowski, & Pass, 1982), a number of overall measures believed to help maintain

vaginal health can be followed by all women. These are in addition to the specific preventive and curative measures discussed in the sections devoted to individual disorders. The following information should be shared with women; it can be made into a handout. It is adapted from The Boston Women's Health Book Collective (1984), Horos (1975), Cherniak (1983), Friedrich (1985a), and Stone (1986).

1. General health may be a key to frequent infections. Poor diet, lack of sleep, and life stresses may all lower resistance. A diet high in refined sugars in particular may increase the likelihood of infection.
2. Vulvar and vaginal irritants should be avoided. Harsh deodorant and perfumed soap, deodorant sprays, and perfumed douches may irritate the vaginal area. Moreover, vaginal douches may alter the pH of the vagina and wash out the naturally occurring secretions and flora that protect the vagina's health.
3. Wiping should always be from the front to the back. Wiping in the opposite direction may increase the chance of fecal contamination of the vagina and urinary tract.
4. Excessive vaginal secretions and heat may create an environment that favors vaginal infections. The genital area should be washed daily with mild soap and water. Absorbent underpants—preferably 100 percent cotton or, less preferably, some other fabric with an all-cotton crotch—are recommended. Panties should be changed daily. Clothing that is too tight in the crotch or thighs should not be worn as it restricts the flow of air to the vaginal area. Sleeping without underwear allows for a daily period when the genitalia can "breathe."
5. Washcloths, towels, douche bags, contraceptive diaphragms or cervical caps, and underwear should not be shared. Bathtubs should be washed after use.
6. Sexual partners should practice good hygiene as well. Daily bathing, particularly before intercourse, is a good idea.
7. Partners should be checked for abnormal discharge or obvious lesions such as blisters, warts, sores, or reddened or raised areas on the penis. Sexual contact should be avoided until all abnormalities have been diagnosed and treated if necessary.
8. Condoms provide some protection against vaginal infections and STDs. They can be used as a method of birth control or as a protective adjunct to any contraceptive method. Vaginal spermicides, contained in foams, creams, and jellies, and used with the diaphragm, cervical cap, vaginal sponge, or contraceptive film, also provide some protection.
9. If a woman or a woman and her partner(s) are being treated for a vaginal infection, intercourse should be avoided or condoms used until treatment is complete. Intercourse during the course of treatment may reinfect the woman or her partner. Whenever possible, treatment should be simultaneous for the woman and her partner(s). All prescribed treatment regimens should be completed even if symptoms subside.
10. Any sexual practice that is painful or abrasive to the vagina should be avoided.
11. Sanitary napkins and internal tampons should be changed frequently during menstruation. Tampons may be a particular risk when worn to bed. Tampons should be avoided on days with scant flow as

they may become adherent to the vagina or cervix and cause trauma when removed.

12. Current public health recommendations caution against all anal–genital intercourse. The mucosa of the anus is more delicate than the vagina; breaks and tears in the mucosa can be the portal of entry for systemic sexually transmitted diseases (see Chapter 12). A condom may provide some protection if couples choose this type of contact. Vaginal penetration after anal intercourse without first removing the condom or washing the male's genitals can be a significant source of infection.

Data Collection. In the sections that follow, each type of vaginal infection is described in detail; etiology, prevalence, risk factors, clinical presentation, and management, including data collection and appropriate interventions, are discussed. This section outlines components of the data collection appropriate whenever *any* vaginal infection is suspected.

Typically, women with a vaginal infection present with one or more of the following symptoms: unusual vaginal discharge, odor, pruritis, burning, dyspareunia. Whenever one or more of these symptoms are reported, complete data collection must follow. The differential diagnosis of vaginitis and the correlation of findings to the specific disorder are outlined in Table 11–1 and discussed under each disorder. Appendix III provides a more complete differential diagnosis for the complaints of vaginal discharge and pelvic pain.

TABLE 11–1. VAGINITIS: DIFFERENTIAL DIAGNOSIS

	Diagnosis					
	Normal	Bacterial Vaginosis	Candidiasis	Trichomoniasis	Atrophic Vaginitis	Chemical or Allergic Vaginitis
Color of discharge	Slate gray/ white/clear	Gray/white	White/Yellow	Yellow-green/ green/gray/ yellow	Gray/yellow	Normal
Odor of discharge	Normal body odor	Fishy	None/yeasty, musty	Foul	Normal	Normal
Consistency of discharge	Thin/homogeneous/mucoid	Thin/homogeneous/milky/ frothy or nonfrothy	Thick plaques; may be adherent to vaginal walls/ creamy/thin, watery	Thin/frothy/may be nonfrothy	Watery/homogeneous/purulent/serosanguineous/ sticky	Normal
Presenting complaint(s)	None	Odor Increased discharge Minimal or no pruritus Occasional irritation	Pruritus Burning Dyspareunia External dysuria Increased discharge or dryness	Pruritis Burning Dyspareunia External dysuria Increased discharge	Spotting Burning Dyspareunia Pruritis External dysuria Increased discharge	Pruritis Tenderness/ pain Burning External dysuria Dyspareunia
Physical findings	Absence of abnormality	Absence of inflammation Pooling of discharge at introitus Positive whiff test	Erythema of vulva, vagina Excoriations secondary to scratching Possible tissue friability	Erythema Petechiae especially of cervix Cervical friability Occasional lower abdominal pain, inguinal lymphadenopathy	Pale, pink vaginal, cervical mucosa/ absence of rugation Sparse, brittle pubic hair Inflammation Ecchymosis Petechiae Excoriation	Erythema Edema Vesicles or blisters Oozing Ulcerations Thickened skin White patches Lymphadenopathy
pH	≤4.5	>4.5	≤4.5 or slightly higher	5.2–7.0	5.5–7.0	≤4.5
Microscopic findings	Squamous epithelial cells Lactobacilli Few WBCs	Rare WBCs Clue cells Decreased lactobacilli Increased bacteria, especially thin, curved, crescent-shaped rods	Pseudohyphae Yeast buds WCBs Lactobacilli	Motile trichomonads with flagellae/ WBCs	Decreased lactobacilli Increased WBCs and bacteria/ RBCs Absence of pathogens Increased number of parabasal cells on maturation index	Absence of pathogens/ WBCs
Relationship of symptoms to menses	Increases around ovulation	Not applicable	Increased before menses Relief with after menses	Increased during, after menses	Not applicable	Not applicable

HISTORY. Ask about associated symptoms including any of the classic symptoms mentioned earlier, dysuria or other urinary tract symptomatology, pelvic or groin pain, fever, abnormal vaginal bleeding or spotting, or any lesions or adenopathy noted by the woman.

Find out about the onset of symptoms, their relationship to menses, their course to date, that is, worsening, improving, or remaining the same.

Discuss factors such as sex or urination that bring on or increase symptoms.

Ask the woman to describe relief measures used and their effects.

Discuss life-style or habits, particularly those that affect vaginal health, and recent changes in these. Include the use of a new detergent, vaginal deodorant or perfume, type of underwear worn, or douching, particularly an increase in the frequency of douching or a change in the solution used.

Obtain the following histories:

- Complete sexual history including number of partners; new partners; number of partners of sexual partners; symptoms in sexual partners; known exposure to vaginitis or STDs; contraception used; and sexual practices such as anal-to-vaginal intercourse
- Complete medical history including systemic illnesses, such as diabetes, and recent or ongoing treatment with antibiotics, including metronidazole (e.g., Flagyl)
- Menstrual history, particularly to rule out pregnancy and to correlate symptoms and their onset and severity to the cycle
- Gynecologic history, particularly past episodes of similar symptoms, their diagnosis, course, treatment or treatments, and results of each treatment
- Diet history, especially recent changes in diet, focusing particularly on intake of sugar

PHYSICAL EXAMINATION. Physical examination must always include these components:

- Abdominal palpation and palpation for costovertebral angle tenderness (CVAT) to rule out gastrointestinal or urinary tract problems
- Palpation for lymphadenopathy and tender lymph nodes
- Inspection of the entire vulva and vagina for parasites, lesions, irritations, excoriations, discharge, and signs of atrophy
- Inspection by speculum of the vaginal walls and cervix, especially for redness, petechial hemorrhages, lesions, discharge and its characteristics, and signs of atrophy
- Analysis of odor of any discharge
- Palpation of the vulva and entire vagina for masses and tenderness

LABORATORY TESTING. Laboratory testing may include vaginal pH testing; wet smears with normal saline and potassium hydroxide (KOH); whiff test with KOH; Pap smear; Gram stain; cultures or monoclonal antibody testing; serologic testing; and urinalysis and/or urine culture and sensitivity. Detailed discussions of the techniques for these tests are found in Chapter 4.

Bacterial Vaginosis. Bacterial vaginosis (BV) is the most common type of vaginal infection in the United States today (Centers for Disease Control, 1979). This entity was originally known as *nonspecific vaginitis*, a term most experts

have now discarded and replaced with a series of names describing the organism thought to be responsible for the disease. Gardner and Dukes (1955) called the disorder *hemophilus vaginitis* after the Gram-negative rod *Hemophilus vaginalis*; it was later renamed *gardnerella* when the organism *Gardnerella vaginalis* was discovered to be distinct from other hemophilic bacteria. It has also been called *corynebacterium vaginale* by some investigators who believe *Hemophilus vaginalis* is a corynebacterium. The current terminology is believed to more accurately describe the pathology of the disease—an increased number of anaerobes in the vaginal flora, including *Gardnerella*, the newly defined *Mobiluncus* sp., and others. *Vaginosis* (as opposed to vaginitis) denotes the lack of inflammation or white blood cells (WBCs) seen in the disorder. The name *bacterial vaginosis* was accepted at a 1984 Stockholm symposium (Spiegel, Amsel, Eschenbach, et al., 1980; Symposium, 1986; Taylor, Blackwell, Barlow, & Phillips, 1982).

PREVALENCE. The prevalence of BV has been cited to be as high as 25 percent among university students, with about one half of those cases being asymptomatic (Amsel, Totten, Spiegel, et al., 1983). Other estimates of its prevalence are about 15 percent of women in gynecologic, STD, and student health clinics and about 10 percent of women in the "average gyn private practice" (Symposium, 1986, p. 203). Amsel and associates (1983) found an increase in this type of vaginitis among IUD wearers, although type of IUD was not specified in their report.

ETIOLOGY. The main etiologic agent in BV is an increase in anaerobes in the vagina. The reason this occurs is unknown. Organisms commonly found include *Bacteroides, Peptococcus,* and a newly described bacterium, *Mobiluncus* sp. The last-named organism is a small, crescent-shaped motile bacterium (Symposium, 1986). These organisms may be accompanied by *Gardnerella vaginalis,* but *Gardnerella* can be found in 40 percent of women without BV (Symposium, 1986). There is a decrease in the normal lactobacilli of the vagina but it is not known whether this is a cause or effect of the disease (Symposium, 1986).

Vaginal pH is increased in BV. The organisms present in BV cause the level of vaginal amines to be high. These amines are volatilized when the pH is increased, causing a characteristic odor.

CLINICAL PRESENTATION. Most women with BV complain of vaginal odor, often described as "fishy." They may complain of an increased vaginal discharge, usually described as thin, white or gray, or milky. Less commonly, vaginal irritation may be noted (Amsel et al., 1983). Vulvar itching, burning, pain, and dyspareunia are uncommon. The odor may be noted after heterosexual intercourse (or by the woman's sexual partner), as semen releases the amines produced by the anaerobes present in the vagina (Amsel et al., 1983; Symposium, 1986).

DIFFERENTIAL DIAGNOSIS. BV must be differentiated from other types of vaginitis—candidiasis, trichomoniasis, and allergic, chemical, or atrophic vaginitis. It must be differentiated from STDs that may present with increased discharge, especially chlamydia and gonorrhea. Odor may also be caused by a foreign body, such as a tampon, in the vagina.

MANAGEMENT

Data Collection. *History.* A careful history can often help distinguish this type of vaginal infection from others. A fishy odor and increased thin discharge are most significant. An increase in odor after intercourse may be an important clue. The absence of pruritus is helpful in diagnosis. Previous occurrences, diagnoses, and treatments should be elicited; often women with BV have been improperly treated.

Physical Examination. The first physical examination clue to diagnosis of BV is often a thin discharge on the vulva or pooling of the discharge at the introitus. A normal vaginal discharge does not usually leak out onto the vulva. Visualization with a speculum reveals a thin homogeneous discharge, easily wiped from the vaginal walls and cervix. The discharge may or may not be frothy; this characteristic is not diagnostic. It is usually white or grayish and milky in consistency and has been described as looking like "a cup of milk . . . poured into the vagina" (Thomason in Symposium 1986, p. 188). The vaginal walls and cervix rarely appear inflamed, unless there is a second infection present. The fishy odor may or may not be readily apparent; secretions on the speculum should always be smelled.

Laboratory Testing. A number of simple office laboratory tests can be performed to diagnose BV. Cultures are not generally helpful and may lead to overtreatment, as Gardnerella is often cultured in women without BV (Symposium, 1986, p. 190).

The first laboratory test to perform is a pH of vaginal secretions. Nitrazine paper is sufficiently sensitive for this test. If the pH is 4.5 or greater, BV is possible, although trichomoniasis must also be ruled out (which is not possible by clinical examination alone). If the pH is less than 4.5, usually the vaginal flora are normal or the woman has candidiasis. To obtain an accurate pH reading, the sample must come from the discharge, not the endocervix. Discharge on the vaginal walls can be sampled with a dry cotton swab; lubricant on the swab can increase the pH. The pH alerts the practitioner to what to expect under the microscope.

Both saline and 10 percent potassium hydroxide smears should be made. If the pH is low, the saline smear will reveal lactobacilli—large, thick rods—and possibly Candida if vaginitis is present. If the pH is high, the saline smear may reveal the characteristic signs of BV: decreased numbers of lactobacilli, with background bacteria outnumbering the lactobacilli (these bacteria are often thin, curved or crescent–shaped rods, characteristic of Mobiluncus sp.); few WBCs (fewer than the number of epithelial cells); and clue cells. Clue cells are vaginal epithelial cells coated with bacteria. They differ from normal epithelial cells in that they look speckled rather than translucent. Their borders appear serrated or unclear because of the adherent bacteria. (See Chapter 4, Figure 4–3.) Clue cells make up 10 to 50 percent of epithelial cells in women with BV (Symposium, 1986). Their presence is 85 percent predictive of this infection (Amsel et al., 1983).

The KOH smear should be examined for Candida, but more relevant to the diagnosis of BV is the fishy odor released when KOH is added to vaginal secretions. This odor is characteristic of BV and its presence when secretions are mixed with KOH is called a positive whiff test.

At least two of the previously described signs should be present to diagnose BV: a thin homogeneous vaginal discharge; vaginal pH greater than 4.5; positive whiff test; and 10 to 50 percent of vaginal epithelial cells coated with bacteria (clue cells). Decreased lactobacilli, few WBCs, and multiple, small curved moving rods are also characteristic

of the infection. Mixed infections (BV and candidiasis or trichomoniasis) may be present, however, and confound the latter findings.

Intervention. Treatment. The Centers for Disease Control (1985) recommend metronidazole as the most effective medication for BV. The recommended treatment regimen is 500 mg orally twice a day for 7 days. At least one report shows a high efficacy with a single 2-g oral dose of metronidazole, which is less expensive and easier to use (Minkowski, Baker, Alleyne, et al., 1983). This is not, however, the CDC's current recommendation for BV treatment. Ampicillin or amoxicillin, 500 mg by mouth, four times daily for 7 days, is a less effective treatment that can be used during pregnancy or in women for whom metronidazole is contraindicated.

The CDC does not advocate treatment for male sexual partners or for asymptomatic cases of BV. There is some evidence, however, that BV may be associated with premature labor and postpartum endometritis. Many practitioners recommend treating even asymptomatic infections in women planning pregnancy. This area certainly deserves further investigation.

In the past topical vaginal creams containing sulfa medications were widely prescribed for BV; these are not considered effective treatments although they may provide palliative relief for a short period.

Metronidazole, available commercially as Flagyl, Protostat, and Metric, is an antiprotozoal and antibacterial (antianaerobic) agent. It is contraindicated in women with hypersensitivity and during the first trimester of pregnancy. Before prescribing this drug, early pregnancy must be ruled out. Metronidazole is contraindicated in lactation because of the high concentrations found in the infant, although if breastfeeding is temporarily discontinued, the drug can be used. Past or present blood dyscrasias and active central nervous system disease contraindicate use of the drug.

Metronidazole side effects are multiple and include a metallic taste, furry tongue, glossitis, and stomatitis; nausea and vomiting; overgrowth of Candida; central nervous system reactions including convulsive seizures, vertigo, weakness, irritability, peripheral neuropathy, and depression; hypersensitivity reactions; urinary tract manifestations including dark-colored urine, dysuria, pyuria, pelvic pressure, and cystitis; and reversible leukopenia. Plasma clearance of the drug is decreased in patients with decreased liver function. Taking the medication with meals reduces the incidence of some side effects (Robbie & Sweet, 1983).

Alcohol combined with metronidazole causes severe abdominal distress, nausea and vomiting, flushing, and headaches. Alcohol must be avoided during metronidazole therapy and for 24 hours after the last dose.

Carcinogenesis and tumorigenesis have been reported with metronidazole given in high doses to mice and rats. Although its carcinogenic potential in humans is not yet known, some drug manufacturers and authorities recommend avoiding unnecessary use of metronidazole (Physicians' desk reference, 1988, p. 1512; Robbie & Sweet, 1983). One retrospective study showed no evidence of increased numbers of cancers after metronidazole therapy (Beard, Noller, O'Fallon, et al., 1979); the study, however, did not account for dosage or the long latent period often seen between exposure and development of cancer (Mirer & Silverstein, 1980).

Some practitioners routinely prescribe a short course of an anticandidal agent (see Candidiasis) with metronidazole or ampicillin to be used prophylactically at the end of and after the course of treatment to prevent overgrowth of Candida.

Treatment for Recurrences. The reported recurrence rate for BV is as high as 30 percent (Symposium, 1986, p. 191). Of course, as with any disease, examination is important to establish the diagnosis. Recurrence should *not* be assumed via the telephone.

Re-treatment with metronidazole cures most recurrences. When metronidazole therapy is repeated, a WBC count is recommended to rule out leukopenia (Symposium, 1986, p. 197), with the medication withheld until the count has returned to normal values.

Some practitioners advise treating male partners when BV is recurrent, although it is not universally agreed that this is effective (Elsner & Hartmann, 1987; Symposium, 1986). The male ejaculate can be cultured for *Gardnerella*, but a positive culture does not mean that this is the woman's source of infection or that the male needs to be treated. Use of a condom for a prolonged period may be just as effective as treating the partner with antibiotic therapy.

Acidification of the vagina is helpful for recurrences as well. Vinegar and water douches (one to two tablespoons of plain vinegar in a quart of water), Aci-Jel, or lactobacillus tablets can be used. Some practitioners have reported success with the use of garlic suppositories over several weeks. The garlic should be peeled and wrapped in gauze with a tail for retrieval and changed every 12 hours. This does not cause an odor.

Additional Self-Help Measures. In addition to vinegar douches, recommended self-help measures include yogurt, goldenseal, or bayberry bark douches along with increased amounts of vitamins B and C (The Boston Women's Health Book Collective, 1984, p. 520). Acidophilus vaginal tablets may be helpful in maintaining vaginal pH.

Additional Teaching and Counseling. Women need to understand the etiology of BV. Because an odor may be associated with a feeling of "uncleanliness," women need reassurance that the disorder is not caused by poor hygiene. As the odor may increase with heterosexual intercourse, they need to understand that sex is not causing the infection. A woman with any vaginal infection, particularly a resistant or recurrent one, needs emotional support as these infections may affect body and self-image.

Women must understand the nature of the treatment for BV and be involved in the choice of a drug like metronidazole. Some women may choose a more "natural" treatment like garlic suppositories. Although the infection is troublesome, it is not now considered to have systemic complications, except possibly in pregnancy or the postpartum period. When prescribing metronidazole, the practitioner must give a thorough explanation of the treatment regimen, including the need to continue the medication even if symptoms abate quickly. Special instructions for this drug, including taking it with meals and avoiding alcohol, must be given, in writing if necessary. Women planning a pregnancy should be told of the possible risks of BV and advised to have the infection treated before pregnancy.

Candidiasis. Caused by an overgrowth of a fungus (or yeast) found in the vaginal flora even in many asymptomatic women, candidiasis (monilial vulvovaginitis or candidal vaginitis) is the second most common form of vaginal infection in the United States (Gardner, 1981a).

ETIOLOGY AND TRANSMISSION. *Candida albicans* is the pathogen responsible for 80 to 95 percent of yeast infections (Paavonen & Stamm, 1987). Other species of *Candida* and *Torulopsis glabrata* are implicated in the remainder of vaginal yeast infections (Odds, 1979, p. 107). Whether or not colonization with a yeast organism causes infection depends on the number of colonies present and the tolerance of the host tissues to the organism (Catterall, 1971).

Some evidence suggests that vaginal candidal infection is due to candidal infection of the digestive tract or is secondary to sexual transmission; however, neither of these has been proven as a route of transmission (Odds, 1979, p. 108). Many women with vaginal yeast colonization have been found to harbor rectal yeasts, pointing to a possible intestinal reservoir (Hilton & Warnock, 1975; Miles, Olsen, & Rogers, 1977). An association between genital yeast infections and known STDs has been demonstrated in 39 percent of women diagnosed with yeast, suggesting, but not proving, the possibility of sexual transmission (Thin, Leighton, & Dixon, 1977). Additional evidence comes from the demonstration of yeasts on the penis; Rodin and Kolator (1976) identified yeasts in 18 percent of circumcised and uncircumcised males, with the uncircumcised men more likely to be symptomatic. Davidson (1977) found equivalent rates of *Candida* among asymptomatic males and a 40 percent culture-positive rate among males with penile balanitis (inflammation of the glans). The length of time that yeasts persist on the penis is unknown, although Rodin and Kolator demonstrated positive cultures in men who reported no sexual intercourse for up to 3 months.

PREVALENCE. The reported prevalence of vulvovaginal candidiasis has risen since the 1940s (Gardner, 1981a). The Centers for Disease Control (1979, p. 62) found that 2.5 to 7.9 percent of women seeking care in a family planning or STD clinic were infected with *Candida*. Up to two times the number who are infected are colonized with a yeast organism (Paavonen & Stamm, 1987). In pregnancy, rates of 15 to 31 percent of yeast infections have been reported, whereas rates in the postpartum period are low (Gillespie, Inmon, & Slater, 1960). This is due to the increased glycogen content of the vagina during pregnancy, especially in its later stages, and to the stimulatory effects of estrogen and progesterone on candidal growth, which occurs because receptors for these hormones are present in candidal organisms (Sobel, 1985a). A small but unknown number of women have recurrent frequent attacks of candidal vaginitis (Sobel, 1985a) or persistent chronic symptoms, mostly affecting the vulva.

PREDISPOSING FACTORS. A number of factors have been implicated as predisposing to yeast infection. These include antibiotic therapy, particularly with broad-spectrum antibiotics such as tetracycline, ampicillin, cephalosporins, and metronidazole; diabetes mellitus, especially uncontrolled diabetes; diets high in refined sugars (Horowitz, Edelstein, & Lippman, 1984); pregnancy; use of corticosteroids and exogenous hormones; obesity; and immunosuppressed states (Paavonen & Stamm, 1987).

Oral contraceptive use is often cited as a predisposing factor (Neeson & Stockdale, 1981; Smith & Lauver, 1984), but the literature is conflicting on this point. Several anecdotal reports (Catterall, 1971; Porter & Lyle, 1966; Yaffee & Grots, 1965) as well as case-control and prospective studies (Jackson & Spain, 1968; Jensen, Hansen, & Blom, 1970; Walsh, Hildebrandt, & Prystowsky 1965, 1968) have shown an association; other studies, however, have not found a statistically significant relationship (Davis, 1969; Hilton & Warnock, 1975; Lapan, 1970; Morris & Morris, 1967; Spellacy, Zaias, Buhi, & Birk, 1971), although some trends toward association have been noted.

Diddle, Gardner, Williamson, and O'Connor (1969) found an increased rate of candidal vaginitis with increased duration of oral contraceptive use; this may explain why some of the studies found no association: in some investigations women were followed only 12 months. Studies on whether newer lower-dose pills are associated with candidal infections are currently unavailable.

Tight clothing and underwear or pantyhose made of nonabsorbent synthetic materials are usually cited as creating a vaginal environment conducive to fungal growth. This conclusion has been based mainly on clinical observation (Breen, 1971; Bull, 1969; Sauer, 1974; Stallworthy, 1971; Tann, 1968). One prospective study was conducted in which women without risk factors were assigned for 2 months either to a control group wearing loose-fitting clothing or to an experimental group wearing tight dresses, jeans, or pants and silk or nylon underwear; the researchers found that two thirds of cultures were positive for *Candida* among the experimental group (Elegbe & Botu, 1982).

Some nutritional factors, in addition to excess sugar intake, may be associated with susceptibility or resistance to *Candida*, although evidence for these associations is sparse. Implicated nutrient deficiencies include vitamin A (Cohen & Elin, 1974; Montes, Krumdieck, & Cornwell, 1973) and iron (Davidson, Hayes, & Hussein, 1977; Fletcher, Mather, Lewis, & Whiting, 1975).

Interestingly, most women with persistent or recurrent yeast infections have no known predisposing factors, leading to the hypothesis that multiple undetermined factors are implicated in the development of vaginal fungal infections. These include both host susceptibility and fungal pathogenicity (Gardner, 1981a, pp. 221–222).

CLINICAL PRESENTATION. The most notable symptom of candidiasis is vulvar and perhaps vaginal pruritus. Itching may be mild or intense and may interfere with activities or rest. Itching and burning may occur with or after intercourse.

Women may or may not complain of a discharge with a yeast infection. If they do, it may be thick and curdlike or thin and watery. Sometimes a feeling of dryness is experienced (Gardner, 1981a, p. 226). Women may report painful urination as the urine passes over the vulva. This occurs most often in women who have vulvar excoriations secondary to scratching.

Symptoms may occur just before menstruation in response to the increased levels of hormone at this time. Relief may be experienced during and after menses.

Vulvar erythema is the most common sign of candidal vaginitis and often corresponds to the degree of itching. The most common place for erythema is the mucocutaneous surfaces between the labia minora (Gardner, 1981a, p. 226). Edema of the labia minora may be present (particularly with candidal infection during pregnancy). Scratching may cause excoriations and fissures. Rarely, these excoriations become secondarily infected, leading to inguinal lymphadenitis.

Vaginal discharge in yeast infections is variable. Many practitioners expect a cottage cheese–like discharge. In fact, discharge may be thick and white; it may, however, be creamy or thin and watery (Odds, 1979, p. 101). Adherent white or yellow patches may be noted (Figure 11–25). They may form a pseudomembranous covering over the vaginal walls (Figure 11–26). Gardner (1981a) reports thrush patches in only 20 percent of women with candidal infections. Sometimes leukoplakia of the cervix is mistaken for thrush patches, but leukoplakia does not readily wipe away. Vaginal erythema may be present beneath the adherent patchy discharge. Some friability of the tissues is occa-

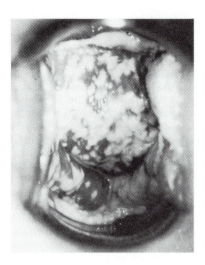

Figure 11–25. Thrush patches of the vaginal wall. *(From Gardner, H. L. [1981]. Candidiasis. In H. L. Gardner & R. H. Kaufman [Eds.], Benign diseases of the vulva and vagina. [2nd ed.]. Boston: G. K. Hall Medical Publishers. Reprinted with permission.)*

sionally seen. An odor is not usually present, although sometimes there may be a yeasty or musty smell.

DIFFERENTIAL DIAGNOSIS. Candidiasis must be differentiated from other forms of vaginitis—trichomoniasis and BV; atrophic and allergic or chemical vaginitis. It must also be differentiated from urinary tract infection and the many vulvar dermatoses and dystrophies described previously in this chapter. Excoriations and abrasions from scratching may look like herpetic lesions (see Chapter 12).

MANAGEMENT

Data Collection. *History.* In addition to a careful history of clinical symptoms and their onset and course (see Clinical Presentation), the woman's risk factors should be assessed: use of antibiotics, oral contraceptives, or corticosteroids; personal or family history of diabetes and clinical signs of diabetes; nutritional intake, focusing on simple sugars; hygienic practices including type of underwear and the wear-

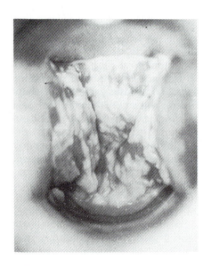

Figure 11–26. Pseudomembrane covering the vaginal wall. *(From Gardner H. L. [1981]. Candidiasis. In H. L. Gardner & R. H. Kaufman [Eds.], Benign diseases of the vulva and vagina. [2nd ed.]. Boston: G. K. Hall Medical Publishers. Reprinted with permission.)*

ing of tight clothing. Note the woman's age and rule out the possibility of pregnancy. It is important to note the woman's history of yeast infections to determine whether the current problem is a persistent or recurrent infection. Note too her history of other types of vaginitis.

Symptoms in the male occurring after intercourse may indicate a hypersensitivity to *Candida albicans* and should be asked about. These include burning, itching, and generalized erythema of the glans and prepuce (Waugh, 1982).

Physical Examination. Physical examination must include a thorough vulvar and vaginal inspection. Discharge should be evaluated and smelled. A speculum examination is essential. Inguinal lymph nodes should be palpated for enlargement and/or tenderness.

Laboratory Testing. Laboratory testing must always be employed to diagnose candidal infections. Even experienced practitioners cannot rely solely on clinical diagnosis to distinguish candidiasis from other forms of vaginitis. Even an adherent, patchy vaginal discharge cannot be considered 100 percent confirmatory because such patches may be masses of desquamated epithelial cells (Figure 11–27).

Vaginal pH is usually normal with candidiasis. Knowing the pH can help rule out other infectious processes and alert the practitioner to what to expect on wet smear. The *Candida* organism is characterized on microscope examination by its filaments, or *pseudohyphae* (see Chapter 4, Figure 4–5). Yeast cells surround the filaments. These often can be seen on a thinly prepared wet mount made with normal saline, but may be confused with other cells and artifacts seen on the wet smear. Cotton fibers particularly may be mistaken for pseudohyphae; cotton, however, usually appears as single strands, larger on the field than pseudohyphae, and without the surrounding yeast buds. White blood cells may be present in the smear and many lactobacilli are observed. A preparation with 10 to 20 percent potassium hydroxide (KOH) causes dissolution of white and red blood cells and transparency of the epithelial cells, making the pseudohyphae more apparent.

Because symptoms may be misleading and clinical diagnosis incorrect, we do not advocate examining a KOH preparation without first looking at a saline slide. A KOH slide may be made in addition to the saline preparation, or the KOH solution can be added under the coverslip after the wet mount has been studied under the microscope.

Candida can be demonstrated on Gram stains (see Chapter 4). Yeast cells and pseudohyphae are Gram positive. Yeast may also be observed on routine Pap smears.

A culture is the most reliable test for *Candida* as a negative KOH smear does not definitely rule out infection (Schnell, 1982). Van Slyke, Michel, and Rein (1981) report a 6.2 percent false-negative rate in KOH smears compared with cultures in symptomatic women.

Appropriate culture media include Sabouraud's or modified Sabouraud's medium, Nickerson's medium, and Pagano-Levin medium. Positive cultures on Sabouraud's and Nickerson's media show a dark brown to jet black color after incubation for 48 to 72 hours at room temperature or in an incubator. Positive cultures on Pagano–Levin medium show varying shades of pink after a comparable incubation period (Mendel, Haberman, & Hall, 1960).

Intervention. A number of standard treatments exist for nonrecurrent vulvovaginal yeast infections. Persistent or recurrent infections pose a more difficult treatment problem and are discussed separately. Many authors agree that in the absence of signs and symptoms in the nonpregnant woman, *Candida* colonization need not mandate treatment (Gardner, 1981a, p. 230).

A variety of antifungal preparations are highly effective against *Candida albicans*. Most are applied intravaginally and have few side effects. The earliest used effective treatment for vulvovaginal candidiasis was gentian violet, still sometimes prescribed. More commonly used today is nystatin or one of the imidazole synthetics—miconazole nitrate, clotrimazole, and butoconazole nitrate. A triazole antifungal—terconazole—has recently been marketed as well. These medications are available in cream or tablet form, to be applied intravaginally. Tablets often are preferred by women over creams as they are less messy. Boric acid has also been found to be effective against *Candida*. Systemic nystatin and, more recently, ketoconazole have been used for recurrent or persistent infections. Many self-help measures can be used in conjunction with treatment regimens and for prevention. These should be taught to women suffering from a yeast infection and to everyone as preventive measures.

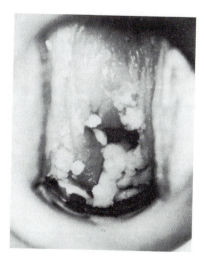

Figure 11–27. Masses of desquamated epithelial cells forming ''pseudo'' thrush patches. *(From Gardner, H. L. [1981]. Candidiasis. In H. L. Gardner & R. H. Kaufman [Eds.], Benign diseases of the vulva and vagina. [2nd ed.]. Boston: G. K. Hall Medical Publishers. Reprinted with permission.)*

Treatment Regimens. *Gentian violet* is used as a topical application in a 0.25 to 2.0 percent aqueous solution, which is usually applied to the vulva and vagina by the practitioner. The tablet form of gentian violet may be less messy and does not require practitioner application. Women should be advised to carefully follow the manufacturer's directions for use. Side effects of gentian violet include staining of clothes and linens and a chemical vulvovaginitis reaction. Chemical vulvovaginitis usually develops when the solutions used are too strong (1 to 2 percent) or are applied too frequently (more than every 2 to 3 days) (Gardner, 1981a, p. 231). Sometimes, the reaction to the gentian violet can be misdiagnosed as an exacerbation of the fungal infection.

Nystatin is available commercially as Mycostatin, Nilstat, or Nystex in cream, vaginal tablet, and ointment form. Recommended doses are one tablet or applicatorful of cream (100,000 units) vaginally for 14 days, twice a day or at bedtime only. Until the introduction of miconazole nitrate and clotrimazole, this was the most effective treatment against vulvovaginal *Candida*.

Miconazole nitrate, a newer drug, is marketed as Monistat cream or tablets. It is reported to be more effective than nystatin as a 14-day treatment. It is also effective in shorter regimens—3 to 7 days, used only at bedtime. This has the important advantage of increased compliance with the medication regimen. Some authors, however, do not advocate shorter treatments for recurrent episodes of candidal vaginitis (Granitzka, 1982).

Three to four percent of women using miconazole report minor local irritations (Gardner, 1981, p. 231) for which discontinuation of the medication provides effective relief. A small amount of medication is absorbed from the vagina; therefore, use of the drug is not advised in the first trimester of pregnancy. Caution is recommended in lactating women.

Miconazole nitrate also comes in a dermatologic preparation, Monistat derm, which can be used externally for candidal vulvitis or for treatment of the male. It can be applied twice a day for 1 to 2 weeks.

Clotrimazole, sold as Gyne-Lotrimin or Mycelex-G, is available in tablet or cream form. The 100-mg tablets are recommended for 6 or 7 nights' use; a 200-mg tablet is recommended for 3 nights' use (Stettendorf, Benijts, Vignali & Kreysing, 1982); and a 500-mg tablet has compared favorably in a 1-night regimen (Cohen, 1985; Fleury, Hughes, & Floyd, 1985; Krause, 1982; Lebherz, Guess, & Wolfson, 1985).

Ritter (1985) found the 1-night treatment to be equivalent to a 3-night regimen because the medication is found in the vagina for at least 3 days. Some authors, however, advise against 1 to 3 days of treatment for recurrent vaginitis (Mendling & Plempel, 1982) and generally, in pregnancy, a 6- or 7-day treatment is advised, after the first trimester.

Clotrimazole cream rarely causes local irritation (Goormans, Bergstein, Loendersloot, & Branolte, 1982). A minimal amount of medication is absorbed from the vaginal mucosa. Clotrimazole is available as Lotrimin cream for external use.

Butoconazole nitrate, an imidazole derivative, is marketed as Femstat and Femstat Prefill. It is a vaginal cream effective in nonpregnant women in a 3-day regimen and in pregnant women in a 6-day regimen.

Vulvovaginal itching and burning have been reported by a few patients using this medication, and discharge, soreness, swelling, and itching of the fingers have been noted in less than 1 percent of users (Syntex Laboratories, 1987). Some absorption of the drug occurs with intravaginal use and usage in the first trimester of pregnancy is not recommended; caution is advised during nursing.

Terconazole, marketed in 1988 by Ortho Pharmaceuticals as Terazol, is available in cream or tablet form. The cream (0.4 percent) is administered intravaginally at night for 7 days; the vaginal tablets (80 mg) are used for 3 nights.

Vulvovaginal burning and itching have been reported rarely in users of terconazole. Some absorption has been noted with this medication, and there may be adverse effects in nursing infants. The base may interact with rubber or latex products, and therefore it should not be used concurrently with vaginal diaphragms or condoms (Ortho Pharmaceutical Corporation, 1988). Use in the first trimester of pregnancy is not advised.

A double-blind comparison of *boric acid powder* with nystatin showed the boric acid to be more effective after a 14-day regimen in nonpregnant women (Van Slyke et al., 1981). Capsules can be made by the pharmacist or patient by filling size 0 gelatin capsules with 600 mg of boric acid. The main advantage of this treatment is its reduced cost. It is also reported to be less messy than vaginal creams, although it is probably not less messy than vaginal tablets. Toxicity has not been found with this treatment; blood boron levels are lower than what is considered toxic. This regimen is not recommended during pregnancy.

Treatment of Recurrent Vulvovaginal Candidiasis.   Persistent or recurrent vulvovaginal candidiasis poses a difficult treatment problem for women and practitioners. The causes of recurrent vulvovaginal candidiasis are not entirely understood.

Resistance of *Candida* to antifungal preparations has not been reported (Warnock, Speller, Milne, et al., 1979), although insufficient treatment may be a factor in recurrence with organisms lying in a dormant stage in the vaginal mucosa for weeks or even months (Sobel, 1985a). The role of an intestinal reservoir of *Candida* leading to perianal infection is controversial, as is the role of sexual transmission of the organism. Both of these may account for some, but probably not all, recurrences. Witkin, Yu, and Ledger (1983) suggest an impaired immune response to *Candida* among women with repeated candidal infections. This theory deserves further investigation; its elucidation may someday lead to more effective therapies for recurrent infections. A mild zinc deficiency may lead to an impaired immune response to the organism causing recurrence (Edman, Sobel, & Taylor, 1986). Horowitz, Edelstein, and Lippman (1985) suggest that in some resistant cases of candidiasis the offending organism is *Candida tropicalis*, a more difficult fungus to eradicate. Testing for diabetes mellitus can be carried out in women with persistent or recurrent candidiasis; *Candida*, however, is almost never the sole presenting symptom of diabetes.

The first step in treating a recurrent infection is correct diagnosis. Sobel (1984) reports that two thirds of women referred to him for recurrent vulvovaginal candidiasis did not in fact have this infection. Telephone diagnosis is obviously inappropriate.

A number of therapeutic measures have been suggested for recurrent vulvovaginal candidiasis. Longer therapies with miconazole or clotrimazole have been advocated. External treatment with a cream applied to the labial folds and beneath the foreskin of the clitoris may kill organisms harbored in these folds. Application of the cream to the perianal area may reduce transfer of rectal yeasts to the vagina (Forssman & Milsom, 1985). Treatment of sexual partners with a candicidal cream applied to the penis for 7 to 10 days may be useful. Condoms or abstinence during treatment is recommended (Gardner, 1981a, p. 233). Davidson and Mould (1978) suggest making sure that no concomitant infections exist whose presence may make eradication of the yeast more difficult.

If possible, antibiotic therapy should be discontinued. If antibiotics must be used for short-term therapy, an intravaginal candicidal agent can be used during and for several days after treatment (Gardner, 1981a, p. 233). Finding an alternative to oral contraceptives for birth control may be beneficial (Horowitz, Edelstein, & Lippman, 1987).

Prophylactic measures for women prone to recurrences include an intravaginal anticandidal medication for one or several nights before the onset of menses, when recurrences are most likely, or anytime irritation or flaring of symptoms is perceived (Cohen, 1985). Gardner (1981a) recommends using an intravaginal candicidal tablet every 2, 3, or 4 nights for up to 3 or 4 months.

Two types of oral anticandidal preparations have been tried for relief of persistent and recurrent candidiasis. Nystatin (Mycostatin, Nilstat, Nystex) is available in oral form as a tablet, liquid, oral suspension, or powder. A newer preparation, ketoconazole, is available in tablet form. Marketed commercially as Nizoral, it is an imidazole antifungal structurally related to miconazole nitrate and clotrimazole. The difference between these two oral medications is that nystatin is not absorbable; it works only on the digestive tract. Ketoconazole is absorbable and therefore works on the vaginal site (and anywhere else in the body where *Candida* may be harbored).

If the source of candidal reinfection were the intestinal tract, then theoretically oral nystatin would be effective in preventing recurrent vaginal candidiasis by wiping out this reservoir of infection. Recommended doses are 500,000 units (one tablet or one eighth of a teaspoon of powder dissolved in liquid) three times a day for 10 to 14 days. Such treatments, however, have not been shown to be effective in preventing vulvovaginal candidiasis (Gardner, 1981a, p. 233; Milne & Warnock, 1979). Nystatin is considered a benign drug without significant side effects (*Physicians' desk reference*, 1988).

Treatment with oral ketoconazole, 400 mg for 14 days, has been shown in prospective, placebo-controlled studies to be more effective against recurrent episodes of candidiasis, but relapses occur after withdrawal of the drug (Sobel, 1985b, 1986). A 3-month regimen, 400 mg daily for 5 days each menstrual cycle, has been shown to be more effective (Sobel, 1984). The optimal duration of prophylactic therapy is being studied. Although approved for use against oral thrush, mucocutaneous candidiasis, and other fungal infections, ketoconazole is still experimental as a treatment for vaginal candidiasis (Sobel, 1988).

Unfortunately, ketoconazole is a potent medication. It has been implicated in causing liver damage. Although the incidence of serious hepatic injury is low (estimated at one in 15,000 exposed persons), the incidence of mild, asymptomatic, reversible elevations in serum transaminases is estimated to be between 5 and 10 percent (Lewis, Zimmerman, Benson, & Ishak, 1984). Lewis and associates recommend periodic biochemical testing and monitoring for signs of hepatitis during therapy with this drug. Nausea and vomiting have been reported in 3 percent of users, and abdominal pain and pruritus in over 1 percent. Other side effects occur in less than 1 percent of users and include other gastrointestinal, dermatologic, musculoskeletal, nervous system, metabolic, nutritional, and ocular effects (Heel, Brogden, Carmine, et al., 1982). Medical consultation and/or referral should be initiated whenever this drug is considered.

SELF-HELP MEASURES. A number of self-help measures have been proposed to prevent fungal infection and recurrence of infection. These have not been subject to adequate scientific testing but are not harmful and may be preventive for many women. Decreasing the amount of simple sugars in the diet while increasing B-complex and vitamin A foods may be helpful.

The following self-help remedies, reported successful by some women for treating candidal infections, are adapted from The Boston Women's Health Book Collective (1984, p. 519) and Neeson and Stockdale (1981, p. 133):

- Daily yogurt douches or intravaginal applicatorfuls of yogurt twice a day for one week (Women must use plain yogurt with active cultures; advise them to read the container label.)
- Acidophilus tablets (These presumably have the same effect as yogurt: restoring *Lactobacillus acidophilus* in the vagina. One tablet has been advised at bedtime for 1 to 2 weeks. Interestingly, however, lactobacilli have been found to be present in excess amounts in the presence of vaginal candidiasis.)
- Douches of goldenseal–myrrh (one tablespoon of each in three cups of water, cooled and strained)
- Garlic suppositories, peeled and wrapped in gauze with a tail for retrieval, used two times a day for about 2 weeks, changed every 12 hours (Women can be reassured that this does not cause an unpleasant odor.)
- Aci-Jel, which acidifies the vaginal environment, used prior to menses or at the first signs of symptoms (Whether this is effective is doubtful as yeast grow in an acid environment.)

Some health practitioners believe that certain people have a particular sensitivity to yeast and advocate a diet low in foods that grow yeasts. These include many fruit and fruit juices, especially melon and dried fruit; breads and pastries; cheeses; alcoholic beverages; condiments, sauces, and vinegar; malt products; edible fungi; processed and smoked meats; teas and coffees; and leftovers in general. Obviously, such a diet is often difficult to maintain, but may be helpful for some individuals (Crook, 1986, pp. 83–84).

Diaphragms, douche bags, and bathtubs should be disinfected after an infection, although their role in reinfection is unknown (Gardner, 1981a, p. 219).

If the external irritation in a yeast infection is very uncomfortable, warm sitz baths may be soothing, and addition of Aveeno powder—a commercially available oatmeal solution—to the bath may increase the woman's comfort. Hygiene is important—wearing cotton fabrics, especially for underwear, avoiding rectovaginal contamination during sex and when wiping after urination or a bowel movement, and generally avoiding tight clothing and douching (Smith & Lauver, 1984).

Additional Teaching and Counseling. Women need to understand the nature of their infection. Careful instructions on use of prescribed treatments must be given and every effort made to ascertain that the woman understands proper medication usage. Women should be told to continue medication for the prescribed duration even if symptoms subside, and the reason for this should be explained carefully. With treatments of short duration, however, women need to be warned that symptoms may not subside during treatment or immediately after the treatment is completed. Vaginal creams and tablets should be kept at room temperature and placed in the vagina after the woman is in bed. Instructions for vaginal insertion should be given. A sanitary pad may help with secretions in the morning. Women should be advised to continue treatment even if menses intervenes but to avoid tampon use during treatment. Condoms or abstinence from sexual intercourse should be strongly advised during any course of treatment.

Trichomoniasis. Trichomoniasis is almost always a sexually transmitted disease. It is also the third most common cause of vaginal infection in women and is therefore included in this chapter. Its effects generally are limited to the vagina and cervix.

ETIOLOGY AND TRANSMISSION. *Trichomonas vaginalis* is the organism that causes trichomoniasis. It is an anaerobic one-celled protozoan with characteristic flagellae. The protozoa live in a moist environment and attach easily to mucous membranes. They can be harbored in the urethra, Skene's glands, and the urine as well as the vagina (Whittington, 1957).

Most often trichomoniasis is transmitted through sexual contact, with an incubation period varying from 4 to 28 days (Catterall, 1972). A number of other routes of infection are possible although likely to account for only a small number of cases. Trichomonads have been found to survive 90 minutes on a wet sponge and 24 hours in water maintained at 32°C centigrade or warmer and on wet cloths used by infected women. The latter finding may account for the occurrence of some cases among institutionalized women (Rein & Müller, 1984). *T. vaginalis* has also been found to survive in vaginal secretions, semen, and urine for 48, 6, and 3 hours, respectively. It survives 45 minutes on toilet seats and in toilet water. The water that splashes after defecation could presumably infect the genital area, although transmission via public toilets has never been documented (Rein & Müller, 1984). Transmission through chlorinated swimming pools or communal bathtubs is unlikely but possible.

PREVALENCE. Trichomoniasis (often call trichomonas) has been estimated to occur in 5 to 33 percent of women, depending on the population studied. The higher rates have been found in women attending STD clinics; the lower rates among married women employees and women attending family planning clinics. The incidence of trichomoniasis peaks at ages 16 to 35, but the infection is relatively prevalent among women aged 30 to 40 and even among women aged 40 to 50 (Rein & Müller, 1984).

CLINICAL PRESENTATION. Trichomoniasis may be asymptomatic, acute, or chronic. In asymptomatic infection, the vaginal pH is 3.8 to 4.2 with organisms present. Women with asymptomatic infections often give a history of clinical symptomatology and may in the future become symptomatic (Gardner, 1981e). Approximately 50 percent of women with trichomonal infection may be asymptomatic (Fouts & Kraus, 1980; Wisdom & Dunlop, 1965).

In chronic infection, vulvar and vaginal tissues are not affected, although vaginal secretions are of abnormal amount, odor, consistency, or pH. Irritation may or may not be present.

Acute infection is characterized by abnormal vaginal discharge, classically yellow green and frothy, although it may be gray and nonfrothy; inflammation of the vulva, vagina, or both; feelings of irritation; and, most especially, pruritus. A foul odor is often noted. Dysuria and dyspareunia may be present. Secretions may be noted from the urethra or Skene's glands. The vagina may be erythematous, swollen, excoriated, abraded, or ecchymotic, with a granular appearance in severe cases. Petechiae may be noted in the vagina or on the cervix. The latter is commonly referred to as a "strawberry" cervix (Figure 11–28). Tender inguinal lymph nodes are present in a small number of women with *T. vaginalis*. Lower abdominal pain may be experienced by a few women, possibly as a result of lymphadenitis. Exacerbation of symptoms often occurs during or shortly after menses. Menstrual pain may occur as a result of congestion (Catterall, 1972; Jirovec & Petrü, 1968). Occasionally a woman with trichomoniasis may present with multiple gasfilled cystoid cavities in the vagina and cervix (called *vaginitis emphysematosa*). These give the vagina a granular feel. Sometimes, when they rupture, which usually happens after intercourse or speculum examination, bleeding occurs.

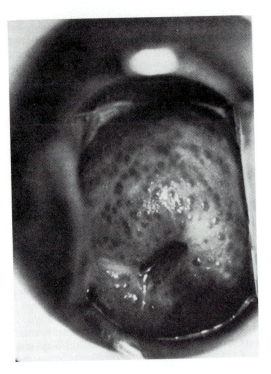

Figure 11–28. Strawberry cervix. *(From Kaufman, R. H. & Faro, S. [1987]. Infectious diseases of the vulva and vagina. In E. J. Wilkinson [Ed.].* Pathology of the vulva and vagina. *New York: Churchill Livingstone. Reprinted with permission.)*

DIFFERENTIAL DIAGNOSIS. Trichomoniasis must be differentiated from other forms of vaginitis. The symptoms of increased discharge and odor may confuse it with BV, whereas the intense itching may be mistaken for candidiasis. Other STDs that may present with discharge must be considered, including gonorrhea and chlamydia (see Chapter 12).

MANAGEMENT

Data Collection. *History.* A careful description of symptoms, their onset and course, and their relationship to menses should be elicited. A sexual history is important as the disease is most often sexually transmitted. Ascertain whether the woman has shared towels with other women. Whether the woman has had similar symptoms in the past may help differentiate chronic from acute infections, although reinfection should be ruled out. Previous treatments and their results should be discussed; if the woman reports treatment, find out if her partner was similarly treated or if she has subsequently had relations with a new partner.

Physical Examination. The inguinal area should be palpated for adenopathy. The vulva, vagina, and cervix must be visually inspected and the urethra gently milked for discharge. A speculum examination is necessary, although it may be uncomfortable. Relaxation techniques and gentle pressure can help the woman accept the speculum.

Practitioners should bear in mind that any of the classic signs may or may not be present on physical examination and cannot be used for definitive diagnosis. Researchers have shown that if a purulent frothy discharge is used as the sole diagnostic criterion, trichomonal infection will be missed 88 percent of the time. A strawberry cervix can be considered diagnostic but is found in only approximately 2 percent of women with trichomoniasis (Fouts & Krause, 1980; Rein & Müller, 1984).

Laboratory Testing. Testing of vaginal pH is a diagnostic aid. The pH in women with acute trichomoniasis is generally 5.2 to 6.0. Definitive diagnosis must be made through demonstration of the organism, however. This is most easily done via a wet smear prepared with normal saline. Discharge from the anterior and posterior fornices is taken on a cotton swab, either placed into a test tube containing 1 mL of saline and transferred to a slide or mixed directly on the slide with a drop of saline. The slide should be examined immediately under the microscope using low and high power. Some authors advise warming the slide first to increase motility of the organisms by passing a match under it.

With trichomonal infection, epithelial cells are present; polymorphonuclear neutrophils (PMNs) are increased and may equal or exceed the number of epithelial cells (Rein & Müller, 1984). Bacterial rods may be present and other pathogens, such as *Candida*, may be concomitantly noted. The diagnostic finding is the presence of *trichomonads*. These organisms are usually larger than the PMNs and smaller than the epithelial cells, although in some women they may be smaller or larger than usual. Protruding from each trichomonad are four flagellae, which are never visible under low power and only sometimes visible under high power see Chapter 4, Figure 4–4.

Healthy trichomonads appear on the wet mount as motile ovoids, usually moving in the direction of the flagellae. Their characteristic motion has been described as jerky or twitching (Gardner, 1981e). Unhealthy trichomonads assume a rounded shape and are more difficult to identify. They may be present in urinary sediment or in the vagina after the woman has douched with a medicated solution, or when the vagina is more acidic, as it may be in asymptomatic cases. These trichomonads are sluggish and may be seen only under high magnification (Gardner, 1981d).

Unfortunately, reports show that wet mounts identify trichomonads in only approximately 60 to 75 percent of cases (Ackers, Lumsden, Catterall, & Coyle, 1975; Hipp, Kirkwood, & Gaafar, 1979; Spence, Hollander, Smith, et al., 1980; Whittington, 1957). Trichomonads may not be seen in early stages of an acute infection. In a woman reporting typical trichomoniasis symptoms for only a day or two, with a negative wet mount, a reexamination is warranted in the next several days (Gardner, 1981e).

A smear stained with Giemsa or acridine orange can also be used to identify *T. vaginalis*. This has no advantages, however, over a wet smear. Gram stains are not recommended because the trichomonads are difficult to distinguish from PMNs by this method (Rein & Müller, 1984).

A number of serologic tests for *T. vaginalis* have been developed; most recently, an enzyme-linked immunosorbent assay for the detection of antibody has been made available. Sensitivity, however, is only 66 percent and specificity, 79 percent, limiting the clinical usefulness of the assay (Jirovec & Petrü, 1968; Sibau, Bebb, Proctor, & Bowie, 1987).

Trichomoniasis can be identified on Pap smears. The characteristic features of a Pap smear in a woman with trichomoniasis are a dirty or smudged background and an increased number of WBCs and parabasal and intermediate cells. The false-negative rate by Pap smear is equivalent to that by the wet smear (Hipp et al., 1979; Mason, Super, &

Fripp, 1976; Spence et al., 1980). The Pap smear also may mistakenly identify trichomonads. Perl (1972) found a 48.4 percent error rate in a sample of Pap smears from 1,199 women; more than half of the errors were false positives. Some experts recommend clinical examination with either wet smear or culture to confirm a diagnosis reported on Pap smear before treatment is initiated (Gardner, 1981e). Trichomoniasis can also lead to cytologic changes that may be confused on Pap smear with cervical neoplasia. Such changes regress after treatment (Gardner, 1981e).

Culture media suitable for trichomonal growth include simplified trypticase serum of Kupferberg, Wittington–Feinberg medium, and Trichosel broth (Gardner, 1981c, 1981e). Cultures usually show growth within 48 hours but should be held for 7 days. Culture is not needed when trichomonads are identified on wet mount.

Intervention. *Treatment*. The CDC-recommended treatment for trichomoniasis is metronidazole 2.0 g by mouth in a single dose (Centers for Disease Control, 1985, p. 99s). An alternate regimen is 250 mg of metronidazole by mouth three times daily for 7 days. The two regimens are comparable in effectiveness (Thin, Symonds, Booker, et al., 1979). Advantages of the single-dose regimen include increased patient compliance and an overall lower dose. It is unknown whether the single-dose regimen might lower or increase the possible carcinogenecity of the drug (Beard et al., 1979).

Treatment with the 2.0-g single-dose regimen is recommended for asymptomatic women and for sexual partners of women with trichomoniasis. Examining the male partner for trichomonal infection is not advised although the CDC recommends examining women and sexual partners for coexisting STDs.

Metronidazole is contraindicated in the first trimester of pregnancy, and CDC recommends avoiding its use throughout pregnancy if possible. Clotrimazole 100 mg per vagina for 7 days has been reported to provide symptomatic relief and cures in some cases; it is a good first-choice treatment during pregnancy. Lactating women can be treated with the 2.0-g single dose, but breastfeeding must be stopped during treatment and for at least 24 hours afterward. Side effects of metronidazole therapy and additional contraindications are discussed under Bacterial Vaginosis.

Some practitioners may be uncomfortable treating sexual partners of their patients. If partners are not treated, however, the likelihood is that the infection will recur. Female partners can be given appointments for examination or referred to their own gynecologic practitioners. Their pregnancy status should be ascertained before treatment is initiated. The history of any person to be treated with metronidazole should be checked for convulsive disorders or leukopenia. An alternative to treating a male sexual partner is to refer him to his health care provider, an STD clinic, a dermatologist, or a urologist for treatment. Treatment of both partners should be simultaneous if possible, and sexual contact should be avoided during its course. If simultaneous treatment is not possible, then sexual contact should be avoided until both partners have completed treatment although a condom may be protective.

Resistant Trichomoniasis. A rare problem in the treatment of trichomoniasis is the metronidazole-resistant infection. Resistance, of course, must be evaluated by examination and, by history, distinguished from reinfection (Hager, Spence, & Mead, 1985).

Although trichomonads resistant to metronidazole have been demonstrated in the laboratory, researchers have found that 85 percent of resistant infections are readily cured with a second course of treatment (Müller, Lossick, & Gorrell, 1988). The Centers for Disease Control (1985) recommends re-treatment with the same regimen. Metronidazole 2.0 g by mouth for 3 days may be effective in mildly resistant cases but the CDC reports limited experience with this regimen. They recommend consultation with an expert for persistent treatment failures. See Bacterial Vaginosis for guidelines on using repeat doses of metronidazole.

Authorities have reported an increased number of treatment failures in patients on phenobarbital and phenytoin, probably because these drugs increase the rapidity with which the liver detoxifies the drug (Hager, et al., 1985). These patients may need increased doses of metronidazole. Their treatment should be managed in consultation with a physician.

Self-Help Measures. Self-help measures may facilitate the treatment of trichomoniasis or relieve symptoms before treatments can be initiated. These include measures to acidify the vagina, for example, vinegar douches. Goldenseal–myrrh douches have been suggested (see Bacterial Vaginosis for instructions on their use) as have chickweed douches. Chickweed douches are made by boiling one quart of water, adding three tablespoons of chickweed, covering the solution, seeping it 5 to 10 minutes, and then straining. Daily douches should be continued for 1 week. Garlic suppositories may also be helpful [see Bacterial Vaginosis (The Boston Women's Health Book Collective, 1984)].

Additional Teaching and Counseling. Women with trichomoniasis need to understand the sexual transmission of this disease. Counseling must be provided in a sensitive manner, as the infection can exist for long periods and it is not possible to tell the woman when she became infected. The woman must be given the opportunity to ask questions and ventilate her feelings. Women should be informed that all sexual partners should be treated. A preferred method of questioning is to ask how many partners need to be treated, rather than to ask if the woman has more than one partner. She may want to discuss how to raise the issue with her partner or partners. She needs information to give to her partners who may resist treatment because they are likely to be asymptomatic. She should be provided with literature for herself and her partner(s) and the partner invited to call the practitioner or clinic or given an appointment to talk. Partners should be treated at the same time as the woman and they should refrain from intercourse or use condoms before and during treatment. Reassurance can be offered the woman that trichomoniasis does not become a systemic infection and is not known to be a cause of infertility. Sharing of towels among women should be discouraged.

Atrophic Vaginitis. Anything that lowers estrogen levels after puberty can result in a loss of vaginal thickness and rugation and a decrease in the elasticity of the vaginal tissues. The pH of the vagina rises, growth of lactobacilli is discouraged, and other bacteria tend to multiply, leading at times to vaginitis. This estrogen-deficient condition, referred to as *atrophic vaginitis*, most commonly occurs among breastfeeding women and women who have undergone natural or surgical menopause. The Boston Women's Health Book Collective (1984) points out that ''atrophic'' is an unfortunate designation to refer to a process that is part of the normal life cycle; this terminology, however, is widely used.

ETIOLOGY. Vaginitis in the postmenopausal woman is rarely due to any of the organisms responsible for vaginitis in the premenopausal woman; candidiasis, trichomoniasis, and bacterial vaginosis are uncommon after the menstruating years. Gardner (1981f) reports some vaginitis caused by various streptococci, including beta streptococci and *Streptococcus faecalis*. He contends, however, that although bacteria play a role in atrophic vaginitis, they may not be the essential cause of the clinical manifestations of the problem. The cause is the depletion of estrogen and the overall effects of the aging process.

CLINICAL PRESENTATION. The woman with atrophic vaginitis may report a small amount of vaginal bleeding after intercourse. She may have dysuria, external burning, pruritus, tenderness, and dyspareunia. She may note a thin, often watery discharge, variable in amount. Bladder symptoms may be present as there may be changes in the bladder as well (see Chapter 24).

Sparse and brittle pubic hair, shrinking of the labia minora, and inflammation of the vulva may be noted in menopausal women. The vulva may appear erythematous and there may be labial edema. Excoriation may be present especially if the woman had complained of pruritus. The vagina may appear pale and without rugation. There may be patches of inflammation along the vaginal wall and on the cervix and possibly petechiae or ecchymosis. Vaginal discharge may be watery, purulent, serosanguineous, or sticky. It may be yellow or gray. Speculum or digital examination may cause spotting from the mucosa.

DIFFERENTIAL DIAGNOSIS. Other forms of vaginitis must be excluded before a diagnosis of atrophic vaginitis is made. Gonorrhea and chlamydia should be excluded as well. If bleeding is a symptom in a postmenopausal woman, the practitioner *must* rule out bleeding of uterine origin. If there is *any* doubt, consultation for endometrial biopsy or dilation and curettage (D&C) must be obtained (see Chapter 24).

MANAGEMENT

Data Collection. *History*. In addition to a complete medical history of symptoms, the most important historic data are the woman's age and menstrual status. Ascertain whether she has stopped menstruating or has had a surgically induced menopause. Find out whether other menopausal symptoms such as hot flashes or flushes are present. If she is premenopausal, ascertain whether she is lactating. Some women continue to nurse several years after birth so do not make assumptions about this.

Physical Examination. Complete pelvic examination including inspection of the external genitalia and speculum and bimanual examinations are necessary. Observe for the signs of atrophy described previously and for sites of bleeding if it has been reported.

Laboratory Testing. The vaginal pH should be tested; it usually is 5.5 to 7.0. A wet mount should be prepared; this usually reveals decreased lactobacilli and increased white blood cells and bacteria. Organisms involved in other forms of vaginitis may be present. Spotting or blood-tinged discharge always indicates the need for a Pap smear and possibly an endometrial biopsy or D&C if it is uterine in origin. A maturation index taken with a spatula from the upper lateral third of the vaginal wall can indicate decreased estrogenization of the vagina by demonstrating an increase in parabasal cells and a decrease in intermediate and superficial cells (Cutler & Garcia, 1984). Gonorrhea and chlamydia cultures are also indicated if white blood cells are present on the wet smear, if bleeding is a presenting complaint, or if sexual history reveals exposure or infection in any partner.

Intervention.   Referral of the perimenopausal woman with vaginal spotting or bleeding is necessary. Cancer of the cervix or endometrium must be ruled out.

Once the diagnosis of atrophic vaginitis has been made, water-soluble lubrication may be recommended for intercourse. Hormonal replacement in the form of vaginal or systemic estrogens may be warranted for the postmenopausal woman. The use of estrogen, which should always be supplemented with cyclic progesterone, is discussed fully in Chapter 24. This discussion includes the indications for usage, the advantages and disadvantages of the therapy including risks, the initial workup required before initiation of therapy, appropriate treatment regimens, and recommended follow-up. Hormonal replacement requires medical consultation or referral, depending on specific institutional or practice protocols.

A number of self-help measures can be recommended for both perimenopausal and breastfeeding women. Kegel exercises to improve muscle tone and elasticity of the vagina may be helpful and are described in Chapters 3 and 17. An open, sensitive discussion of sexuality should be initiated by the practitioner. The woman should be reassured that this problem is physical, not emotional. Lubrication for intercourse may be extremely helpful. Water-soluble jel, available over-the-counter in a number of commercial preparations, or vegetable oil such as olive oil can be used. Masturbation without penetration may be suggested as a gratifying form of sexual expression in the initial lactation period. Masturbation also facilitates the natural resumption of the production of lubricating secretions by the body (The Boston Women's Health Book Collective, 1984). In the female-superior position, the woman can control the depth of thrusting and this may prove to be a more comfortable position during lactation. Women should be counseled to discuss the problem with their partners and explain to them its physical cause. They should be given support for determining their own sexuality. Of course, treatment of any secondary infection is necessary.

Additional Self-Help Measures.   The Boston Women's Health Book Collective (1984) recommends topical applications of bancha tea or vitamin E oil for vulvar dryness. Vinegar douches or Aci-Jel can help restore vaginal pH.

Additional Teaching and Counseling.   Women need explanations of the etiology of atrophic vaginitis. They should understand that it is a natural part of a woman's life cycle. It does not mean that the sexual organs are truly "atrophying." Sexuality can continue throughout life; indeed, the best method for ensuring continuing comfort with sexual intercourse is to maintain an active sex life.

Menopause may be an emotional issue for some women. Ascertain what each woman knows about the menopause and explore with her any misconceptions she may have. Chapter 24 provides detailed discussion of the physical and psychological changes associated with menopause as well as hormonal replacement therapy and self-help measures for enhancing all aspects of health during this life stage.

Contact Vulvovaginitis: Chemical and Allergic Vaginitis.
Vulvovaginitis may result from reactions to exogenous agents, most often medications used to treat infections or to maintain vaginal hygiene (Gardner, 1981b). Two types of reactions may be seen: primary irritant reactions and allergic reactions. A primary irritant is a substance that can produce irritation on first exposure. It may be a chemical such as an acid. Sometimes this reaction is not seen until prolonged exposure and is called cumulative primary irritation. Use over time of intravaginal medications for vaginitis may produce a cumulative primary irritation.

Allergic reactions are known as contact dermatitis or allergic eczema. These differ from primary irritant reactions because they occur only in persons with susceptibility and after previous exposure. Allergic reactions may take several days or weeks to manifest themselves and may follow local or systemic administration of the allergen.

CLINICAL PRESENTATION.   Primary irritant and allergic reactions may not be clinically distinguishable from each other. The signs usually include erythema, edema, vesicles or blisters, and oozing. Ulceration may occur and, over time, scaling. Thickening of the skin and white patches may develop. Women with these problems present most commonly with pruritus. Other symptoms include tenderness, pain, and burning. External dysuria may occur, and some women report an inability to urinate secondary to the discomfort. Adenitis may be present.

DIFFERENTIAL DIAGNOSIS.   Allergic or irritant vulvovaginitis must be differentiated from other forms of vulvar and vaginal disorders many of which have been described previously in this chapter. Some of the more common diagnoses with which irritant or allergic reactions may be confused are candidiasis, trichomoniasis, tinea cruris, seborrheic dermatitis, psoriasis, and herpes genitalis. The diagnosis may be especially difficult when the reaction is to a medication used to treat vulvovaginitis. It is important to distinguish a resistant or recurrent infection from a medication reaction.

MANAGEMENT

Data Collection.   *History.* A careful history is the most important part of data collection. Exposure to possible irritants or allergens should be determined. Possible agents include chemicals or douches; vaginal medications; vaginal spermicides or the base used in their manufacture, including spermicides in the vaginal contraceptive sponge; rubber (as in condoms, diaphragms, or cervical caps); copper in copper IUDs; plants such as poison ivy or poison oak; vaginal deodorants or perfumes; toilet paper dye; noncotton underwear or the elastic in underwear, especially in the summer, or bleach or detergent in which underwear is washed; potassium permanganate (no longer widely used); local or systemic antibiotics; and topical anesthetics (Gardner, 1981b). Some of these substances act as allergens in some women and as irritants in other women. Recent changes in vaginal hygiene practices and use of soaps and detergents or contraceptive methods should be explored; all medication usage and local therapies should be determined.

Physical Examination.   The vulva and vagina should be visually inspected for signs of erythema, edema, and lesions. A speculum examination is necessary. Signs of other types of vaginitis should be noted.

Laboratory Testing.   A wet smear must be made to rule out offending organisms, and Pap smears and cultures taken as necessary. A patch test, described under Contact Dermatitis, in the section on The Vulva, may help determine whether a woman is sensitive or allergic to a particular agent. An immediate reaction indicates an irritant response, whereas a delayed reaction suggests an allergy; however, a positive reaction may not be seen on skin because it is not damp like the vulva or vagina. Consultation with a dermatologist or allergist may be necessary for diagnosis and should be undertaken when all gynecologic diagnoses have been ruled out.

Intervention.   *Treatment.* Most often, removal of the offending substance is all that is needed to alleviate the chemical or allergic reaction. Topically applied wet compresses of Burrow's or boric acid solution may bring relief. After 1 to 2 days of wet compresses, cortisone cream can be applied if necessary. Antihistamines such as diphenhydramine may not be helpful except for certain reactions such as penicillin allergies. Topical antihistamines may themselves induce an allergic reaction and are not recommended (Gardner, 1981b).

Referral.   Referral is warranted for severe allergic reactions. Treatment with systemic corticosteroids may be necessary. Referral is also necessary whenever other causes of the disorder are ruled out and removal of the presumed irritant along with topical relief measures do not cure the problem.

Self-Help Measures.   In instances of suspected contact vulvovaginitis when the offending substance cannot be easily identified by history, a woman may need to become aware of possible exposures and keep careful track of them to identify and eliminate the cause of her problem. She should avoid vaginal medications, douches, deodorants, perfumes and perfumed toilet paper, sanitary pads, and tampons. She can be advised to try different types or brands of barrier contraceptives or to have a copper IUD removed. She should use detergents without perfumes, bleaches, or fabric softeners and avoid adding bleach or softener to her laundry, especially to underwear washes. She can put her laundry through a double rinse. She should wear cotton underwear and keep the vaginal area as dry as possible as sometimes the moisture in the environment encourages the reaction.

Additional Teaching and Counseling.   As with any vaginal problem, the woman with a chemical or allergic reaction needs reassurance. Because a cause for the disorder may not be readily apparent, she needs patient and sensitive care. Recognition that she has a problem, even if the cause is not easily identified, is therapeutic. For some women who react to vaginal contraceptives, the problem can be particularly devastating if she has exhausted other methods of birth control or is opposed to their use. Although ultimately, the woman herself must find a solution to this problem, the help of a caring practitioner can be invaluable.

REFERENCES

Ackers, J. P., Lumsden, W. H. R., Catterall, R. D., & Coyle, R. (1975, October). Antitrichomonal antibody in the vaginal secretions of women infected with *T. vaginalis*. *British Journal of Venereal Diseases, 51*(5), 319–323.

Al-Kurdi, M., & Monaghan, J. M. (1981, November). Thirty-two years experience in management of primary tumours of the vagina. *British Journal of Obstetrics and Gynaecology, 88*(11), 1145–1150.

Altchek, A. (1985). Pediatric and adolescent gynecology. In D. H. Nichols and J. R. Evrard (Eds.), *Ambulatory gynecology*. Philadelphia: Harper & Row.

American Cancer Society. (1987). *Cancer facts and figures.* New York: American Cancer Society.

Amsel, R., Totten, P. A., Spiegel, C. A., et al. (1983, January). Nonspecific vaginitis: Diagnostic criteria and microbial and epidemiologic associations. *American Journal of Medicine, 74*(1), 14–22.

Beard, C. M., Noller, K. L., O'Fallon, W. M., et al. (1979, September 6). Lack of evidence for cancer due to use of metronidazole. *New England Journal of Medicine, 301*(10), 519–522.

Benedet, J. L., Murphy, K. J., Fairey, R. N., & Boyes, D. A. (1983, December). Primary invasive carcinoma of the vagina. *Obstetrics and Gynecology, 62*(6), 715–719.

The Boston Women's Health Book Collective. (1984). *The new our bodies, ourselves.* New York: Simon & Schuster.

Breen, J. T. (1971, March 18). Vaginitis and tights [Letter]. *British Medical Journal, 1*(5749), 610.

Bull, M. J. V. (1969, January 11). Wearing tights. *British Medical Journal, 1*(5636), 120.

Buttram, V. C. (1983, August). Müllerian anomalies and their management. *Fertility and Sterility, 40*(2), 159–163.

Catterall, R. D. (1971, February). Influence of gestogenic contraceptive pills on vaginal candidosis. *British Journal of Venereal Diseases, 47*(1), 45–47.

Catterall, R. D. (1972, September). Trichomonal infections of the genital tract. *Medical Clinics of North America, 56*(5), 1203–1209.

Centers for Disease Control. (1979, February 16). Nonreported sexually transmissible diseases—United States. *Morbidity and Mortality Weekly Report, 28*(6), 61–63.

Centers for Disease Control. (1985, October 18). 1985 STD treatment guidelines. *Morbidity and Mortality Weekly Report, 34*(4, Suppl.), 75S–108S.

Cherniak, D. (1983). *A book about sexually transmitted diseases.* Montreal, Canada: Montreal Health Press.

Cohen, B. E., & Elin, R. J. (1974, August). Enhanced resistance to certain infections in vitamin A-treated mice. *Plastic and Reconstructive Surgery, 54*(2), 192–194.

Cohen, L. (1969, September). Influence of pH on vaginal discharges. *British Journal of Venereal Diseases, 45*(3), 241–247.

Cohen, L. (1985, August 1). Is more than one application of an antifungal necessary in the treatment of acute vaginal candidiasis? *American Journal of Obstetrics and Gynecology, 152*(7, Part 2), 961–964.

Copeland, L. J., Sneige, N., Gershenson, D. M., et al. (1986, June). Bartholin gland carcinoma. *Obstetrics and Gynecology, 67*(6), 794–801.

Crafts, R. C. (1986). The female reproductive tract. In D. N. Danforth & J. R. Scott (Eds.), *Obstetrics and gynecology* (5th ed.). Philadelphia: J. B. Lippincott.

Crook, W. G. (1986). *The yeast connection* (3rd ed.). Jackson, TN: Professional Books.

Cutler, W. B., & Garcia, C.-R., (1984). *The medical managemenet of menopause and premenopause: Their endocrinologic basis.* Philadelphia: J. B. Lippincott.

Davidson, F. (1977, February). Yeasts and circumcision in the male. *British Journal of Venereal Diseases, 53*(1), 121–122.

Davidson, F., Hayes, J. P., & Hussein, S. (1977, April). Recurrent genital candidosis and iron metabolism. *British Journal of Venereal Diseases, 53*(2), 123–125.

Davidson, F., & Mould, R. T. (1978, June). Recurrent genital candidosis in women and the effect of intermittent prophylactic treatment. *British Journal of Venereal Diseases, 54*(3), 176–183.

Davis, B. A. (1969, July). Vaginal moniliasis in private practice. *Obstetrics and Gynecology, 34*(1), 40–45.

Davis, P. C., & Franklin, E. W. (1975, October). Cancer of the vagina. *Southern Medical Journal, 68*(10), 1239–1242.

Diddle, A. W., Gardner, W. H., Williamson, P. J., & O'Connor, K. A. (1969, September). Oral contraceptive medications and vulvovaginal candidiasis. *Obstetrics and Gynecology, 34*(3), 373–377.

DiSaia, P. J. (1987, October 15). The case against the surgical concept of en bloc dissection for certain malignancies of the reproductive tract. *Cancer, 60*(8, Suppl.), 2025–2034.

Edman, J., Sobel, J. D., & Taylor, M. L. (1986, November). Zinc status in women with recurrent vulvovaginal candidiasis. *American Journal of Obstetrics and Gynecology, 155* (5), 1082–1085.

Elegbe, I. A., & Botu, M. (1982, February) A preliminary study on dressing patterns and incidence of candidiasis. *American Journal of Public Health, 72*(2), 176–177.

Elsner, P. & Hartmann, A. A. (1987, April–June). *Gardnerella vaginalis* in the male upper genital tract: A possible source of reinfection of the female partner. *Sexually Transmitted Diseases, 14*(2), 122–123.

Ervin, C. T., Komaroff, A. L., Baranowski, K., & Pass, T. M. (1982, February). Behavioral factors and vaginitis. *Nurse Practitioner, 7*(2), 20–21.

Fairey, R. N., MacKay, P. A., Benedet, J. L., et al. (1985, March 1). Radiation treatment of carcinoma of the vulva, 1950–1980. *American Journal of Obstetrics and Gynecology, 151*(5), 591–597.

Figge, D. C., Tamini, H. K., & Greer, B. E. (1985, June 15). Lymphatic spread in carcinoma of the vulva. *American Journal of Obstetrics and Gynecology, 152*(4), 387–394.

Fisher, S. G. (1979, June). Psychosexual adjustment following total pelvic exenteration. *Cancer Nursing, 2*(3), 219–225.

Fletcher, J., Mather, J., Lewis, M. J., & Whiting, G. (1975, January). Mouth lesions in iron-deficient anemia: Relationship to *Candida albicans* in saliva and to impairment of lymphocyte transformation. *Journal of Infectious Diseases, 131*(1), 44–50.

Fleury, F., Hughes, D., & Floyd, R. (1985, August 1). Therapeutic results obtained in vaginal mycoses after single-dose treatment with 500 mg clotrimazole vaginal tablets. *American Journal of Obstetrics and Gynecology, 52*(7, Part 2), 968–970.

Forssman, L., & Milsom, I. (1985, August 1). Treatment of recurrent vaginal candidiasis. *American Journal of Obstetrics and Gynecology, 152*(7, Part 2), 959–960.

Fouts, A. C., & Kraus, S. J. (1980, February). *Trichomonas vaginalis*: Reevaluation of its clinical presentation and laboratory diagnosis. *Journal of Infectious Diseases, 141*(2), 137–143.

Friedrich, E. G. (1985a, June 1). Vaginitis. *American Journal of Obstetrics and Gynecology, 152* (3), 247–251.

Friedrich, E. G. (1985b, March). Vulvar dystrophy. *Clinical Obstetrics and Gynecology, 28*(1), 178–187.

Friedrich, E. G., & MacLaren, N. K. (1984, September 15). Genetic aspects of vulvar lichen sclerosus. *American Journal of Obstetrics and Gynecology, 150*(2), 161–166.

Gardner, H. L. (1981a). Candidiasis. In H. L. Gardner & R. H. Kaufman (Eds.), *Benign diseases of the vulva and vagina* (2nd ed.). Boston: G. K. Hall.

Gardner, H. L. (1981b). Contact vulvovaginitis: Primary irritant and allergic reactions. In H. L. Gardner & R. H. Kaufman (Eds.), *Benign diseases of the vulva and vagina* (2nd ed.). Boston: G. K. Hall.

Gardner, H. L. (1981c). Interpretation of common signs, symptoms, and laboratory findings. In H. L. Gardner & R. H. Kaufman (Eds.), *Benign diseases of the vulva and vagina* (2nd ed.). Boston: G. K. Hall.

Gardner, H. L. (1981d). Pyodermas of the vulva. In H. L. Gardner & R. H. Kaufman (Eds.), *Benign diseases of the vulva and vagina* (2nd ed.). Boston: G. K. Hall.

Gardner, H. L. (1981e). Trichomoniasis. In H. L. Gardner & R. H. Kaufman (Eds.), *Benign diseases of the vulva and vagina* (2nd ed.). Boston: G. K. Hall.

Gardner, H. L. (1981f). Vulvovaginal atrophism and atrophic vaginitis. In H. L. Gardner & R. H. Kaufman (Eds.), *Benign diseases of the vulva and vagina* (2nd ed.). Boston: G. K. Hall.

Gardner, H. L., & Dukes, C. D. (1955, May) *Haemophilus vaginalis* vaginitis: A newly defined specific infection previously classified nonspecific vaginitis. *American Journal of Obstetrics and Gynecology, 69*(5), 962–976.

Gardner, H. L., & Kaufman, R. H. (1981). *Benign diseases of the vulva and vagina* (2nd ed.). Boston: G. K. Hall.

Gillespie, H. L., Inmon, W. B., & Slater, V. (1960, August). Incidence of *Candida* in the vagina during pregnancy. *Obstetrics and Gynecology, 16*(2), 185–188.

Gomez-Carrion, Y., Kaufman, R. H., & Richart, R. J. (1988, February). Treatment priorities for vulvar neoplasia. *Contemporary Ob/Gyn, 31*(2), 79–94.

Goormans, E., Bergstein, N. A. M., Loendersloot, E. W., & Branolte, J. H. (1982). One-dose therapy of *Candida* vaginitis. *Chemotherapy, 28*(Suppl. 1), 106–109.

Granitzka, S. (1982). Efficiency of various therapeutic concepts in genital mycoses. *Chemotherapy, 28*(Suppl. 1), 92–98.

Green, T. H. (1977). *Gynecology* (3rd ed.). Boston: Little, Brown.

Hager, W. D., Spence, M. R., & Mead, P. B. (1985, June). Trichomoniasis: Reinfection or resistance? *Contemporary Ob/Gyn, 25*(6), 141–148.

Heel, R. C., Brogden, R. N., Carmine, A., et al. (1982, January–February). Ketoconazole: A review of its therapeutic efficacy in superficial and systemic fungal infections. *Drugs, 23*(1/2), 1–36.

Hilborne, L. E., & Fu, Y. S. (1987). Intraepithelial, invasive, and metastatic neoplasms of the vagina. In E. J. Wilkinson (Ed.), *Pathology of the vulva and vagina*. New York: Churchill Livingstone.

Hilton, A. L. & Warnock, D. W. (1975, November). Vaginal candidiasis and the role of the digestive tract as a source of infection. *British Journal of Obstetrics and Gynaecology, 82*(11), 922–926.

Hipp, S. S., Kirkwood, M. W., & Gaafar, H. A. (1979, October–November). Screening for *Trichomonas vaginalis* infection by use of acridine orange fluorescent microscopy. *Sexually Transmitted Diseases, 6*(4), 235–238.

Horos, C. (1975). *Vaginal health*. New Canaan, CT: Tobey.

Horowitz, B. J., Edelstein, S. W., & Lippman, L. (1984, July). Sugar chromatography studies in recurrent *Candida* vulvovaginitis. *Journal of Reproductive Medicine, 29*(7), 441–443.

Horowitz, B. J., Edelstein, S. W., & Lippman, L. (1985, August). *Candida tropicalis* vulvovaginitis. *Obstetrics and Gynecology, 66*(2), 229–232.

Horowitz, B. J., Edelstein, S. W., & Lippman, L. (1987, June). Sexual transmission of *Candida*. *Obstetrics and Gynecology, 69*(6), 883–886.

Iversen, T. (1985, March). New approaches to treatment of squamous cell carcinoma of the vulva. *Clinical Obstetrics and Gynecology, 28*(1), 204–210.

Jackson, J. L. & Spain, W. T. (1968, August 15). Comparative study of combined and sequential antiovulatory therapy on vaginal moniliasis. *American Journal of Obstetrics and Gynecology, 101*(8), 1134–1135.

Jensen, H. K., Hansen, P. A., & Blom, J. (1970). Incidence of *Candida albicans* in women using oral contraceptives. *Acta Obstetricia et Gynecologica Scandinavica, 49*(3), 293–296.

Jirovec, O., & Petrü, M. (1968). *Trichomonas vaginalis* and trichomoniasis. *Advances in Parasitology, 6*, 117–188.

Johnston, G. A., Klotz, J., & Boutselis, J. G. (1983, January). Primary invasive carcinoma of the vagina. *Surgery, Gynecology, and Obstetrics, 156*(1), 34–39.

Jones, R. W., & McLean, M. R. (1986, October). Carcinoma in situ of the vulva: A review of 31 treated and five untreated cases. *Obstetrics and Gynecology, 68*(4), 499–503.

Kaplan, A. L. (1985, March). Vulvar reconstruction. *Clinical Obstetrics and Gynecology, 28*(1), 211–219.

Kaufman, R. H. (1981a). Cystic tumors. In H. L. Gardner & R. H. Kaufman (Eds.), *Benign diseases of the vulva and vagina* (2nd ed.). Boston: G. K. Hall.

Kaufman, R. H. (1981b). Solid tumors. In H. L. Gardner & R. H. Kaufman (Eds.), *Benign diseases of the vulva and vagina* (2nd ed.). Boston: G. K. Hall.

Kaufman, R. H. & Faro, S. (1987). Infectious diseases of the vulva and vagina. In E. J. Wilkinson (Ed.), *Pathology of the vulva and vagina*. New York: Churchill Livingstone.

Krause, U. (1982). Results of single-dose treatment of vaginal mycoses with 500 mg Canesten vaginal tablets. *Chemotherapy, 28*(Suppl. 1), 99–105.

Lamb, M. A., & Woods, N. F. (1981, April). Sexuality and the cancer patient. *Cancer Nursing, 4*(2), 137–144.

Lapan, R. (1970, April 15). Is the "pill" a cause of vaginal candidiasis? *New York State Journal of Medicine, 70*(8), 949–951.

Lebherz, T., Guess, E., & Wolfson, N. (1985, August 1). Efficacy of single- versus multiple-dose clotrimazole therapy in the management of vulvovaginal candidiasis. *American Journal of Obstetrics and Gynecology, 152*(7, Part 2), 965–968.

Lenehan, P. M., Meffe, F., & Lickrish, G. M. (1986, September). Vaginal intraepithelial neoplasia: Biologic aspects and management. *Obstetrics and Gynecology, 68*(3), 333–337.

Lewis, J. H., Zimmerman, H. J., Benson, G. D. & Ishak, K. G. (1984, March). Hepatic injury associated with ketoconazole therapy. *Gastroenterology, 86*(3), 503–513.

Liu, L.-Y., Hou, Y.-J., & Li, J.-,Z. (1987, October). Primary malignant melanoma of the vagina: A report of seven cases. *Obstetrics and Gynecology, 70*(4), 569–572.

Malinak, R. L., & Franklin, R. R. (1981). Developmental anomalies of the vulva and vagina. In H. L. Gardner & R. H. Kaufman (Eds.), *Benign diseases of the vulva and vagina* (2nd ed.). Boston: G. K. Hall.

Mason, P. R., Super, H., & Fripp, P. J. (1976, February). Comparison of four techniques for the routine diagnosis of *Trichomonas vaginalis* infection. *Journal of Clinical Pathology, 29*(2), 154–157.

McKay, M. (1985, March). Vulvodynia versus pruritus vulva. *Clinical Obstetrics and Gynecology, 28*(1), 123–133.

Mendel, E. B., Haberman, S., & Hall, D. K. (1960, August). Isolation of *Candida* from clinical specimens: Comparative study of Pagano–Levin and Nickerson's culture media. *Obstetrics and Gynecology, 16*(2), 180–184.

Mendling, H., & Plempel, M. (1982). Vaginal secretion levels after 6 days, 2 days and 1 day of treatment with 100, 200 and 500 mg vaginal tablets of clotrimazole and their therapeutic efficacy. *Chemotherapy, 28*(Suppl. 1), 43–47.

Michael, H., & Roth, L. M. (1987). Congenital and acquired cysts, benign and malignant skin adnexal tumors, and Paget's disease of the vulva. In E. J. Wilkinson (Ed.), *Pathology of the vulva and vagina*. New York: Churchill Livingstone.

Miles, M. R., Olsen, L., & Rogers, A. (1977, October). Recurrent vaginal candidiasis: Importance of an intestinal reservoir. *Journal of the American Medical Association, 238*(17), 1836–1837.

Milne, J. D., & Warnock, D. W. (1979, October). Effect of simultaneous oral and vaginal treatment on the rate of cure and relapse in vaginal candidosis. *British Journal of Venereal Diseases, 55*(5), 362–365.

Minkowski, W. L., Baker, C. J., Alleyne, D., et al. (1983, June). Single oral dose metronidazole therapy for *Gardnerella vaginalis* in adolescent females. *Journal of Adolescent Health Care, 4*(6), 113–116.

Mirer, F. E., & Silverstein, M. A. (1980, February 28). Cancer after metronidazole [Letter]. *New England Journal of Medicine, 302*(9), 519–520.

Monif, G. R. G. (1982). *Infectious diseases in obstetrics and gynecology.* Philadelphia: Harper & Row.

Montes, L. F., Krumdieck, C., & Cornwell, P. E. (1973, August). Hypovitaminosis A in patients with mucocutaneous candidiasis. *Journal of Infectious Diseases, 128*(2), 227–230.

Morley, G. W. (1981, July 15). Cancer of the vulva: A review. *Cancer, 48*(2, Suppl.), 597–601.

Morris, C.A., & Morris, D. F., (1967, July). "Normal" vaginal microbiology of women of childbearing age in relation to the use of oral contraceptives and vaginal tampons. *Journal of Clinical Pathology, 20*(4), 636–640.

Müller, M., Lossick, J. G., & Gorrell, T. E. (1988, January- March). In vitro susceptibility of *Trichomonas vaginalis* to metronidazole and treatment outcome in vaginal trichomoniasis. *Sexually Transmitted Diseases, 15*(1), 17–24.

Neeson, J. D., & Stockdale, C. R. (1981). *The practitioner's handbook of ambulatory ob/gyn.* New York: John Wiley & Sons.

Nichols, D. H., & McGoldrick, K. L. (1985). Minor and ambulatory surgery. In D. H. Nichols & J. R. Evrard (Eds.), *Ambulatory gynecology*. Philadelphia: Harper & Row.

Odds, F. C. (1979). *Candida and candidosis.* Baltimore: University Park Press.

Ortho Pharmaceutical Corporation (1988). Terazol [package insert].

Paavonen, J., & Stamm, W. E. (1987, March). Lower genital tract infection in women. *Infectious Disease Clinics of North America, 1*(1), 179–198.

Peckham, B. M., Maki, D. G., Patterson, J. J., & Hafez, G.-R. (1986, April). Focal vulvitis: A characteristic syndrome and cause of dyspareunia. *American Journal of Obstetrics and Gynecology, 154*(4), 855–864.

Perez, C., DiSaia, P. J., Knapp, R. C., & Young, R. C. (1985). Gynecologic tumors. In V. T. DaVita, S. Hellman, & S. A. Rosenberg (Eds.), *Cancer: Principles and practice of oncology* (2nd ed.). Philadelphia: J. B. Lippincott.

Perl, G. (1972, January). Errors in the diagnosis of *Trichomonas vaginalis* infection: As observed among 1199 patients. *Obstetrics and Gynecology, 39*(1), 7–9.

Peters, W. A., Kumar, N. B., & Morley, G. W. (1985, November). Microinvasive carcinoma of the vagina: A distinct clinical entity? *American Journal of Obstetrics and Gynecology, 153*(5), 505–507.

Physicians' desk reference (42nd ed.). (1988). Oradell, NJ: Medical Economics Company.

Pierson, K. K. (1987). Malignant melanomas and pigmented lesions of the vulva. In E. J. Wilkinson (Ed.), *Pathology of the vulva and vagina*. New York: Churchill Livingstone.

Pincus, S. H., & Stadecker, M. J. (1987). Vulvar dystrophies and noninfectious inflammatory conditions. In E. J. Wilkinson (Ed.), *Pathology of the vulva and vagina*. New York: Churchill Livingstone.

Porter, P. S., & Lyle, J. S. (1966, April). Yeast vulvovaginitis due to oral contraceptives. *Archives of Dermatology, 93*(4), 402–403.

Pride, G. L., Schultz, A. E., Chuprevich, T. W., & Buchler, D. A. (1979, February). Primary invasive squamous carcinoma of the vagina. *Obstetrics and Gynecology, 53*(2), 218–225.

Pritchard, J. A., MacDonald, P. C., & Gant, N. F. (1985). *Williams obstetrics* (17th ed.). Norwalk, CT: Appleton–Century–Crofts.

Rein, M. F., & Müller, M. (1984). *Trichomonas vaginalis*. In K. K. Holmes, P.-A. Mårdh, P. F. Sparling, & P. J. Weisner (Eds.), *Sexually transmitted diseases*. New York: McGraw–Hill.

Richart, R. M., Gomez-Carrion, Y., & Kaufman, R. H. (1988, February). Treatment priorities for vulvar neoplasia. *Contemporary Ob/Gyn, 31*(2), 79–80, 82–83, 87–88, 91, 94.

Ritter, W. (1985, August 1). Pharmacokinetic fundamentals of vaginal treatment with clotrimazole. *American Journal of Obstetrics and Gynecology, 152*(7, Part 2), 945–947.

Robbie, M. O., & Sweet, R. L. (1983, April 1). Metronidazole use in obstetrics and gynecology: A review. *American Journal of Obstetrics and Gynecology, 145*(7), 865–881.

Rodin, P., & Kolator, B. (1976, May 8). Carriage of yeasts on the penis. *British Medical Journal, 1*(6018), 1123-1124.

Sauer, G. C. (1974, February 25). Monilial vaginitis [Letter]. *Journal of the American Medical Association, 227*(8), 941.

Schnell, J. D. (1982). Investigations into the pathoaetiology and diagnosis of vaginal mycoses. *Chemotherapy, 28*(Suppl. 1), 14–21.

Sibau, L., Bebb, D., Proctor, E. M., & Bowie, W. R. (1987, October-December). Enzyme-linked immunosorbent assay for the diagnosis of trichomoniasis in women. *Sexually Transmitted Diseases, 14*(4), 216–220.

Smith, L. S., & Lauver, D. (1984, June). Assessment and management of vaginitis and cervicitis. *Nurse Practitioner, 9*(6), 34–67.

Sobel, J. D. (1984, September). Vulvovaginal candidiasis—What we do and do not know. *Annals of Internal Medicine, 101*(3), 390–392.

Sobel, J. D. (1985a, August 1). Epidemiology and pathogenesis of recurrent vulvovaginal candidiasis. *American Journal of Obstetrics and Gynecology, 152*(7, Part 2), 924–935.

Sobel, J. D. (1985b, March). Management of recurrent vulvovaginal candidiasis with intermittent ketoconazole prophylaxis. *Obstetrics and Gynecology, 65*(3), 435–440.

Sobel, J. D. (1986, December 4). Recurrent vulvovaginal candidiasis: A prospective study of the efficacy of maintenance ketoconazole therapy. *New England Journal of Medicine, 315*(23), 1455–1458.

Sobel, J. D. (1988, February). When candidal vaginitis warrants systemic treatment. *Contemporary Ob/Gyn, 31*(2), 73–77.

Spellacy, W. N., Zaias, N., Buhi, W. C., & Birk, S. A. (1971, September). Vaginal yeast growth and contraceptive practices. *Obstetrics and Gynecology, 38*(3), 343–349.

Spence, M. R., Hollander, D. H., Smith, J., et al. (1980, October-December). The clinical and laboratory diagnosis of *Trichomonas vaginalis* infection. *Sexually Transmitted Diseases, 7*(4), 168–171.

Spiegel, C. A., Amsel, R., Eschenbach, D., et al (1980, September 11). Anaerobic bacteria in nonspecific vaginitis. *New England Journal of Medicine, 303*(11), 601–607.

Stage, A. H., Humeniuk, J. M, & Easley, W. K. (1984, September 1). Bullous pemphigoid of the vulva: A case report. *American Journal of Obstetrics and Gynecology, 120*(2), 169–170.

Stallworthy, J. (1971, April 10). Vaginitis and tights [Letter]. *British Medical Journal, 2*(5753), 108.

Stettendorf, S., Benijts, G., Vignali, M., & Kreysing, W. (1982). Three-day therapy of vaginal candidiasis with clotrimazole vaginal tablets and econazole ovules: A multicenter comparative study. *Chemotherapy, 28*(Suppl. 1), 87–91.

Stone, K. M. (1986, April 4). Primary prevention of sexually transmitted disease: A primer for clinicians. *Journal of the American Medical Association, 225*(14), 1763–1766.

Sutton, G. P., Stehman, F., Ehrlich, C. E., & Roman, A. (1987, October). Human papillomavirus deoxyribonucleic acid in lesions of the female genital tract: Evidence for type 6/11 in squamous carcinoma of the vulva. *Obstetrics and Gynecology, 70*(4), 564–568.

Symposium: Establishing bacterial vaginosis. (1986, February). *Contemporary Ob/Gyn, 27*(2), 186–203.

Syntex Laboratories. (1987). Butoconazole nitrate [package insert].

Tancer, M. L., Rosenberg, M., & Fernandez, D. (1956, June). Cysts of the vulvovaginal (Bartholin's) gland. *Obstetrics and Gynecology, 7*(6), 608–610.

Tann, L. (1968, December 21). Wearing tights [Letter]. *British Medical Journal, 4*(5633), 776.

Taylor, E., Blackwell, A. L., Barlow, D., & Phillips, I. (1982, June 19). Gardnerella Vaginalis, Anaerobes, and Vaginal Discharge, *Lancet, 1*(8286), 1376–1379.

Thin, R. N., Leighton, M., & Dixon, M. J. (1977, July 9). How often is genital yeast infection sexually transmitted? *British Medical Journal, 2*(6078), 93–94.

Thin, R. N., Symonds, A. E., Booker, R., et al. (1979, October). Double-blind comparison of a single dose and a five-day course of metronidazole in the treatment of trichomoniasis. *British Journal of Venereal Diseases, 55*(5), 354–356.

Tovell, H. M. M., & Danforth, D. N. (1986). Structural defects and relaxations. In D. N. Danforth & J. R. Scott (Eds.), *Obstetrics and Gynecology* (5th ed.). Philadelphia: J. B. Lippincott.

Townsend, D. E. (1984, January). Examining the vulva and the vagina. *Contemporary Ob/Gyn, 23*(1), 161–168.

Van Slyke, K. K., Michel, V. P., & Rein, M. F. (1981, September 15). Treatment of vulvovaginal candidiasis with boric acid powder. *American Journal of Obstetrics and Gynecology, 141*(2), 145–148.

Wagner, G., & Levin, R. J. (1978). Vaginal fluid. In E. S. E. Hafez & T. N. Evans (Eds.), *The human vagina*. New York: Elsevier/North-Holland Biomedical Press.

Walsh, H., Hildebrandt, R. J., & Prystowsky, H. (1965, November 15). Candidal vaginitis associated with the use of oral progestational agents. *American Journal of Obstetrics and Gynecology, 93*(6), 904–905.

Walsh, H., Hildebrandt, R. J., & Prystowsky, H. (1968, August 1). Oral progestational agents as a cause of *Candida* vaginitis. *American Journal of Obstetrics and Gynecology, 101*(7), 991–993.

Warnock, D. W., Speller, D. C. E., Milne, J. D., et al. (1979, October). Epidemiological investigation of patients with vulvovaginal candidosis. *British Journal of Venereal Diseases, 55*(5), 357–361.

Waugh, M. A. (1982). Clinical presentation of candidal vaginitis—Its differential diagnosis and treatment. *Chemotherapy, 28*(Suppl. 1), 56–60.

Whittington, M. J. (1957, June). Epidemiology of infections with *Trichomonas vaginalis* in the light of improved diagnostic methods. *British Journal of Venereal Diseases, 33*(2), 80–91.

Wisdom, A. R., & Dunlop, E. M. C. (1965, June). Trichomoniasis: Study of the disease and its treatment. *British Journal of Venereal Diseases, 41*(2), 90–96.

Witkin, S. S., Yu, I. R., & Ledger, W. J. (1983, December 1). Inhibition of *Candida albicans*-induced lymphocyte proliferation by lymphocytes and sera from women with recurrent vaginitis. *American Journal of Obstetrics and Gynecology, 147*(7), 809–811.

Wolcott, H. D., & Gallup, D. G. (1984, November 15). Wide local incision in the treatment of vulvar carcinoma in situ: A reappraisal. *American Journal of Obstetrics and Gynecology, 150*(6), 605–608.

Woodruff, J. D. (1985). Noninfectious diseases of the vulva. In D. H. Nichols, & J. R. Evrard (Eds.), *Ambulatory gynecology*. Philadelphia: Harper & Row.

Woodruff, J. D. (1986). Lesions of the vulva and vagina. In D. N. Danforth and J. R. Scott (Eds.), *Obstetrics and Gynecology* (5th ed.). Philadelphia: J. B. Lippincott.

Yaffee, H. S., & Grots, I. (1965, March 25). Moniliasis due to norethynodrel with mestranol [Letter]. *New England Journal of Medicine, 272*(12), 647.

12

Sexually Transmitted Diseases

Ronnie Lichtman and Paula Duran

As knowledge about sexually transmitted diseases (STDs) has increased, and more organisms and diseases have been identified as sexually transmitted, the field has grown. As both the health care community and the general public become more aware of these diseases and their consequences, it behooves all practitioners to become as knowledgeable as possible about STDs, their mode of transmission, incubation periods, epidemiology, diagnosis, therapies, and preventive measures—at all levels of prevention. This applies both to diseases that the primary care practitioner can manage independently and those for which referral is necessary.

More than 20 organisms have been implicated to date in causing STDs (Table 12–1). More than 25 specific infections, syndromes, or complications caused by these organisms have been identified (Table 12–2). A number of these have been discussed in Chapter 11. Certain complications of STDs, including cervicitis and cervical intraepithelial neoplasia (CIN), pelvic inflammatory disease (PID) or salpingitis, ectopic pregnancy, cystitis, urethritis, the acute urethral syndrome, and infertility, are covered in subsequent chapters (13, 15, 17, and 27). Several others are male diseases or relate to pregnancy and/or the newborn and are outside the scope of this textbook. The remainder of the listed disorders are discussed in this chapter.

The chapter begins with a discussion of the epidemiology and prevention of STDs relevant to many of the diseases covered. Included is information that should be part of routine patient teaching and counseling. Then, a section is devoted to each sexually transmitted disease that the woman's health care practitioner may encounter in practice, with varying degrees of frequency. Each section includes a discussion of the etiology and transmission of the disease, its epidemiology, clinical presentation, consequences, and sequelae as relevant, and management. Management refers to data collection needed for diagnosis and interventions including medical and surgical therapies, self-help measures, and teaching and counseling.

We caution all readers to bear in mind that knowledge about STDs increases at a phenomenal speed. New and improved diagnostic techniques, preventive measures, and treatments continue to be developed. We advise all practitioners to stay abreast of new developments by reading up-to-date journals, attending conferences, and being particularly aware of recommendations of the Centers for Disease Control (CDC).

EPIDEMIOLOGY

Certain overall observations regarding the epidemiology of STDs in general can be made. Data, however, are limited by the fact that not all STDs are reportable; many of the generalizations made are based on the reportable sexually transmitted diseases: syphilis, gonorrhea, lymphogranuloma venereum, chancroid, and granuloma inguinale. The following discussion is adapted from Aral and Holmes (1984).

In order, STDs can be expected in the following age groups: 20- to 24-year-olds, 25- to 29-year-olds, and 15- to 19-year-olds, with the incidence being higher in 18- to 19-year-olds than in 15- to 17-year-olds. This latter finding is influenced by the fact that the rates of sexual activity are lower among the younger adolescents; for sexually active adolescents, the incidence of STDs is inversely related to age.

STDs tend to occur at earlier ages in women than men; however, age-specific incidence rates are higher for men than women. This difference may reflect the fact that manifestations of certain STDs in males lead to better diagnosis and therefore more reporting. Disease severity of STDs is greater for women than men, except for homosexual males.

Among racial groups, the highest morbidity is seen in blacks, the lowest in Orientals, with whites in-between. This distribution may reflect socioeconomic, rather than racial, differences, but the data apparently do not allow such a conclusion to be drawn. In general, morbidity rates are higher among unmarried persons and persons of lower socioeconomic groups. Rates of STDs are higher among urban than rural dwellers. Some question exists, however, as to the extent that reporting differences between private and public health facilities affects these statistics.

The most rapidly increasing STDs in recent years have been herpes genitalis and nongonococcal urethritis, largely attributable to *Chlamydia trachomatis*. Chlamydial infection, herpes genitalis, and gonorrhea are the three most prevalent STDs among heterosexuals today.

Overall, rates of STDs are increasing. Only trichomoniasis (covered in Chapter 11) and perhaps scabies are declining. Gonorrhea recently declined in incidence, but this trend may be reversing, and syphilis has been increasing in recent years. Clearly, these diseases constitute a major individual and public health problem today, leading to significant morbidity and even mortality. Mortality from these

TABLE 12-1. ORGANISMS CAUSING STDS

Bacteria

Calymmatobacterium granulomatis
Campylobacter fetus
Chlamydia trachomatis
Hemophilus ducreyi
Mycoplasma hominis
Neisseria gonorrhoeae
Salmonella
Shigella species
Treponema pallidum
Ureaplasma urealyticum

Viruses

Cytomegalovirus
Hepatitis virus
Herpes simplex virus
Human immunodeficiency virus
Human papillomavirus
Molluscum contagiosum

Protozoa

Entamoeba histolytic
Giardia lamblia
Trichomonas vaginalis

Ectoparasites

Phthirus pubis
Sarcoptes scabiei

TABLE 12-2. INFECTIONS, SYNDROMES, AND COMPLICATIONS CAUSED BY SEXUALLY TRANSMITTED ORGANISMS

Infections

Amebiasis
Cervicitis
Chancroid
Condylomata acuminata (genital warts)
Cystitis
Dermatitis
Enteritis
Epididymitis
Giardiasis
Gonorrhea
Granuloma inguinale
Hepatitis
Lymphogranuloma venereum (LGV)
Molluscum contagiosum
Pediculosis pubis
Proctitis
Proctocolitis
Scabies
Shigellosis
Syphilis
Urethritis
Ulcerative warts
Vaginitis

Syndromes

Acquired immune deficiency syndrome
Acute urethral syndrome
Gay bowel syndrome

Complications

Cervical intraepithelial neoplasia (CIN)/cervical cancer
Ectopic pregnancy
Infertility
Perinatal infection
Prematurity (possibly)
Salpingitis (pelvic inflammatory disease)

diseases is largely accounted for by syphilis, the complications of PID, cervical cancer (Grimes, 1986), and, most recently, acquired immune deficiency syndrome (AIDS).

PREVENTION

The prevention of STDs should be a national priority. Practitioners must become familiar with both primary and secondary preventive measures and make dissemination of information about such measures a part of *routine* care. Currently available preventive measures include treatment of current cases (if treatment exists), identification and treatment of all sexual partners of the infected person, and minimization of risk behaviors for contracting and transmitting STDs.

Effective prevention must involve individual efforts and concerted institutional and governmental efforts. The latter include widespread screening, contact tracing, accessible and sensitive clinic services, education, and surveillance (e.g., reporting cases and identifying organism resistance) (Cates & Wiesner, 1984).

Primary Prevention

Primary preventive measures refer to those aimed at avoiding infection. The main thrusts of primary prevention of STDs include modifying selection of sexual partners, avoiding certain sexual practices, and using barrier methods of birth control, particularly the condom and methods that are used with vaginal spermicides (Stone, Grimes, & Magder, 1986a). Other preventive methods such as prophylactic antibiotics are not routinely recommended; postcoital hygienic practices such as urination, washing, and/or douching have not been studied.

Choice of Sex Partner. Although abstinence has been cited as the only guaranteed method of prevention against STDs

(Stone, Grimes, & Magder, 1986b), limiting the number of partners and partners known to have many partners decreases the chances of acquiring an STD. Avoiding sexual contact with people known only casually may be advisable; it is reasonable to assume that a casually met partner has frequent casual encounters. Mutual monogamy is highly protective, assuming neither partner has an infection at the time sexual activity is initiated (Curran, 1984).

Although many STDs can be asymptomatic (including, for example, gonorrhea, herpes, hepatitis B, syphilis, chlamydia, enteric infections, and AIDS), examining partners for lesions, sores, ulcerations, rashes, redness, discharge, swelling, and odor before initiating sexual activity is recommended with sexual intercourse avoided if any unusual findings are noted. Partners should be asked about exposure to STDs and about their sexual practices, including their number of partners.

Sexual Practices. Anal–genital intercourse, anal–oral contact, and anal–digital activity are considered high-risk sexual behaviors (Stone et al., 1986b). The epithelium of the rectum is delicate and penetration can easily result in abrasions of the mucosa, providing a portal of entry for such organisms as human immunodeficiency virus (HIV). Enteric infections may be transmitted by oral–fecal contact; these include hepatitis A, giardiasis, amebiasis, and shigellosis. Vaginal or oral intercourse should never follow anal contact without first washing. Other sexual practices, such as fisting, that may increase the likelihood of damage to body tissues should be avoided.

Barrier Contraceptive Methods. Condoms and spermicides have been shown to be effective against many sexually transmitted organisms including *N. gonorrhoeae, Treponema pallidum,* herpes simplex virus, cytomegalovirus, human papillomavirus, *mycoplasma hominis,* HIV, and the presumed causative agent(s) in cervical cancer (Asculai, Weis, Rancourt, & Kupferberg, 1978; Conant, Spicer, & Smith, 1984; Conant, Hardy, Sernatinger, et al., 1986, Feldblum & Fortney, 1988; Jick, Hannan, Stergachis, et al., 1982; Singh, Cutler, & Utidjian, 1972; Singh, Postic, & Cutler 1976). Condoms and spermicides can be used as protection even by women and couples who use other methods of contraception. Diaphragms used with spermicides are protective; diaphragms without spermicides may offer some protection but this has not been verified (Stone et al., 1986a). Condoms and spermicides, however, are not to be considered absolutely protective against all STDs (Kappus & Quinn, 1986) and are most effective when used with low-risk behaviors.

Secondary Prevention

Secondary prevention involves the prompt identification and effective treatment of persons infected with a sexually transmitted organism. Immediate diagnosis and treatment should be sought by any person who believes that she or he may have contracted an STD, demonstrates symptoms of an STD, has had sexual relations with someone who has symptoms of an STD, or has a partner who has been diagnosed with an STD. Many state and local health departments have free STD [or VD (venereal disease)] clinics or offer free treatment in hospital emergency rooms. Any person diagnosed with an STD should be tested for other STDs, particularly the infections that can be asymptomatic such as gonorrhea, chlamydia, syphilis, and trichomoniasis. A Pap smear should be taken as well.

Infected persons should identify and notify all partners who have possibly been exposed to the disease. The practitioner may need to help prepare women to do this by suggesting ways of informing partners, providing literature, and role playing with the woman. Patients can be assured that although it may be embarrassing to talk to partners about exposure to an STD, most people appreciate being given the opportunity for treatment, rather than having the information withheld. Reportable diseases should be reported so that contact tracing can be offered.

All treatments must be carefully and thoroughly explained and the patient's understanding of treatment regimens assessed. A vital component of treatment is the completion of all medication regimens, regardless of whether symptoms subside. Women should be advised to refrain from intercourse until all treatment is completed and tests-of-cure have shown the treatment to be effective. Follow-up appointments should be provided as necessary.

Routine STD screening—particularly for asymptomatic infections—should be recommended as frequently as every 3 to 6 months for women who are at high risk for contracting STDs or who consider themselves at high risk. Such women include those with multiple casual sexual partners or partners with numerous partners or those engaging in prostitution. Criteria for risk for HIV infection and recommendations for testing are covered in the section on the acquired immune deficiency syndrome.

MANAGEMENT CONSIDERATIONS

The framework for management presented in Chapter 11 provides an applicable approach for dealing with STDs as well. Indeed, the symptoms of vulvar or vaginal disorders may not be immediately distinguishable from those of STDs, so data collection proceeds in the same manner for either type of disease. The caveats discussed in the section on treatments in Chapter 11 apply as well, including indications for prescribing, consultation, and referral. Treatments outlined here are for adult, nonpregnant women. A comprehensive referral network must be built that includes gynecologists, internists, dermatologists, infectious disease specialists, rheumatologists, counselors and therapists, and support groups.

Practitioners must be ever cognizant of the emotional and social consequences of an STD diagnosis. In addition to providing factual information, they must demonstrate extreme sensitivity to the psychosocial needs of patients.

THE "CLASSIC" STDS

Five diseases have been classically known as STDs or "venereal diseases": gonorrhea, syphilis, lymphogranuloma venereum, chancroid, and granuloma inguinale. All are bacterial infections. Syphilis and gonorrhea can be considered "major" STDs; the other three are relatively uncommon in the United States today and can be considered "minor" infections (Krieger, 1984).

Gonorrhea

Gonorrhea was the first bacterial infection to be documented, although, in early descriptions, it was often seen as the same disease as syphilis. The diseases were recognized as separate entities in the eighteenth century; in 1879, the causative agent of gonorrhea was identified (Kampmeier, 1984).

Etiology and Transmission. Gonorrhea is caused by the bacteria *Neisseria gonorrhoeae,* a Gram-negative diplococcus. Several strains of *N. gonorrhoeae* have been defined according to a complex system called auxotyping which is based on the growth response of the organisms on certain chemical media and is dependent on varying nutritional requirements of differing strains. Gonococci grow only on rich culture media. Heated blood (chocolate agar) and other supplements are added to the medium to support the growth of *N. gonorrhoeae* (Swanson & Mayer, 1984). Initiation of growth of the organism depends on the addition of carbon dioxide or bicarbonate ion. A candle jar or CO_2 incubator is generally used.

Sensitivity and resistance to antibiotics of gonococci are of major clinical importance. Originally treated with sulfonamides, the organism developed resistance to these drugs by the mid-1940s and penicillin then became the treatment of choice (Swanson & Mayer, 1984). As early as the 1950s, however, penicillin resistance was seen among gonococci, leading to the need for increased doses of medication for effective treatment.

In the 1970s, strains of gonococci were isolated that were totally resistant to penicillin. These strains contained genes for *β-lactamase,* an enzyme that inactivates penicillin. They are known as penicillinase-producing *N. gonorrhoeae* (PPNG). These strains are also resistant to other antibiotics such as the tetracyclines (Krieger, 1984). They were at first most commonly seen in cases originating in the Far East and parts of West Africa. By the early 1980s, however, the incidence of these resistant strains had increased rapidly in the United States and ceased to be associated with foreign travel (Centers for Disease Control, 1987a).

Other resistant gonococcal strains exist that do not produce β-lactamase. CMRNG demonstrates chromosomal resistance to penicillin and may also be resistant to tetracycline, the cephalosporins, spectinomycin, and aminoglycosides. To date, however, CMRNG has not generally been associated with treatment failure because the level of resistance is not high enough or because an appropriate antibiotic can be found (CDC, 1987a). A third type of resistant organism identified in 1985, TRNG, is resistant to tetracycline, but not to penicillin.

Gonorrhea is transmitted by sexual contact, including genital, anal–genital, and oral–genital intercourse. It has been transmitted via donor semen in artificial insemination (Mascola & Guinan, 1987).

The risk of acquiring gonorrhea increases with increased exposure. Male-to-female transmission is higher than female-to-male. About 90 percent of female partners of men with *gonococcal urethritis* have been reported to become infected, although data do not account for numbers of exposures (Handsfield, 1984).

The incubation period for gonorrhea in women is variable and less certain than that in men (which is 1 to 14 days, usually 2 to 5), but generally women who become symptomatic do so within 10 days (Handsfield, 1984).

Infection with *N. gonorrhoeae* does not confer immunity. Repeat infections are possible.

Epidemiology. Gonorrhea is the most common among reported STDs. After a steady increase in the number of reported cases from 1965 to 1975, the next 10 years showed a decline in incidence. In 1984, 878,556 cases were reported to the CDC representing a 12 percent decline from 1975 (Rice, Aral, Blount, & Zaidi, 1987). The absolute number of cases of gonorrhea declined most in the adolescent population, but number of cases per population actually declined the *least* in this group, explainable by its shrinking size. Data for 1985, however, show a reversal in the declining trend with a concomitant increase in the proportion of resistant strains. The future pattern remains to be seen.

Demographic risk factors for gonorrhea include black race (which may be an artifact of blacks utilizing public clinics with a greater likelihood of case reporting); low socioeconomic status; urban residence; early onset of sexual activity; unmarried status; male homosexuality; and history of prior gonorrhea infection (Handsfield, 1984). Morbidity rates for gonorrhea are highest in the southeastern states and Alaska. In males, the peak incidence occurs in 20- to 24-year-olds; in women, the peak occurs between ages 18 and 24 (Dallabetta & Hook, 1987). More males are diagnosed with gonorrhea than females, but screening programs can significantly reduce the male-to-female ratio of diagnosed infection (Felman, Synder, Giordano, & Griffin, 1978). A high prevalence of other STDs is found in women with gonorrhea including chlamydial infections, trichomoniasis, bacterial vaginosis, and herpes genitalis (Handsfield, 1984).

Clinical Presentation. Gonorrhea infection may be asymptomatic, symptomatic, or complicated by infection of several sites. In women, asymptomatic infection may exist in the endocervix, urethra, rectum, and/or pharynx; symptomatic infection may cause urethritis, cervicitis, pharyngitis, Bartholinitis, and/or conjunctivitis (Handsfield, 1984). Local complications include salpingitis (see Chapter 15), Bar-

tholin's gland abscess (see Chapter 11), lymphangitis, and periurethral abscess. The infection can also become disseminated.

Because of the affinity of gonococci for columnar epithelial cells, the primary site of gonorrheal infection in women is the endocervical canal, except in prepubescent girls. Before puberty, the cervix is less susceptible to gonorrheal infection because of its lack of endocervical glands; the infection in young girls usually resides within the vagina. The thinness of the vaginal walls, absence of estrogenic effect, and the alkaline pH make it susceptible (Bolton, 1983). Infection of the urethra is common (seen in 70 to 90 percent of infected women) as is infection of Skene's glands and Bartholin's ducts. Except in women with prior hysterectomies, however, urethral or Skene's glands infections are rarely seen without endocervical infection.

When gonorrheal symptoms exist, they include vaginal discharge, intermenstrual bleeding, and menorrhagia. Discharge may be purulent or mucopurulent and seen from the cervix, Skene's glands, or Bartholin's gland ducts.

Anorectal infection is present in 35 to 50 percent of women with gonorrhea. It is the only site of infection in approximately 5 percent of infected women (Kinghorn & Rashid, 1979; Thin & Shaw, 1979). This area can be infected without anogenital sexual contact; its prevalence is related to duration of infection, suggesting contamination with cervical and vaginal discharge (Handsfield, 1984). Symptoms of anorectal infection may be absent, minimal, or severe and include pruritus, mucopurulent discharge, rectal bleeding, pain, tenesmus, and constipation. External anal examination rarely shows changes. The prevalence of symptoms is undetermined (Handsfield, 1984).

Pharyngeal infection is found in 10 to 20 percent of women with gonorrhea. The pharnyx is the only site of infection in less than 5 percent of the infected (Tice & Rodriguez, 1981; Wiesner, Tronca, Bonin, et al., 1973). Pharyngeal infection is transmitted through oral–genital contact with greater transmissibility from males to females. More than 90 percent of pharyngeal infections are asymptomatic. Rare symptoms include acute pharyngitis or tonsillitis, fever, and lymphadenopathy.

Complications and Sequelae. The most common complications of gonorrheal infection in women are salpingitis or PID and Bartholin's gland abscess (see Chapters 11 and 15). Gonococci may pass directly into the uterine cavity, where they may cause superficial endometritis. Perinatal complications may include prematurity, chorioamnionitis, ophthalmia neonatorum, pharyngeal infection, or other problems of the newborn.

Ascent of gonococci into the fallopian tubes generally occurs during or after menstruation (McGee, 1984). Sequelae of gonococcal salpingitis result from inflammatory reactions involving the fallopian tubes, leakage of exudate into the peritoneal cavity, or resulting scar tissue. Specific sequelae include tuboovarian abscesses (see Chapter 16), most likely to occur after a repeat episode of PID; ectopic pregnancy; involuntary infertility (Arya, Taber, & Nsanze, 1980; Weström 1975); perihepatitis, also called Fitz–Hugh–Curtis syndrome (Semchyshyn, 1979); pyosalpinx, hydrosalpinx, and intraabdominal adhesions with chronic pelvic or abdominal pain; recurrent menstrual pain and abnormal bleeding (Curran, Rendtorff, Chandler, et al., 1975); and sacroiliitis (McGee, 1984).

Conjunctivitis occurs rarely in adults with gonorrhea, usually in people with anogenital gonorrhea, secondary to autoinoculation (Thatcher & Pettit, 1971). Skin infections, presenting as localized ulcers of the genitals, perineum, lower extremities, or fingers have been reported (Scott & Scott, 1982).

Disseminated gonococcal infection (DGI) is a complication with diverse clinical manifestations. Approximately 1 percent of patients with untreated mucosal gonorrhea infection are estimated to develop DGI (Barr & Danielsson, 1971; Holmes, Wiesner, & Pedersen, 1971). Its incidence may be higher in whites than blacks for unknown reasons.

Host factors predisposing to DGI are a lack of one of the complement components or an abnormality of the component (Brooks, Israel, & Petersen, 1976; Lee, Utsinger, Synderman, et al., 1978; Petersen, Graham, & Brooks, 1976). In females, many cases of DGI occur close to menstruation or during pregnancy, suggesting that hormonal factors in women may be important (Holmes, Counts, & Beaty, 1971; Keiser, Ruben, Wolinsky, & Kushner, 1968). DGI is rarely coexistent with gonococcal PID; they may be caused by different strains of the organism (Thompson & Hager, 1977).

Clinical manifestations of DGI commonly include fever, leukocytosis, skin lesions, tenosynovitis, polyarthralgias, oligoarthritis, hepatitis, and mild myopericarditis (Brogadir, Schimmer, & Myers, 1979; Keiser et al., 1968). Less common syndromes are endocarditis, meningitis, and perihepatitis. Rarely, pneumonia, adult respiratory distress syndrome, and osteomyelitis are seen (Black & Cohen, 1984; Mills & Brooks, 1984).

Skin lesions in DGI begin as erythematous macules, becoming pustules, possibly with hemorrhagic or necrotic centers. They are usually found on the upper extremities, and often near the small joints of the hands or feet. Tenosynovitis may occur at one or several sites, most often involving the tendons and tendon sheaths of the knees, ankles, and wrists (Holmes et al., 1971; Keefer & Spink, 1937). Erythema, swelling, and tenderness with pain on motion of the involved tendon are present. Arthritis rarely causes severe problems at its onset. Joint involvement is migratory. Later, septic oligoarthritis may occur, most commonly associated with involvement of the knee, elbow, ankle, and small hand joints (Mills & Brooks, 1984).

Differential Diagnosis. Gonorrhea must be differentiated from other STDs. When a woman reports exposure to a male with urethritis, the diagnosis is usually gonorrhea or nongonococcal urethritis (NGU), most often caused by *Chlamydia trachomatis*. When she presents with vaginal discharge or other symptoms of gonorrhea, the disease must be differentiated from vaginitis (Chapter 11) and from other STDs including chlamydia. PID caused by gonorrhea must be differentiated from PID caused by other organisms and from appendicitis; septic abortion; endometritis; endometriosis; ectopic pregnancy; ovarian tumors, cysts, or hematomas; torsion or rupture of an ovarian cyst; and adnexal torsion (see Chapters 14, 15, 16, and 18).

Management

DATA COLLECTION

History. Although a history of symptoms is always important, it may not yield information specific enough to point to a diagnosis of gonorrhea, especially because of the high rate of asymptomatic infections in women. Because women with gonorrhea may not become symptomatic until infection has ascended, symptoms of salpingitis should be sought, including chills, fever, anorexia, nausea and vomiting, and lower abdominal pain, usually bilateral, but possibly with more pain on one side than the other. Sudden motion may increase the pain. Abnormal vaginal bleeding or prolonged menstruation may occur secondary to endometritis (McGee, 1984). Onset of symptoms may be gradual or sudden, reaching a severe level within 24 to 48 hours. Symptoms often occur during or just after menses.

A history of exposure or symptoms in the woman's male partner or partners is significant. Males infected with gonorrhea most commonly complain of acute dysuria and urethral discharge (Handsfield, 1984). Discharge begins scant and mucoid and within 24 hours is purulent and frank. Infected males may also have acute epididymitis and penile and lymph edema. Symptoms of gonorrheal urethritis are usually more pronounced than those of NGU; nevertheless, laboratory data should confirm the diagnosis. A small number of infected males do not develop symptoms. Spontaneous resolution usually occurs within several weeks to 6 months if the infection is left untreated, but, rarely, a carrier state may persist (Handsfield, 1984).

A diagnosis of gonorrhea in a sexual partner is sufficient for treatment (CDC, 1985b, p. 82s). If a partner is known to have symptoms of urethritis, the woman should try to find out the man's definitive diagnosis if he has sought care; she should urge him to seek care if he has not. In any case, symptoms in a male partner or a history of his being treated for "painful peeing," "a drip," or "the clap," should prompt laboratory testing for gonorrhea and chlamydia and treatment for both.

As the likelihood of acquiring any STD increases with increased numbers of sexual partners, increased numbers of partners of partners, and increased numbers of casual contacts, this information should be included in the routine history. Questions regarding such sexual practices should be asked matter-of-factly. "How many partners do you and your partner have?" is perceived as less judgmental than setting up the dichotomy, "Do you have one or more than one partner?"

Exposed women should be asked about anal- or oral-genital intercourse to ascertain appropriate sites for gonorrhea culture. All medication allergies must be noted, especially to penicillin, tetracycline, and other antibiotics used in the treatment of gonorrhea (see later).

Physical Examination. Whenever gonorrhea is suspected, or another STD has been diagnosed, the practitioner should examine the woman for local signs of infection as well as signs of salpingitis. The abdomen should be lightly and deeply palpated for pain, including rebound tenderness. The inguinal lymph area should be palpated for enlargement and tenderness. Skene's glands and the urethra should be milked for discharge, and Bartholin's glands viewed and palpated for swelling, tenderness, and exudate. Cervical erythema, friability, purulent or mucopurulent discharge, and ectopy (see Chapter 13) should be noted. Bimanual examination should be used to rule out cervical motion tenderness, uterine tenderness or fixation, and/or adnexal tenderness and masses.

Laboratory Testing. Laboratory tests provide the only definitive diagnosis of gonorrhea. Laboratory diagnosis can be accomplished via culture, microscopic examination of stained smears, or immunoassay; culture is the most sensitive of these, particularly for women. Serologic tests have been developed but are not sensitive or specific enough to be clinically useful (Handsfield, 1984).

Culture media selective for *N. gonorrhoeae* show a sensitivity rate between 75 and 93 percent (Judson & Werness, 1980; Schmale, Martin, & Domescik, 1969; Thin & Shaw,

1979). Because the cervix is almost always infected, this is the main site to culture; posthysterectomy, the urethra is the best site to culture (Handsfield, 1984). Before puberty, the vagina is most likely to harbor the infection.

The urethra, gland ducts, anal canal, and pharynx can be cultured, depending on symptoms, physical findings, and history of exposure, although without culturing the cervix as well, the positive yield from such cultures would be low (Handsfield, 1984). The technique for gonorrhea culture is described in Chapter 4. The usual culture medium is Thayer–Martin medium and results take up to 48 hours. Other media used include Transgrow and Neigon (JEMBEC) media. JEMBEC is convenient in a private office setting because it uses a CO_2-generating tablet in a culture plate sealed in a plastic bag rather than the more cumbersome candle jar (Riccardi & Felman, 1979). Practitioners must remember to use culture plates at room temperature and to incubate the culture immediately. Incubation overnight at 35 to 37°C is sufficient. Cooler temperatures kill the gonococci so it is important not to refrigerate cultures or specimens.

Romanowski, Harris, Wood, and Kessock-Philip (1986) recommend that two endocervical cultures and a rectal culture be taken on two occasions, a day apart, to increase the yield of positive results. Judson and Werness (1980) point out the cost effectiveness of placing the cervical and anal cultures on the same culture plate.

A variety of stains have been used for microscopic examination including the Gram stain, methylene blue, and acridine orange (Handsfield, 1984). The Gram stain has been the most widely used. It is considered positive when typical Gram-negative diplococci are identified within or near polymorphonuclear leukocytes. In women, however, the sensitivity of Gram stain is only 41 to 70 percent (D'Angelo, Mohla, Sneed, & Woodward, 1987; Handsfield, 1984; Thin & Shaw, 1979), making this an unreliable test for women. There is also a possibility of false-positive results with the Gram stain (Lossick, Smeltzer, & Curran, 1982). Gonozyme^R, an enzyme immunoassay, has been tested and compared with culture in a number of studies. Its advantage over culture would be the rapidity with which results could be obtained. Lossick et al. (1982) showed that treatment delays of even 48 to 72 hours can result in development of PID in 7.3 percent of infected women. Gonozyme sensitivity rates for women range from 80 to 92 percent, however, making this a particularly poor test in populations with low rates of disease (D'Angelo et al., 1987; Lieberman & Wheelock, 1987; Martin, Coopes, Neagle, et al. 1986; Nasello, Callihan, Menegus, & Steigbigel, 1985).

Additional laboratory procedures include tests of the organism for β-lactamase and susceptibility to penicillin, tetracycline, spectinomycin, cefoxitin, and ceftriaxone. In vitro testing, however, does not replace tests-of-cure after treatment (Centers for Disease Control, 1987a).

Concomitant laboratory tests to be performed include syphilis serology, chlamydial culture, and wet mounts with saline and potassium hydroxide for microscopic examination for trichomoniasis and other forms of vaginitis (see Chapter 11). A complete blood count is part of the workup whenever symptoms of pelvic infection are present. In addition to culturing for gonorrhea in women with reported exposure, reported symptoms in their partner(s), or symptoms themselves (including vaginal, urethral, or Skene's gland discharge and/or cervicitis), all persons with other diagnosed STDs, including trichomoniasis, should be cultured. Women with multiple sex partners should be rou-

tinely cultured at annual gynecologic examinations. Women presenting for prenatal care or women in the third trimester of pregnancy should be routinely cultured (because of the risk of ophthalmia neonatorum).

INTERVENTION. Intervention strategies for gonorrhea include prompt initiation of effective antibiotic regimens; examination and treatment of all sexual partners; reporting of cases for public health surveillance; teaching and counseling regarding medication regimens, avoidance of intercourse until all treatments are complete, and preventive measures for the future; and follow-up for test-of-cure.

Treatment Regimens. The Centers for Disease Control (1985b) recommends the following treatments: amoxicillin 3.0 g or ampicillin 3.5 g PO, OR aqueous procaine penicillin G (APPG) 4.8 million units IM, OR ceftriaxone 250 mg IM. Amoxicillin, ampicillin, and penicillin (but not ceftriaxone) are accompanied by probenecid 1.0 g PO. In addition, patients should receive tetracycline HCl 500 mg PO four times daily for 7 days or doxycycline 100 mg PO twice daily for 7 days. If tetracyclines are contraindicated, the single-dose regimen may be followed by erythromycin base or stearate 500 mg PO four times daily for 7 days or erythromycin ethylsuccinate 800 mg PO four times daily for 7 days.

The reason for the addition of tetracycline or doxycycline is the high rate of coexistent chlamydial infection, reported to occur in 45 percent of all gonorrhea cases. The tetracyclines are not used alone because of the increased likelihood of treatment failure resulting from noncompliance when medication must be taken over a period of time and because of the possibility of tetracycline resistance.

These regimens are adequate for women with pharyngeal and rectal infections as well as urogenital infection. Disadvantages of these regimens include the risk of secondary vulvovaginal candidiasis and the potential for masking a chlamydial infection if compliance is poor (Centers for Disease Control 1985b).

Recommended treatment for persistent infections consists of spectinomycin 2.0 g IM or ceftriaxone 250 mg IM. Documented PPNG or gonorrhea in patients who acquired the infection in areas with a high prevalence of PPNG prevalence should be treated with spectinomycin 2.0 g IM or ceftriaxone 250 mg IM, both followed by tetracycline, doxycycline, or erythromycin in the doses outlined earlier. Major cities where resistant strains exist are New York, San Francisco, Miami, Los Angeles, and San Diego (Monif, 1982). For pharyngeal infection caused by PPNG, recommended treatment is ceftriaxone 250 mg IM or nine tablets of trimethoprim/sulfamethoxazole (720 mg/3,600 mg) per day in one daily dose for 5 days.

Adverse effects of aqueous procaine penicillin therapy include gastrointestinal complications, local reactions, and allergic and toxic nonallergic reactions, the latter occurring within seconds after injection. These include visual, auditory, and taste disturbances; fear of death; agitation; and grand mal seizures (Judson, 1986). Allergic reactions occur in 0.004 to 0.04 percent of patients receiving parenteral penicillin. Death ensues in one to two cases per 100,000 (Russo & Thompson, 1984). A history of previous reaction precludes the use of this drug. Penicillin-allergic reactions can be immediate, accelerated, or delayed, as outlined in Table 12–3.

Adverse reactions to cephalosporins are similar to those of the penicillins. Allergic reactions occur in approximately 5 percent of persons treated with cephalosporins. A small

TABLE 12-3. ALLERGIC REACTIONS TO PENICILLIN

Immediate Reaction

Time:	Characteristics:
2–20 min after administration	Diffuse (giant) urticaria; laryngeal edema; wheezing, rhinitis; hypoxia; hypotension; tachycardia; nausea; vomiting; abdominal pain; diarrhea; rigors; vascular collapse

Accelerated Reaction

Time:	Characteristics:
30 min to 48 h after administration	Urticaria; laryngeal edema (infrequently)

Delayed Reaction

Time:	Characteristics:
Usually greater than 3 days after administration	Skin rashes (erythema, urticaria, exfoliative dermatitis, Stevens-Johnson syndrome, fixed drug eruption, contact dermatitis, bullous eruptions); serum sickness; hematologic reactions; lupus-like syndrome; vasculitis; drug fever; hepatitis; nephropathy

From Russo, M. E., & Thompson, M. I. B. (1984). Pharmacology of drugs used in venereology. In K. K. Holmes, P.-A. Mårdh, P. F. Sparling, & P. J. Wiesner [Eds.], Sexually Transmitted Diseases. New York: McGraw-Hill. Reprinted with permission.

percentage of people with an allergy to penicillin have been reported to exhibit hypersensitivity to the cephalosporins (Weinstein & Kaplan, 1970).

In comparison to penicillin, ceftriaxone has several advantages including decreased amount of medication injected and less pain at the injection site. Allergic reactions may occur as with penicillin and the drug is not advised in patients with a true allergy to penicillin. It is a more expensive drug as well (Judson, 1986), but only one injection is needed compared with two for aqueous penicillin.

The tetracyclines are discussed in the treatment section under *Chlamydia trachomatis*. Specific treatment for PID is covered in Chapter 15. Recommended treatments for disseminated gonococcal infection include (1) aqueous crystalline penicillin G 10 million units intravenously per day for at least 3 days followed by amoxicillin or ampicillin 500 mg by mouth four times daily for at least 7 days of total therapy; (2) amoxicillin 3.0 g or ampicillin 3.5 g each with probenecid 1.0 g by mouth, followed by amoxicillin or ampicillin 500 mg by mouth four times daily for at least 7 days; (3) cefoxitin 1.0 g intravenously four times daily for at least 7 days; (4) cefotaxime 500 mg intravenously four times daily for at least 7 days; or (5) ceftriaxone 1.0 g intravenously once for 7 days. Tetracycline or doxycycline can be used for patients allergic to penicillins or cephalosporins. Obviously, DGI requires referral to a medical practitioner for hospital admission and management (CDC, 1985b).

Follow-up. Follow-up cultures should be taken from the infected site or sites 3 to 7 days, or 4 to 7 days if doxycycline was used, after completion of treatment. Rectal cultures should be included in the test-of-cure (CDC, 1987a).

Self-Help Measures. Depending upon the nature and site of symptoms, if any, warm sitz baths, keeping the vulva clean and dry, and salt water gargles may afford some relief (Neeson & Stockdale, 1981).

Additional Teaching and Counseling. The practitioner must stress the importance of completely following all medication regimens regardless of whether symptoms were present or subside quickly. Patients must be told to inform all sexual partners of the previous 2 or 3 months of the need for treatment (regardless of whether they are symptomatic or not), and refrain from intercourse until all treatment is completed and until tests-of-cure have proven both partners to be free of disease. All persons treated for gonorrhea must be given appropriate follow-up appointments and understand the value of tests-of-cure even if they are feeling well.

Because gonorrhea has its onset shortly after exposure, and spontaneous resolution occurs within weeks or months, patients need to face the irrefutable fact of recent sexual transmission. They must be helped to identify and air their feelings. They may need help in determining how to discuss the issue with their partner or partners. The importance of this must be stressed. The CDC (1985b) reports that most recurrences after appropriate treatment are due to reinfection, indicating the need for improved tracing of partners and education of patients. Patients should be informed that the disease is reportable. Written information for the woman and her partner or each of her partners should be provided. Partners must be given appropriate referrals for diagnosis and treatment.

Syphilis

The lesions of syphilis are among the earliest described sexually transmitted lesions. The origin of the disease, however, was not identified until 1905 (Kampmeier, 1984).

Etiology and Transmission. Syphilis is caused by *Treponema pallidum*, one of a small group of treponemes. Other treponemes cause yaws, pinta, and endemic syphilis. Because of its cell wall and response to treatment with antibiotics, this spirochete organism is considered a bacterium (Monif, 1982). *T. pallidum* is not readily grown in vitro, however, and cannot be seen by light microscopy.

The skin and mucous membranes provide barriers against the organism's entry into the body; it is thought to enter the subcutaneous tissue through microscopic abrasions that occur secondary to sexual intercourse (Musher, 1984). Transmission can also occur via kissing, biting, or oral–genital sex (Monif, 1982; Faro, 1985). After the first few years of infection, transmission is ordinarily no longer possible (see Clinical Presentation). In utero transmission is also possible up to approximately 8 years after initial infection (Sparling, 1984).

Approximately one third of persons exposed via sexual relations to *T. pallidum* become infected. The incubation period varies according to the number of organisms present, with the first signs of infection appearing as early as 5 to 7 days or as late as 3 weeks to 90 days. The average incubation period is 3 weeks (Sparling, 1984).

Epidemiology. Between 1977 and 1981, the rate of syphilis infections increased slightly in the United States. After this, it demonstrated a steady decline until 1987, when the Centers for Disease Control (1987c) reported an increase from 10.9 cases per 100,000 (in 1986) to 13.3 cases per 100,000 population. The greatest increases were reported in California, Florida, and New York City. The current increase, unlike the pattern seen in the 1970s, reflects an increase among heterosexuals. The rate of congenital syphilis, highest in the areas of the largest increases in primary and secondary syphilis, also began to increase in the 1980s, after an 8-year decline.

The frequency of syphilis is higher in males than females, blacks than whites. The highest rates of syphilis occur in the 20- to 24-year-old age group. Infection with syphilis does not confer immunity; reinfection can occur.

Clinical Presentation. The clinical course of untreated syphilis is long, variable, and *unlike most other diseases*. The disease progresses through a number of stages—primary, secondary, latent, and tertiary syphilis. The latent period has been divided into early and late latency.

PRIMARY SYPHILIS. Primary syphilis presents with a typical lesion—the primary chancre—which appears from 5 to 90 days after infection. The lesion (Fig. 12–1) is usually single, although it may be multiple. It is generally painless and may be associated with inguinal adenopathy. The lesions appear at the site of infection, most commonly the genital area. In women, the chancre is most likely to occur on the vulva, labia, fourchette, clitoris, or cervix. As it heals spontaneously after 2 to 8 weeks, it may be missed by the woman and the practitioner.

The chancre classically appears as a dull red macule at its onset, then develops into a papule with erosion at its surface. It is round or oval with a clearly defined border. The base of the lesion when it first appears is smooth and shiny, later gray. The chancre feels firm, like a button (Knox & Rudolph, 1984). Atypical chancres may be found and chancres may be secondarily infected, causing pain and tender lymphadenopathy. Extragenital chancres may appear on fingers, anus, mouth, tongue, lips, tonsils, breasts, axillae, and umbilicus with varying appearances. The chancre may reappear at its original site as a manifestation of tertiary syphilis.

SECONDARY SYPHILIS. Secondary syphilis occurs as a result of treponemal multiplication and usually appears within a few weeks or months of the original chancre (although on occasion it may occur with the primary lesion) (Sparling, 1984). The usual time of appearance is about 6 weeks after the first appearance of the chancre. Typically, secondary syphilis presents with variable symptoms of systemic illness, including low-grade fever, malaise, sore throat, hoarseness, headache, anorexia, generalized adenopathy, and skin or mucous membrane lesions (Fig. 12–2) and rashes. Skin rashes typically are papulosquamous, although macular, maculopapular, papular, follicular, papulopustular, or pustular lesions may be seen (Knox & Rudolph, 1984). Lesions are called maculopapular when they are slightly raised, and when a papule becomes scaly, it is called papulosquamous. Often, the rash appears on the palms and soles, a helpful diagnostic aid (Fig. 12–3).

An early manifestation of secondary syphilis is a rash called *macular syphilis* or *roseola syphilitica*, characterized by flat, erythematous, round to oval, rose to pale pink lesions on the trunk. The lesions become more apparent after a warm bath or physical activity, especially in the fair-skinned. Lesions vary in size and color from light to dark red, to yellowish, brownish, or grayish.

Mucous membrane lesions are common, particularly in the mouth (Fig. 12–4). They are round, flat, shiny, gray or pinkish to whitish with a dull red surrounding and are called *mucous patches*. Condylomata lata may appear on the vulva or perineum (Fig. 12–5). These are hypertrophied, flat, moist wartlike lesions (Eschenbach, 1986). They may be confused with condylomata acuminata, but condylomata acuminata are not moist (see later). Condylomata lata are highly contagious.

Alopecia may be present; hair loss in secondary syphilis is patchy (Fig. 12–6) and may involve the eyebrows, eyelashes, and beard. Up to 10 percent of patients have mild hepatitis with hepatomegaly and occasionally splenomegaly.

Manifestations of secondary syphilis heal within 2 to 10 weeks even if untreated. Hair grows back, although some hyperpigmentation, especially on the soles and palms of dark-skinned persons, may remain. Relapses of secondary syphilis may occur within the first 2 years of infection and rarely up to 4 years.

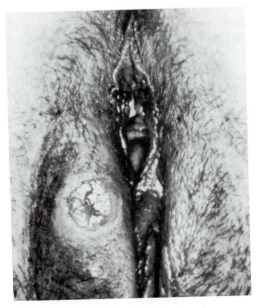

Figure 12–1. Primary syphilis chancre. *(From Kaufman, R. H. & Faro, S. [1987]. Infectious diseases of the vulva and vagina: In E. J. Wilkinson [Ed.], Pathology of the vulva and vagina. New York: Churchill Livingstone. Reprinted with permission.)*

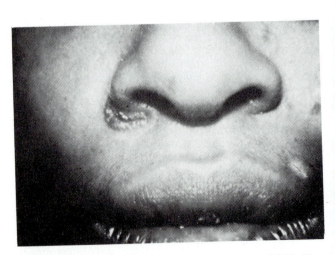

Figure 12–2. Secondary syphilis: papule of the nasal fold. *(From Knox, J. M. & Rudolph, A. H. [1984]. Acquired infectious syphilis. In K. K. Holmes, P.-A. Mårdh, P. F. Sparling, & P. J. Wiesner [Eds.], Sexually transmitted diseases. New York: McGraw–Hill. Reprinted with permission.)*

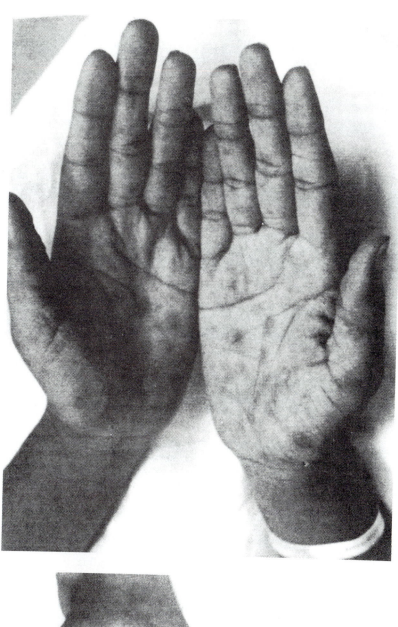

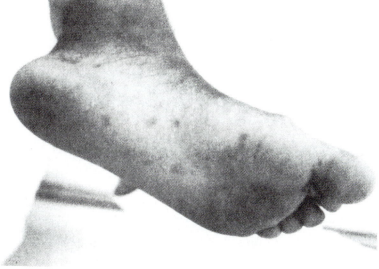

Figure 12–3. (Top) Secondary syphilis: Papular rash of the palms. **(Bottom)** Secondary syphilis: Papular rash of the sole. *(From Faro, S. [1985]. Sexually transmitted diseases. In S. Faro [Ed.], Diagnosis and management of female pelvic infections in primary care medicine. Baltimore: Williams & Wilkins. Reprinted with permission.)*

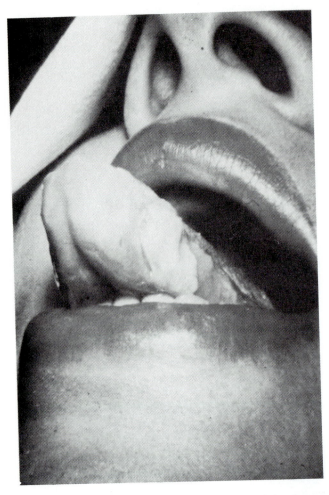

Figure 12-4. Secondary syphilis: Mucous patch of the tongue. *(From Knox, J. M. & Rudolph, A. H. [1984]. Acquired infectious syphilis. In K. K. Holmes, P.-A. Mårdh, P. F. Sparling, & P. J. Wiesner [Eds.], Sexually transmitted diseases. New York: McGraw–Hill. Reprinted with permission.)*

LATENT SYPHILIS. Latent syphilis has no clinical symptoms, although relapses of secondary disease may occur in up to 25 percent of untreated persons, particularly in the first year.

Early latency is potentially infectious and defined by the U.S. Public Health Service as 1 year from the onset of infection although some authors extend this period. *Late latent* syphilis follows and persists until symptoms of tertiary syphilis become manifest.

TERTIARY SYPHILIS. Tertiary syphilis is the main cause of morbidity and mortality from syphilis in adults. It has manifestations in the skin, bones, central nervous system, and/or heart and blood vessels. Manifestations of tertiary syphilis can appear from 1 to 2 years after onset of infection or as late as 30 to 40 or more years later.

Cutaneous bone lesions are called *gumma*. They are amenable to treatment, but can cause destruction of soft tissue and bone. Neurologic syphilis may be asymptomatic, defined as abnormalities in the cerebrospinal fluid without clinical symptoms. When symptomatic, neurosyphilis may present as acute syphilitic meningitis, vascular neurosyphilis, syphilis of the spinal cord, general paresis, tabes dorsalis (characterized by a weakening or loss of ankle and bone reflexes), optic atrophy, or intracranial masses (Swartz, 1984). Untreated neurosyphilis causes clinical symptomatology in up to 87 percent of the infected over a 5- to 18-year period. The disorder is often responsive to treatment, however. Cardiovascular syphilis can cause aortic aneurysm, coronary artery disease, aortic valve disease, and, rarely, myocarditis (Bulkley, 1984). Congenital syphilis has a particular course, a description of which is beyond the scope of this book.

The clinical presentation of the person with tertiary syphilis depends on the body system or systems affected. She may have impaired speech, concentration, and memory with tremors of the hands or lips. She may have personality changes and manic/euphoric states. Absence or weakening of the deep tendon reflexes of the knees or ankles may be noted.

Differential Diagnosis. The differential diagnosis of syphilis varies according to its stage. Primary syphilis must be differentiated from other STDs including herpes, chan-

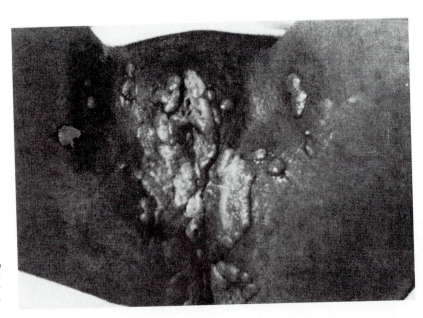

Figure 12-5. Condylomata lata of secondary syphilis. *(From Faro, S. [1985]. Sexually transmitted diseases. In S. Faro [Ed.], Diagnosis and management of female pelvic infections in primary care medicine. Baltimore: Williams & Wilkins. Reprinted with permission.)*

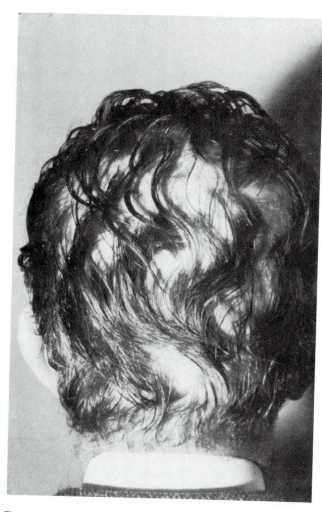

Figure 12–6. Secondary syphilis: Patchy alopecia. *(From Knox, J. M. & Rudolph, A. H. [1984]. Acquired infectious syphilis. In K. K. Holmes, P.-A. Mårdh, P. F. Sparling, & P. J. Wiesner [Eds.], Sexually transmitted diseases. New York: McGraw–Hill. Courtesy of E. Stolz.)*

croid, granuloma inguinale, and lymphogranuloma venereum, as well as from tumors and a great variety of skin and mucous membrane disorders, many of which are discussed in Chapter 11. Secondary syphilis must be differentiated from dermatologic and infectious diseases such as measles, infectious mononucleosis, erythema multiforme, leukemia, lymphoma, tinea, and a host of others (Knox & Rudolph, 1984). Condylomata lata must be differentiated from condylomata acuminata. Latent syphilis generally goes undetected, except by laboratory testing. The differential diagnosis of tertiary syphilis depends on the organs or systems that it affects; it must obviously be differentiated from other pathologic conditions affecting those systems. A full discussion of the differential diagnosis of tertiary syphilis is beyond the scope of this book.

The laboratory examinations for syphilis are not necessarily specific for the disorder. The differential diagnosis of a positive serologic test is discussed under Data Collection.

Management

DATA COLLECTION

History. A sexual history including numbers of partners, numbers of partners of partners, and numbers of casual

partners provides information revealing a woman's likelihood of acquiring any STD and should be routinely included in the history. Any history of a lesion on the patient's or her partner's genitalia should lead to a suspicion of syphilis, particularly if it was nontender, followed sexual relations by 5 to 90 days, and healed within 2 to 8 weeks. Any undiagnosed lesions or rashes, especially on the mucous membranes and/or soles or palms, should be discussed, particularly if they have healed spontaneously. Patchy hair loss is a significant historic finding.

Any history of exposure to syphilis or other STD should prompt immediate diagostic testing. Previous diagnosed episodes of syphilis, the treatment regimen followed, and results of follow-up testing should be fully discussed. This is especially important in the interpretation of serologic tests. Although syphilis infection does not result in immunity, sometimes a seeming positive test for the disease actually indicates a previously treated infection (see later).

Physical Examination. A careful examination of the genitals, including vulva, vagina, labia, clitoris, and cervix, anal area, other mucous membranes, and soles and palms, should be performed, looking for signs of primary and secondary syphilis as described earlier. Palpation of the liver and spleen on abdominal examination may reveal organomegaly, occasionally seen in secondary syphilis. Palpation of firm inguinal lymph nodes should arouse suspicion of an STD or vaginal infection.

Laboratory Testing. Laboratory testing and correct interpretation of tests are key to appropriate diagnosis of syphilis. Darkfield microscopic examination and serologic testing are the standard diagnostic tests in use today. Examination of cerebrospinal fluid (CSF) is part of a diagnostic workup for patients suspected of having neurosyphilis. It is imperative that the practitioner be able to judge when to implement these tests as screening or diagnostic measures, know how to interpret them, and decide when additional testing and when consultation or referral are required for diagnosis. A positive darkfield microscopic examination is a definitive test for syphilis. Darkfield can identify *T. pallidum* in lesions associated with primary, secondary, relapsing, and early congenital syphilis. All suspicious lesions should be subjected to a darkfield examination (Larsen, McGrew, Hunter, & Creighton, 1984). A properly equipped laboratory and trained personnel must be available for this specialized test. Before a specimen is collected for darkfield, the practitioner must make certain that the laboratory can perform this test or refer the patient to a facility where such an examination can be carried out. A positive test is one in which the syphilis spirochetes are demonstrated with their characteristic morphology and motility.

The serous fluid in the lesion provides the best darkfield specimen; it is rich in *T. pallidum* with few red blood cells that can obscure the organism. Rubber gloves should be worn when obtaining the specimen. Eating, drinking, and smoking should be avoided while the specimen is being taken. The procedure is as follows (Larsen et al., 1984):

1. Remove scabs or crusts from the lesion.
2. Using a gauze wet with water or saline, remove tissue debris and superficial bacteria.
3. Dry and gently abrade the lesion with a dry gauze sponge until there is slight bleeding and exudation of fluid.
4. Wipe away the first drops of blood and wait for the exudate to appear clear. Pressure may be applied if

necessary at the base of the lesion to cause exudation.

5. Apply a clean slide to the lesion or use a sterile bacteriologic loop to place exudate from the lesion onto the slide. The loop is used for vaginal and cervical lesions.
6. Place a coverslip over the specimen.
7. Make several slides if enough exudate is available.

Skin lesions, or healing lesions, may be sampled by making a superficial abrasion of the lesion with a needle or scalpel or by aspirating fluid with a small-gauge needle or syringe.

Specimens with serous fluid oozing from the coverglass should be discarded in a suitable container with disinfectant and replaced with another specimen with less fluid. Seventy percent ethyl alcohol should be used to clean up any areas contaminated by exudate.

The darkfield examination should be done *immediately*; before the specimen is taken, the laboratory must be notified that a slide is coming or asked to send laboratory personnel with the microscope to the examining room. In some institutions, the patient is sent to the laboratory and laboratory personnel take the specimen.

A positive darkfield is indicative of syphilis. A negative examination, however, does not provide a definite diagnosis. A negative examination can be repeated within 3 days, or the patient can be referred for aspiration of lymph nodes. Serologic testing is required when suspicion persists despite a negative darkfield examination. It should be performed in 1 week, 1 month, and 3 months. If the 3-month serology remains negative, the diagnosis can then be excluded.

The Wasserman test was the first of the nontreponemal serologic tests developed for syphilis; it was widely used in the first part of this century. Later, a number of other nontreponemal tests were developed and are used more widely today. The treponemal tests are more specific, but more difficult to perform, and are used to confirm diagnosis when the nontreponemal test is positive.

Nontreponemal serologic tests are used on serum to demonstrate the presence of *reagin*, a group of antibodies present in syphilis. Examples of nontreponemal tests include the VDRL (Venereal Disease Research Laboratory) slide test, the USR (unheated serum reagin) test, the RPR (rapid plasma reagin) card test, and the ART (automated reagin test). The newest test is the RST (reagin screen test). The tests most commonly used today are the VDRL and RPR.

Sensitivity of these tests is highest in secondary syphilis; the VDRL and other nontreponemal tests have a sensitivity of 59 to 87 percent in primary disease, 100 percent in secondary disease, 73 to 91 percent in latent disease, and 37 to 94 percent in late-stage disease (Jaffe, 1984). Laboratory testing must therefore be correlated closely with historic information and physical examination findings. When a test is negative in any suspected stage other than secondary, it should be repeated after 1 to 3 months; if the suspicion is of latent or late syphilis, then a treponemal test should be ordered.

Conditions other than syphilis can result in a positive nontreponemal test. These include acute bacterial or viral infections such as infectious mononucleosis and malaria; aging; drug addiction; autoimmune disease such as systemic lupus erythematosus and arthritis; and pregnancy.

Treponemal tests detect an antibody more specific for the genus *Treponema*. The standard treponemal test is the fluorescent treponemal antibody absorption (FTA-ABS).

Two newer tests may also be used: the microhemagglutination assay for *T. pallidum* (MHA-TP) and the hemagglutination treponemal test for syphilis (HATTS). They are less expensive and easier to perform than the FTA-ABS but, today, less widely available (Jaffe 1984).

The FTA-ABS is 56 to 100 percent sensitive in primary syphilis, 99 to 100 percent sensitive in secondary syphilis, 96 to 99 percent sensitive in latent disease, and 96 to 100 percent sensitive in late-stage disease.

Treponemal tests have a 99 percent specificity rate, which means they rarely show false-positive results, occurring mainly in women with systemic lupus erythematosus. False-positive results are often transient. Because of this high specificity, treponemal tests can be used to confirm the results of a positive nontreponemal test.

Patients with multiple sex partners and those with other STDs should be screened for syphilis. Routine screening is done on all pregnant women. Premarital screening is mandated in some states by law and must be implemented where required before a marriage licence is granted.

Diagnostic testing is implemented in patients with a history of exposure or any suspicious lesions, or a history of suspicious lesions, in themselves or their partners. Sexual partners must also be tested for syphilis whenever the disease is diagnosed or suspected.

A positive nontreponemal test should always be followed by a treponemal test; if both are positive the diagnosis is generally assumed. If the second test is negative, a search for another cause of a positive nontreponemal test should be undertaken. Medical consultation or referral is required. A positive nontreponemal test should be serially quantified to help determine whether the positive test indicates current infection or previously treated infection; the former is characterized by a high titer or a fourfold increase in titer; the latter is characterized by a low titer that does not increase. The stage of the disease can also be inferred from the quantitative results, with high titers in secondary syphilis and low titers in primary or late-stage disease; when available, however, historic and physical examination data provide better information regarding disease stage.

Primary syphilis is most easily diagnosed by the presence of the treponemal spirochetes under darkfield microscopy. Nontreponemal tests may be nonreactive in about 25 percent of persons with primary disease. The nontreponemal test should then be repeated at 1 week, 1 month, and 3 months. If it remains negative, the diagnosis is excluded. Although the treponemal test has a higher sensitivity at this stage of disease, it is usually not done.

Lesions of *secondary syphilis* should correlate with both nontreponemal and treponemal testing. If nontreponemal testing is positive, both a quantitative nontreponemal assay and a treponemal test should be performed. If the treponemal test is negative, the practitioner must search for a cause other than syphilis. Titers of the nontreponemal test are usually 1:16 or greater with secondary syphilis. By late syphilis, however, titers may fall to 1:16 or 1:8 (Faro, 1985).

Nontreponemal tests are relatively insensitive in *late syphilis*; all patients with suspected late syphilis should have a treponemal test. With a suspicion of neurosyphilis, a lumbar puncture for analysis of cerebrospinal fluid (CSF) should be performed. For syphilis of more than 1 year's duration there is controversy about whether routine tests of CSF are necessary; however, as routine treatments may not be effective for neurosyphilis after disease has persisted more than 1 year, this test is often recommended (Graman, Trupei, & Reichman, 1987; Jaffe, 1984).

Tests for other STDs including gonorrhea, chlamydia,

and trichomoniasis should be implemented for anyone diagnosed with syphilis or in whom the suspicion exists.

INTERVENTION

Treatment. Treatment must be initiated for anyone diagnosed with syphilis by laboratory examination. Although lesions associated with primary and secondary syphilis heal spontaneously, the potential for tertiary syphilis is too great to allow the disease to go untreated. Treatment is determined by stage of disease, based on historic, physical examination, and laboratory information. In the absence of physical findings, without a history that pinpoints exposure, the practitioner must assume late latent disease and treat accordingly.

The CDC (1985b) recommends the following treatments:

- *Syphilis of less than 1 year's duration:* Benzathine penicillin G 2.4 million units total IM at one session or tetracycline HCl 500 mg by mouth four times daily for 15 days for penicillin-allergic patients. Erythromycin 500 mg by mouth four times daily for 15 days is an alternative for patients unable to tolerate tetracycline.
- *Syphilis of more than 1 year's duration:* Benzathine penicillin G 2.4 million units IM once a week for 3 successive weeks (7.2 million units total) or tetracycline HCl or erythromycin 500 mg by mouth four times daily for 30 days for penicillin- or tetracycline-allergic persons.

These regimens may be insufficient for neurosyphilis. Neurosyphilis should be managed in coordination with an expert; hospitalization for intravenous or daily intramuscular penicillin may be necessary.

Pregnant women with demonstrated syphilis should be treated with penicillin or erythromycin. Congenital syphilis requires treatment effective for neurosyphilis, even in the absence of positive cerebrospinal fluid findings.

In addition to allergic or toxic reactions to penicillin (Table 12–2), patients treated with penicillin for syphilis can develop a reaction to the rapid destruction of spirochetes in their bodies. This is known as the Jarisch–Herxheimer reaction. Within hours of treatment, the patient develops chills, fever, headache, myalgia, and arthralgia. The syphilitic lesions become edematous, prominent, and bright in color. The reaction, which lasts a few hours, is seen most often in the treatment of secondary syphilis (about 9 percent of these cases). Patients should be made more comfortable with sedation. Treatment must not be withheld or discontinued because of the reaction (Monif, 1982).

Follow-up. Follow-up must be provided for all persons treated for syphilis. Those with early or congenital syphilis should have quantitative nontreponemal tests at 3, 6, and 12 months after treatment. Titers should decline to nonreactive or low reactive levels. Test results may decline more slowly after treatment of disease of longer duration; persons treated for syphilis of longer duration should have a repeat test at 24 months. Patients with neurosyphilis need CSF examinations for at least 3 years and more frequent serologic testing.

Re-treatment should be considered when clinical signs or symptoms of syphilis persist or recur, there is a fourfold increase in the titer of a nontreponemal test, or an initially high-titer nontreponemal test fails to decrease fourfold within a year. For retreatment, doses recommended for syphilis of more than 1 year's duration should be used.

Patients may continue to have low reactive nontreponemal titers for life. The treponemal test will always remain positive.

Teaching and Counseling. The nature of syphilis and its mode of transmission must be explained. The need for treatment, even in the absence of symptoms, must be carefully discussed. When patients need to have treatment over several weeks, the need to return to complete the full course must be made extremely clear. It is imperative that the practitioner ascertain each woman's understanding of the disease and treatment regimen as adequate therapy depends on follow-up. Sometimes people without symptoms are reluctant to subject themselves to treatment, particularly if injections are painful or a reaction ensues. The signs of the Jarisch–Herxheimer reaction should be explained and patients told to call if symptoms occur.

Intercourse should not be resumed until all evidence of primary or secondary syphilis is gone. It is advisable to wait until serologic evidence of cure is demonstrated.

Women must be told to notify all sexual partners who might have been exposed to the infection to be tested and treated if necessary. They should be informed that the disease is reportable. Names of sex partners can be reported to the Department of Health for tracing if the woman agrees. Women should also have their children screened if it is possible that they had the infection during pregnancy. Women should be given the opportunity to be tested for other STDs, including gonorrhea and chlamydia.

Preventive measures outlined in the early part of this chapter should be discussed. Women should understand that syphilis infection does not afford immunity and that they can be reinfected.

Extreme sensitivity is essential when discussing the diagnosis of syphilis; the disease carries many negative connotations. It may instill a sense of dread, shame, or fear; practitioners must demonstrate objectivity in providing information while showing sensitivity to each patient's feelings and emotional needs. All women must be given ample opportunity to air their feelings, ask any questions, and call the practitioner with any concerns that surface later. As always, literature should be provided for patients and their partners.

Lymphogranuloma Venereum

Lymphogranuloma venereum (LGV) was recognized as a separate venereal disease in 1915, and a skin test was developed for diagnosis in 1924 (Krieger, 1984). This disease has also been called *bubo, strumous bubo, poradenitis inguinalis, Durand–Nicolas–Favre disease,* and *lymphogranuloma inguinale.* It has often been confused clinically with syphilis, genital herpes, and chancroid. Unlike these diseases, however, it is primarily a disorder of lymph tissue.

Etiology and Transmission. LGV is caused by three specific types of *Chlamydia,* designated L1, L2, and L3. The chlamydial organism is discussed more thoroughly under *Chlamydia trachomatis.*

These organisms enter the skin or mucous membranes, most likely through tiny lacerations and abrasions (Perine & Osoba, 1984). The infectivity of the disease is not known. The primary lesion of LGV usually appears at the site of infection 3 to 12 or more days after exposure. Infection does not confer immunity.

Epidemiology. LGV is endemic in east and west Africa, India, parts of Southeast Asia, South America, and the Caribbean. In the United States, where LGV is a reportable disease, it is uncommon, with 600 to 1,000 cases reported annually (Faro, 1985). Many of these cases occur in people who have traveled to endemic areas. The disease is more common in urban than rural areas, among persons with multiple sex partners, and in the lower socioeconomic groups. Of interest is that large segments of the population have been found to have positive serologic or skin tests without historic or physical evidence of the disease (Perine & Osoba, 1984).

LGV peaks in persons in their twenties, although it has been seen in adolescents. It is more common in men than women, although this may be because early symptomatic infection is less common in females.

Clinical Presentation. LGV has three clinical stages. The primary disease manifestation may be a papule, a shallow ulcer or erosion, a small herpeslike lesion, or nonspecific urethritis. Primary lesions are symptomatic and appear in only 3 to 53 percent of infected persons. In women, the lesion is most often seen on the posterior vaginal wall, the fourchette, the posterior cervical lip, or the vulva. Primary disease may cause cervicitis. Lesions may occur in the mouth and pharynx secondary to oral–genital sex. The primary lesion heals within days without treatment.

In its secondary stage, apparent 1 to 3 weeks after healing of the lesion, LGV causes two main syndromes: the inguinal syndrome and/or the anal–genital–rectal syndrome. The inguinal syndrome is characterized by inflammation of the lymph nodes in the inguinal area, but only 20 to 30 percent of women show inguinal adenopathy. The enlarging nodes are called *inguinal buboes*. Infected women in this stage may complain of lower back and abdominal pain, indicating involvement of the deep pelvic and lumbar lymph nodes. The anal–genital–rectal syndrome is characterized by proctocolitis and hyperplasia of intestinal and perirectal lymphatics. In women, rectal manifestations are secondary to either anal intercourse or contamination of the anal area by vaginal secretions or through spread via the lymphatics from the cervix and posterior vaginal wall. Symptoms of proctocolitis include fever, rectal pain, and tenesmus. The left upper quadrant of the abdomen is tender and the pelvic colon may feel thickened on examination. Rectal examination reveals granular rectal mucosa. Most patients recover from second-stage disease without problems.

Late-stage manifestations include perirectal abscesses, ischiorectal and rectovaginal fistulas, anal fistulas, and rectal strictures or stenosis. Other chronic LGV symptoms include ulcerations, particularly of the labia majora, crural folds, and perineum, and papillary growths on the urethra, which may cause urinary tract symptoms. Elephantiasis of the labia and clitoris may develop in late-stage disease, 1 to 20 years after infection (Coutts, 1950, p. 552).

Differential Diagnosis. Early-stage LGV must be differentiated from other vulvar and vaginal problems causing ulcerations or papular lesions, including herpes genitalis, secondary syphilis, chancroid, granuloma inguinale, and allergic or contact vulvovaginitis. The lower abdominal and back pain associated with the second stage of LGV may be mistaken for acute gastroenteritis or appendicitis, salpingitis, or a tuboovarian abscess. Other diseases causing lymphadenopathy include plague, tularemia, tuberculosis, genital herpes, syphilis, chancroid, and Hodgkin's disease. Proctocolitis mimics inflammatory bowel disease. Rectal stricture is often mistaken for rectal cancer. Late-stage elephantiasis must be differentiated from filariasis and mycosis.

Management

DATA COLLECTION

History. A history of travel to or immigration from areas endemic for LGV or of sexual relations with a partner with recent travel is significant. A lesion appearing up to 1 month after intercourse and healing spontaneously is another clue, although because of the rarity of this diagnosis, the suspicion of LGV is rarely aroused. If the lesion is followed by symptoms of inguinal or anal–genital–rectal syndrome, then the likelihood of the diagnosis increases.

Physical Examination. Physical examination should include abdominal and inguinal palpation and complete visualization of the external and internal genitalia, including the urethra and cervix. Rectal examination is important if anorectal symptoms are reported.

Laboratory Testing. Diagnosis of LGV is made by laboratory examination. Several types of diagnostic tests exist. The original Frei skin test is no longer in use because it is nonspecific and may remain positive long after the infection is gone, even for life (Perine & Osoba, 1984). Newer tests include the complement fixation test, the neutralizing antibody test, the microimmunofluorescent (MICRO-IF) test, and other serologic tests. Cytology may be used and later disease stages must be differentiated from other diagnoses by a variety of medical tests. Definitive diagnosis, however, can only be made through isolation of the organism from infected tissue.

The complement fixation (CF) test measures antibodies in serum. Active infections show reactivity with titers of 1:40 or greater (Wall, Heyman, & Beeson, 1947). High titers may be found, however, in patients with other chlamydial infections and asymptomatic individuals. Titers may persist many years at high or low levels (Greaves & Taggart, 1953). Titers may or may not vary at different stages of acute infection and up to 6 weeks of convalescence.

The neutralizing antibody test is another test of serum less commonly performed. The microimmunofluorescent (Micro-IF) test is more sensitive than the CF test but less widely available. Other serologic tests under investigation involve the use of serotype-specific monoclonal antibodies. These include enzyme-linked immunosorbent assay (ELISA) testing, which will make the diagnosis much more specific (Perine & Osabo, 1984).

LGV is caused by a chlamydial organism. Cytology and cultures for chlamydial organisms are discussed later in this chapter. Specimens can be taken from lesions or aspirated from enlarged lymph nodes.

Tests for other STDs should be performed as other STDs commonly coexist with LGV (Coutts, 1950).

INTERVENTION

Treatment. Although many patients with LGV become asymptomatic during the secondary period, the disease may be protracted, relapse, or progress to the tertiary stage (Coutts, 1950). The recommended treatment for LGV is tetracycline HCl 500 mg by mouth four times daily (Centers for Disease Control, 1985b). Alternative regimens with less confirmatory results include doxycycline 100 mg by mouth twice daily; erythromycin 500 mg by mouth four times daily; and sulfamethoxazole 1.0 g by mouth twice daily. All treatments must continue at least 2 weeks. Sex partners should be treated as well. More information about tetracycline is provided under *Chlamydia trachomatis*.

Consultation and Referral. LGV should be managed with consultation or referral to a physician experienced in its diagnosis and treatment. Complications of second- and third-stage disease certainly need medical evaluation and management. Fluctuant lymph nodes may require needle aspiration for diagnosis or to prevent rupture, although incision and drainage are contraindicated (Centers for Disease Control 1985b; Perine & Osaba, 1984).

Teaching and Counseling. The sexual transmission of LGV needs to be discussed with patients. Sexual partners must be notified, examined, and treated and intercourse avoided until all treatment regimens are completed.

Chancroid

Chancroid, also called *soft chancre* to differentiate it from hard chancre (syphilis), was first described in the midnineteenth century (Ronald & Albritton, 1984). It has been called one of the lesser STDs (Schwarz, 1983) because its effects are localized, not systemic, and because it is uncommon in this country.

Etiology and Transmission. Chancroid is caused by *Hemophilus ducreyi*, a Gram-negative facultative anaerobic bacillus. The organism has very rigid requirements for growth. It is transmitted through abrasions of the skin with an incubation period from 3 to 10 days, most commonly 4 to 7 days. The likelihood of being infected after sexual contact is unknown. Immunity is not conferred by infection and reinfection is relatively common (Schwarz, 1983).

Epidemiology. Chancroid is uncommon in the United States; a mean of 878 cases a year were reported between 1971 and 1980 (Schmid, 1986). In recent years, however, the number of cases in the United States has increased dramatically. In 1985, for the first time since 1956, more than 2,000 cases were reported; in 1986, 3,418 cases were reported (Schmid, Sanders, Blount, & Alexander, 1987). This increased prevalence is thought to be associated with the patronizing of prostitutes and travel outside the country to endemic areas. Cases have been clustered in New York, Texas, California, Florida, and Georgia, with these five states reporting 94.8 percent of the cases in 1986. Specific clusters of cases have also been reported in Winnipeg, Canada (between 1975 and 1977), Seattle (in 1978), and Orange County, California (between 1980 and 1982) (D'Costa, Bowmer, Nsanze, et al., 1986; Hammond, Slutchuk, Scatliff, et al., 1980). In some countries, particularly in the third world, the disease is one of the most commonly reported STDs (Faro, 1985; Ronald & Albritton, 1984). Males, particularly uncircumcized men, have higher rates of infection than females.

Clinical Presentation. The presenting symptom of chancroid is a soft, nonindurated genital ulcer, beginning as a tender papule with an erythematous surrounding. Over a 24- to 48-hour period, the lesion becomes a pustule and is eroded and ulcerated (Fig. 12–7). In women, the ulcer may or may not be painful. It is often friable and its base covered with a gray or yellow purulent exudate. Several ulcers may be present and may form one large lesion. Ulcers usually

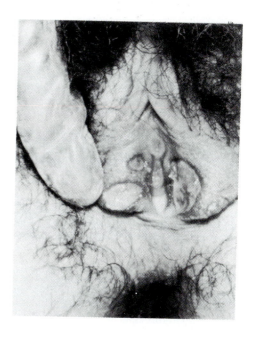

Figure 12–7. Chancroid of the female genitalia: Multiple, well-defined ulcers with gray, necrotic bases. *(From Gardner, H. L. [1981]. Venereal diseases. In H. L. Gardner & R. H. Kaufman [Eds.], Benign diseases of the vulva and vagina [2nd ed.]. Boston: G. K. Hall Medical Publishers. Reprinted with permission.)*

appear at the vaginal entrance; other common sites include the labia, vestibule, clitoris, and periurethral area. Perianal ulcers may be present (Hammond et al., 1980). Extragenital lesions may occur where there are abrasions on the skin. Ulcers may persist weeks to months without treatment. Superinfection of the ulcers may cause severe tissue destruction.

Presenting symptoms in women may not relate directly to the ulcer. Women often complain of dysuria, even to the extent of urinary retention; pain with defecation; rectal bleeding; dyspareunia; or vaginal discharge. Prickling or itching has been described (Lao & Trussell, 1947). Mild systemic symptoms may be present although the organism does not cause disease in distant sites.

Complications. Complications of chancroid include rectovaginal fistulas and painful inguinal adenopathy, often one sided with redness of the overlying skin. Rupture of these "inguinal buboes" may occur. The buboes can be differentiated from those of LGV because with LGV they are bilateral and multiple.

In Africa, there is evidence that the open lesions of chancroid and other ulcerative diseases have contributed to the rapid spread of human immunodeficiency virus (see later in this chapter) (Schmid et al., 1987).

Differential Diagnosis. Chancroid must be differentiated from other diseases that present with genital ulcers. These include syphilis, genital herpes, and granuloma inguinale. Inguinal buboes may be mistaken for the buboes of LGV.

Management

Data Collection. History. An onset of genital symptoms after recent travel to or immigration from the tropics or sexual contact with a partner from the tropics may precede the onset of symptoms. Engaging in prostitution or sexual contact with a partner who has had contact with a prostitute can be considered a risk factor and should be queried about. Additional historic data in women may not help much with diagnosis as symptoms may be nonspecific. If a genital ulcer is reported, the absence of a prodrome helps to differentiate it from herpes genitalis (see later), and the presence of pain, from primary syphilis (see earlier).

Physical Examination. The entire genital and anal areas should be carefully examined for a tender lesion as described earlier. The inguinal area should be palpated for tender lymphadenopathy.

Laboratory Testing. *H. ducreyi* must be isolated from the genital ulcer or bubo for definitive diagnosis. The organism can be cultured on gonococcal chocolate agar medium or Mueller–Hinton agar base (D'Costa et al., 1986). Cultures should be allowed to grow up to 7 days. The specimen is best taken from scrapings from the edges of the ulcer or aspirated from the bubo. A Gram stain of exudate may be difficult to interpret because other bacteria are usually present; however, an aspirate from a bubo that demonstrates Gram-negative rods in chains without other bacteria may be considered diagnostic (Faro, 1985). Diagnostic testing for chancroid may require referral so that an aspirate can be taken from the bubo. Tests to rule out syphilis, herpes, and LGV should be performed and testing for other STDs such as gonorrhea and chlamydia is appropriate.

INTERVENTION

Treatment. The CDC-recommended treatment for chancroid is erythromycin 500 mg by mouth four times daily for 7 days or ceftriaxone 250 mg intramuscularly in a single dose. Alternative regimens include trimethoprim/sulfamethoxazole, one double-strength tablet by mouth twice daily for a minimum of 7 days or a single oral dose of four double-strength or eight single-strength tablets. Amoxicillin 500 mg plus clavulanic acid 125 mg three times daily for 7 days constitute another alternative. The alternative treatments have not been evaluated in the United States, however.

The CDC points out that susceptibility of the organism *H. ducreyi* varies. If treatment is not successful within 7 days, antimicrobial susceptibility testing should be initiated and an alternative medication regimen prescribed.

Follow-Up. Sexual contacts should be treated even if asymptomatic (Schmid, 1986). Follow-up at frequent intervals is important to assess response to medication and reinfection; reinfection has been noted within 2 months of treatment (Lao & Trussell, 1947).

Consultation and Referral. Referral to a medical expert with experience treating chancroid should always be made. Fluctuant lymph nodes may require aspiration. Incision and drainage is contraindicated.

Self-Help Measures. Soaking with saline or dilute potassium permanganate may promote healing of the genital ulcers (Monif, 1982). Keeping the area clean to avoid secondary infection is important. Washing with soap and water and general hygienic practices should be encouraged.

Additional Teaching and Counseling. Patients must understand the sexually transmitted nature of this disease and make certain that their sex partners receive treatment. Condoms have not been proven effective in prevention, but minimal data exist on their role (Ronald & Albritton, 1984). Patients should be provided with follow-up appointments within 2 months of treatment for reevaluation.

Granuloma Inguinale

Also known as *donovanosis*, granuloma inguinale was described in the late nineteenth century and its causative agent identified by Donovan in 1905 (Hart, 1984). It is a chronic, bacterial infection of the genitals that can lead to progressive destruction of the genital area.

Etiology and Transmission. Granuloma inguinale is caused by *Calymmatobacterium granulomatis*, a Gram-negative bacteria. The disease, formerly called *Donovania granulomatis*, is generally considered sexually transmitted, although lesions have not always been detected in sexual partners of the infected (Hart, 1984). This may be a result of the disease's long incubation period—8 to 80 days—or the existence of inconspicuous lesions. Disease is known to occur after nonsexual trauma, however.

Granuloma inguinale is not highly infective; repeated exposure is necessary for infection. Presumably, the organism enters through breaks in the skin or mucosa (Schwarz, 1983). Anal intercourse is a major cause of transmission, and vaginal infection may follow autoinoculation from the rectum (Goldberg, 1964). Immunity is not conferred by infection.

Epidemiology. Granuloma inguinale is one of the most prevalent STDs in the Third World. It is endemic among certain aboriginal groups in Australia and common in India, the Caribbean, Africa, and other tropical areas (Bhagwandeen & Naik, 1977; Hart, 1984). In 1974, 51 cases were reported in the United States (Schwarz, 1983), with clustering of the few reported cases among the black population of the southeastern United States.

Clinical Presentation. Granuloma inguinale begins with single or multiple subcutaneous nodules that erode through the skin. The skin lesions are granulomatous, are sharply defined, and usually produce no pain. They bleed easily on contact and grow slowly. Beefy red granulation tissue may be seen. Secondary infection may produce necrosis on or around the lesion. There may be inguinal enlargement.

Complications and Sequelae. Massive edema of the vulva (elephantiasis) may occur. Systemic disease is rare, although Monif (1982) reports a possible association between granuloma inguinale and cancer of the vulva in young women in Jamaica, even after treatment. The liver, thorax, and bones may be involved.

Differential Diagnosis. Early lesions may be confused with primary syphilis or with condylomata lata of secondary syphilis. The lesion may be confused with herpes, chancroid, or LGV, and amebiasis and cancer in males, but its granulomatous nature should differentiate it from ulcers associated with these other STDs. Inguinal enlargement may lead to confusion of the disease with LGV or chancroid (Hart, 1984).

Management

DATA COLLECTION

History. Travel to the tropics or immigration from a tropical country may give a clue to the presence of this disease. A careful history of symptoms in the patient and sexual partners should be elicited.

Physical Examination. A complete examination of the inguinal, anal, and genital areas, externally and internally, is essential.

Laboratory Testing. Diagnosis of granuloma inguinale is made by a smear stained with Wright's or Giemsa's stain showing Donovan bodies—clusters of blue or black organisms with a safety pin appearance in the cytoplasm of large mononuclear cells (Hart, 1984). The ulcer should be scraped near its base to obtain the specimen. Biopsy can confirm diagnosis. Obviously, someone experienced in identifying the lesions should examine the specimen; referral is therefore necessary.

Darkfield microscopy should be performed to distinguish the lesions from syphilis (see earlier) and a serology taken after 1 week, 2 months, and 3 months if diagnosis has not been made. Tests for other STDs, including gonorrhea and chlamydia, should be performed.

INTERVENTION

Treatment. Antibiotics effective against the disease include chloramphenicol (0.5 g every 8 hours by mouth for 21 days), gentamycin (1 mg/kg twice daily for 21 days), streptomycin (1 g twice a day intramuscularly), and erythromycin (500 mg every 6 hours for 10 days) (Hart, 1984; Lal, 1971; Robinson & Cohen, 1953). Oral ampicillin (250 to 500 mg four times daily) is effective but may require use up to 12 weeks (Thew, Swift, & Heaton, 1969). Cotrimoxazole (two tablets every 12 hours for 10 days) has been found effective (Latif, Mason, & Paraiwa, 1988). Tetracycline is often the first choice for treatment: 500 mg every 6 hours for at least 3 weeks.

Resistance has sometimes been seen (Breschi, Goldman, & Shapiro, 1975). Treatment must be continued as long as the lesions persist. Treatment stopped before 3 weeks is associated with higher rates of recurrence (Hart, 1984). Clinical response, however, is usually seen within 7 days if treatment is effective. Lesions become paler and less friable, and shrink shortly afterward. A depigmented area may persist at the border of the healed lesion.

Follow-up. Follow-up is essential during treatment and should be weekly once treatment is initiated until it is completed and lesions are healed. Examinations should then be scheduled every 3 to 4 months with immediate follow-up if lesions recur.

Self-Help Measures. Breschi et al. (1975) recommend local treatment consisting of thorough washing with soap twice daily. Warm sitz baths with 1:10,000 potassium permanganate three times a day have proven helpful as well (Monif, 1982).

Additional Teaching and Counseling. The patient should understand the nature of the disease and its treatment. She should be able to explain the treatment regimen and receive appointments for follow-up visits. All issues regarding the prevention of STDs should be discussed, stressing particu-larly the risks of anal–genital intercourse. All sexual partners within the previous 3 to 6 months should be notified, examined, and treated as necessary. Patients should be informed that granuloma inguinale is a reportable disease.

OTHER BACTERIAL INFECTIONS

Chlamydia Trachomatis

Genital infections caused by *Chlamydia trachomatis* are the most prevalent of the STDs in the United States today (Centers for Disease Control, 1985a). Although their clinical course may be silent, their complications and sequelae can be serious. Therefore, the detection and treatment of this organism are of primary importance in well-woman gynecologic care. Various diseases caused by a form of this organism, including LGV, have been described since antiquity, although it was not until this century that the chlamydial organism was identified (Schachter, 1984).

Etiology and Transmission. Chlamydial organisms are classified as bacteria although they share properties with both bacteria and viruses. They are obligate intracellular parasites, like viruses; however, like bacteria, they contain both deoxyribonucleic acid (DNA) and ribonucleic acid (RNA), divide by binary fission, and have cell walls similar to Gram-negative bacteria. Because of the difficulty involved in growing the organism in culture medium, it was only relatively recently that chlamydial-caused infections were able to be diagnosed.

Two species of chlamydial organisms exist (*C. trachomatis* and *C. psittaci*), and a number of serotypes of *C. trachomatis* have been identified. These cause a variety of diseases including LGV, blinding trachoma, conjunctivitis, nongonococcal urethritis, cervicitis, salpingitis, proctitis, epididymitis, and newborn pneumonia (Schachter, 1984). Types D through K cause genital infections (Loucks, 1987). Strains other than those causing LGV seem to grow only in squamocolumnar cells.

C. trachomatis can be transmitted sexually, and, in industrialized Western society, all clinical infections of *C. trachomatis* are acquired this way or through perinatal transmission. The organism has been transmitted in donor semen through artificial insemination (Mascola & Guinan, 1987). Trachoma, an infection of the eye caused by *C. trachomatis* and resulting in blindness, is endemic in many parts of the Third World and is often acquired through child-to-child transmission; whether there is a genital tract reservoir for this infection is unknown (Schachter, 1984).

The incubation period for *C. trachomatis* infection is 1 to 2 weeks after exposure; infection, however, often is clinically inapparent. Although some degree of immunity may be conferred after one or more infections, this is usually not strong enough to keep individuals from becoming reinfected, and repeat infections are, in fact, common (Schachter, 1984).

Epidemiology. Chlamydial genital infections are the most prevalent STD in the United States today. It is estimated that three to four million people contract chlamydia annually (Centers for Disease Control, 1985a). More than half of women infected with *C. trachomatis* have no clinical signs or symptoms (Schachter, Stoner, & Moncada, 1983). In men, *C. trachomatis* is found in 30 to 60 percent of nongonococcal urethritis (NGU) and is responsible for 70 percent of postgonococcal urethritis (Schachter, 1978). Fifty to seventy percent of female sexual partners of men with chlamydial

NGU are found to harbor *C. trachomatis* in the cervix (Stamm & Holmes, 1984). Prevalence studies have found infection rates in asymptomatic women varying from 3 to 5 percent to over 20 percent in STD clinics (Bowie, Borrie-Hume, Manzon, et al., 1981; Brunham, Irwin, Stamm, & Holmes, 1981; Hilton, Richmond, Milne, et al., 1974; Johannisson, Lowhagen, & Lycke, 1980; Oriel, Johnson, Barlow, et al., 1978; Oriel, Powis, Reeve, et al., 1974; Paavonen, Saikku, Vesterinen, et al., 1978; Richmond, Paul, & Taylor, 1980; Ripa, Svensson, Mårdh, & Weström, 1978; Schachter et al., 1983).

Rates of chlamydial infection in adolescents have been reported between 15 and 28 percent, with some studies showing higher rates among blacks and persons from lower socioeconomic groups (Chacko & Lovchik, 1984; Eagar, Beach, Davidson, & Judson, 1985; Saltz, Linnemann, Brookman, & Rauh, 1981; Shafer, Chew, Kromhout, et al., 1985). Rates in sexually active women less than 20 years old are two to three times higher than rates in women 20 years old or older. Women in their twenties have higher rates of infection than those in their thirties (Schachter et al., 1983). Use of oral contraceptives has been associated with chlamydial infection (see Chapter 7).

Predictors of *C. trachomatis* infection are young age, increased numbers of sexual partners, and low socioeconomic status. In one study, the following demographic, behavioral, and clinical characteristics were predictive of chlamydial infection: age 24 or less; intercourse with a new partner within the preceding 2 months; examination results showing purulent or mucopurulent cervical exudate; bleeding induced by swabbing the endocervical mucosa; and use of no contraception or a nonbarrier method (Handsfield, Jasman, Roberts, et al., 1986).

Clinical Presentation. In women, chlamydial infections are often asymptomatic. Infection in men is more likely to be symptomatic, but up to 30 percent of males with chlamydial urethritis have few or no symptoms (CDC, 1985a). Three clinical syndromes exist in women with chlamydial infection: mucopurulent cervicitis, urethral syndrome or urethritis, and pelvic inflammatory disease (PID or salpingitis). These various syndromes are described in Chapters 13, 15, and 17.

Thirty to fifty percent of women with a mucopurulent cervical exudate are found to harbor *C. trachomatis* (Brunham, Holmes, & Eschenbach, 1984). Hypertrophic ectopy has been found in women with chlamydia; this is defined as an edematous, congested, and friable area of the cervix. Ectopy may not be appreciated, however, without the benefit of colposcopy. Ectopy may, in fact, predispose women to chlamydial infection because it exposes a greater number of susceptible columnar epithelial cells to infection. This may explain why oral contraceptive use is associated with chlamydial infection; use promotes ectopy (Harrison, Costin, Meder, et al., 1985; Stamm & Holmes, 1984).

Complications and Sequelae. Acute or chronic salpingitis (PID) followed by subsequent infertility or possibly ectopic pregnancy may be associated with chlamydial infection of the fallopian tubes even more commonly than with gonorrheal infection (Mårdh, Ripa, Svensson, & Westrom, 1977; Osser & Persson, 1982; Thompson & Washington, 1983). Postabortion salpingitis and endometritis have been shown to be associated with chlamydial infection (Mårdh, Moller, Ingerslev, et al., 1981; Osser & Persson, 1984). Perihepatitis (Fitz-Hugh-Curtis syndrome) is a complication of chlamydia (Dalaker, Gjonnaess, Kvile, et al., 1981; Wølner-Hanssen, Weström, & Mårdh, 1980). Proctitis and pharyn-

gitis may occur (Goldmeier & Darougar, 1977; Schachter & Atwood, 1975).

Chlamydial infection may be passed to the newborn through the birth canal and cause newborn conjunctivitis and/or pneumonia (Chandler, Alexander, Pheiffer, 1977; Frommell, Rothenberg, Wang, & McIntosh, 1979; Hammerschlag, Anderka, Semine, et al., 1979). Other perinatal complications including prematurity have been suggested (Martin, Koutsky, Eschenbach, et al., 1982) and are being investigated. *Chlamydia* has been hypothesized to have a potentiator role in the development of cervical cancer (Cardillo, 1985; Harnekar, Leiman, & Markowitz, 1985), but this remains unproven.

Differential Diagnosis. Chlamydial and gonorrheal infections may be impossible to distinguish clinically. Other causes of cervical discharge including vaginitis (see Chapter 11) must be considered. The differential diagnoses of salpingitis and urinary tract infections are discussed in Chapters 15 and 17, respectively.

Management

Data Collection. History History of known exposure through sexual contact is most important; a history of exposure to NGU or to any male with urethritis is presumptive of chlamydia. Exposure to gonorrhea is also significant as the two infections frequently coexist. A sexual history should be thorough and include numbers of sexual partners and numbers of their partners, a new partner within the previous 2 months, and nonuse of contraception or use of nonbarrier methods, particularly oral contraceptives. Young age also is a significant risk factor.

Symptoms of urethritis in the female (Stamm, Wagner, Amsel, et al., 1980), of PID, and of vaginal discharge, particularly without irritation, pruritis, or odor may signify chlamydia; certainly this diagnosis should be considered.

Physical Examination. Thorough abdominal and pelvic examinations should be completed, with an especially careful cervical inspection. The most important physical examination finding in chlamydial infection is purulent or mucopurulent cervical discharge. Hypertrophic cervical ectopy should be noted although this may not be visible without magnification. Bartholin's glands should be examined and milked for discharge; *C. trachomatis* may cause infection of these glands. Chapters 15 and 17 provide a description of physical findings in salpingitis and urethritis, respectively.

Laboratory Testing. Because chlamydial infection cannot be distinguished from gonorrhea through clinical signs and symptoms, and because the infection is so often asymptomatic, laboratory testing constitutes the only definitive way to establish the diagnosis (although history of certain exposures and presence of gonorrhea presume infection and justify treatment).

Screening and diagnostic tests for *C. trachomatis* consist of cytology; antigen detection including fluorescent antibody examination of a direct smear and enzyme immunoassay; serologic testing; and culture.

In the past, stained smears were used to detect chlamydial infections but these are very insensitive. Today, other techniques have largely replaced them for diagnosing chlamydia (CDC, 1985a); however, the presence of five or more polymorphonucleocytes (PMNs) per high-power field may be an indication for further testing (Moscicki, Shafer, Millstein, et al., 1987). Pap smear may have some use as a screening test to identify women for whom further diagnostic testing would be worthwhile (Kiviat, Paavonen, Brockway, et al., 1985a; Kiviat, Peterson, Kinney-Thomas, et al., 1985b). The smear cannot be considered diagnostic, however (Dorman, Danos, Wilson, et al., 1983; Forster, Cookey, Munday, et al., 1985; Geerling, Nettum, Lindner, et al., 1985).

Several criteria have been proposed for interpretation of possible chlamydial infection on Pap smear. Pap smears showing a moderate to severe level of inflammation in the exudate, particularly with moderate to large numbers of transformed lymphocytes, were found in several studies to correlate with cultures positive for *C. trachomatis* (Kiviat et al., 1985a, 1985b; Lindner, Geerling, Nettum, et al., 1985; Shafer et al., 1985). In one study, intracytoplasmic coccoid inclusion bodies within metaplastic cells had a sensitivity of 54 percent and specificity of 71 percent when compared with cell culture for *C. trachomatis* (Quinn, Gupta, Burkman, et al., 1987). Other criteria have included nuclear alterations in cells with granular cytoplasm, inclusion bodies or eosinophilic chlamydial particles, or dense aggregates seen in vacuolated cytoplasmic inclusions (Dorman, Danos, Caron, et al., 1985; Gupta, Lee, Erozan, et al., 1979).

Antigen Detection. Material for a direct smear for fluorescent antibody examination is obtained by swab and placed on a slide. It is incubated with a fluorescein-conjugated monoclonal antibody and then examined under a fluorescence microscope. The sensitivity and specificity of this test are high; the former is 90 percent or higher and the latter 98 percent or higher. An additional advantage is the rapid processing time for the test. A commercially available direct fluorescent antibody test is the Microtrak. The test's usefulness is limited, however, by the need for specialized equipment and highly experienced personnel (CDC, 1985a; Tam, Stamm, Handsfield, et al., 1984).

Enzyme immunoassay measures antigen–antibody responses through an enzyme-linked immunosorbent assay (ELISA). Sensitivity and specificity for the detection of *C. trachomatis* using an ELISA test vary from 67 to 90 percent and 92 to 97 percent, respectively. The test takes about 4 hours. A widely available commercial test for enzyme immunoassay is the chlamydiazyme (Abbott Laboratories) (Jones, Smith, Houglum, & Herrmann, 1984).

Isolation of *C. trachomatis* in tissue culture provides the most reliable diagnosis but requires special antibiotic-treated medium and a well-collected and -transported specimen. Cell scrapings provide better specimens than purulent discharges or secretions; the cervix should therefore be swabbed after mucus and debris are removed from the os (Stamm & Holmes, 1984). Cotton or rayon swabs are advised as swabs with calcium alginate may depress recovery of *C. trachomatis* and Dacron swabs may cause false-positive readings (Stamm & Holmes, 1984). Specimens should be immediately placed into a special medium, refrigerated, transported on ice, and inoculated within 24 hours if possible. If rapid inoculation is not possible, the specimen should be frozen until it can be inoculated, although this may reduce the culture yield (Ngeow, Munday, Evans, & Taylor-Robinson, 1981).

Chlamydia culture testing is not universally available. Cost varies from $15 to $40 and results take at least 4 days (Loucks, 1987). Antibody tests are generally less expensive.

Although serologic testing has been used in some epidemiologic studies, it is too nonspecific for clinical use.

Tests for other STDs, particularly gonorrhea, should be instituted for all patients diagnosed with *C. trachomatis* or known exposure (Osser & Persson, 1984).

Obviously, exposure and clinical signs and symptoms warrant the initiation of laboratory testing. Screening is also appropriate for high-risk women because of the large proportion of women with infection who are asymptomatic and because of the possibility of transmission from an asymptomatic partner.

Handsfield and associates (1986) recommend testing of all women with two or more of the following risk factors: age 24 years or less; intercourse with a new partner within the preceding 2 months; examination results showing purulent or mucopurulent cervical exudate; bleeding induced by swabbing the endocervical mucosa; use of no contraception or a nonbarrier method. These authors maintain that such a screening program would detect 90 percent of all infections.

INTERVENTION

Treatment. The CDC-recommended treatment for uncomplicated urethral, endocervical, or rectal infection with *C. trachomatis* is tetracycline HCl 500 mg by mouth four times daily for 7 days OR doxycycline 100 mg by mouth twice daily for 7 days. If tetracyclines are contraindicated or not tolerated, an alternative regimen is erythromycin base or stearate 500 mg by mouth four times daily for 7 days OR erythromycin ethyl succinate 800 mg by mouth four times daily for 7 days.

Sulfonamides are also effective for treatment of chlamydia; sulfamethoxazole 1 g by mouth twice daily for 10 days is recommended by CDC (1985b, p. 78s) as ''probably effective.''

All exposed sexual partners must be treated.

Treatment for salpingitis is outlined in Chapter 15.

Cure rates with tetracycline, doxycycline, and erythromycin are greater than 95 percent. Although test-of-cure cultures are recommended 3 to 6 weeks after treatment, because of the high rate of cure, the CDC notes that they can be omitted in situations of limited laboratory resources.

Re-treatment with one of the preceding regimens should be instituted if test-of-cure cultures are positive.

Tetracycline is a broad-spectrum antibiotic. Doxycycline is a longer-acting drug in the same class as tetracycline with the same contraindications and side effects. These drugs are contraindicated in persons with hypersensitivity, in pregnant women, and during lactation. They must not be used in children 8 years of age and under because they discolor developing teeth. Persons with renal impairment require lower-dose therapy and monitoring of serum levels of the drug. Patients on anticoagulant therapy may need downward adjustment of their dose as the drug depresses prothrombin activity. Consultation or referral must be obtained for all persons with medical problems or those taking other medications before antibiotic treatment is initiated.

Photosensitivity has been described and patients on tetracycline should avoid direct sunlight or ultraviolet light. Other adverse reactions include gastrointestinal problems: anorexia, nausea and vomiting, diarrhea, glossitis, dysphagia, enterocolitis, and inflammation; candidal overgrowth in the anogenital region; skin rashes; dose-related renal toxicity; blood disorders including hemolytic anemia, thrombocytopenia, neutropenia, and eosinophilia; pericarditis; purpura; exacerbation of systemic lupus erythematosus; and hypersensitivity reactions including urticaria, edema, and anaphylaxis (*Physician's desk reference*, 1988).

Antacids and dairy and food products interfere with tetracycline absorption. Oral tetracycline should be given 1 hour before or 2 hours after meals.

Teaching and Counseling. Because chlamydial infection is often asymptomatic, the patient requires a careful explanation of the infection and its possible sequelae should it go untreated. The treatment schedule must be understood and special instructions regarding taking tetracyclines between meals should be discussed. Erythromycin can also cause gastric upsets; patients should be instructed to call if these occur.

Sexual partners need to be treated, preferably at the same time as the patient. Intercourse should be avoided or condoms used until treatment is complete. In one study, the spermicide nonoxynol-9 was shown *not* to inhibit *C. trachomatis* (Kappus & Quinn, 1986). Patients with STDs often want to know when they were infected. Because of the asymptomatic nature of a chlamydial infection, it is not always possible to provide this information. The emotional consequences of the diagnosis must always be borne in mind.

Follow-up appointments should be made for tests-of-cure. A discussion of prevention of future STDs should be initiated.

The Genital Mycoplasmas

The first mycoplasma discovered in a human being was isolated from a Bartholin's gland abscess in 1937 (McCormack & Taylor-Robinson, 1984).

Etiology and Transmission. Three mycoplasma species have been shown to cause human disease: *Mycoplasma pneumoniae* causes an unusual form of pneumonia; *Mycoplasma hominis* and *Ureaplasma urealyticum* cause anogenital disease. These organisms are most often thought to be transmitted sexually, but individuals without sexual contact are colonized infrequently (McCormack & Taylor-Robinson, 1984). Transmission through the birth canal occurs as well, but tends not to persist. Mycoplasmas have been transmitted in donor semen via artificial insemination (Mascola & Guinan, 1987).

Epidemiology. Colonization with mycoplasma is related to increased numbers of sexual partners, particularly in women, suggesting increased susceptibility in females compared with males (Taylor-Robinson & McCormack, 1980a). Black women have a higher rate of colonization than white women, even when controlling for sexual experience (McCormack, Rosner, Alpert, et al., 1986). Persons of lower socioeconomic status have higher rates of colonization; studies have shown prevalence rates of 53.6 to 76.3 percent among clinic patients compared with rates of 21.3 to 52 percent for private gynecologic and obstetric patients. The prevalence rates of both mycoplasma organisms decreases after menopause. The mycoplasmas have been found with increased frequency among persons with other STDs including *C. trachomatis, Trichomonas vaginalis,* and *N. gonorrhoeae* (Persson, Persson, Hansson, et al., 1979).

Clinical Presentation. There is no specific condition associated with the genital mycoplasmas. Rather, they have a possible role in the following disorders (Cassell, Waites, Gibbs, & Davis, 1986; Gravett & Eschenbach, 1986; Mårdh & Weström, 1970; McCormack, Lee, & Zinner, 1973; Platt, Lin, Warren, et al., 1980; Rosene, Eschenbach, Tompkins, et al, 1986; Stray-Pedersen, Eng, & Reikvam 1978; Taylor-Robinson & McCormack, 1980a; 1980b; Watts & Eschenbach, 1987):

- in Males
  Nongonococcal urethritis (*U. urealyticum* only)
  Prostatitis (possibly associated with *M. hominis*)
- in Females
  Bartholin's gland abscess (possibly caused by *M. hominis*)
  PID (associated with *M. hominis,* possibly caused by *U. urealyticum*)
  Postabortion fever (associated with *M. hominis*)
  Postpartum fever (*M. hominis* and *U. urealyticum*)
- in Males and females
  Urinary calculi (possibly associated with *U. urealyticum*)
  Pyelonephritis (associated with *M. hominis*)
- Reproductive disorders
  Infertility (possibly associated with *U. urealyticum*);
  Spontaneous abortion and stillbirth (possibly associated with *M. hominis*);
  Low birth weight (associated with *U. urealyticum*);
  Premature rupture of membranes (possibly associated with *U. urealyticum*).

Further research is needed on the exact role of the mycoplasmas in causing many of these problems (Sweet, 1986). Although *M. hominis* has been found in association with vaginal pathogens (Dattani, Gerken, & Evans, 1982), mycoplasmas are not considered to cause vaginitis (Mendel, Rowan, Graham, & Dellinger, 1970), although *U. urealyticum* may play a role in bacterial vaginosis (McCormack & Taylor-Robinson, 1984).

Management

DATA COLLECTION

History. NGU not known to be caused by *C. trachomatis* may be due to mycoplasma; any exposure to NGU of unknown etiology may be significant. A history of recent abortion or birth is significant in patients presenting with symptoms of endometritis or salpingitis. History taking should include discussion of symptoms of the syndromes listed earlier.

Physical Examination. There are no physical examination findings specific to mycoplasma-caused infection but examination should be specific to signs of the syndromes listed earlier.

Laboratory Testing. Although mycoplasmas are Gram-negative organisms, they do not take up stain well enough for Gram stains to be useful for diagnosis. They can be grown on special culture media; *Ureaplasma* grows in 1 to 2 days; *M. hominis* needs up to 1 week to grow (McCormack & Taylor-Robinson, 1984). Samples should be taken with a rayon-tipped plastic swab from the posterior vaginal fornix (Mårdh, 1984). Because of the prevalence of these organisms, however, cultures are rarely done; a positive culture does not prove causality.

INTERVENTION

Treatment. The tetracyclines and erythromycin are usually effective against mycoplasmas, although resistance has been shown (Bowie & Willetts, 1987; Klotsky, Stamm, Brunham, et al., 1983). As mycoplasma-caused infection is difficult to prove, treatment for mycoplasma is not generally justified, but because these medications are broad-spectrum agents and also effective against *C. trachomatis,* treatment with one of these antibiotics is appropriate for a number of problems including NGU or exposure to it, pelvic inflammatory disease (as part of a multiple-therapy regimen), and postabortion fever or prophylaxis. Clindamycin is also effective against the mycoplasmas.

VIRAL INFECTIONS

Herpes Genitalis

Infection of the genitalia with herpes simplex virus has become a major STD. First described in the eighteenth century, the number of patient visits for primary herpes infections increased 15-fold in the 15 years from 1966 to 1984 (Centers for Disease Control, 1986). Because there is no known cure for the virus, the disease can be devastating to sufferers, with psychological, sexual, and social implications.

Etiology and Transmission. Two strains of herpesvirus are responsible for sexually transmitted herpes infections—herpesviruses type 1 (HSV-1) and type 2 (HSV-2). Infection with HSV-1 is acquired in most people during the first year and a half of life, usually via the respiratory tract (Rapp, 1984), with manifestations in the oral mucosa. HSV-2 is generally acquired during sexual activity, and its lesions classically occur in the genital area. In recent years, however, type 1 virus has been seen in genital herpes and type 2 in oral lesions, presumably as a result of changes in sexual practices.

After the herpesvirus enters the body, it eventually comes to reside in the cells of the nervous system, where it remains latent. Clinical attacks of varying frequency may or may not occur. Herpesviruses affecting the oral mucosa generally live in the trigeminal ganglion; genital herpesviruses reside in the sacral dorsal root ganglia.

Transmission of the herpesvirus occurs through close contact of a susceptible mucosal surface, such as the oropharynx, cervix, or conjunctiva, with the shedding virus. The virus can also enter the body through small cracks in the skin. The incubation period is 1 to 26 days, with a median of 6 to 8 days (Corey & Spear, 1986a). The risk of infection from single or repeated exposures to herpesvirus is not known. Although it is known that active herpes lesions are infective, the extent to which transmission can occur during asymptomatic periods via asymptomatic viral shedding is unknown, but certainly lower than transmission during active outbreaks (Mertz & Corey, 1984). The rates of asymptomatic viral shedding in infected persons is not known either, but probably infrequent (Stenzel-Poore, Hallick, Fendrick, et al., 1987). The extent to which a person infected with one strain of herpesvirus may become infected with another is also unknown, but the risk may be reduced (Mertz & Corey, 1984).

Epidemiology. HSV is increasing in the United States. Because the disease is not reportable, prevalence data are based largely on symptomatic patients who seek medical care. These data are thought to underestimate the actual number of individuals with genital herpes infections (Webb & Fife, 1987).

The 15-fold increase in physician consultations for genital herpes from 1966 to 1984 may not result entirely from an actual increase in the number of cases but, in part, from media publicity and the recent availability of a medical treatment for the disease (see Intervention); however, because persons with asymptomatic infection may not present for care, prevalence estimates may understate the actual number of persons infected with herpesvirus. Measurements of antibody to herpesvirus in the blood show the virus to be ubiquitous in the population (Mertz & Corey, 1984).

In some populations, such as college students, the prevalence of HSV greatly exceeds that of either gonorrhea or syphilis (Sumaya, Marx, & Ullis, 1980). Prevalence is higher among women with multiple sexual partners than those with fewer partners. The prevalence of clinically diagnosed infections is higher in whites than others (Corey 1984). The greatest number of new cases occur between the ages of 15 and 35 years. Estimates of new cases in the United States are as high as 724,000 annually, with a prevalence of over 20 million (Guinan, Wolinsky, & Reichman, 1985). Among these, an unknown portion are asymptomatic.

Clinical Presentation. Infection with HSV-1 is indistinguishable from infection with HSV-2; however, the first herpes episode presents a clinical picture very different from recurrences. Differences in the severity of first episodes depend on whether the episode represents a primary infection. This is determined by whether there was a prior infection with HSV-1 or HSV-2 that may have been asymptomatic. In the literature, the distinction is made by referring to *primary first-episode* disease and *nonprimary first-episode* disease (Mertz & Corey, 1984).

PRIMARY FIRST EPISODES. Primary first episodes of genital HSV infection are characterized by both systemic and local symptoms, lasting, on the average, up to 3 weeks. The clinical course of the primary infection is generally more severe in women than men. Systemic symptoms usually appear early in the course of the infection, peak on about day 3 or 4 after onset of lesions, and subside over 3 to 4 days. More than half of women with primary disease report fever, headache, malaise, and myalgias (Corey, 1984). Local symptoms include pain; itching; vaginal or urethral discharge; internal and external dysuria, even to the extent of urinary retention; and tender inguinal lymphadenopathy. Pain at the site of the lesions increases during the first week of illness, intensifies between days 7 and 11, and gradually subsides during weeks 2 and 3. Lymphadenopathy occurs late in the clinical course of infection, week 2 or 3, and is often the last persisting symptom.

The typical lesions of a primary HSV infection start as papules or vesicles (Fig. 12–8). They spread rapidly over the entire genital area. By the time the patient presents to the practitioner, they may appear as pustules with large ulcerated areas. The ulcerative lesions last 4 to 15 days and then crust over. New lesions can form up to day 10 of the disease course. Severe vulvar edema may be present and the woman may complain of difficulty sitting down. Painless lesions have been reported in males (Silber & Burgess, 1985).

HSV cervicitis is common in primary first-episode infections, particularly with HSV-2 infection, although it may be present in HSV-1 infection and in nonprimary first-episode disease. The cervix may appear normal or be reddened and friable, ulcerated, or necrotic (Barton, Kinghorn, Walker, et al., 1981) (Fig. 12–9). A heavy, watery or mucoid discharge is common (Harger, Pazin, & Breinig, 1986).

The mean duration of viral shedding with primary infections is about 12 days, although abstinence from sexual

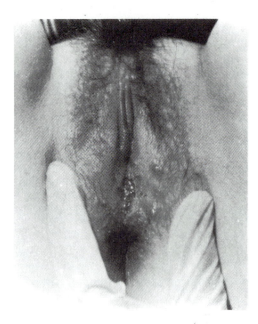

Figure 12–8. Primary herpetic lesions: Vesicles and ulcerations. *(From Webb, D. H. & Fife, K. H. [1987, March]. Genital herpes simplex virus infections. Infectious Disease Clinics of North America, 1 (1), 104. Reprinted with permission.)*

contact is advised until all lesions are reepithelialized; the average time of reepithelialization in women is 19.5 days (Corey, 1984).

RECURRENT EPISODES. Recurrent episodes of HSV produce only local symptoms. The recurrent episodes are shorter than primary episodes, lasting an average of 8 to 12 days, with a mean duration of viral shedding of 4 days from the onset of lesions and complete reepithelialization within 10 days. Pain and itching are less severe than in primary infections.

Recurrent episodes of HSV infection are more severe in women than men. In addition to pain and itching, women may experience external dysuria. Lesions usually occur on one side of the genitalia, most often in the same area with

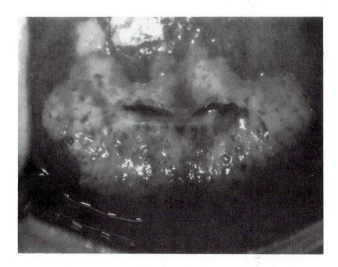

Figure 12–9. Herpetic cervicitis. *(From Webb, D. H. & Fife, K. H. [1987, March]. Genital herpes simplex virus infections. Infectious Disease Clinics of North America, 1 (1), 105. Reprinted with permission.)*

each recurrence. Sometimes only one or two lesions are present, although up to 15 or 20 lesions have been noted. Lesions begin as vesicles and quickly rupture to form ulcerations. A small number of women with recurrent disease have cervicitis compared with the vast majority with primary disease.

About 50 percent of herpes sufferers experience a prodromal phase with recurrent infection—a period of some symptoms before lesions erupt. The prodrome may last from one-half hour to 2 days before the lesions appear. Prodromal symptoms may be as mild as a tingling sensation or as severe as shooting pains in the buttocks, legs, or thighs (Corey, 1984). Some people experience prodromal symptoms without the eruption of lesions or viral shedding (Harger et al., 1986).

The rate of recurrence for persons infected with HSV-1 is lower than that for patients with HSV-2 (Corey & Spear, 1986b; Reeves, Corey, Adams, et al., 1981). More severe first episodes are associated with greater likelihood of recurrence. Recurrences do not follow a pattern; they vary from person to person and over time in any one person. One study showed the median annual number of episodes to be between five and eight (Knox, Corey, Blough, & Lerner, 1982). Studies on recurrences, however, may be skewed by a selection bias against individuals without recurrences or with few recurrences. Whether the frequency of recurrence changes in a predictable way with the duration of infection is not known (Mertz & Corey, 1984).

Various stressors are believed to stimulate the activation of HSV. The stimuli vary and include emotional stress, heat, moisture, changes in climate, fever, pregnancy, oral contraceptive use, anesthesia, and trauma (Corey, 1984; Guinan, MacCalman, Kern, et al., 1981). In women, episodes have been found to cluster around the time of menses (Guinan et al., 1981) although not consistently (Rattray, Corey, Reeves, et al., 1978).

The mechanism for recurrence is unknown; two theories are currently postulated. In the "ganglion trigger" theory, latent virus is stimulated to replicate by changes in the environment; the virus then migrates through sensory nerves. In the "skin trigger" theory, virus is continually replicating and becomes symptomatic when host immune factors change (Guinan et al., 1985).

Complications and Sequelae. Herpetic lesions may form at extragenital sites, including the buttocks, groin, or thigh, and, less commonly, the finger and eye. Herpes of the fingers is called herpetic whitlow. Central nervous system complications can occur (Craig & Nahmias, 1973), including meningitis, manifested by headache, nuchal rigidity, fever, photophobia, and vomiting. Meningitis usually has a spontaneous resolution. Autonomic nervous system dysfunction has been reported (Caplan, Kleeman, & Berg, 1977; Klastersky, Cappel, Snoeck, et al., 1972). This is temporary, causing urinary retention, constipation, perineal and lower back hyperesthesia or anesthesia, and, in men, erectile dysfunction (Harger et al., 1986). Encephalitis, which can be fatal, rarely occurs (Ross & Stevenson, 1961). Dissemination via the bloodstream can occur and is evidenced by multiple lesions over the thorax and extremities. Endometritis (Schneider, Behm, & Mumaw, 1982), arthritis (Friedman, Pincus, Gibilisco, et al., 1980), hepatitis (Hamory, Luger, & Kobberman, 1981), and thrombocytopenia (Corey, 1984) are seen rarely. Proctitis is a complication occurring in homosexual males (Mertz & Corey, 1984). In immunosuppressed individuals, the virus can spread to multiple organs. Superinfection, particularly with fungi, may occur.

A particularly serious complication of HSV infection is

neonatal herpes, a potentially fatal or disabling disease. Most neonatal infections are believed to be caused by passage of primary infections through the placenta. Recurrent infection is transmissible through the birth canal from an active lesion and, possibly, though less likely, through asymptomatic viral shedding. Asymptomatic viral shedding was shown in a study of 147 pregnant women to be more common when the first symptomatic episode occurred during the pregnancy (Brown, Vontver, Benedetti, et al., 1985). The risk of neonatal acquisition of HSV from a recurrent infection with symptomatic or asymptomatic viral shedding is considered to be low, with a maximum infection rate thought to be about 8 percent (Prober, Sullender, Yasukawa, et al., 1987). Viral titer, antibody in serum and/or amniotic fluid, immune response of the neonate, and use of internal fetal monitoring equipment may influence the likelihood of acquisition of neonatal infection (Goldkrand, 1982; Parvey & Ch'ien, 1980; Tejani, Klein, & Kaplan, 1979; Yeager, Arvin, Urbani, & Kemp, 1980). A full discussion of the disease course, consequences, prevention, and treatment of neonatal herpes, and of the management of HSV infection in pregnancy, is beyond the scope of this book.

An association between cervical cancer and HSV-2 has been demonstrated in many epidemiologic reports (Rapp, 1984), with biologic evidence from animal studies supporting a possible association. There are, however, several variables related to both conditions that make a cause-and-effect relationship uncertain in humans (Nahmias, Naib, & Josey, 1974), including early sexual activity, early pregnancy, and multiple sex partners (see Chapter 13). Zur Hausen (1982) has suggested an interaction between human papillomavirus (HPV) and herpes simplex virus in the etiology of cervical cancer, with HSV thought to be an initiator, and HPV a promoter, of carcinogenesis. More information is needed to establish a definite etiologic link between cervical cancer and herpes simplex virus or to clarify their relationship.

Differential Diagnosis. Herpetic infection must be differentiated from other STDs and vulvovaginal syndromes that present with ulcerative lesions. These include syphilis, chancroid, vaginal trauma or irritation, folliculitis, focal vulvitis, and the lesions of Behcet's syndrome. Any type of vulvovaginitis that causes pruritus with excoriations secondary to scratching, such as candidiasis or allergic vulvovaginitis, may be confused with herpes (Kaufman, 1981). These diseases are described in other sections in this chapter and in Chapter 11.

Management

DATA COLLECTION

History. A careful history often provides extensive clues to the diagnosis of herpes. In primary infection, exposure via oral–genital or genital intercourse is important, although infection from asymptomatic persons is possible. The history of symptoms and their severity may often lead to a high suspicion, particularly extensive vulvar pain, dysuria, and/or urinary retention, experienced with systemic symptoms. In recurrent infections, patients may report painful "pimples," "bumps," or "blisters," most often on the labia, which they may have had intermittently in the past with spontaneous healing. Questions regarding a prior history of primary infection symptoms and prodromal symptoms help pinpoint the diagnosis, although the absence of either does not exclude the diagnosis of herpes.

Physical Examination. The inguinal area should be palpated for tender lymph nodes, often a lingering symptom in primary infection. The entire vulvar, perineal, vaginal, and cervical areas should be carefully inspected. Classic vesicular lesions may not be present at the time of examination; ulcerated or crusted areas may instead be present. Because of the exquisite tenderness associated with herpes infections, particularly primary first episodes, a speculum examination may be difficult and have to be postponed. If it is thought essential, Faro (1985) suggests placing lidocaine gel or ointment on the vulva before inserting the instrument.

Laboratory Testing. Four types of laboratory tests are currently used to diagnose HSV with varying degrees of sensitivity, specificity, expense, availability, and clinical usefulness: the Pap or Tzanck smear, immunologic detection of antigen, viral culture, and serum viral antibody titration (serologic testing).

The advantage of using either the Pap or Tzanck smear for diagnosis is that it can be done relatively rapidly. The Tzanck preparation involves the use of Wright–Giemsa stain. Both tests are less expensive than the other available tests (Kellum & Loucks, 1982). The cytologist looks for enlarged cells with intranuclear inclusions and fusions of cells into multinucleated giant cells. The detection rates for these two methods, however, are low—approximately 40 to 60 percent (Brown, Jaffe, Zaidi, et al., 1979).

Immunologic tests include immunofluorescence tests and enzyme-linked immunosorbent assay (ELISA). Immunofluoresence tests are more sensitive than smears, provided the specimens contain a sufficient number of cells. Scrapings from the specimens must be transported to a laboratory in an appropriate herpes transport medium, which is not always available. Sensitivity of this method varies from 70 to 90 percent (Fife & Corey, 1984). ELISA tests are being studied for their usefulness in HSV diagnosis.

Cultures for HSV must be sent to the laboratory in an appropriate viral medium. Fife and Corey recommend using distilled water for transport if a herpes medium is not available. Specimens should not be frozen, but should be kept at 4°C (refrigerator temperature) until inoculated into tissue culture. Specimens are viable for 48 hours, although there is a loss of titer over time. The median time needed for culture growth is 4 days; 65 percent of positive cultures can be identified within 5 days and 90 percent by 10 days. Cultures should be observed for up to 14 days.

For both smears and cultures, cells should be collected by vigorously swabbing the lesions with a cotton- or Dacron-tipped swab after opening the vesicles with the swab or with a small-gauge needle. If lesions are large, vesicular fluid can be aspirated. The patient must be forewarned that this will be uncomfortable for a few moments. Cervical specimens should be obtained from the ectocervix rather than the endocervix (Fife & Corey, 1984).

One problem with laboratory testing for herpes is that in recurrent disease, cultures are rarely positive after about 4 days of infection (Harger et al., 1986). Even early in recurrences, 15 to 40 percent of lesions may not show positive cultures. In recurring disease, a negative culture taken from an ulcerative lesion does not rule out HSV infection. Primary first episodes have longer periods of viral shedding. The best time to culture is in the vesicular or pustular stage of disease; the early stage (maculopapular) and later stages (ulceration and crusted lesions) have lower yields, although in primary first episodes, virus can often be cultured from ulcers.

Serologic studies of serum for antibody to herpes are

most useful in epidemiologic studies evaluating disease prevalence, because most persons with prior infection have high antibody levels. In primary infection, titers showing a fourfold rise in the convalescent phase may be diagnostic. A fall in antibody may later be demonstrated. In persons with prior HSV infection, however, the antibody level may not be diagnostic (Fife & Corey, 1984). Less than 10 percent of persons with recurrent disease show a rise in titer between acute and convalescent sera (Reeves et al., 1981). Some serologic tests differentiate between HSV-1 and HSV-2; others do not.

In addition to tests for herpes, testing for syphilis, gonorrhea, and chlamydia should be carried out. If lesions persist, a test for chancroid should be considered.

INTERVENTION. Intervention for HSV infections includes specific therapy for primary and recurrent infection, treatment of complications, self-help measures to increase comfort during attacks, prevention of recurrent infections, prevention of spread of infection including neonatal infection, and early detection of cervical cancer.

Treatment.   There currently is no cure for herpes simplex virus infection. It must be considered a chronic disease. The only FDA-approved medication is acyclovir (Zovirax), an antiviral agent that shortens the mean duration of primary eruptions by between 3 and 5 days and may reduce systemic symptoms (CDC, 1985b). It also reduces the duration of viral shedding (Guinan, 1986).

If signs, symptoms, and a careful history establish an attack as a primary episode, the recommended treatment is acyclovir 200 mg by mouth 5 times daily (every 4 hours when awake), for 7 to 10 days, initiated within 6 days from onset of lesions. Topical acyclovir ointment has some benefit in decreasing viral shedding but is not considered to have a significant effect on symptoms or healing time. Treatment with acyclovir for a primary or nonprimary first episode has no effect on subsequent recurrence rate (Corey, Mindel, Fife, et al. 1985; Guinan, 1986). For patients with severe primary symptoms or complications, hospitalization for treatment with intravenous acyclovir for five to seven days may be necessary.

The effect of acyclovir on recurrent episodes is minimal, shortening the duration of symptoms by about one day. The CDC recommends use of oral acyclovir only for patients with severe recurrence symptoms. Treatment should be started at the beginning of the prodrome or within two days of the onset of lesions. The recommended dose is 200 mg orally 5 times daily for 5 days (every 4 hours when awake). Intravenous and topical acyclovir are not recommended for recurrent HSV attacks.

Other possible treatments under study include additional antiviral agents and interferon. Interferon, in comparison with placebo, has been shown to reduce the duration of recurrent episodes when given as a subcutaneous injection but often brings on flu-like symptoms (Lassus, Bergelin, Paloranta, et al., 1987).

Treatment of concomitant vaginal infections is important. If they go untreated, the duration and severity of genital HSV infection are greater (Monif, 1982).

The most common side effect of oral acyclovir is mild gastrointestinal intolerance. Hypersensitivity reactions are rare (Webb & Fife, 1987). Toxicity of acyclovir for 5- to 120-day therapy is minimal (Guinan, 1986). Headache, dizziness, diarrhea, fatigue, anorexia, edema, and medication taste have been reported in less than 4 percent of users (Pepper, 1985). The long-term toxicity is unknown. The

drug is not teratogenic in animal studies. It has not been used in pregnancy, however, and is not recommended for pregnant women. Whether resistant strains will develop is unknown.

Consultation/Referral.   Consultation and/or referral are warranted in patients with severe symptoms in a primary infection or with clinical evidence of complications including fever, significant headache with visual changes, stiff neck, and severe abdominal pain. Hospitalization for intravenous therapy may be indicated. Urinary retention may require the placement of an indwelling catheter for the duration of infection.

Prevention.   Treatment with oral acyclovir may help reduce transmission of disease to sexual contacts by reducing the duration of viral shedding. Acyclovir also can be used to suppress outbreaks of herpes in patients with frequent attacks. Prophylactic dosage is 200 mg three times a day up to 6 months. This has not been shown to reduce asymptomatic viral shedding or to reduce the frequency of attacks once therapy is discontinued.

People with herpes should refrain from sexual contact from the onset of prodrome to complete healing of lesions, regardless of whether they are taking acyclovir. Many authorities recommend consistent condom use for all persons with genital herpes (CDC, 1985b). Depending on the location of lesions, however, condoms may not prevent transmission, particularly in female-to-male transmission. Ultimately, a vaccine would provide the best protection. More must be learned about HSV, however, before an effective vaccine is developed (Kit & Kit, 1985).

Self-Help Measures.   Although acyclovir reduces duration of infection, it does not provide comfort for the patient while lesions are present. The following measures, adapted principally from The Boston Women's Health Book Collective (1984), have been advocated for increasing patient comfort:

- Practice good hygiene. Lesions should be kept clean and dry; cotton underwear should be worn and changed often. Wiping from front to back is important. Perineal care with betadine solution in water may be helpful for extensive ulcers. Careful handwashing is important to avoid autoinoculation of the face or eyes with the virus.
- Urinate in a bath, shower, or sitz bath. (Patients must be informed to notify their care provider if they are unable to urinate.)
- Apply drying aids after rupture of vesicles. These include hydrogen peroxide, Burrow's solution, Aveeno baths, warm sitz baths with baking soda, a cool hair dryer to keep away moisture. Application of Camphophenique or Listerine followed by a thin layer of aloe vera gel has helped control pain and burning in some women with herpes.
- Take aspirin, two tablets by mouth four times a day. This may relieve pain and systemic symptoms associated with primary first episodes. Pain may be so severe that codeine becomes necessary.
- Apply a thin layer of lidocaine ointment or an antiseptic spray, especially if walking is difficult. Loosefitting clothing or long dresses without underpants may be more comfortable.

A variety of herbal and nutritional preparations have been recommended either to increase comfort, to prevent recurrences, or to reduce duration of episodes. Most of these have not been subjected to controlled, randomized studies, but are not deemed to be harmful:

- Cold milk compresses.
- Echinacea, a plant reported to be a blood strengthener, taken in capsule form every 3 hours, made into a tincture and applied every 2 hours for 3 to 4 days, or brewed as a tea, four cups daily.
- Echinacea (2 droppersful)—mixed with calendula and burdock root (1 dropperful each), taken orally in juice or herbal tea, 3 times daily.
- Chlorophyll powder with wheatgrass made into a drink with warm water.
- Compresses made of black tea with cloves (for the anesthetic effect of tannic acid) or bearberry tea.
- Poultices of pulverized calcium, powdered slippery elm, goldenseal, myrrh, or comfrey root. Any of these can be made into a paste with warm water and applied.
- Vitamin C 2,000 mg or two capsules of Kelp followed by sarsaparilla tea, four to five cups per day.
- Zinc 5 to 60 mg daily to prevent recurrences.
- Acupuncture at the onset of prodromal symptoms to prevent outbreaks.

The amino acid L-lysine has been recommended in doses of 750 to 1,000 mg daily while lesions are present, and of 500 mg during asymptomatic periods. Lysine competes with arginine (also an amino acid) which favors the replication of HSV. Foods of high lysine content include potatoes, meat, milk, brewer's yeast, fish, liver, and eggs. Foods with arginine can be limited; these include nuts, chocolate, cola, rice, cottonseed meal, and oil. L-Lysine has been shown to have an inhibitory effect on the multiplication of herpes simplex virus in cell cultures; controlled studies, however, have not demonstrated reduced duration of symptoms or frequency of recurrences in doses of 500 mg twice daily (Milman, Scheibel, & Jessen, 1978, 1980).

Additional Teaching and Counseling. The woman with herpes needs to understand the mode of transmission of the disease. She must know to avoid both oral and genital intercourse while she or her partner have lesions or even a prodrome. She should understand, however, that asymptomatic viral shedding is possible and be advised to consider using condoms prophylactically.

The role of stress in bringing on herpes attacks can be discussed and referrals made for stress reduction therapy, yoga, exercise, or meditation classes. Women may want to keep diaries to try to discover what stresses seem to be associated with herpes attacks for them and to learn to avoid them, if possible. Some helpful suggestions might be to avoid excessive heat and sun, tight-fitting clothing, and hot baths, and to use a lubricant during sex to reduce friction.

Women with herpes can be reassured that the disease does not cause systemic damage, although it may be associated with cervical cancer. All herpes sufferers must have annual Pap smears for cervical cancer. Women should be told that if they become pregnant, they should inform their midwife or care provider of this diagnosis so appropriate management can be implemented to avoid congenital HSV infection in the newborn. They can be reassured, however, that most congenital herpes infections are due to primary disease and that most women with herpes genitalis infections have normal vaginal births.

The emotional impact of acquiring an HSV infection is substantial and must be addressed. The publicity surrounding this disease has made receiving the diagnosis a devastating experience for many people. Patients cannot be offered cures and most will experience recurrences. Women must be given the opportunity to ventilate feelings and helped to learn to live with the disease. Most people develop ways to cope with recurrences.

Herpes affects a woman's sexuality and can affect a current or future relationship. There may be feelings of anger, shame, embarrassment, denial, and guilt. The woman may need to work out feelings toward her sexual partner, although, if a first episode is not a primary episode, it cannot be conclusively determined when she contracted the disease. She may need to discuss how to raise the issue with her partner or with prospective partners.

An understanding practitioner can be instrumental in easing adjustment to this condition and promoting acceptance of it. Patients who feel isolated can be assured of the widespread prevalence of herpes virus and referred to support groups. The American Social Health Association (ASHA) provides information about local community resources and publishes *The Helper*, a quarterly newsletter. The organization can be contacted at P.O. Box 100, Palo Alto, CA 94302.

Human Papillomavirus/Condylomata Acuminata

Genital warts, venereal warts, or condylomata acuminata have been described since antiquity, but it was not until the eighteenth century that they were recognized as an entity separate from syphilis and not until the following century were they perceived to be distinct from gonorrhea (Oriel, 1984). In 1949, the viral etiology of warts was confirmed by electron microscopy.

Etiology and Transmission

Condylomata acuminata are caused by the human papillomavirus (HPV), part of the papovirus family. These viruses have been difficult to study because they have not been grown in cell culture (Oriel, 1984). Recently, however, scientists have been able to characterize the virus and identify multiple species of HPV by a technique called DNA hybridization. Some anogenital warts have been found to be caused by HPV types 1 and 2, which commonly cause skin warts such as plantar warts, but more often, anogenital warts are caused by distinct HPV types, most notably HPV types 6, 11, 16, 18, and 31, or a combination of types (Koss, 1987).

Condylomata acuminata are sexually transmitted. The incubation period for HPV infection is usually long but very variable (Lynch, 1985). In an early study of the wives of infected servicemen, warts developed 4 to 6 weeks after exposure (Barrett, Silbar, & McGinley, 1954). Other studies have shown an average incubation period of 3 months with a range of 3 weeks to 8 or 9 months (Lynch, 1985; Margolis, 1984). New warts may appear months after treatment through previous autoinoculation or the long-term existence of the virus in latent phase, so that what appears to be a recent infection may actually be the result of a prior exposure (Ferenczy, Silverstein, & Crum, 1987; Lynch, 1985).

The infectivity of HPV is considered high (Meisels, Morin, & Casas-Cordero, 1982). It is unknown whether there are different rates of transmission, however, for different viral types or for clinically apparent versus subclinical warts (Kirby & Corey, 1987).

Epidemiology. Condyloma acuminatum is not a reportable STD and until relatively recently was thought to be rather unimportant as a cause of significant morbidity. National data are, therefore, unavailable. Nevertheless, recent reports indicate a dramatic increase in the number of cases (CDC, 1983a; Chuang, Perry, Kurland, & Ilstrup, 1984). Between 1966 and 1981, the number of private physician visits for genital warts increased by 459 percent (CDC, 1983a). The greatest number of visits were among 20- to 24-year-olds. Data from surveys of several STD clinics showed similar recent increases (Becker, Stone, & Alexander, 1987). In 1981, there were 946,000 visits to private physicians for condylomata acuminata (CDC, 1983a). In a small study of 49 women with condylomata acuminata and 196 age-matched controls without disease, Daling, Sherman, and Weiss (1986) found increased risks associated with the presence of other STDs, increased numbers of sexual partners, cigarette smoking, and use of oral contraceptives for 5 or more years. In the data from STD clinic surveys, the disease was twice as frequent among white women than black women (Becker et al., 1987).

Clinical Presentation. Condylomata acuminata may be clinically apparent or subclinical. Clinical warts usually appear first at the posterior part of the introitus and the labia minora; they may spread to other parts of the vulva or appear elsewhere first, including the clitoral region and mons pubis. Sometimes warts involve the perineum and anus. Vaginal warts usually affect the upper and lower portions (Oriel, 1984). Condylomata acuminata may also be seen on the cervix. Often, however, these lesions can be visualized only under magnification. Cervical and/or vaginal lesions may be present in up to 70 percent of women infected with vulvar warts (Roy, Meisels, Fortier, et al., 1981). In a study of 169 women with vulvar condylomata, Greenberg, Mann, Chumas, and associates (1987) found cervical involvement in 42.6 percent and vaginal and cervical involvement in 17.1 percent. Condylomata acuminata may occur in nongenital sites including the lip, nipple, umbilicus, and, most commonly, the anus.

Vulvar condylomata appear as soft, pink, whitish, flesh-colored, or hyperpigmented vascular growths with multiple fine finger-like projections (Fig. 12–10). They are most likely to be seen on moist areas, especially areas exposed to friction during sexual relations (Campion, 1987). Multiple lesions may eventually coalesce, forming larger lesions that look like the top of cauliflower.

Vaginal condylomata are usually multiple and may cause discharge or pruritus, or both. Bleeding may occur after coitus. The lesions are raised, white, and elevated (Campion, 1987). Cervical lesions, which may be single or multiple, are not usually seen by the unaided eye. One variety of cervical lesion, called the *flat condyloma* does not resemble the classical proliferative condyloma, but does contain HPV virus (Oriel, 1984).

Many women with condylomata also present with other STDs or vaginal infections (Oriel, 1984; Roy et al. 1981).

Complications and Sequelae. Long thought to be a relatively benign disease, HPV has been shown in recent data to have a definite association with genital cancer. The association exists for both clinically overt and subclinical lesions. Of the 40 types of HPV identified to date by molecular virology techniques, the most common viruses associated with genital disease are types 6, 11, 16, 18, and 31. Currently, experts believe that types 16, 18, and 31 are most likely to be related to cancer and that types 6 and 11

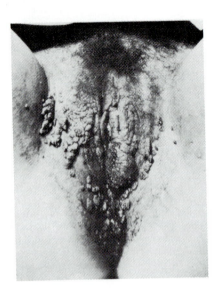

Figure 12–10. Vulvar condylomata acuminata. *(From Eschenbach, D. A., [1986]. Pelvic infections. In D. N. Danforth & J. R. Scott [Eds.], Obstetrics and gynecology [5th ed.]. Philadelphia: J. B. Lippincott Co. Reprinted with permission.)*

have low oncogenic potential (Bergeron, Ferenczy, Shah, & Naghashfar, 1987; Reid, Greenberg, Jenson, et al., 1987). Viral types 6 and 11 are more likely to be found in vulvar than cervical lesions; types 16, 18, and 31 are more likely to be found in cervical condylomata (Reid et al., 1987). The association has been most extensively studied for cervical cancer, but associations also exist between HPV infection and vulvar, vaginal, anal, and penile neoplasia (Kirby & Corey, 1987).

Not all persons infected with HPV types 16 and 18 develop cancer, however, suggesting that the virus is in itself not a sufficient condition for the development of cancer. The development of HPV-associated carcinoma may be related to young age at first exposure, repeated infections, immune status, and other unknown factors, possibly herpesvirus type 2 (Koss, 1987; zur Hausen, 1982) or in utero diethylstilbestrol (DES) exposure (Bornstein, Kaufman, Adam, & Adler-Storthz, 1987).

Condylomata may also become large, uncomfortable, and embarrassing. They may ulcerate, become secondarily infected, and bleed (Oriel, 1984). In pregnancy, lesions tend to grow and may become quite extensive. Laryngeal papillomata may develop in some children born to mothers infected with genital HPV, usually via passage through the birth canal (Quick, Watts, Krzyzek, & Faras, 1980). These lesions narrow the airway (Kashima & Shah, 1987). There may be a long latency period before papillomata develop, making estimates of risk difficult. Schwartz, Greenberg, Daoud, and Reid (1987) cite the occurrence of laryngeal papillomata to be between 1:30 and less than 1:1,000 in children born to infected mothers, compared with an overall risk of 1:2,000.

Differential Diagnosis. Condylomata acuminata must be differentiated from *condylomata lata* found in secondary syphilis. Condylomata lata (Fig. 12–5) are found in the vulva and anus and are broader and flatter than condylomata acuminata. Granuloma inguinale and, occasionally, molluscum contagiosum may be confused with warts. Several benign neoplasms and malignancies of the anogenital area may also be mistaken for condylomata acuminata (see Chapter 11).

Management

DATA COLLECTION

History. Although condylomata acuminata are usually asymptomatic, women may occasionally complain of discomfort, itching, or postcoital bleeding. More often, they report "bumps" on the vulva. A known exposure is significant; however, because of the possible long period of latency and the possibility of subclinical infection in males, the absence of known exposure cannot be used to rule out condylomata.

Physical Examination. Inspection of the vulva, perineum, anus, vagina, and cervix is important whenever condylomata acuminata are suspected or visualized in one area. Routine speculum examination may obscure some vaginal lesions; the blades must be rotated so all areas of the vagina seen (Campion, 1987). Unfortunately, many cervical lesions are not visible and some vaginal and vulvar infections may also be subclinical (Paavonen, 1985). For visible lesions, the characteristic appearance is considered diagnostic of condylomata acuminata. Because of the potential of spread of vulvar or vaginal lesions to the anus, change of gloves is now recommended between vaginal and anal examinations (Gusberg, 1986).

Laboratory Testing. A number of laboratory tests have been advocated to help diagnose HPV and its sequelae, including cytology (Pap smear), colposcopy, and, at times, biopsy. Although vulvar lesions are most often diagnosed by appearance alone, cervical, and possibly vaginal, lesions are often not visible. Physical examination cannot distinguish types of HPV or precancerous or cancerous cellular changes. Minimally, a Pap smear of the cervix should be taken to rule out cytologic evidence of HPV infection(Centers for Disease Control, 1985b). The classic cytologic finding in HPV is the *koilocyte* or "balloon cell" (Drake, Medley, & Mitchell, 1987). This is a squamous cell, possibly enlarged, frequently binucleate or multinucleate, with dense and opaque nuclear material.

Some authorities, citing high rates of cervical involvement and relatively high false-negative rates on cytology, suggest colposcopic examination of the vagina and cervix in any woman with vulvar condylomata (Greenberg et al., 1987). Acetic acid application followed by magnification often reveals clinically inapparent lesions. Sometimes, it is difficult to distinguish condylomata acuminata from dysplasia by colposcopy. Biopsy is then needed to confirm the findings (Kirby & Corey, 1987). Classic histologic findings in genital warts are basal cell hyperplasia, acanthosis, papillomatosis, koilocytosis, parakeratosis, and mild nuclear atypia. Not all of these features are always present, however, and DNA hybridization provides a more specific diagnosis of HPV infection (Kirby & Corey, 1987). When possible, referral for diagnosis should be to a facility with the capability of performing this test. Recently, tests have been developed to simplify DNA hybridization. The Food and Drug Administration has approved at least one kit for this purpose, the ViraPap (Life Technologies, Inc., Gaithersburg, MD). These tests have high specificity and sensitivity. In the near future, screening for HPV using DNA hybridization may become routine in sexually active women, particularly women with multiple partners (Richart, Becker, Ferenczy, et al., 1989).

Additional diagnostic tests in the presence of warts should include gonorrhea and chlamydia cultures, syphilis serology, and microscopic examination of saline and potassium hydroxide slides.

INTERVENTION

Consultation and Referral. Extensive condylomata and/or cervical lesions mandate referral for treatment. Whether all patients with condylomata acuminata should be referred for colposcopy is controversial at this time and will depend on institutional and practice protocols and improved future knowledge about the course of the disease and its sequelae. In 1985, the CDC stated, "Colposcopy in consultation with an expert should be considered," for women with external genital warts (Centers for Disease Control, 1985b, p. 100S). As research continues to be carried out regarding HPV infection, the value of routine colposcopic examination should become more apparent. Referrals must be to a colposcopist familiar with the classic signs of HPV; optimally, laboratory facilities should be available for DNA hybridization studies of specimens, although it is not unreasonable to assume that any cervical lesion has malignant potential, even if viral type is unknown.

Treatment. Although infections with HPV types 6 and 11 often regress spontaneously, treatment is recommended because of the infectivity of the virus and the possibility of coexisting infection with the more oncogenic viral types. Current chemical and surgical treatments include local applications of podophyllin, trichloracetic acid, and 5-Fluorouracil; local, intralesional, and systemic interferon; and destructive techniques including scissor excision, cautery or coagulation, cryosurgery, and laser surgery. Initial treatment of external warts may be carried out by the primary care provider; treatment for vaginal and/or cervical lesions requires consultation and/or referral (Centers for Disease Control, 1985b, p. 100s).

Podophyllin is a resin mixture obtained from the dried rhizome and roots of podophyllin plants. CDC recommends the use of a 10 percent solution in tincture of benzoin, which should be applied to each wart, taking care to avoid the normal surrounding tissue. If necessary, the surrounding area can be protected with petrolatum before the podophyllin application (Silva, Micha, & Silva, 1985). The solution should be washed off thoroughly 1 to 4 hours after the initial treatment. Once patient tolerance is established, this period can be extended, even to 24 hours (Oriel, 1984), although the usual time is 4 to 6 hours. Treatment can be repeated once or twice weekly. The CDC recommends alternative therapies if warts do not regress after four applications. Some authors advise use of a 25 percent solution, with 0.5 mL as the maximum advisable dose at one session.

Podophyllin cannot be used during pregnancy or for cervical or oral warts. Many consultants avoid the use of podophyllin for anal warts (Centers for Disease Control, 1985b).

Unfortunately, podophyllin has a number of local and systemic side effects. Local side effects include inflammatory reactions, chemical burns in patients given podophyllin for self-treatment, necrosis and scarring of the anogenital region, and allergic reactions (Miller, 1985). Systemic side effects have been seen when the medication has been applied to extensive areas and has remained in contact for extended periods. These include nausea and vomiting, respiratory stimulation, peripheral neuropathy, fever, confusion, tachycardia, oliguria, anuria, adynamic ileus, coma, and even death (Miller, 1985).

Fisher (1981, pp. 248, 266) recommends the following guidelines for podophyllin use:

- Treatment should be an office procedure.
- The initial application should remain in place only 1 hour.
- If the initial application does not cause undue inflammation or pain, then subsequent applications can be kept on 4 to 6 hours.
- If pruritic dermatitis occurs, an allergic reaction should be considered. This is usually to the benzoin. Podophyllin may then be made into a solution with mineral oil.
- Old, discolored, or gritty preparations of podophyllin should be avoided.
- Podophyllin resin should be used in tincture of benzoin prepared without Indian podophyllin (which is stronger and more irritating) and guaiacum gum (which may be a sensitizer).

Other investigators have made the following additional recommendations (Miller, 1985):

- Limit applications to small areas of intact skin.
- Avoid extended periods of contact.
- Avoid alcoholic beverages for several hours after treatment (alcohol may increase absorption).
- Avoid use of podophyllin resin on the buccal mucosa and tongue.

Trichloracetic acid can be used in a 50 percent solution for vulvar, vaginal, or anal warts. It is usually used when podophyllin treatment fails. The medication can be applied twice a week and has been recommended for up to 6 weeks (Ferenczy, 1986). It need not be washed off. Accidental spills on unaffected skin, however, can cause severe burns. A solution of sodium bicarbonate can counteract these burning effects. Extensive use of trichloracetic acid should be avoided as it can cause burning and swelling. Some authors advise self-application of trichloracetic acid; it can be applied by the patient with a Q-tip; this makes treatment more convenient and less expensive (Ferenczy, 1986).

5-Fluorouracil (5-Fu) is a pyrimidine antimetabolite that causes necrosis and sloughing of rapidly growing tissues. It can be used on vulvar, vaginal, intraurethral, and perianal warts (Dretler & Klein, 1975). Patients can apply the medication themselves. In one study of 20 women with vaginal condylomata using one third of an applicatorful (1.5 g) of 5 percent 5-Fu cream at bedtime once a week for 10 weeks, 85 were disease free 3 months later. Twice weekly application to the vulva for resistant or extensive condylomata is also well tolerated but is less effective.

Mild vulvar irritation and vaginal discharge have been noted with 5-Fu therapy (Krebs, 1987b). At recommended dosages, systemic toxicity is not seen. With more frequent usage, pain and burning may occur (Krebs, 1987a). This treatment should not be used in pregnant women.

Interferons are proteins with antiviral properties. They can be applied topically, injected directly into lesions, or given as intramuscular or subcutaneous injections in a variety of dosage schedules. In a placebo-controlled study, Friedman-Kein, Eron, Conant, and associates (1988) showed a 62 percent cure rate compared with a 21 percent cure rate for the placebo group in 86 patients receiving interferon-α injections into lesions twice a week up to 8 weeks. Interferon treatment is currently reserved for patients with persistent and recurrent disease for whom conventional therapy has failed (Trofatter, 1987).

In addition to being very expensive, interferons are associated with a number of side effects, most notably flulike symptoms including fever, chills, headaches, myalgias, and arthralgias. Long-term use is associated with additional side effects including malaise, fatigue, anorexia, muscle weakness, and, occasionally, weight loss. Significant gastrointestinal complaints, hair loss, and psychiatric problems are seen less often, and, at high doses, vomiting, diarrhea, and hypotension may occur (Trofatter, 1987).

A variety of destructive techniques have been advocated for treatment of condylomata including scissor excision, cautery, electrocoagulation, cryosurgery, and CO_2 laser therapy (Baggish, 1985; Bekassy & Weström, 1987; Reid, 1985a, 1985b, 1987). High cure rates have been demonstrated with both cryosurgery and laser therapy. Both are appropriate for cervical lesions. Cryosurgery takes 4 to 6 weeks to heal and results in a profuse vaginal discharge for several weeks. Laser therapy may cause bleeding (Micha & Silva, 1986). Choice of therapy often depends on the physician's preference and experience.

Patients with extensive, cervical, or resistant condylomata should be referred for one of the destructive therapies to a physician experienced in treating these lesions.

In addition to treatment for condylomata acuminata, all concurrent vaginal infections and STDs must be treated to effect cure (Powell, 1972).

Self-Help. For patients with discomfort from condylomata or their treatment, some relief may be obtained by bathing with Aveeno oatmeal solution and drying the area with a cool hair dryer. Patients must understand their role in effective treatment (such as washing off podophyllin, appropriately using 5-Fu, returning for follow-up visits, etc.).

Additional Teaching and Counseling. Women must understand the nature of transmission of HPV infection. They should advise their partners to be checked, even if apparently asymptomatic. Seventy-three to seventy-seven percent of male partners of women with condylomata acuminata have evidence of HPV at initial examination or within 6 months (Sedlacek, Cunnane, & Carpiniello, 1986). Colposcopic examination of the penis after the application of acetic acid or vinegar has been advocated to locate subclinical lesions (Krebs & Schneider, 1987; Rosemberg 1985; Rosemberg, Greenberg, & Reid, 1987). Referrals can be made to urologists, dermatologists, or gynecologists with expertise in this area.

Condoms are protective against HPV and should be advised for all women infected with HPV or women with infected partners. They should be used until all warts are completely resolved (Bourcier & Seidler, 1987) and even up to 9 months after appearance of lesions as subclinical condylomata may be infectious. Instructions for all medications and treatments must be extensive. Women must understand the advisability of treatment before pregnancy, and the need for lifetime annual gynecologic checkups with screening for cervical cancer.

Cytomegalovirus

Etiology and Transmission. Cytomegalovirus (CMV) is a member of the herpesvirus group. It shares the capacity with other herpesviruses to remain latent and be active in the presence of host antibody (Lang, 1984).

Sexual contact is considered one means of transmission of CMV. Evidence for this comes from recovery of the virus from genital sites (Lang, 1984); seropositivity and positive cultures for the virus found in significant numbers of male sex partners of infected women (Handsfield, Chandler, Caine, et al., 1985); association of the virus with numbers of lifetime sex partners, young age at first sexual intercourse, and infection with *C. trachomatis* (Chandler, Holmes, Wentworth, et al., 1985); and demonstration of a higher prevalence of CMV virus in women attending STD clinics compared with women attending other clinics (Embil, Garner, Pereira, et al., 1985). The importance of the sexual route for transmission of the virus is debated, however (Knox, 1983).

Epidemiology. CMV is most common in children, the young, unmarried, and those with multiple sexual partners. In pregnancy, young, primiparous women are most likely to be infected. Cervical isolation of virus is increasingly common as pregnancy advances, suggesting suppression in early gestation (Stagno, Reynolds, Tsiantos, et al., 1975).

Clinical Presentation. In most healthy adults, infection with CMV is asymptomatic. Some mild cases of anicteric hepatitis, heterophil-negative mononucleosis, interstitial pneumonia, Guillain-Barre ascending paralysis, hemolytic anemia, and thrombocytopenia purpura are associated with CMV (Lemon, 1984). In immunocompromised persons, the virus may cause devastating disease.

Complications and Sequelae. The major consequences of CMV infections are in newborns infected pre- or postnatally through the placenta or through other body secretions, including breast milk, urine, saliva, blood, and, at times, stool (Lang, 1984). Severe fetal involvement occurs in at least 31 percent of newborns born to women with primary CMV infections (Brunham et al., 1984). Approximately 1 percent of infants born in the United States are infected with CMV; 10 to 20 percent of these infants eventually manifest adverse effects on central nervous system development, possibly including deafness (Hanshaw, Scheiner, Moxley, et al., 1976).

Management

DATA COLLECTION

History. Because most infections are asymptomatic or non-specific, few women are aware of exposure.

Physical Examination. Physical examination does not reveal symptoms of CMV infection in healthy adults except in the presence of the diseases mentioned earlier, in which case CMV should be ruled out as a possible cause. Full discussion of the signs and symptoms of these disorders is beyond the scope of this book. The interested reader is referred to a general medical text.

Laboratory Testing. CMV can be identified by serologic testing; the complement fixation test is most widely used (Lang, 1984). Seroconversion or a fourfold rise in titers indicates recent infection. Because this test is relatively nonsensitive, indirect immunofluorescence antibody testing has been used to enhance sensitivity. CMV-specific IgM antibody can also be detected. Cultures for CMV can be taken.

INTERVENTION

Treatment. Several antiviral agents are in the experimental stage as treatments for CMV. At present, no treatment is available.

Teaching and Counseling. As the major consequences of CMV are in the newborn, teaching and counseling need to be geared to pregnant women or those planning pregnancy. Postponement of pregnancy should be discussed if recent infection is evidenced by serologic tests. Pregnant women should not be exposed to infants or children with known CMV infections. It is possible that a vaccine will be available in the future, but because of the persistence of infection even in the presence of antibody, much work needs to be done before this is possible.

Molluscum Contagiosum

Molluscum contagiosum is a benign viral disease of the skin.

Etiology and Transmission. Molluscum contagiosum virus is a poxvirus. In children, the disease is transmitted either by direct contact or possibly through vehicles such as shared towels and gymnasium equipment and benches (Brown, 1984). Childhood lesions occur on the face, trunk, and limbs. In young adults, the disease is considered to be sexually transmitted, based on the location of lesions, numbers of sexual partners of infected persons, presence of the disease in sexual partners, and existence of other STDs among the infected (Cobbold & MacDonald, 1970; Gudgel, 1954; Lynch & Minkin, 1968; Snell & Fox, 1961; Wilkin, 1977).

The incubation period for molluscum contagiosum in clinical reports ranges from 1 week to 6 months (Brown, Nalley, & Kraus, 1981), and in experimental studies, from 14 to 50 days (Brown 1984).

Epidemiology. Molluscum contagiosum is relatively rare in the United States. In one report from a number of STD clinics, it was seen in one in every 190 patients; this equals one case for every 42 cases of gonorrhea (Brown, 1984). Becker and associates (1986), however, analyzed data from national surveys and from two STD clinics from 1966 to 1983 and 1977 to 1981, respectively. They reported an 11-fold increase in private physicians visits for this disease from 1966 to 1983 although clinic visits remained stable from 1977 to 1981. Clinic patients aged 15 to 24 and private patients aged 20 to 29 are most likely to be infected.

Clinical Presentation. Molluscum contagiosum presents with papules, generally seen on the lower abdomen, pubis, genitalia, and inner thighs in adult infections. The lesions are rarely seen on the palms and soles. Papules are typically smooth, firm, and spherical with a central depression (Fig. 12-11). A curdy white material can be expressed from the central area (Postlethwaite, 1970). Lesions usually range from 2 to 5 mm in diameter but lesions as large as 1.5 cm have been seen. They are flesh-colored, white, translucent, or yellow. Usually 1 to 20 lesions occur, but more than 100 may occur.

Most patients with molluscum contagiosum are asymptomatic but a few may complain of pruritus, tenderness, and pain (Postlethwaite, Watt, Hawley, et al., 1967). The lesions may become inflamed or infected and resemble furuncles (see Chapter 11) (Lynch & Minkin, 1968).

Differential Diagnosis. Molluscum contagiosum must be differentiated from any other disease causing skin lesions including condylomata acuminata, syphilis, herpes simplex virus, and various vulvar dermatoses (see Chapter 11).

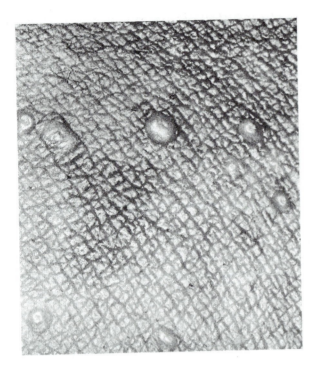

Figure 12-11. Molluscum contagiosum *(From Kaufman, R. H. [1981]. Viral infections. In H. L. Gardner & R. H. Kaufman [Eds.], Benign diseases of the vulva and vagina. Boston: G. K. Hall Medical Publishers. Reprinted with permission.)*

Management

DATA COLLECTION

History. A history of multiple sex partners or new partners is important in the diagnosis of molluscum contagiosum, as it is for any STD. The presence of similar lesions on the body of a sex partner often points to an STD. Except for the lesions, symptoms of this disease are usually nonexistent or nonspecific but any associated symptoms should be noted.

Physical Examination. Diagnosis is usually made by inspection. The abdomen, pubis, genitalia, and thighs should all be carefully examined.

Laboratory Testing. Diagnosis can be confirmed by Pap smear or smears stained with Wright, Giemsa, or Gram stain, identifying the inclusion bodies characteristic of molluscum contagiosum (Brown, 1984). Obviously, interpretation by a practitioner or technician with experience in identifying this lesion is necessary, and dermatologic referral may be required. Tests for gonorrhea, syphilis, chlamydia, and herpes should be carried out.

INTERVENTION. Without treatment, molluscum contagiosum persists 6 months to 2 years; each lesion may remain about 2 months (Hawley, 1970). Treatment is provided to decrease the possibility of autoinoculation and/or transmission of infection and for aesthetic reasons.

Treatment. Treatments for molluscum contagiosum include curettage with local anesthesia as necessary or cryotherapy with liquid nitrogen. A variety of chemical irritants have been used including podophyllin, phenol, silver nitrate, or tretinoin (Margolis, 1984). Laser therapy has been tried, but has resulted in keloid scarring (Friedman & Gal, 1987).

Teaching and Counseling. Aspects of teaching and counseling discussed previously regarding STD prevention apply to any person with molluscum contagiosum. Patients can be reassured that this disease is not associated with systemic spread or sequelae. Support should be given for the possible psychological consequences of perceived disfigurement caused by the lesions, which can be extensive. Patients should be warned that new lesions may develop after treatment. Sex partners should be examined.

Viral Hepatitis

Sexual contact is one possible route of transmission of viral hepatitis. For this reason, the disease is covered in this chapter. Well-woman gynecologic practitioners may be involved in screening for and counseling about hepatitis infection, but management requires medical intervention and follow-up.

Etiology and Transmission. Viral hepatitis can be caused by hepatitis A virus (HAV), hepatitis B virus (HBV), and several types of non-A, non-B (NANB) viruses. Hepatitis B virus, of the most concern as a sexually transmitted organism in women, is a complex organism with three antigenic structures: hepatitis B surface antigen (HBsAg; formerly called the Australia antigen), which is the outer surface coat; hepatitis B core antigen (HBcAg), which is within the surface coat; and HBeAg, which is associated with the core of the virus (Lemon, 1984). Familiarity with these is important because screening for active or chronic disease or disease immunity is based on testing for these antigens and their antibodies.

Sexual transmission is considered the major means of transmission of hepatitis B virus and a lesser means of transmission of HAV and, possibly, of NANB (Lemon, 1984). Hepatitis B surface antigen has been found in blood, saliva, sweat, tears, vaginal secretions, and semen. Intrauterine transmission or transmission to infants shortly after birth is possible. Transmission also has occurred through artificial insemination (Berry, Gottesfeld, Alter, & Vierling, 1987). HBV can also be transmitted via blood transfusion, but the incidence of such transmission has decreased with the testing of blood for hepatitis surface antigen (see later). Drug abusers, however, are subject to hepatitis B infection via shared needles as are health care workers who are exposed to blood and at risk for needle sticks.

Hepatitis A is transmitted via fecal–oral spread including sex practices involving oral–anal contact, although sexual transmission is considered an infrequent source of transmission (Szmuness, Dienstag, Purcell, et al., 1976). Common-source outbreaks resulting from contaminated food or water and the ingestion of uncooked shellfish are associated with hepatitis A.

Non-A, non-B hepatitis can be waterborne or transmitted via blood transfusions and other percutaneous means. It may possibly be sexually transmitted.

The incubation period for hepatitis B is 29 to over 100 days but may be shorter (as short as 6 days) with parenteral exposure (Krugman, Overby, Mushahwar, et al., 1979). The incubation period for hepatitis A infection is 23 to 50 days, with an average of 33 days (Boggs, Melnick, Conrad, & Felsher, 1970). Non-A, non-B hepatitis has an incubation period of 2 weeks to 6 months.

Epidemiology. The prevalence of hepatitis A is related to age and socioeconomic status; when living conditions are poor, it is seen more often in children (Szmuness et al., 1976). Hepatitis B accounts for approximately 50 percent of cases of fulminating hepatitis (Rakela, Redeker, Edwards, et al., 1978). Non-A, non-B hepatitis is thought to account for a large number of acute cases as well (Dienstag, Alaama, Mosley, et al., 1977). Hepatitis B is prevalent in parts of Asia and Africa and in immigrants from these countries (Sobeslavsky, 1978; Szmuness, 1978). In New York City, in a study of several thousand blood donors, approximately 5 percent had past exposure and less than 1 percent, current or chronic infection (Szmuness, 1978). Evidence of infection was associated with age and inversely related to socioeconomic status, higher among blacks and Orientals than whites, and higher in males than females, presumably because of increased promiscuity and male homosexuality (Szmuness, Much, Prince, et al., 1975). Health care workers are at increased risk (Segal, Llewellyn, Irwin, et al., 1976).

Clinical Presentation. Hepatitis is a disease of the liver with clinical symptoms indistinguishable among the three types of infections. Hepatitis B, however, is often a silent infection, whereas hepatitis A causes symptoms in nine out of ten infected adults (Lemon, 1984). Nevertheless, hepatitis B is a more serious illness, leading more frequently to acute hepatic failure and death. Chronic hepatitis occurs with HBV infection and with NANB hepatitis but not with hepatitis A.

Early symptoms of hepatitis infection include skin eruptions, urticaria, arthralgias, arthritis, lassitude, anorexia, nausea, vomiting, headache, fever, and mild abdominal pain. Later symptoms include clay colored stool, dark urine, increase in abdominal pain, and jaundice.

Jaundice is a late finding and seen in only one fourth of patients with hepatitis infection (Judson, 1984). Often, by the time it occurs, the patient is feeling better.

Complications and Sequelae. Complications of hepatitis infection include chronic persistent active hepatitis or a chronic carrier state, cirrhosis of the liver, hepatocellular carcinoma, hepatic failure, and death.

Management. Hepatitis must be managed by a physician. The primary care provider, however, can offer screening for the disease.

DATA COLLECTION

History. A history of blood transfusion, known exposure via sexual intercourse or close personal contact, work in the health care field, particularly with blood or blood products as in surgery or dentistry, male homosexuality, and immigration from parts of the world with high rates of hepatitis, such as Southeast Asia and Africa, are all significant risk factors. The symptoms outlined earlier should be part of the history taking.

Physical Examination. Physical examination includes inspection of the skin for rashes, inspection of the skin and conjunctivae for jaundice, and palpation of the liver for enlargement. Weight loss and overall debility may be significant.

Laboratory Testing. Hepatitis A and B can be diagnosed by blood studies, whereas NANB hepatitis is diagnosed by exclusion of these and other viral syndromes such as CMV and Epstein–Barr virus. Hepatitis A is diagnosed by serologic testing for anti-HAV. Acute infection can be diagnosed by a significant rise in anti-HAV titer or the demonstration of IgM specific to HAV.

Testing for hepatitis B is more complex (Table 12–4). Patients with acute hepatitis B have detectable HBsAg levels in the serum. These levels generally become detectable in the late incubation phase of the disease, 2 to 5 weeks before the development of symptoms (Hoofnagle, 1981). Tests for antibody can also be helpful. Anti-HBs with a negative HBsAg test denotes immunity. This means the antigen is no longer present and the antibody is protective. Anti-HBs with a positive antigen denotes a chronic carrier state which poses a risk for future liver disease, including cancer; during this time the disease may be transmitted. Although HBcAg cannot be found in the serum, anti-HBc can be detected; it may be present in acute infection, diagnosed when antigen (HBsAg) is also present; in recovery from acute infection, diagnosed when no other markers are present; or in immunity, diagnosed when anti-HBs is also present. During the recovery period, the patient may continue to be infectious even though HBsAg has disappeared. This is called the *window phase* and is denoted by anti-HBc in the

TABLE 12–4. LABORATORY TESTING FOR HBV

Antigen	Antibody	Denotes	Comments
HBsAg +	NEG.	Active infection.	With HBeAg, denotes high degree of infection.
HBsAg +	Anti-HBc +	Active infection.	
HBsAg +	Anti-HBs +	Chronic carrier state.	Anti-HBc may or may not be present.
NEG.	Anti-HBs +	Immunity.	Anti-HBc may or may not be present.
NEG.	Anti-HBc +	Recovery: May be infectious in "window phase" or past period of infectivity.	IgM specific for Anti-HBc denotes recent infection with infectivity. Once Anti-HBs develops, immunity is denoted; no longer infectious.

absence of anti-HBs (which, if immunity is to be developed, will become detectable at a later stage). Anti-HBc alone does not, however, definitely mean the patient is infective; this antibody can persist for many years after infectivity had passed, and surface antibody, granting immunity, may simply never develop. The presence of IgM specific for anti-HBc denotes infection within 6 to 24 months and means that the potential for infectivity exists. IgM is tested for only if anti-HBc is the only marker present and history does not clarify when the patient was infected.

The presence of HBeAg can also be tested for. This is done in the person with HBsAg. Presence of HBeAg suggests a high degree of infectivity. Table 12–4 outlines the interpretation of laboratory tests for HBV.

Laboratory tests should be performed serially and post-infection in patients with hepatitis and for screening purposes in persons at risk. Patients with current or past hepatitis should have liver function tests performed unless previous postdisease testing had been normal.

INTERVENTION

Treatment. There is no specific therapy for hepatitis. Recovery from hepatitis B is usually spontaneous in 3 to 16 weeks. As with any infectious process, supportive therapy can shorten the course and decrease the severity of the illness.

Good nutrition, including a high-calorie diet, is the cornerstone of therapy. Bedrest also enhances recovery. The patient with hepatitis should avoid alcohol and drugs, which can further compromise liver function. In severe cases hospitalization may be necessary.

Teaching and Counseling. All nonimmune persons at high or moderate risk of hepatitis should be aware of the existence of hepatitis B vaccine (Centers for Disease Control, 1987g). Persons for whom hepatitis B vaccine is recommended or should be considered are listed in Table 12–5. Individuals can be reassured that receiving vaccine does not carry a risk of contracting human immunodeficiency vi-

rus (Centers for Disease Control, 1984, 1983c). Vaccination is not associated with serious side effects; soreness at the injection site and mild systemic symptoms may be experienced. The vaccine is given in a series of three doses over a 6-month period, with the first two doses given within 1 month of each other. To increase efficacy, vaccine should be given in the deltoid muscle whenever possible.

Anyone with hepatitis must be aware of the need to follow their antigen–antibody status and have liver function tests performed periodically until they revert to normal. The follow-up varies in length depending on test results and symptoms exhibited.

All infectious persons should be counseled to avoid sexual contact involving exchange of body fluids, to avoid sharing personal articles such as toothbrushes and razors, not to donate blood, and to have family members or sexual partners tested for hepatitis and offered vaccine if testing is negative. Intravenous drug users should be made aware of the risks to themselves and others of sharing needles. Referral to appropriate drug rehabilitation services is timely for a patient with recently diagnosed hepatitis.

Human Immunodeficiency Virus/Acquired Immune Deficiency Syndrome

In recent years, the acquired immune deficiency syndrome (AIDS) has become a major focus of public health concern, investigation, and preventive efforts. This concern is matched by the general public; in 1985, public opinion polls showed AIDS to rank number 2 among health concerns of Americans, with only cancer being of greater concern (Minkoff, 1986).

AIDS was first identified in 1981 as a clinical entity after four male homosexuals developed illnesses known to occur only in individuals with immunosuppression (Gottlieb, Schroff, Schanker, et al., 1981).

Etiology and Transmission. AIDS is caused by a retrovirus, now called the human immunodeficiency virus (HIV), previously known as human T-cell lymphotropic virus type III (HTLV-III) or lymphadenopathy-associated virus (LAV). Discovered in 1983, the virus is thought to have been found originally in primates in central Africa (Minkoff, 1986).

Retroviruses grow slowly. Infection wth the virus may persist for the lifetime of the infected, whether or not disease symptoms become manifest (Symposium, 1986). What triggers the virus to initiate its effects on the immune system and allow the diseases that form the acquired immune deficiency syndrome to occur is one of the key issues under investigation by AIDS researchers.

Transmission of the virus causing AIDS occurs by sexual contact or direct exposure to an infected body fluid. The virus has been identified in semen, saliva, urine, blood or blood products, vaginal secretions, tears, serum, cerebrospinal fluid, and alveolar fluid (Friedland & Klein, 1987). Only blood and semen, however, have been directly implicated in transmission, although transmission through breast milk and vaginal fluids is likely.

Transmission is known to occur in a number of ways:

- Homosexual sexual intercourse, most commonly receptive anal intercourse
- Sharing of needles and syringes
- Heterosexual intercourse, male-to-female (Friedland & Klein, 1987; Padian, Marquis, Francis, et al., 1987) or female-to-male (Redfield, Markham, Salahuddin, et al., 1985)

TABLE 12–5. PERSONS FOR WHOM HEPATITIS B VACCINE IS RECOMMENDED OR SHOULD BE CONSIDERED

Preexposure

Persons for whom vaccine is recommended:
  Health-care workers having blood or needle-stick exposures
  Clients and staff of institutions for the developmentally disabled
  Hemodialysis patients
  Homosexually active men
  Users of illicit injectable drugs
  Recipients of certain blood products
  Household members and sexual contacts of HBV carriers
  Special high-risk populations
Persons for whom vaccine should be considered:
  Inmates of long-term correctional facilities
  Heterosexually active persons with multiple sexual partners
  International travelers to HBV endemic areas

Postexposure

Infants born to HBV positive mothers
Health-care workers having needle-stick exposures to human blood

From Centers for Disease Control (1987, June 19) Update on hepatitis B antibody to human immunodeficiency virus. Morbidity and Mortality Weekly Report, 36 (23), 357.

- Blood or blood product transfusion of infected blood (Peterman, Jaffe, Feorino, et al., 1985)
- Transplacentally from mother to child (Minkoff, Nanda, Menez, & Fikrig, 1987; Mok, Giaquinto, De-Rossi, et al., 1987) or during birth
- Postnatally via breast milk or other maternal–infant contact (Lepage, Van de Perre, Carael, et al., 1987; Ziegler, Cooper, Johnson, & Gold, 1985)
- Artificial insemination by donor (Stewart, Tyler, Cunningham, et al., 1985)
- Very rarely, needle sticks or other exposure of health care workers to infected blood (Centers for Disease Control, 1987f; Weiss, Saxinger, Rechtman, et al., 1985)

Transmission is not known to occur via casual physical contact even among household members of AIDS sufferers or those caring for AIDS patients (Fischl, Dickinson, Scott, et al., 1987; Friedland, Saltzman, Rogers, et al., 1986; Gerberding, Bryant-LeBlanc, Nelson, et al., 1987; Henderson, Saah, Zak, et al., 1986; McCray, 1986).

AIDS appears to be less transmissible than many other STDs for which a single encounter poses risk. In a number of studies examining heterosexual transmission, couples in long-term relationships with repeated sexual encounters over years showed a rate of infection of partners of the infected ranging from 7 to 68 percent (Friedland & Klein, 1987). Engaging in receptive anal intercourse increases the risk of transmission for both homosexual males and heterosexual women (Padian et al., 1987).

The time from HIV exposure to a detectable antibody response is unknown and may vary (Ranki, Valle, Krohn, et al., 1987), although CDC reports that detectable antibody usually occurs within 6 to 12 weeks of infection (Centers for Disease Control, 1987d). The CDC estimates the median incubation period between infection and development of disease as 7 years (Centers for Disease Control, 1987b, p. 2).

Epidemiology. Information on the prevalence of AIDS comes from surveys and studies conducted by state and local health departments, medical centers, the U.S. Public Health Service, and other federal agencies with varying degrees of accuracy and bias (Centers for Disease Control, 1987b). Although information on prevalence rates is extensive, incidence rates (i.e., new cases) and disease trends are less clear. Groups recognized at risk for HIV infection in the United States include homosexual and bisexual men, intravenous drug users, hemophiliacs, and heterosexual partners of persons with HIV infection or at recognized risk (Centers for Disease Control, 1987b).

Among these risk groups are the following CDC-estimated prevalence rates:

- Homosexual men: 20 to 25 percent infection with the highest rates in San Francisco (CDC suggests this may be an overestimate as statistics are based largely on males seen at STD clinics.)
- IV drug users: great geographic variation; 50 to 60 percent in New York City, New Jersey, and Puerto Rico, less than 5 percent in areas other than the East Coast (This may be an underestimate because data have been derived largely from surveys at drug treatment centers.)
- Hemophiliacs: 35 percent with hemophilia B and 70 percent with hemophilia A (This largely represents infection before 1985 when screening of blood and

plasma and heat treatment of clotting factor concentrates were initiated routinely.)
- Heterosexual partners of persons with HIV infection or recognized risk: infection rates varying from 10 to 60 percent. (More data are needed to evaluate the relative efficiency of male-to-female versus female-to-male transmission.)

Among groups not at risk but routinely tested for HIV infection, the following rates have been identified:

- 0.432 percent for first-time blood donors from 1985 to 1987
- 0.15 percent among military applicants between October 1985 and September 1987
- 0.33 percent among job corps applicants, which represents a 16- to 21-year-old, economically disadvantaged population
- 0.21 percent for childbearing women (based on Massachusetts data), with 0.80 percent prevalence among women in inner-city hospitals compared with 0.09 percent at suburban and rural hospitals (This rate is 2.6 percent in New York City and Puerto Rico with rates up to 30 percent among pregnant drug users.)
- 0 to 45 percent among prostitutes with highest rates in inner-city areas where IV drug use is common (It is not currently possible to review the importance of IV drug use versus sexual exposure as the important factor in prevalence among prostitutes, but the CDC considers prostitution a significant means for heterosexual transmission.)

The actual risk of disease among newborns born to women infected with HIV is not yet known but appears to be approximately 30 to 50 percent (Centers for Disease Control, 1987b).

Rates of AIDS increase rapidly among persons in their late twenties and thirties, where they peak, then decline in the forties and fifties. The disease is 13 times more prevalent among males than females; if male homosexuals are removed from this analysis, however, the ratio is only 2.9 to 1, male to female. Among IV drug abusers, the prevalence does not significantly differ between males and females. The disease shows a disproportionately high rate among blacks (3:1) and Hispanics (2.6:1) compared with whites, particularly when homosexuals and bisexuals are excluded (12:1 for blacks; 9.3:1 for Hispanics). The reasons for this are not known; IV drug use may account for some of this difference, but the racial disproportion holds even *among* IV drug users.

Although hard data are difficult to accumulate and assess, evidence exists that new infection may be slowed in some groups, including homosexual and bisexual men. HIV infection rates among IV drug users and in inner-city areas, however, may be increasing. The total number of reported AIDS cases has been approximately 50,000 in the United States with estimates of 250,000 to 300,000 cases by 1991 (Allen & Curran, 1988).

As of 1986, heterosexual transmission in the United States accounted for only 1 percent of AIDS cases, but among partners of IV drug abusers, one study found a 40 percent rate of infection (Drucker, 1986). As of 1987, 74 percent of AIDS cases in U.S. adults had been among homosexual men; of these, 8 percent also used IV drugs. As of January 1987, only 6.7 percent of all AIDS cases in the United States had been among women. Worldwide studies, however, show heterosexual transmission to be more important than homosexual transmission (Friedland & Klein, 1987). The proportion of cases that are attributable to heterosexual transmission is increasing more rapidly than the proportion of cases in any other risk category (Friedland & Klein, 1987). Among heterosexual cases, minority groups are overrepresented. Among women acquiring AIDS via heterosexual intercourse, five times as many have been partners of IV drug users than of bisexuals.

Risk factors for AIDS among women include the following:

- Having had a sex partner who is a bisexual male
- IV drug use or a partner with IV drug use
- Having received a transfusion of blood or blood products before April 1985, or being a partner of someone who received blood or a blood product before April 1985
- Being a prostitute
- Having or having had a partner or partners whose sexual or drug history is unknown
- Being born in a country where heterosexual transmis-

sion is believed to play a major role in transmission or being a sex partner of men from these countries (State of New York, 1987)

Pathology and Clinical Presentation. Infection with HIV affects primarily T4 cells, which are surface markers or receptors on lymphocytes. T4 cells are helper cells that are important in the overall function of the immune system. HIV is lymphotrophic for T4 cells. Infection causes a reversal of the ratio of these helper cells to suppressor cells (T8 cells). This defect, however, is not specific to AIDS as it occurs in infection with CMV, Epstein–Barr virus, and hepatitis virus (Minkoff, 1986). Other AIDS-induced immune defects include anergy (impaired or absent ability to react to specific antigens), lymphopenia, poor mitogen response, decreased interferon production, and decreased B-cell activity. None of these is pathognomonic for AIDS (Minkoff, 1986).

The definition of AIDS was revised in 1987 by the CDC and appears as Table 12–6. Because there is no single clinical syndrome indicative of AIDS infection, this definition is

TABLE 12–6. 1987 REVISION OF CASE DEFINITION FOR AIDS

For national reporting, a case of AIDS is defined as an illness characterized by one or more of the following "indicator" diseases, depending on the status of laboratory evidence of HIV infection, as shown below.

I. **Without Laboratory Evidence Regarding HIV Infection**
If laboratory tests for HIV were not performed or gave inconclusive results and the patient had no other cause of immunodeficiency listed in Section I.A below, then any disease listed in Section I.B indicates AIDS if it was diagnosed by a definitive method
   A. **Causes of immunodeficiency that disqualify diseases as indicators of AIDS in the absence of laboratory evidence for HIV infection**
      1. high-dose or long-term systemic corticosteroid therapy or other immunosuppresive/cytotoxic therapy ≤ 3 months before the onset of the indicator disease
      2. any of the following diseases diagnosed ≤3months after diagnosis of the indicator disease: Hodgkin's disease, non-Hodgkin's lymphoma (other than primary brain lymphoma), lymphocytic leukemia, multiple myeloma, any other cancer of lymphoreticular or histiocytic tissue, or angioimmunoblastic lymphadenopathy
      3. a genetic (congenital) immunodeficiency syndrome or an acquired immunodeficiency syndrome atypical of HIV infection, such as one involving hypogammaglobulinemia
   B. **Indicator diseases diagnosed definitively**
      1. candidiasis of the esophagus, trachea, bronchi, or lungs
      2. cryptococcosis, extrapulmonary
      3. cryptosporidiosis with diarrhea persisting >1 month
      4. cytomegalovirus disease of an organ other than liver, spleen, or lymph nodes in a patient >1 month of age
      5. herpes simplex virus infection causing a mucocutaneous ulcer that persists longer than 1 month; or bronchitis, pneumonitis, or esophagitis for any duration affecting a patient >1 month of age
      6. Kaposi's sarcoma affecting a patient <60 years of age
      7. lymphoma of the brain (primary) affecting a patient <60 years of age
      8. lymphoid interstitial pneumonia and/or pulmonary lymphoid hyperplasia (LIP/PLH complex) affecting a child <13 years of age
      9. *Mycobacterium avium* complex or *M. kansasil* disease, disseminated (at a site other than or in addition to lungs, skin, or cervical or hilar lymph nodes)
      10. *Pneumocystis carinii* pneumonia
      11. progressive multifocal leukoencephalopathy
      12. toxoplasmosis of the brain affecting a patient >1 month of age

II. **With Laboratory Evidence for HIV Infection**
   Regardless of the presence of other causes of immunodeficiency (I.A.), in the presence of laboratory evidence for HIV infection any disease listed above (I.B.) or below (II.A or II.B) indicates a diagnosis of AIDS.
   A. **Indicator diseases diagnosed definitively**
      1. bacterial infections, multiple or recurrent (any combination of at least two within a 2-year period), of the following types affecting a child <13 years of age:
         septicemia, pneumonia, meningitis, bone or joint infection, or abscess of an internal organ or body cavity (excluding otitis media or superficial skin or mucosal abscesses), caused by *Haemophilus, Streptococcus* (including pneumococcus), or other pyogenic bacteria
      2. coccidioidomycosis, disseminated (at a site other than or in addition to lungs or cervical or hilar lymph nodes)
      3. HIV encephalopathy (also called "HIV demenia," "AIDS dementia," or "subacute encephalitis due to HIV")
      4. histoplasmosis, disseminated (at a site other than or in addition to lungs or cervical or hilar lymph nodes)
      5. isosporiasis with diarrhea persisting >1 month
      6. Kaposi's sarcoma at any age
      7. lymphoma of the brain (primary) at any age

TABLE 12–6. CONTINUED

8. other non-Hodgkin's lymphoma of B-cell or unknown immunologic phenotype and the following histologic types:
   a. small noncleaved lymphoma (either Burkitt or non-Burkitt type)
   b. immunoblastic sarcoma (equivalent to any of the following, although not necessarily all in combination: immunoblastic lymphoma, large-cell lymphoma, diffuse histiocytic lymphoma, diffuse undifferentiated lymphoma, or high-grade lymphoma)

   Note: Lymphomas are not included here if they are of T-cell immunologic phenotype or their histologic type is not described or is described as ''lymphocytic,'' ''lymphoblastic,'' ''small cleaved,'' or ''plasmacytoid lymphocytic''
9. any mycobacterial disease caused by mycobacteria other than *M. tuberculosis,* disseminated (at a site other than or in addition to lungs, skin, or cervical or hilar lymph nodes)
10. disease caused by *M. tuberculosis,* extrapulmonary (involving at least one site outside the lungs, regardless of whether there is concurrent pulmonary involvement)
11. *Salmonella* (nontyphoid) septicemia, recurrent
12. HIV wasting syndrome (emaciation, ''slim disease'')

B. Indicator diseases diagnosed presumptively

Note: Given the seriousness of diseases indicative of AIDS, it is generally important to diagnose them definitively, especially when therapy that would be used may have serious side effects or when definitive diagnosis is needed for eligibility for antiretroviral therapy. Nonetheless, in some situations, a patient's condition will not permit the performance of definitive tests. In other situations, accepted clinical practice may be to diagnose presumptively based on the presence of characteristic clinical and laboratory abnormalities.

1. candidiasis of the esophagus
2. cytomegalovirus retinitis with loss of vision
3. Kaposi's sarcoma
4. lymphoid interstitial pneumonia and/or pulmonary lymphoid hyperplasia (LIP/PLH complex) affecting a child < 13 years of age
5. mycobacterial disease (acid-fast bacilli with species not identified by culture), disseminated (involving at least one site other than or in addition to lungs, skin, or cervical or hilar lymph nodes)
6. *Pneumocystis carinii* pneumonia
7. toxoplasmosis of the brain affecting a patient > 1month of age

III. With Laboratory Evidence Against HIV Infection
With laboratory test results negative for HIV infection, diagnosis of AIDS for surveillance purposes is ruled out *unless:*
A. all the other causes of immunodeficiency listed above in Section I.A are excluded: AND
B. the patient has had either:
   1. *Pneumocystis carinii* pneumonia diagnosed by a definitive method
   OR
   2. a. any of the other diseases indicative of AIDS listed above in Section I.B diagnosed by a definitive method; AND
      b. a T-helper/inducer (CD4) lymphocyte count <400/mm³.

From *Centers for Disease Control. (1987, August 14). Revision of the CDC surveillance case definition for acquired immunodeficiency syndrome. Morbidity and Mortality Weekly Report. 36 (1 Supplement): 45–65.*[a]
[a]More information on diagnosis of the above disorders can be found in this reference.

---

based on laboratory evidence (see below) and/or the presence of certain diseases known to be rare or nonexistent in young, healthy individuals.

Symptoms suggestive of AIDS infection include (Centers for Disease Control, 1983b; LaCamera, 1985) night sweats, fever (either low-grade or spikes to 39°C), anorexia, unexplained weight loss, extreme fatigue, lymph node enlargement persisting longer than 1 month, cough, shortness of breath, mild infections such as colds that persist longer and are more severe than usual, severe watery diarrhea, and neurologic dysfunction (acute meningitis or progressive dementia). Eventually, patients may develop a specific disease commonly associated with AIDS such as Kaposi's sarcoma or *Pneumocystis carinii* pneumonia (PCP).

Women with AIDS differ from men in their presenting complaints. According to the International Conference on AIDS in Paris, 1986, women commonly present with the complaint of persistent, severe, unresponsive vulvovaginitis (Minkoff, 1986; Symposium, 1986). Women may also develop esophageal candidiasis and present with severe dysphagia. Women are much less likely to develop Kaposi's sarcoma or central nervous system involvement (Symposium, 1986). As a large percentage of women with AIDS are IV drug users, they are more likely to present for treatment late in the disease and require longer hospitalizations than do homosexual men, for example.

AIDS-related complex (ARC) is a syndrome characterized by nonspecific symptoms suggestive of AIDS but without opportunistic infections. This classification, however, is no longer used by CDC for surveillance purposes.

Complications and Sequelae. The most serious complication of AIDS is death. The case fatality rate is high; 60 percent of patients diagnosed for 1 year have died; 80 percent of individuals with known cases have died within 2 years of diagnosis (Minkoff, 1986). PCP is the cause of death in approximately one half of AIDS victims.

Many factors have been identified as affecting length of survival after contracting AIDS. Patients already debilitated, such as IV drug users, have a higher incidence of opportunistic infections and a higher mortality rate (Maayan, Wormser, Hewlett, et al., 1985). According to a CDC and New York State Department of Health study, the number of manifestations of AIDS (the number of different opportunistic infections at the time of diagnosis) is the most important predictor of length of survival. Age is also an important predictor of length of survival; people 35 years of age or older have a statistically significant shorter survival than younger patients. Homosexual males aged 30 to 34 with Kaposi's sarcoma only have demonstrated the best survival rate; more than 80 percent have survived beyond a year from diagnosis. Black IV drug abusers have lower survival rates. Historically, they have been outside the medical establishment and may seek treatment later in the disease, but nutrition may also play a role in length of survival. A yet unpublished set of data from the University of Medicine and Dentistry of New Jersey demonstrates clearly the overall impact of good nutrition on the functioning of the immune system and survival with AIDS (Symposium on AIDS, University of Medicine and Dentistry, New Jersey, December 4, 1987).

Management. The main role of the primary care practitioner in the management of AIDS is screening and teaching and counseling regarding risk factors, indications for being tested, and preventive measures (''safer'' sex practices). Of course, the primary care provider should always be available for emotional support to any patient testing positive for and/or manifesting clinical signs and symptoms of AIDS.

DATA COLLECTION

History. Significant historic data in women include a known history of exposure or any of the risk factors outlined earlier. Sexual practices such as anal intercourse may increase risk. It is important to know whether a woman is planning a pregnancy so that AIDS testing can be offered before pregnancy is attempted.

Physical Examination. There are no definitive physical signs associated with AIDS. A complete physical examination including evaluation of the oral cavity, the chest, and the lymph nodes is appropriate for all patients.

Laboratory Testing. Currently available laboratory tests for AIDS are based on the presence of antibody to HIV and therefore provide indirect evidence of infection. It is not known how many persons infected with HIV will eventually develop AIDS but all such persons should be considered infective.

Currently, two laboratory tests are used for diagnosis of HIV infection: an enzyme immunoassay (EIA) screening test and a Western blot (WB) or immunofluorescence assay. Tests are considered positive for AIDS only when the EIA test is repeatedly reactive and the WB test validates the results. The sensitivity and specificity of these tests together are high; this is discussed further in Chapter 4. False-negative rates may be a result of recent exposure or the presence of such overwhelming infection that antibody is unavailable. When a negative result is obtained in a person with recent exposure or at high risk, the test should be repeated in 6 months (Centers for Disease Control, 1988).

Additional diseases to test for in a person suspected of having AIDS include tuberculosis, mononucleosis, Epstein–Barr virus, cytomegalovirus, hepatitis, and secondary syphilis (Centers for Disease Control, 1983b). Of course, these tests should be carried out by a practitioner experienced in diagnosing and treating AIDS. Referral is mandatory.

INTERVENTION

Consultation and Referral. Anyone with a known diagnosis of AIDS or HIV infection based on laboratory findings or the existence of clinical syndromes consistent with the disease (Table 12–6) or with symptoms suggestive of the disorder, particularly in the presence of identified risk factors, deserves referral. Referral should be to a medical practitioner or facility with expertise in the care of persons with AIDS. Referral for psychological care may also be warranted; this can include both individual therapy and/or an AIDS support group. Additional referrals may include counseling for death and dying, suicide prevention, financial assistance (both medical and general), food stamps, and legal advocacy. Referral to a substance abuse program should be offered to all AIDS patients who are drug users.

Treatment. No cure is currently available for this disease. For now, the presenting diseases are vigorously managed with treatment specific to the disease. Along with supportive treatment of opportunistic infections, emotional support is an integral part of an AIDS patient's care. The vast majority of AIDS patients are facing its mortality statistics at a young age. At the same time they must deal with the consequences of a disease that carries a tremendous social stigma (Salisbury, 1986) and catastrophic costs for individuals and families.

A number of experimental drugs are under investigation as treatment for AIDS, most notably AZT (Retrovir), which appears to retard progress of the disease. Ways of enhancing the immune system are also being studied (Mariman, 1986). Such therapies may someday be more readily available and widely used in AIDS treatment. As of this writing, an effective vaccine has not been developed.

Alternative treatments should be made available to AIDS sufferers as well. These include visualization, chiropractic, and holistic remedies. Of utmost importance is some type of group involvement with other people with AIDS. This kind of support has been cited by AIDS patients as of key emotional value to them in their illness. Within the gay community, a buddy system has been established in which healthy individuals help with tasks of daily living and provide emotional support for people with AIDS.

Self-Help. The keys to preventing further spread of AIDS are education and the implementation of preventive measures. It is the clear responsibility of all health care providers to discuss risk behaviors with *all* recipients of care regardless of their current sexual practices. Safer sex practices include limiting the number of sex partners, particularly casual partners whose histories are unknown, avoiding anal sex, and using condoms for both oral and genital relations (and anal sex if it is still practiced). Spermicides may also provide some protection and spermicidally lubricated condoms may provide increased protection. Some authorities suggest that latex condoms provide more protection than natural skin condoms although this is not agreed upon (Feldblum & Fortney, 1988). Sexual practices that increase the likelihood of mucous membrane abrasions should be avoided.

Additional Teaching and Counseling. Careful and sensitive counseling must be provided persons deciding whether to be tested for AIDS. Although the test has potential value in aiding preventive efforts, AIDS differs from most diseases for which screening is widely advocated because no treatment can be offered to those testing positive. A positive test may carry a social stigma even to the extent of economic consequences. There is currently no way of knowing whether a person who tests positive will go on to develop AIDS or how long it will be before disease symptoms are apparent; however, there are support groups available and ways, through nutrition and healthful living, of possibly boosting the immune system in the presence of HIV infection. Persons being tested need to understand all these factors before a final decision is made. Ultimately, the decision belongs to each individual, although it is the responsibility of the practitioner to see that the decision is based on complete information, including the potential emotional, social, and financial consequences of a positive test. The practice of safer sex should be encouraged regardless of a person's current risk factors, whether she chooses to be tested or not, and, indeed, regardless of the results of the test. All persons should be provided with CDC's AIDS hotline number: 1–800–342–AIDS. Many state and local departments of health provide AIDS information and testing. Practitioners should become familiar with resources in their individual states.

Intravenous drug users should be counseled to avoid sharing of needles and other drug paraphernalia. Some state or local departments of health have initiated needle exchange programs. Referrals to such programs should be made as appropriate.

Women in risk categories who are in the first trimester of pregnancy or are considering pregnancy are encouraged to be tested because of the potential transmission of infection to the fetus. Indeed, some groups and authorities recommend suggesting testing for all pregnant women. The option of abortion or postponement of pregnancy should be raised for women testing positive (Symposium, 1986). Even in these circumstances, however, the decision belongs to the individual. It is imperative that these suggestions not become a source of discrimination against women and that their rights to full disclosure, complete confidentiality, and unbiased health care are strictly maintained.

People with AIDS may be able to affect their length of survival and quality of life. They can be encouraged to make life-style changes that make them as healthy as possible: good nutrition, enough sleep, proper hygiene, and avoidance of drugs and alcohol may all improve the quality and length of their lives.

As care providers it is very difficult to keep up with the constantly changing picture of AIDS. *AIDS Alert* is one helpful resource. Information regarding subscription is available from American Health Consultants, Department 4543, 67 Peachtree Park Drive, Atlanta, GA 30309.

ENTERIC INFECTIONS

Enteric infections may be transmitted sexually although the organisms are usually thought of as food- or waterborne. These include the bacterial pathogens *Shigella*, *Campylobacter*, and *Salmonella* and the protozoa *Giardia lamblia* and *Entamoeba histolytica*. These are discussed very briefly; the practitioner should be aware of the broad range of STDs, but as these organisms are almost exclusively sexually transmitted in the male homosexual, the diseases they cause are not a focus of well-woman practice.

Transmission. Sexual transmission of enteric pathogens generally occurs through oral–anal or genital–anal contact (Quinn & Holmes, 1984).

Epidemiology. Enteric infections with these organisms are seen in increasing numbers in homosexual men.

Clinical Presentation. Enteric clinical syndromes produced by sexual contact include proctitis, proctocolitis, and enteritis. Symptoms depend on the organism and include diarrhea, fever, nausea, cramps, or abdominal pain. Stool may contain mucus or blood. The reader is referred to Quinn

and Holmes (1984) or to more specific medical textbooks for a delineation of symptoms associated with specific pathogens.

Management

DATA COLLECTION

History. History should include a discussion of sexual practices, exposures, symptoms in sexual partners, and details of experienced symptoms.

Physical Examination. Physical examination includes inspection of the anus, digital rectal examination, and anoscopy to look for friability, exudate, polyps, ulcerations, or fissures. Sigmoidoscopy may be necessary. Obviously, referral to an internist, gastroenterologist, or infectious disease specialist is required.

Laboratory Testing. Diagnosis of an enteric pathogen is confirmed by Gram stain of rectal exudates or stool, culture of the stool, and darkfield microscopy of suspicious lesions. Tests for gonorrhea, syphilis, herpesvirus, and *Chlamydia trachomatis* should be carried out.

INTERVENTION

Treatment. Treatment consists of appropriate antimicrobial medications and is beyond the scope of this chapter.

Teaching and Counseling. Anal intercourse carries the risk for a number of diseases and is considered a risky sexual practice. If individuals continue to participate in anal intercourse, condoms should be strongly encouraged.

ECTOPARASITES

Pediculosis

Etiology and Transmission. Three species of lice infest humans: *Phthirus pubis*, the crab louse; *Pediculus humanus humanus*, the body louse; and *Pediculus humanus capitis*, the head louse. Of these, *P. pubis* is sexually transmitted and is the focus of this section. Like all lice, the crab louse goes through five life-cycle stages: the egg or nit, three nymphal stages, and the adult stage. The female louse lays approximately four eggs per day, which hatch 5 to 10 days after incubation in the host's body. After hatching, the louse requires frequent meals of blood to stay alive. Off the host, therefore, pubic lice survive only up to 24 hours. Because of the short life span off the host, they are rarely transmitted through routes other than sexual contact, although transmission can occur via toilet seats, beds, loose hairs dropped by infected persons, or shared objects. Head and body lice are more often transmitted by sharing personal articles such as combs, towels, hairbrushes, and clothing.

Epidemiology. Based on sales figures of pediculocides, an estimated three million cases of pediculosis occur annually in the United States (Billstein, 1984). Most are due to head and pubic lice. Epidemics occur under conditions of unsanitary crowding such as famine, disaster, and war and are therefore rare in this country today. Single persons aged 15 to 25 are most likely to be infected. Pubic lice is rare in persons over age 35 (Billstein, 1984).

Clinical Presentation. Pubic lice can be found in the pubic area and on eyelashes, eyebrows, beards, and in the axillae.

Pruritus is the main presenting symptom of pubic lice. At first, there may be no symptoms or only a slight sting, itching, or redness. After about 5 days, allergic sensitization occurs and erythema, irritation, and inflammation are seen secondary to scratching. Fever, malaise, and irritability may be experienced with large infestations. Over time, either insensitivity to the louse bites occurs or superinfection may develop secondary to extensive scratching.

P. pubis is 2 to 3 cm long, sedentary, translucent, and difficult to see unless it has recently ingested blood. It is difficult to dislodge as its grasp on the hair is tight. Nits appear as white flakes. Patients may present without symptoms but have seen the nits or lice or have a sex partner who has seen them.

Differential Diagnosis. Lice must be differentiated from other forms of vulvovaginitis and vulvar dystrophies (see Chapter 11). Nits may be mistaken for seborrheic dermatitis, hair sprays, and hair casts.

Complications and Sequelae. There is some evidence that crab lice harbor organisms associated with endemic typhus and trench fever and may play a role in transmission of these diseases (Crissey, 1984). Superinfection may occur over time.

Management

DATA COLLECTION

History. Sexual history of known exposure is important. Patients may report seeing insects on the vulva or a partner may have noticed them.

Physical Examination. Good light and a magnifying glass help in visualization of the lice, although both shiny nits and lice can be seen with the naked eye. The nits may be seen more easily.

Laboratory Testing. Plucking a hair or removing the crust of a bite for microscopic examination usually reveals a nit or organism, possibly just as the specimen is placed on a slide, even before looking under the microscope. Testing for other STDs is appropriate.

INTERVENTION

Treatment. Several prescription and nonprescription drugs are effective against pubic lice. RID and Triple X are available in liquid and shampoo form; containing pyretrins and piperonyl butoxide, these are usually effective after one application. RID comes with a fine-tooth comb, helpful in combing out the nits after treatment. A-200 Pyrinate shampoo contains lesser concentrations of the same medications and requires two applications, 7 days apart, to kill all the nits.

Kwell and Scabene (Lindane) consist of 1 percent γ-benzene hexachloride. Kwell is available as lotion, shampoo, or cream; Scabene as a lotion. These must be applied for 8 hours, showered off, and reapplied for two more 8-hour periods. Kwell and Scabene may be associated with absorption and have caused neurotoxicity if not washed off or if used on large areas of excoriated skin (Billstein, 1984). They should be avoided in small children and pregnant women.

Follow-up visits should be scheduled 4 to 7 days after treatment.

Self-Help Measures. Patients must be instructed to wash all clothes and linen in hot water or have them dry cleaned. Nonwashable items can be disinfected with commercially available disinfectants such as R&D spray, Black Flag, and Raid. Items such as quilts and blankets can be stored for 2 weeks; this will kill all lice and nits.

Additional Teaching and Counseling. Patients must be advised that sexual and household contacts should be examined and treated as necessary. Treatment regimens must be carefully explained and the patient's understanding assessed, as the medications are applied by the patient at home.

Scabies

Etiology and Transmission. Scabies is caused by *Sarcoptes scabiei*, identified in the seventeenth century. The male of the tiny mite measures 0.2 × 0.15 mm, and the female, which is responsible for the clinical manifestations of the disease, measures 0.4 × 0.3 mm. The parasite burrows into the epidermis where the female lays 10 to 25 eggs. The eggs develop into adults in 10 days. Transmission occurs by close personal contact, including sexual contact, particularly when partners spend a night together (Orkin & Maibach, 1984). In primary infection, symptoms do not appear for several weeks.

Epidemiology. Scabies is seen in all segments of the population, most commonly in male homosexuals and less commonly in blacks than whites (Alexander, 1978; Orkin & Maibach, 1984). The disease decreased during the 1950s, revived in the 1960s, and increased by 1980, although it has decreased slightly since then. Reasons for the increase include increased sexual promiscuity, greater opportunity to travel, and failure of medical practitioners to recognize a disease that had been uncommon (Crissey, 1984).

Clinical Presentation. Itching is the main symptom of scabies. It increases at night. Lesions appear as tiny papules, often excoriated with a bloody crust. The *burrow* is a pathognomonic sign, but not always present, or obscured by secondary infection. It is a thin, grayish or dirty, straight, wavy, or zig-zag line about 2 to 14 mm long, most commonly seen on the finger webs, wrists, elbows, and penis. Body parts most often affected by scabies include the hands, mainly on the finger webs and sides of the digits, the flexor surface of the wrists, the extensor surface of the elbows, and the anterior axillary folds. The abdomen, lower buttocks, and female breasts may be involved. The head, back, face, soles, and palms are rarely involved. An alternate form of scabies causes nodules to form as a hypersensitivity reaction (Orkin & Maibach, 1984). Frequent bathing may remove many mites, and, when lesions are not obvious, the diagnosis may be difficult to make.

Differential Diagnosis. Scabies must be differentiated from other dermatologic disorders, such as contact dermatitis, urticaria, pruritic dermatoses of pregnancy, insect bites, and secondary syphilis. Because secondary skin infections are common with scabies, the parasites must be considered as a primary cause in the presence of disorders such as impetigo and furuncles (Crissey, 1984).

Complications and Sequelae. Secondary bacterial infections may complicate scabies. Infection with strains of streptococci with nephrotoxic potential can result in glomerulonephritis (Orkin & Maibach, 1984). This occurs mostly, but not exclusively, in tropical areas.

Management

DATA COLLECTION

History. A history of nocturnal itching, particularly on the hands, wrists, elbows, axillary folds, buttocks, breasts, abdomen, and genitals is highly suggestive of scabies. The practitioner should ask about known exposure or similar symptoms in sexual partners or household members.

Physical Examination. The classical burrow and lesions should be looked for in the appropriate places. Although the female mite is large enough to be visualized without aids, because of its burrowing habits, it is rarely observed.

Laboratory Testing. Several laboratory tests can be utilized to identify scabies. Specimens for microscopic examination can be obtained from skin scrapings, needle extraction of the mite, curettage of burrows, epidermal shave biopsy, or punch biopsy. The lesion can be swabbed with clear cellophane tape which is transferred to a slide. The burrow ink test involves rubbing the papule with ink from a fountain pen to demonstrate the burrow; it is painless, but may show false-negative results. Topical tetracycline can be applied to the lesion and wiped off, and the lesion then examined with a Woods light. Obviously, these tests should be performed by a practitioner with experience in the area, usually a dermatologist.

INTERVENTION

Consultation and Referral. Referral to a dermatologist is appropriate for diagnosis and treatment when scabies is suspected.

Treatment. Lindane, crotamiton, and sulfur are all effective against scabies; their relative efficacy has not been tested. Sulfur in petrolatum is messier and more odorous than the other treatments. Sulfur ointment is applied for three consecutive nights, and can be repeated weekly without side effects. Lindane, available in cream or lotion form, is left on 8 to 12 hours and then washed off. This may be absorbed and cause central nervous system toxicity if misused. Repeat applications should only be done if the initial treatment fails. Crotamiton cream is massaged into the skin for two consecutive nights. It is washed off 24 hours after the second application.

An antipruritic medication such as antihistamine or salicylate may be used with the initial treatment, and a hydrocortisone preparation may be prescribed for pruritus that persists after treatment. Sometimes, antibacterial agents are used for secondary infection.

Self-Help Measures. Clothing and linen must be washed in hot water or dry cleaned. Storage of blankets and quilts for 1 to 2 weeks should kill all mites.

Additional Teaching and Counseling. Patients should be informed that itching may persist after treatment. Sexual partners and household members should be examined and treated as necessary. Sexual or close contact must be avoided until all infected persons are treated.

REFERENCES

Alexander, A. M. (1978, April). Role of race in scabies infestation [Letter]. *Archives of Dermatology, 114*(4), 627.

Allen, J. R., & Curran, J. W. (1988, April). Prevention of AIDS and HIV infections: Needs and priorities for epidemiologic research. *American Journal of Public Health, 78*(4), 381–386.

Aral, S. O., & Holmes, K. K. (1984). Epidemiology of sexual transmitted diseases. In K. K. Holmes, P.-A. Mårdh, P. F. Sparling, & P. J. Wiesner (Eds.), *Sexually transmitted diseases.* New York: McGraw-Hill.

Arya, O. P., Taber, S. R., & Nsanze, H. (1980, December 1). Gonorrhea and female infertility in rural Uganda. *American Journal of Obstetrics and Gynecology, 138*(7, Part 2), 929–931.

Asculai, S. S., Weis, M. T., Rancourt, M. W., & Kupferberg, A. B. (1978, April). Inactivation of herpes simplex viruses by nonionic surfactants. *Antimicrobial Agents and Chemotherapy, 13*(4), 686–690.

Baggish, M. S. (1985, November 1). Improved laser techniques for the elimination of genital and extragenital warts. *American Journal of Obstetrics and Gynecology, 153*(5), 545–550.

Barr, J., & Danielsson, D. (1971, February 27). Septic gonococcal dermatitis. *British Medical Journal, 1* (5747), 482–485.

Barrett, T. J., Silbar, J. D., & McGinley, J. P. (1954, January 23). Genital warts—A venereal disease. *Journal of the American Medical Association, 154*(4), 333–334.

Barton, I. G., Kinghorn, G. R., Walker, M. J., et al. (1981, November 14). Association of HSV-1 with cervical infection [Letter]. *Lancet, 2* (8255), 1108.

Becker, T. M., Blount, J. H., Douglas, J., & Judson, F. N. (1986, April-June). Trends in molluscum contagiosum in the United States, 1966–1983. *Sexually Transmitted Diseases, 13*(2), 88–92.

Becker, T. M., Stone, K. M., & Alexander, E. R. (1987, June). Genital human papillomavirus infection: A growing concern. *Obstetrics and Gynecology Clinics of North America, 14*(2), 389–396.

Bekassy, Z., & Weström, L. (1987, October-December). Infrared coagulation in the treatment of condyloma accuminata in the female genital tract. *Sexually Transmitted Diseases, 14*(4), 209–212.

Bergeron, C., Ferenczy, A., Shah, K. V., & Naghashfar, Z. (1987, May). Multicentric human papillomavirus infections of the female genital tract: Correlation of viral types with abnormal mitotic figures, colposcopic presentation, and location. *Obstetrics and Gynecology, 69*(5), 736–742.

Berry, W. R., Gottesfeld, R. L., Alter, H. J., & Vierling, J. M. (1987, February 28). Transmission of hepatitis B virus by artificial insemination. *Journal of the American Medical Association, 257*(8), 1079–1081.

Bhagwandeen, B. S., & Naik, K. S. (1977, November). Granuloma venereum (granuloma inguinale) in Zambia. *East African Medical Journal, 54*(11), 637–642.

Billstein, S. (1984). Human lice. In K. K. Holmes, P.-A. Mårdh, P. F. Sparling, & P. J. Wiesner (Eds.), *Sexually transmitted diseases.* New York: McGraw-Hill.

Black, J. R., & Cohen, M. S. (1984, April-June). Gonococcal osteomyelitis: A case report and review of the literature. *Sexually Transmitted Diseases, 11*(2), 96–99.

Boggs, J. D., Melnick, J. L., Conrad, M. E., & Felsher, B. F. (1970, November 9). Viral hepatitis: Clinical and tissue culture studies. *Journal of the American Medical Association, 214*(6), 1041–1046.

Bolton, G. C. (1983). Venereal disease in adolescents. In A. M. Bongiovanni (Ed.), *Adolescent gynecology: A guide for clinicians.* New York: Plenum.

Bornstein, J., Kaufman, R. H., Adam, E., & Adler-Storthz, K. (1987, July). Human papillomavirus associated with vaginal intraepithelial neoplasia in women exposed to diethylstilbestrol in utero. *Obstetrics and Gynecology, 70*(1), 75–80.

The Boston Women's Health Book Collective. (1984). *The new our bodies, ourselves.* New York: Simon & Schuster.

Bourcier, K. M., & Seidler, A. J. (1987, January/February). Chlamydia and condylomata acuminata: An update for the nurse practitioner. *Journal of Obstetric, Gynecologic, and Neonatal Nursing, 16*(1), 17–22.

Bowie, W. R., Borrie-Hume, C. J., & Manzon, L. M. et al. (1981, June 1). Prevalence of *Chlamydia trachomatis* and *Neisseria gonor-*

rhoeae in two different populations of women. *Canadian Medical Association Journal, 124*(1), 1477–1479.

Bowie, W. R., & Willetts, V. (1987, April–June). Suboptimal efficacy of erythromycin and tetracycline against vaginal *Ureaplasma urealyticum. Sexually Transmitted Diseases, 14*(2), 88–91.

Breschi, L. C., Goldman, G., & Shapiro, S. R. (1975, March). Granuloma inguinale in Vietnam: Successful therapy with ampicillin and lincomycin. *Journal of the American Venereal Disease Association, 1*(3), 118–120.

Brogadir, S. P., Schimmer, B. M., & Myers, A. R. (1979, February). Spectrum of the gonococcal arthritis–dermatitis syndrome. *Seminars in Arthritis and Rheumatism, 8*(3), 177–183.

Brooks, G. F., Israel, K. S., & Petersen, B. H. (1976, November). Bactericidal and opsonic activity against *Neisseria gonorrhoeae* in sera from patients with disseminated gonococcal infection. *Journal of Infectious Diseases, 134*(5), 450–460.

Brown, S. T. (1984). Molluscum contagiosum. In K. K. Holmes, P.-A. Mårdh, P. F. Sparling, & P. J. Wiesner (Eds.), *Sexually transmitted diseases.* New York: McGraw-Hill.

Brown, S. T., Jaffe, H. W., & Zaidi, A., et al. (1979, January–March). Sensitivity and specificity of diagnostic tests for genital infection with herpesvirus hominis. *Sexually Transmitted Diseases, 6*(1), 10–13.

Brown, S. T., Nalley, J. F., & Kraus, S. J. (1981, July–September). Molluscum contagiosum. *Sexually Transmitted Diseases, 8*(3), 227–234.

Brown, Z. A., Vontver, L. A., & Benedetti, J., et al. (1985, September 1). Genital herpes in pregnancy: Risk factors associated with recurrences and asymptomatic viral shedding. *American Journal of Obstetrics and Gynecology, 153*(1), 24–30.

Brunham, R. C., Holmes, K. K., & Eschenbach, D. (1984). Sexually transmitted diseases in pregnancy. In K. K. Holmes, P.-A. Mårdh, P. F. Sparling, & P. J. Wiesner (Eds.), *Sexually transmitted diseases.* New York: McGraw-Hill.

Brunham, R., Irwin, B., Stamm, W. E., & Holmes, K. K. (1981, February). Epidemiological and clinical correlates of *Chlamydia trachomatis* (CT) and *Neisseria gonorrhoeae* (GC) infection among women attending a clinic for sexually transmitted disease (STD). *Clinical Research, 29*(1), 47A.

Brunham, R. C., Paavonen, J., & Stevens, C. E., et al. (1984, July 5). Mucopurulent cervicitis—The ignored counterpart in women of urethritis in men. *New England Journal of Medicine, 311*(1), 1–6.

Bulkley, B. H. (1984). Cardiovascular syphilis. In K. K. Holmes, P.-A., Mårdh, P. F. Sparling, & P. J. Wiesner (Eds.), *Sexually transmitted diseases.* New York: McGraw-Hill.

Campion, M. J. (1987, June). Clinical manifestations and natural history of genital human papillomavirus infection. *Obstetrics and Gynecology Clinics of North America, 14*(2), 363–388.

Caplan, L. R., Kleeman, F. J., & Berg, S. (1977, October 27). Urinary retention probably secondary to herpes genitalis. *New England Journal of Medicine, 297*(17), 920–921.

Cardillo, M. R. (1985). Association of human papilloma virus and *Chlamydia trachomatis* infections with incidence cervical neoplasia. *European Journal of Gynaecologic Oncology, 6*(3), 218–221.

Cassell, G. H., Waites, K. B., Gibbs, R. S., & Davis, J. K. (1986, November/December). Role of *Ureaplasma urealyticum* in amnionitis. *Pediatric Infectious Disease, 5*(6, Suppl.), S247–S252.

Cates, W., & Wiesner, P. J. (1984). National strategies for control of sexually transmitted diseases: A U.S. perspective. In K. K. Holmes, P.-A. Mårdh, P. F. Sparling, & P. J. Wiesner (Eds.), *Sexually transmitted diseases.* New York: McGraw-Hill.

Centers for Disease Control (CDC). (1983a, June 17). Condyloma acuminatum—United States, 1966–1981. *Morbidity and Mortality Weekly Report, 32*(23), 306–308.

Centers for Disease Control (CDC). (1983b, May 13). Human T-cell leukemia virus infection in patients with acquired immunodeficiency syndrome: Preliminary observations. *Morbidity and Mortality Weekly Report, 32*(18), 233–234.

Centers for Disease Control (CDC). (1983c, March 18). The safety of hepatitis B virus vaccine. *Morbidity and Mortality Weekly Report, 32*(10), 134–136.

Centers for Disease Control (CDC). (1984, December 14). Hepatitis B. vaccine: Evidence confirming lack of AIDS transmission. *Morbidity and Mortality Weekly Report, 33*(56), 73–74.

Centers for Disease Control (CDC). (1985a, August 23). *Chlamydia trachomatis* infections. *Morbidity and Mortality Weekly Report, 34*(3, Suppl.), 53S–74S.

Centers for Disease Control (CDC). (1985b, October 18). 1985 STD treatment guidelines. *Morbidity and Mortality Weekly Report, 34*(4, Suppl.), 75S–108S.

Centers for Disease Control (1986, June 20). Genital herpes infection—United States, 1966–1984. *Morbidity and Mortality Weekly Report, 35*(24), 402–404.

Centers for Disease Control (1987a, September 11). Antibiotic-resistant strains of *Neisseria gonorrhoeae. Morbidity and Mortality Weekly Report, 36*(5, Suppl.), 1S–18S.

Centers for Disease Control. (1987b, December 18). Human immunodeficiency virus infection in the United States: A review of current knowledge. *Morbidity and Mortality Weekly Report, 36*(6, Suppl.), 1–48.

Centers for Disease Control. (1987c, July 13). Increases in primary and secondary syphilis—United States. *Morbidity and Mortality Weekly Report, 36*(25), 393–397.

Centers for Disease Control. (1987d, August 14). Public Health Service guidelines for counseling and antibody testing to prevent HIV infection and AIDS. *Morbidity and Mortality Weekly Report, 36*(31), 509–515.

Centers for Disease Control. (1987e, August 14). Revision of the CDC surveillance case definition for acquired immunodeficiency syndrome. *Morbidity and Mortality Weekly Report, 36*(1, Suppl.), 1S–15S.

Centers for Disease Control. (1987f, May 22). Update: Human immunodeficiency virus infections in health-care workers exposed to blood of infected patients. *Morbidity and Mortality Weekly Report, 36*(19), 285–289.

Centers for Disease Control. (1987g, June 19). Update on hepatitis B prevention. *Morbidity and Mortality Weekly Report, 36*(23), 353–366.

Centers for Disease Control. (1988, January 8). Update: Serologic testing for antibody to human immunodeficiency virus. *Morbidity and Mortality Weekly Report, 36*(52), 833–840.

Chacko, M. R., & Lovchik, J. C. (1984, June). *Chlamydia trachomatis* infection in sexually active adolescents: Prevalence and risk factors. *Pediatrics, 7*(6), 836–840.

Chandler, J. W., Alexander, E. R., Pheiffer, T. A., et al. (1977, March–April). Ophthalmia neonatorum associated with maternal chlamydial infections. *Transactions of the American Academy of Ophthalmology and Otolaryngology, 83*(2), 302–308.

Chandler, S. H., Holmes, K. K., & Wentworth, B. B., et al. (1985, September). The epidemiology of cytomegaloviral infection in women attending a sexually transmitted disease clinic. *Journal of Infectious Diseases, 152*(3), 597–605.

Chuang, T.-Y., Perry, H. O., Kurland, L. T., & Ilstrup, D. M. (1984, April). Condyloma acuminatum in Rochester, Minn, 1950–1978. *Archives of Dermatology, 120*(4), 469–475.

Cobbold, R. J. C., & MacDonald, A. (1970, March). Molluscum contagiosum as a sexually transmitted disease. *The Practitioner, 204*(1221), 416–419.

Conant, M., Hardy, D., & Sernatinger, J., et al. (1986, April 4). Condoms prevent transmission of AIDS-associated retrovirus [Letter]. *Journal of the American Medical Association, 255*(13), 1706.

Conant, M. A., Spicer, D. W., & Smith, C. D. (1984, April–June). Herpes simplex virus transmission: Condom studies. *Sexually Transmitted Diseases, 11*(2), 94–95.

Corey, L. (1984). Genital herpes. In K. K. Holmes, P.-A. Mårdh, P. F. Sparling, & P. J. Wiesner, (Eds.), *Sexually transmitted diseases.* New York: McGraw-Hill.

Corey, L., Mindel, A., & Fife, K. H., et al. (1985, October–December). Risk of recurrence after treatment of first-episode genital herpes with intravenous acyclovir. *Sexually Transmitted Diseases, 12*(4), 215–218.

Corey, L., & Spear, P. G. (1986a, March 13). Infections with herpes simplex viruses (first of two parts). *New England Journal of Medicine, 314*(11), 686–691.

Corey, L., & Spear, P. G. (1986b, March 20). Infections with herpes simplex viruses (second of two parts). *New England Journal of Medicine, 314*(12), 749–757.

Coutts, W. E. (1950). Lymphogranuloma venereum: A general review. *Bulletin of the World Health Organization, 2*(4), 545–562.

Craig, C. P., & Nahmias, A. J. (1973, April). Different patterns of neurologic involvement with herpes simplex virus types 1 and 2: Isolation of herpes simplex virus type 2 from the buffy coat of two adults with meningitis. *Journal of Infectious Diseases, 127*(4), 365–372.

Crissey, J. T. (1984). Scabies and pediculosis pubis. *Urologic Clinics of North America, 11*(1), 171–176.

Curran, J. W. (1984). Prevention of sexually transmitted diseases. In K. K. Holmes, P.-A. Mårdh, P. F. Sparling, & P. J. Wiesner (Eds.), *Sexually transmitted diseases.* New York: McGraw–Hill.

Curran, J. W., Rendtorff, R. C., Chandler, R. W., et al. (1975, February). Female gonorrhea: Its relation to abnormal uterine bleeding, urinary tract symptoms, and cervicitis. *Obstetrics and Gynecology, 45*(2), 195–198.

Dalaker, K., Gjonnaess, H., & Kvile, G., et al. (1981, February). *Chlamydia trachomatis* as a cause of acute perihepatitis associated with pelvic inflammatory disease. *British Journal of Venereal Diseases, 57*(1), 41–43.

Daling, J. R., Sherman, K. J., & Weiss, N. S. (1986, January-March). Risk factors for condyloma acuminatum in women. *Sexually Transmitted Diseases, 13*(1), 16–18.

Dallabetta, G., & Hook, E. W., III, (1987, March). Gonococcal infections. *Infectious Disease Clinics of North America, 1*(1), 25–54.

D'Angelo, L. T., Mohla, C., Sneed, J., & Woodward, K. (1987, July). Diagnosing gonorrhea; A comparison of standard and rapid techniques. *Journal of Adolescent Health Care, 8*(4), 344–347.

Dattani, I. M., Gerken, A., & Evans, B. A. (1982, February). Aetiology and management of non-specific vaginitis. *British Journal of Venereal Diseases, 58*(1), 32–35.

D'Costa, L. J., Bowmer, I., & Nsanze, H., et al. (1986, July-September). Advances in the diagnosis and management of chancroid. *Sexually Transmitted Diseases, 13*(3, Suppl.), 189–191.

Dienstag, J. L., Alaama, A., & Mosley, J. W., et al. (1977, July). Etiology of sporadic hepatitis B surface antigen-negative hepatitis. *Annals of Internal Medicine, 87*(1), 1–6.

Dorman, S. A., Danos, L. M., & Caron, B. L., et al. (1985, September-October). Detection of *Chlamydia trachomatis* in Papanicolaou-stained cervical smears by an indirect immunoperoxidase method. *Acta Cytologica, 29*(5), 665–669.

Dorman, S. A., Danos, L. M., & Wilson, D. J., et al. (1983, April). Detection of chlamydial cervicitis by Papanicolaou stained smears and culture. *American Journal of Clinical Pathology, 79*(4), 421–425.

Drake, M., Medley, G., & Mitchell, H. (1987, June). Cytologic detection of human papillomavirus infection. *Obstetrics and Gynecology Clinics of North America, 14*(2), 431–450.

Dretler, S. P., & Klein, L. A. (1975, February). The eradication of intraurethral condyloma acuminata with 5 per cent 5-Fluorouracil cream. *Journal of Urology, 113*(2), 195–198.

Drucker, E. (1986, March/June). AIDS and addiction in New York City. *American Journal of Drug and Alcohol Abuse, 12*(1/2), 165–181.

Eagar, R. M., Beach, R. K., Davidson, A. J., & Judson, F. N. (1985, July). Epidemiologic and clinical factors of *Chlamydia trachomatis* in black, hispanic and white female adolescents. *Western Journal of Medicine, 143*(1), 37–41.

Embil, J. A., Garner, J. B., Pereira, L. H., et al. (1985, October-December). Association of cytomegalovirus and herpes simplex virus infections of the cervix in four clinic populations. *Sexually Transmitted Diseases, 12*(4), 224–227.

Eschenbach, D. A. (1986). Pelvic infections. In D. N. Danforth & J. R. Scott (Eds.), *Obstetrics and gynecology* (5th ed.). Philadelphia: J. B. Lippincott.

Faro, S. (1985). Sexually transmitted diseases. In S. Faro (Ed.), *Diagnosis and management of female pelvic infections in primary care medicine.* Baltimore: Williams & Wilkins.

Feldblum, P. J., & Fortney, J. A. (1988, January). Condoms, spermicides, and the transmission of human immunodeficiency virus: A review. *American Journal of Public Health, 78*(1), 52–54.

Felman, Y., Snyder, R., Giordano, R., & Griffin, J. (1978, July). Gonorrhea screening. *New York State Journal of Medicine, 78*(7), 1267–1270.

Ferenczy, A. (1986, June). To contain spread of condyloma—Treat your patient's partner. *Contemporary Ob/Gyn, 27*(6), 51–70.

Ferenczy, A., Silverstein, S., & Crum, C. P. (1987, November). Importance of latency in HPV infections. *Contemporary Ob/Gyn, 30*(5), 71–84.

Fife, K. H., & Corey, L. (1984). Viral agents: Herpes simplex virus, cytomegalovirus, hepatitis A and B. In K. K. Holmes, P.-A. Mårdh, P. F. Sparling, & P. J. Wiesner (Eds.), *Sexually transmitted diseases.* New York: McGraw–Hill.

Fischl, M. A., Dickinson, G. M., Scott, G. B., et al. (1987, February 6). Evaluation of heterosexual partners, children, and household contacts of adults with AIDS. *Journal of the American Medical Association, 257*(5), 640–644.

Fisher, A. A. (1981, September). Severe systemic and local reactions to topical podophyllum resin. *Cutis, 28*(3), 233–266.

Forster, G. E., Cookey, I., & Munday, P. E., et al. (1985, April). Investigation into the value of Papanicolaou stained cervical smears for the diagnosis of chlamydial cervical infection. *Journal of Clinical Pathology, 38*(4), 399–402.

Friedland, G. H., & Klein, R. S. (1987, October 29). Transmission of the human immunodeficiency virus. *New England Journal of Medicine, 317*(18), 1125–1135.

Friedland, G. H., Saltzman, B. R., Rogers, M. F., et al. (1986, February 6). Lack of transmission of HTLV-III/LAV infection to household contacts of patients with AIDS or AIDS-related complex with oral candidiasis. *New England Journal of Medicine, 314*(6), 344–349.

Friedman, M., & Gal, D. (1987, September). Keloid scars as result of CO_2 laser for molluscum contagiosum. *Obstetrics and Gynecology, 70*(3, Part 1), 394–395.

Friedman, H. M., Pincus, T., & Gibilisco, P., et al. (1980, August). Acute monoarticular arthritis caused by herpes simplex virus and cytomegalovirus. *The American Journal of Medicine, 69*(2), 241–247.

Friedman-Kien, A. E., Eron, L. J., & Conant, M., et al. (1988, January 22/29). Natural interferon alfa for treatment of condylomata acuminata. *Journal of the American Medical Association, 259*(4), 533–538.

Frommell, G. T., Rothenberg, R., Wang, S., & McIntosh, K. (1979, July). Chlamydial infection of mothers and their infants. *The Journal of Pediatrics, 95*(1), 28–32.

Gardner, H. L. (1981). Venereal diseases. In H. L. Gardner & R. H. Kaufman (Eds.), *Benign diseases of the vulva and vagina* (2nd ed.). Boston: G. K. Hall.

Geerling, S., Nettum, J. A., Lindner, L. E., et al. (1985, September-October). Sensitivity and specificity of the Papanicolaou-stained cervical smear in the diagnosis of *Chlamydia trachomatis* infection. *Acta Cytologica, 29*(5), 671–675.

Gerberding, J. L., Bryant-LeBlanc, C. E., & Nelson, K., et al. (1987, July). Risk of transmitting the human immunodeficiency virus, cytomegalovirus, and hepatitis B virus to health care workers exposed to patients with AIDS and AIDS-related conditions. *Journal of Infectious Diseases, 156*(1), 1–8.

Goldberg, J. (1964, June). Studies on granuloma inguinale: VII. Some epidemiological considerations of the disease. *British Journal of Venereal Diseases, 40*(2), 140–145.

Goldkrand, J. W. (1982, February). Intrapartum inoculation of herpes simplex virus by fetal scalp electrode. *Obstetrics and Gynecology, 59*(2), 263–265.

Goldmeier, D., & Darougar, S. (1977, June). Isolation of *Chlamydia trachomatis* from the throat and rectum of homosexual men. *British Journal of Venereal Diseases, 53*(3), 184–185.

Gottlieb, M. S., Schroff, R., Schanker, H. M., et al. (1981, December 10). *Pneumocystis Carinii* pneumonia and mucosal candidiasis in previously healthy homosexual men. *New England Journal of Medicine, 305*(24), 1425–1431.

Graman, P. S., Trupei, M. A., & Reichman, R. C. (1987, October-December). Evaluation of cerebrospinal fluid in asymptomatic late syphilis. *Sexually Transmitted Diseases, 14*(4) 205–208.

Gravett, M. G., & Eschenbach, D. A. (1986, November-December). Possible role of *Ureaplasma urealyticum* in preterm premature rupture of the fetal membranes. *Pediatric Infectious Disease, 5*(6, Suppl.), 253–257.

Greaves, A. B., & Taggart, S. R. (1953, May). Serology, Frei reaction, and epidemiology of lymphogranuloma venereum. *American Journal of Syphilis, Gonorrhea, and Venereal Diseases, 37*(3), 273–282.

Greenberg, H., Mann, W. J., & Chumas, J., et al. (1987, November). Cervical and vaginal pathology in women with vulvar condylomata. *Journal of Reproductive Medicine, 32*(11), 801–804.

Grimes, D. A. (1986, April 4). Deaths due to sexually transmitted disease: The forgotten component of reproductive mortality. *Journal of the American Medical Association, 255*(13), 1727–1729.

Gudgel, E. (1954, August). Can molluscum contagiosum be a venereal disease? *United States Armed Forces Medical Journal, 5*(8), 1207–1208.

Guinan, M. E. (1986, April 4). Oral acylcovir for treatment and suppression of genital herpes simplex virus infection: A review. *Journal of the American Medical Association, 255*(13), 1747–1749.

Guinan, M. E., MacCalman, J., & Kern, E. R., et al. (1981, March 26). The course of untreated recurrent genital herpes simplex infection in 27 women. *New England Journal of Medicine, 304*(13), 759–763.

Guinan, M. E., Wolinsky, S. M., & Reichman, R. C. (1985). Epidemiology of genital herpes simplex virus infection. *Epidemiologic Reviews, 7*, 127–146.

Gupta, P. K., Lee, E. F., & Erozan, Y. S., et al. (1979, July-August). Cytologic investigations in *Chlamydia* infection. *Acta Cytologica, 23*(4), 315–320.

Gusberg, S. B. (1986, January). Human papilloma virus and the gynecologist [Editorial]. *Gynecologic Oncology, 23*(1), iii.

Hammerschlag, M. R., Anderka, M., & Semine, D. Z., et al. (1979, August). Prospective study of maternal and infantile infection with *Chlamydia trachomatis*. *Pediatrics, 64*(2), 142–148.

Hammond, G. W., Slutchuk, M., & Scatliff, J., et al. (1980, November-December). Epidemiologic, clinical, laboratory, and therapeutic features of an urban outbreak of chancroid in North America. *Reviews of Infectious Diseases, 2*(6), 867–879.

Hamory, B., Luger, A., & Kobberman, T. (1981, August). Herpesvirus hominis hepatitis of mother and newborn infant. *Southern Medical Journal, 74*(8), 992–995.

Handsfield, H. H. (1984). Gonorrhea and uncomplicated gonococcal infection. In K. K. Holmes, P.-A. Mårdh, P. F. Sparling, & P. J. Wiesner (Eds.), *Sexually transmitted diseases*. New York: McGraw-Hill.

Handsfield, H. H., Chandler, S. H., & Caine, V. A., et al. (1985, February). Cytomegalovirus infection in sex partners: Evidence for sexual transmission. *Journal of Infectious Diseases, 151*(2), 344–348.

Handsfield, H. H., Jasman, L. L., & Roberts, P. L., et al. (1986, April 4). Criteria for selective screening for *Chlamydia trachomatis* infection in women attending family planning clinics. *Journal of the American Medical Association, 255*(13), 1730–1734.

Hanshaw, J. B., Scheiner, A. P., Moxley, A. W., et al. (1976, August 26). School failure and deafness after "silent" congenital cytomegalovirus infection. *New England Journal of Medicine, 295*(9), 468–470.

Harger, J. H., Pazin, G. J., & Breinig, M. C. (1986, May). Current understanding of the natural history of genital herpes simplex. *Journal of Reproductive Medicine, 31*(5, Suppl.), 365–373.

Harnekar, A. B., Leiman, G., & Markowitz, S. (1985, September-October). Cytologically detected chlamydial changes and progression of cervical intraepithelial neoplasia: A retrospective case-control study. *Acta Cytologica, 29*(5), 661–664.

Harrison, H. R., Costin, M., & Meder, J. B., et al. (1985, October 1). Cervical *Chlamydia trachomatis* infection in university women: Relationship to history, contraception, ectopy, and cervicitis. *American Journal of Obstetrics and Gynecology, 153*(3), 244–251.

Hart, G. (1984). Donovanosis. In K. K. Holmes, P.-A. Mårdh, P. F. Sparling, & P. J. Wiesner (Eds.), *Sexually transmitted diseases*. New York: McGraw-Hill.

Hawley, T. G. (1970, December). The natural history of molluscum contagiosum in Fijian children. *Journal of Hygiene, 68*(4), 631–632.

Henderson, D. K., Saah, A. J., & Zak, B. J., et al. (1986, May). Risk of nosocomial infection with human T-cell lymphotropic virus type III/lymphadenopathy-associated virus in a large cohort of intensively exposed health care workers. *Annals of Internal Medicine, 104*(5), 644–647.

Hilton, A. L., Richmond, S. J., & Milne, J. D., et al. (1974, February). *Chlamydia* A in the female genital tract. *British Journal of Venereal Diseases, 50*(1), 1–10.

Holmes, K. K., Counts, G. W, & Beaty, H. N. (1971, June). Dis-

seminated gonococcal infection. *Annals of Internal Medicine, 74*(6), 979–991.

Holmes, K. K., Wiesner, P. J., & Pedersen, A. H. B. (1971, September). The gonococcal arthritis–dermatitis syndrome. *Annals of Internal Medicine, 75*(3), 470–471.

Hoofnagle, J. H. (1981). Serologic markers of hepatitis B virus infection. *Annual Review of Medicine, 32*, 1–11.

Jaffe, H. W. (1984). Management of the reactive serology. In K. K. Holmes, P.-A. Mårdh, P. F. Sparling, & P. J. Wiesner (Eds.), *Sexually transmitted diseases*. New York: McGraw-Hill.

Jick, H., Hannan, M. T., & Stergachis, A., et al. (1982, October 1). Vaginal spermicides and gonorrhea. *Journal of the American Medical Association, 248*(13), 1619–1621.

Johannisson, G., Lowhagen, G.-B., & Lycke, E. (1980, December). Genital *Chlamydia trachomatis* infection in women. *Obstetrics and Gynecology, 56*(6), 671–675.

Jones, M. F., Smith, T. F., Houglum, A. J., & Herrmann, J. E. (1984, September). Detection of *Chlamydia trachomatis* in genital specimens by the chlamydiazyme test. *Journal of Clinical Microbiology, 20*(3), 456–467.

Judson, F. N. (1984, February). Sexually transmitted viral hepatitis and enteric pathogens. *Urologic Clinics of North America, 11*(1), 177–185.

Judson, F. N. (1986, July-September). Treatment of uncomplicated gonorrhea with ceftriaxone: A review. *Sexually Transmitted Diseases, 13*(3, Suppl.), 199–202.

Judson, F. N., & Werness, B. A. (1980, August). Combining cervical and anal-canal specimens for gonorrhea on single culture plate. *Journal of Clinical Microbiology, 12*(2), 216–219.

Kampmeier, R. H. (1984). Late benign syphilis. In K. K. Holmes, P.-A. Mårdh, P. F. Sparling, & P. J. Wiesner (Eds.), *Sexually transmitted diseases*. New York: McGraw-Hill.

Kappus, E. W., & Quinn, T. C. (1986, July-September). The spermicide nonoxynol-9 does not inhibit *Chlamydia trachomatis* in vitro. *Sexually Transmitted Diseases, 13*(13), 134–137.

Kashima, H. K., & Shah, K. (1987, June). Recurrent respiratory papillomatosis: Clinical overview and management principles. *Obstetrics and Gynecology Clinics of North America, 14*(2), 581–588.

Kaufman, R. H. (1981). Viral infections. In H. L. Gardner and R. H. Kaufman (Eds.), *Benign diseases of the vulva and vagina* (2nd ed.). Boston: G. K. Hall.

Kaufman, R. H., & Faro, S. (1987). Infectious diseases of the vulva and vagina. In E. J. Wilkinson (Ed.), *Pathology of the vulva and vagina*, New York: Churchill Livingstone.

Keefer, C. S., & Spink, W. W. (1937, October 30). Gonococci arthritis: Pathogenesis, mechanism of recovery and treatment. *Journal of the American Medical Association, 109*(18), 1448–1453.

Keiser, H., Ruben, F. L., Wolinsky, E., & Kushner, I. (1968, August 1). Clinical forms of gonococcal arthritis. *New England Journal of Medicine, 279*(5), 234–240.

Kellum, M. D., & Loucks, A. L. (1982, February). Genital herpes infections: Diagnosis and management. *Nurse Practitioner, 7*(2), 14–21.

Kinghorn, G. R., & Rashid, S. (1979, December). Prevalence of rectal and pharyngeal infection in women with gonorrhea in Sheffield. *British Journal of Venereal Diseases, 55*(6), 408–410.

Kirby, P., & Corey, L. (1987, March). Genital human papillomavirus infections. *Infectious Disease Clinics of North America, 1*(1), 123–143.

Kit, S., & Kit, M. (1985, March). Herpes simplex virus vaccines—Where are we? *Clinical Obstetrics and Gynecology, 28*(1), 164–177.

Kiviat, N. B., Paavonen, J. A., & Brockway, J., et al. (1985a, February 15). Cytologic manifestations of cervical and vaginal infections. I. Epithelial and inflammatory cellular changes. *Journal of the American Medical Association, 253*(7), 989–996.

Kiviat, N. B., Peterson, M., & Kinney-Thomas, E., et al. (1985b, February 15). Cytologic manifestations of cervical and vaginal infections: II. Confirmation of *Chlamydia trachomatis* infection by direct immunofluorescence using monoclonal antibodies. *Journal of the American Medical Association, 253*(7), 997–1000.

Klastersky, J., Cappel, R., & Snoeck, J. M., et al. (1972, July 27). Ascending myelitis in association with herpes-simplex virus. *New England Journal of Medicine, 287*(4), 182–184.

Klotsky, L. A., Stamm, W. E., & Brunham, R. C., et al. (1983,

October-December). Persistence of *Mycoplasma hominis* after therapy: Importance of tetracycline resistance and of coexisting vaginal flora. *Sexually Transmitted Diseases, 11*(4, Suppl.), 374–381.

Knox, G. E. (1983, March). Cytomegalovirus: Import of sexual transmission. *Clinical Obstetrics and Gynecology, 26*(1), 173–177.

Knox, J. M., & Rudolph, A. H. (1984). Acquired infectious syphilis. In K. K. Holmes, P.-A. Mårdh, P. F. Sparling, & P. J. Wiesner (Eds.), *Sexually transmitted diseases.* New York: McGraw–Hill.

Knox, S. R., Corey, L., Blough, H. A., & Lerner, A. M. (1982, January-March). Historical findings in subjects from a high socioeconomic group who have genital infections with herpes simplex virus. *Sexually Transmitted Diseases, 9*(1), 15–20.

Koss, L. G. (1987, October 15). Cytologic and histologic manifestations of human papillomavirus infection of the female genital tract and their clinical significance. *Cancer, 60*(8, Suppl.), 1942–1950.

Krebs, H.-B. (1987a, June). The use of topical 5-Fluorouracil in the treatment of genital condylomas. *Obstetrics and Gynecology Clinics of North America, 14*(2), 559–566.

Krebs, H.-B. (1987b, July). Treatment of vaginal condylomata acuminata by weekly topical application of 5-Fluorouracil. *Obstetrics and Gynecology, 70*(1), 68–71.

Krebs, H.-B., & Schneider, V. (1987, September). Human papillomavirus-associated lesions of the penis: Colposcopy, cytology, and histology. *Obstetrics and Gynecology, 70*(3, Part 1), 299–304.

Krieger, J. N. (1984, February). Biology of sexually transmitted diseases. *Urologic Clinics of North America, 11*(1), 15–25.

Krugman, S., Overby, L. R., & Mushahwar, I. K., et al. (1979, January 10). Viral hepatitis, type B: Studies on natural history and prevention re-examined. *New England Journal of Medicine, 300*(3), 101–105.

LaCamera, D. J. (1985, March). The acquired immunodeficiency syndrome. *Nursing Clinics of North America, 20*(1), 241–252.

Lal, S. (1971, December). Continued efficacy of streptomycin in the treatment of granuloma inguinale. *British Journal of Venereal Diseases, 47*(6), 454–455.

Lang, D. J. (1984). Cytomegalovirus infections. In K. K. Holmes, P.-A. Mårdh, P. F Sparling, & P. J. Wiesner (Eds.), *Sexually transmitted diseases.* New York: McGraw–Hill.

Lao, D. G., & Trussell, R. E. (1947, May). Chancroid in women in Manila. *American Journal of Syphilis, Gonorrhea, and Venereal Diseases, 31*(3), 281.

Larsen, S. A., McGrew, B. E., Hunter, E. F., & Creighton, E. T. (1984). Syphilis serology and dark field microscopy. In K. K. Holmes, P.-A. Mårdh, P. F. Sparling, & P. J. Wiesner (Eds.), *Sexually transmitted diseases.* New York: McGraw–Hill.

Lassus, A., Bergelin, I., & Paloranta, A., et al. (1987, October-December). Efficacy of interferon and placebo in the treatment of recurrent genital herpes: A double-blind trial. *Sexually Transmitted Diseases, 14*(4), 185–190.

Latif, A. S., Mason, P. R., & Paraiwa, E. (1988, January-March). The treatment of donovanosis (granuloma inguinale). *Sexually Transmitted Diseases, 15*(1), 27–29.

Lee, T. J., Utsinger, P. D., & Snyderman, R., et al. (1978, September). Familial deficiency of the seventh component of complement associated with recurrent bacteremic infections due to *Neisseria. Journal of Infectious Diseases, 138*(3), 359–366.

Lemon, S. M. (1984). Viral hepatitis. In K. K. Holmes, P.-A. Mårdh, P. F. Sparling, & P. J. Wiesner (Eds.), *Sexually transmitted diseases.* New York: McGraw–Hill.

Lepage, P., Van de Perre, P., & Carael, M., et al. (1987, August 15). Postnatal transmission of HIV from mother to child [Letter]. *Lancet, 2*(8555), 400.

Lieberman, R. W., & Wheelock, J. B. (1987, May). The diagnosis of gonorrhea in a low-prevalence female population: Enzyme immunoassay versus culture. *Obstetrics and Gynecology, 69*(5), 743–746.

Lindner, L. E., Geerling, S., & Nettum, J. A., et al. (1985, September-October). The cytologic features of chlamydial cervicitis. *Acta Cytologica, 29*(5), 676–682.

Lossick, J. G., Smeltzer, M. P., & Curran, J. W. (1982, July-September). The value of the cervical Gram stain in the diagnosis and treatment of gonorrhea in women in a venereal disease clinic. *Sexually Transmitted Diseases, 9*(3), 124–127.

Loucks, A. (1987, July). Chlamydia: An unheralded epidemic. *American Journal of Nursing, 87*(7), 920–922.

Lynch, P. J. (1985, March). Condylomata acuminata (anogenital warts). *Clinical Obstetrics and Gynecology, 28*(1), 142–151.

Lynch, P. J., & Minkin, W. (1968, August). Molluscum contagiosum of the adult. *Archives of Dermatology, 98*(2), 141–143.

Maayan, S., Wormser, G. P., & Hewlett, D., et al. (1985, September). Acquired immunodeficiency syndrome (AIDS) in an economically disadvantaged population. *Archives of Internal Medicine, 145*(9), 1607–1612.

Mårdh, P.-A. (1984). Bacteria, chlamydiae, and mycoplasmas. In K. K. Holmes, P.-A. Mårdh, P. F. Sparling, & P. J. Wiesner (Eds.), *Sexually transmitted diseases.* New York: McGraw–Hill.

Mårdh, P.-A., Moller, B. R., & Ingerselv, H. J., et al. (1981, June). Endometritis caused by *Chlamydia trachomatis. British Journal of Venereal Diseases, 57*(3), 191–195.

Mårdh, P.-A., Ripa, T., Svensson, L., & Weström, L. (1977, June 16). *Chlamydia trachomatis* infection in patients with acute salpingitis. *New England Journal of Medicine, 296*(4), 1377–1379.

Mårdh, P.-A., & Weström, L. (1970, October). Antibodies to *Mycoplasma hominis* in patients with genital infections and in healthy controls. *British Journal of Venereal Diseases, 46*(5), 390–397.

Margolis, S. (1984, February). Genital warts and molluscum contagiosum. *Urologic Clinics of North America, 11*(1), 163–170.

Mariman, E. C. M. (1986). The AIDS combat: A survey. *Biomedicine and Pharmacotherapy, 40*(10), 399–407.

Martin, D. H., Koutsky, L., & Eschenbach, D. A., et al. (1982, March 19). Prematurity and perinatal mortality in pregnancies complicated by maternal *Chlamydia trachomatis* infections. *Journal of the American Medical Association, 247*(11), 1585–1588.

Martin, R., Coopes, S., & Neagle, P., et al. (1986, April-June). Comparison of Thayer-Martin, transgrow, and gonozyme for detection of *Neisseria gonorrhoeae* in a low-risk population. *Sexually Transmitted Diseases, 13*(2), 108–110.

Mascola, L., & Guinan, M. E. (1987, February 27). Semen donors as the source of sexually transmitted diseases in artificially inseminated women: The saga unfolds. *Journal of the American Medical Association, 257*(8), 1093–1094.

McCormack, W. M., Lee, Y.-H., & Zinner, S. H. (1973, May). Sexual experience and urethral colonization with genital mycoplasmas: A study in normal men. *Annals of Internal Medicine, 78*(5), 696–698.

McCormack, W. M., Rosner, B., & Alpert, S., et al. (1986, April-June). Vaginal colonization with *Mycoplasma hominis* and *Ureaplasma urealyticum. Sexually Transmitted Diseases, 13*(2), 67–70.

McCormack, W. M., & Taylor-Robinson, D. (1984). The genital mycoplasmas. In K. K. Holmes, P.-A. Mårdh, P. F. Sparling, & P. J. Wiesner (Eds.), *Sexually transmitted diseases.* New York: McGraw–Hill.

McCray, E. (1986, April 24). Occupational risk of the acquired immunodeficiency syndrome among health care workers. *New England Journal of Medicine, 314*(17), 1127–1132.

McGee, Z. A. (1984). Gonococcal pelvic inflammatory disease. In K. K. Holmes, P.-A. Mårdh, P. F. Sparling, & P. J. Wiesner (Eds.), *Sexually transmitted diseases.* New York: McGraw–Hill.

Meisels, A., Morin, C., & Casas-Cordero, M. (1982). Human papillomavirus infection of the uterine cervix. *International Journal of Gynecological Pathology, 1*(1), 75–94.

Mendel, E. B., Rowan, D. F., Graham, J. H. M., & Dellinger, D. (1970, January). *Mycoplasma* species in the vagina and their relation to vaginitis. *Obstetrics and Gynecology, 35*(1), 104–108.

Mertz, G., & Corey, L. (1984, February). Genital herpes simplex virus infections in adults. *Urologic Clinics of North America, 11*(1), 103–113.

Micha, J. P., & Silva, P. D. (1986, August). Condyloma acuminata and related HPV infections: Assessing their malignant potential. *The Female Patient, 11*(8), 43–58.

Miller, R. A. (1985, October). Podophyllin. *International Journal of Dermatology, 24*(8), 491–498.

Mills, J., & Brooks, G. F. (1984). Disseminated gonococcal infection. In K. K. Holmes, P.-A. Mårdh, P. F. Sparling, & P. J.

Wiesner (Eds.), *Sexually transmitted diseases*. New York: Mc-Graw–Hill.

Milman, N., Scheibel, J., & Jessen, O. (1978, October 28). Failure of lysine treatment in recurrent herpes simplex labialis [Letter]. *Lancet, 2*(8096), 942.

Milman, N., Scheibel, J., & Jessen, O. (1980). Lysine prophylaxis in recurrent herpes simplex labialis: A double-blind, controlled crossover study. *Acta Dermatovener (Stockholm), 60*(1), 85–87.

Minkoff, H. (1986, July/August). Acquired immunodeficiency syndrome. *Journal of Nurse-Midwifery, 31*(4), 189–193.

Minkoff, H., Nanda, D., Menez, R., & Fikrig, S. (1987, March). Pregnancies resulting in infants with acquired immunodeficiency syndrome or AIDS-related complex: Follow-up of mothers, children, and subsequently born siblings. *Obstetrics and Gynecology, 69*(3, Part 1), 288–291.

Mok, J. Q., Giaquinto, C., & DeRossi, A., et al. (1987, May 23). Infants born to mothers seropositive for human immunodeficiency virus: Preliminary findings from a multicentre European study. *Lancet, 1*(8543), 1164–1168.

Monif, G. R. G. (1982). *Infectious diseases in obstetrics and gynecology* (2nd ed.). Philadelphia: Harper & Row.

Moscicki, B., Shafer, M.-A., & Millstein, S. G., et al. (1987, July). The use and limitation of endocervical Gram stains and mucopurulent cervicitis as predictors for *Chlamydia trachomatis* in female adolescents. *American Journal of Obstetrics and Gynecology, 157*(1), 65–71.

Musher, D. M. (1984). Biology of *Treponema pallidum*. In K. K. Holmes, P.-A. Mårdh, P. F. Sparling, & P. J. Wiesner (Eds.), *Sexually transmitted diseases*. New York: McGraw–Hill.

Nahmias, A. J., Naib, Z. M., & Josey, W. E. (1974, May). Epidemiological studies relating genital herpetic infection to cervical carcinoma. *Cancer Research, 34*(5), 1111–1117.

Nasello, M. A., Callihan, D. R., Menegus, M. A., & Steigbigel, R. T. (1985, October-December). A solid-phase enzyme immunoassay (Gonozyme®) test for direct detection of *Neisseria gonorrhoeae* antigen in urogenital specimens from patients at a sexually transmitted disease clinic. *Sexually Transmitted Diseases, 12*(4), 198–202.

Neeson, J. D., & Stockdale, C. R. (1981). *The practitioner's handbook of ambulatory ob/gyn*. New York: Wiley.

Ngeow, Y. F., Munday, P. E., Evans, R. T., & Taylor-Robinson, D. (1981, February). Taking cell cultures to the patient in an attempt to improve chlamydial isolation. *British Journal of Venereal Diseases, 57*(1), 44–46.

Oriel, J. D. (1984). Genital warts. In K. K. Holmes, P.-A. Mårdh, P. F. Sparling, & P. J. Wiesner (Eds.), *Sexually transmitted diseases*. New York: McGraw–Hill.

Oriel, J. D., Johnson, A. L., & Barlow, D., et al. (1978, April). Infection of the uterine cervix with *Chlamydia trachomatis*. *Journal of Infectious Diseases, 137*(4), 443–451.

Oriel, J. D., Powis, P. A., & Reeve, P., et al. (1974, February). Chlamydial infections of the cervix. *British Journal of Venereal Diseases, 50*(1), 11–15.

Orkin, M., & Maibach, H. I. (1984). Scabies. In K. K. Holmes, P.-A. Mårdh, P. F. Sparling, & P. J. Wiesner (Eds.), *Sexually transmitted diseases*. New York: McGraw–Hill.

Osser, S., & Persson, K. (1982, February). Epidemiologic and serodiagnostic aspects of chlamydial salpingitis. *Obstetrics and Gynecology, 59*(2), 206–209.

Osser, S., & Persson, K. (1984, November 15). Postabortal pelvic infection associated with *Chlamydia trachomatis* and the influence of humoral immunity. *American Journal of Obstetrics and Gynecology, 150*(6), 699–703.

Paavonen, J. (1985, April). Colposcopic findings associated with human papillomavirus infection of the vagina and cervix. *Obstetrical and Gynecological Survey, 40*(4), 185–189.

Paavonen, J., Saikku, P., & Vesterinen, E., et al. (1978, August). Genital chlamydial infections in patients attending a gynaecological outpatient clinic. *British Journal of Venereal Diseases, 54*(4), 257–261.

Padian, N., Marquis, L., & Francis, D. P., et al. (1987, August 14). Male-to-female transmission of human immunodeficiency virus. *Journal of the American Medical Association, 258*(6), 788–790.

Parvey, L. S., & Ch'ien, L. T. (1980, June). Neonatal herpes simplex virus infection introduced by fetal-monitor scalp electrodes. *Pediatrics, 65*(6), 1150–1153.

Pepper, G. A. (1985, December). Oral acyclovir (Zovirax®): Major or minor miracle? *Nurse Practitioner, 10*(12), 50–51.

Perine, P. L., & Osoba, A. O. (1984). Lymphogranuloma venereum. In K. K. Holmes, P.-A. Mårdh, P. F. Sparling, & P. J. Wiesner (Eds.), *Sexually transmitted diseases*. New York: McGraw–Hill.

Persson, K., Persson, K., & Hansson, H., et al. (1979, December). Prevalence of nine different microorganisms in the female genital tract. *British Journal of Venereal Diseases, 55*(6), 429–433.

Peterman, T. A., Jaffe, H. W., & Feorino, P. M., et al. (1985, November 22/29). Transfusion-associated acquired immunodeficiency syndrome in the United States. *Journal of the American Medical Association, 254*(20), 2913–2917.

Petersen, B. H., Graham, J. A., & Brooks, G. F. (1976, February). Human deficiency of the eighth component of complement. *Journal of Clinical Investigation, 57*(2), 283–289.

Physicians' desk reference (PDR) (42nd ed.). (1988). Oradell, NJ: Medical Economics Company.

Platt, R., Lin, J.-S., Warren, J. W, et al. (1980, December 6). Infection with *Mycoplasma hominis* in postpartum fever. *Lancet, 2*(8206), 1217–1221.

Postlethwaite, R. (1970, September). Molluscum contagiosum: A review. *Archives of Environmental Health, 21*(3), 432–448.

Postlethwaite, R., Watt, J. A., & Hawley, T. G., et al. (1967, September). Features of molluscum contagiosum in the north-east of Scotland and in Fijian village settlements. *Journal of Hygiene, 65*(3), 281–291.

Powell, L. C. (1972, December). Condyloma acuminatum. *Clinical Obstetrics and Gynecology, 15*(4), 948–965.

Prober, C. G., Sullender, W. M., & Yasukawa, L. L., et al. (1987, January 29). Low risk of herpes simplex virus infections in neonates exposed to the virus at the time of vaginal delivery to mothers with recurrent genital herpes simplex virus infections. *New England Journal of Medicine, 316*(5), 240–244.

Quick, C. A., Watts, S. L., Krzyzek, R. A., & Faras, A. J. (1980, July-August). Relationship between condylomata and laryngeal papillomata: Clinical and molecular virological evidence. *Annals of Otology, Rhinology, and Laryngology, 89*(4, Part 1), 467–471.

Quinn, T. C., Gupta, P. K., & Burkman, R. T. et al. (1987, August). Detection of *Chlamydia trachomatis* cervical infection: A comparison of Papanicolaou and immunofluorescent staining with cell culture. *American Journal of Obstetrics and Gynecology, 157*(2), 394–399.

Quinn, T. C., & Holmes, K. K. (1984). Proctitis, proctocolitis, and enteritis in homosexual men. In K. K. Holmes, P.-A. Mårdh, P. F. Sparling, & P. J. Wiesner (Eds.), *Sexually transmitted diseases*. New York: McGraw–Hill.

Rakela, J., Redeker, A. G., & Edwards, V. M., et al. (1978, May). Hepatitis A virus infection in fulminant hepatitis and chronic active hepatitis. *Gastroenterology, 74*(5, Part 1), 879–882.

Ranki, A., Valle, S.-L., & Krohn, M., et al. (1987, September 12). Long latency precedes overt seroconversion in sexually transmitted human-immunodeficiency-virus infection. *Lancet, 2*(8559), 589–593.

Rapp, F. (1984). Herpes simplex viruses. In K. K. Holmes, P.-A. Mårdh, P. F. Sparling, & P. J. Wiesner (Eds.), *Sexually transmitted diseases*. New York: McGraw–Hill.

Rattray, M. C., Corey, L., & Reeves, W. C., et al. (1978, August). Recurrent genital herpes among women: Symptomatic v. asymptomatic viral shedding. *British Journal of Venereal Diseases, 54*(4), 262–265.

Redfield, R. R., Markham, P. D., & Salahuddin, S. Z., et al. (1985, October 10). Heterosexually acquired HTLV-III/LAV disease (AIDS-related complex and AIDS): Epidemiologic evidence for female-to-male transmission. *Journal of the American Medical Association, 254*(15), 2094–2096.

Reeves, W. C., Corey, L., & Adams, H. G., et al. (1981, August 6). Risk of recurrence after first episodes of genital herpes: Relation to HSV type and antibody response. *New England Journal of Medicine, 305*(6), 315–319.

Reid, R. (1985a, April 15). Superficial laser vulvectomy. I. Efficacy of extended superficial ablation for refractory and very extensive condylomas. *American Journal of Obstetrics and Gynecology, 151*(8), 1047–1052.

Reid, R. (1985b, July 1). Superficial laser vulvectomy. III. A new surgical technique for appendage-conserving ablation of refractory condylomas and vulvar intraepithelial neoplasia. *American Journal of Obstetrics and Gynecology, 152*(5), 504–509.

Reid, R. (1987, June). Physical and surgical principles governing expertise with the carbon dioxide laser. *Obstetrics and Gynecology Clinics of North America, 14*(2), 513–535.

Reid, R., Greenberg, M., & Jenson, A. B., et al. (1987, January). Sexually transmitted papillomaviral infections. I. The anatomic distribution and pathologic grade of neoplastic lesions associated with different viral types. *American Journal of Obstetrics and Gynecology, 156*(1), 212–222.

Riccardi, N. B., & Felman, Y. M. (1979, December 14). Laboratory diagnosis in the problem of suspected gonococcal infection. *Journal of the American Medical Association, 242*(24), 2703–2705.

Rice, R. J., Aral, S. O., Blount, J. H., & Zaidi, A. A. (1987, April-June). Gonorrhea in the United States 1975–1984: Is the giant only sleeping?'' *Sexually Transmitted Diseases, 14*(2), 83–87.

Richart, R. M., Becker, T. M., Ferenczy, A. M., et al. (1989, April). HPV DNA: quicker ways to discern viral types. *Contemporary Ob/Gyn 33*(4):112–114, 117–119, 123–124, 129–133.

Richmond, S. J., Paul, I. D., & Taylor, P. K. (1980, February). Value and feasibility of screening women attending STD clinics for cervical chlamydial infections. *British Journal of Venereal Diseases, 56*(1), 92–95.

Ripa, K. T., Svensson, L., Mårdh, P.-A., & Weström, L. (1978, December). *Chlamydia trachomatis* cervicitis in gynecologic outpatients. *Obstetrics and Gynecology, 52*(6), 698–702.

Robinson, H. M., & Cohen, M. M. (1953, June). Treatment of granuloma inguinale with erythromycin. *Journal of Investigative Dermatology, 20*(6), 407–409.

Romanowski, B., Harris, J. R. W., Wood, H., & Kessock-Philip, S. (1986, June). Improved diagnosis of gonorrhea in women. *Sexually Transmitted Diseases, 13*(2), 93–96.

Ronald, A. R., & Albritton, W. L. (1984). Chancroid and *Haemophilus ducreyi*. In K. K. Holmes, P.-A. Mårdh, P. F. Sparling, & P. J. Wiesner (Eds.), *Sexually transmitted diseases*. New York: McGraw-Hill.

Rosemberg, S. K. (1985, December). Subclinical papilloma viral infection of male genitalia. *Urology, 26*(6), 554–557.

Rosemberg, S. K., Greenberg, M. D., & Reid, R. (1987, June). Sexually transmitted papillomaviral infection in men. *Obstetrics and Gynecology Clinics of North America, 14*(2), 495–511.

Rosene, K., Eschenbach, D. A., & Tompkins, L. S., et al. (1986, June). Polymicrobial early postpartum endometritis with facultative and anaerobic bacteria, genital mycoplasmas, and *Chlamydia trachomatis*: Treatment with piperacillin or cefoxitin. *Journal of Infectious Diseases, 153*(6), 1028–1037.

Ross, C. A. C., & Stevenson, J. (1961, September 23). Herpes-simplex meningoencephalitis. *Lancet, 2*(7204), 682–685.

Roy, M., Meisels, A., & Fortier, M., et al. (1981, June). Vaginal condylomata: A human papillomavirus infection. *Clinical Obstetrics and Gynecology, 24*(2), 461–483.

Russo, M. E., & Thompson, M. I. B. (1984). Pharmacology of drugs used in venereology. In K. K. Holmes, P.-A. Mårdh, P. F. Sparling, & P. J. Wiesner (Eds.), *Sexually transmitted diseases*. New York: McGraw-Hill.

Salisbury, D. B. (1986, December). AIDS: Psychosocial implications. *Journal of Psychosocial Nursing, 24*(12), 13–16.

Saltz, G. R., Linnemann, C. V., Brookman, R. R., & Rauh, J. L. (1981, June). *Chlamydia trachomatis* cervical infections in female adolescents. *Journal of Pediatrics, 98*(6), 981–985.

Schachter, J. (1978, February 23). Chlamydial infections (first of three parts). *New England Journal of Medicine, 298*(8), 428–435.

Schachter, J. (1984). Biology of *Chlamydia trachomatis*. In K. K. Holmes, P.-A. Mårdh, P. F. Sparling, & P. J. Wiesner (Eds.), *Sexually transmitted diseases*. New York: McGraw-Hill.

Schachter, J., & Atwood, G. (1975, September). Chlamydial pharyngitis? *Journal of the American Venereal Disease Association, 2*(1), 12.

Schachter, J., Stoner, E., & Moncada, J. (1983, March). Screening for chlamydial infections in women attending family planning clinics. *Western Journal of Medicine, 138*(3), 375–379.

Schmale, J. D., Martin, J. E., Jr., & Domescik, G. (1969, October 13). Observations on the culture diagnosis of gonorrhea in women. *Journal of the American Medical Association, 210*(2), 312–314.

Schmid, G. P. (1986, April 4). The treatment of chancroid. *Journal of the American Medical Association, 255*(13), 1757–1762.

Schmid, G. P., Sanders, L. L., Blount, J. H., & Alexander, E. R. (1987, December 11). Chancroid in the United States: Reestablishment of an old disease. *Journal of the American Medical Association, 258*(22), 3265–3268.

Schneider, V., Behm, F. G., & Mumaw, V. R. (1982, February). Ascending herpetic endometritis. *Obstetrics and Gynecology, 59*(2), 259–262.

Schwartz, D. B., Greenberg, M. D., Daoud, Y., & Reid, R. (1987, June). The management of genital condylomas in pregnant women. *Obstetrics and Gynecology Clinics of North America, 14*(2), 589–599.

Schwarz, R. H. (1983, March). Chancroid and granuloma inguinale. *Clinical Obstetrics and Gynecology, 26*(1), 138–142.

Scott, M. J., Jr., & Scott, M. J., Sr. (1982, May). Primary cutaneous *Neisseria gonorrhoeae* infections. *Archives of Dermatology, 118*(5), 351–352.

Sedlacek, T. V., Cunnane, M., & Carpiniello, V. (1986, March). Colposcopy in the diagnosis of penile condyloma. *American Journal of Obstetrics and Gynecology, 154*(3), 494–496.

Segal, H. E., Llewellyn, C. H., & Irwin, G., et al. (1976, July). Hepatitis B antigen and antibody in the U.S. army: Prevalence in health care personnel. *American Journal of Public Health, 66*(7), 667–671.

Semchyshyn, S. (1979, January). Fitz-Hugh and Curtis syndrome. *Journal of Reproductive Medicine, 22*(1), 45–48.

Shafer, M-A., Chew, K. L., & Kromhout, L. K., et al. (1985, March 15). Chlamydial endocervical infections and cytologic findings in sexually active female adolescents. *American Journal of Obstetrics and Gynecology, 151*(6), 765–771.

Silber, T. J., & Burgess, G. R. (1985, January). Painless primary herpes. *Journal of Adolescent Health Care, 6*(1), 40–42.

Silva, P. D., Micha, J. P., & Silva, D. G. (1985, September). Management of condyloma acuminatum. *Journal of the American Academy of Dermatology, 13*(3), 457–463.

Singh, B., Cutler, J. C., & Utidjian, H. M. D. (1972, February). Studies on the development of a vaginal preparation providing both prophylaxis against venereal disease and other genital infections and contraception. II. Effect *in vitro* of vaginal contraceptive and non-contraceptive preparations on *Treponema pallidum* and *Neisseria gonorrhoeae*. *British Journal of Venereal Diseases, 48*(1), 57–64.

Singh, B., Postic, B., & Cutler, J. C. (1976, October 15). Virucidal effect of certain chemical contraceptives on type 2 herpesvirus. *American Journal of Obstetrics and Gynecology, 126*(4), 422–425.

Snell, E., & Fox, J. G. (1961, November 18). Molluscum contagiosum venereum. *Canadian Medical Association Journal, 85,* 1152–1154.

Sobeslavsky, O. (1978). HBV as a global problem. In G. N. Vyas, S. N. Cohen, & R. Schmid (eds.), *Viral hepatitis: A contemporary assessment of etiology, epidemiology, pathogenesis, and prevention.* Philadelphia: The Franklin Institute Press.

Sparling, P. F. (1984). Natural history of syphilis. In K. K. Holmes, P.-A. Mårdh, P. F. Sparling, & P. J. Wiesner (Eds.), *Sexually transmitted diseases*. New York: McGraw-Hill.

Stagno, S., Reynolds, D., & Tsiantos, A., et al. (1975, May). Cervical cytomegalovirus excretion in pregnant and nonpregnant women: Suppression in early gestation. *Journal of Infectious Diseases, 131*(5), 522–527.

Stamm, W. E., & Holmes, K. K. (1984). *Chlamydia trachomatis* infections of the adult. In K. K. Holmes, P.-A. Mårdh, P. F. Sparling, & P. J. Wiesner (Eds.), *Sexually transmitted diseases*. New York: McGraw-Hill.

Stamm, W. E., Wagner, K. F., & Amsel, R., et al. (1980, August 21). Causes of the acute urethral syndrome in women. *New England Journal of Mecicine, 303*(8), 409–415.

State of New York. (1987, March 3). Department of Health Memorandum: Human immunodeficiency virus infections and women. Public Health Series: H-11, HMD-6, D&TC-8, PH-4.

Stenzel-Poore, M. P., Hallick, L. M., & Fendrick, J. L., et al. (1987, January-March). Herpes simplex virus shedding in genital secretions. *Sexually Transmitted Diseases, 14*(1), 17–22.

Stewart, G. J., Tyler, J. P. P., & Cunningham, A. L., et al. (1985, September 14). Transmission of human T-cell lymphotropic virus type III (HTLV-III) by artificial insemination by donor. *Lancet, 2*(8455), 581–584.

Stone, K. M., Grimes, D. A., & Magder, L. S. (1986a, July). Personal protection against sexually transmitted diseases. *American Journal of Obstetrics and Gynecology, 155*(1), 180–188.

Stone, K. M., Grimes, D. A., & Magder, L. S. (1986b, April 4). Primary prevention of sexually transmitted diseases: A primer for clinicians. *Journal of the American Medical Association, 255*(13), 1763–1766.

Stray-Pedersen, B., Eng, J., & Reikvam, T. M. (1978, February 1). Uterine T-mycoplasma colonization in reproductive failure. *American Journal of Obstetrics and Gynecology, 130*(3), 307–311.

Sumaya, C. V., Marx, J., & Ullis, K. (1980, January-March). Genital infections with herpes simplex virus in a university student population. *Sexually Transmitted Diseases, 7*(1), 16–20.

Swanson, J. & Mayer, L. W. (1984). Biology of *Neisseria gonorrhoeae*. In K. K. Holmes, P.-A. Mårdh, P. F. Sparling, & P. J. Wiesner (Eds.), *Sexually transmitted diseases.* New York: McGraw–Hill.

Swartz, M. N. (1984). Neurosyphilis. In K. K. Holmes, P.-A. Mårdh, P. F. Sparling, & P. J. Wiesner (Eds.), *Sexually transmitted diseases.* New York: McGraw–Hill.

Sweet, R. L. (1986, November/December). Colonization of the endometrium and fallopian tubes with *Ureaplasma urealyticum*. *Pediatric Infectious Disease, 5*(6, Suppl.), S244–S246.

Symposium: AIDS: Not just a man's problem anymore. (1986, October). *Contemporary Ob/Gyn, 28*(4), 128–138.

Szmuness, W. (1978). Sociodemographic aspects of the epidemiology of hepatitis B. In G. N. Vyas, S. N. Cohen, & R. Schmid (Eds.), *Viral hepatitis: A contemporary assessment of etiology, epidemiology, pathogenesis, and prevention.* Philadelphia: The Franklin Institute Press.

Szmuness, W., Dienstag, J. L., & Purcell, R. H., et al. (1976, September 30). Distribution of antibody to hepatitis A antigen in urban adult populations. *New England Journal of Medicine, 295*(14), 755–759.

Szmuness, W., Much, I., & Prince, A. M., et al. (1975, October). On the role of sexual behavior in the spread of hepatitis B infection. *Annals of Internal Medicine, 83*(4), 489–494.

Tam, M. R., Stamm, W. E., & Handsfield, H. H., et al. (1984, May 3). Culture-independent diagnosis of *Chlamydia trachomatis* using monoclonal antibodies. *New England Journal of Medicine, 310*(18), 1146–1150.

Taylor-Robinson, D., & McCormack, W. M. (1980a, May 1). The genital mycoplasmas (first of two parts). *New England Journal of Medicine, 302*(18), 1003–1010.

Taylor-Robinson, D., & McCormack, W. M. (1980b, May 8). The genital mycoplasmas (second of two parts). *New England Journal of Medicine, 302*(19), 1063–1067.

Tejani, N., Klein, S. W., & Kaplan, M. (1979, October 15). Subclinical herpes simplex genitalis infections in the perinatal period. *American Journal of Obstetrics and Gynecology, 135*(4), 547.

Thatcher, R. W., & Pettit, T. H. (1971, March 1). Gonorrheal con-

junctivitis. *Journal of the American Medical Association, 215*(9), 1494–1496.

Thew, M. A., Swift, J. T., & Heaton, C. L. (1969, November 3). Ampicillin in the treatment of granuloma inguinale. *Journal of the American Medical Association, 210*(5), 866–867.

Thin, R. N., & Shaw, E. J. (1979, February). Diagnosis of gonorrhea in women. *British Journal of Venereal Diseases, 55*(1), 10–13.

Thompson, S. E., & Hager, W. D. (1977, July-September). Acute pelvic inflammatory disease. *Sexually Transmitted Diseases, 4*(3), 105–111.

Thompson, S. E., & Washington, A. F. (1983). Epidemiology of sexually transmitted *Chlamydia trachomatis* infections. *Epidemiologic Reviews, 5*, 96–123.

Tice, A. W., & Rodriguez, V. L. (1981, December 11). Pharyngeal gonorrhea. *Journal of the American Medical Association, 246*(23), 2717–2719.

Trofatter, K. F., Jr. (1987, June). Interferon. *Obstetrics and Gynecology Clinics of North America, 14*(2), 569–679.

Wall, M. J., Heyman, A., & Beeson, P. B. (1947, May). Studies on the complement fixation reaction in lymphogranuloma venereum. *American Journal of Syphilis, Gonorrhea, and Venereal Diseases, 31*(3), 289–299.

Watts, D. H., & Eschenbach, D. A. (1987, March). Sexually transmitted diseases in pregnancy. *Infectious Disease Clinics of North America, 1*(1), 253–275.

Webb, D. H., & Fife, K. H. (1987, March). Genital herpes simplex virus infections. *Infectious Disease Clinics of North America, 1*(1), 97–122.

Weinstein, L., & Kaplan, K. (1970, May). The cephalosporins: Microbiological, chemical, and pharmacological properties and use in chemotherapy of infection. *Annals of Internal Medicine, 72*(5), 729–739.

Weiss, S. H., Saxinger, C., & Rechtman, D., et al. (1985, October 18). HTLV-III infection among health care workers: Association with needle-stick injuries. *Journal of the American Medical Association, 254*(15), 2089–2093.

Weström, L. (1975, March 1). Effect of acute pelvic inflammatory disease on fertility. *American Journal of Obstetrics and Gynecology, 121*(5), 707–713.

Wiesner, P. J., Tronca, E., & Bonin, P., et al. (1973, January 25). Clinical spectrum of pharyngeal gonococcal infection. *New England Journal of Medicine, 288*(4), 181–185.

Wilkin, J. K. (1977, July 1). Molluscum contagiosum venereum in a women's outpatient clinic: A venereally transmitted disease. *American Journal of Obstetrics and Gynecology, 128*(5), 531–535.

Wølner-Hanssen, P., Weström, L., & Mårdh, P.-A. (1980, April 26). Perihepatitis and chlamydial salpingitis. *Lancet, 1*(8174), 901–903.

Yeager, A. S., Arvin, A. M., Urbani, L. J., & Kemp, J. A., III. (1980, August). Relationship of antibody to outcome in neonatal herpes simplex virus infections. *Infection and Immunity, 29*(2), 532–538.

Ziegler, J. B., Cooper, D. A., Johnson, R. O., & Gold, J. (1985, April 20). Postnatal transmission of AIDS-associated retrovirus from mother to infant. *Lancet, 1*(8434), 896–897.

zur Hausen, H. (1982, December 18). Human genital cancer: Synergism between two virus infections or synergism between a virus infection and initiating events? *Lancet, 2*(8311), 1370–1372.

13

The Cervix

Ronnie Lichtman

Although part of the uterus, the cervix warrants a separate discussion. Because cervical cancer is seen in otherwise healthy young women, screening for this disorder is a major focus of gynecologic practice. Indeed, the desire for routine Pap testing (Papanicolaou smear) is the motivation for many women to seek regular gynecologic care. The well-woman gynecologic practitioner must be able to perform the Pap smear, interpret its results, and determine the need for further workup. In addition, the cervix can harbor many sexually transmitted organisms. The practitioner must be able to assess the general health of the cervix and know when to implement screening and diagnostic testing for disease, when to treat, and when to refer for diagnosis and treatment.

This chapter briefly reviews the anatomy of the cervix, outlines congenital anomalies of the cervix, describes pathology commonly seen, and provides an intensive discussion of cervical cancer and its precursors, summarizing appropriate screening, diagnosis, and intervention.

ANATOMY

The cervix is often called the neck of the uterus. Extending from the uterus into the posterior portion of the vagina, it is approximately 2.0 to 2.5 cm long in the adult, premenopausal woman. The cervical canal is open at both ends; these openings are called the *external os* and *internal os*. The external os appears as a small oval opening before childbirth and is often referred to as a "dimple" os. After childbirth, it appears as a transverse slit and has been called a "smile" os (see Fig. 1–9). The *ectocervix* is the cervical portion extending outward from the external cervical os; the portion of the cervix above the os is called the anterior lip; the portion below is the posterior lip. The *endocervix* extends upward from the external os to the internal os, where the cervical epithelium meets the uterine endometrium.

Cervical epithelium is composed of squamous and columnar cells. Squamous epithelium, appearing smooth and pink, lines the vagina and continues upward to cover variable amounts of the ectocervix (Singer, 1975). The stratified squamous epithelium of the cervix can be divided into four layers: basal, parabasal, intermediate, and superficial. The basal layer lies on a thin basement membrane. The middle two layers—parabasal and intermediate—are comparable to the middle layers of the skin. The superficial layer varies in thickness, in response to fluctuating amounts of estrogen.

Superficial cells are continually sloughed off into the vagina (Edmundson, 1982). Columnar epithelium, darker red and more granular appearing, lines the endometrium and continues downward to the cervix, lining the endocervical canal. The boundary between squamous and columnar epithelium is called the *squamocolumnar junction* and may occur anywhere on the ecto- or endocervix. Rarely, it is located in the vaginal fornix. Sometimes, the insertion of a speculum causes the cervical lips to retract, and the portion of the endocervix containing the squamocolumnar junction becomes visible, appearing to be on the ectocervix. When the speculum blades are pulled back or closed, however, the squamocolumnar junction returns to its actual location on the endocervix. These two views have been referred to as "apparent" and "real" (Edmundson, 1982).

The squamocolumnar junction may regress at various times as a result of hormonal variation, particularly with sexual activity and during pregnancy, through processes known as *epidermialization* and *squamous metaplasia*. Epidermialization is an upward growth of squamous cells that replace columnar cells. Squamous metaplasia is the differentiation of columnar cells into squamous cells (Merrill, 1986). The area between the original and new squamocolumnar junction is called the *transformation zone*.

When columnar epithelium is visible on the ectocervix, appearing as a granular red area, it is referred to as *eversion*, *ectropion*, or *ectopy*. This is often seen in pregnancy or with oral contraceptive use. The term *erosion* has been used interchangeably with these other terms, although erosion literally means "a wearing away or eroding of tissue" or a loss of surface epithelium (Mukherjee, Dutta, & Dawn, 1984) and is more precisely used to refer to a pathologic process usually caused by trauma. The term, however, is not specific and is widely interpreted by various observers (Purola & Paavonen, 1982).

In the cervix, numerous glands extend from the surface of the endocervical mucosa into adjacent connective tissue. These glands secrete into the cervical canal. Cyclic changes occur in the glands and cervical mucus changes at various times of the menstrual cycle (described in Chapter 5). At the time of ovulation, the mucus exhibits the properties of *spinnbarkeit*, the ability to be drawn out in long strands, and *ferning*, a characteristic pattern resembling fern leaves seen in dried mucus under microscopic magnification. Ferning is due to crystallization of sodium chloride, which increases in response to estrogen (Pritchard, MacDonald, & Gant, 1985).

CONGENITAL ABNORMALITIES

Congenital anomalies of the cervix result from lack of fusion or incomplete fusion of the müllerian ducts or incomplete or absent development of one duct (Pritchard et al., 1985). As a result of these abnormalities of development, the cervix may be septate, double, or incomplete (hemicervix). In the septate cervix, the septum may be confined to the cervix or, more often, be continuous with a uterine and/or longitudinal vaginal septum (see Chapters 11 and 14). A double cervix may also exist in conjunction with a longitudinal vaginal septum, making the clinical distinction between the double and septate cervix difficult.

The septate cervix may rupture during labor with subsequent hemorrhage. Major obstetric difficulties, however, are due to uterine abnormalities, described in Chapter 14. Diagnosis of cervical abnormalities depends on careful visual and digital examination. Diagnosis and treatment of coexisting uterine abnormalities are outlined in Chapter 14.

Other congenital anomalies of the cervix are related to in utero diethylstilbestrol (DES) exposure, described in Chapter 18.

BENIGN DISORDERS

Cysts

Nabothian Cysts. A Nabothian cyst is an obstructed endocervical gland that becomes distended with mucus (Merrill, 1986). Nabothian cysts appear on the cervical surface as slightly raised blue or yellowish nodules, 1 to 3 mm in diameter. They are not clinically significant and require no treatment.

Endometriomas. Endometriomas—the cysts caused by endometriosis—occasionally appear on the cervix. These cysts may resemble Nabothian cysts. Primary cervical endometriosis often develops after surgical trauma; secondary endometriosis of the cervix is spread from other sites (Gardner, 1981).

Women with cervical endometriosis may experience premenstrual, intermenstrual, or postcoital bleeding. On physical examination, the lesions are seen as superficial submucosal round spots, red or dark blue in color and usually 2 to 3 mm in diameter. Detailed information on endometriosis is found in Chapter 18.

Tumors

Myomas. Myomas of the cervix are rare. If they grow large, they may cause pressure symptoms. They cause most problems in pregnancy, where they have the potential to obstruct vaginal delivery. Myomas are diagnosed on bimanual examination, with sonogram used for confirmation when the diagnosis is in question or to document growth. Myomas are discussed in detail in Chapter 14.

Polyps. Polyps are the most common tumors of the cervix. They are most often found in women in the menstruating years. Polyps are soft, red lesions, usually pedunculated with a narrow base. They often protrude from the cervical os and vary from several millimeters to 2 cm in diameter (Fig. 13–1).

Usually polyps are asymptomatic, but they may cause bleeding, especially after intercourse or douching. Diagnosis is made by inspection. Referral for removal of the polyp is recommended. This is usually an in-office procedure. The polyp should be sent for laboratory diagnosis of possible malignancy, although this is rare. If the patient had complained of abnormal bleeding, an endometrial biopsy or curettage is recommended to rule out other conditions that more often cause bleeding (Merrill, 1986).

Condylomata Acuminata. Cervical condylomata acuminata, caused by the human papillomavirus (HPV), are an increasing problem associated with cervical intraepithelial neoplasia (see later) (Boon & Kok, 1985; Cardillo, 1985; Meisels, Morin, & Casas-Cordero, 1982). Cervical condylomata acuminata are often subclinical, and diagnosis depends on cytology and colposcopy (see later). Their clinical presentation, diagnosis, and treatment are discussed fully in Chapter 12.

Hemangiomas. Occasional reports of cervical hemangiomas have appeared in the literature. The lesions are usually small and deep wine red in color. All reported lesions have been benign; conservative therapy is recommended (Ahern & Allen, 1978).

Other Benign Conditions

Cervicitis. Cervicitis is a vague term used in the literature to denote a number of conditions. Because the cervix is continuously exposed to trauma and irritation, it is commonly

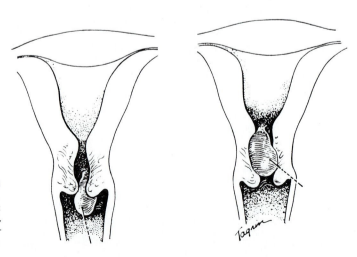

Figure 13–1. (Left) Ectocervical polyp. (Right) Endocervical polyp. *(From Green, T. H. [1977]. Gynecology: Essentials of clinical practice [3rd ed.], Boston: Little, Brown and Company. Reprinted with permission.)*

inflamed (Merrill, 1986). Clinically significant inflammation, however, can be difficult to diagnose. The practitioner must differentiate between the exposure of normal columnar epithelial cells (eversion or ectopy, see earlier text) and inflammatory changes. Once inflammation is identified, its cause, either an infectious process or physical or chemical trauma, must be determined. Acute cervicitis must then be differentiated from chronic cervicitis.

ETIOLOGY. Among the infectious processes that may cause acute cervicitis are those associated with vaginitis and a number of sexually transmitted organisms. The most common of these is *Chlamydia trachomatis* (Brunham, Paavonen, Stevens, et al., 1984; Paavonen, Vesterinen, Meyer, & Saksela, 1982; Paavonen, Critchlow, DeRouen, et al., 1986). Other organisms involved in acute cervicitis include *Neisseria gonorrhoeae*, herpes simplex virus, *Ureaplasma urealyticum*, and *Trichomonas vaginalis* (which may cause typical ''strawberry'' spots on the cervix). Detailed information on these organisms, their diagnosis, and their management is found in Chapters 11 and 12. Oral contraceptive use has also been associated with cervicitis (Paavonen et al., 1986). Additional possible causes include vaginal medications, tampons, or surgical trauma to the cervix including cryo- and laser surgery.

Chronic cervicitis, a condition disputed in the literature (Selim & Shalodi, 1985), is related to trauma and lacerations occurring with childbirth, instrumentation, infection, or atrophy associated with decreased estrogen levels (Merrill, 1986).

CLINICAL PRESENTATION. The most common presenting symptom of cervicitis is a mucopurulent discharge. Patients may complain of discharge and/or pain, bleeding, or dysuria, but often they may be asymptomatic. On physical examination, the cervix may be edematous and erythematous, and may show exposed columnar epithelium. It may be friable to touch. Reddened areas may be seen around the os. Their irregularity and friability sometimes differentiate them from eversion; other times, colposcopy is required to make this distinction.

DIAGNOSIS. A mucopurulent cervical discharge is a key indicator of infection with *C. trachomatis*, often otherwise asymptomatic. Cultures or other diagnostic tests for this organism are required to confirm the diagnosis (described in Chapter 12). A wet smear should be examined under the microscope to rule out *T. vaginalis* and/or other vaginal pathology. Tests for *N. gonorrhoeae* may be appropriate as this organism has an affinity for the cervix and often coexists with *C. trachomatis*. Vesicular or ulcerated cervical lesions warrant testing for herpes simplex virus, syphilis, and/or chancroid. Complete information on screening indications and the historic, physical, and laboratory data to be collected in diagnosing these conditions appears in Chapter 12.

Inflammatory changes may be identified on Pap smear; if organisms are identified, the patient should be examined and further diagnostic testing and treatment initiated as warranted. Inflammation on Pap smear may be seen with oral contraceptive use and pregnancy. If atypia is also present on the smear, identified organisms should be treated and the Pap smear repeated after 3 months (see later).

INTERVENTION. Cervical inflammation caused by identified organisms should be treated appropriately, with referral and consultation as necessary. Whether cervicitis without an identifiable cause should be treated is controversial. If the cervix has a suspicious lesion, the patient should be referred for colposcopy and/or biopsy regardless of cytology results (see later). If the patient is symptomatic or has a cervix that appears grossly abnormal to the practitioner, referral for possible treatment is warranted. Treatments include acid douches and jellies (e.g., Aci-Jel), topical or systemic estrogens for menopausal women (see Chapter 24), silver nitrate application, or cryo- or laser surgery (Merrill, 1986).

Cervical Stenosis. Cervical stenosis occurs after trauma to the cervix, including infection, cauterization, conization, cryosurgery, and radiation therapy. Stenosis may cause abnormal bleeding, dysmenorrhea, and infertility. If stenosis is complete, the uterine cavity may become distended with blood, fluid, or other exudate. Eventually, cramping may be experienced. The condition is diagnosed by history and the inability of the practitioner to pass a sound or probe into the cervical canal, with fluid escaping when the canal is opened. Anesthesia may be needed to open the cervix, with cervical dilation preceding the sounding (Merrill, 1986); gynecologic referral is required.

CERVICAL INTRAEPITHELIAL NEOPLASIA: CERVICAL CANCER AND ITS PRECURSORS

Cervical cancer is a progressive disease with a number of histologically definable stages, diagrammed in Figure 13-2. Together with its precursors, the cancerous lesion, which can be in situ or invasive, is called *cervical intraepithelial neoplasia* (CIN) (Nelson, Averette, & Richart, 1984). The precancerous lesions have also been called *dysplasia,* which can be broken down into mild, moderate, and severe.

Among cervical cancers, 90 percent are squamous cell carcinomas, which are further subdivided into three types: small cell; intermediate, large cell, or nonkeratinizing; and keratinizing. Approximately 5 percent are adenocarcinomas, which arise from the mucosa of the endocervix in the mucus-secreting glands (Perez, DiSaia, Knapp, & Young, 1985). Another 1 to 2 percent are clear cell type, most of which are related to in utero DES exposure (see Chapter 18). Other cancers rarely reported include adenosquamous carcinoma, primary sarcoma (including leiomyosarcoma, rhabdomyosarcoma, stromal sarcoma, and carcinosarcoma), and lymphoma.

Etiology and Epidemiology. Invasive cancer of the cervix is the third most common genital malignancy in women in the United States (American Cancer Society, 1987). The American Cancer Society estimated 12,800 cases of invasive carcinoma of the cervix in 1987. In recent years, the diagnosis of cancer precursors has increased, most likely as the result of increased screening, whereas the diagnosis of more advanced lesions, including cancer in situ (CIS), has decreased, because of increased screening, diagnosis, and treatment (Cashavelly, 1987; Parkin, Nguyen-Dinh, & Day, 1985). Indeed, cervical cancer is now considered a preventable disease (Chow, Greenberg, & Liff, 1986).

The average age of diagnosis of precancerous lesions in the United States is 33 to 38 years, whereas the average age of diagnosis of invasive cancer is 43 to 48 (Lovejoy, 1987). Rates of abnormal cervical cytology in adolescents and women under age 25 have been increasing, presumably because of increased sexual activity and increased infection with HPV (Delke, Veridiano, Russell, & Tancer, 1981; Raymond, 1987). Incidence rates are higher in blacks than

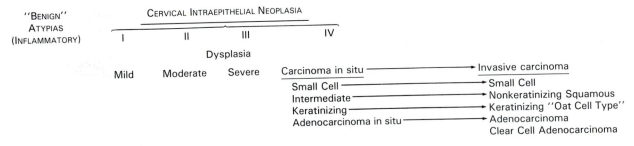

Figure 13–2. Histogenesis of Carcinoma of the Cervix *(From Perez, C. A., DiSaia, P. J. Knapp, R. C. & Young, R. C. [1985]. Gynecologic tumors. In V. T. Davita, S. Hellman, & S. A. Rosenberg [Eds.]. Cancer: Principles and practice of Oncology, [2nd ed.], Philadelphia: J. B. Lippincott. Reprinted with permission.)*

whites and in women of low socioeconomic status (Gusberg, DiSaia, & Deppe, 1986).

The causative agents of cervical cancer are not known. Increasingly, however, evidence is pointing to an association between cervical cancer and HPV; HPV has been detected in cervical carcinomas (Lancaster, Castellano, Santos, et al., 1986; Smotkin, Berek, Fu, et al., 1986). Herpes simplex virus type 2 (HSV-2) has been named as another possible etiologic agent. Zur Hausen (1982) has hypothesized an interaction of these viruses in the etiology of cervical cancer, with HSV an initiator and HPV a promoter of cancer, although this hypothesis remains speculative. Recent controlled studies, however, have refuted the etiologic role of HSV in cervical cancer (Richart, 1987; Vonka, Kǎnka, Hirsch, et al., 1984a; Vonka, Kǎnka, Jelinek, et al., 1984b), pointing out that the association does not represent cause and effect but rather shared risk factors for both diseases. These viruses are discussed more extensively in Chapter 12.

Neither squamous cell carcinoma nor its precursors occur in virgins, and the risk of developing cervical cancer increases with the number of male sexual partners a woman has ever had and with the numbers of partners her male partner has had (Richart, 1987). A male factor, which may be the transmission of HPV, has been postulated in the etiology of cervical cancer (Kessler, 1977; Singer, Reid, & Coppleson, 1976). Women whose male partners have had vasectomies may have lower rates of cervical cancer than other women, suggesting exposure to sperm itself as the possible male factor (Swan & Brown, 1979). Certain proteins of the sperm head—histones—may interact with cervical cells in a cancer-promoting manner (Singer et al., 1976). Several studies of female partners of men with cancer of the penis have shown an increased rate of cervical cancer among the women (Cartwright & Sinson, 1980; Graham, Priore, Graham, et al., 1979; MacGregor & Innes, 1980; Martínez, 1969; Smith, Kinlen, White, et al., 1980).

Male circumcision had been believed to be protective against cervical cancer in the female partners of circumcised men, based largely on the low incidence of cervical cancer in Jewish women; however, as the disease has a high incidence in Moslem women, whose partners are also circumcised, this theory is no longer considered valid (Briggs & Paavonen, 1984; Terris, Wilson, & Nelson, 1973). Early age at first intercourse (usually cited as before age 20) has been associated with cervical cancer in some studies, but when numbers of partners have been controlled, this variable has ceased to be significant (Harris, Brinton, Cowdell, et al., 1980), although most authors still cite it as a risk factor.

Cigarette smoking has been associated with cervical cancer (Winkelstein, Shillitoe, Brand, & Johnson, 1984). The greatest risk from smoking may be during adolescence (Lyon, Gardner, West, et al., 1983). Hypothesized reasons

for this association include an effect of an agent in cigarettes on the immune system (Clarke, Hatcher, McKeown-Eyssen, & Lickrish, 1985), an interaction between smoking and endocrine factors, and the secretion of absorbed metabolic products of cigarette smoke by vaginal or endometrial cells (Lyon et al., 1983).

Nutritional deficiencies, particularly of vitamin A, β-carotene, and vitamin C, have been implicated in cervical cancer (Romney, Palan, Duttagupta, et al., 1981), as have other sexually immunosuppressive agents (Lovejoy, 1987). Other sexually transmitted diseases (STDs) have been investigated in relation to cervical cancer, but it is generally believed that they coexist with cervical cancer secondary to the same risk factors, rather than being causative (Briggs & Paavonen, 1984). Barrier contraceptives have been shown to be protective and may even facilitate regression of precancerous lesions (Richardson & Lyon, 1981; Thomas, 1973).

Clinical Presentation. Invasive cancer of the cervix and its precursors are detectable by cytology before becoming symptomatic and before gross clinical signs appear; a small superficial ulceration of the central cervix may be the only abnormality seen in CIN, including CIS (Figure 13–3). When symptoms are present they usually include (in order of frequency) postcoital spotting, intermenstrual bleeding, especially after exertion, and increased menstrual bleeding. Patients with invasive cancer may experience serosangui-

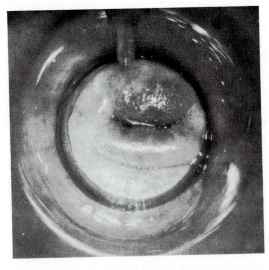

Figure 13–3. Cervical intraepithelial neoplasia. *(From Gusberg, S. B., DiSaia, P. J., & Deppe, G. [1986]. Malignant lesions of the cervix uteri. In D. N. Danforth & J. R. Scott [Eds.], Obstetrics and gynecology [5th ed.]. Philadelphia: J. B. Lippincott. Reprinted with permission.)*

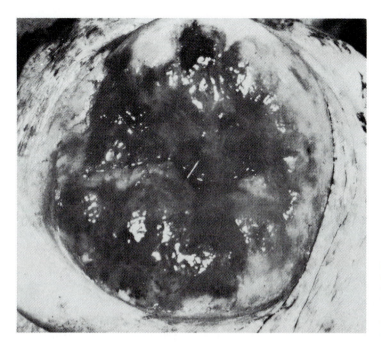

Figure 13–4. Squamous cell carcinoma of the cervix. *(From Gusberg, S. B. DiSaia, P. J., & Deppe, G. Malignant lesions of the cervix uteri. In D. N. Danforth & J. R. Scott [Eds.], Obstetrics and gynecology [5th ed.]. Philadelphia: J. B. Lippincott. Reprinted with permission.)*

neous or yellowish vaginal discharge, which may be foul smelling and intermixed with blood. Symptoms of anemia may ensue when bleeding is severe. Pelvic or epigastric pain is experienced only with large lesions. Advanced disease may cause urinary or rectal symptoms including bleeding (Perez et al., 1985). On speculum examination, advanced lesions appear as necrotic ulcers (Figure 13–4); in invasive disease they may extend upward or protrude into the vagina.

Disease Course. Cancer of the cervix is a relatively slow-growing lesion. Richart and Barron (1969) followed 557 patients with abnormal cervical cytologies for 10 years. The median time for dysplasia to progress to CIS was 12 months for severe dysplasia (CIN grade III) and 85 months for mild dysplasia (CIN grade I). Some lesions did not progress. Nasiell, Roger, and Nasiell (1986) followed 555 women with mild dysplasia. Regression to normal occurred in 62 percent over 39 months; progression to severe dysplasia, CIS, or invasive cancer occurred in 16 percent, and persistent dysplasia was seen in 22 percent. Overall, a woman with mild dysplasia had a risk of developing severe dysplasia, CIS, or invasive cancer 560 times greater than that of a woman without dysplasia.

Staging, Metastasis, and Prognosis. Because of its slow growth and available treatments (see below), cervical intraepithelial neoplasia is a curable lesion and should not result in serious sequelae or mortality if diagnosed and treated early in its course. When the lesion breaks through the basement membrane and invades the cervical stroma, metastasis becomes possible. If the invasion is less than 3 mm without vascular involvement, the lesion is called microinvasive (Perez et al., 1985). The incidence of metastasis is directly related to the depth of invasion. The lesion can also extend into the lower uterine segment or endometrial cavity.

Prognosis is related to stage and volume of tumor (Table 13–1), depth of stromal invasion, and lymph node metastasis. Overall, pelvic lymph nodes are involved in 5 to 8 percent of invasive cancer lesions. The literature is not in

TABLE 13–1. CLINICAL STAGING OF CERVICAL CANCER

Preinvasive carcinoma

Stage 0	Carcinoma in situ, intraepithelial carcinoma. Cases of stage 0 should not be included in any therapeutic statistics for invasive carcinoma.

Invasive carcinoma

Stage I	Carcinoma is strictly confined to the cervix (extension to the corpus should be disregarded).
IA	Microinvasive carcinoma (early stromal invasion).
IB	All other cases of stage I. Occult cancer should be marked "occ."
Stage II	The carcinoma extends beyond the cervix, but has not extended to the pelvic wall. The carcinoma involves the vagina but not the lower third.
IIA	Parametrial involvement is not obvious.
IIB	Parametrial involvement is obvious.
Stage III	The carcinoma has extended to the pelvic wall. On rectal examination there is no cancer-free space between the tumor and the pelvic wall. The tumor involves the lower third of the vagina. All cases with a hydronephrosis or nonfunctioning kidney should be included, unless they are known to have other causes.
IIIA	Tumor extends to the pelvic wall.
IIIB	Tumor extends to the pelvic wall and hydronephrosis or nonfunctioning kidney is present.
Stage IV	The carcinoma has extended beyond the true pelvis or has clinically involved the mucosa of the bladder or rectum. A bullous edema as such does not permit a case to be allotted to stage IV.
IVA	Growth has spread to adjacent organs.
IVB	Growth has spread to distant organs.

Adopted in 1976 by the International Federation of Gynecology and Obstetrics (FIGO). Adapted from Perez, C. A., DiSaia, P. J., Knapp, R. C., & Young, R. C. (1985). Gynecologic tumors. In V. T. DaVita, S. Hellman, & S. A. Rosenberg (Eds.), Cancer: Principles and practice of oncology (2nd ed.). Philadelphia: J. B. Lippincott. Reprinted with permission.

agreement on whether age at diagnosis affects prognosis. The American Cancer Society estimated 6,800 deaths from invasive cervical cancer in 1987.

Management

DATA COLLECTION

History.   The focus of historic data in the diagnosis of cervical cancer is on risk factors, as symptoms are rare and usually seen only in advanced disease. Symptoms include abnormal bleeding—postcoital, intermenstrual, and/or menstrual—serosanguineous foul-smelling vaginal discharge, and pelvic or epigastric pain. Risk factors to be discussed routinely include numbers of male sexual partners and numbers of partners of partners, age at first intercourse, and smoking. A history of genital HPV is most significant, and a history of other STDs important. A contraceptive history should be taken as barrier methods are protective. A diet history, focusing on intake of vitamin A, β-carotene, and vitamin C may be significant. The use of immunosuppressant medications should be noted. The woman's last gynecologic checkup and the results of any previous Pap smears and previous cervical pathology and treatment should be discussed. Additional information needed by the laboratory performing cytology includes the patient's age, parity and gravidy, last menstrual period, previous gynecologic surgery, use of hormones, radiation therapy, and current pregnancy or postpartum status if relevant (Baldwin & Goodwin, 1985).

Physical Examination.   Physical examination must include abdominal and lymph node palpation and complete inspection and palpation of the external genitalia, a careful speculum examination with visualization of the cervix and vaginal walls, and a thorough bimanual examination. Any abnormal findings of the cervix, including cysts, polyps, erosion, friability, vesicles, white patches (leukoplakia), granularity, and mucopurulent discharge, should be noted and reported to the pathologist reading the Pap smear (Baldwin & Goodwin, 1985).

Laboratory Testing.   Because the precursors of cervical cancer are neither symptomatic nor visible, laboratory testing is the crux of early diagnosis. The Pap smear is the standard screening test; colposcopy, biopsy, endocervical curettage, and, at times, conization are the mainstays of diagnosis.

The *Pap smear* is the basic screening test for cervical cancer. Although it does not afford definitive diagnosis, and abnormal findings must be confirmed and clarified by more definitive diagnostic testing, the smear is easy, rapid, and inexpensive to perform and is not associated with morbidity or mortality (Richart & Barron, 1981). The technique was developed in the 1920s and widely introduced in the 1940s (Papanicolaou & Traut, 1941). Although interpretation of the smear has changed as understanding of the disease has increased, the basic concept remains valid.

The technique for Pap smear testing is described in detail in Chapter 4. All women should be advised to avoid douching, intercourse, and vaginal medications, including contraceptives, for 24 to 48 hours before the Pap test. Ideally, to increase accuracy, the smear should not be taken during menses (Lovejoy, 1987).

Unfortunately, random controlled clinical trials to determine the efficacy of Pap smear screening have never been carried out (Eddy, 1981); case control studies, however, have found it to be highly effective (Clarke & Anderson, 1979). All women should be screened periodically by Pap smear for cervical cancer, although there is controversy regarding recommended screening frequency. Table 13–2 outlines the recommendations of various groups. Many practitioners continue to advocate yearly Pap smears (Beal, 1987). Because of the high prevalence of risk factors [including multiple lifetime male sexual partners (greater than three), partners with multiple partners, intercourse initiated at age 20 or younger, history of other STDs, smoking, and in utero DES exposure], and because of the relatively high rate of false-negative reports on Pap smears, practitioners apply the most frequent guidelines to all women (Morell, Taylor, Synder, et al., 1982). False-negative reports are estimated to occur in 1 to 69 percent of smears (Yobs, Swanson, & Lamotte, 1985), with an average in clinical practice of 33 percent (Richart & Barron, 1981). False-negative rates are related to errors in sampling technique and misread smears (Eddy, 1980). Other facts are taken into consideration in recommending frequent Pap smear testing: many women prolong the recommended interval, and additional health screening takes place at visits initiated for the purpose of obtaining a Pap smear. Further discussion of this issue is provided in Chapter 4.

TABLE 13–2. RECOMMENDATIONS ON THE FREQUENCY OF PAP TESTING

	ACOG 1980	American Cancer Society 1980	Canadian Task Force 1982	International Academy of Cytology 1980	National Cancer Institute 1980
Start	Age 18 or when sexually active	Age 20 or when sexually active	When sexually active	Age 18 or when sexually active	When sexually active
Ages 18–35	Annually	Annually, until two negative tests, then continue every 3 yr	Annually, if sexually active	Annually	After two negative tests, continue every 1 to 3 yr
Ages 36–60	Annually	At least every 3 yr, more frequently if high risk; pelvic exam annually after age 40	After two negative tests, continue every 5 yr	Annually	Every 1 to 3 yr
Over age 60	Annually	At least every 3 yr, more frequently if high risk; pelvic exam annually	After two negative tests, testing may be stopped	Annually	After two negative tests, testing may be stopped

From the American College of Obstetricians and Gynecologists. (1984) "Cervical cancer screening—How often?" ACOG Newsletter, 28. Reprinted with permission.

TABLE 13-3. CLASSIFICATION OF PAP SMEARS[a]

Findings inadequate for diagnosis
Findings essentially normal
Atypical cells present suggestive of (specify)
Cytologic findings consistent with
  Cervical intraepithelial neoplasia
    Grade I (mild dysplasia)
    Grade II (moderate dysplasia)
    Grade III (severe dysplasia to carcinoma in situ)
  Invasive squamous cell carcinoma
  Endometrial carcinoma
  Other cancer (specify)

[a]Other abnormal findings, such as vaginal pathogens or endometrial cells, even if benign, should be reported as well.
From Richart, R. M. (1981, February 7). Current concepts in obstetrics and gynecology: The patient with an abnormal Pap smear—Screening techniques and management. New England Journal of Medicine, 302(6), 332. Reprinted with permission.

The original classification of Pap smears comprised classes 1 to 5. Class 1 was normal; class 2, normal with abnormal or atypical cells; class 3, suspicious cells; class 4, signs of malignancy; and class 5, malignant. This system has been replaced by a classification using the newer terminology of cervical intraepithelial neoplasia and more description of atypical cells. This new classification appears as Table 13-3. Richart (1979) points out that all laboratories with adequate quality control should occasionally report inadequate smears.

The various grades of CIN are defined in the following way (Koss, 1978, pp. 122–125):

- *CIN grade I:* Isolated abnormal (enlarged and hyperchromatic) nuclei within the framework of orderly epithelium; usually seen in the transformation zone of the squamocolumnar junction
- *CIN grade II:* 50 percent of abnormal cells, without loss of the basic characteristics of normal epithelium
- *CIN grade III:* Cancer cells of one of three types

1. Keratinizing-type cells, which show keratin formation on the epithelial surface
2. Large-cell–type lesions, which are generally composed of nonkeratinizing, large cells that replace the entire thickness of the epithelium
3. Small-cell–type lesions, which are similar to large-cell–type lesions, except that the cells are smaller (This lesion is thought to derive from the endocervical epithelium and may contain mucus-forming cells; it often involves endocervical glands.)

Richart (1987) more recently proposed an alternative classification for cervical lesions, replacing the terms dysplasia and CIS completely. His classification scheme includes condylomata as a separate category, with lesions with HPV types 16 or 18 considered CIN. This classification appears as Table 13-4.

Pap smear findings can also suggest the presence of certain infectious organisms including herpes simplex virus, *Chlamydia trachomatis,* human papillomavirus, *Trichomonas vaginalis, Candida albicans,* and *Actinomyces israelii.* Sometimes, the presence of these organisms can lead to atypical smears. More information about these organisms and the Pap smear findings that suggest them is provided in Chapters 8 (for *Actinomyces*), 11, and 12.

The Pap smear, when taken from the inner third of the lateral vaginal wall, can also be used to assess endocrine function (Richart, 1979). It is called a maturation index and is described in Chapter 24.

In pregnant women and in women using oral contraceptives, the cellular pattern of the cervix changes; there is an increased incidence of eversion early in pregnancy (Singer, 1975) and of cervical congestion and hypertrophy in the third trimester (Kopan, Beckman, Bigelow, et al., 1980). These changes make cytologic evaluation more difficult in pregnancy and cause a greater-than-normal false-positive rate.

The primary care practitioner must be able to evaluate when repeat Pap testing or referral for further diagnostic

TABLE 13-4. TERMINOLOGY AND MANAGEMENT OF CERVICAL LESIONS

Diagnosis	Criteria	Clinical Implications
Normal and its variants	Diploid, cytologically benign. Includes squamous metaplasia, inflammation, and repair.	No evidence of cancer or cancer precursors. Patient continues in follow-up pool for periodic screening.
Condyloma acuminatum	Acuminate lesions. Papillomatosis, acanthosis, cytologic atypia (polyploidy), and koilocytosis. HPV types 6 and 11.[a]	Treat for condyloma with podophyllin, trichloracetic acid, cautery, CO_2 laser, or surgical removal. Biopsy lesions resistant to therapy before ablative therapy to rule out invasion.
Flat condyloma	Flat, white, or pigmented lesions. Koilocytosis, cytologic atypia, binucleated cells. Normal mitotic figures, tripolar mitoses, or tetraploid dispersed metaphases (polyploidy). HPV types 6 and 11.	Colposcopy and biopsy to rule out invasive cancer. Treat with cryotherapy, CO_2 laser therapy, 5-FU, or local surgery depending on size and distribution of lesion(s).
CIN	Minimal or no koilocytosis, high degree of cytologic atypia, mitoses, and poorly differentiated cells in upper 33 percent of epithelium and abnormal mitotic figures (aneuploidy). HPV 16/18 group.	Colposcopy and biopsy to rule out invasive cancer. Treat with cryotherapy, CO_2 laser therapy, 5-FU, or local surgery depending on size and distribution of lesion(s).
Microinvasion	One or more tongues of neoplastic epithelium extending through the plane of the basement membrane into the stroma to a depth of 3 mm or less.	Simple hysterectomy or conization in selected cases.
Invasive carcinoma	Tongues of invasion extending more than 3 mm into stroma.	Radical hysterectomy or radiation therapy.

[a]HPV, human papillomavirus; 5-FU, 5-Fluorouracil; CIN, cervical intraepithelial neoplasia.
From Richart, R. M. (1987, October 15). Causes and management of cervical intraepithelial neoplasia. Cancer, 60(8, Suppl.), 1955. Reprinted with permission.

testing and possibly treatment is warranted. This is discussed later under Intervention.

Because a Pap smear does not offer definitive diagnosis, any smear showing inflammation or changes suggestive of any type of vaginitis or STD should be followed up with testing for these conditions, described in Chapters 11 and 12, and treatment as appropriate. If tests do not confirm the Pap smear results, and the original smear reported atypia, a repeat Pap can be performed after 3 to 6 months. Repeat Pap smears performed before 3 months may show false-negative results because the cells removed in the first smear have not had adequate time to regenerate.

The *Schiller test* was widely used to locate abnormal cervical cells before colposcopy became standard. It is rarely used today, essentially replaced by colposcopy (see later). In the Schiller test the cervical mucosa is stained with Schiller's iodine solution. Normal cells pick up the stain because of a reaction with the glycogen in their cytoplasm. In CIN, cells contain less glycogen and therefore do not stain with the iodine. This test is not diagnostic but can indicate areas appropriate for biopsy. It is, however, quite nonspecific, and the majority of areas that fail to pick up stain are benign lesions, including cervical erosions (Gusberg et al., 1986).

Cervicography was introduced in 1981 (Stafl, 1981) in an effort to improve the sensitivity of screening methods for premalignant disease of the cervix. In this technique, speculum examination is performed, acetic acid applied to the cervix, and a special cervicograph camera used to take magnified photographs (cervicograms) of the cervix. Advantages of cervicography are that the cervicogram can be taken by a physician or nonphysician after brief training and sent to an expert for evaluation and that the photograph provides a permanent document. In a study of 97 patients with atypical Pap smears, cervicography was found to be more sensitive than repeat Pap smears, but not as good as colposcopy, in identifying patients with both CIN and HPV infection (Spitzer, Krumholz, Chernys, et al., 1987). Another study of 3,271 women confirmed these findings: the cervicogram was more sensitive than the Pap smear, but less specific, meaning more false-positive results were reported, necessitating further workup; however, fewer false-negative results were seen (Tawa, Forsythe, Cove, et al., 1988). Further evaluation of cervicography is needed before it is widely accepted.

Colposcopy offers more precise information than Pap smear. A colposcope is a set of binoculars with a magnification of 10- to 15-fold mounted on a stand (Perez et al., 1985) (Figure 13–5). The examination is done with a speculum. Prior to colposcopic examination, 3 percent acetic acid (or plain vinegar) is applied to the cervical epithelium. This helps to remove mucus and causes dehydration of the surface cells. The dehydration enhances the nuclear-to-cytoplasmic ratio in dysplastic cells and creates the white epithelium when light is reflected off these cells (Perez et al., 1985). It is this white epithelium as well as various vascular patterns that allow identification of potentially malignant areas.

The colposcopist is most interested in the transformation zone. Abnormal findings suggestive of neoplasia include white epithelium, punctation, mosaic, hyperkeratosis, and abnormal blood vessels. These are defined in Table 13–5. Other important variables in colposcopic examination include vascular pattern, intercapillary distance, surface pattern, color tone, and clarity of demarcation. From these findings, the colposcopist can infer the histologic diagnosis. For a complete description of abnormal colposcopic findings, the reader is referred to specialized textbooks.

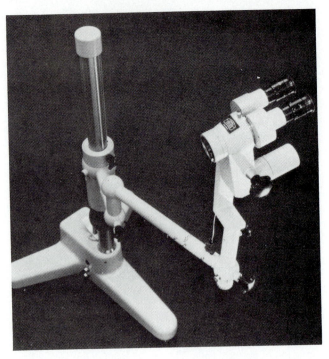

Figure 13–5. The colposcope. *(From Stafl, A. [1986]. Colposcopy. In D. N. Danforth & J. R. Scott [Eds.], Obstetrics and gynecology [5th ed.]. Philadelphia: J. B. Lippincott. Reprinted with permission.)*

Proficiency in colposcopic examination and interpretation requires training and practice. Whenever possible, referral should be made to an experienced colposcopist.

Colposcopy is indicated for all women with Pap smears showing dysplasia. Authors vary on their recommendations regarding the use of colposcopy after Pap smears showing atypia. Žarković (1985) found no difference in the rate of progression to dysplasia from normal Pap smears and Pap smears with atypical cells over a 7- to 8-year period. Some clinicians ignore atypical results, others repeat the smear in 3 months, and others treat with a variety of antibacterial agents (Noumoff, 1987). Noumoff (1987) recommends subdividing atypical smears into three categories: inflammatory atypia, squamous atypia, and endocervical atypia. He recommends colposcopy for squamous or endocervical atypia and inflammatory atypia that persists after treatment with therapy appropriate for the identified organism. In his study of 375 women with these findings, 29 percent were shown on colposcopy to have CIN; of these, 35 percent had lesions of severity greater than grade I. Davis, Hernandez, Davis, and Miyazawa (1987) found similar results evaluating patients with squamous atypia: 18.7 percent of 406 patients with atypical squamous cells had CIN. These authors advocate colposcopy for women with squamous atypia; when this is not available, they recommend serial repeat Pap smears, at least every 3 to 6 months.

Multiple punch biopsies are recommended for cervical lesions that appear abnormal on inspection (Perez et al., 1985) and for areas of suspected malignancy on colposcopy. Biopsy is done on an outpatient basis during colposcopic examination; specimens must be sent to the laboratory for histologic analysis. At least one specimen must be obtained from each suspicious area and from nonsuspicious areas. The biopsies are usually somewhat painful.

Richart, Crum, and Townsend (no date) recommend

TABLE 13–5. CORRELATION OF COLPOSCOPIC AND HISTOLOGIC FINDINGS

Colposcopic Term	Colposcopic Appearance	Histologic Correlate
Original squamous epithelium	Smooth, pink Indefinitely outlined vessels No change after application of acetic acid	Squamous epithelium
Columnar epithelium	Grapelike structures after application of acetic acid	Columnar epithelium
Transformation zone	Tongues of squamous metaplasia ''Gland openings'' Nabothian cysts	Metaplastic squamous epithelium
White epithelium	White, sharp-bordered lesion visible only after application of acetic acid No vessels visible	From minimal dysplasia to carcinoma in situ
Punctation	Sharp-bordered lesion Red stippling Epithelium whiter after application of acetic acid	From minimal dysplasia to carcinoma in situ
Mosaic	Sharp-bordered lesion Mosaic pattern Epithelium whiter after application of acetic acid	From minimal dysplasia to carcinoma in situ
Hyperkeratosis	White patch Rough surface Already visible before application of acetic acid	Usually hyperkeratosis or parakeratosis; seldom carcinoma in situ or invasive carcinoma
Atypical vessels	Horizontal vessels running parallel to surface Constrictions and dilations of vessels Atypical branching, winding course	From carcinoma in situ to invasive carcinoma

From Stafl, A. (1986). Colposcopy. In D. N. Danforth and J. R. Scott (Eds.), Obstetrics and gynecology (5th ed.) Philadelphia: J. B. Lippincott. Reprinted with permission.

the combination of colposcopy, colposcopically directed multiple punch biopsies, and *endocervical curettage* (ECC) as the diagnostic procedures of choice for abnormal Pap smears, although ECC is contraindicated in pregnancy and other specific clinical situations. The ECC is rapid, has no side effects, is inexpensive, and causes discomfort for only a short period. It can confirm the colposcopist's impression of a negative endocervical canal or can detect neoplasms of the endocervical epithelium or squamous neoplasia if the colposcopic examination was incorrect.

A *cone biopsy (conization)* encompasses the entire squamocolumnar junction and lower portion of the cervical canal. This was previously the primary diagnostic modality for women with abnormal Pap smears. The advantage of the conization procedure is that it removes a large amount of tissue, increasing the likelihood that areas important for diagnosis can be assessed. The entire transformation zone can be examined and invasive cancer ruled out. Conization, however, is an invasive procedure, requiring hospitalization and general anesthesia. Significant side effects are experienced by up to 15 percent of women undergoing the procedure (Richart et al., no date). These include uterine perforation during the procedure, early or delayed hemorrhage, postoperative pelvic infection (Green, 1977), cervical stenosis, and cervical incompetence or infertility (Luesley, Wade-Evans, Mylotte, & Emens, 1985).

Today, colposcopy, biopsy, and endocervical curettage have largely replaced conization as primary diagnostic methods. To guarantee that invasive cancer is not missed, however, conization may be indicated after these other procedures. Richart et al. (no date) recommend conization in the following circumstances:

- A diagnosis of invasive cancer cannot be made or ruled out by endocervical curettage.
- The limits of the lesion cannot be seen and therefore cannot be sampled adequately.

- Invasive cancer is not detected on histologic examination but the cytologist or colposcopist believes that invasive cancer is present.
- The endocervical curettage detects neoplastic epithelium.
- A diagnosis of microinvasion is made on punch biopsy and frankly invasive cancer cannot be ruled out.
- The patient is thought to be unreliable with a high likelihood that she will not return for follow-up.

These authors suggest making the conization therapeutic as well as diagnostic whenever possible to obviate the subsequent need for further surgery when it is not indicated.

INTERVENTION FOR ATYPIA AND CIN

Consultation and Referral. Any woman with cytologic findings showing squamous or endocervical atypia, persistent inflammatory atypia after treatment, suggestions of HPV, or any degree of CIN deserves referral to an experienced colposcopist. The results of further testing determine treatment to be implemented, if any.

Treatment. When atypical Pap smears identify an organism amenable to treatment, treatment should be initiated and the smear then repeated after 3 to 6 months. Further workup or treatment depends on the findings of additional diagnostic testing outlined previously. When CIN has been confirmed by the tests outlined earlier, intervention is warranted. The extent of appropriate treatment for CIN grade I (mild dysplasia) is controversial as many of these lesions regress. Richardson and Lyon (1981) recommend use of condoms for women with CIN. For more than 6 months, they studied 136 women with varying degrees of CIN who received no treatment; none had progression of the disease while condoms were used and 136 showed disease regression. Topical application of retinoids and folic acid is being studied for their effect on precancerous lesions (Lovejoy, 1987).

Treatments for CIN, microinvasive cancer, and frankly invasive cancer include excisional biopsy, conization, hot cautery, cryosurgery, carbon dioxide laser surgery, hysterectomy, radiation, and chemotherapy. A comprehensive nutritional evaluation with nutritional support has been recommended for women being treated for cervical cancer (Orr, Wilson, Bodiford, et al., 1985a, 1985b).

Whether or not conservative treatment is appropriate depends on the extent of the lesion; conservative treatment has been advocated for patients with less than 3 mm of invasion if fertility is desired (Creasman, Fetter, Clarke-Pearson, et al., 1985). Therapy for women with 3 to 5 mm of invasion must be individualized.

Among the conservative treatments suitable for patients with precancerous lesions and CIS, cure rates are usually reported as comparable among electrocautery, cryotherapy, and laser surgery (Deigan, Carmichael, Ohlke, & Karchmar, 1986). Richart et al. (no date) recommend cryosurgery; they point out that electrocautery is painful without anesthesia and results in high rates of cervical stenosis, particularly in older women. Cryosurgery has equivalent results with less morbidity, although in more advanced lesions, such as marked dysplasia and CIS, the failure rate of cryosurgery has been reported to increase (Creasman, Hinshaw, & Clarke-Pearson, 1984; Ostergard, 1980; Wright & Davies, 1981). Most of these persistent lesions, however, can be successfully retreated with a second cryosurgery (Creasman et al., 1984). The carbon dioxide laser can be applied more precisely but is more expensive and time consuming. Cryotherapy leads to vaginal discharge for up to 6 weeks (Winer, 1982); laser therapy may result in vaginal bleeding (Wright, Davies, & Riopelle, 1984). Ultimately, the choice depends on the surgeon's preference and experience.

Both radiation and radical hysterectomy have been advocated for patients with stage IB and IIA cervical cancer (Averette, Girtanner, & Sevin, 1985). Five-year survival rates have been reported as between 87 and 92 percent after either therapy. Recurrences have been documented in patients with stage IB cervical carcinoma; treatment for recurrences includes radiation therapy, pelvic exenteration, systemic chemotherapies, or a combination of these. Survival after recurrences, however, is reported as only between 2 and 9 percent (Burke, Hoskins, Heller, et al., 1987). Adjuvant radiotherapy has been advocated as decreasing recurrence rates in patients with pelvic node metastases treated with radical hysterectomy (Larson, Stringer, Copeland, et al., 1987).

Hysterectomy carries the risks of anesthesia accidents, hemorrhage, and postoperative infection. Radiation therapy can result in bladder symptoms, including frequency, urgency, and dysuria (Farquharson, Shingleton, Sanford, et al., 1987), and bowel and intestinal complications (Jones, 1987).

Patients with stage IIB and III cervical cancer are usually treated with radiation alone. Patients with stage IVA are treated with either high doses of radiation or pelvic exenteration (Perez et al., 1985).

A discussion of the treatment of CIN and cervical cancer in pregnancy is beyond the scope of this chapter. Treatment depends on the extent of disease and gestational age at the time of diagnosis. Generally, early lesions can be followed until pregnancy is over, with vaginal delivery considered safe (Hacker, Berek, Lagasse, et al., 1982).

Follow-Up. Long-term follow-up should be provided for patients treated for CIN or cancer. Benedet, Miller, Nickerson, and Anderson (1987) follow patients treated with cryosurgery for CIN grades I to III without endocervical involvement with repeat Pap smears and colposcopic examination at 3- to 4-month intervals for 1 year posttreatment. If all findings remain negative, patients are then referred to their practitioners for cytologic evaluation at 6-month intervals. Follow-up, of course, depends on institutional or practice protocols.

Teaching and Counseling. All women deserve a complete explanation of screening and diagnostic tests for cervical cancer, including the Pap smear and its follow-up procedures. Results must be carefully explained. The benefit of condoms should be discussed for women with CIN, although the extent of treatment is determined by the findings on colposcopy, biopsy, ECC, and conization, as appropriate. Pre- and postprocedure instructions should be provided, including no douching, intercourse, or tampon use for at least 2 to 3 weeks after treatments, or until discharge or bleeding ceases. Appropriate follow-up appointments must be provided and their importance stressed.

Any diagnosis of cancer—or precancerous lesions—prompts an emotional reaction. Most women with cervical abnormalities can be assured of cure; however, those facing extensive surgeries, radiation, or chemotherapy deserve supportive counseling and possibly referral for more intensive therapy. Family members and significant others should be included in the counseling to the extent the woman wishes.

REFERENCES

Ahern, J. K., & Allen, N. H. (1978, October). Cervical hemangioma: A case report and review of the literature. *Journal of Reproductive Medicine, 21*(4), 228–231.

American Cancer Society. (1987). *Cancer facts and figures 1987.* New York: American Cancer Society.

American College of Obstetricians and Gynecologists. (1984). Cervical cancer screening—How often? *ACOG Newsletter, 28.*

Averette, H. E., Girtanner, R. E., & Sevin, B. (1985, October). Radical hysterectomy for cervical Ca—When is it indicated? *Contemporary Ob/Gyn, 26*(4), 139–155.

Baldwin, K. A., & Goodwin, K. (1985, November/December). The Papanicolaou smear. *Journal of Nurse-Midwifery, 30*(6), 327–332.

Beal, M. W. (1987, March). Understanding cervical cytology. *Nurse Practitioner, 12*(3), 8–22.

Benedet, J. L., Miller, D. M., Nickerson, K. G., & Anderson, G. H. (1987, August). Results of cryosurgical treatment of cervical intraepithelial neoplasia at one, five, and ten years. *American Journal of Obstetrics and Gynecology, 157*(2), 268–273.

Boon, M. E., & Kok, L. P. (1985). Koilocytotic lesions of the cervix: The interrelation of morphometric features, the presence of papillomavirus antigens, and the degree of koilocytosis. *Histopathology, 9*, 751–763.

Briggs, R. M., & Paavonen, J. (1984). Cervical intraepithelial neoplasia. In K. K. Holmes, P.-A. Mårdh, P. F. Sparling, & P. J. Wiesner (Eds.), *Sexually transmitted diseases.* New York: McGraw-Hill.

Brunham, R. C., Paavonen, J., Stevens, C. E., et al. (1984, July 5). Mucopurulent cervicitis—The ignored counterpart in women of urethritis in men. *New England Journal of Medicine, 311*(1), 1–6.

Burke, T. W., Hoskins, W. J., Heller, P. B., et al. (1987, March). Clinical patterns of tumor recurrence after radical hysterectomy in stage 1B cervical carcinoma. *Obstetrics and Gynecology, 69*(3, Part 1), 382–385.

Cardillo, M. R. (1985). Association of human papilloma virus and *Chlamydia trachomatis* infections with incidence of cervical neoplasia. *European Journal of Gynaecologic Oncology, 6*(3), 218–221.

Cartwright, R. A., & Sinson, J. D. (1980, January 12). Carcinoma of penis and cervix [Letter]. *Lancet, 1*(8159), 97.

Cashavelly, B. J. (1987, August). Cervical dysplasia: An overview of current concepts in epidemiology, diagnosis, and treatments. *Cancer Nursing, 10*(4), 199–206.

Chow, W., Greenberg, R. S., & Liff, J. M. (1986, November). Decline in the incidence of carcinoma in situ of the cervix. *American Journal of Public Health, 76*(11), 1322–1324.

Clarke, E. A., & Anderson, T. W. (1979, July 7). Does screening by "Pap" smears help prevent cervical cancer? *Lancet, 2*(8132), 1–4.

Clarke, E. A., Hatcher, J., McKeown-Eyssen, G. E., & Lickrish, G. M. (1985, March 1). Cervical dysplasia: Association with sexual behavior, smoking and oral contraceptive use? *American Journal of Obstetrics and Gynecology, 151*(5), 612–616.

Creasman, W. T., Fetter, B. F., Clarke-Pearson, D. L., et al. (1985, September 15). Management of stage IA carcinoma of the cervix. *American Journal of Obstetrics and Gynecology, 153*(2), 164–172.

Creasman, W. T., Hinshaw, W. M., & Clarke-Pearson, D. L. (1984, February). Cryosurgery in the management of cervical intraepithelial neoplasia. *Obstetrics and Gynecology, 63*(2), 145–149.

Davis, G. L., Hernandez, E., Davis, J. L., & Miyazawa, K. (1987, January). Atypical squamous cells in Papanicolaou smears. *Obstetrics and Gynecology, 69*(1), 43–46.

Deigan, E. A., Carmichael, J. A., Ohlke, I. D., & Karchmar, J. (1986, February). Treatment of cervical intraepithelial neoplasia with electrocautery: A report of 776 cases. *American Journal of Obstetrics and Gynecology, 154*(2), 255–259.

Delke, I. M., Veridiano, N. P., Russell, S., & Tancer, M. L. (1981, June). Brief clinical and laboratory observations: Abnormal cervical cytology in adolescents. *Journal of Pediatrics, 98*(6), 985–987.

Eddy, D. (1980, July/August). ACS report on the cancer-related health checkup. *Ca—A Cancer Journal for Clinicians, 30*(4), 194–223.

Eddy, D. (1981, October). Appropriateness of cervical cancer screening. *Gynecologic Oncology, 12*(2, Part 2), S168–S185.

Edmundson, M. A. (1982). Conditions of the cervix. In L. J. Sonstegard, K. M. Kowalski, & B. Jennings (Eds.), *Women's health: Ambulatory care.* New York: Grune & Stratton.

Farquharson, D. I. M., Shingleton, H. M., Sanford, S. P., et al. (1987, July). The short-term effect of pelvic irradiation for gynecologic malignancies on bladder function. *Obstetrics and Gynecology, 70*(1), 81–84.

Gardner, H. L. (1981). Endometriosis. In H. L. Gardner & R. H. Kaufman (Eds.), *Benign diseases of the vulva and vagina* (2nd ed.). Boston: G. K. Hall.

Graham, S., Priore, R., Graham, M., et al. (1979, November). Genital cancer in wives of penile cancer patients. *Cancer, 44*(5), 1870–1874.

Green, T. H. (1977). *Gynecology: Essentials of clinical practice* (3rd ed.). Boston: Little, Brown.

Gusberg, S. B., DiSaia, P. J., & Deppe, G. (1986). Malignant lesions of the cervix uteri. In D. N. Danforth & J. R. Scott (Eds.), *Obstetrics and gynecology* (5th ed.). Philadelphia: J. B. Lippincott.

Hacker, N. F., Berek, J. S., Lagasse, L. D., et al. (1982, June). Carcinoma of the cervix associated with pregnancy. *Obstetrics and Gynecology, 59*(6), 735–746.

Harris, R. W. C., Brinton, L. A., Cowdell, R. H., et al. (1980, September). Characteristics of women with dysplasia or carcinoma in situ of the cervix uteri. *British Journal of Cancer, 42*(3), 359–369.

Jones, W. B. (1987, October 15). Surgical approaches for advanced or recurrent cancer of the cervix. *Cancer, 60*(8, Suppl.), 2094–2101.

Kessler, I. I. (1977, April). Venereal factors in human cervical cancer. *Cancer, 39*(4, Suppl.), 1912–1918.

Kopan, S., Beckman, E. M., Bigelow, B., et al. (1980, November). The role of colposcopy in the management of cervical intraepithelial neoplasia during pregnancy and postpartum. *Journal of Reproductive Medicine, 25*(5), 279–284.

Koss, L. (1978, February). Nomenclature of precancerous and early cancerous lesions of the uterine cervix. *Contemporary Ob/Gyn, 11*(2), 119–126.

Lancaster, W. D., Castellano, C., Santos, C., et al. (1986, January). Human papillomavirus deoxyribonucleic acid in cervical carci-

noma from primary and metastatic sites. *American Journal of Obstetrics and Gynecology, 154*(1), 115–119.

Larson, D. M., Stringer, C. A., Copeland, L. J., et al. (1987, March). Stage IB cervical carcinoma treated with radical hysterectomy and pelvic lymphadenectomy: Role of adjuvant radiotherapy. *Obstetrics and Gynecology, 69*(3, Part 1), 378–381.

Lovejoy, N. C. (1987, February). Precancerous lesions of the cervix: Personal risk factors. *Cancer Nursing, 10*(1), 2–14.

Luesley, D. M., Wade-Evans, T., Mylotte, M. J., & Emens, J. M. (1985, February). Complications of cone biopsy related to the dimensions of the cone and the influence of prior colposcopic assessment. *British Journal of Obstetrics and Gynaecology, 92*(2), 158–163.

Lyon, J. L., Gardner, J. W., West, D. W., et al. (1983, May). Smoking and carcinoma in situ of the uterine cervix. *American Journal of Public Health, 73*(5), 558–562.

MacGregor, J. E., & Innes, G. (1980, June 7). Carcinoma of penis and cervix. [Letter]. *Lancet, 1*(8180), 1246–1247.

Martínez, I. (1969, October). Relationship of squamous cell carcinoma of the cervix uteri to squamous cell carcinoma of the penis. *Cancer, 24*(4), 777–780.

Meisels, A., Morin, C., & Casas-Cordero, M. (1982). Human papillomavirus infection of the uterine cervix. *International Journal of Gynecological Pathologists, 1*(1), 75–94.

Merrill, J. A. (1986). Benign lesions. In D. N. Danforth & J. R. Scott (Eds.), *Obstetrics and gynecology* (5th ed.). Philadelphia: J. B. Lippincott.

Morell, N. D., Taylor, J. R., Snyder, R. N., et al. (1982, July) False-negative cytology rates in patients in whom invasive cervical cancer subsequently developed. *Obstetrics and Gynecology, 60*(1), 41–45.

Mukherjee, C., Dutta, S. K., & Dawn, C. S. (1984, April). A clinicopathological study of cervical erosion cases. *Journal of the Indian Medical Association, 82*(4), 124–127.

Nasiell, K., Roger, V., & Nasiell, M. (1986, May). Behavior of mild cervical dysplasia during long-term follow-up. *Obstetrics and Gynecology, 67*(5), 665–669.

Nelson, J. H., Averette, H. E., & Richart, R. M. (1984, November/December). Dysplasia, carcinoma in situ, and early invasive cervical carcinoma. *Ca—A Cancer Journal for Clinicians, 34*(6), 306–327.

Noumoff, J. S. (1987, March). Atypia in cervical cytology as a risk factor for intraepithelial neoplasia. *American Journal of Obstetrics and Gynecology, 156*(3), 628–631.

Orr, J. W., Wilson, K., Bodiford, C., et al. (1986a, March 1). Nutritional status of patients with untreated cervical cancer. I. Biochemical and immunologic assessment. *American Journal of Obstetrics and Gynecology, 151*(5), 625–631.

Orr, J. W., Wilson, K., Bodiford, C., et al. (1985b, March 1). Nutritional status of patients with untreated cervical cancer. II. Vitamin assessment. *American Journal of Obstetrics and Gynecology, 151*(5), 632–635.

Ostergard, D. R. (1980, August). Cryosurgical treatment of cervical intraepithelial neoplasia. *Obstetrics and Gynecology, 56*(2), 231–234.

Paavonen, J., Critchlow, C. W., DeRouen, T., et al. (1986, March). Etiology of cervical inflammation. *American Journal of Obstetrics and Gynecology, 154*(3), 556–564.

Paavonen, J., Vesterinen, E., Meyer, B., & Saksela, E. (1982, June). Colposcopic and histologic findings in cervical chlamydial infection. *Obstetrics and Gynecology, 59*(6), 712–714.

Papanicolaou, G. N., & Traut, H. F. (1941, August). Diagnostic value of vaginal smears in carcinoma of the uterus. *American Journal of Obstetrics and Gynecology, 42*(2), 193–205.

Parkin, D. M., Nguyen-Dinh, X., & Day, N. E. (1985, February). The impact of screening on the incidence of cervical cancer in England and Wales. *British Journal of Obstetrics and Gynaecology, 92*(2), 150–157.

Perez, C. A., DiSaia, P. J., Knapp, R. C., & Young, R. C. (1985). Gynecologic tumors. In V. T. DaVita, S. Hellman, & S. A. Rosenberg (Eds.), *Cancer: Principles and practice of oncology.* Philadelphia: J. B. Lippincott.

Pritchard, J. A., MacDonald, P. C., & Gant, N. F. (1985). *Williams Obstetrics* (17th ed.). East Norwalk, CT: Appleton-Century-Crofts.

Purola, E., & Paavonen, J. (1982). Routine cytology as a diagnostic aid in chlamydial cervicitis. *Scandinavian Journal of Infectious Diseases, 32*(Suppl.), 55–58.

Raymond, C. A. (1987, May 8). Cervical dysplasia upturn worries gynecologists, health officials. *Journal of the American Medical Association, 257*(18), 2397–2398.

Richardson, A. C., & Lyon, J. B. (1981, August 15). Effect of condom use on squamous cell cervical intraepithelial neoplasia. *American Journal of Obstetrics and Gynecology, 140*(8), 909–913.

Richart, R. M. (1979, September). Screening techniques for cervical neoplasia. *Clinical Obstetrics and Gynecology, 22*(3), 701–710.

Richart, R. M. (1981, February 7). Current concepts in obstetrics and gynecology: The patient with an abnormal Pap smear—Screening techniques and management. *New England Journal of Medicine, 302*(6), 332–334.

Richart, R. M. (1987, October 15). Causes and management of cervical intraepithelial neoplasia. *Cancer, 60*(8, Suppl.), 1951–1959.

Richart, R. M., & Barron, B. A. (1969, October 1). A follow-up study of patients with cervical dysplasia. *American Journal of Obstetrics and Gynecology, 105*(3), 386–393.

Richart, R. M., & Barron, B. A. (1981, March 1). Screening strategies for cervical cancer and cervical intraepithelial neoplasia. *Cancer, 47*(5, Suppl.), 1176–1181.

Richart, R. M., Crum, C. P., & Townsend, D. E. (no date). Workup of the patient with an abnormal Papanicolaou smear. Unpublished manuscript.

Romney, S. L., Palan, P. R., Duttagupta, C., et al. (1981, December 15). Retinoids and the prevention of cervical dysplasias. *American Journal of Obstetrics and Gynecology, 141*(8), 890–894.

Selim, M. A., & Shalodi, A. D. (1985, July). Benign diseases of the uterine cervix. *Postgraduate Medicine, 78*(1), 141–150.

Singer, A. (1975, February). Uterine cervix from adolescence to the menopause. *British Journal of Obstetrics and Gynaecology, 82*(2), 81–99.

Singer, A., Reid, B. L., & Coppleson, M. (1976, September 1). A hypothesis: The role of a high-risk male in the etiology of cervical carcinoma. *American Journal of Obstetrics and Gynecology, 126*(1), 110–115.

Smith, P. G., Kinlen, L. J., White, G. C., et al. (1980, March). Mortality of wives of men dying with cancer of the penis. *British Journal of Cancer, 41*(3), 422–428.

Smotkin, D., Berek, J. S., Fu, Y. S., et al. (1986, August). Human papillomavirus deoxyribonucleic acid in adenocarcinoma and adenosquamous carcinoma of the uterine cervix. *Obstetrics and Gynecology, 68*(2), 241–244.

Spitzer, M., Krumholz, B. A., Chernys, A. E., et al. (1987, May). Comparative utility of repeat Papanicolaou smears, cervicography, and colposcopy in the evaluation of atypical Papanicolaou smears. *Obstetrics and Gynecology, 69*(5), 731–735.

Stafl, A. (1981, April 1). Cervicography: A new method for cervical cancer detection. *American Journal of Obstetrics and Gynecology, 139*(7), 815–825.

Stafl, A. (1986). Colposcopy. In D. N. Danforth & J. R. Scott (Eds.), *Obstetrics and gynecology* (5th ed.). Philadelphia: J. B. Lippincott.

Swan, S. H., & Brown, W. L. (1979, July 5). Vasectomy and cancer of the cervix. [Letter]. *New England Journal of Medicine, 301*(1), 46.

Tawa, K., Forsythe, A., Cove, J. K., et al. (1988, February). A comparison of the Papanicolaou smear and the cervigram: Sensitivity, specificity, and cost analysis. *Obstetrics and Gynecology, 71*(2), 229–235.

Terris, M., Wilson, F., & Nelson, J. H. (1973, December 15). Relation of circumcision to cancer of the cervix. *American Journal of Obstetrics and Gynecology, 117*(8), 1056–1066.

Thomas, D. B. (1973, July). An epidemiologic study of carcinoma in situ and squamous dysplasia of the uterine cervix. *American Journal of Epidemiology, 98*(1), 10–28.

Vonka, V., Kǎnka, J., Hirsch, I., et al. (1984a, January). Prospective study on the relationship between cervical neoplasia and herpes simplex type-2 virus. II. Herpes simplex type-2 antibody presence in sera taken at enrollment. *International Journal of Cancer, 33*(1), 61–66.

Vonka, V., Kǎnka, J., Jelinek, J., et al. (1984b, January). Prospective study on the relationship between cervical neoplasia and herpes simplex type-2 virus. I. Epidemiological characteristics. *International Journal of Cancer, 33*(1), 49–60.

Winer, W. K. (1982, September). Laser treatment of cervical neoplasia. *American Journal of Nursing, 82*(9), 1384–1387.

Winkelstein, W., Shillitoe, E. J., Brand, R., & Johnson, K. K. (1984, January). Reviews and commentary: Further comments on cancer of the uterine cervix, smoking, and herpesvirus infection. *American Journal of Epidemiology, 119*(1), 1–7.

Wright, V. C., & Davies, E. M. (1981, June). Conservative management of cervical intraepithelial neoplasia: The use of cryosurgery and the carbon dioxide laser. *British Journal of Obstetrics and Gynaecology, 88*(6), 663–668.

Wright, V. C., Davies, E., & Riopelle, M. (1984, November 15). Laser cylindrical excision to replace conization. *American Journal of Obstetrics and Gynecology, 150*(6), 704–709.

Yobs, A. R., Swanson, R. A., & Lamotte, L. C., Jr. (1985, February). Laboratory reliability of the Papanicolaou smear. *Obstetrics and Gynecology, 65*(2), 235–244.

Žarković, G. (1985). Alterations of cervical cytology and steroid contraceptive use. *International Journal of Epidemiology, 14*(3), 369–377.

zur Hausen, H. (1982, December 18). Human genital cancer: Synergism between two virus infections or synergism between a virus infection and initiating events? *Lancet, 2*(8311), 1370–1372.

14

The Uterus

Virginia Jackson

The uterus is a unique organ. Its musculature has the potential for tremendous growth, and its lining is shed and regenerated many times during a woman's lifetime. Disorders of this organ are largely treatable when diagnosis is prompt. Screening for uterine disorders is an important component of well-woman gynecologic care.

This chapter reviews the anatomy and physiology of the uterus and discusses abnormalities and pathology of the uterine body including congenital defects, myomas, endometritis, and cancer. In each section, the clinical presentation and diagnosis of the particular condition and the treatment options are outlined. Guidelines regarding the role of the primary woman's health care practitioner are offered, although this role varies with the specific problem, its severity, and clinic or practice protocols and consultation arrangements. Disorders of the uterine cervix are discussed in Chapter 13.

ANATOMY AND PHYSIOLOGY

The uterus is a pear-shaped muscular organ located between the rectum and the bladder. Its interior is hollow, flat, and triangular. The muscular uterine wall is composed of three layers: the innermost layer or endometrium is thin and mucosal; the middle layer or myometrium is thick and smooth; the outer layer or peritoneum is serosal.

In a mature, nulliparous woman the uterus is approximately 3 in. (6.6 cm) long. The *fundus*, or top of the uterus, is above the insertion of the fallopian tubes and measures 2 to $2\frac{1}{2}$ in. (4.4 to 5.5 cm) wide. The *corpus*, or body of the uterus, gradually narrows to the isthmus, where the *cervix* begins. At this level the uterus is only 1 in. (2.2 cm) wide. The cervix extends into the vagina about 1 to $1\frac{1}{2}$ in. (2.2 to 3.3 cm). The cervical *os* is the opening of the uterine cavity. In a nulliparous woman, the os appears as a small dimple; in a parous woman, it is slitlike. After childbirth, the uterus is slightly larger in all dimensions. After menopause, it is smaller.

During bimanual examination the normal uterus can be found in the midline of the pelvis, feels symmetric in shape, and is movable in all directions. The uterus is normally smooth, nontender, and firm. The entire corpus may not be palpable, depending on the uterine position. Consequently, it may be necessary to evaluate it only with respect

to a part, although sometimes more of it can be appreciated rectally. Abnormal findings include asymmetry, enlargement in a nongravid woman, lateral displacement, limited mobility or fixation, masses, induration, nodularity, or tenderness to touch or movement (Wallach, Hammond, Goldfarb, & Kempers, 1983).

Physiologically, the uterine endometrium has been described as "remarkable" because of its ability to shed and regenerate on a continuous basis (Pritchard, MacDonald, & Gant, 1985, p. 65). During each menstrual cycle, the endometrium undergoes several phases in response to hormonal changes associated with the cycle. The following discussion of these phases is adapted from Pritchard et al. (1985, pp. 67–69).

The four phases of the endometrial cycle are proliferation, secretion, premenstrual ischemia, and menstruation. The proliferative and secretory phases can be divided further into early and late stages.

The endometrium proliferates under the influence of estrogen, primarily 17 β-estradiol. In the early proliferative stage, the endometrium is thin with narrow, tubular glands. Mitosis of glands occurs during the proliferative stage. In the late proliferative stage, the endometrium becomes somewhat thicker secondary to glandular hyperplasia and an increase in stromal ground substance. The proliferative phase varies in length among women, whereas the secretory phase is constant. The early secretory phase of the endometrial cycle occurs after ovulation, primarily under the influence of progesterone. In the absence of ovulation, proliferation continues, leading eventually to endometrial hyperplasia. In the secretory stage, the endometrium becomes slightly thinner and three zones are delineated: the basal zone, closest to the myometrium; the compact or superficial zone, just beneath the surface; and the spongy, or intermediate, zone. The late secretory phase is characterized by extreme vascularity and hypertrophic changes of the stromal cells. This phase is ideal for implantation. Premenstrually, with regression of the corpus luteum (see Chapter 1) and a decrease in estrogen and progesterone secretion, the framework of the stroma in the superficial zone disintegrates and the endometrial thickness decreases; the endometrial stroma are infiltrated by leukocytes, giving the endometrium an inflammatory appearance. Four to twenty-four hours before menstruation, vasoconstriction occurs. During the menstrual phase, the endometrium is shed.

CONGENITAL ABNORMALITIES

At 5 to 6 weeks of embryonic development the müllerian ducts appear. These duplicate structures are the precursors of the fallopian tubes, uterus, and upper vagina. At the end of 3 months of fetal life, distinct muscle and connective tissue layers are seen in the uterus; at the end of the sixth month, endometrium appears. Deviations in the normal fusion of the müllerian duct buds can result in duplication of all or part of the uterus, cervix, and/or upper vagina. There are degrees of fusion failure. As fusion of the ducts begins in the most caudal portion and extends upward, incomplete or partial fusion results in duplication of the upper uterus. The most common congenital müllerian abnormality—septate uterus—results from failure of absorption of the medial aspects of the fused müllerian system. Deviations also can occur in duct development and growth, resulting in an absent or incomplete uterus. Uterine deformities may be a result of teratogenesis.

Prevalence

The prevalence of congenital abnormalities of the uterus is difficult to determine as most are completely asymptomatic. It is estimated that müllerian duct defects occur in about one in 700 women. Of these, 80 percent are septate uteri (Farber, Noumoff, Freedman, & Oberkotter, 1984). Most cases of uterine anomaly present with a complaint of infertility or reproductive failure, although some may cause primary amenorrhea, thus presenting as a problem during adolescence.

Classification

Uterine congenital defects include the septate uterus, the bicornuate uterus, the uterus didelphys, the absent uterus, the unicornuate uterus, and the T-shaped uterus (Figs. 14–1 through 14–5).

Septate Uterus. The uterine septum that results from failure of absorption of the medial aspects of the fused müllerian system is composed of fibromuscular tissue similar to myometrium but more collagenous with little vascular supply. The septum can be incomplete and limited to the fundus, or complete, involving the upper and lower uterine segment (Fig. 14–1). On pelvic examination the uterus is grossly normal. The woman usually presents with a complaint of two or more second-trimester spontaneous abortions not explainable by other factors. These often occur in the latter part of the second trimester.

Although diagnosis of a septate uterus may be suggested by ultrasound, sonograms may not differentiate this condition from bicornuate uterus (Romero & Horgan, 1985, p. 267). Diagnosis can be further aided by a hysterosalpingogram (HSG), but this too may be imprecise. Firm diagnosis may depend on laparoscopy and hysteroscopy (Siegler, 1983, p. 150). Treatment, necessary only when a term pregnancy cannot be achieved, is surgical correction—metroplasty. After metroplasty, a repeat HSG should be done after 6 months with a laparoscopy and hysteroscopy after 1 year, if the woman has not become pregnant, to assess the success of the procedure and rule out adhesions. Traditional abdominal metroplasty carries a 5 to 10 percent rate of infertility secondary to complications of the surgery (Farber et al., 1984). After the procedure, cesarean section is the recommended mode of delivery, although the dehiscence rate of the uterine scar is not known. Recently, septal incision has been performed by operative hysteroscopy

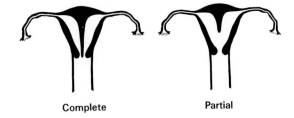

Figure 14–1. Septate uterus. *(From Buttram, V. C. & Gibbons, W. E. [1979, July]. Müllerian anomalies: A proposed classification [an analysis of 144 cases]. Fertility and Sterility, 32[1]. Reprinted with permission.)*

(Daly, Walters, Soto-Albors, & Riddick, 1983); this eliminates the need for cesarean section and has fewer operative complications.

Bicornuate Uterus and Uterus Didelphys. Bicornuate uterus and uterus didelphys (Figs. 14–2 and 14–3) result from incomplete or absent fusion of müllerian ducts. A bicornuate uterus is one with two separate cavities; a mildly bicornuate uterus is also called an arcuate uterus. On bimanual examination, the uterus may be palpated as large and heart-shaped, with an external indentation in the midline of the fundus. Sonogram may be useful but may not be able to differentiate a bicornuate uterus from a septate uterus. Confirmatory diagnosis may be made by HSG, but HSG may also confuse the bicornuate uterus with the septate uterus. Laparoscopy may become necessary (Siegler, 1983, p. 150).

Classically, the bicornuate uterus is associated with prematurity, abnormal fetal presentation, and late second-trimester spontaneous abortion in first pregnancies. Subsequent pregnancies often achieve a longer gestation but continue to carry a risk of malpresentation and/or prematurity. Surgical intervention is rarely necessary.

Uterus didelphys is the presence of a double uterus, that is, two separate structures. It can be identified by ultrasound and is frequently associated with a double or septate vagina, identifiable on pelvic examination. When the vagina is normal, however, one of the uterine structures is obstructed and severe dysmenorrhea may result. This may occur shortly after menarche and cause the adolescent to seek gynecologic care. A lateral vaginal bulging may be seen or felt on pelvic examination (Altchek, 1985, p. 57). Obstruction requires intervention, although generally there is no indication for treatment for a didelphic uterus as its obstetric risk is low.

Absent or Unicornuate Uterus. Uterine *agenesis* or *dysgenesis* is the failure of duct development and growth. Agen-

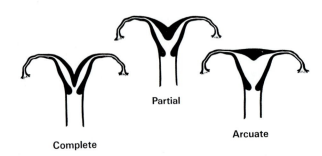

Figure 14–2. Bicornuate uterus. *(From Buttram, V. C. & Gibbons, W. E. [1979, July]. Müllerian anomalies: A proposed classification [an analysis of 144 cases]. Fertility and Sterility, 32[1]. Reprinted with permission.)*

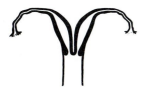

Figure 14–3. Uterus didelphys. *(From Buttram, V. C. & Gibbons, W. E. [1979, July]. Müllerian anomalies: A proposed classification [an analysis of 144 cases]. Fertility and Sterility, 32[1]. Reprinted with permission.)*

esis or bilateral failure leads to a blind vaginal pouch with a variety of müllerian remnants, although vaginal agenesis may coexist (Fig. 14–4). Müllerian remnants may have functional endometrial tissue that causes cyclic pain. The ovaries and fallopian tubes typically are normal. Dysgenesis refers to unilateral duct failure and results in a unicornuate uterus (Fig. 14–5).

The absence of the uterus causes primary amenorrhea and is easily identified at the time of pelvic examination. When no vagina is present, uterine absence can be appreciated on rectal examination. Sonogram is not always reliable for diagnosis because stool and gas in the rectum may be misinterpreted as a uterus with obstructed menstrual flow (Altchek, 1985, p. 47). Laparoscopy is indicated when the diagnosis is not clear. Karyotyping is needed to clarify diagnosis and to rule out the presence of the Y chromosome. Obviously, uterine agenesis precludes pregnancy; the major aim of its treatment is the establishment of a functional vagina. A woman can accomplish this through a carefully taught, self-administered regimen in which she applies gradually increasing pressure to the urogenital dimple between the urethra and rectum, with dilators if necessary. Intensive family support and counseling have been recommended to assist women utilizing this therapy (Rock, Reeves, Retto, et al., 1983). A vagina can be created surgically for women unwilling or unable to attempt dilation or when dilation fails (Altchek 1985, p. 49).

A unicornuate uterus may sometimes be felt lateral to the midline or identified on sonogram. It may be associated with an absent kidney on the contralateral side (Siegler, 1983) and with a number of adverse pregnancy outcomes including malpresentation, incompetent cervix, and small-for-gestational-age infants. There is no treatment for such a defect. Increased vigilance should be maintained during pregnancy to provide the best outcome.

A variation of the unicornuate uterus is a uterus with a

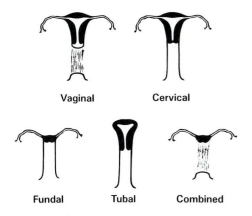

Figure 14–4. Müllerian agenesis. *(From Buttram, V. C. & Gibbons, W. E. [1979, July]. Müllerian anomalies: A proposed classification [an analysis of 144 cases]. Fertility and Sterility, 32[1]. Reprinted with permission.)*

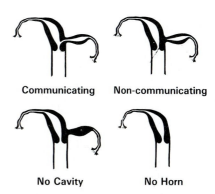

Communicating   Non-communicating

No Cavity   No Horn

Figure 14–5. Uterine dysgenesis—Unicornuate uterus with and without rudimentary horn. *(From Buttram, V. C. & Gibbons, W. E. [1979, July]. Müllerian anomalies: A proposed classification [an analysis of 144 cases]. Fertility and Sterility, 32[1]. Reprinted with permission.)*

rudimentary horn (Fig. 14–5). If this horn has an endometrial cavity and does not communicate with the uterine cavity, a hematoma develops one to several cycles after menarche, the woman has severe cyclic pain, and an abdominal pelvic mass is palpable. Treatment is excision of the horn (Buttram & Gibbons, 1979).

T-Shaped Uterus. A T-shaped uterus (Fig. 14–6) is associated with diethylstilbestrol (DES) exposure in utero. This defect, detectable on sonogram, may interfere with childbearing. See Chapter 18 for more discussion of this and other abnormalities identified with DES exposure.

Management

Diagnosis. Medical consultation should be sought for women with a history of repeated reproductive failure suggestive of uterine anomaly, with abnormal findings on bimanual examination as outlined earlier, or with delayed menarche. Chapter 21 provides a diagnostic framework for adolescents presenting with amenorrhea and describes the role of the progestin or estrogen-plus-progestin challenge in the amenorrheic adolescent.

HSG is the single most useful diagnostic procedure in the investigation of uterine anomalies, although sonogram can demonstrate some of these abnormalities. Few false-positive or false-negative results were demonstrated in a recent blinded study of 89 women whose sonograms were compared with other diagnostic modalities (Nicolini, Bellotti, Bonazzi, et al., 1987). Laparoscopy may be necessary to distinguish septate from bicornuate uteri. Women with congenital uterine malformations have an increased incidence of renal anomalies, although renal effects have not

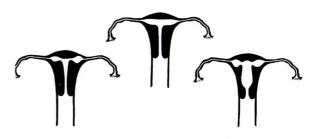

Figure 14–6. DES exposure: T-shaped uterus. *(From Buttram, V. C. & Gibbons, W. E. [1979, July]. Müllerian anomalies: A proposed classification [an analysis of 144 cases]. Fertility and Sterility, 32[1]. Reprinted with permission.)*

been demonstrated with anomalies caused by DES exposure. Intravenous pyelogram (IVP) or sonographic evaluation of the renal fossae is indicated in these women (Romero & Horgan, 1985; Siegler, 1983).

Intervention. Whether specific interventions are necessary in the presence of uterine congenital anomalies depends on the specific abnormality, existing complications, and a woman's plans for childbearing. Interventions range from careful monitoring during childbearing to surgical correction of defects. Their indications have been discussed earlier under each anomaly. The primary care practitioner may be involved in providing contraception for women with anomalies and, of course, in meeting their educational and counseling needs.

CONTRACEPTION. The intrauterine device (IUD) is contraindicated as a method of birth control in the presence of structural uterine defects. The diaphragm may be difficult to fit if the uterine anomaly is accompanied by vaginal or cervical defects.

TEACHING AND COUNSELING. Prior to diagnosis, women with suspected uterine anomalies need preparation for the diagnostic workup. Each test must be explained and informed consent obtained. Once diagnosis is confirmed, counseling about the nature of the defect with prognosis for future pregnancies and prospective management should be given (Daly et al., 1983; Farber et al., 1984). Women may need extensive support to adjust to their diagnosis. Abnormalities may be detected during adolescence and interfere with the development of a positive body image. Diagnosis may follow the loss of a pregnancy and may exacerbate the grieving process. In some cases, an anomaly may preclude childbearing and requires acceptance of this reality. The possible need for intensive counseling should always be considered and appropriate referrals made whenever necessary.

MYOMAS

Myomas (or leiomyomata) are the most common tumors of the female pelvis. Although called fibroids, they actually arise from muscle cells. Myomas are almost always benign. Their etiology is unknown, although evidence suggests that estrogen, particularly estradiol, and possibly growth hormone or human placental lactogen (hPL) may cause tumor growth (Buttram & Reiter, 1981).

Uterine myomas arise from the proliferation of smooth muscle cells and all begin in the same part of the uterus—the central area of the myometrium. Over time, however, the location of the myoma may change. Myomas are thus identified by name according to location (at the time of diagnosis) as follows (Fig. 14–7):

- *Interstitial (intramural):* staying within the uterine wall as it grows; most common form of myoma
- *Submucosal:* protruding into the uterine cavity; accounting for 5 percent of all myomas
- *Subserosal (Subperitoneal):* bulging through the outer uterine wall
- *Intraligamentous:* within the broad ligament
- *Pedunculated:* any myoma that has developed a thin pedicle attachment to a uterine base
- *Parasitic:* completely extruding from the uterus with a developed accessory blood supply

Interstitial myomas have a rounded shape as they are subjected to relatively equal pressure from all sides. As the uterus contracts, however, the originally interstitial tumors are squeezed either inward or outward from their central location. Myomas that are pushed into the uterine cavity are termed *submucosal.* Those that migrate in the opposite direction and appear on the outer surface of the uterus are called *subserosal.* As myomas migrate, they change in shape, becoming irregular; their blood supply within their connective attachment may become quite thin and attenuated, resulting in pedunculation. Myomas extruded into the broad ligament may develop an entirely new blood supply within the ligament, becoming parasitic. Parasitic and pedunculated myomas are difficult to distinguish from ovarian masses.

Prevalence

In the United States, it is estimated that myomas occur in 10 percent of white and 30 percent of black women by the age of 30. By age 50, this prevalence increases to 30 and 50 percent, respectively (Wallach et al., 1983), although the prevalence in postmenopausal women is lower, as preexisting myomas often regress after menopause while new myomas do not develop.

Clinical Presentation

The majority of uterine myomas cause no discomfort or awareness of their existence; however, myomas can be the cause of common gynecologic complaints including abnormal bleeding, pain, and pressure (Appuzzio, Pelosi, Kaminetzky, & Louria, 1985). It has been estimated that 20 to 50 percent of myomas cause symptoms (Buttram & Reiter, 1981).

When abnormal bleeding occurs secondary to a myoma, it tends to be with menses (menorrhagia or hypermenorrhea). Commonly, concern about the increase in amount and duration of menstrual flow prompts a gynecologic visit. Submucous and interstitial myomas are usually implicated. Such myomas increase endometrial surface area, impair myometrial contraction around spiral arterioles (Green, 1977, p. 389), and compress the venous plexi of the adjacent myometrium and endometrium (Buttram & Reiter, 1981).

Intermenstrual bleeding (metrorrhagia) or irregular bleeding cycles usually do not result from myomas. Although myomas may be present, simply because of their prevalence, this type of bleeding should prompt an investigation for other causes (Goldfarb, 1984). See Chapter 21.

Pressure symptoms result from large myomas and/or myomas located on the cervix or near the bladder or rectosigmoid colon. Those near the bladder may cause bladder pressure, urinary frequency, or incontinence. Myomas near the rectosigmoid colon may cause rectal pressure or constipation (Buttram & Reiter, 1981).

Pain is not typical of myomas; it may signify a coexisting pelvic problem. When it does occur, submucous and interstitial myomas are often the cause. The pain usually is crampy and felt with menses. It may be caused by pressure on the small bowel (Green, 1977, p. 349). If acute, it may be a result of torsion of a pedunculated myoma or sudden degeneration (Dawood, 1984; Ranney & Frederick, 1979).

Complications

Uterine myomas are implicated in some cases of infertility, although their precise effect is controversial. Myomas aris-

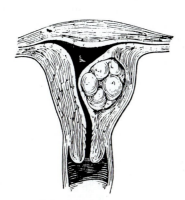

Submucous Leiomyomas

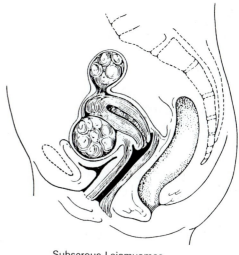

Subserous Leiomyomas

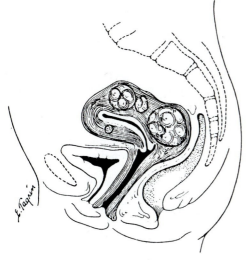

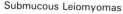

Intramural Leiomyomas

Figure 14–7. Leiomyomata uteri (fibroids). *(From Kistner, R. W. [1986]. Gynecology: Principles and practice. Chicago: Year Book Medical Publishers, p. 226. Reprinted with permission.)*

ing from or near the cervix lead to difficulty in sperm capture or travel and may be obstructive during pregnancy. Occasionally a myoma interferes with the contractile mechanisms at the uterotubal junction or obstructs the intramural portion of the fallopian tube. Submucous myomas can interrupt the vascularity of the endometrium, lead to atrophy or ulceration of the endometrium at the site of the myoma, and distort or elongate the endometrial cavity, thus impeding implantation (Buttram & Reiter, 1981). Depending on size and location, some myomas may present obstructive problems during pregnancy or compel the fetus to assume a malpresentation.

Degenerative changes in myomas—identifiable on sonogram—may occur over time. Often, calcification of myomas is seen in older, postmenopausal women. This can cause pressure or uterine prolapse. Red or carneous degeneration most often occurs during pregnancy and is part of the differential diagnosis for acute abdominal pain in pregnancy. In this situation the myoma undergoes rapid growth under stimulation from estrogen, outgrowing the available blood supply. Vascular impairment results in infarction. The resultant uterine irritability may lead to pain, sponta-

neous abortion, or premature labor (Benson, 1983). Low-grade fever and moderate leukocytosis may be present with red degeneration. Symptoms usually abate within a few days, and, in the absence of premature labor, treatment is confined to analgesia (Pritchard et al., 1985, p. 689).

A very rare complication is the development of a gas abscess within a degenerated myoma. This occurs when organisms such as coliforms, streptococci, or staphylococci enter a degenerated myoma. Gas formation can be seen on x-ray; however, if the gas abscess is unrecognized and untreated, it can rupture into the peritoneal cavity (Green, 1977, p. 387).

Obstruction of omental vessels is an infrequent complication of myomas. Occurring with parasitic myomas, the obstruction may lead to ascites. Postpartum bleeding may also occur secondary to myomas (Buttram & Reiter, 1981).

Whether sarcomatous degeneration or the development of malignant change in a myoma can occur is controversial. Some practitioners insist that a malignant growth was never, in fact, a myoma. Others, however, cite malignant occurrence in some patients, with sudden rapid growth of tumors that had been followed without change for many years. The majority of reports put the incidence of malignant development at about 0.5 percent (Buttram & Reiter, 1981; Green, 1977, p. 387; Wallach et al., 1983).

Differential Diagnosis

Suspicion that a myoma exists may be based on reported symptoms or, more commonly, physical examination findings. Differential diagnosis includes pregnancy, [missed menses spontaneous abortion,] endometriosis, adenomyosis, uterine anomaly, adnexal mass, endometrial hyperplasia, endometrial polyps, endometrial or ovarian cancer, and pelvic inflammatory disease.

Management

Data Collection

HISTORY. Reported pelvic or bladder pressure or heavy or prolonged bleeding with menses should alert the practitioner to the possibility of a myoma, especially in the premenopausal woman over 30. Most myomas, however, are asymptomatic. If a woman knows that a myoma had been diagnosed previously, information should be obtained about its duration, the modalities utilized in diagnosis, prior size and possible growth, associated symptoms, and any treatment undergone and its results.

PHYSICAL EXAMINATION. Myomas are usually recognized through bimanual pelvic examination. Uterine irregularity and/or enlargement with unusually firm, mobile, nontender, smooth nodules is characteristic. If the uterus is soft, pregnancy must be suspected. Fixation or tenderness during the exam should alert the examiner to the possibility of infection or endometriosis. Ovarian dysfunction or cancer should be suspected if the adnexae cannot be distinguished clearly (Carlson, Allegra, Day, & Wittliff, 1984; Wallach et al., 1983).

LABORATORY TESTING. Laboratory studies and procedures help both in making the diagnosis and in evaluating the possible consequences of myomas. Their implementation is based on whether a myoma is symptomatic, the specific symptoms present, and the need to rule out other conditions. The first time an enlarged uterus is palpated, a Pap test must be obtained and a pregnancy test performed. A baseline blood count (CBC) can help to rule out an infectious process and assess the progressive severity of anemia resulting from blood loss. An erythrocyte sedimentation rate (ESR) also helps to rule out infection. If pressure symptoms are present, a urinalysis and culture and sensitivity are warranted. Referral for an IVP may be considered to rule out structural urinary tract problems.

A sonogram may be of use in baseline measurement of myomas and remeasurement in 3 to 4 months (Gross, Silver, & Jaffe, 1983), although overall performance of ultrasound has been found to be inferior to clinical examination (O'Brien, Buck, & Nash, 1984). Examination, however, may miss masses smaller than 5 cm. If a woman's symptoms suggest a myoma, but none is felt, a sonogram is indicated (Wallach et al., 1983). A hysteroscopy is useful for confirmation and visualization of myomas within the uterine cavity (Neuwirth, 1983) and to evaluate other possible etiologies for bleeding. It is indicated in the presence of serious clinical problems such as menorrhagia and anemia.

Intervention

TREATMENT. Most women with myomas can be followed quite conservatively (Buttram & Reiter, 1981; Wallach et al., 1983). Initially, the woman is seen twice, 3 months apart, to check growth, and then every 6 months. Documentation should include when the myoma appeared, how long it has been followed, and how rapidly it is growing. Overall, management is based largely on the severity of symptoms and plans for childbearing or contraception. Any anemia should be corrected. The use of aspirin should be discouraged for women with excessive bleeding because of its effect on platelets.

If heavy and prolonged bleeding persists, gynecologic referral is warranted. Rapid growth (particularly after or at menopause), difficulty in adnexal palpation, and any tenderness or fixation are causes for referral for laparoscopic examination. If the uterus is 12 to 14 weeks size or larger, and the woman is symptomatic, intervention is indicated. A dilation and curettage may provide temporary relief, but is not curative. There is some suggestion that progesterone can reduce the size of myomas. A newer treatment involves gonadotropin-releasing hormone (GnRH) analogs that can shrink myomas by inhibiting ovulation and inducing pseudomenopause. These agents can be administered subcutaneously or intranasally, with the latter route demonstrating less severe menopausal side effects such as hot flushes (Maheux, Lemay, & Merat, 1987). Although myomas grow back when treatment is stopped, long-term therapy is not recommended because of the adverse effects on bones and blood vessels of hypoestrogenicity. The most likely use of GnRH analogs in the treatment of myomas will be to shrink tumors preoperatively when surgery is necessary.

If the potential for childbearing is to be preserved, a myomectomy is the surgical intervention of choice. A myomectomy may also be indicated in some cases of infertility, although surgery may substitute one cause of infertility for another, as scar tissue, adhesions, or Asherman's syndrome may result (Berkley, DeCherney, & Polan, 1983; Wallach et al., 1983). Indications for myomectomy in women with otherwise unexplained infertility are not clear, but successful results have been demonstrated (Babaknia, Rock, & Jones, 1978; Garcia & Tureck, 1984; Rosenfeld, 1986), although controlled studies are lacking. Before surgery in anemic women, a progestational agent such as Depo-Provera may be used to render the patient amenorrheic. Anemia can then be treated with iron supplementation and nutritional intervention.

Fifteen percent of patients have recurrence of some symptoms after a myomectomy, and 15 to 30 percent require reoperation (Babaknia et al., 1978). Febrile morbidity is higher with myomectomy than with hysterectomy (Ranney & Frederick, 1979; Wallach et al., 1983). Myomectomy is especially difficult if multiple myomas are to be removed; it is a lengthier procedure and predisposes to more intraoperative bleeding. Most practitioners consider the uterine scarring from a myomectomy to be an indication for future cesarean delivery.

Some physicians perform hysteroscopic resection of myomas for pedunculated submucous myomas, which can be shaved off and brought through the cervical canal (Richart & Neuwirth, 1985). Advantages include the maintenance of uterine integrity with a chance for subsequent labor and vaginal delivery. Contraindications to the hysteroscopic approach include a large pelvic mass, adnexal tumor, malignant or premalignant tissue, and a uterus so large that inspection and control of distension from bleeding during and after surgery would be difficult.

In some circumstances, hysterectomy is the treatment of choice for myomas. Although a major operation, hysterectomy is very common in the United States. More than 400,000 are performed every year in women aged 15 to 44 (Galask, 1985). There has been considerable controversy among practitioners regarding justifiable indications for hysterectomy. Data from the Collaborative Review of Sterilization show that only about one half of the preoperative diagnostic indications are amenable to pathologic confirmation; of these, 80 percent are confirmed (Lee, Dicker, Rubin, & Ory, 1984). The use of hysterectomy in the treatment of myomas is reserved for women who do not desire future pregnancies or women with severe symptoms.

CONTRACEPTION. The contraceptive needs of women with diagnosed myomas must be met. Intrauterine devices are not advisable as such devices may cause or compound the problem of blood loss. Their effectiveness may be reduced in women with distortions of the uterine cavity (Buttram & Reiter, 1981). Because uterine myomas are sensitive to estrogen, oral contraceptives may contribute to their growth and increase the occurrence of symptoms. A woman with a myoma who takes oral contraceptives requires a bimanual vaginal examination every 6 months. The location of myomas may make the diaphragm uncomfortable and this method may exacerbate pressure symptoms. It also has been recommended that women with known myomas not receive estrogen at menopause (Wallach et al., 1983), although this recommendation is not universally accepted.

THE PRIMARY CARE ROLE. The role of the primary woman's health practitioner in management of the care of a woman with a myoma varies with the tumor's severity, related symptomatology, and institutional or practice protocols. Certainly, the primary care provider can follow the woman with a newly or previously diagnosed myoma that exists for a period without growth or symptoms. Rapid growth or the development of symptoms, including infertility, warrants referral for further assessment and possible treatment. In some institutions, protocols require referral anytime a previously undiagnosed myoma is suspected. Of course, if the practitioner has any doubt about the diagnosis, consultation or referral should be initiated. The extent to which diagnostic tests, such as sonograms, can be ordered before referral varies with protocols and practitioner experience.

TEACHING AND COUNSELING. Although the diagnosis of myoma may be commonplace to the practitioner, it may be quite distressing to the woman. She should receive full information on the characteristics of uterine myomas, with emphasis on their benign nature. Her concerns should never be dismissed as trivial; all her questions need to be answered. Informed consent must be obtained for all treatments; women facing surgery need to understand its benefits and risks. See Chapter 27 for further discussion of the needs of women and couples for whom myomas are related to infertility.

ENDOMETRITIS

Endometritis is an infection of the uterus representing an invasion of the endometrium by vaginal flora that occurs after pregnancy. It may also occur, although less commonly, with pelvic tuberculosis (tuberculous endometritis) (Green, 1977) or IUD use, or secondary to genital cancer (Mickal, Faro, & Pastorek, 1985, p. 462). The latter is seen in elderly women. This section concentrates on postpartum endometritis.

The principal responsible organisms are Gram-negative aerobic bacilli (*Escherichia coli, Klebsiella,* or *Proteus mirabilis*), Gram-negative anaerobic bacilli, group B streptococci, Gram-positive anaerobic cocci (peptostreptococci), and enterococci (*Bacteroides fragilis*). Group A streptococcus infection is rare (American College of Obstetricians and Gynecologists, 1986; Mead, 1984). Occasionally, *Neisseria gonorrhoeae* or *Chlamydia trachomatis* is the causative organism (Mickal et al., 1985, p. 462).

Incidence

Endometritis follows 5 to 85 percent of all cesarean deliveries, with the higher incidences occurring in large teaching institutions; postvaginal delivery incidence is 0.9 to 3.9 percent; the postabortion rate is 0.5 to 1 percent (Elliot, 1984; Mead, 1984).

Risk Factors

Women of low socioeconomic status are considered to be at substantial risk for endometritis after both vaginal and cesarean delivery. Additional risk factors include anemia and/or malnutrition, prolonged rupture of membranes, prolonged labor, young maternal age, multiple vaginal examinations in labor, extended duration of internal monitoring, forceps delivery, and maternal soft tissue trauma (Duff, 1986; Mead, 1984).

Prevention

Prophylaxis with an antibacterial agent may be undertaken to reduce the incidence of postoperative and postdelivery endometritis. The use of cephalosporins has reduced the number of patients with endometritis; however, selection of resistant bacteria does occur (Galask, 1985). The widespread use of broad-spectrum antibiotics alters the genital tract flora, affecting the types of organisms isolated from prophylactic failures and their resistant characteristics. One study used irrigation lavage of the operative site with cefanamdole and resulted in a 1.7 percent infection rate in 298 patients undergoing cesarean section (Elliot, 1984).

Clinical Presentation

Endometritis presents with fever of 100.4°F or greater 24 hours postdelivery, tachycardia, uterine tenderness, subinvolution of the uterus, adnexal tenderness, lower abdominal pain, general malaise, pelvic peritoneal irritation, and possibly foul lochia. Five percent of women with endometritis have concurrent wound infections; 5 to 10 percent have concurrent urinary tract infections. Ten percent have bacteremia; less than 2 percent develop septic shock, pelvic abscess, or pelvic thrombophlebitis.

Nonpuerperal endometritis may cause abnormal vaginal bleeding and uterine tenderness, often mild. IUD use or history of recent intrauterine manipulation should alert the practitioner to the possibility of endometritis. In the elderly, a purulent foul discharge with vaginal bleeding may be indicative of endometritis secondary to genital cancer (Mickal et al., 1985, p. 463).

Differential Diagnosis

Endometritis must be differentiated from urinary tract infection, appendicitis, atelectasis, pneumonia, viral syndrome, and acute pyelonephritis. If the patient does not respond to antibacterial treatment, then pelvic abscess, collagen vascular disease, venous thromboembolism, drug fever, septic pelvic thrombophlebitis, or wound infection with an exudate requiring drainage must be considered.

Management

Data Collection

HISTORY AND PHYSICAL EXAMINATION. Any patient with a postpartum fever deserves a thorough history taking and complete physical examination with particular attention to those systems in which symptoms are reported. Historic data should include previous infections and exposures to rule out other conditions or infectious processes. When history or chart review reveals factors predisposing to endometritis, a high suspicion of this disorder should be maintained. Bimanual pelvic examination is usually unnecessary for initial assessment and may exacerbate the condition. A sterile speculum examination, however, is necessary to obtain cervical cultures.

LABORATORY TESTING. A specimen for aerobic culture should be taken with a transcervical swab. Additional laboratory tests to exclude other diagnoses or confirm endometritis include blood cultures in aerobic and anaerobic bottles; CBC with differential; erythrocyte sedimentation rate; urine culture and sensitivity; wound culture, if discharge is present; chest x-ray if pneumonia, atelectasis, or pulmonary embolism is suspected; ultrasound, computerized tomography, or gallium-67 scanning if pelvic abscess is suspected (Duff, 1986; Mead, 1984).

Intervention

TREATMENT. When patients present with symptoms of endometritis, consultation is necessary as antibiotic therapy is indicated. The primary care practitioner, however, can obtain many of the necessary diagnostic tests. Most women with endometritis are in-hospital postpartum patients, although with early discharge after delivery, this condition may be seen increasingly in the office or outpatient setting.

The following discussion of treatments for endometritis is based on the recommendations of Mead (1984) and the American College of Obstetricians and Gynecologists (1986). A regimen of clindamycin 600 mg IV every 6 hours plus gentamycin 1.5 mg/kg IV every 8 hours has proven to be significantly more effective than penicillin plus gentamycin. Clindamycin plus gentamycin is currently the standard against which other regimens should be compared; however, this combination is ineffective against enterococci and has the potential for nephrotoxicity and ototoxicity as well as for diarrhea. The addition of ampicillin extends the spectrum of coverage to include enterococci.

Regimens with favorable coverage and clinical experience include cefoxitan 2 g IV every 6 hours; piperacillin 2 to 3 g IV every 4 to 6 hours; and mezlocillin 4 g IV every 6 hours or 3 g every 4 hours.

Regimens with less favorable antibacterial coverage but with good clinical effects are metronidazole 15 mg/kg loading dose followed by 7.5 mg/kg IV every 6 hours plus gentamycin; cefamandole 2 g IV every 4 to 6 hours; and cefoperazone 2 g IV every 12 hours.

All antibiotic therapies should be continued intravenously at least 4 to 5 days and at least 24 hours after defervescence. Most specialists in infectious diseases believe that additional oral therapy is not needed. Rest and fluids should be encouraged during therapy. For patients receiving aminoglycosides, creatinine should be measured every other day; peak (6 to 10 μg/mL) and trough (2 μg/mL) levels may help adjust dosage.

If fever continues after treatment, particularly with spikes and tachycardia and without abscess, pelvic thrombophlebitis must be considered. An arterial PO_2 of less than 88 mm in a nonsmoker supports a diagnosis of thrombophlebitis. Pelvic thrombophlebitis is treated with intravenous heparin anticoagulation; this should decrease fever within 48 hours if the problem has been correctly identified. Any abscess usually requires appropriate drainage. The most frequent location for a pelvic abscess is the posterior cul-de-sac (Duff, 1986; Mead, 1984).

TEACHING AND COUNSELING. Women with postpartum endometritis need supportive care and counseling. In hospital, they may be separated from their infants. If diagnosed after discharge, they may face readmission for intravenous antibiotic therapy. For more information on postpartum needs, see Chapter 23.

UTERINE PROLAPSE

Uterine prolapse or descensus is the descent of the uterus from its usual position in the pelvis as a result of the loss of the uterine supports. The cardinal ligaments are the primary uterine supports, whereas the round, broad, and uterosacral ligaments are necessary for maintaining the uterine position. The uterus usually forms an acute angle with the axis of the vagina that also helps prevent prolapse.

When the cardinal ligaments are injured or stretched during childbirth and do not return to normal, the uterus can sag backward and downward into the vagina. If there is relaxation of the other supporting ligaments and vaginal walls, as can occur with advancing age, the pressure of the abdominal organs forces the uterus down through the vagina. Gradually, the vagina inverts and carries the bladder and rectum with it as the uterus descends further.

Although uterine prolapse is most commonly seen in older, multiparous women, it can also occur in nulliparous women, children, and infants. Prolapse in these groups is caused by defects in innervation and in the basic integrity of the uterine supports (Willson, 1983).

Uterine descensus is described in degrees:

First degree	The cervix lies between the level of the ischial spines and the introitus.
Second degree	The cervix protrudes through the introitus.
Third degree	Both the cervix and the uterus have come through the introitus and the vagina is inverted.

Clinical Presentation

Symptoms of uterine prolapse may include pressure sensations and disruption of bladder and bowel function. There may be bleeding if the cervix has prolapsed through the introitus and has ulcerated.

Management

Diagnosis. Diagnosis of uterine prolapse is made by physical examination (see Chapter 3). It may be necessary to examine the woman in the standing position as a uterine prolapse may reduce spontaneously when she lies down.

Differential diagnosis includes hypertrophy and elongation of the cervix without loss of support.

Intervention

TREATMENT. Treatment of uterine prolapse is primarily surgical. Procedures can be performed that return the uterus to an anterior position, shorten the cardinal ligaments, and repair accompanying cystocele and rectocele. Alternatively, a vaginal hysterectomy can be performed. If age or the general medical condition of the woman precludes surgery, a pessary can be tried although it may not be helpful if there is no support at the vaginal outlet (Tovell & Danforth, 1986). There are a number of different types of pessaries, and the choice of an appropriate device must be individualized. Tovell and Danforth (1986) recommend estrogen therapy to improve vaginal tone and resistance to infection for all postmenopausal women wearing pessaries (see Chapter 24).

REFERRAL. Operative success may depend on the skill of the surgeon. Whenever possible, the woman should be referred to a surgeon with experience in these operations. If the woman is to use a pessary, it must be carefully fit and checked periodically by someone comfortable in fitting the device.

TEACHING AND COUNSELING. Uterine prolapse may interfere with body image, daily activities, and sexuality. Patients with the problem need emotional support and information. Treatment options should be discussed fully with each woman and instructions given regarding postprocedure care. The woman wearing a pessary must report any discomfort to her care provider. A discussion of sexual functioning may be important. Sexual intercourse can be resumed 3 weeks after a vaginal hysterectomy. Sexual functioning may present more difficulties after reparative surgery. The vagina may become narrowed and shortened or vulvar and vaginal stenosis may occur. Intercourse can usually be resumed 6 weeks after reparative surgery and may be helpful in reducing stenosis. Dilators and water-soluble lubricants may be useful in relieving vaginal tightness (Lowdermilk, 1981, p. 298).

ENDOMETRIAL HYPERPLASIA AND CANCER

Malignant tumors of the uterine body include adenocarcinoma, adenoacanthoma, adenosquamous carcinoma, squamous cell carcinoma, endometrial stroma and myometrial sarcoma, carcinosarcoma, mixed mesodermal tumors, and some rare tumors including osteogenic sarcoma and malignant lymphoma (Gompel & Silverberg, 1985). The uterus also may be the site for metastasis of other malignancies. Most cancers of the uterine body, however, develop in the endometrium, and 95 percent of these are adenocarcinomas. The discussion that follows, therefore, focuses on endometrial adenocarcinoma.

Incidence

Most carcinomas of the uterine body occur in women aged 50 to 70. They represent 10 to 15 percent of malignancies seen in women (Gompel & Silverberg, 1985). The overall incidence of endometrial cancer in postmenopausal women who have not taken estrogens is 1 in 1,000, increasing to 4 in 1,000 among women who have taken estrogen (The British Gynecological Cancer Group, 1981; Jelovsek, Hammond, Woodard, et al., 1980; Richart, Ferenczy, Fu, & Kurman, 1983; Richart, Ferenczy, Koss, & Weid, 1984). An estimated 2.9 million women were taking exogenous estrogens in the United States in 1983 (Peterson, Lee, & Rubin, 1985). Endometrial cancer occurs more frequently in white than black women (Mahboubi, Eyler, & Wynder, 1982).

Risk Factors

It is generally agreed that there is a relationship between unopposed estrogen and endometrial cancer. Although the mechanism regulating ovarian steroid action in target tissues is still not defined and the exact role played by estrogen and progesterone in carcinogenesis is not known, current data suggest that estrogen may be a tumor promoter rather than a carcinogen (Richart et al., 1983). Estrogen promotes mitotic growth of the endometrium, causing proliferation. Abnormal progression of growth through cystic hyperplasia, adenomatous hyperplasia, atypia, and early carcinoma have been associated with unopposed estrogen activity. Progesterone at normal levels inhibits the proliferative activity of estrogen on the endometrium by differentiating the endometrial lining to a secretory state.

Nulliparity or low parity, early menarche, late menopause, irregular menses, and obesity are factors responsible for prolonged exposure of the uterus to endogenous estrogens without the counterbalancing protective effect of progesterone (Coulam, 1984). A panel of experts at the National Institutes of Health (NIH) concluded in February 1985 that obesity in women is linked to higher mortality from cancer of the gallbladder, biliary passages, breast, cervix, uterus, endometrium, and ovaries, with the obesity link most pronounced for endometrial cancer. The NIH panel concluded that markedly obese women are five times more likely to develop endometrial cancer than are nonobese women (Eastman, 1985). The American Cancer Society research shows that women who are at least 40 percent overweight have a 55 percent greater risk of developing cancer than women of normal weight (Eastman, 1985; Schneider, Bradlow, Strain, et al., 1983). Diabetes, hypertension, and infertility are also risk factors for endometrial cancer. It is possible that the effects of diabetes and hypertension are related to their association with obesity (Berg & Lampe, 1981), although the evidence is unclear (Mahboubi et al., 1982).

The use of combination oral contraceptives (OCs) is protective against endometrial cancer. Risk is decreased by one half after use of OCs for 1 year, particularly for nulliparous women (Centers for Disease Control, 1982; Kaufman, Shapiro, Slone, et al., 1980).

Prevention

Treatment of amenorrhea or prolonged menstrual cycles that suggest unopposed estrogen stimulation of the endometrium may prevent the development of endometrial cancer. Of course, other causative factors must first be ruled out. See Chapter 21 for more discussion of the management of bleeding abnormalities.

For menopausal therapy, a combination of estrogen and progesterone is greatly preferred to the administration of estrogen alone (Collins, Donner, Allen, & Adams, 1980). Prior to the initiation of estrogen replacement therapy, an endometrial sampling should be done. See Chapter 24 for detailed discussion of hormonal replacement therapy.

Diagnosis and Classification

Irregular vaginal bleeding after menopause is commonly associated with endometrial cancer; 90 percent of women with cancer have painless irregular bleeding (Jones & Jones, 1981). *Whenever a perimenopausal woman presents with abnormal bleeding, medical consultation and immediate endometrial sampling are mandatory.*

Pathologists have difficulty diagnosing endometrial lesions (Richart et al., 1983). Classifications vary but generally are described as hyperplasia, atypical hyperplasia, and carcinoma. Mild hyperplasia, also called cystic hyperplasia, is used to characterize persistent and proliferative endometrium; the moderate form is often referred to as adenomatous hyperplasia without significant atypia; severe hyperplasia is used to specify adenomatous hyperplasia with severe cytologic atypia. Carcinoma is divided into typical endometrial adenocarcinoma, adenocarcinoma with squamous differentiation, squamous carcinoma, clear cell adenocarcinoma, mucinous adenocarcinoma, papillary serous carcinoma, undifferentiated carcinoma, and miscellaneous or rare types (Richart et al., 1984).

After diagnosis, staging should be done by means of a fractional dilation and curettage according to criteria established by the International Federation of Gynecology and Obstetrics (FIGO) (Jones & Jones, 1981):

Stage 0   Carcinoma in situ
Stage I   Carcinoma confined to the uterine corpus
   IA   Uterine cavity 8 cm or shorter
   IB   Uterine cavity longer than 8 cm
(also subgrouped by histologic type)
   G1   Highly differentiated adenomatous carcinoma
   G2   Differentiated adenomatous carcinoma with partly solid areas
   G3   Predominantly solid or entirely undifferentiated carcinoma
Stage II   Carcinoma involving the uterine corpus and cervix
Stage III   Carcinoma extending outside the uterus but not outside the pelvis
Stage IV   Carcinoma extending outside the true pelvis or obviously involving mucosa of the bladder or rectum

Prognosis and Management

As adenocarcinoma of the uterus remains localized for a long time, it has a favorable prognosis (Gompel & Silverberg, 1985). Five-year survival rates have been reported to be 80 percent, and 10-year survival rates, 68 percent (Webb & Lagios, 1987). Prognosis, of course, is related to stage of disease and degree of differentiation of tumor.

In stage I disease, total abdominal hysterectomy and bilateral salpingo-oophorectomy are performed (Kurman, 1984; Richart et al., 1984). Stage II disease is treated with combined radiation and surgery. Advanced endometrial malignancy receives individualized treatment. Surgery may be palliative and chemotherapy of some benefit (Averette, 1985). Referral should be made to a gynecologic oncologist.

TROPHOBLASTIC DISEASE/CHORIOCARCINOMA

Trophoblastic tumors are most often seen after a molar pregnancy, when they may be cancerous or noncancerous.

Cancerous trophoblastic tumors are called choriocarcinoma. Trophoblastic disease may also occur after term or ectopic pregnancy or abortion. After a nonmolar pregnancy, the disease is always cancerous (Perez, DiSaia, Knapp, & Young, 1985). The practitioner of well-woman gynecology, therefore, may occasionally encounter women with this disease.

Pathology

Choriocarcinoma consists of anaplastic trophoblastic tissue that cannot form the villous structure that occurs in normal pregnancy (Perez et al., 1985). Trophoblastic tumors produce human chorionic gonadotropin (hCG) in large quantities. The tumors are located within the uterus, with distant dissemination in 5 percent of women with molar pregnancy and in 1 in 40,000 abortions or term or ectopic pregnancies. Sites of dissemination include lungs, pelvis, brain, liver, bowel, kidney, and spleen.

Epidemiology

Trophoblastic tumors are most common in Asia, with nutritional deficiencies a possible etiologic factor. The tumor is seen with increased frequency in women over the age of 40.

Clinical Presentation

Trophoblastic disease may cause abnormal vaginal bleeding. An early pregnancy with bleeding, uterine size large-for-dates, and early signs of pregnancy-induced hypertension should lead to a high degree of suspicion.

Diagnosis. Patients with suspected trophoblastic disease, based on history of current or recent pregnancy and symptoms of abnormal vaginal bleeding not attributable to other causes (see Chapter 21), should be referred for diagnosis and treatment. Diagnosis is made by ultrasound, isotope scan, hCG determinations, and tissue pathology (Perez et al., 1985).

Intervention. Chemotherapy is generally the treatment of choice for trophoblastic disease. Whether single or combination chemotherapy is used depends on risk factors which include metastasis, levels of serum β-hCG, previous unsuccessful treatment, duration of symptoms greater than 4 months, and development of the disease after a term pregnancy. Obviously, women and families facing this diagnosis and its treatments need psychosocial support and possible referral for more intensive counseling.

OTHER UTERINE CONDITIONS

Other uterine disorders include endometrial polyps, vascular abnormalities, adenomyosis, and Asherman's syndrome. An endometrial polyp is a mass of tissue held onto the mucosa by a pedicle. Endometrial polyps can occur at any age, may be single or multiple, and are usually 0.5 to 3 cm in diameter (Gompel & Silverberg, 1985). They may be asymptomatic or cause irregular, often heavy, bleeding. Diagnosis and treatment usually consist of endometrial biopsy or dilation and curettage (D&C), although hysteroscopic treatment has been used as well (DeCherney & Friedman, 1985, p. 289).

Vascular abnormalities of the endometrium may also cause bleeding, usually after biopsy or curettage (Mickal et

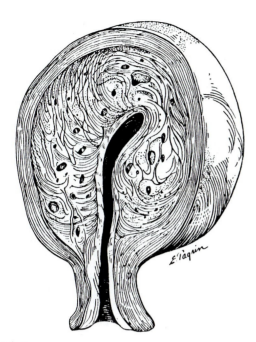

Figure 14–8. Adenomyosis. *(From Kistner, R. W. [1986].* Gynecology: Principles and practice. *Chicago: Year Book Medical Publishers, p 223. Reprinted with permission.)*

al., 1985, p. 470). This may result in an emergency situation.

Adenomyosis is the presence of endometrial glands and stroma within the uterine myometrium (Fig. 14–8). It most commonly develops during the late reproductive years, with the highest incidence among women in their forties. Adenomyosis is associated with abnormal menstrual bleeding, dysmenorrhea, uterine enlargement, uterine tenderness during menstruation, and, on occasion, infertility, although it also may be asymptomatic. It is thought rarely to undergo malignant change (Gompel & Silverberg, 1985). Treatment, when necessary, is surgical: resection of localized areas of adenomyosis or hysterectomy if severe (Green, 1977, p. 396).

Asherman's syndrome is characterized by intrauterine synechiae or adhesions. This syndrome usually follows a D&C for abortion. Symptoms include postabortion amenorrhea or oligomenorrhea. Diagnosis usually is made by hysterography. Treatment involves D&C, often with insertion of an IUD to keep the uterine walls separated until healing occurs.

REFERENCES

American College of Obstetricians and Gynecologists. (1986, October). *Antimicrobial therapy for gynecologic infections.* Technical Bulletin No. 97.

Altchek, A. (1985). Pediatric and adolescent gynecology. In D. H. Nichols & J. R. Evrard (Eds.), *Ambulatory gynecology.* Philadelphia: Harper & Row.

Appuzzio, J. J., Pelosi, M. A., Kaminetzky, H. A., & Louria, D. B. (1985, December). Comparative clinical evaluation of ceftizoxime with clindamycin and gentamycin and cefoxitin in the treatment of post cesarean section endomyometritis. *Surgery, Gynecology and Obstetrics, 161* (6), 518–522.

Averette, H. E. (1985, October). How pelvic nodes predict endometrial cancer outcomes. *Contemporary Ob/Gyn, 26*(4), 158–172.

Babaknia, A., Rock, J. A., & Jones, H. W. (1978, December). Pregnancy success following abdominal myomectomy for infertility. *Fertility and Sterility, 30*(6), 644–647.

Benson, R. (1983). *Handbook of obstetrics and gynecology.* Los Altos, CA: Lange.

Berg, J. W., & Lampe, J. G. (1981, July 15). High-risk factors in gynecologic cancer. *Cancer, 48*(2, Suppl.), 429–441.

Berkley, A. S., DeCherney, A. H., & Polan, M. L. (1983, March). Abdominal myomectomy and subsequent fertility. *Surgery, Gynecology and Obstetrics, 156*(3), 319–322.

The British Gynecological Cancer Group. (1981, June 20). Oestrogen replacement and endometrial cancer. *Lancet, 1*(8234), 1359–1360.

Buttram, V. C., & Gibbons, W. E. (1979, July). Müllerian anomalies: A proposed classification (an analysis of 144 cases). *Fertility and Sterility, 32*(1), 40–55.

Buttram, V. S., & Reiter, R. C. (1981, October). Uterine leiomyoma: Etiology, symptomatology and management. *Fertility and Sterility, 36*(4), 433–445.

Carlson, J. A., Allegra, J. C., Day, T. G., & Wittliff, J. L. (1984, May). Tamoxifen and endometrial carcinoma: Alterations in estrogen and progesterone receptors in untreated patients and combination hormonal therapy in advanced neoplasia. *American Journal of Obstetrics and Gynecology, 149*(2), 149–153.

Centers for Disease Control. (1982, July 30). Oral contraceptives and cancer risk. *Morbidity and Mortality Weekly Report, 31*(29), 393–394.

Collins, J., Donner, A., Allen, L. H., & Adams, O. (1980, November 1). Oestrogen use and survival in endometrial cancer. *Lancet, 2*(8201), 961–963.

Coulam, C. (1984, May). Why Ca risk is higher in anovulatory women. *Contemporary Ob/Gyn, 23*(5), 85–100.

Daly, D. C., Walters, C. A., Soto-Albors, C. E., & Riddick, D. (1983, May). Hysteroscopic metroplasty: Surgical technique and obstetric outcome. *Fertility and Sterility, 39*(5), 623–628.

Dawood, M. Y. (1984, June). An update on dysmenorrhea. *Contemporary Ob/Gyn, 23*(6), 73–94.

DeCherney, A. H., & Friedman, A. J. (1985). Endoscopy. In D. H. Nichols & J. R. Evrard (Eds.), *Ambulatory gynecology.* Philadelphia: Harper & Row.

Duff, P. (1986, February). Pathophysiology and management of post cesarean section endomyometritis. *Obstetrics and Gynecology, 67*(2), 269–276.

Eastman, P. (1985, August). The case for the anticancer diet. *Contemporary Ob/Gyn, 26*(Special Issue), 71–90.

Elliot, J. P. (1984, May). Lavage to prevent post cesarean infection. *Contemporary Ob/Gyn, 23*(5), 43–48.

Farber, G., Noumoff, J., Freedman, M., & Oberkotter, L. (1984, December). Understanding and correcting genital anomalies. *Contemporary Ob/Gyn, 24*(6), 113–129.

Galask, R. P. (1985, September). Combating the menace of post-hysterectomy infection. *Contemporary Ob/Gyn, 26*(3), 131–136.

Garcia, C.-R., & Tureck, R. W. (1984, July). Submucosal leiomyomas and infertility. *Fertility and Sterility, 42*(1), 16–19.

Goldfarb, A. F. (1984, September). Controlling dysfunctional uterine bleeding. *Contemporary Ob/Gyn, 24*(3), 77–82.

Gompel, C., & Silverberg, S. G. (1985). *Pathology in gynecology and obstetrics* (3rd ed.). Philadelphia: J.B. Lippincott.

Green, T. H. (1977). *Gynecology: Essentials of clinical practice* (3rd ed.). Boston: Little, Brown.

Gross, B. H., Silver, T. M., & Jaffe, M. H. (1983, September). Sonographic features of uterine leiomyomas: Analysis of 41 proven cases. *Journal of Ultrasound Medicine, 2*(9), 401–406.

Jelovsek, F. R., Hammond, C. B., Woodard, B. H., et al. (1980, May). Risk of exogenous estrogen and endometrial cancer. *American Journal of Obstetrics and Gynecology, 137*(1), 85–91.

Jones, H. W., & Jones, G. S. (1981). *Novak's textbook of gynecology* (10th ed.). Baltimore: Williams & Wilkins.

Kaufman, D. W., Shapiro, S., Slone, D., et al. (1980, October 30). Decreased risk of endometrial cancer among oral-contraceptive users. *New England Journal of Medicine, 303*(18), 1045–1047.

Kistner, R. W. (1986). *Gynecology: Principles and practice.* Chicago: Year Book Medical Publishers.

Kurman, R. J. (1984, January). Diagnosing and treating the intermediate endometrial neoplasia. *Contemporary Ob/Gyn, 23*(1), 144–157.

Lee, N. C., Dicker, R. C., Rubin, G. L., & Ory, H. W. (1984, October 1). Confirmation of the preoperative diagnoses for hysterectomy. *American Journal of Obstetrics and Gynecology, 150*(3), 283–287.

Lowdermilk, D. L. (1981). Reproductive surgery. In C. I. Fogel & N. F. Woods (Eds.), *Health care of women: A nursing perspective.* St. Louis, MO: C.V. Mosby.

Mahboubi, E., Eyler, N., & Wynder, E. L. (1982, March). Epidemiology of cancer of the endometrium. *Clinical Obstetrics and Gynecology, 25*(1), 5–17.

Maheux, R., Lemay, A., & Merat, P. (1987, February). Use of intranasal luteinizing hormone–releasing hormone agonist in uterine leiomyomas. *Fertility and Sterility, 47*(2), 229–233.

Mead, P. (1984, May). When your patient has postpartum endometritis. *Contemporary Ob/Gyn, 23*(5), 38–40.

Mickal, A., Faro, S., & Pastorek, J. G., II. (1985). Emergency care. In D. H. Nichols & J. R. Evrard (Eds.), *Ambulatory gynecology.* Philadelphia: Harper & Row.

Neuwirth, R. S. (1983, October). Hysteroscopic management of symptomatic submucous fibroids. *Obstetrics and Gynecology, 62*(4), 509–511.

Nicolini, U., Bellotti, M., Bonazzi, B., et al. (1987, January). Can ultrasound be used to screen uterine malformations? *Fertility and Sterility, 47*(1), 89–93.

O'Brien, W. F., Buck, D. R., & Nash, J. D. (1984, July 15). Evaluation of sonography in the initial assessment of the gynecologic patient. *American Journal of Obstetrics and Gynecology, 149*(6), 598–612.

Perez, C. A., DiSaia, P. J., Knapp, R. C., & Young, R. C. (1985) Gynecologic tumors, In V. T. DeVita, S. Hellman, & S. A. Rosenberg (Eds.), *Cancer: Principles and practice of Oncology* (2nd ed.). Philadelphia: J. B. Lippincott.

Peterson, H. B., Lee, C., & Rubin, G. L. (1985, October). ERT: What are the cancer risks? *Contemporary Ob/Gyn, 26*(4), 55–81.

Pritchard, J. A., MacDonald, P. C., & Gant, N. F. (1985). *Williams obstetrics* (17th ed.). East Norwalk, CT: Appleton–Century–Crofts.

Ranney, B., & Frederick, I. (1979, April). The occasional need for myomectomy. *Obstetrics and Gynecology, 53*(4), 437–441.

Richart, R. M., Ferenczy, A. M., Fu, Y., & Kurman, R. (1983, September). Detecting endometrial cancer and precursor lesions. *Contemporary Ob/Gyn, 22*(3), 231–250.

Richart, R. M., Ferenczy, A., Koss, L., & Weid, G. (1984, June). Screening for endometrial cancer. *Contemporary Ob/Gyn, 23*(6), 103–123.

Richart, R. M., & Neuwirth, R. S. (1985, January). Hysteroscopic resection of submucous leiomyomas. *Contemporary Ob/Gyn, 25*(1), 103–125.

Rock, J. A., Reeves, L. A., Retto, H., et al. (1983, June). Success following vaginal creation for müllerian agenesis. *Fertility and Sterility, 39*(6), 809–813.

Romero, R., & Horgan, J. G. (1985). Diagnostic ultrasound in gynecology. In D. H. Nichols & J. R. Evrard (Eds.), *Ambulatory gynecology.* Philadelphia: Harper & Row.

Rosenfeld, D. L. (1986, August). Abdominal myomectomy for otherwise unexplained infertility. *Fertility and Sterility, 46*(2), 238–330.

Schneider, J., Bradlow, H. L., Strain, G., et al. (1983, May). Effect of obesity on estradiol metabolism: Decreased formation of nonuterotropic metabolites. *Journal of Clinical Endocrinology and Metabolism, 56*(5), 973–978.

Siegler, A. M. (1983, August). Hysterosalpingography. *Fertility and Sterility, 40*(2), 139–157.

Tovell, H. M. M., & Danforth, D. N. (1986). Structural defects and relaxations. In D. N. Danforth & J. R. Scott (Eds.), *Obstetrics and gynecology* (5th ed.). Philadelphia: J.P. Lippincott.

Wallach, E. E., Hammond, C., Goldfarb, A., & Kempers, R. (1983, November). Problems linked to uterine myomas. *Contemporary Ob/Gyn, 22*(5), 265–279.

Webb, G. A., & Lagios, M. D. (1987, June). Clear cell carcinoma of the endometrium. *American Journal of Obstetrics and Gynecology, 156*(6), 1486–1491.

Willson, J. R. (1983). Immediate and remote effects of childbirth injury: Uterine retrodisplacement. In J. R. Willson, E. R. Carrington, & W. Ledger (Eds.), *Obstetrics and gynecology.* St. Louis, MO: C.V. Mosby.

15

The Fallopian Tubes

Virginia Jackson

Problems involving the fallopian tubes must be viewed as serious. Both ectopic pregnancy and salpingitis—the two most commonly encountered tubal disorders—pose a potential threat to a patient's future fertility and even to her life. These conditions demand medical consultation and referral for treatment. Nevertheless, the primary care practitioner has a vital role in screening for and diagnosing fallopian tube problems; in offering teaching, counseling, and support before and during treatment; and in providing follow-up care. Essential knowledge, therefore, for all gynecologic practitioners includes the etiology and risk factors associated with these diagnoses; their presenting symptoms and differential diagnosis; screening and diagnostic procedures, including history taking, physical examination, and laboratory tests; current treatment modalities; and possible sequelae. This chapter covers each of these areas.

ANATOMY AND PHYSIOLOGY

Anatomically, the fallopian tubes are bilateral connecting tunnels between each ovary and the uterus. They are the site of fertilization. Each hollow tube features a varying diameter and lining—the endosalpinx—and is covered by muscle. The *interstitial* portion of each tube, joining the uterine wall pathways, has a lumen only 0.4 mm in diameter. The *isthmus* has a thick muscle wall, with few longitudinal foldings of endosalpinx and a very contracted lumen approximately 1 mm in diameter. The thin-walled *ampulla*, with a 1- to 2-cm-wide lumen and an endosalpinx with complex, extensive foldings, is the longest section of the tube, about two thirds of the total length of 10 to 12 cm. The most distal portion of the tube, the last 1 to 2 cm, consists of the *infundibulum* with its fimbria.

The epithelial lining of the tube is composed of four types of cells: secretory cells, ciliated cells, peg cells, and small "indifferent" cells. Secretory cells are thought to provide nutrients to the ovum while it is in the tube. The ciliated cells, with microvilli extending from their edges, carry the ovum toward the uterus. To reach the ovum, sperm must move against their action. These two types of cells are responsive to the hormonal changes of the menstrual cycle. During the proliferative phase, the tubal epithelium is raised and the cells are at the same height. During the luteal phase, the ciliated cells decrease and the secretory cells increase in number. Peg cells are "placed between" cells and

appear to be old cells on their way to removal from the tube. The small indifferent cells have no known function.

There are three layers of tubal musculature: inner longitudinal, middle circular, and outer longitudinal. Some evidence indicates that the isthmus of the tube is subject to spasm and may act as a sphincter.

The fallopian tube is an essential element in human reproduction. After being swept in by the fimbria, the ovum enters the tube through the infundibulum. This ovum may then be fertilized by sperm in the ampulla. Achievement of a pregnancy depends on the combination of the following factors: ovulation and its accompanying hormonal support; patency of the tube; ability of sperm to reach the tubal ampulla; movement of the fertilized egg into the uterus by action of the tube's ciliated cells; and presumed secretion of proper levels of nutrients. When the normal process of reproduction is altered, the result may be an ectopic pregnancy. Anatomic or chronic tubal abnormalities, however, are most often discovered in the course of a workup for infertility (Green, 1977; Muckle, 1985a, 1985b).

The normal fallopian tube is not palpable on examination. Any enlargement, therefore, warrants investigation; however, adnexal masses may not be distinguishable as specifically tubal or ovarian. Patient discomfort may prevent adequate differentiation. Fortunately, physical examination is not the clinician's only assessment tool. Problems of tubal origin may be uncovered through a thorough history. General physical examination elicits specific areas of pain. Laboratory data may be required for appropriate diagnosis. Consultation and referral are generally necessary in the light of tubal abnormalities, but many components of a diagnostic workup can be initiated before referral is made or in consultation with a backup physician. A conscientious and safe practitioner, however, should err in the direction of overconsulting in the face of a potentially life-threatening tubal disorder.

SALPINGITIS

In assessing a woman with lower abdominal pain, with or without other symptoms of salpingitis, the practitioner is confronted by a diagnostic challenge. Although acute salpingitis, or pelvic inflammatory disease (PID), may offer definitive symptoms, the chronic and subacute stages of this disease are much more difficult to distinguish from other disorders. Studies of laparoscopically confirmed salpingitis, for example, show that only 35 to 40 percent of cases cause fever (Jacobson & Weström, 1969). In fact, there are a great variety of clinical presentations of salpingitis. The danger in the unchecked progress of this disease is the impairment of future fertility or, perhaps, severe peritonitis.

Etiology and Pathophysiology

In the past, the most frequent causative agent of salpingitis was thought to be *Neisseria gonorrhoeae*; however, salpingitis caused by *Chlamydia trachomatis* is of increasing concern. The Centers for Disease Control (CDC, 1985a) estimate that *C. trachomatis* is responsible for one fourth to one half of all cases of PID. This organism is most frequently found in those patients with serious sequelae (Svensson, Weström, Ripa, & Mårdh, 1980).

Salpingitis is the result of infection by an organism that is capable of ascending from the lower to the upper genital tract. This ascent usually occurs toward the end of or just after the menstrual period following acquisition of the infectious agent. During menses, the cervical os is slightly open and the cervical mucous barrier is absent; in addition, menstrual blood provides an excellent medium for growth. Salpingitis may also occur after abortion, pelvic surgery, or delivery. The infection rises by surface spread from the vagina to the uterus, to the tubes. In the fallopian tubes an inflammatory response is initiated, resulting in edema, fluid accumulation, loss of tubal function, possible formation of purulent material with subsequent formation of a tubo-ovarian abscess, pyosalpinx, or hydrosalpinx and possible peritonitis.

It is postulated that in infections caused by *N. gonorrhoeae*, the gonococcus merely starts the infectious process, causing tubal damage and making the tubes more vulnerable to subsequent invasion by a variety of organisms. *Escherichia coli, Bacterioides, Peptostreptococcus, Ureaplasma urealyticum,* and *Mycoplasma hominis* have been cultured from infected tubes (Eschenbach, Buchanen, Pollack, et al., 1975).

Incidence and Risk Factors

The CDC (1985a) estimates that at least one million diagnosed cases of pelvic inflammatory disease occur in the United States each year, in addition to unrecognized infection of the tube. Risk factors for the development of salpingitis include having more than one sexual partner, being under the age of 25, being economically disadvantaged, having a history of previous salpingitis, and/or using an intrauterine device (IUD) for contraception. The rising incidence of salpingitis is related to the increase in sexually transmitted diseases (STDs) and abortions. It has been commonly reported that approximately 10 to 17 percent of women with a gonococcal infection of the lower genital tract develop salpingitis (Dougherty & Pastorek, 1985).

Clinical Presentation

Acute Salpingitis. The patient with acute salpingitis presents with complaints of abdominal pain. She may complain of metrorrhagia. The timing of patient complaints may add to the confusion in diagnosis, because the onset of salpingitis generally occurs during or just after menses. On physical exam, abdominal tenderness is elicited with or without rebound. There is adnexal tenderness and tenderness with motion of the cervix/uterus. A urethral or cervical discharge may be present. Pelvic tenderness is usually bilateral. There may or may not be a palpable adnexal swelling or thickening. A high temperature, 102°F or above, without much appearance of illness, is characteristic. In spite of the leukocytosis (20,000 to 30,000 with a left shift), salpingitis may be differentiated from appendicitis by the lack of generalized "sickness" of the patient. Usually, there is no gastrointestinal upset or appetite loss. The erythrocyte sedimentation rate (ESR) is markedly elevated to above 50 mm/hr.

Fever and peritonitis are more typical of gonococcal salpingitis than of the nongonococcal variety, which is more likely to be "silent" and therefore result in tubal obstruction, because of either delayed diagnosis or inadequate treatment.

Subacute Salpingitis. The patient with subacute salpingitis complains of vague lower abdominal pain. On abdominal examination, there is usually no rebound tenderness. There is slight adnexal tenderness on cervical motion. A hydrosalpinx is common, giving the fallopian tubes a thickened, hoselike feel. Cervical and/or urethral discharge may be noted. There is usually no elevation in either temperature or white blood cell count (Green, 1977; Sweet, 1981).

A grading system, designed as a guide for evaluating the need for laparoscopy, has been proposed for salpingitis (Hager, Eschenbach, Spence, & Sweet, 1983, p. 113). Because, in theory, a laparoscopy may spread the disease, patients with classic symptoms may be treated without this procedure (Mead, Faro, Gibbs, & Gomel, 1984). Laparoscopy may facilitate diagnosis for patients with atypical symptoms or frequent recurrences, although there are conflicting opinions in the literature on the value of this procedure and on its appropriate use. The following grading system is proposed:

Grade I   Uncomplicated, limited to tube or ovary or both

Grade II   Complicated, inflammatory mass or abscess involving tube and/or ovary

Grade III   Spread to structures beyond pelvis (ruptured tubo-ovarian abscess)

Differential Diagnosis

Salpingitis must be differentiated from ectopic pregnancy, ruptured corpus luteum cyst, twisted ovarian cyst, twisted or degenerative fibroid, and nongynecologic problems that may be associated with similar symptoms. These problems include appendicitis, diverticulitis, and bladder infection. *Mittleschmerz*, dysmenorrhea, premenstrual pain, and adenomyosis should also be considered. The three problems most often confused with salpingitis are appendicitis, ectopic pregnancy, and endometriosis.

Management

Data Collection

HISTORY. The initial phase in any diagnostic workup is history taking. Certain symptomatology is more characteristic of disorders other than salpingitis and is very valuable to rule out these conditions. Timing and onset, location, nature, frequency, duration, and intensity of pain are basic to a history of the complaint. A menstrual history helps a woman pinpoint the onset of symptoms in relation to her cycle. Other associated factors also may be relevant. Appendicitis pain is most often unilateral and accompanied by gastrointestinal upset and appetite loss. Unilateral pain without gastrointestinal symptoms suggests ectopic pregnancy or ovarian cyst. Suprapubic pain suggests a bladder infection. Endometriosis usually causes the patient a longer history of cyclic pain occurring in the first 1 to 2 days of menses. Temperature is usually less than 101°F in both appendicitis and bladder infection and is not elevated at all in endometriosis and unruptured ectopic pregnancy.

History of recent pelvic operation, delivery, or abortion is significant. A sexual history is an aid in diagnosis, as salpingitis is rare in non–sexually active women, unless it is a long-standing, chronic problem relating to prior sexual experiences (Martin, 1978). Possible exposure to an STD, especially gonorrhea or nongonococcal urethritis, or the likelihood of such exposure based on the sexual behavior of the woman and/or her partner(s) is an important piece of data. Symptoms of STDs in the patient's partner or partners should be noted (Loucks, 1983). Contraceptive use is relevant as salpingitis may be associated with IUD use, and chlamydial infections, with oral contraceptive use (see Chapters 7 and 8).

PHYSICAL EXAMINATION. A complete physical examination should follow the history taking. Vital signs are important. A careful abdominal examination can provide valuable diagnostic information. In a patient with salpingitis, abdominal examination reveals tenderness on palpation. There may be guarding with deep—or even light—palpation, depending on the acuity and severity of the infection. Tenderness is more likely to be bilateral than with appendicitis or ectopic pregnancy. There may or may not be rebound tenderness, although this is generally characteristic of appendicitis. Tenderness of the costovertebral angle should be evaluated to rule out pyelonephritis.

Pelvic examination should be thorough and careful. Uterine sources of pain must be ruled out. An adnexal mass may represent an ectopic pregnancy, ovarian cyst, tubo-ovarian abscess, hydrosalpinx, or pyosalpinx. The latter three may accompany salpingitis. A rectal examination may help localize the pain.

Whether or not a primary care practitioner should perform a pelvic examination on a woman for whom there is a strong suspicion of salpingitis is a serious question. Without a pelvic assessment, the diagnosis cannot be made; however, as therapy requires medical management and often even hospitalization, it is quite likely that the pelvic examination will be repeated by the physicians involved in treatment. Unfortunately, this diagnostic tool may exacerbate the problem as well as cause great pain for the woman; all authors advise the minimum number of necessary examinations. If the diagnosis of salpingitis seems rather clear from history and abdominal examination findings and the referring physician is available, it may be prudent to defer the pelvic examination.

LABORATORY TESTING. Laboratory data, however, can be ordered before or concurrently with a consultation and/or referral. An ESR greater than 50 mm/hr and a CBC with differential showing leukocytosis and a left shift are consistent with a diagnosis of salpingitis. Cultures of the endocervix and any periurethral exudate should be taken for *N. gonorrhoeae* and *C. trachomatis* (see Chapter 4 for further discussion of these tests). Culturing for other microorganisms is considered largely a waste because correlation between endocervical and intraperitoneal organisms is poor (Mead et al., 1984). Noninflammatory adnexal conditions seldom yield the laboratory changes of salpingitis. The laboratory

changes may, however, be delayed, and appear after clinical manifestations. Microscopic urinalysis and urine culture and sensitivity are necessary to rule out a urinary tract infection or to discover a coincident infection. Serum tests for syphilis should be performed on all patients with salpingitis, as 3 to 10 percent of patients positive for gonorrhea are also positive for syphilis (Martin, 1978, p. 270).

Sonography is another useful diagnostic tool. It can detect uterine causes of pain and, perhaps, reveal ovarian cysts or an ectopic pregnancy. In salpingitis, sonography may reveal an adnexal mass, which, in acute cases, may be a pyosalpinx or a tubo-ovarian abscess. In subacute cases of salpingitis such a mass may be a hydrosalpinx. If a culdocentesis is performed by a physician to rule out an ectopic pregnancy, purulent material may be recovered in the case of salpingitis. This should be cultured.

Laparoscopy is extremely useful in diagnosis and evaluation of the extent of tubal damage. Laparoscopy is routinely carried out in all suspected cases of salpingitis in Scandinavia (Jacobson & Weström, 1969); however, the procedure is invasive and, at this time, is not used as readily here as in Scandinavia because of the fear of peritoneal spread of the infection (Hager et al., 1983, p. 113).

Intervention

TREATMENT. Physician consultation and referral are mandatory for the treatment of salpingitis. Although some experts recommend hospitalization for all women with PID, the CDC (1985b, p. 92S) recommends hospitalization in the following situations: "(1) the diagnosis is uncertain, (2) surgical emergencies such as appendicitis and ectopic pregnancy cannot be excluded, (3) a pelvic abscess is suspected, (4) the patient is pregnant, (5) the patient is a prepubertal child, (6) severe illness precludes outpatient management, (7) the patient is unable to follow or tolerate an outpatient regimen, (8) the patient has failed to respond to outpatient therapy, and (9) clinical follow-up within 72 hours of starting antibiotic treatment cannot be arranged." The CDC also recommends considering hospitalization for adolescents because of unpredictable compliance with therapy and the severity of the long-term sequelae in this age group. Subacute salpingitis may be managed on an outpatient basis, but also in conjunction with a gynecologist.

The CDC (1985b) has issued guidelines for the treatment of salpingitis. The therapy is aimed at gonorrhea, chlamydia, and a variety of aerobic and anaerobic bacteria. Either regimen A or regimen B is recommended for in-hospital treatment of acute salpingitis.

Regimen A
- Doxycycline, 100 mg IV twice daily *plus*
- Cefoxitin, 2.0 g IV four times daily
- Continue drugs IV for at least 4 days and at least 48 hours after the patient shows improvement
- Continue doxycycline 100 mg by mouth twice a day, after discharge from the hospital to complete 10 to 14 days of total therapy.

Regimen B
- Clindamycin 600 mg IV four times daily *plus*
- Gentamycin 2.0 mg/kg IV followed by 1.5 mg/kg IV three times daily in patients with normal renal function
- Continue drugs IV for at least 4 days and at least 48 hours after the patient shows improvement.
- Continue clindamycin 450 mg by mouth four times daily to complete 10 to 14 days of therapy.

The CDC has also made recommendations for ambulatory patients.

- Cefoxitin 2.0 g IM, or amoxicillin 3 g by mouth, *or* ampicillin 3.5 g by mouth, *or* aqueous procaine penicillin G 4.8 million units IM at two sites, *or* ceftriaxone 250 mg IM. Each of these regimens, except ceftriaxone, is accompanied by probenecid 1.0 g by mouth, followed by doxycycline 100 mg by mouth, twice daily for 10 to 14 days.
- Tetracycline HCl 500 mg by mouth four times daily is less active against certain anaerobes and requires more frequent dosing.
- Treatment with penicillin, ampicillin, amoxicillin, or a cephalosporin alone is not recommended.
- Tetracycline or a derivative covers better for *Chlamydia*. Doxycycline given by mouth causes nausea.

FOLLOW-UP CARE AND TEACHING AND COUNSELING. All male sexual partners of patients with salpingitis should be examined for STDs and promptly treated. Green (1977) recommends bedrest in low or medium Fowler's position and few pelvic examinations during the disease's acute phase. Care during the recovery phase includes prolonged restriction of activities with adequate rest and nutrition for several months. When the patient is completely asymptomatic and has a totally negative pelvic exam, regular activities may be resumed subsequent to several normal menstrual cycles. Follow-up laboratory work after treatment for salpingitis should include endocervical cultures for a test-of-cure. Sonography after treatment may be useful for the detection of resultant tubal abnormalities (Spirtos, Bernstine, Crawford, & Fayle, 1982).

Contraceptive counseling must be provided. Condoms provide some protection from STDs. IUDs in place at the time of salpingitis should be removed, and such a patient is a poor risk for reinsertion. A woman with a history of salpingitis needs to understand this risk before she chooses this method of birth control. Oral contraceptive users have been found to carry only one fourth the risk of developing salpingitis secondary to gonorrhea as those using IUDs and are one half as likely to develop salpingitis as women who use no contraception (Ory, 1982); however, they have been found to have an increased risk of developing chlamydial infections (Washington, Gove, Schachter, & Sweet, 1985). Diaphragm users should have a new diaphragm prescribed and discard the one used at the time of infection.

Fertility may be compromised by salpingitis secondary to pelvic adhesions, impaired ciliary action, or scarred tubal lumen. It is important to remember that a pelvic or adnexal mass is not necessary for an infection to cause sterility. In Weström's epidemiologic study among Swedish women, it was shown that after one episode of salpingitis, 11 percent of those affected are rendered infertile; after two episodes, 24 percent; and after three, 54 percent (Mead et al., 1984). Subacute salpingitis results in more disruption of tubal function, highlighting the importance of correct early diagnosis and the insidiousness of the *Chlamydia* organism.

The discovery of infertility secondary to salpingitis may not occur until a woman attempts to become pregnant. After salpingitis, a woman should be advised that if she encounters this difficulty in the future, she should inform her health care provider of her previous salpingitis. Pinpointing this as a probable cause may help ease an infertility workup.

Because any disease related to the reproductive system is so intimately tied up with sexuality, and with body image and self-image, women diagnosed with salpingitis need supportive care. Feelings need to be discussed and partners included in the care, both because they require diagnosis and treatment for themselves in the case of either gonococcal or nongonococcal infections and because they are involved in the emotional aspects of this disease. All care, of course, must be provided in a nonjudgmental fashion with consideration given to possible psychological sequelae. Short- or long-term counseling may be indicated and appropriate referrals should be offered as needed.

ECTOPIC PREGNANCY

The failure of a fertilized ovum to implant within the uterus yields an ectopic pregnancy. Such pregnancies can be fatal. The skill and alertness of the clinician are vital, as early diagnosis of this condition is the best assurance of its safe and satisfactory resolution.

Most ectopic pregnancies are the result of implantation in the fallopian tube; indeed, this accounts for approximately 97 percent of all ectopic pregnancies. The remaining 3 percent of ectopic pregnancies occur at ovarian sites, in a rudimentary uterine horn, in the broad ligament, in the abdomen itself, and, most uncommonly, at the cervix. Abdominal pregnancies have extremely rarely been completed with a viable fetus (Birnbaum, 1981).

Among tubal implantations, the most frequent site is the ampulla, possibly because it is the normal site of fertilization. Interstitial pregnancy, however, is very difficult to diagnose in its early stages and, therefore, represents a significant danger. Awareness of such a pregnancy often occurs after spontaneous rupture at 12 to 16 weeks of gestation, with severe intraabdominal bleeding and shock as its consequences (Benson, 1980).

Etiology

The leading single predisposing factor for ectopic pregnancy is salpingitis. About 25 percent of the cases of ectopic pregnancy are associated with previous or coexisting salpingitis. The inflammatory disease process results in partial obstruction and narrowing and twisting of the tubal lumen, which leads to the formation of tubal pockets that may entrap a fertilized ovum. Damage to the cilia or the tube impedes its ability to effect ovum migration. Although prompt recognition of inflammatory disease with effective therapy prevents total tubal obstruction, some impairment of tubal function is usually sustained (Weström & Mårdh, 1981).

Previous tubal or abdominal surgery resulting in the formation of adhesions that can cause partial tubal occlusion is implicated in ectopic pregnancy. Congenital anomalies featuring atresia, diverticula, or accessory ostia (openings), as well as benign tubal tumors and cysts, interfere with migration of the ovum from the tube to the uterus. An ectopic pregnancy may occasionally be a complication of a tubal ligation, particularly if the technique used involves extensive destruction, such as occurs with unipolar coagulation (Halka, 1985). It is also possible that a fistula may be created in some women at the site of the ligation scar, providing a passageway for sperm to fertilize the egg which may then lodge in the distal stump of the tube (Halka, 1985).

Slightly more than half of all ectopic pregnancies are not associated with any of these predisposing factors. In tubes that are anatomically and histologically normal, a number of factors may be involved in an ectopic pregnancy. Any fluctuation in the regular cycle of hormonal output may lead to delay in the proper function of ciliated cell, secretory cell, and smooth muscle activity, which is quite dependent on ovarian hormonal stimulation. Instead of being transported, the fertilized ovum continues its development in the tubes beyond its usual 3-day stay and tubal implantation results. An interesting finding in a number of ectopic pregnancies is the formation of a contralateral corpus luteum, suggesting either migration of the ovum to the opposite tube rather than to the uterus or fertilization in the peritoneal space. Tubal spasm, seen on hysterosalpingogram, has been postulated as interfering with transport. Such spasms are thought to be the result of disturbance of the normal autonomic nervous system regulation of tubal muscular activity caused by an emotional or psychological disturbance (Green, 1977). Finally, if ovulation and fertilization are delayed so that they do not coincide with uterine conditions necessary for adequate uterine implantation and support, the fertilized ovum may be transported back into the tube through a reflux mechanism.

Incidence, Risk Factors, and Sequelae

The incidence of ectopic pregnancy is rising dramatically (DeVore & Baldwin, 1986). This increase may be related to the concurrent rise in the incidence of PID (salpingitis). Between the years 1978 and 1983 the yearly rise in ectopic pregnancies averaged over 11 percent. The rate of ectopic pregnancy per 1,000 live births tripled over 11 years, from 4.8 in 1970 to 14.5 in 1980. When all reported pregnancies are considered, the rate increased from 4.5 per 1,000 in 1970 to 10.5 per 1,000 in 1980 (CDC, 1984). There has, however, been an almost sevenfold decline in deaths from nonuterine pregnancy, from 3.5 per 1,000 in 1970 to 0.53 per 1,000 in 1983 (Atrash, Friede, & Hogue, 1987). This is due to an increase in earlier diagnosis and the widespread use of effective treatment (Dorfman, 1983). Mortality rates are significantly higher for black and other minority women than for whites, particularly among adolescents. This difference may be a result of inadequate access to care (Atrash et al., 1987).

Current treatment of ectopic pregnancy concerns itself with the preservation of as much of the fallopian tube as possible to protect the patient's future reproductive capability. Again, the earlier the diagnosis, the better the outlook for subsequent fertility.

Women who have had a previous ectopic pregnancy, salpingitis, or tuboplasty or who are in a low socioeconomic group all have a higher-than-average risk of ectopic pregnancy. The ectopic pregnancy rate is highest in women aged 35 to 44 and in black women of all age groups (Benson, 1980; Green, 1977).

Clinical Presentation

A woman with an unruptured ectopic pregnancy presents with amenorrhea, lower abdominal pain (often unilateral), and slight vaginal bleeding. Classic physical findings include a normal or slightly softened uterus and a unilateral tender adnexal mass. If the ectopic pregnancy has ruptured, the patient presents with severe generalized—or at least bilateral—abdominal pain, referred shoulder pain secondary to intraabdominal bleeding, vertigo, fainting, and shock. There is exquisite tenderness on cervical motion, cul-de-sac fullness, and a severely painful adnexal mass. The clinical picture is not always clear, however. A very early ectopic pregnancy may not yet be palpable and a normal intrauterine pregnancy may appear with a corpus luteum cyst mistaken for an adnexal mass and staining from

physiologic placental growth mistaken for bleeding from an ectopic implantation.

The majority of patients, in fact, present with subacute manifestations of ectopic pregnancy. About a fourth of women with diagnosed ectopic pregnancies have no history of amenorrhea. Abdominal pain is usually vague and of a "crampy" nature. Uterine enlargement is another very variable feature. The indefinite symptomatology, in combination with the value of early diagnosis, creates a clinical management challenge (Altchek, 1984).

Symptoms may depend on the site of ectopic implantation. Tubal implantations in the interstitial portion of the tube may become symptomatic at a later stage of pregnancy than other tubal pregnancies (14 to 16 weeks compared with 5 to 10 weeks) and may be associated with a larger degree of hemorrhage (Johns, 1984).

Differential Diagnosis

The frequent lack of specific symptoms in ectopic pregnancy makes the list of differential diagnoses rather long:

- Normal intrauterine pregnancy with implantation bleeding
- Intrauterine pregnancy with an accompanying cause for abdominal pain
    Painful, normal corpus luteum
    Ruptured, bleeding corpus luteum
    Ovarian cyst
    Torsion of the ovary containing the corpus luteum
    Torsion of the fallopian tube
    Round ligament pain
    Degeneration or torsion of pedunculated fibroid
- Intrauterine pregnancy with threatened abortion
- Intrauterine pregnancy with missed or incomplete abortion
- Appendicitis
- Endometriosis
- Pelvic inflammatory disease (salpingitis)
- Ovarian tumors or cysts
- Pedunculated fibroids
- Tubo-ovarian abscess
- Diverticular abscess

Management

Data Collection

HISTORY. Because of the ambiguity in the presenting picture of an ectopic pregnancy, this diagnosis should be considered in any woman with lower abdominal pain and/or unusual vaginal bleeding. A careful history is the first essential step in determining the likelihood of this diagnosis. A thorough history of risk and predisposing factors is helpful. The presenting complaint should be described precisely. Onset, type, duration, and frequency of pain are all important. Presence of referred pain, especially to the shoulder, presence of any associated factors, such as dizziness and fatigue, and increase in pain are all important to assess. Factors that may bring on the pain, such as sex, diet, and activity, as well as all episodes of unusual bleeding, should be documented. Sometimes a patient interprets unusual bleeding as a normal variation in her menstrual cycle, so a complete menstrual history is necessary, including usual frequency, duration, amount, and character of blood, associated pain, and recent variations in any of these. Again, factors associated with or preceding bleeding should be elicited. A sexual and contraceptive history are obviously important in ruling out ectopic pregnancy.

PHYSICAL EXAMINATION. Physical examination is the next step in diagnosis. Traditional findings in a tubal pregnancy include a normal or slightly softened or enlarged uterus with a tender adnexal mass on one side; however, these may not be present and findings may more closely approximate those of a normal nonpregnant examination or even an early intrauterine pregnancy.

LABORATORY TESTING. If, after history and physical examination, the suspicion of an ectopic pregnancy still exists, laboratory data are essential and can generally be ordered by the primary care practitioner, although institutional protocols and/or practice agreements with consultants and laboratories may necessitate that the physician order some of these tests.

The most useful laboratory tools for conservative management of suspected ectopic pregnancy in the absence of signs of rupture are determination of the β subunit of human chorionic gonadotropin (hCG) and sonogram (Holman, Tyrey, & Hammond, 1984). Radioimmunoassay (RIA) for β-hCG with a sensitivity of 5 mIU/mL should be used to avoid the false-negative results obtained with less sensitive tests (Berry, Thompson, & Hatcher, 1979; Romero & Horgan, 1985, p. 270). The concentration of serum hCG doubles every 2 to 3 days through the first 6 weeks of pregnancy (8 weeks from last menstrual period), at which time it levels off. At 6.5 weeks from the last menstrual period, the mean hCG is 10,000 mIU/mL. Failure to reach this level at the appropriate gestational age or failure of hCG to double in 48 hours is suggestive of ectopic pregnancy. In most ectopic pregnancies, hCG is above the normal nonpregnant level of 10 mIU/mL, but below 6,000 mIU/mL (Ackerman, Deutsch, & Krumholtz, 1982).

Ultrasound is able to identify an intrauterine pregnancy 6 weeks after the last menstrual period or when the β-hCG titer is 6,000 to 6,500 mIU/mL or greater (Kadar, DeVore, & Romero, 1981), as the gestational sac is then visible. Prior to this time, a sonogram to document pregnancy or detect an ectopic pregnancy is unreliable. It is most useful to document or rule out other conditions. A sonogram may, however, reveal tubal enlargement, although it may not be able to differentiate such an enlargement from other adnexal masses (Pedersen, 1980).

Once ectopic pregnancy has been strongly suggested or confirmed, medical management is necessary for its prompt treatment. There are also several additional diagnostic tests that fall into the realm of medical procedures.

Culdocentesis may be done to determine the presence of free blood in the pelvis; however, the information provided by culdocentesis is limited and its use in diagnosing ectopic pregnancy has decreased in recent years. Failure to obtain bloody fluid does not rule out ectopic pregnancy, as a false-negative culdocentesis occurs in at least 10 percent of cases, apparently as a result of early, nonleaking ectopic pregnancies. Furthermore, blood obtained from the tap may originate from a leaking ovarian cyst, a miscarriage, or retrograde menstruation. The accuracy of culdocentesis is therefore only about 75 to 80 percent. Any blood obtained from this procedure should be observed for coagulation for 10 minutes; absence of clotting indicates that free-lying intraperitoneal fluid was aspirated, whereas clotting signifies accidental pelvic venipuncture (Altchek, 1984).

Dilation and curettage (D&C) may be performed for diagnosis if the patient does not desire a pregnancy. Recovery of decidua and villi confirms intrauterine pregnancy. An empty gestational sac with an hCG greater than 6,500 mIU/mL suggests a missed abortion.

Laparoscopy yields very reliable diagnoses. An unruptured ectopic pregnancy looks like an oval, smooth, egg-shaped dusky blue tubal enlargement. Combined false-negative and false-positive rates of laparoscopy total less than 3 percent (DeCherney, Minkin, & Spangler, 1981). It is, however, an invasive procedure, carrying with it the risks of surgery and anesthesia.

Intervention

TREATMENT. A ruptured ectopic pregnancy with accompanying hemorrhage and shock is an emergency. A woman presenting in this condition should be brought to the hospital for surgery as soon as possible. The patient should be advised of what she can expect in the hospital. Blood will be drawn for a complete blood count (CBC), type, Rh, antibody screen, prothrombin time (PT), and partial thromboplastin time (PTT), fibrinogen, and chemistries. She may need to receive blood and general anesthesia for emergency surgery.

A suspected ectopic pregnancy may be managed expectantly (Altchek, 1984; DeCherney, et al., 1981), in consultation with a physician. The more invasive diagnostic procedures may be deferred depending on the acuity of the symptoms and the availability of laboratory and sonographic facilities. The practitioner, however, must always be aware of the danger of a missed diagnosis.

A CBC should be obtained for a baseline hemoglobin and hematocrit and to monitor possible blood loss. An ESR may be useful as it is markedly elevated in salpingitis, to levels greater than 50 mm/mL, higher than the elevation seen in pregnancy. Quantitative hCG levels should be obtained. CBC and quantitative hCG should be repeated in 24 hours. Depending on the time from the last menstrual period, a sonogram can rule out intrauterine pregnancy and may identify an adnexal mass. Blood type and Rh must be known in anticipation of possible surgery and administration of RhoGAM.

If hCG and sonographic results point to an extrauterine pregnancy, the investigation may advance to culdocentesis. A positive culdocentesis necessitates laparotomy; a negative one, laparoscopy. Laparoscopy may be preferred without prior culdocentesis. Culdocentesis should not be done if the uterus is sharply retroflexed. If the possibility of an incomplete abortion still exists, a D&C may be done before laparoscopy, with a frozen section for identification of villi if necessary.

Conservative surgery with the aim of preserving future childbearing ability is recommended, if feasible. Careful technique, microcautery, atraumatic handling of tissue, and use of fine nonreactive suture provide the patient with the best chance of intact tubal function (Schenker & Evron, 1983). Approximately 50 percent of patients who experience ectopic pregnancy subsequently achieve a normal intrauterine pregnancy. Unfortunately, 10 percent incur repeat ectopic pregnancies. Infertility results in the remaining 40 percent, with 30 percent rendered sterile (Benson, 1980). The occurrence of salpingitis increases the chances of a subsequent ectopic pregnancy (Nagamani, London, & St. Amand, 1984).

TEACHING AND COUNSELING. Throughout the procedures, tests, and examinations described earlier, the patient should be informed of the working diagnosis, the nature of the tests, the information gained, and the plan of management. After surgery, the patient should receive RhoGAM if Rh negative. She should be counseled regarding contraception, with the risks of the IUD to reproductive capability made clear. The outlook for future childbearing should be discussed. The patient should be fully informed, in writing if necessary, of the extent of her surgery in terms she can understand. She may need a description of anatomy and physiology, with an explanation that even the most radical surgery—unilateral salpingectomy—does not necessarily interrupt the reproductive process; however, such women should also receive thorough counseling regarding the symptoms of another ectopic pregnancy as they are at increased risk for a recurrence. The symptoms of salpingitis should also be reviewed so, if an episode should occur, she can receive prompt treatment to minimize further tubal damage.

Many women experience a severe sense of loss after an ectopic pregnancy. They may go through the grieving process, especially if the ectopic pregnancy was a planned, wanted pregnancy. Fear is a normal reaction, particularly if future childbearing is desired. Sympathetic, compassionate, and supportive counseling should be provided, with the woman's partner and family included to the extent she desires. Guilt may be present and needs to be dispelled. Referrals to social services, grieving teams, and psychological counseling services may be necessary.

For women who wish to become pregnant again, the general advice is to await postoperative healing (approximately 6 to 8 weeks) and the resumption of six normal menstrual cycles. This allows for the resolution of the grieving process (see Chapter 23) (DeVore & Baldwin, 1986). Patients should be aware of the significant increased risk of a repeat ectopic pregnancy and be taught its signs and symptoms. Early pregnancy testing is recommended. Predisposing factors such as salpingitis must be treated prior to a pregnancy attempt. Anomalies should be corrected if possible. Counseling and referral for in vitro fertilization should be considered if total bilateral loss of the tubes or of tubal function occurs and if pregnancy is desired.

OTHER TUBAL PROBLEMS

Other tubal problems are most often found coincidental with another gynecologic disorder. Some are discovered during a workup for infertility.

Congenital Anomalies

Etiology. Tubal formation occurs late in the sixth week of gestation. Anomalies may result from genetic or environmental factors. Failure of müllerian duct fusion may result in the absence of fallopian tubes, in the development of rudimentary tubes, or in extra ostia.

Symptoms. There are no symptoms specific to tubal anomalies. The absence of tubes almost always occurs in conjunction with the absence of a uterus. Infertility obviously is a consequence. Accessory tubes and ostia are factors predisposing to ectopic pregnancy.

Treatment. If pregnancy is desired and tubal function is inadequate, in vitro fertilization may be suggested. Accessory tubes can be removed and ostia closed surgically.

Torsion of the Fallopian Tube

Torsion of the fallopian tube is a rare condition. It may occur with or without associated tubal disease, in pregnancy,

or after tubal ligation. It is seen most commonly during the menstruating years. Because pain is often the only symptom, the diagnosis is almost always made at surgery. Pain may be sharp and coliclike or intermittent; it may radiate to the thigh or the flank and loin. Nausea and vomiting are occasionally present. Temperature and pulse are usually normal or slightly elevated, and the patient generally feels otherwise well. Localized abdominal tenderness is present and a tender adnexal mass can be palpated on pelvic examination. Differential diagnoses include appendicitis, twisted ovarian cyst, ectopic pregnancy, ruptured ovarian follicle, pelvic inflammatory disease, and renal or ureteral colic, because of the radiating pain to the flank (Filtenborg & Hertz, 1981).

Tubal Masses

There are many types of benign neoplasms of the fallopian tubes, but they are extremely rare. Malignancies are more common. Benign neoplasms usually do not produce problems for the patient and are almost never diagnosed preoperatively. A description of several benign neoplasms follows.

Tumors

ADENOMATOID TUMORS. Adenomatoid tumors constitute the most common type of benign tubal neoplasm, with an incidence of only 0.4 percent in one study involving examination of 7,485 tubes (Bolton & Hunter, 1958). They are quite small and asymptomatic, appearing as firm grayish white or yellow nodules within the muscle of the tube. These tumors are chiefly significant for their association with uterine leiomyomas.

LEIOMYOMA. Only 75 cases of tubal leiomyoma have been reported (Klein & Smith, 1965; Roberts & Marshall, 1961). In the very rare instance when these leiomyomas are large, they can cause torsion of the tube and result in pain; however, tubal leiomyomas are usually small and single. Degeneration, similar to that seen in uterine leiomyomas, may also occur (see Chapter 14).

TERATOID TUMORS. *Teratoid tumors* are solid tumors, usually small, often pedunculated from the tubal mucosa, and found in the middle of the tube. There have been only 46 reported cases, 50 percent of which have occurred in nulliparous women (Mazzarella, Okagaki, & Richart, 1972). Large teratomas produce a palpable mass and symptoms of pressure, pain, and secondary infection. Torsion may occur.

Cysts. There are two types of paraovarian cysts: paramesonephric and mesonephric. Pregnancy exacerbates the growth of these cysts.

PARAMESONEPHRIC CYSTS. Paramesonephric cysts develop in the mesosalpinx and are interligamentous in the broad ligament. They are unilocular, filled with clear fluid, and tend to be large, usually 10 cm in diameter. Such cysts are palpable and cause pressure and pain. With acute torsion or rupture, the resultant symptoms are suggestive of ectopic pregnancy and lead to surgical intervention.

MESONEPHRIC CYSTS. Mesonephric cysts are the second most common paraovarian cyst and develop from vestigial remnants of the mesonephric (or wolffian) ductal system of the fetus, particularly of structures known as the epoophoron and paraoophoron, which lie in the broad ligaments, the mesosalplinx, and the meso-ovarium. Gartner's duct cysts (of the vagina), wolffian cysts, and uterine cysts all fall into this category, as do *hydatid cysts of Morgagni*, which are small pedunculated structures that occur at the fimbriated end of the tube and are symptomatic only with torsion.

Carcinoma. Adenocarcinoma is the most common malignant lesion of the fallopian tube. Rarely occurring malignancies include lymphoma, sarcoma, carcinosarcoma, and choriocarcinoma. Primary fallopian tube carcinoma is the rarest of all female pelvic malignancies; its incidence has been reported as between 0.1 and 1.0 percent (Green, 1977).

Postmenopausal women who report a history of infertility are at highest risk for these malignancies. Frequently, salpingitis, uterine fibroids, and tubal carcinoma are coexistent, although a history of salpingitis alone is not a significant risk factor.

CLINICAL PRESENTATION. Tubal carcinoma may be quite advanced before the patient experiences signs of disease. Women in their fifties and sixties may present with vague pelvic discomfort or pain, particularly with abnormal vaginal bleeding or discharge. Frequently associated with tubal carcinoma is *hydrops tubal profluens*, which is the intermittent occurrence of profuse, watery, yellow or bloody vaginal discharge that is abrupt in onset with colicky pain. This occurs, however, in a minority of patients. The lesions remain nonpalpable in the early stages of disease when chance for resection would be greatest. Vaginal cytologic findings are positive in less than half of patients with tubal carcinoma (Green, 1977). Persistent bleeding after negative endometrial curettage in postmenopausal women should alert a practitioner to the possibility of tubal malignancy.

TREATMENT AND PROGNOSIS. Because of the rarity of primary tubal carcinoma, its optimal treatment remains unclear (Boronow, 1973). Prognosis is related to the clinical stage of the carcinoma at the time of treatment. Staging is based on the extent of disease. A variety of staging criteria have been proposed, but, in all, early stages describe disease confined to the tubes or with extension only to the pelvic region; later stages involve intraperitoneal or distant metastases (Raju, Barker, & Wiltshaw, 1981; Roberts & Lifshitz, 1982; Schiller & Silverberg, 1971). Five-year survival rates in the literature show a wide variation: for patients diagnosed with early-stage tubal cancer, survival rates have been reported as high as 76.5 percent (Roberts & Lifshitz, 1982); later-stage disease is associated with survival rates up to 25 percent (Raju et al., 1981) and 33 percent (Tamimi & Figge, 1981), although much lower rates have been noted (Wong, Tindall, Wagstaff, et al., 1985). Overall survival rates have been reported at between 5 and 48 percent (Raju et al., 1981; Wong et al., 1985). All reports are based on studies involving small numbers of patients.

Treatment generally consists of total abdominal hysterectomy with bilateral ooporectomy and salpingectomy, although debulking may be the only surgery possible with very large tumors. Chemotherapy and radiation have both been used in the treatment of primary tubal carcinoma, but their benefits are unclear. Guthrie and Cohen (1981) report a case of inoperable tubal carcinoma that became operable after combination chemotherapy with Adriamycin, cyclophosphamide, and a progestogen. Other recent authors agree that chemotherapy needs further investigation (Raju et al., 1981; Tamimi & Figge, 1981). Several authors (Roberts & Lifshitz, 1982; Wong et al., 1985) have found no

value in pelvic irradiation. In a literature review, Tamimi and Figge (1981) conclude that it is not possible to evaluate the role of radiation therapy because of a lack of consistency concerning disease staging and radiation modalities. The difficulty in determining the most efficacious treatments for primary tubal carcinoma lies in the rarity of this tumor.

REFERENCES

Ackerman, R., Deutsch, S., & Krumholtz, B. (1982, July). Levels of human chorionic gonadotropin in unruptured and ruptured ectopic pregnancy. *Obstetrics and Gynecology, 60*(1), 13–15.

Altchek, A. (1984, September). Ectopic pregnancy in young patients. *Contemporary Ob/Gyn, 24*(3), 120–152.

Atrash, H. K., Friede, A., & Hogue, C. J. R. (1987, December). Ectopic pregnancy mortality in the United States. *Obstetrics and Gynecology, 70*(6), 817–822.

Benson, R. (1980). *Current obstetric and gynecologic diagnosis and treatment.* San Mateo, CA: Lange Medical Publications.

Berry, C. M. Thompson, J. D., & Hatcher, R. (1979, July). The radioreceptor assay for hCG in ectopic pregnancy. *Obstetrics and Gynecology, 54*(1), 43–46.

Birnbaum, S. J. (1981). Ectopic pregnancy. In G. Schaefer & E. A. Graber (Eds.), *Complications in obstetrics and gynecology.* New York: Harper & Row.

Bolton, R. N., & Hunter, W. C. (1958, September). Adenomatoid tumors of the uterus and adnexa. *American Journal of Obstetrics and Gynecology, 76*(3), 647–652.

Boronow, R. C. (1973, July). Chemotherapy for disseminated tubal cancer. *Obstetrics and Gynecology, 42*(1), 62–66.

Centers for Disease Control (CDC). (1984, April 20). Current trends: Ectopic pregnancies—United States 1970–1980. *Morbidity and Mortality Weekly Report, 33*(15), 201–202.

Centers for Disease Control (CDC). (1985a, August 23). Chlamydia trachomatis infections: Policy guidelines for prevention and control. *Morbidity and Mortality Weekly Report, 34*(3, Suppl.), 53S–74S.

Centers for Disease Control (CDC). (1985b, October 18). Sexually transmitted diseases: Treatment guidelines. *Morbidity and Mortality Weekly Report, 34*(4, Suppl.), 75S–108S.

DeCherney, A. H., Minkin, M. J., & Spangler, S. (1981, October). Contemporary management of ectopic pregnancy. *The Journal of Reproductive Medicine, 26*(10), 519–523.

DeVore, N., & Baldwin, K. (1986, June). Ectopic pregnancy on the rise. *American Journal of Nursing, 86*(6), 674–678.

Dorfman, S. F. (1983, September). Deaths from ectopic pregnancy, United States 1970–1980. *Obstetrics and Gynecology, 62*(3), 334–338.

Dougherty, C., & Pastorek, J. (1985). Sexually transmitted diseases and miscellaneous pelvic infections. In W. Droegemueller & J. Sciarra (Eds.), *Gynecology and Obstetrics* (Vol. I). Philadelphia: Harper & Row.

Eschenbach, D. A., Buchanen, T. M., & Pollack, H. M., et al. (1975, July 24). Polymicrobial etiology of acute pelvic inflammatory disease. *New England Journal of Medicine, 293*(4), 166–171.

Filtenborg, T. A., & Hertz, J. B. (1981, September). Case report: Torsion of the fallopian tube. *European Journal of Obstetrics, Gynecology and Reproductive Biology, 12*(3), 177–181.

Green, T., Jr. (1977). *Gynecology: Essentials of clinical practice.* (3rd ed.). Boston: Little, Brown.

Guthrie, D., & Cohen, S. (1981, October). Carcinoma of the fallopian tube treated with a combination of surgery and cytotoxic chemotherapy. *British Journal of Obstetrics and Gynaecology, 88*(10), 1051–1053.

Hager, W. D., Eschenbach, D. A., Spence, M., & Sweet, R. L. (1983, January). Criteria for diagnosis and grading of salpingitis. *Obstetrics and Gynecology, 61*(1), 113–114.

Halka, J. (1985). Gynecologic laparoscopy. In W. Droegemueller & J. Sciarra (Eds.), *Gynecology and obstetrics* (Vol. I). Philadelphia: Harper & Row.

Holman, J. F., Tyrey, E. L., & Hammond, C. B. (1984, September 15). A contemporary approach to suspected ectopic pregnancy with use of quantitative and qualitative assays for the β subunit of human chorionic gonadotropin and sonography. *American Journal of Obstetrics and Gynecology, 150*(2), 151–157.

Jacobson, L., & Weström, L. (1969, December 1). Objectivized diagnosis of acute pelvic inflammatory disease. *American Journal of Obstetrics and Gynecology, 105*(7), 1088–1098.

Johns, J. L. (1984, June). Ectopic pregnancy. *Nurse Practitioner, 9*(6), 17–22.

Kadar, N., DeVore, G., & Romero, R. (1981, August). Discriminatory hCG zone: Its use in the sonographic evaluation of ectopic pregnancy. *Obstetrics and Gynecology, 58*(2), 156–161.

Klein, H. Z., & Smith, R. L. (1965, October). Fibromyoma of the uterine tube. *Obstetrics and Gynecology, 26*(4), 515–517.

Loucks, A. (1983, October). Pelvic inflammatory disease: A review of therapy. *Nurse Practitioner, 8*(9), 13, 16–18.

Martin, L. (1978). *Health care of women.* Philadelphia: J. B. Lippincott.

Mazzarella, P., Okagaki, T., & Richart, R. M. (1972, March). Teratoma of the uterine tube: A case report and review of literature. *Obstetrics and Gynecology, 39*(3), 381–388.

Mead, P. B., Faro, S., Gibbs, R., & Gomel, V. (1984, January). Symposium: Modern management protocols for PID. *Contemporary Ob/Gyn, 23*(1), 225–244.

Muckle, C. W. (1985a). Clinical anatomy of the uterus, fallopian tubes, and ovaries. In W. Droegemueller & J. Sciarra (Eds.), *Gynecology and obstetrics* (Vol. I). Philadelphia: Harper & Row.

Muckle, C. (1985b). Developmental abnormalities of the female reproductive organs. In W. Droegemueller & J. Sciarra (Eds.), *Gynecology and Obstetrics* (Vol. I). Philadelphia: Harper & Row.

Nagamani, M., London, S., & St. Amand, P. (1984, July 1). Factors influencing fertility after ectopic pregnancy. *American Journal of Obstetrics and Gynecology, 149*(5), 533–535.

Ory, H. W. (1982, March 15). The non-contraceptive health benefits of oral steroid contraceptives. *American Journal of Obstetrics and Gynecology, 142*(6, Part 2), 809–816.

Pedersen, J. F. (1980, January). Ultrasonic scanning in suspected ectopic pregnancy. *British Journal of Radiology, 53*(625), 1–4.

Raju, K. S., Barker, G. H., & Wiltshaw, E. (1981, November). Primary carcinoma of the fallopian tube: Report of 22 cases. *British Journal of Obstetrics and Gynaecology, 88*, 1124–1129.

Roberts, J. A., & Lifshitz, S. (1982, June). Primary adenocarcinoma of the fallopian tube. *Gynecologic Oncology, 13*(3), 301–308.

Roberts, C. L., & Marshall, H. K. (1961, August). Fibromyoma of the fallopian tube. *American Journal of Obstetrics and Gynecology, 82*(2), 364–366.

Romero, R., & Horgan, J. G. (1985). Diagnostic ultrasound in gynecology. In D. H. Nichols & J. R. Evrard (Eds.), *Ambulatory gynecology.* Philadelphia: Harper & Row.

Schenker, J. G., & Evron, S. (1983, December). New concepts in the surgical management of tubal pregnancy and the consequent postoperative results. *Fertility and Sterility, 40*(6), 709–723.

Schiller, H. M., & Silverberg, S. G. (1971, August). Staging and prognosis in primary carcinoma of the fallopian tube. *Cancer, 28*(2), 389–395.

Spirtos, N. J., Bernstine, R. L., Crawford, W. L., & Fayle, J. (1982, June). Sonography in acute pelvic inflammatory disease. *Journal of Reproductive Medicine, 27*(6), 312–320.

Svensson, L., Weström, L., Ripa, K. T., & Mårdh, P.-A. (1980, December 1). Differences in some clinical and laboratory parameters in acute salpingitis related to culture and serologic findings. *American Journal of Obstetrics and Gynecology, 138*(7, Part 2), 1017–1021.

Sweet, R. L. (1981, October–December). Pelvic inflammatory disease: Etiology, diagnosis and treatment. *Sexually Transmitted Diseases, 8*(4, Suppl.), 308–315.

Tamimi, H. K., & Figge, D. C. (1981, September 15). Adenocarcinoma of the uterine tube: Potential for lymph node metastases. *American Journal of Obstetrics and Gynecology, 141*(2), 132–137.

Washington, A. E., Gove, S., Schachter, J., & Sweet, R. L. (1985, April 19). Oral contraceptives, *Chlamydia trachomatis* infection, and pelvic inflammatory disease. *Journal of the American Medical Association, 253*(15), 2246–2250.

Weström, L., & Mårdh, P.-A. (1981). Impact of sexually transmitted diseases on human reproduction: Swedish studies of infertility and ectopic pregnancy. *Sexually Transmitted Diseases 1980 Status Report*, NIH Study Group NIH Publications, 43.

Wong, W. S., Tindall, V. R., & Wagstaff, J., et al. (1985, August). Surgery and radiation in the treatment of primary carcinoma of the fallopian tube—Report of 18 cases. *Australian and New Zealand Journal of Obstetrics and Gynaecology, 25*(3), 211–215.

16

The Ovaries

Virginia Jackson and Ronnie Lichtman

The ovaries provide an unusually large number of opportunities for pathologic expression, because they comprise a variety of cell types and perform many functions. The primary care practitioner must screen for ovarian abnormalities and make decisions regarding the need for consultation and referral.

This chapter prepares the practitioner for these tasks by briefly reviewing the anatomy and physiology of the ovary and describing selected ovarian disorders. These include congenital and developmental disorders, abnormalities of ovarian function, and a variety of ovarian enlargements and tumors, including cancer. Inflammatory disease of the ovary and ovarian pregnancy are briefly discussed. Because most ovarian pathology is not managed independently by primary care providers, discussions of management focus on the screening role.

ANATOMY AND PHYSIOLOGY

The normal ovary is approximately 3.5 × 2 × 1.5 cm in the postmenarcheal, premenopausal woman. After menopause, the ovary atrophies and is usually about 2 × 1 × 0.5 cm. There are two ovaries, one on each side of the uterus, in the upper part of the pelvic cavity. They are held in the broad ligament by the mesoovarium and attached to the uterus by the ovarian ligament. The infundibulopelvic ligament anchors each ovary to the pelvic wall. The ovary itself is composed of several layers: the *germinal epithelium*, or covering, is a thin layer of columnar cells whose name is somewhat of a misnomer, as germ cells do not arise from this layer as was originally believed; the *cortex*, or outer layer, and the *medulla*, or central layer. Tiny follicles are located within the cortex of each ovary; ova develop within the follicles. The medulla consists of connective tissue, blood vessels, and smooth muscle fibers.

The ovaries produce two main hormones—estrogen and progesterone—as well as androgens and relaxin. Estrogen, particularly estradiol, is secreted mainly by the graafian follicles, and progesterone is secreted by the corpus luteum, which is formed each menstrual cycle at the site of the ruptured follicle. The corpus luteum also produces a small amount of estrogen. Androstenedione, an androgen, is secreted chiefly by the ovarian stroma. A normal menstrual cycle involves a complex series of stimulation/inhibition responses among the cerebral cortex, hypothalamus,

pituitary gland, endometrium, and ovaries, which is described in Chapter 1. Therefore, ovarian dysfunction may result not only from ovarian pathology, but from pathology in any of the other organs associated with reproductive function.

In addition to being an endocrine gland, the ovary is the repository of a lifetime's worth of immature ova or egg cells. Some ova mature and undergo division by meiosis; these are released from the ovary for possible fertilization. Others undergo atresia and are resorbed. An understanding of the stages of oogenesis—the production of ova—is necessary for an appreciation of the development of ovarian enlargements and some ovarian neoplasms. The following summary of oogenesis is adapted primarily from Marrs (1986) and Pritchard, MacDonald, and Gant (1985).

Primary oocytes are formed in the fetus and increase in number by mitosis, a process that results in replication of identical cells. The first phase of cellular meiosis, or the division into cells with half the number of chromosomes (23), also occurs during fetal life. Oocytes remain in this phase of meiotic development, called the germinal vesicle stage, until stimulated by the gonadotropins follicle-stimulating hormone (FSH) and luteinizing hormone (LH). In each menstrual cycle, under the influence of these two hormones, one follicle matures to become the *graafian* follicle. FSH is necessary for selection of primary ovarian follicles—up to 20 or more each cycle—that will undergo the changes necessary for the maturation of a single dominant follicle. After stimulation by gonadotropins, especially FSH, follicular (or granulosa) cells expand and increased fluid secretions create an *antrum* or large pool of fluid. Differentiation also occurs in ovarian stromal cells and a layer of specialized connective tissue is formed, the *theca folliculi*, which consists of an outer and inner portion, the *theca externa* and *theca interna* (Fig. 16-1). A mucoid band, the *zona pellucida*, also develops around the ovum and persists until the fertilized ovum reaches the uterus. FSH stimulates the follicular cells to form receptors for FSH and LH, and, as a result, estradiol is produced and secreted. This has a positive feedback on the hypothalamus and pituitary gland and more FSH and LH are secreted, causing further growth of the dominant follicle. LH stimulates completion of the first meiotic division before oocyte release. Completion of all phases of meiosis does not occur, however, until penetration by spermatozoa.

As the graafian follicle grows to 10 or 12 mm in diameter, it reaches the ovarian surface from which it protrudes

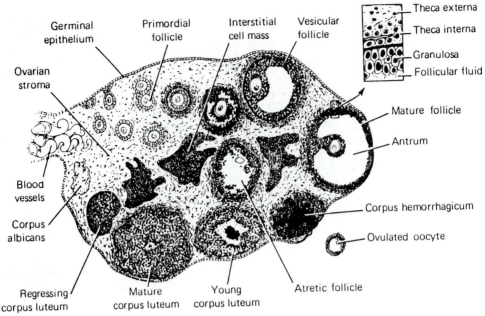

Figure 16–1. Maturation of dominant follicle. *(From Pernoll, M. L. & Benson R. C. (1987).* Current obstetric & gynecologic diagnosis & treatment. *East Norwalk, CT. Appleton & Lange.)*

and ultimately ruptures. The ovum is thus released. Immediately after ovulation, the *corpus luteum* is formed at the site of the ruptured follicle. The corpus luteum undergoes four developmental stages—proliferation, vascularization, maturity, and regression. During vascularization, bleeding occurs from thin-walled capillaries and fills the central cavity of the corpus luteum with blood. This is known as the *corpus hemorrhagicum.* A mature progesterone-secreting corpus luteum is usually 1 to 3 cm in diameter and is characteristically bright yellow. Its degeneration begins about 10 days after ovulation and 4 days before the onset of menstruation. When fertilization occurs, corpus luteum degeneration is postponed up to 2 to 4 weeks. In the absence of fertilization, degenerated lutein cells are resorbed and replaced by new connective tissue resembling the surrounding ovarian tissue.

STRUCTURAL, DEVELOPMENTAL, AND FUNCTIONAL ABNORMALITIES

Structural Abnormalities

Supernumerary and Accessory Ovaries. Supernumerary and accessory ovaries are formed during embryonic development (Jones & Jones, 1981). Supernumerary ovaries are extranormal ovaries found separate from the regularly located ovaries. There may be one or more. This condition is extremely rare. When extraovarian tissue is found near the normal ovary, connected to it, or has developed from it, it is termed an *accessory ovary.* Such ovaries are small, usually less than 1 cm in diameter. Generally, they are attached to the broad ligament near the ovary. Most often, they are found only at surgery, when they are mistaken for lymph nodes, and discovered to be ovarian tissue only on microscopic examination. Ovaries also may be malpositioned. This may be associated with müllerian anomalies described in Chapter 14 (Rock, Parmley, Murphy, & Jones 1986).

Tubal and Ovarian "Absence." Torsion of the ovarian pedicle may cause an ovary to separate from its normal at-

tachments and become parasitic to abdominal structures. The ovary and tube may appear absent but, most often, a small stump of tube and tiny nodule indicate a mechanical, rather than embryonic, etiology for this condition (Jones & Jones, 1981, pp. 208–209).

Developmental Abnormalities

Developmental abnormalities present with a failure in secondary sexual development (usually by age 14) or with the beginning of development followed by a cessation in its progress (Riddick, 1986). These problems are often a focus of adolescent health care (see Chapter 22).

Developmental disorders can result from dysfunction in a number of organs including the hypothalamus, pituitary, and ovary. Chapters 21 and 27 discuss the differential diagnosis of reproductive system dysfunction and present diagnostic approaches. This chapter briefly outlines ovarian causes of absent or arrested sexual development.

Ovarian Agenesis or Dysgenesis. Embryonic agenesis or dysgenesis leads to problems in sexual development. Ovarian agenesis, also called Turner's syndrome, is congenital absence of the ovaries. The müllerian ducts are present, but immature in this condition. The ovaries are represented by fibrous bands and are referred to as streak ovaries. Women with ovarian agenesis show an absence of one of the X chromosomes in all body cells (Riddick, 1986). The etiology of this disorder is nondisjunction of the sex chromosomes.

Clinically, women with Turner's syndrome are short with webbing of the neck, a "shield-type" chest with nipples placed laterally, and absence of breast development. Axillary and pubic hair is scanty or lacking. Coarctation of the aorta and absence of one kidney may be associated. A given woman with the syndrome, however, may not have all or any of these typical features. Laboratory findings include elevated gonadotropin levels and abnormal chromatin pattern in most patients. Treatment of this syndrome is hormonal: estrogen and progesterone to induce vaginal bleeding and secondary sexual characteristics. Ovarian transplants may become the treatment of the future (Jones & Jones, 1981).

Androgen insensitivity syndrome (also called testicular feminization) is a disorder inherited as a sex-linked recessive trait. These individuals, with 45 XY karyotypes, may have feminine or ambiguous genitalia along with intraabdominal testes. At puberty, changes associated with estrogen stimulation are seen. Breasts, therefore, develop fully. Development requiring androgen stimulation is absent; the woman has no pubic or axillary hair. Vaginal examination shows a blind vaginal pouch; the uterus and ovaries are absent (Riddick, 1986).

Women with pure gonadal dysgenesis have an XX chromosomal pattern. Gonadal dysgenesis results from oocyte damage prior to the eighth week of embryonic development. Women with mosaics or 45 XY chromosomal patterns (Swyer's syndrome) may have similar manifestations, but the etiology is different. Clinically, these women have normal-appearing female genitalia, but they do not undergo puberty or menarche (Riddick, 1986). The latter also may present with hypertrophy of the clitoris or with almost normal testicular development and male external genitalia with hypospadias (Jones & Jones, 1981, pp. 761–762). Neoplastic changes occur in the gonads of 20 to 30 percent of women with XY gonadal dysgenesis. Therefore, the gonadal tissue is usually removed and cyclical hormonal therapy instituted when an XY chromosomal pattern is detected (Sarto, 1986, p. 38).

Functional Abnormalities

Ovarian Failure. Ovarian failure occurs when the follicles do not produce estradiol in response to gonadotropin stimulation. It may result from a loss of follicles during embryonic development, at puberty, or in the years after puberty. Ovarian failure also may be the result of radiation or chemotherapy. The latter is often reversible (Riddick, 1986).

Premature Ovarian Failure. Premature ovarian failure (POF) is defined as failure of ovarian estrogen production anytime between menarche and age 35 or 40 (Alper & Garner, 1985; Davajan & Kletzky, 1986). It may present with amenorrhea, signs and symptoms of estrogen deficiency (menopausal signs and symptoms), and elevated levels of FSH and LH. On biopsy, ovaries show changes consistent either with a postmenopausal state or with a lack of follicular development. Women with POF have elevated gonadotropin levels. A serum FSH determination above 30 to 50 mIU/mL is usually diagnostic. No uterine bleeding follows progesterone administration. Thyroid and adrenal insufficiency should be screened for in women under age 35 with POF. Estrogen/progesterone replacement is usually the recommended treatment for POF. Women with POF are considered sterile, although rarely ovulation can be induced (Aiman & Smentek, 1985; Davajan and Kletzsky, 1986).

The Insensitive Ovarian Syndrome. The insensitive ovarian syndrome (also called Savage syndrome) is an extremely rare disorder of increased gonadotropin levels but with follicular development to the antrum stage (see Anatomy and Physiology). The ovaries in this syndrome are resistant to gonadotropin stimulation. A case report, however, has appeared documenting a viable pregnancy in a woman with this syndrome treated with estrogen and progesterone (Shangold, Turksoy, Bashford, & Hammond, 1977).

Luteal Phase Defects. Luteal phase defects are responsible for some cases of infertility or recurrent abortion. These defects have a variety of etiologies, among which are ovarian disorders. The corpus luteum may function poorly, leading to inadequate progesterone production. This may be caused by defective or insufficient numbers of ovarian LH receptors, possibly resulting from inadequate FSH stimulation of ovarian granulosa cells (March, 1986). Inadequate follicular development or premature atresia of follicles may also lead to luteal phase defects. Luteal phase defects present with infertility despite normally occurring ovulation. Luteal phase defects can be diagnosed by endometrial biopsy in the luteal phase and possibly treated with progesterone therapy. Therapy is administered after ovulation by rectal suppository (Darland, 1985).

The *luteinized unruptured follicle syndrome* (LUF) refers to a condition in which a follicle matures but never ruptures, although the cells around the oocyte contained in the follicle show luteal phase changes (Katz, 1987). No cause has been identified for this syndrome (LeMaire, 1987); evidence is uncertain whether LUF is associated with endometriosis or pelvic inflammatory disease. LUF can be demonstrated by ultrasound. It is possible that it is implicated in some cases of infertility, but LUF occurs intermittently in some fertile women.

Polycystic Ovarian Syndrome. Polycystic ovarian syndrome (PCOS) is a disorder characterized by amenorrhea, hirsutism, and obesity, originally thought to be caused by enlarged polycystic ovaries. In fact, the ovaries are not inherently abnormal in this syndrome. Enlarged or polycystic ovaries are neither necessary for, nor specific to PCOS. Although the ovaries may be enlarged and/or polycystic in PCOS, they may be grossly normal. Enlarged, polycystic ovaries also may be associated with Cushing's syndrome, congenital adrenal hyperplasia, and some ovarian or adrenal tumors, and, on occasion, they may be seen in normal young girls. The main hormonal abnormality in PCOS is increased LH levels with normal or low FSH levels and elevated androgens. The increased ovarian androgen secretion may lead to premature follicular atresia and thus ovarian dysfunction. This dysfunction, however, is not a result of an ovarian pathology. Lobo (1986, p. 320) has suggested renaming the syndrome hyperandrogenism with chronic anovulation (HCA).

When history suggests PCOS, referral should be made for a complete hormonal workup for diagnosis, including, for example, levels of FSH and LH, androgens, and 17-ketosteroids. Thyroid function tests can be initiated to rule out hypothyroidism.

Clinical Presentation. Structural ovarian defects such as supernumerary and accessory ovaries cause no problems and need no treatment. Developmental disorders present as intersex or endocrine problems noted in infancy or adolescence. Functional disorders lead to bleeding problems, infertility, or both. They offer a challenge in diagnosis because of the variety of organs that are involved in menstrual and reproductive control.

Management

Data Collection

HISTORY. Complete history taking, including menstrual, gynecologic, sexual, contraceptive, medical, and family histories, is of extreme importance in making diagnostic decisions and in selecting appropriate management for ovarian disorders. The age of the woman is an integral component of this history. Chapters 21 and 27 provide detailed information on historical data necessary in the evaluation of women with abnormalities of bleeding and infertility.

PHYSICAL EXAMINATION. A thorough physical and pelvic examination is essential. Chapter 22 describes specific components of physical assessment necessary to evaluate adolescent development. Chapter 21 provides further discussion of physical examination findings that help the practitioner determine the organ responsible for developmental and menstrual dysfunctions.

LABORATORY TESTING. Most often, ovarian disorders require consultation and referral for diagnosis and treatment. Karyotyping is important in any abnormality presenting with disorders of development or sexuality. Chapters 21 and 27 discuss laboratory testing appropriate for women with problems related to menstrual function and fertility.

Intervention. Treatment for ovarian disorders generally involves hormonal manipulation. Additional interventions may include manual or surgical creation of a functional vagina and/or surgical removal of testes. Primary care management requires referral to a gynecologic endocrinologist or to a specialist in adolescent medicine or infertility.

TUMORS

This section begins with a description of the classification of ovarian enlargements and tumors and symptoms shared by most types of tumors. Then, selected benign enlargements and tumors are described. A brief discussion of ovarian cancer follows. All components of management are outlined within the description of each type of tumor. The specific management role of the primary care provider is highlighted at the conclusion of the entire section.

Classification

Tumors can arise in the many different types of ovarian connective tissue or cells with specific differentiation and function, as well as from ovarian embryonic remnants. Nonneoplastic ovarian enlargements result from the processes of follicular development and atresia (Merrill, 1986).

Tumors or neoplasms of the ovary are classified according to cell type and whether or not growth is cystic. The degree of fibrous stroma also is considered. Within each category, the tumor is then designated as benign, of low malignant potential, also called borderline malignant, or malignant. Degree of malignancy is most important in evaluating prognosis (Colgan & Norris, 1983).

The most common neoplasms of the ovary arise from the germinal or surface epithelium of the ovary. Most ovarian tumors are seen during the reproductive years and are most common among women in their forties. In children and postmenopausal women, ovarian tumors are likely to be malignant.

Symptoms

Many ovarian tumors are asymptomatic. When symptoms are present, they tend to occur late in the tumor's development and are not specific to a particular type of tumor. Pressure, an increase in abdominal girth, pain, gastrointestinal symptoms, menstrual abnormalities, and hormonal changes are among the usual presenting symptoms. The following descriptions are adapted from Merrill (1986).

Pressure. A large tumor may lead to a feeling of heaviness or generalized pressure in the pelvic area. As the tumor grows, it may press on the bladder leading to urinary frequency or incontinence. Occasionally, the urethra or ureters may be obstructed. Large tumors also may interfere with lymphatic and venous drainage of the legs, resulting in edema or varicosities. They can cause venous distension over the abdomen and elevate the diaphragm so that shortness of breath occurs.

Increased Girth. When a tumor attains a large size, it may produce an increase in girth, which may be the only symptom associated with the tumor. This may be obscured in the obese woman. In a young child, tumor growth may be noted by parents while bathing or dressing the child.

Pain. Pain is a rare symptom of an ovarian tumor. When it does occur, it is usually associated with tumor rupture, torsion of its pedicle, or rapid distension, possibly from hemorrhage. Pain of ovarian origin is described as a constant aching. It may be referred to the iliac or inguinal region on the same side and the inner aspect of the upper thigh. Occasionally, it radiates to the vulva. A tumor may cause dyspareunia.

Gastrointestinal Symptoms. Mild nausea, epigastric discomfort, and anorexia may occur with ovarian tumors. These symptoms, however, are quite nonspecific and may not arouse suspicion of a problem of ovarian origin.

Menstrual Abnormalities. Tumors may lead to menstrual abnormalities, particularly if they are hormone secreting. Estrogen-secreting tumors can cause oligomenorrhea or amenorrhea followed by irregular, heavy, or long menstrual periods.

Hormonal Changes. Ovarian tumors may be associated with feminization or masculinization. An ovarian tumor should be considered in the young girl with precocious sexual development (Brenner, 1986) and in the postmenopausal woman with a return of uterine bleeding. Signs of Cushing's syndrome and hyperthyroidism may be related to an ovarian tumor (see Chapter 21). Although these changes are among the most obvious symptoms of ovarian tumors, tumors that produce them are not common.

Complications

Complications of ovarian tumors include hemorrhage, torsion, rupture, and, rarely, infection. These may create emergency situations.

Hemorrhage. Hemorrhage into a cyst usually is gradual and associated with minimal symptoms. If it is sudden, however, and of a large amount, acute radiating abdominal pain will occur. If blood escapes into the peritoneal cavity, abdominal distension, tenderness, and rebound tenderness will be present. Once the cyst has ruptured, diagnosis is difficult if its presence had not been detected previously.

Torsion. Both cystic and solid tumors may develop a weak pedicle. Complete or partial torsion of the pedicle may result. The latter produces congestion and enlargement of the tumor with thrombosis of vessels. The former may lead to obstruction of the arterial blood supply with necrosis. The resulting pain may be sudden or gradual.

Torsion occurs more frequently with benign tumors

than with malignant neoplasms, which are often larger, heavier, less mobile, and more often adherent to adjacent structures. Among the specific tumors discussed in the subsequent section, torsion is seen most commonly with dermoid cysts, cystadenomas, and fibromas.

Rupture. An ovarian cyst may rupture after hemorrhage, torsion, or trauma, including intercourse or bimanual examination. Its contents may be spilled into the peritoneal cavity. Symptoms may be increased or actually lessened temporarily, if they had been secondary to distension. Symptoms depend on the contents of the cyst, with serous fluid causing few or none. Chemical peritonitis may result, particularly after rupture of a dermoid cyst (see Dermoid Cysts).

Infection. Ovarian tumors rarely become infected, although infection may occur secondary to hemorrhage, necrosis, or concomitant salpingitis. An infected ovarian tumor may be indistinguishable from a tubo-ovarian abscess (see Tubo-ovarian Abscess later in this chapter).

Specific Types of Benign Ovarian Enlargements or Tumors

There are more than 50 different histologic variants of primary ovarian neoplasm (Katsube, Berg, & Silverberg, 1982). This chapter cannot discuss each variety of ovarian enlargement or tumor. Indeed, many of the distinctions are clinically insignificant in terms of the primary care role. Therefore, this chapter presents brief descriptions of the more common types of enlargements and tumors, particularly those that the primary care practitioner may manage conservatively. This section focuses on providing the practitioner with the information necessary to distinguish such functional cysts from more pathologic varieties and to determine when consultation and referral are warranted.

Follicular Cysts. Follicular cysts are the most frequently encountered type of ovarian cyst. Follicular cysts are formed during the first half of the menstrual cycle if the dominant follicle fails to ovulate and continues to grow or if any of the other follicles fail to undergo atresia. The largest follicular cysts are about the size of a lemon, although most are much smaller. Very large, and possibly multiple, follicular cysts may be seen occasionally with hyperstimulation from exogenous gonadotropins used to induce ovulation (Kilgore & Younger, 1984) (see Chapter 27). The most frequent outcome of a follicular cyst is spontaneous resorption, just as in the normal process of atresia.

SYMPTOMS. There are no symptoms specific to follicular cysts; however, they may have some effects on menses. The estrogen-rich fluid of the cysts may cause irregular menses, particularly when the cysts are large. Large cysts also may cause feelings of pelvic heaviness, congestion, and aching on the affected side. Torsion of the pedicle or the very rare spontaneous rupture with bleeding produces sudden abdominal pain. This clinical picture resembles ectopic pregnancy.

MANAGEMENT

Data Collection: History. Because of the asymptomatic nature of follicular cysts, a history may yield no specific data; however, the woman's age and menstrual status are important in evaluating the potential significance of any ovarian

enlargement or growth. Last menstrual period and recent menstrual pattern should be noted to correlate with development of the cyst, or to evaluate whether there is menstrual irregularity. Sexual and contraceptive histories should be taken and subjective symptoms of pregnancy asked about to help rule out ectopic pregnancy.

Physical Examination. Follicular cysts normally are noted during pelvic examination. They are small, rarely achieving a diameter greater than 3 cm, often multiple, and commonly bilateral. It is, however, difficult to base a diagnosis on one examination. A follicular cyst commonly disappears within 8 weeks, whereas a neoplastic growth persists or enlarges.

Laboratory Testing. Laboratory testing generally is not required. Ultrasound is not very useful, with the information obtained no better, or worse, than that obtained via clinical examination (O'Brien, Buck, & Nash, 1984). A pregnancy test should be performed to rule out ectopic pregnancy (see Chapter 15).

Intervention. Unless a woman is postmenopausal, the initial intervention when a follicular cyst is suspected is expectancy. The woman should be reexamined in 6 to 10 weeks. If the adnexal mass is still present, or larger, referral for laparotomy should be made.

If follicular cysts are found during surgery, they may be treated by needling and draining or excision, depending on their size. No treatment is required, however, for small follicular cysts.

Lutein (Corpus Luteum) Cysts. Lutein cysts usually are formed by a hematoma or unusual growth of the corpus luteum. They are less common, but more clinically significant, than follicular cysts. They form in the latter part of the menstrual cycle.

The normal corpus luteum of menstruation and pregnancy does not exceed 2 cm and is not cystic. The mechanism of cyst formation is excessive physiologic bleeding into the central cavity during the second or vascularization stage of corpus luteum development (see Anatomy and Physiology). Rupture may occur as well from a normal-sized corpus luteum in the vascularization stage (Hallatt, Steele, & Snyder, 1984). Multiple corpus luteum cysts may result from hyperstimulation of the ovary after the use of fertility drugs (Kilgore & Younger, 1984). Most often, corpus luteum cysts disappear spontaneously, as in the normal regression stage of the corpus luteum.

SYMPTOMS. Persistent corpus luteum cysts produce menstrual irregularities; generally, delay in onset of the next menses is seen, usually up to 3 or 4 weeks, but uncommonly up to 6 months. Subsequent flow is irregular and prolonged. Ovarian distension causes crampy pain, usually unilateral and dull. A ruptured corpus hemorrhagicum may occur any time during the luteal phase of the cycle, usually about 1 week before menses, causing generalized, severe abdominal pain. Depending on the amount of bleeding, the pain may radiate to the back, shoulders, or legs, with rectal and/or bladder discomfort. A ruptured corpus luteum cyst usually occurs either late in the cycle or during or after the delayed menses. Actual rupture may be preceded by several days of slow bleeding into the cyst capsule, resulting in adnexal discomfort. Bleeding is often extensive. This entity may almost precisely mimic ruptured ectopic pregnancy.

Differential Diagnosis. Differential diagnosis includes ectopic pregnancy, ovarian cyst with torsion, pyosalpinx, hydrosalpinx, tubo-ovarian abscess, and other ovarian masses. With rupture, the clinical picture may be confused with appendicitis or ruptured ectopic pregnancy.

MANAGEMENT

Data Collection. History. A painstaking menstrual history is needed to determine when in the cycle symptoms appeared, whether menses is or has been delayed, and whether the last period was prolonged with unusual, unilateral pain. The possibility of ectopic or intrauterine pregnancy must also be ruled out, requiring a thorough sexual and contraceptive history. Whether the woman is on any anticoagulant therapy is important, as this has been known to lead to a bleeding corpus luteum (Hallatt, Steele, & Snyder 1984).

Physical Examination. With a corpus luteum cyst, pelvic examination usually reveals a small tender swelling on the side of the pelvis corresponding to the pain.

Laboratory Testing. Because corpus luteum cysts are difficult to distinguish from ectopic pregnancy, a pregnancy test must be done. If there is no pregnancy, the cyst yields no β human chorionic gonadotropin (hCG). A complete blood count (CBC) should be performed and repeated if management is expectant. When the diagnosis is unclear, referral for culdoscopy or laparotomy, or both, should be made. Serosanguineous fluid on culdocentesis is consistent with a ruptured corpus luteum cyst (Hallatt et al., 1984).

Intervention. The treatment of lutein cysts or hematomas consists of observation and expectant management, as most of them will disappear spontaneously. Once bleeding from a corpus luteum stops, no treatment is required, provided the diagnosis is certain. In the case of hemorrhagic cysts of considerable size or where there is evidence of active intraperitoneal bleeding, excision is necessary. Before removal of the cyst, the possibility of very early gestation should be considered. Then the corpus luteum should be preserved, if possible, or exogenous hormonal therapy given immediately. A rupture with subsequent hemoperitoneum can result in massive blood loss. Treatment consists of laparotomy and hemostasis.

Dermoid Cysts. A dermoid cyst is a benign cystic teratoma. It is the most common ovarian germ cell neoplasm and constitutes approximately 18 to 25 percent of all ovarian tumors (Katsube et al., 1982; Merrill, 1986). It is the most frequently encountered type of ovarian tumor in women less than 20 years old (Woodruff, Protos, & Peterson, 1968). It peaks in incidence among women aged 20 to 40 years old.

The dermoid consists of tissue from all three embryonic germ cell layers: ectoderm, mesoderm, and endoderm. It has a thick, formed capsule that is lined with squamous epithelium, beneath which are found sweat, apocrine, and sebaceous glands. Cartilage, nervous tissue, and hair may be present. The most notable content of this cyst is teeth. Dermoid cysts usually are found on a long ovarian pedicle. The incidence of torsion varies but has been estimated to be about 16 percent (Woodruff et al., 1968).

SYMPTOMS. There are no symptoms specific to a dermoid cyst. A feeling of pelvic heaviness and ache may be present. Symptoms may occur with torsion. When torsion is slight,

the resulting pain is moderately severe and transitory. The pain may resolve spontaneously if the cyst untwists. Torsion may be sudden, with more dramatic symptoms and excruciating pain.

MANAGEMENT

Data Collection. History and Physical Examination. Any ovarian or related symptomatology should be elicited when the history is taken. A dermoid cyst is often palpated in the abdomen or anterior to the uterus because of its long pedicle. Dermoids are bilateral approximately 12 percent of the time (Merrill, 1986), and most measure 5 to 10 cm in diameter. Their consistency on physical examination is tensely cystic.

Laboratory Testing. An X-ray examination may be useful in diagnosing a dermoid cyst because the teeth, found in 30 to 50 percent of dermoids, can be visualized. A pregnancy test should be ordered to rule out ectopic pregnancy whenever an adnexal mass is palpated (see Chapter 15).

Intervention. Excision is the treatment of choice for a dermoid cyst. Approximately 1 to 3 percent of these cysts become malignant (Green, 1977). Whether the opposite ovary should be incised and inspected for a second tumor is controversial (Merrill, 1986). Prognosis is related to the intactness of the capsule and the absence of extraovarian extension. Among those rare tumors with malignant change, 80 percent are squamous cell cancers, 7 percent are adenocarcinoma, and the remainder are sarcomas of various types: melanomas, carcinoids, and thyroid carcinomas (Jones & Jones, 1981).

Other Benign Ovarian Masses

COMMON SURFACE EPITHELIAL NEOPLASMS. Surface epithelial neoplasms include *mucinous cystadenomas* and *serous cystadenomas*. The difference between these lies in whether they resemble tissues of the fallopian tube or of the endocervix. Serous tumors resemble the tube and mucinous tumors resemble the endocervix (Jones & Jones, 1981, p. 509).

Mucinous cystadenomas account for 16 to 30 percent of all benign ovarian tumors (Merrill, 1986). They occur most commonly among women in their twenties to forties. They grow rather large, often up to 30 cm in diameter, and at times up to 50 cm. These adenomas are rarely bilateral. Inadvertent rupture during dissection may result in a complication known as *pseudomyxoma peritonei* in which diffuse implants develop on the peritoneal surfaces and mucinous material accumulates within the peritoneal cavity. This condition leads to intestinal obstruction with subsequent malnutrition and has a high mortality rate.

Serous cystadenomas are less common, but together with mucinous cystadenomas, they comprise the most common ovarian tumors. These masses occur most commonly in women aged 20 to 50. They may grow from 5 to 15 cm in diameter. They are reported to be bilateral between 12 and 50 percent of the time. Occasionally, they may fill the abdomen. At times, these tumors may lead to excessive production of androgens (Bernhisel & Hammond, 1986). Their potential malignancy is reported at 32 to 45 percent (Merrill, 1986). A variant of the serous cystadenoma is the *cystadenofibroma*. It is a less common tumor, partially cystic and partially solid, and most often unilateral.

OVARIAN RETENTION CYSTS. Retention cysts are seen in menstruating women. They can be quite large and often disappear spontaneously.

ENDOMETRIAL CYSTS. Endometrial cysts, known as endometriomas, arise from endometriosis and are discussed in Chapter 18.

BENIGN SOLID TUMORS. Benign solid tumors consist of *fibromas, Brenner's tumors,* and *thecomas.* Complications of these include torsion and degeneration. Fibromas occur most frequently in middle age; the average age of occurrence is 48 years. They are occasionally bilateral and average about 6 cm in diameter; rarely, fibromas as large as 20 cm have been found. Ascites and hydrothorax (Meig's syndrome) may occur in association with fibromas. Brenner's tumors are seen most commonly in postmenopausal women and may be associated with postmenopausal bleeding. These tumors may be androgenic (Bernhisel & Hammond, 1986). A thecoma may secrete estrogens (Young & Scully, 1982).

SEX CORD–MESENCHYMAL TUMORS (GONADAL STROMAL TUMORS). Sex cord tumors demonstrate endocrine function. They include *granulosa cell tumors, Sertoli–Leydig cell tumors,* and some *thecomas.*

The granulosa cell tumor is a unilateral estrogen-secreting neoplasm that may grow as large as 30 cm. It may cause precocious puberty if it occurs in a prepubertal girl, although only approximately 5 percent of these tumors are in this age group (Brenner, 1986). About 50 percent occur in the postmenopausal years (Merrill, 1986, p. 1125). Malignancy is reported as between 10 and 35 percent (Piver, 1984).

Sertoli–Leydig cell tumors, also called *androblastomas,* are rare tumors, accounting for less than 0.2 percent of ovarian neoplasms. They are usually unilateral, androgen secreting, and found in women between 20 and 40 years old. Their peak incidence occurs at age 25, although these tumors can be seen at any age (Bernhisel & Hammond, 1986). Virilism or hirsutism occurs in about 50 percent of all cases. Amenorrhea may be present. Occasionally, these tumors are estrogenic (Young & Scully, 1982). Torsion, hemorrhage, and degeneration are common. The malignancy rate is about 25 percent (Merrill, 1986).

Ovarian Cancer

Ovarian cancer is actually a collection of malignancies and is impossible to describe as a single entity because of the variety of histogenic types originating in the ovary. Each type of ovarian cell has the potential to develop a tumor. The ovary also is a site for metastasis of other cancers, both genital and extragenital (Mazur, Hsueh, & Gersell, 1984).

Most primary ovarian malignancies, however, fall into one of three categories (Zaloudek, Tavassoli, & Kurman, 1986): neoplasms derived from the ovarian surface epithelium, called *epithelial tumors;* neoplasms derived from the gonadal stroma, called *gonadal stromal tumors;* and neoplasms derived from germ cells, called *germ cell tumors.* A few rare tumors do not fit any of the categories, for example, soft tissue sarcomas, which arise from mesenchymal elements that make up the supportive framework of the ovary; others contain elements of more than one type of tissue. Epithelial tumors are the most common among adult women. Highly malignant solid teratomas, embryonal carcinomas, dysgerminomas, and sarcomas most frequently appear at puberty or during adolescence.

Incidence and Mortality. In 1987, the American Cancer Society (ACS) estimated 19,000 new cases of ovarian cancer, representing over 26 percent of all female genital cancer, although only 4 percent of all cancer seen in women. Ovar-

ian cancer is the leading cause of death among gynecologic cancers, estimated in 1987 to cause more than 50 percent of deaths from cancer of the genital tract. It is responsible for approximately 5 percent of deaths from cancer in women, following only lung, breast, and colorectal cancer in female cancer mortality. In 1987, ACS estimated 11,700 deaths from ovarian cancer in the United States.

Most ovarian cancers appear at or shortly after menopause; 60 percent are in women 40 to 60 years old. Twenty percent develop in women over 60 years old, and the remaining 20 percent occur in women under 40 years of age. Incidence per population increases with age, with 70 cases per 100,000 population seen at age 75 (Zaloudek et al., 1986).

Etiology and Risk Factors. The etiology of ovarian cancer is largely unknown. Environmental factors or diet may play a role in its development; asbestos, talc, and intake of animal fat have been postulated as causative agents, but insufficient data exist to prove causality (Piver, 1986; Zaloudek et al., 1986). Epidemiologic studies indicate several risk factors, however. Risks include nulliparity, family history of ovarian cancer, history of breast, endometrial, or colorectal cancer, early menopause (before age 45) or late menarche (after age 14), or history of other ovarian dysfunction or malfunction (Larson 1983; Szamborski, Czerwinski, & Gadomska, 1981). Rare genetic disorders and Peutz–Jeghers syndrome, characterized by polyps of the gastrointestinal tract and mucocutaneous melanin pigmentation, predispose to ovarian tumors (Young et al., 1985; Zaloudek et al., 1986). Ovarian cancer rates are highest for Jewish women, nuns, and never-married women; the latter two may be related to nulliparity. Ovarian cancer is seen most often in North America and Europe and least often in Asia and Africa. Ovarian cancer is most common in developed nations with the exception of Japan. Japanese immigrants to the United States and their offspring, however, have rates higher than those of women in Japan (Young et al., 1985). It is not known whether the low rate of ovarian cancer in underdeveloped countries is real or due to underdiagnosis.

Oral contraceptive (OC) use is protective against ovarian cancer. This protective effect persists for years after discontinuation of OCs (Centers for Disease Control, 1982).

Symptoms. Unfortunately, symptomatology specific to ovarian cancer is lacking. Although the importance of early diagnosis is clear, the infrequency and inexactness of early symptoms hinder diagnosis. Ovarian cancer should be considered whenever any woman over 40 years old has complaints of vague abdominal or pelvic discomfort, increased flatulence, a sense of bloating, and/or indigestion (Barber, 1984). Menstrual disorders may occur with a hormone-producing tumor. Although most postmenopausal bleeding is associated with endometrial cancer, some instances are the result of ovarian cancer and this diagnosis must be ruled out. Abdominal swelling, pain, discomfort, abnormal uterine bleeding, and gastrointestinal and urinary complaints may occur with ovarian cancer (Dugan, 1985). Hemorrhage into the tumor or torsion of the ovary may produce sudden pain and other symptoms of acute abdomen (Zaloudek et al., 1986). Ascites is a late symptom.

Prognosis. Prognosis in ovarian cancer depends on cell type and stage and grade at the time of diagnosis. Staging of ovarian cancer helps predict survival and determine treatment. It is valuable in assessing which patients need therapy adjuvant to surgery and which do not. As adjuvant radiation and chemotherapy have serious side effects and have been associated with a small but significant risk of secondary malignancies, this is most important (Tucker & Fraumeni, 1987; Young, 1987). Staging is carried out by laparotomy. The stages of ovarian cancer, defined by the Federation of Gynecology and Obstetrics (FIGO) in 1974, appear in Table 16–1.

Women with stage I epithelial cancers have long-term survival rates of 60 to 70 percent (Zaloudek et al., 1986). This has been hypothesized to indicate the existence of occult metastasis. Unfortunately, less than 20 percent of women with ovarian cancer present with stage I and stage II disease (Brady, Markoe, DeEulis, & Lewis, 1987). Overall, 5-year survival in ovarian cancer is 29 to 32 percent (Lewis 1987).

It has been suggested that tumors be graded as well as staged; grading is determined according to degree of differentiation of cells in the tumor. This gives additional prognostic information and guidelines for treatment (Ozols, Garvin, & Costa, et al., 1980).

Metastasis. Metastasis of ovarian cancer occurs via a number of pathways: through direct invasion, peritoneal fluid, the lymphatics, and the venous system. These pathways are shown in Figures 16–2 and 16–3.

Data Collection

HISTORY. History may reveal vague symptoms or none at all. Age of the woman and menstrual status are most important in evaluating the likelihood of malignancy. Family history of ovarian cancer is highly significant.

PHYSICAL EXAMINATION. Pelvic examination reveals a mass in the adnexa; the mass is generally irregular and nontender, with immobility resulting from adhesions and fixation. Palpation of a mass, however, may be difficult in obese women. Bilaterality is an important finding; 70 percent of ovarian cancer is bilateral compared with only 5 percent of benign adnexal masses (Barber, 1984). A rectal examination should be done to better appreciate the mass. The examiner should note bilaterality, contour, fixation, tenderness, texture, size, and cul-de-sac nodules. A complete physical examination is warranted to rule out manifestations of endocrine-producing tumors and of possible metastases.

In a postmenopausal woman, the ovaries should not be palpable. A palpable ovary must lead to a suspicion of malignancy (Young et al., 1985).

TABLE 16–1. FIGO STAGING: COMMON EPITHELIAL OVARIAN CANCER

Stage I	Growth limited to the ovaries
IA	Growth limited to one ovary; no ascites
	1. No tumor on the external surface; capsule intact
	2. Tumor present on the external surface and/or capsule ruptured
IB	Growth limited to both ovaries; no ascites
	1. No tumor on the external surface; capsules intact
	2. Tumor present on the external surface and/or capsule(s) ruptured
IC	Tumor either stage IA or stage IB, but with ascites or positive peritoneal washings
Stage II	Growth involving one or both ovaries with pelvic extension
IIA	Extension and/or metastases to the uterus and/or tubes
IIB	Extension to other pelvic tissues
IIC	Tumor either stage IIA or IIB, but with ascites or positive peritoneal washings
Stage III	Growth involving one or both ovaries with intraperitoneal metastases outside the pelvis and/or positive retroperitoneal nodes; tumor limited to the true pelvis with histologically proven malignant extension to the small bowel or omentum.
Stage IV	Growth involving one or both ovaries with distant metastases. (If pleural effusion is present, there must be positive cytology to allot a case to stage IV; parenchymal liver metastases are classified in stage IV.)
Special Category	Unexplored cases thought to be ovarian carcinoma

From Dugan, K. K. The bleak outlook on ovarian cancer. American Journal of Nursing. 1985, 85(2), 146. Reprinted with permission.

LABORATORY TESTING. Laboratory testing may include Pap smear to rule out coexisting cervical cancer, a CBC, and a variety of possible tumor markers. These markers may be specific for particular tumors and include carcinoembryonic antigen (CEA), which has been reported in 58 percent of women with stage III epithelial ovarian cancer (Young et al., 1985); CA125, which has been isolated from more than 80 percent of women with epithelial ovarian malignancies (Averette et al., 1987); α=fetoprotein (AFP), which is elevated in endodermal sinus tumors (Barber, 1984); lactic dehydrogenase (LDH), which may be a tumor marker for dysgerminomas (Lurain, 1985) and which is elevated in women with extensive hepatic metastases (Barber, 1984); and hCG, which is produced by choriocarcinoma and em-

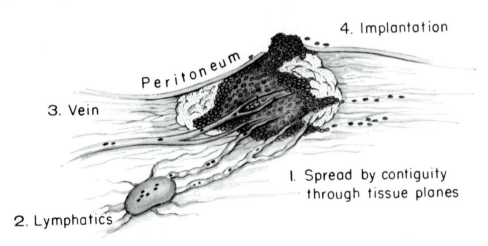

Figure 16–2. Schematic mechanisms of spread of ovarian cancer cells. *(From Cole, W. H., McDonald, G. O., Roberts, S. S. & Southwick, H. W. [1961] Dissemination of cancer. New York: Appleton-Century-Crofts. Reprinted with permission.)*

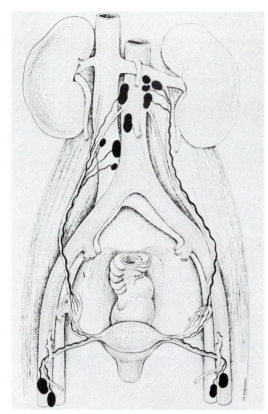

Figure 16–3. Lymphatics of the ovaries: The para-aortic and external iliac nodes. *(From Zaloudek, C., Tavassoli, F. A., & Kurman, R. J. [1986]. Lesions of the ovary: Malignant lesions. In D. N. Danforth, & J. R. Scott (Eds.), Obstetrics and gynecology [5th ed.]. Philadelphia: Lippincott. 1137. Reprinted with permission.)*

bryonal carcinoma and germ cell tumors with choriocarcinomatous elements (Young et al., 1985; Zaloudek et al., 1986). Other tests used to investigate complications and consequences of cancer include renal functions tests, liver chemistries, electrolyte studies, blood coagulation studies, chest X-ray, electrocardiogram (ECG), intravenous pyelogram (IVP), and barium enema (Helewa, Krepart, and Lotocki, 1986). Computerized axial tomography (CT scanning) and ultrasound are more useful in recurrent or advanced cancer (Zaloudek et al., 1986), although some authors advise their use in initial diagnosis (Lewis, 1987). Ultimately, laparotomy is necessary. Surgical staging and grading must be carried out.

Intervention

TREATMENT. Treatment of ovarian cancer almost always involves a combination of therapies. It always includes the surgical staging of the disease as well as removal of all tumor found and, most often, ovaries, fallopian tubes, uterus, and omentum—total abdominal hysterectomy (TAH) and bilateral salpingo-oophorectomy (BSO). After surgery, radiation therapy, chemotherapy, or both may be used. Sonography is useful in monitoring the effects of treatment. Measurement of CEA, CA125, AFP, LDH, and hCG is helpful in monitoring response to therapy, if levels had been elevated at the start of treatment.

Newer treatments, using biologic therapy, with such agents as interferon, monoclonal antibodies, immunotoxins, and antitumor antibodies, are in various stages of experiment (Hamilton, Ozols, & Longo, 1987). These agents are both immunologic and nonimmunologic. They act either directly on the tumor, on a physiologic process on which the tumor depends, or as a boost to the immune system.

A "second-look" laparotomy is often advised as part of treatment for ovarian cancer for restaging, tumor debulking, if it had not been possible prior to medical therapies, or evaluation of treatment (Averette et al., 1987; Stuart et al., 1982).

In young women, preservation of childbearing potential may be a consideration. Dysgerminomas appear most frequently in young women. Although all dysgerminomas are malignant, the degree is highly variable. The bilateral lesions fall into the highly malignant category in both histologic findings and clinical manifestations. In the case of young women with well-encapsulated unilateral tumors that contain no other aggressive cancer cells and are no larger than 10 cm, conservative operation, consisting of unilateral salpingo-oophorectomy, is justified by good survival rates at 5 and 10 years (Piver, 1984). These tumors do, however, have a high incidence of recurrence, approximately 43 percent (Thoeny, 1961). In stage II, III, or IV, the decision for total abdominal hysterectomy and bilateral salpingo-oophorectomy is clear-cut.

PREVENTIVE MEASURES. Avoiding exposure to talc and asbestos and reducing the fat content of the diet should be advised, particularly for women with a family history of ovarian cancer. High intake of vitamin A also has been advocated as preventive (Heintz, 1987). Some authors (Piver, 1986) advocate prophylactic oophorectomy for women with two or more first-degree relatives (mother, sister, aunt, first cousin) with a history of ovarian cancer and for postmenopausal women undergoing hysterectomy. In the former case, the risks of removing the ovaries while they are still functioning must be weighed against the potential benefits associated with oophorectomy.

TEACHING, COUNSELING, AND SUPPORTIVE CARE. Women with ovarian cancer need information and supportive care for themselves and their families or significant others (Dugan, 1985). In one study, Mishel and co-investigators (1984) found that among women with gynecologic cancer, uncertainty about the disease and its treatment was found to be related to pessimism and adjustment problems.

Women receiving radiotherapy need information regarding skin care: the avoidance of all irritants, including soap, heat, lotion, creams, ointments, massage, or friction from tight-fitting clothing. Loose-fitting cotton clothing is advisable during therapy. Women need to be reassured that they are not radioactive or dangerous to others.

Good nutrition, including small, frequent meals, adequate hydration, rest, and antispasmodics and antiemetics may be needed to combat the side effects of cramps, diarrhea, anorexia, upset stomach, vomiting, fatigue, and malaise. Women need to know that symptoms are temporary. Women receiving chemotherapy may experience the same or similar effects. In addition, they need to be helped to cope with alopecia, which they may not realize is temporary, and increased susceptibility to infection.

Women and their partners need to discuss feelings about body image and sexuality, and to be encouraged to participate in alternative expressions of sexuality when intercourse is not possible, such as in the postoperative period or when a woman is overly fatigued from radio- or chemotherapy. Women and their partners may have many misconceptions about sexual functioning and the effect of surgery such as TAH and BSO on sexuality (Holmes, 1987).

The helpful provider must initiate discussion of perceptions, fears, and anxieties. The woman and her family must be given ample opportunity to vent feelings and ask questions. Patients and families may benefit from referral to individual, family, or group counseling, relaxation programs, or peer support groups. Information about these is available from the American Cancer Society.

Management Approach to Ovarian Enlargements and Tumors

Prior sections have provided information on the management of specific types of ovarian enlargements and tumors. A woman with an ovarian mass, however, presents with a symptom or physical finding, not a confirmed diagnosis. The following section provides a framework for dealing with an ovarian growth suspected from reported symptoms or found on physical examination.

General Diagnosis. The problems and approach are essentially the same for all ovarian masses. The goals of management are threefold: first, to establish that the mass is actually ovarian in origin; second, to distinguish between physiologic cysts, which resolve spontaneously, and true neoplastic cysts and tumors, which require treatment; and third; to determine, prior to laparotomy, whether a given mass is benign or malignant. Obviously, not all of these can be accomplished by the primary care provider.

Data Collection

HISTORY. Careful and complete menstrual, contraceptive, gynecologic, sexual, medical, and family histories must be obtained. The woman's age is a highly significant factor. In one large epidemiologic study of ovarian neoplasms, 95 percent of those found in women under age 20 were benign and more than 86 percent of those in women presenting between ages 20 and 40 were benign (Katsube et al., 1982). History of onset and nature of any symptoms must be ascertained.

PHYSICAL EXAMINATION. The following characteristics should be assessed and correlated with knowledge of different types of ovarian enlargements and masses: location of the lesion with respect to the uterus; mobility or adherence; consistency (cystic, doughy, firm and solid, partially cystic and partially solid); contour (smoothly rounded, irregular, or nodular); size and weight; and presence or absence of bilateral masses. Benign tumors generally are unilateral, separate from the uterus, and movable. Most are cystic and pedunculated. They are smooth and tense and may move from one side of the pelvis to the other. Some tumors may be most easily palpated by rectal examination. Malignant tumors may be firm, irregular in shape, and fixed. They are likely to be bilateral.

If abdominal swelling is present and is obviously fluid, a large fluid-filled cyst can usually be differentiated from ascites by abdominal percussion. Dullness over the cyst with tympany in the flanks and no change in tone with position changes are typical of cysts, in contrast to the shifting dullness in the flanks characteristic of ascites. The umbilicus is invariably protruding and everted in the presence of ascites, remaining flat if abdominal distension is due to an ovarian cyst. Large ovarian cysts may cause the lower abdominal veins to become distended. With ascites, the mass usually proves to be malignant; however, the possibility of Meig's syndrome with an ovarian fibroma must be kept in mind, as must cirrhosis and other less common causes of ascites.

LABORATORY TESTING. A plain x-ray of the abdomen may establish the diagnosis of a dermoid cyst as its teeth show up on the x-ray. Diffuse calcification on x-ray may be associated with malignancy, but is not diagnostic. If definite ascities is present, a chest x-ray is indicated to reveal any associated pleural effusion or to demonstrate possible pulmonary metastases. Paracentesis and cytologic examination may settle the question.

An IVP distinguishes a pelvic kidney or low-lying renal tumor. An IVP also reveals any displacement or distortion of the ureters by the mass. This is indicated before surgery.

Ultrasound studies are advocated by some authors, whereas others believe that they add little to physical examination findings for initial diagnosis. In one study, O'Brien et al. (1984) found ultrasound to be less accurate than clinical examination in diagnosing uterine or ovarian masses, with a high number of false-positive results. Sonograms may be helpful in distinguishing the nature and location of pelvic masses and differentiating between solid tumors, cysts, and ascites. Ovarian cancer has several sonographic manifestations, but absolute diagnosis of malignancy cannot be made by sonogram. Ultrasound generally can be reserved for cases of uncertain physical findings. It may be useful in recurrent and advanced cancer.

Magnetic resonance imaging (MRI) is an attractive means of diagnosing gynecologic pathology because it is noninvasive and utilizes neither ionizing radiation nor intravenous contrast medium. Its use in the diagnosis of ovarian tumors has not yet been clarified (Lewis, 1987). It cannot distinguish benign from malignant masses (McCarthy, 1986).

Primary Care Management. Large, bilateral, or symptomatic masses require immediate consultation or referral for diagnosis and possible intervention. An asymptomatic mass no more than 5 cm in diameter in women under age 40 can be followed expectantly for 1 to 3 months to evaluate whether the mass regresses (Zaloudek et al., 1986). If it is still felt at the follow-up visit, consultation or referral is indicated. A further diagnostic workup generally requires testing, as outlined earlier, beyond the scope of the nonphysician care provider. Of course, the practitioner must meet the teaching and counseling needs of both women being followed expectantly and women referred for further diagnostic testing. Their fears and concerns must be listened to attentively and addressed and their feelings respected. What may seem a routine follow-up to a practitioner may be quite traumatic for a woman.

INFECTIONS OF THE OVARY

Infections of the ovary are not common; they rarely are seen without salpingitis. This disorder is discussed fully in Chapter 15.

Tubo-ovarian Abscess

A tubo-ovarian abscess may be a complication of untreated or inadequately treated salpingo-oophoritis, also called pelvic inflammatory disease (PID). Such an abscess may be unilateral or bilateral. It can be relatively small or as large as 30 to 40 cm in diameter. The rectosigmoid, uterus, pelvic sidewall, and loops of bowel may be involved (Green, 1977, pp. 254–255).

Diagnosis. Suspicion of an abscess should be high in the woman who fails to respond to antibiotic therapy for pelvic infection. An abscess may be felt as an adnexal mass on pelvic examination or demonstrated by ultrasound.

Complications. Rupture of a tubo-ovarian abscess can be a serious complication as its purulent contents spill into the peritoneal cavity. It presents an acute emergency with the need for immediate intervention and should be suspected whenever signs and symptoms of an acute abdomen appear in a woman with a known or suspected pelvic infection. These include severe abdominal pain, fever, tachycardia and tachypnea, abdominal rigidity, and signs of shock. Fluctuation of the cul-de-sac may be present.

Obviously, the primary care role in tubo-ovarian abscess is immediate consultation and referral. Treatment includes hospitalization and intravenous broad-spectrum antibiotic therapy; surgical intervention is necessary, when medical management fails or rupture occurs. Conservative surgery may be possible, although often TAH and BSO are performed (Ginsburg, Stern, & Hamod, 1980).

OVARIAN PREGNANCY

Rarely, a pregnancy occurs in the ovary (Grimes, Nosal, & Gallagher 1983; Hallatt, 1982). Most such pregnancies rupture at an early gestational age, but a few have gone to term and, on occasion, have resulted in a viable infant (Williams, Malver, & Kraft, 1982). Alternatively, the products of conception may degenerate and form an ovarian tumor (Pritchard et al., 1985, p. 437). A pregnancy also may be tubo-ovarian; in this case, the fetal sac is adherent to both the fallopian tube and ovary.

Ovarian pregnancies follow a course similar to that of tubal pregnancies, which are, by far, the most common of ectopic pregnancies. Chapter 15 offers a complete discussion of the management of ectopic pregnancies.

REFERENCES

Aiman, J., & Smentek, C. (1985, July). Premature ovarian failure. *Obstetrics and Gynecology, 66*(1), 9–14.

Alper, M. M., & Garner, P. R. (1985, July). Premature ovarian failure: Its relationship to autoimmune disease. *Obstetrics and Gynecology, 66*(1), 27–30.

American Cancer Society. (1987). *Cancer Facts and Figures—1987.* New York: American Cancer Society.

Averette, H.E., Donato, D.M., Lovecchio, J.L., & Sevin, B. (1987, October). Surgical staging of gynecologic malignancies. *Cancer, 60*(8, Suppl.), 2010–2020.

Barber, H.R.K. (1984, December). Ovarian cancer: Diagnosis and management. *American Journal of Obstetrics and Gynecology, 150*(8), 910–916.

Bernhisel, M.A., & Hammond, C.B., (1986). Androgen excess. In D. N. Danforth & J. R. Scott (Eds.), *Obstetrics and gynecology* (5th ed.). Philadelphia: J. B. Lippincott.

Brady, L. W., Markoe, A.M., DeEulis, T. & Lewis, Jr. G.C., (1987, October). Treatment of advanced and recurrent gynecologic cancer, *Cancer 60*(8, Suppl.), 2081–2093.

Brenner, P.F., (1986). Precocious puberty in the female. In D.R. Mishell, & V. Davajan, (Eds.), *Infertility, Contraception and Reproductive Endocrinology.* (2nd ed.) Oradell, NJ: Medical Economics Books.

Centers for Disease Control. (1982, July). Oral contraceptives and cancer risk. *Morbidity and Mortality Weekly Reports. 31*(29), 393–394.

Cole, W. H., McDonald, G. O., Roberts, S. S. & Southwick, H. W. (1961) *Dissemination of Cancer.* New York, NY: Appleton-Century-Crofts.

Colgan, T.J. & Norris, H.F. (1983). Ovarian epithelial tumors of low malignant potential: A review. *International Journal of Gynecological Pathology. 1*(4), 367–382.

Darland, N. W. (1985, May/June). Infertility associated with luteal phase defect. *Journal of Obstetric, Gynecologic, and Neonatal Nursing,* 212–217.

Davajan, V., and Kletzky, O. A. (1986). Secondary amenorrhea. In D. R. Mishell, & V. Davajan (Eds.), *Infertility, Contraception and Reproductive endocrinology* (2nd ed.). Oradell, NJ: Medical Economics Books.

Dugan, K.K. (1985, February). The bleak outlook on ovarian cancer. *American Journal of Nursing, 85*(2), 144–147.

Ginsburg, D. S., Stern, J. L., Hamod, K. A. et al. (1980, December). Tubo-ovarian abscess: A retrospective review. *American Journal of Obstetrics and Gynecology 138*(7, Part 2), 1055–1058.

Green, T. H. (1977). *Gynecology: Essentials of clinical practice* (3rd ed.). Boston: Little, Brown.

Grimes, H. G., Nosal, R. A., & Gallagher, J. C. (1983, February). Ovarian pregnancy: A series of 24 cases. *Obstetrics and Gynecology, 61*(2), 174–180.

Hallatt, J. G. (1982, May). Primary ovarian pregnancy: A report of twenty-five cases. *American Journal of Obstetrics and Gynecology, 143*(1), 55–58.

Hallatt, J. G., Steele, C. H., & Snyder, M. (1984, May). Ruptured corpus luteum with hemoperitoneum: A study of 173 surgical cases. *American Journal of Obstetrics and Gynecology, 149*(1), 5–9.

Hamilton, T. C., Ozols, R. F., & Longo, D. L. (1987, October). Biologic therapy for the treatment of malignant common epithelial tumors of the ovary. *Cancer, 60*(8, Suppl.), 2054–2063.

Heintz, A. P. M. (1987, March). What causes ovarian cancer? *Contemporary Ob/Gyn, 29*(3), 25–30.

Helewa, M. E., Krepart, G. V., & Lotocki, R. (1986, February). Staging laparotomy in early epithelial ovarian cancer. *American Journal of Obstetrics and Gynecology, 154*(2), 282–286.

Holmes, B. C. (1987, October). Psychological evaluation and preparation of the patient and family. *Cancer, 60*(8, Suppl.), 2021–2024.

Jones, H. W., & Jones, G. S. (1981). *Novak's textbook of gynecology* (10th ed.). Baltimore: Williams & Wilkins.

Katsube, Y., Berg, J. W., & Silverberg, S. G. (1982). Epidemiologic pathology of ovarian tumors: A histopathologic review of primary ovarian neoplasms diagnosed in the Denver standard metropolitan statistical area, 1 July–31, December 1969 and 1 July–31, December 1979. *International Journal of Gynecological Pathology, 1*(1), 3–16.

Katz, E. (1987, December). Luteinized unruptured follicle syndrome. *Contemporary Ob/Gyn, 39*(6), 97–100, 103.

Kilgore, L. C., & Younger, J. B. (1984, November). When fertility drugs overstimulate the ovaries. *Contemporary Ob/Gyn, 24*(5), 59–69.

Larson, E. (1983, August). Epidemiologic correlates of breast, endometrial, and ovarian cancers. *Cancer Nursing, 6*(4), 295–301.

LeMaire, G. S. (1987, March/April). The luteinized unruptured follicle syndrome: Anovulation in disguise. *Journal of Obstetric, Gynecologic, and Neonatal Nursing,* 116–120.

Lewis, E. (1987, October). The use and abuse of imaging in gynecologic cancer. *Cancer, 60*(8, Suppl.), 1993–2009.

Lobo, R. A. (1986). Polycystic ovary syndrome. In D. R. Mishell & V. Davajan (Eds.), *Infertility, contraception and reproductive endocrinology* (2nd ed.). Oradell, NJ: Medical Economics Books.

Lurain, J. R. (1985, March). Confronting nongestational ovarian choriocarcinoma. *Contemporary Ob/Gyn, 25*(3), 67–75.

March, C. M. (1986). Luteal phase defects. In D. R. Mishell & V. Davajan (Eds.), *Infertility, contraception and reproductive endocrinology* (2nd ed.). Oradell, NJ: Medical Economics Books.

Marrs, R. P. (1986). Oocytes. In D. R. Mishell & V. Davajan (Eds.), *Infertility, contraception and reproductive endocrinology* (2nd ed.). Oradell, NJ: Medical Economics Books.

Mazur, M. T., Hsueh, S., & Gersell, D. J. (1984, May). Metastases to the female genital tract: Analysis of 325 cases. *Cancer, 53*(9), 1978–1984.

McCarthy, S. (1986). How MRI is helping diagnose gyn disease. *Contemporary Ob/Gyn, 28*(5), 151–156.

Merrill, J. A. (1986). Lesions of the ovary: Benign lesions. In D. N. Danforth & J. R. Scott, (Eds.), *Obstetrics and gynecology.* (5th ed.). Philadelphia: J. B. Lippincott.

Mishel, M. H., Hostetter, T., King, B., & Graham, V. (1984). Predictors of psychosocial adjustment in patients newly diagnosed with gynecological cancer. *Cancer Nursing, 7*(4), 291–299.

O'Brien, W. F., Buck, D. R., & Nash, J. D. (1984, July). Evaluation of sonography in the initial assessment of the gynecologic patient. *American Journal of Obstetrics and Gynecology, 149*(6), 598–602.

Ozols, R. F., Garvin, A. J., Costa, J., et al. (1980, February). Advanced ovarian cancer: Correlation of histologic grade with response to therapy and survival. *Cancer, 45*(3), 572–581.

Pernoll, M. L. & Benson, R. C. (1987). *Current obstetric & gynecologic diagnosis and treatment.* East Norwalk, CT: Appleton & Lange.

Piver, M. S. (1984, May). Preserving fertility of ovarian Ca patients. *Contemporary Ob/Gyn, 23*(5), 49–68.

Piver, M. S. (1986, February). Alarming trends in the familial ovarian cancer registry. *Contemporary Ob/Gyn, 27*(2), 120–129.

Pritchard, J. A., MacDonald, P. C., & Gant, N. F. *Williams obstetrics* (17th ed.). East Norwalk, CT: Appleton–Century–Crofts.

Riddick, D. H. (1986). Disorders of menstrual function. In D. N. Danforth & J. R. Scott (Eds.), *Obstetrics and gynecology* (5th ed.). Philadelphia: J. B. Lippincott.

Rock, J. A., Parmley, T., Murphy, A. A., & Jones, H. W., Jr. (1986, April). Malposition of the ovary associated with uterine anomalies. *Fertility and Sterility, 45*(4), 561–563.

Sarto, G. E. (1986). Genetic considerations. In D. N. Danforth & J. R. Scott (Eds.), *Obstetrics and Gynecology* (5th ed.). Philadelphia: J. B. Lippincott.

Shangold, M. M., Turksoy, R. N., Bashford, R. A., & Hammond, C. B. (1977, November). Pregnancy following the insensitive ovary syndrome. *Fertility and Sterility, 28*(11), 1179–1181.

Stuart, G. C. E., Jeffries, M., Stuart, J. L., & Anderson, R. J. (1982, March). The changing role of ''second-look'' laparotomy in the management of epithelial carcinoma of the ovary. *American Journal of Obstetrics and Gynecology, 142*(6, Part 1), 612–616.

Szamborski, J., Czerwinski, W., Gadomska, H., et al. (1981, February). Case control study of high-risk factors in ovarian carcinomas. *Gynecological Oncology, 11*(1), 8–16.

Thoeny, R. H., Dockerty, M. B., Hunt, A. B., & Childs, D. S. (1961, December). Study of ovarian dysgerminoma with emphasis on the role of radiation therapy. *Surgery, Gynecology, and Obstetrics, 113*(6), 691–692.

Tucker, M. A., & Fraumeni, J. F. (1987). Treatment-related cancers after gynecologic malignancy. *Cancer, 60*(8, Suppl.), 2117–2122.

Williams, P. C., Malvar, T. C., & Kraft, J. R. (1982, March). Term ovarian pregnancy with delivery of a live female infant. *American Journal of Obstetrics and Gynecology, 142*(5), 589–591.

Woodruff, J. D., Protos, P., & Peterson, W. F. (1968, November). Ovarian teratomas. *American Journal of Obstetrics and Gynecology, 102*(5), 702–715.

Young, R. C., (1987). Initial therapy for early ovarian carcinoma. *Cancer, 69*(8, Suppl.), 2042–2049.

Young, R. C., Fuks, Z., Knapp, R. C., & DiSaia, P. J. (1985). Cancer of the ovary. In V. T. DeVita, S. Hellman, & S. A. Rosenberg (Eds.), *Cancer: Principles and practice of oncology.* Philadelphia: J. B. Lippincott.

Young, R. H., & Scully, R. E. (1982). Ovarian sex cord–stromal tumors: Recent progress. *International Journal of Gynecological Pathology. 1*(1), 101–123.

Zaloudek, C., Tavassoli, F. A., & Kurman, R. J. (1986). Lesions of the ovary: Malignant lesions. In D. N. Danforth, & J. R. Scott (Eds.), *Obstetrics and gynecology* (5th ed.). Philadelphia: J. B. Lippincott.

17

The Urinary Tract

Ronnie Lichtman and Susan Papera

Urinary tract problems are common in women. Indeed, infections of the urinary tract are the second most frequently seen infections today, exceeded in incidence only by respiratory infections (Fair, 1983, p. 91; Roberts, 1984, p. 103; Neu, 1983, p. 130). This chapter discusses a number of urinary tract disorders likely to be encountered in clinical practice, emphasizing the most prevalent among young healthy women—the lower urinary tract infection (cystitis or UTI). Other related entities briefly covered are upper urinary tract infection (pyelonephritis), asymptomatic bacteriuria, the urethral syndrome, and interstitial cystitis. Urinary stress incontinence is discussed separately at the chapter's end.

ANATOMY OF THE URINARY TRACT

The urinary tract consists of a pair of kidneys and ureters, a bladder and urethra. The kidneys are located behind the parietal peritoneum, against the posterior abdominal wall, at the level of T12 and L1, 2, and 3. Each lima bean-shaped kidney is approximately 1 inch thick and measures about 4.5 × 2 to 3 inches, with the left kidney usually slightly larger and located higher than the right. Each has an inner medulla and an outer cortex, surrounded by a fibrous capsule. The microanatomy and function of the kidneys in excretion and in the maintenance of fluid, electrolyte, and acid-base balance are complex; their discussion is beyond the scope of this chapter.

The ureters form a conduit between the kidneys and bladder with peristaltic waves forcing urine through them toward the bladder. Each tube is 10 to 12 inches long and less than 1/2 inch in diameter. The walls of the ureters are lined with mucous membrane. Their inner surface is smooth muscle; their outer coat is fibrous tissue. The ureters enter the bladder at the posterior corners of the trigone, the triangular shaped bladder floor. A valve at the bladder entrance, consisting of a fold of mucous membrane, prevents urinary reflux into the ureters.

The bladder is an expandable sac located behind the symphysis pubis. Its walls are composed of three layers of smooth muscle, together comprising the detrusor muscle. Its lining consists of mucous membrane.

The urethra enters the bladder at the anterior, lower corner of the trigone. It is a small, short tube, in women only about 1 to 1-1/2 inches in length. The urethra is located directly behind the symphysis pubis, above the vagina. It is lined with mucous membrane and carries urine, propelled by bladder contractions, to the outside.

URINARY TRACT INFECTIONS AND RELATED DISORDERS

Definitions and Incidence

Urinary tract infection is defined as the presence of bacteria in the urinary tract (Roberts, 1984, p. 103). The most common type, cystitis, is generally a superficial mucosal infection confined to the lower urinary tract (Neu, 1983, p. 131). Traditionally, 100,000 (10^5) or more colony-forming units per milliliter (CFUs/mL) of urine has been considered indicative of UTI; however, many experts agree that in the presence of symptoms, a lower bacterial colony count is significant. This is particularly true when *pyuria*, pus or white blood cells in the urine, can be demonstrated on microscopic urinalysis (Roberts, 1984, pp. 103–104; Stamm et al., 1980).

UTI is seen in up to 20 percent of women at some time in their lives (Roberts, 1984, p. 103; Neu, 1983, p. 130). Up to 5 percent of school-age girls have UTIs between grades 1 and 12 (Neu, 1983, p. 132). UTIs are the most commonly acquired infections in hospitals, usually secondary to catheterization (Neu, 1983, pp. 130, 132; Madsen, Larsen, & Dorflinger, 1985).

Upper urinary tract infection, or *pyelonephritis*, is a serious infection of the kidney involving the renal parenchyma and associated with systemic manifestations such as chills, fever, and leukocytosis. Pyelonephritis can lead to sepsis and renal failure (Abraham, Brenner, & Simon, 1983, p. 228). Chronic pyelonephritis, causing kidney destruction, may occur secondary to infection (Braude, 1984, p. 68) or as a result of vascular disease of the kidney, analgesic abuse, or uric acid nephropathy (Neu, 1983, p. 130).

Asymptomatic bacteriuria is the presence of 10^5 CFUs mL of bacteria in the urine in the absence of symptoms (Neu, 1983, p. 130; Roberts, 1984, p. 104). This is significant in pregnant women, in those with certain chronic illnesses such as diabetes and sickle cell anemia, and in women being followed for cure of a diagnosed UTI, but otherwise is not considered to be pathologic or to predispose the healthy, nonpregnant woman to either the development of a UTI or to renal damage. It is seen in approximately 5 percent of women aged 16 to 65 (O'Dowd, 1984).

The acute urethral syndrome (AUS) or *chronic urethral syn-*

drome (CUS) is the presence of urinary tract symptoms—most commonly dysuria, frequency, and urgency—in the absence of bacteria on urine culture and without bladder or urethral abnormalities. Recent studies, however, have demonstrated that many cases of AUS are in fact the result of infection, with colony counts lower than 10^5 bacteria/mL or organisms that do not regularly grow in routine culture media (Curran, 1977; Stamm et al., 1980; Fihn & Stamm, 1983; Scotti & Ostergard, 1984). It has been suggested that in approximately one third of women with frequency and dysuria, no apparent cause is found and the diagnosis of acute or chronic urethral syndrome is made. Although the incidence is not known, the urethral syndrome has been estimated to occur in as many as 20 to 30 percent of adult women (Scotti & Ostergard, 1984, p. 516). A number of etiologies for the syndrome have been proposed, including hormonal or vitamin deficiencies, developmental abnormalities, urethral spasm or stenosis, inflammation of the urethral glands, trauma, cold weather, allergy, and neurosis or psychiatric disturbance (Scotti & Ostergard, 1984, p. 515).

Interstitial cystitis, called by Reid (1985) "the other cystitis," is a rare condition, seen mostly in women between the ages of 30 and 50 (Parivar & Bradbrook, 1986, p. 239). This disease is chronic and debilitating, characterized by urinary urgency and frequency, often nocturnal, and associated with a decreased bladder capacity and pinpoint hemorrhages or ulcerations on the bladder mucosa (Messing & Stamey, 1978).

Although the cause of interstitial cystitis is unknown, several proposed etiologies have appeared in the literature, including autoimmune disease, psychiatric disease, and neurogenic disorders. A viral etiology was proposed but ruled out by Fall, Johansson, and Vahlne (1985). Studies to date have been unable to show definitive causality (Brown 1983; Rosin, Griffiths, Sofras, et al., 1979).

Pathogenesis

Anatomy. The anatomy of the female urologic system helps explain its predisposition to infection. The short urethra of females and its proximity to the anal area make bladder colonization with pathogens more likely in women than in men (Neu, 1983, p. 130; Schaeffer, 1983, p. 106).

Microbiology. The rectal flora is the primary reservoir for bacteria infecting the urinary tract. Although anaerobes are more prevalent in the bowel than aerobes, they are not usually responsible for UTIs (Sabath & Charles, 1980, p. 162s). Gram-negative rods of the family Enterobactericeae account for between 80 and 90 percent of bacterial UTIs (Ronald, 1983, p. 114). Of these, *Escherichia coli* is the most common pathogen, causing over 70 percent of UTIs (Sabath & Charles, 1980, p. 162s; Roberts, 1984, p. 105). Some strains of this organism are more likely to be involved in UTIs than others.

Proteus mirabilis is the second main urinary pathogen. This organism has an affinity for the upper urinary tract, causing pyelonephritis and possible renal damage (Sabath & Charles, 1980, p. 162s). Roberts (1984, p. 110) reports that pyelonephritis with a *Proteus* infection is most likely to occur in the presence of renal obstruction caused by stones. Interestingly, *Staphylococcus epidermidis*, most often thought of as normal flora, has been known to cause infection in the urinary tract. See Table 17–1 for a list of disease-causing bacteria found in the urinary tract and those that tend not to cause infection.

TABLE 17–1. ORGANISMS FOUND IN THE URINARY TRACT THAT ARE AND ARE NOT ASSOCIATED WITH INFECTION

Organisms Commonly Found in the Absence of Disease	Organisms Associated with Urinary Tract Infections[a]
Lactobacillus spp	*Escherichia coli*
Corynebacterium spp	*Klebsiella*
Micrococci	Indole-positive *Proteus* spp
Neisseria spp	*Proteus mirabilis*
	Pseudomonas aeruginosa
	Staphylococcus epidermidis

[a]These organisms cause urinary tract infection when present in significant numbers.
From Sabath, L. D., and Charles, D. (1980). Urinary tract infections in the female. Obstetrics and Gynecology, 55(5 Suppl.), 163s. Reprinted with permission.

Organisms associated with sexually transmitted diseases that do not appear on routine bacterial cultures also cause UTI—*Chlamydia trachomatis, Neisseria gonorrhoeae,* herpes simplex virus, and, less commonly, *Mycoplasma hominis* and *Ureaplasma urealyticum* (Curran, 1977; Stamm et al., 1980; Paavonen & Vesterinen, 1982; Berg et al., 1984; Hedelin et al., 1983).

Natural Resistance. The urinary tract has a number of defense mechanisms against infections. Schaeffer (1983, p. 106) divides these into those extrinsic to the bladder and those intrinsic to it.

Several extrinsic mechanisms are active in the vaginal introitus. Vaginal epithelial cells ordinarily have a low receptivity to bacterial colonization (Schaeffer, 1983, pp. 107–108); bacteria adhere more readily to the uroepithelial and vaginal cells in women with recurrent UTIs. This receptivity may be genetically determined. The low pH of the vagina has been postulated to inhibit vaginal colonization with urinary tract pathogens (Stamey & Timothy, 1975; Neu, 1983, p. 131), although this remains in dispute (Schaeffer, 1983, p. 108). In addition, cervicovaginal antibody may play a role; it has been shown to be reduced in women with recurrent UTIs (Stamey, Wehner, Mihara, & Condy, 1978).

Intrinsic bladder defenses include primary, secondary, and tertiary mechanisms. The primary mechanism is voiding or the mechanical elimination of bacteria from the bladder. Secondary mechanisms cause the bladder to resist bacterial colonization and infection. Uroepithelial cells are not highly receptive to bacterial adherence, and the bladder mucosa demonstrates antibacterial action against microorganisms on its surface (Schaeffer, 1983, p. 110). Tertiary resistance comes from antibacterial properties of the urine itself (Schaeffer, 1983, p. 111). These are related to urine osmolarity and concentration of urea and ammonium. Normal urine is most inhibitory to normal vaginal flora and less so to enterobacteria and enterococci, explaining the microbial pathology of most UTIs (Schaeffer, 1983, p. 111). It has been reported that overnight concentrated urine provides the most defense against UTIs (Cicmanec, Shank, & Evans, 1985).

Predisposing Factors. Specific factors predisposing to UTI include perineal hygienic practices that bring fecal bacteria toward the urethra (Quinlan, 1984, p. 42) and sexual practices in which vaginal contact follows anal contact. Sexual intercourse itself has been implicated as a predisposing factor to the development of UTIs (Buckley et al., 1978; Elster et al., 1981; Nicolle et al., 1982). Trauma to the urethra, which occurs with intercourse, is thought to explain why bacteria enter the bladder during sex, although trauma does not always lead to infection (Bran, Levison, & Kaye, 1972).

Use of the vaginal diaphragm as a contraceptive method has been associated with the occurrence of bacteriuria and/or UTI (Gillespie, 1984; Fihn, Latham, Roberts, et al., 1985a; Fihn, Running, Pinkstaff, et al., 1985; Peddie, Gorrie, & Bailey, 1986). Although one study failed to confirm the association (Wall & Baldwin-Johnson, 1984), this was a case-control study, utilizing chart review for data in only 98 women, which neglected to specify size and type of diaphragm worn or to standardize prospectively for fit. Explanations for the diaphragm's effect on UTI include urethral obstruction (Fihn et al., 1985b) and elevation of the posterior bladder neck necessitating increased bladder pressure for voiding and leading to urinary retention. Retention provides a pool of residual urine with bacteria that are not washed away by voiding; the increase in intravesical pressure may also increase the susceptibility of the bladder mucosa to bacterial action (Gillespie, 1984, pp. 27, 29). These findings all have been demonstrated by urinary flow studies and corroborated by patient histories.

Changes that occur after menopause predispose to the development of UTIs. The postmenopausal vaginal epithelial cells and vaginal pH increase the chances of symptomatic UTI (Roberts, 1984, p. 109). See Chapter 24 for more discussion of these changes, their significance, diagnosis, and treatment.

The use of whirlpool baths and spas contaminated with *Pseudomonas aeruginosa* has been identified as a possible risk factor (Salmen, Dwyer, Vorse, & Kruse, 1983). Bubble bath and perfumed soap have been reported clinically to be related to inflammation of the lower urinary tract in children, without bacterial growth, although this association has not been confirmed by research (Marshall, 1965).

Diabetes mellitus predisposes to UTI, particularly in women (Roberts, 1984, p. 109). Any urinary tract instrumentation such as catheterization increases the risk of urinary tract infection (Madsen et al., 1985).

Clinical Presentation. A woman with a lower urinary tract problem typically presents with a triad of symptoms—urinary urgency, frequency, and dysuria (Abraham et al., 1983, p. 228). Dysuria is commonly felt at the end of urination, as a suprapubic "burning." Although urgency and frequency are experienced, the actual flow of urine may be diminished in volume. Lower back pain may be present (Quinlan, 1984, p. 39). Patients may notice blood in the urine, and the urine itself may be cloudy, concentrated, and odorous. On occasion, systemic symptoms such as fever, chills, nausea, and vomiting may occur, although most often these are associated with upper tract infection. Onset of symptoms may be rapid or slow. Suprapubic tenderness may be noted on physical examination.

The woman with an upper urinary tract infection (pyelonephritis) usually presents with a different constellation of symptoms. These are often systemic and include chills, fever, flank pain, rigors, nausea, and vomiting (Abraham et al., 1983, pp. 228, 230). Urine may be cloudy, suggesting pyuria, and gross hematuria may be present. On physical examination, suprapubic tenderness and costovertebral angle tenderness may be elicited. Sometimes, however, an upper urinary tract infection causes no systemic manifestations, whereas a lower tract infection may present with systemic symptoms (Abraham et al., 1983, pp. 228–231). Symptomatology alone is not necessarily diagnostic.

The urethral syndrome is characterized by symptoms resembling a lower tract infection—urgency, frequency, dysuria. Fullness after voiding, urge or apparent stress incontinence, suprapubic tenderness, and dyspareunia may be present (Scotti & Ostergard, 1984, p. 515).

Interstitial cystitis presents with frequency and urgency, often nocturnal. Infra- and suprapubic pain may be present. Hematuria and hesitancy in urination can occur. Other symptoms may be less specific and include generalized abdominal pain and back and rectal pain. With this disorder, symptoms are usually relieved with urination.

Differential Diagnosis. The practitioner must differentiate between upper urinary tract problems (pyelonephritis or kidney stones) and lower urinary tract disorders (cystitis, the urethral syndrome, and interstitial cystitis), as well as nonurinary tract problems such as vaginitis or pelvic infection. Initial diagnostic techniques include those familiar to the primary care women's health practitioner—history taking, physical examination, and some laboratory studies. Other tests, such as cystoscopy, are performed by a gynecologist or urologist. If the problem does not seem to be confined to the lower urinary tract, referral is warranted for further diagnostic workup.

Management

DATA COLLECTION. Historical and physical examination data pertinent to an assessment of urinary tract problems are outlined in Table 17–2 with the diagnoses suggested by the findings listed.

LABORATORY STUDIES. Microscopic urinalysis and urine culture are the standard diagnostic tests for UTIs. Interpretation of these tests determines diagnosis and treatment. Recently, several rapid tests have been developed for office use. In addition, tests to differentiate upper from lower urinary tract infection may be warranted. A complete blood count may be useful, as patients with pyelonephritis often exhibit leukocytosis (Sheldon & Gonzalez, 1984, p. 321). Further testing that may be necessary with recurrent problems indicative of a chronic condition include cystoscopy, cystometry, and bladder biopsy, and require referral to a gynecologist with urologic expertise or a urologist (Brown, 1983, p. 67).

Urinalysis. The most important diagnostic parameter in a urinalysis is the presence of pyuria—white blood cells (WBCs) or pus in the urine. In the absence of symptoms, this is called asymptomatic bacteriuria; in the presence of symptoms, it is diagnostic of UTI (Wright & Matsen, 1984, p. 46). Pyuria has been defined by various authors as from 8 to 50 WBCs per high-power field in a spun urine specimen (Stamm et al., 1982, p. 464; Roberts, 1984, p. 112; Harris, 1983, p. 49), although 8 to 10 WBCs per high-power field is the most widely accepted standard. Often, when an infection is present, red blood cells (hematuria) and bacteria are seen as well (Harris, 1983, p. 49). Bacteria, however, can replicate quickly in urine (Wright & Matsen, 1984, p. 47) so, unless a specimen was immediately looked at, transported to the laboratory, or refrigerated, bacteria could represent contamination. Large numbers of epithelial cells also indicate contamination, and WBCs seen in their presence may not be diagnostic (Brumfitt, 1984, p. 97; Wright & Matsen, 1984, p. 46).

Asymptomatic bacteriuria in healthy nonpregnant

TABLE 17-2. HISTORICAL AND PHYSICAL EXAMINATION DATA IN URINARY TRACT INFECTIONS AND RELATED DISORDERS[a]

	Additional Data Necessary	Suggested Diagnosis or Diagnoses
Symptom or Finding		
Urinary frequency	Recent onset	Lower UTI; AUS
	Onset longer than 1 week, but recent	Lower UTI; Pyelo
	Chronic	CUS; ISC
Urinary urgency	See *Urinary frequency*	See *Urinary frequency*
Dysuria	External (perineal) discomfort	Vaginal infection or trauma; perineal lesion
	Internal (suprapubic) pain described as "burning" at the end of urination	Lower UTI; Pyelo; AUS or CUS; ISC
Suprapubic pain		Pyelo, lower UTI, AUS, or CUS; ISC
Urge or apparent stress incontinence		AUS or CUS
Nocturia		ISC
Postvoid fullness		Lower UTI; Pyelo; AUS or CUS
Symptoms relieved by voiding		ISC
Dyspareunia	Recent onset	Lower UTI; Pyelo; AUS
	Chronic	CUS; ISC
Hematuria		Pyelo; Lower UTI; ISC
Cloudy, concentrated, odorous urine		Lower UTI; Pyelo; AUS or CUS
Hesitancy in urinating	Recent onset	Lower UTI; Pyelo; AUS
	Chronic	CUS; ISC
Lower back or flank pain		Pyelo; occasionally lower UTI; ISC
Fever and chills		Pyelo; occasionally lower UTI
Nausea and vomiting		Pyelo; occasionally lower UTI
Rigors		Pyelo
Abdominal pain or cramping		Pyelo; lower UTI; AUS or CUS; ISC
Previous pelvic trauma or congenital or known urologic abnormalities		May predispose to any condition or itself present a problem
Neurologic disease, diabetes, cardiovascular disease, neoplasms		May predispose to infection, incontinence, or obstruction
Recent intercourse	Intercourse before onset of symptoms	Intercourse may predispose to UTI
	Anal contact before vaginal	May bring fecal bacteria to urethra
Contraceptive use		Diaphragm may be related to UTI
Hygienic practices	Wiping back to front; clothing: not cotton, tight pants, pantyhose	May predispose to UTI
Menopausal status		May predispose to UTI or AUS or CUS
Medications	Include those taken by immunocompromised patients, nephrotoxic antibiotics (including aminoglycosides and tetracyclines)	May be nephrotoxic
Recent catheterization		May predispose to UTI
Physical Sign		
Suprapubic tenderness		Lower UTI; pyelo; AUS or CUS; ISC
Costovertebral angle tenderness		Pyelo
Atrophy of the genital mucosa		Indicates menopause, which may predispose to UTI or AUS or CUS
Urethral discharge		Suggests infection or CUS
Redness or irritation around urethra		Suggests infection or CUS

[a]UTI, urinary tract infection; pyelo, pyelonephritis; AUS, acute urethral syndrome; CUS, chronic urethral syndrome; ISC, interstitial cystitis.

women generally is not a cause for concern, although in pregnant patients it warrants treatment to avoid premature labor (Wright & Matsen, 1984, p. 47) and pyelonephritis, which occurs in 25 to 30 percent of pregnant women with asymptomatic bacteriuria (Harris, 1983, p. 50). Routine screening for bacteriuria in asymptomatic, nonpregnant women is not advised because it is costly and can lead to unnecessary treatment (Roberts, 1984, p. 111).

Culture and Sensitivity. A culture identifies the pathologic bacteria in the urine, and a sensitivity provides an in vitro analysis of which antibiotics will be effective against it.

COLLECTION OF SPECIMEN. An accurate culture requires a midstream, clean-catch urine specimen. Careful patient instruction is essential for collection of a good specimen. The woman must be given two to three perineal wipes, saturated with soap, and a sterile collection container. Although antiseptic wipes containing alcohol or peroxide are often given to patients, these may be irritating and can be bactericidal to organisms in the urine (Quinlan, 1984, p. 41). Instruct the patient to open the specimen container, placing the lid up, and to wash her hands. If she is menstruating or has a heavy vaginal discharge, a tampon in the vagina may help prevent contamination of the specimen. The patient should stand over the toilet with her legs apart and use the fingers of one hand to separate the labia. She should then clean the area around the urinary meatus two or three times, by wiping from front to back, once with each wipe. Instruct the woman to urinate first into the toilet, then into the collection container, and to finish urinating into the toilet. This is done because the first few milliliters of urine are often contaminated with bacteria present in the distal portion of the urethra and because the last part of the urine is expelled with less force and therefore may be contaminated with organisms that commonly are found in the periurethral area (Sabath & Charles, 1980, p. 163s). Make sure the woman understands not to touch the inside of the urinary collection container and to handle the lid only on its outer edge. The specimen should be immediately refrigerated or sent to the laboratory.

Alternate urine transport systems that prevent bacterial growth up to 24 hours at room temperature are available from the laboratory; however, only 96 percent of bacteria resume growing when these specimens are later diluted on routine culture media, sometimes causing false-negative results (Wright & Matsen, 1984, p. 50).

Interpretation of Results. Classically, the demonstration of at least 10^5 CFUs per milliliter of urine has been considered diagnostic of a urinary tract infection (Abraham et al., 1983, p. 228). More recent studies, however, correlating voided cultures with those obtained by suprapubic aspiration or urethral catheterization, have found that a midstream urine showing only 10^2 (100) CFUs per milliliter is diagnostic of a UTI in dysuric women with pyuria (Stamm et al., 1982). Some authorities use 10^3 (1000) or 10^4 (10,000) as the cutoff for diagnosis of infection or repeat the test when culture identifies a prevalent organism but shows a low bacterial count (Smith, Brumfitt, & Hamilton-Miller, 1983). Bacterial counts less than 10^5 may be caused by frequency or diuresis (possibly resulting from advice given at the onset of symptoms to increase fluids) or by self-medication prior to culture (Ronald, 1983, p. 114). Sometimes a sterile urine culture does not rule out a UTI because the offending organism may be one not grown on routine cultures, such as *Chlamydia trachomatis* (Stamm et al., 1981; Berg et al., 1984), *Neisseria gonorrhoeae* (Curran, 1977), and, less often, herpes simplex virus (Stamm et al., 1980), *Mycoplasma hominis*, and *Ureaplasma urealyticum* (Hedelin et al., 1983; Stamm et al., 1980). In the past, women infected with such organisms had been diagnosed as having the idiopathic acute urethral syndrome, but a number of studies have shown symptoms often to be relieved with antibiotics effective against these sexually transmitted organisms, particularly, but not exclusively, when pyuria is present (Stamm et al., 1980, 1981; Wong, Fennell, & Stamm, 1984).

OTHER SCREENING TESTS. Several tests that indirectly detect leukocytes or bacteria recently have become available for quick screening for UTIs. An understanding of their biologic basis and sensitivity and specificity, assessed in light of signs and symptoms, provides guidelines on when and how to use their results for making treatment decisions.

Rapid measurements of leukocytes in urine are based on the fact that esterases contained in neutrophils can be detected by a test that, through a series of chemical reactions, causes a pink-to-lavender color to appear on a specially treated dipstick within 60 seconds (Chernow et al., 1984, p. 151). Urine must be tested within 6 hours of collection. A positive reaction means that there are more than 5 WBCs per high-power field ("A Quick Check for UTI," 1984, p. 60). In correlations of this test with urine culture, it was found to be highly sensitive; a negative test therefore has a high predictive value (97 percent) and reduces the need for urine culture (Chernow et al., 1984, p. 152). The test, however, is relatively nonspecific, and a positive result does not necessarily signify the need for treatment.

A nitrite test, which tests for the reduction of nitrates to nitrite by urinary bacteria (Harris, 1983, p. 49), was found to have a higher specificity, with fewer false positives, but a lower sensitivity. This test, therefore, cannot be used to exclude UTI, but a positive result strongly indicates the need for culture and possibly treatment (Chernow et al., 1984, p. 153). Used in combination, the leukocyte esterase test and the nitrite test give a predictive negative value reported as high as 99 percent (Wright & Matsen, 1984, p. 46). Both tests are available on the same test strip. False negatives can be the result of proteinuria and leukopenia, and false positives may be caused by WBCs from outside the urinary tract (Wright & Matsen, 1984, p. 46).

A rapid screen for bacteria, the Bact-T-Screen, detects bacteria or WBCs or both in about 2 minutes. The sensitivity of this test has been reported at 92 percent (lower than the leukocyte esterase test; higher than the nitrite test), but the specificity is low. This means that like the leukocyte esterase test, this can be used to exclude UTI with high probability (Columbia Presbyterian Medical Center, 1985).

DIFFERENTIATION OF LOWER FROM UPPER URINARY TRACT INFECTIONS. Although symptoms and response to treatment often differentiate lower from upper UTIs, laboratory testing is available to aid in this diagnosis, particularly in the presence of resistant infection (Sabath & Charles, 1980, p. 166s). These tests are invasive (Sheldon & Gonzalez, 1984) and require referral to be ordered and performed. The Stamey test involves bladder irrigation via a cystoscope followed by the passage of catheters through the ureters to obtain renal urine samples. The Fairley test, which is often performed by nurses, involves a "bladder washout" with an antimicrobial drug via a Foley catheter. Specimens are taken for culture before and after the washout. The test is considered diagnostic of upper urinary tract infection if there is greater than a 10 percent rise in the colony count of specimens taken after the washout (Sheldon & Gonzalez, 1984, pp. 322–323).

The antibody-coated bacteria test is an immunofluorescence test for the detection of antibody-coated bacteria in urinary sediment (Thomas, Shelokov, & Forland, 1974). A positive test denotes kidney infection. The physiologic basis for this test is that when organisms infect tissue, the production of specific antibodies is stimulated; these antibodies then adhere to the organisms (Sheldon & Gonzalez, 1984, p. 323). The test is not highly sensitive; its false-negative rate has been reported to be as high as 15 to 25 percent (Ronald, 1983, p. 116; Sheldon & Gonzalez, 1984, p. 323). False positives may occur if the urine is at all contaminated because bacteria normally present in the urethra and vagina have fluorescing antibodies on their surface (Ronald, 1983, p. 116). Therefore, urine must be obtained either by catheterization or by suprapubic aspiration. Clinical use of the test is thus limited.

Intervention

Treatment. The most efficacious treatment for lower UTI involves the use of an antibiotic that is specific to the pathologic organism, has a high urinary concentration and a low serum level, exhibits minimal effects on fecal and vaginal flora, causes little or no gastric distress, is available at reasonable cost, and is effective orally (Parsons, 1985, pp. 489–490; Lindan, 1981, p. 38). The causative organism must therefore always be identified, although some authorities feel that because the great majority of outpatient infections are caused by *E. coli*, a sensitivity is not always necessary (Sabath & Charles, 1980).

A number of available drugs meet the preceding criteria to varying degrees. The organisms for which these antibiotics are effective, their usual dosages, and their common side effects are outlined in Table 17–3. For accuracy, urine for culture must be collected prior to the initiation of antibiotic therapy (Abraham et al., 1983, p. 231). Once a culture is obtained, a broad-spectrum urinary antibiotic (see Table 17–3) can be prescribed; therapy can be adjusted as necessary on the basis of culture results, which should be available within 18 to 48 hours of plating in the laboratory (Lindan, 1981, p. 38). If the urine has a "fishy" odor or an alkaline pH (about 8.0), the infection may be caused by *Proteus*, and an antibiotic likely to be effective against this organism, such as trimethoprim–sulfamethoxazole, should be chosen (Lindan, 1981, p. 40). A UTI involving *Proteus* is cause for referral for diagnostic evaluation of the kidney (Parsons, 1985, p. 491; Roberts, 1984, p. 110).

When a patient is in pain, the urinary analgesic phenazopyridine hydrochloride (Pyridium) can be used before a culture can be obtained and while waiting for antibiotic therapy to provide relief. Usual dosage is 200 mg tid after meals (*Physicians' Desk Reference*, 1986, p. 1387). Phenazopyridine should not affect culture results but may turn the urine reddish orange. In addition, increased fluids may help cleanse the urinary tract, and acid ash fluids, particularly cranberry juice, may aid in bacteriostasis. It should be noted, however, that increasing fluids may dilute the urine and thus lower the concentration of pathogens found on culture (Ronald, 1983, p. 117). Avoidance of irritants such as alcohol and caffeine should be advised (Lindan, 1981, p. 40).

The question of how long to continue antibiotic therapy is somewhat controversial. A number of researchers have found 1-day therapy with amoxicillin, sulfisoxazole, or trimethoprim–sulfamethoxazole (co-trimoxazole or TMP–SMX) to be approximately as effective against lower urinary tract infections as 5- to 10-day regimens. The following doses have been compared favorably with 5- to 7-day courses of therapy (Bailey & Abbott, 1978; Bailey & Blake, 1980; Buckwold et al., 1982; Counts et al., 1982; Prentice et al., 1985): 3 g of amoxicillin; 1 to 2 g of sulfasoxazole; 1.96

TABLE 17–3. SELECTED MEDICATIONS FOR LOWER URINARY TRACT INFECTION[a]

Medication	Activity Effective Against	Usual Dosage	Possible Side Effects[b]	Comments
Trimethoprim–sulfamethoxazole (TMP–SMX, co-trimoxazole, Bactrim, Septra)	*Escherichia coli, Klebsiella–Enterobacter, Proteus mirabilis,* indole-positive species	Regular strength 2 tablets po bid × 5–10 days or 4 to 6 tablets po × 1 Double strength 1 tablet po bid × 5–10 days or 2 to 3 tablets po × 1	Hypersensitivity; hemolysis in G6PD deficiency patients; other blood dyscrasias; skin, GI, CNS reactions; drug fever, chills and toxic nephrosis	Fewer side effects with single-dose therapy; does not potentiate drug-resistant transfer in large bowel; maintain adequate fluids; not recommended in pregnancy
Sulfisoxazole (Gantanol; Gantrisin)	*E. coli, Klebsiella–Aerobacter, Staphylococcus aureus, P. mirabilis,* (some strains of *Klebsiella, Pseudomonas, Proteus,* and *Aerobacter* are resistant)	500 mg po qid × 10 days	Hypersensitivity; hemolysis in G6PD deficiency patients; other blood dyscrasias; skin, GI, CNS reactions; drug fever, chills and toxic nephrosis	Maintain adequate fluid intake; contraindicated in third trimester of pregnancy
Ampicillin	Broad spectrum including staphylococci, *Neisseria gonorrhoeae, P. mirabilis,* (ineffective against *Klebsiella* spp and *Pseudomonas*)	250 mg po qid × 10 days	Low toxicity but may result in hypersensitivity Fungal overgrowth	Contraindicated with previous hypersensitivity to any penicillin
Amoxicillin	Similar to ampicillin	250–500 mg po tid × 10 days or 3 g po × 1	See *Penicillin VK*	See *Penicillin VK*
Penicillin VK	Broad spectrum including staphylococci and *N. gonorrhoeae*	250 mg po tid or qid × 10 days	Hypersensitivity (anaphylactoid) reactions; nausea, vomiting, epigastric distress, diarrhea; black hairy tongue; fungal overgrowth	Contraindicated with previous hypersensitivity
Nitrofurantoin (Macrodantin)	Many gram-positive and gram-negative organisms including *E. coli* (ineffective against *Pseudomonas* and some strains of *Klebsiella*)	50–100 mg po qid × 10 days or 3 g po × 1	Acute and chronic pulmonary reactions; allergic reactions; liver damage; blood dyscrasias; neuropathy	Risk of side effects higher in women, increases with age; lower dose for petite and older women; take with food (unlike others listed) to avoid nausea; best in acidic urine; generic form not well tolerated by GI tract; no effect on fecal or vaginal flora

TABLE 17–3. CONTINUED

Medication	Activity Effective Against	Usual Dosage	Possible Side Effects[b]	Comments
Cephalosporins	*E. coli, P. mirablis, Klebsiella,* some strains of *Enterobacter* and *Enterococcus*	Cephalexin (Keflex) 250 mg po qid × 10 days; Cefadroxil (Duricef) 500 mg po bid × 10 days; Cephradine (Velosef) 250 mg po tid × 10 days	Hypersensitivity; skin reactions; GI upset; fever; blood dyscrasias	Expensive; relatively few side effects but usually used with organisms resistant to other antibiotics
Nalidixic acid (NegGram)	*E. coli, Proteus, Klebsiella, Enterobacter* (not effective against *Pseudomonas*)	1 g qid po × 7–14 days	CNS effects: drowsiness, weakness, visual disturbances; GI symptoms; allergic reactions; overdose can lead to convulsions, psychosis, other side effects	Associated with drug resistance during therapy; works at all urinary pH; avoid direct exposure to sunlight; contraindicated with history of convulsive disorders
Tetracycline	Many gram-positive and gram-negative organisms: *E. coli, Klebsiella, Enterobacter, Staph. aureus; C. trachomatis* (not effective against *Pseudomonas*)	250–500 mg tid po × 7–10 days	Allergic reactions; GI upset; rashes; fungal overgrowth	Not for use during pregnancy, nursing, infancy, early childhood; most active in acidic urine; take 1–2 hours before or 2 hours after meals; dairy products and some antacids interfere with absorption; avoid direct sunlight
Doxycycline	See *Tetracycline*	100 mg po bid × 7–10 days	See *Tetracycline*	See *Tetracycline*
Erythromycin	*Staph. aureus, N. gonorrhoeae, Chlamydia trachomatis*	250 mg po qid × 7–10 days	GI upsets; fungal overgrowth	Few side effects but rarely used for UTI except for *N. gonorrhoeae* or *C. trachomatis* when other therapies contraindicated

[a]References: Abraham et al. (1983); Bailey and Abbott (1978); Bailey and Blake (1980); Holmberg et al. (1980); Lindan (1981); Parsons (1985); *Physician's desk reference* (1986); Prentice et al. (1985); Sabath and Charles (1980).
[b]See *Physicians' desk reference* or other equivalent source for more description of these effects and listings of additional untoward reactions.

to 2.88 g of TMP—SMX (Bactrim or Septra 2 to 3 tablets double strength [D.S.] or 4 to 6 regular-strength tablets, equivalent to .32 to .48 g of trimethoprim and 1.60 to 2.40 g of sulfamethoxazole).

One study (Hooton, Running, & Stamm, 1985) found single-dose amoxicillin and a regimen of single-dose cyclacillin to be less effective than longer treatment, but found single-dose TMP—SMX to be effective.

Advantages of single-dose therapy include fewer and less severe side effects, better patient compliance, and lower cost. Risks include lower cure rates in patients with undetected upper tract infection and resistance to longer-term therapy after treatment failure (Hooton et al., 1985, p. 387). Patients treated with single-dose therapy may complain because symptoms are not always relieved immediately; they can be reassured as long as cultures have reverted to normal (Ronald, 1983, p. 117).

As simple, rapid, and reliable tests for differentiating women with upper from lower tract infection are not available, it has been recommended that single-dose treatment not be used for women with signs or symptoms of pyelonephritis including a duration of symptoms longer than 1 week. Research data derived from use of the antibody-coated bacteria test have suggested that women whose socioeconomic status is low may have a higher incidence of pyelonephritis than other populations; consequently, cau-

tion has been advised in using single-dose therapy for clinic patients (Stamm, 1980, pp. 591–592). It is also not appropriate for women with urologic abnormalities or women with kidney stones (Stamm, 1980, p. 591). Single-dose therapy has not been studied in children or pregnant women and may not be effective for women with previous UTIs caused by antibiotic-resistant organisms. This regimen should be reserved for women who will be likely to return for follow-up cultures to test the cure; the importance of such follow-up must be stressed when prescribing single-dose antibiotics.

Response to 1-day treatment can be used as a means of localizing urinary tract infection, with those whose cultures remain positive considered to have an upper tract infection (Abraham et al., 1983, p. 230).

In patients with negative cultures, but with definite symptoms, particularly pyuria, treatment with tetracycline, doxycycline, or erythromycin (in pregnancy) for 7 days is recommended on the basis that there may be a bacterial cause for the symptoms, often *Chlamydia*. Cervical, urethral, and urine cultures for *C. trachomatis, N. gonorrhoeae, M. hominis,* and *U. urealyticum* can be performed in these patients (Roberts, 1984, p. 112; Stamm et al., 1980), although these tests may have relatively high false-negative rates (see Chapter 12). In populations with low rates of sexually transmitted infections, such as older women, single-dose treatment for AUS with TMP–SMX has been advocated (Fihn & Stamm, 1983, p. 127).

Other organisms, such as *Trichomonas, Candida,* gardnerella and human papillomavirus have been reported as causing urinary tract symptoms in patients without positive cultures (Maskell, Pead, Pead, & Balsdon, 1984). Such organisms should be looked for in the vagina and treated appropriately (Scotti & Ostergard, 1984, p. 521) (see Chapters 11 and 12).

Asymptomatic bacteriuria, except in pregnant women or women with diabetes or sickle cell disease, need not be treated because it has not been shown to lead to urinary tract infection (Asscher et al., 1969).

The role of the primary care practitioner in treating UTIs depends on institutional or practice protocols, state law regarding prescription-writing privileges, presence of risk factors for upper tract infection, condition of the patient, and response to treatment. Certainly, symptoms suggestive of upper tract infection require consultation and/or referral as do recurrent or chronic conditions. Many primary care practitioners routinely treat lower tract infections, using standing orders or consultation for prescribing when state law prohibits their signing prescriptions. Before consultation or referral is initiated, a complete data base, including laboratory testing, should be obtained and appropriate patient teaching and counseling provided.

Follow-up. A urine culture should be repeated 7 days after completion of antibiotic therapy (Abraham et al., 1983, p. 230; Roberts, 1984, p. 112). A positive culture suggests an upper tract infection and calls for consultation or referral for prolonged antibiotic therapy, for as long as 4 to 6 weeks. Hospitalization may be required for intravenous antibiotics in pregnant women, patients with structural abnormalities, diabetes, immunosuppression, sickle cell anemia, or an inability to tolerate oral medications (Abraham et al., 1983, pp. 232–233). Persistent bacteriuria after treatment warrants referral for further urologic investigation for anatomic abnormalities (Abraham et al., 1983).

Resistance and Recurrence. It has been estimated that one half of women with a urinary tract infection will have a second infection within 1 year (Ronald, 1983, p. 117). Ronald (1983, p. 118) describes three patterns of recurrence that should be identified in any woman with more than one recurrence in this time period: persistence, relapse, and reinfection.

Persistence is due to use of an antimicrobial drug to which the organism is resistant, or improper taking of an appropriate medication. Inadequate excretion of the drug in the urine may be responsible for persistence; this occurs with certain drugs, particularly nitrofurantoin. In patients with indwelling catheters or other urinary drainage procedures, a superimposed infection with a second organism may lead to persistence.

Relapse occurs when the medication used fails to eradicate the pathologic organism. Relapse usually is seen within 2 weeks of completion of therapy. It almost always occurs in women with renal stones or chronically scarred kidneys, but may also be seen in patients without kidney damage.

Reinfection accounts for most recurrences. Such infections may appear sporadically or in clusters.

After single-dose therapy, women with a relapse should be treated with 2-week therapy (Ronald, 1983, p. 118). Subsequent relapse requires referral for a workup for renal calculi or other pathology. An intravenous pyelogram may be necessary, although if one has been done in the past and found to be normal, repetition of this test is unnecessary (Ronald, 1983, p. 118). Continuous long-term antibiotic suppression, generally with a trimethoprim–sulfonamide combination, amoxicillin, or cephalexin, may be indicated. Women on such therapy need frequent urologic and renal assessment. Ronald (1983, p. 119) recommends trimethoprim–sulfamethoxazole, 1 tablet, three times a week. This may be ongoing for 6 months to start or for up to 2 years if recurrence occurs within 3 months of stopping prophylaxis. Alternatively, women can be provided with a single-dose regimen to be used when symptoms appear, with follow-up cultures done after 2 weeks to test for cure. Another prophylactic regimen involves single-dose antibiotics after sexual intercourse (Vosti, 1975).

Additional prophylactic measures are discussed in the next section, Teaching and Counseling.

Another type of persistent urinary tract problem that requires referral is the occurrence of symptoms in the presence of sterile urine culture and the absence of pyuria. This may signify the urethral syndrome or interstitial cystitis. The urethral syndrome, diagnosed by exclusion and without known cause, presents a treatment dilemma. Diagnosis of interstitial cystitis is made on the basis of symptoms and exclusion of other pathology by cytology, cystoscopy, and biopsy. Reduced bladder capacity and ulcerations are the classic findings on cystoscopy although not all patients demonstrate either or both of these findings. Pinpoint hemorrhages, called *glomerulations,* seen on the bladder mucosa when the bladder is filled to capacity are diagnostic (Messing & Stamey, 1978, p. 384). The value of immunologic studies for diagnosis is controversial (Messing & Stamey, 1978; Rosin et al., 1979). Unfortunately, treatment for interstitial cystitis has not been highly successful (Messing & Stamey, 1978, p. 388). Bladder instillations (Messing & Stamey, 1978; Brown, 1983), electrical nerve innervation (Fall, Carlsson, & Erlandson, 1980; Fall, 1985), and surgical procedures including denervation of the bladder (Freiha & Stamey, 1980) and urinary diversion (Reid, 1985) all have been used with varying results, often providing temporary relief (Messing & Stamey, 1978; Brown, 1983).

Teaching and Counseling. Because so many women can expect to have at least one urinary tract infection during their lifetime, learning preventive behaviors is valuable for all women and especially important for those with a history of such infections. Preventive behaviors are meant to reduce risk factors and enhance the urinary system's own defenses. Areas amenable to behavioral input include hygienic and sexual practices, fluid intake, diet, and, at times, contraceptive method. In addition, counseling must consider the emotional needs of the woman suffering from a UTI or prone to such infections.

HYGIENIC PRACTICES. After urination or defecation, the urethral, vaginal, and perineal areas should be cleaned, wiping always from front to back to avoid bringing fecal bacteria to the vaginal introitus and urethral meatus. Use of plain, white, unscented tissue is advisable (Nichols & Wisgirda, 1985, p. 203). Washing with soap and water after a bowel movement has been recommended. Women should be encouraged to urinate soon after feeling the urge (Quinlan, 1984, p. 41), as urinary stasis may predispose to bacterial growth. Although the contribution of clothing to the development of UTI is debatable (Lindan, 1981, p. 43), cotton underwear, which absorbs moisture, and panty hose with a cotton, ventilated crotch generally are considered preferable to other types of underclothes. Tight-fitting clothes may lead to the area's being hot and sweaty, creating a medium for bacterial growth (Quinlan, 1984, p. 42). Changing of wet clothes after swimming or exercise should be encouraged. Lindan (1981, p. 43) recommends tampons, except when contraindicated, over sanitary pads, which she points out act as a blood culture medium connecting the urethral opening and the anus.

Bubble bath and vaginal perfumes should be avoided (Quinlan, 1984, p. 42). Because a vaginal pH greater than 4.4 has been shown to favor introital colonization in women with recurrent UTIs (Stamey & Timothy, 1975; Stamey & Kaufman, 1975), vaginal infections that might alter pH should be diagnosed and treated promptly (Quinlan, 1984, p. 42).

SEXUAL PRACTICES. Urinating after intercourse washes out organisms that may have been brought to the urethra during coitus. Drinking a glass of water before intercourse facilitates this (Ronald, 1983, p. 119). Women should be warned against sexual practices that bring fecal organisms to the vagina such as having penile or digital vaginal contact after anal contact without washing.

FLUID INTAKE. Large quantities of fluid intake (up to 10 to 14 glasses per day) increase the force of the urine flow, thus increasing the elimination of bacteria (Quinlan, 1984, p. 41). As concentrated overnight urine has been shown to be bacteriocidal (Cicmanec et al., 1985), fluid intake should be timed to produce frequent daytime voiding only.

Cranberry juice often is advised to acidify the urine, increasing its bacteriostatic properties. It has been reported to be useful for both prevention and treatment of urinary tract infection. Cranberries or cranberry juice has been shown to slightly increase the acidity of urine by increasing its concentration of hippuric acid (Fellers, Redmon, & Parrott, 1933; Bodel, Cotran, & Kass, 1959), although one small study showed only transient effects of cranberry juice on urinary pH (Kahn, Panariello, Saeli, et al., 1967). Cranberry juice has also been found to inhibit bacterial adherence, generally considered a prerequisite for colonization and infection (Sobota, 1984). This may be more responsible for the beneficial effects of cranberry juice on the urinary tract than acidification of urine. Cranberry cocktail, cranberry concentrate, and fresh cranberry juice were all found effective.

DIET. An acid ash diet that includes high intake of meat, nuts, prunes, plums, cranberries (or the same fruit juices), and whole-grain cereals and breads and restricts milk and most fruits and vegetables may be useful in preventing UTIs, although its effect has not been scientifically demonstrated (Lindan, 1981, p. 43; Quinlan, 1984, p. 42). Its value must be weighed against other health risks of this type of diet. Ascorbic acid in doses of 2 to 4 g a day is a urinary acidifier (Lindan, 1981, p. 43).

CONTRACEPTIVE PRACTICES. When history implicates the vaginal diaphragm in recurrent UTIs, a change in birth control method may offer relief. For women not wishing to change contraceptives, a trial using a smaller diaphragm with a less rigid rim may be more acceptable (Gillespie, 1984). See Chapter 6 and Section II for more discussion of this and other methods of birth control.

HOME REMEDIES. Advocates of home remedies for UTI recommend apple cider vinegar, 2 tablespoons, 3 times daily, taken in juice. It may, however, cause intolerable heartburn. The herb, echinacea, is also advocated. The dosage is 1 dropperful, 3 times daily, in juice or herbal tea. As with any remedy, a urinary culture is advised before the initiation of treatment and antibiotics may be necessary.

EMOTIONAL NEEDS. A urinary tract infection is often perceived as a serious problem. Besides the severe and possibly disabling pain that it causes, it can be experienced as an assault on sexuality and body integrity, particularly if it is persistent or recurrent. Sensitivity to the feelings to which such infections may lead is an important aspect of the care of women with UTIs.

URINARY INCONTINENCE

Definitions and Classifications

Urinary incontinence is a symptom (Harrison, 1978, p. 67). It presents in a variety of ways and has a number of causes. Incontinence can be defined as "abnormal leakage of urine" (Green, 1975, p. 368) or "difficulty in voiding control" (Nichols & Wisgirda, 1985, p. 205). Mild degrees of incontinence may not pose a problem for a particular woman, but when it interferes with activity or causes lifestyle changes, it should always be considered abnormal (Duchin, 1984, p. 33).

Incontinence results from an imbalance between the mechanism of urethral closure and the function of the bladder (or detrusor) muscle (Nichols & Wisgirda, 1985, p. 205). Incontinence occurs when intravesical (bladder) pressure exceeds intraurethral pressure (Duchin, 1984, p. 33). A defect could be present in any of the regulatory mechanisms—neurologic, structural, or hormonal. Function may be affected by aging, medications, and infectious processes (Nichols & Wisgirda, 1985, pp. 201, 205). Incontinence, although seen in all age groups, creates a particular problem for elderly women, affecting 5 to 10 percent of the elderly in the community and as much as 50 percent among the institutionalized; it can lead to social isolation, institutionalization, and infection and skin breakdown (Williams & Pannill, 1982, p. 895).

The most common type of incontinence is stress incontinence, accounting for 75 to 80 percent of urinary incontinence in women (Green, 1975, pp. 368, 370). Urinary stress incontinence has been defined by the International Continence Society as a *symptom*, a *sign*, and a *condition* (Harrison, 1978, p. 68):

1. The *symptom* stress incontinence indicates the patient's statement of involuntary loss of urine when exercising physically.
2. The *sign* stress incontinence denotes the observation of involuntary loss of urine from the urethra immediately upon an increase in abdominal pressure.
3. The *condition* (genuine stress incontinence) is involuntary loss of urine when the intravesical pressure exceeds the maximum urethral pressure but in the absence of detrusor activity.

Patients with urinary stress incontinence typically present with loss of urine with "sudden but brief increases in intraabdominal pressure, as with laughing, coughing, sneezing, or changing position" (Nichols & Wisgirda, 1985, p. 207). The pathophysiology of urinary stress incontinence involves a deviation from the normal 90° angle made where the urethra meets the bladder (the posterior urethral vesical, or PUV, angle). This abnormality results from loss of support to the bladder neck and causes a change in the transmission of intraabdominal pressure so that counter-

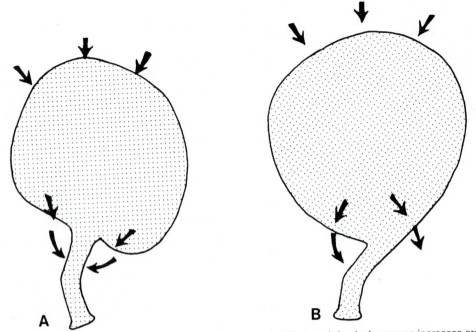

With a 90-degree posterior urethral vesicle (PUV) angle (A), intraabdominal pressure increases are distributed equally in all directions and continence is maintained; when this angle is lost (B), counter-pressure at the proximal urethra is also lost and pressure is distributed unequally leading to leakage of urine.

Figure 17-1. Anatomic abnormality in stress incontinence loss of 90° PUV angle. *(From Hajj, S. N. [1979, July]. Female urinary incontinence: A dynamic evaluation.* The Journal of Reproductive Medicine, *23(1), 34. Reprinted by permission.)*

pressure in the urethra is lost (see Fig. 17–1) (Hajj, 1979, p. 34).

Nichols & Wisgirda (1985, pp. 207–209) describe other causes of incontinence including (1) detrusor muscle hyperactivity (also called detrusor irritability, instability, or dyssynergia [Green, 1975, p. 370] or urge incontinence), resulting from structural weakness, poor tone, sacral reflex activity, or infections; (2) overflow incontinence, occurring when there is loss of urine without contraction of the detrusor muscle and in the presence of neurologic or anatomic abnormalities; (3) neurogenic bladder, encompassing many conditions resulting from central nervous system regulatory defects; and (4) extrinsic causes of incontinence, including congenital abnormalities and problems, such as urinary tract fistulas, secondary to trauma, previous surgery, or radiation therapy. Warwick (1979, pp. 22–23) describes "giggle incontinence," a condition commonly seen in young girls; it can last through adolescence and occasionally into adulthood, and involves loss of a large amount of urine with giggling. This benign reflex condition may lead to great embarrassment, but patients need to be reassured that it is not abnormal.

Women who experience incontinence to the extent that it "becomes a social or a hygienic problem" (Duchin, 1984, p. 33) deserve referral to a gynecologist with interest in this area or to a urologist for a complete diagnostic workup and possible treatment. A neurologic assessment may also be indicated as incontinence may be either a result or a symptom of a neurogenic disorder. A careful history often can be extremely valuable in establishing the type of incontinence experienced, in sorting out the possible cause of this problem, and in choosing an appropriate source of referral. In addition, exercises that prevent or correct urinary stress incontinence can be taught.

Management

Data Collection. History taking should include questions to elicit a careful description of symptoms, including onset, duration, and subjective assessment of severity, change over time, predisposing factors, and relief measures. Whether the condition has caused the use of protective measures ranging from increased frequency of underwear changes to wearing of pads should be discussed (Walter & Olesen, 1982, p. 395). If the problem is true stress incontinence, the woman should report immediate loss of urine with physical stress, usually in small amounts, and only in the standing position. There is usually no history of prior bladder problems, although the symptoms may have occurred during and after a previous pregnancy. There is no urgency, as there is with disorders of the detrusor muscle. Patients with urinary stress incontinence can halt the flow of urine during voiding and this "stop test" may be part of diagnosis (Warwick, 1979, p. 15).

A history of dysuria may indicate an infection and requires laboratory testing as previously outlined. A history of disease related to urinary incontinence should be elicited whenever this symptom is present. Significant conditions include neurologic disorders, chronic problems such as diabetes mellitus or collagen diseases, which may alter the tone or function of the urethra (Duchin, 1984, p. 33), and chronic respiratory disease whose manifestations may cause increases in intraabdominal pressure. Symptoms of undiagnosed neurologic disease such as loss of balance or diplopia should be explored (Nichols & Wisgirda, 1985, pp. 209–210).

Use of certain medications often causes urinary tract problems: diuretics of course may lead to frequency and nocturia; with their use, an inability to get to the toilet in time may be mistaken for true incontinence; β blockers such as propranolol (Inderal) and terbutaline may lead to bladder hypotonia (Nichols & Wisgirda, 1985, p. 209). Methyldopa (Aldomet), doxepin hydrochloride (Adapin, Sinequan), piperacetazine (Quide), phenoxybenzamine hydrochloride (Dibenzyline), reserpine, chlorpromazine (Thorazine), thioridazine (Mellaril), and prazosin hydrochloride (Minipress) may all cause stress incontinence (Duchin, 1984, p. 44). Caffeine may lead to detrusor hyperactivity and/or diuresis (Nichols & Wisgirda, 1985, p. 209).

A menstrual history revealing menopause or its preceding symptoms may explain dysuria, frequency, and incontinence (Nichols & Wisgirda, 1985, p. 209).

Pregnancy (current and past) and previous pelvic surgery or procedures should be reviewed. Constant heavy lifting or wearing of tight abdominal supports such as girdles should be discussed, as they may lead to stress incontinence.

Physical examination should incorporate evaluation for genital prolapse and cystocele and rectocele, which may coexist with incontinence, although they are not necessarily causative (Walter & Olesen, 1982, p. 394). Previous surgical repair may have led to incontinence (Duchin, 1984, p. 46); scarring and fibrosis should be observed for (Harrison, 1978, p. 70). Signs of vaginal atrophy should be noted (see Chapter 24). Any intraabdominal mass such as a uterine myoma or ovarian cyst or enlarged uterus (possibly secondary to pregnancy) can cause stress incontinence (Duchin, 1984, p. 33). Other observations should include the ability to contract the pelvic floor (Harrison, 1978, p. 70) and whether coughing or laughing causes urinary leakage; the latter must be tested for in the standing position.

Other diagnostic testing in the assessment of urinary incontinence may involve a number of urologic studies discussion of which is beyond the scope of this chapter. In addition to urinalysis and culture and sensitivity, these include intravenous pyelography, cystoscopy, urethroscopy, cystometrograms, and urodynamic screening (Green, 1975, p. 380; Warwick & Brown, 1979, p. 215). All these studies are normal in the woman with true stress incontinence (Green, 1975, p. 380).

Intervention. Treatment of urinary stress incontinence includes exercise and surgery. Current authors generally advise surgical treatment once a firm diagnosis is made and abnormalities of the detrusor muscle that are not amenable to surgical repair are ruled out (e.g., Green, 1975; Stanton, 1978; Hajj, 1979; Warwick & Brown, 1979). Physiotherapy, however, has been successful in treating this condition (Kegel, 1956; Jones, 1963). Kegel found that specific exercises of the pubococcygeus muscle led to slight to excellent improvement in over 90 percent of 155 patients after 3 to 6 weeks of diligent exercise following careful instructions and follow-up to ensure correct contraction of the muscle. Jones found a 56 to 69 percent improvement, related to degree of pretreatment incontinence. The well-known Kegel exercise is described in Chapter 2. Dr. Kegel suggested the following regimen for correction of urinary stress incontinence (Kegel, 1956, p. 491):

1. Before arising in the morning, contract the muscles five times, . . . then contract them again five times on first standing up; try to hold the muscles in a contracted position while walking to the toilet.
2. Interrupt the urinary stream several times during each voiding.
3. Repeat contractions of the same muscle five times

every half hour throughout the day. (It is brought to the patient's attention that permitting the muscles to sag for long periods retards progress and that to "bear down" during exercises may aggravate her complaints.)

The early morning exercises are especially important, for the patient begins the day with the perineum in a high position, whereas previously she started out with a sagging pelvic floor.

In the absence of improvement satisfactory to the patient, referral for possible surgical correction of urinary stress incontinence may be indicated.

REFERENCES

Abraham, E., Brenner, B. E., & Simon, R. R. (1983, April). Cystitis and pyelonephritis. *Annals of Emergency Medicine, 12*(4), 228–234.

Asscher, A. W., Sussman, M., & Waters, W. E., et al. (1969, March). Asymptomatic significant bacteriuria in the nonpregnant woman. II. Response to treatment and follow-up. *British Medical Journal,* 804–806.

Bailey, R. R., & Abbott, G. D. (1978, March). Treatment of urinary tract infection with a single dose of trimethoprim-sulfamethoxazole. *Canadian Medical Association Journal, 118,* 551–552.

Bailey, R. R., & Blake, E. (1980, October). Treatment of uncomplicated urinary tract infections with a single dose of co-trimoxazole. *New Zealand Medical Journal,* 285–286.

Berg, A. O., Heidrich, F. E., & Fihn, S. D., et al. (1984, February). Establishing the cause of genitourinary symptoms in women in a family practice. *Journal of the American Medical Association, 251*(5), 620–625.

Bodel, P. T., Cotran, R., & Kass, E. H. (1959, December). Cranberry juice and the antibacterial action of hippuric acid. *Journal of Laboratory and Clinical Medicine, 54*(6), 881–888.

Bran, J. L., Levison, M. E., & Kaye, D. (1972, March). Entrance of bacteria into the female urinary bladder. *The New England Journal of Medicine, 286*(12), 626–629.

Braude, A. (1984, June). Bacterial pyelonephritis. *Comprehensive Therapy, 19*(6), 65–74.

Brown, R. J. (1983, February). Interstitial cystitis. *The Journal of the Kansas Medical Society, 65*–83.

Brumfitt, W. (1984, January). Urology and the family doctor. *The Practitioner, 228,* 97.

Buckley, R. M., McGuckin, M., & MacGregor, R. R. (1978, February). Urine bacterial counts after sexual intercourse. *The New England Journal of Medicine, 298*(6), 321–324.

Buckwold, F. J., Ludwig, P., Harding, G. K. M., et al., (1982, April). Therapy for acute cystitis in adult women: Randomized comparison of single-dose sulfisoxazole vs. trimethoprim-sulfamethoxazole. *The Journal of the American Medical Association, 247*(13), 1839–1842.

Chernow, B., Zaloga, G. P., & Soldano, S., et al. (1984, March). Measurement of leukocyte esterase activity: A screening test for urinary tract infections. *Annals of Emergency Medicine, 13*(3), 150–154.

Cicmanec, J. F., Shank, R. A., & Evans, A. T. (1985, August). Overnight concentration of urine: Natural defense mechanism against urinary tract infection. *Urology, 26*(2), 157–159.

Columbia Presbyterian Medical Center. (1985, October). *Update on Genito-Urinary Infections, 7*(3), 1–4.

Counts, G. W., Stamm, W. E., McKevitt, M., Running, K., Holmes, K. K., & Turck, M. (1982, March/April). Treatment of cystitis in women with a single dose of trimethoprim–sulfamethoxazole. *Reviews of Infectious Diseases, 4*(2), 484–490.

Curran, J. W. (1977, July–September). Gonorrhea and the urethral syndrome [Editorial]. *Sexually Transmitted Diseases, 4*(3), 119–121.

Duchin, H. E. (1984, June). Ways to avoid iatrogenic urinary stress incontinence. *Contemporary OB/GYN, 23*(6), 33–34, 43–52.

Elster, A. B., Lach, P. A., Roghmann, K. J., & McAnarney, E. R. (1981, June). Relationship between frequency of sexual intercourse and urinary tract infections in young women. *Southern Medical Journal, 74*(6), 704–708.

Fair, W. R. (1983, May). Editorial overview: Urinary tract infections—Current status. *Seminars in Urology, 1*(2), 91–96.

Fall, M. (1985, May). Conservative management of chronic interstitial cystitis: Transcutaneous electrical nerve stimulation, and transurethral resection. *The Journal of Urology, 133*(5), 774–778.

Fall, M., Carlsson, C. A., & Erlandson, B. J. (1980, February). Electrical stimulation in interstitial cystitis. *The Journal of Urology, 123*(2), 192–195.

Fall, M., Johansson, S. L., & Vahlne, A. (1985, May). A clinicopathological and virological study of interstitial cystitis. *The Journal of Urology, 133*(5), 771–773.

Fellers, C. R., Redmon, B. C., & Parrott, E. M. (1933, September). Effect of cranberries on urinary acidity and blood alkali reserve. *Journal of Nutrition, 6*(5), 455–463.

Fihn, S., Latham, R. H., Roberts, P., Running, K., & Stamm, W. E. (1985, July). Association between diaphragm use and urinary tract infection. *The Journal of the American Medical Association, 254*(2), 240–245.

Fihn, S. D., Running, K., Pinkstaff, C., Roberts, P., & Stamm, W. E. (1985). Diaphragms cause urinary obstruction in women with prior urinary tract infection. *Clinical Research, 33*(2), 720A.

Fihn, S. D., & Stamm, W. E. (1983, May). The urethral syndrome. *Seminars in Urology, 1*(2), 121–129.

Freiha, F., & Stamey, T. A. (1980, March). Cystolysis: A procedure for the selective denervation of the bladder. *The Journal of Urology, 123*(3), 360–363.

Gillespie, L., (1984, July). The diaphragm: An accomplice in recurrent urinary tract infections. *Urology, 24*(1), 25–30.

Green, T. H. (1975, June). Urinary stress incontinence: Differential diagnosis, pathophysiology, and management. *The American Journal of Obstetrics and Gynecology, 122*(3), 368–400.

Hajj, S. N. (1979, July). Female urinary incontinence: A dynamic evaluation. *The Journal of Reproductive Medicine, 23*(1), 33–41.

Harris, R. E. (1983, August). Causes and treatment of genitourinary tract infections. *Comprehensive Therapy, 9* (8), 48–53.

Harrison, N. W. (1978, April). Stress incontinence—past and present. *Clinics in Obstetrics and Gynecology, 5*(1), 67–81.

Hedelin, H. H., Mårdh, P-A., & Brorson, J-E., et al. (1983, October–December). *Mycoplasma hominis* and interstitial cystitis. *Sexually Transmitted Diseases, 10*(4:Suppl.), 327–330.

Holmberg, L., Boman, G., & Bottiger, L. E., et al. (1980, November). Adverse reactions to nitrofurantoin: Analysis of 921 reports. *The American Journal of Medicine, 69*(5), 733–738.

Hooton, T. M., Running, K., & Stamm, W. E. (1985, January). Single-dose therapy for cystitis in women: A comparison of trimethoprim–sulfamethoxazole, amoxicillin, and cyclacillin. *The Journal of the American Medical Association, 253*(3), 387–390.

Jones, E. G. (1963). Nonoperative treatment of stress incontinence. *Clinical Obstetrics and Gynecology, 6*(1), 220–235.

Kahn, H. D., Panariello, V. A., Saeli, J., Sampson, J. R., & Schwartz, E. (1967, September). Effect of cranberry juice on urine. *Journal of the American Dietetic Association, 51*(3), 251–254.

Kegel, A. H. (1956, April). Stress incontinence of urine in women: Physiologic treatment. *Journal of the International College of Surgeons, 25*(4), 487–499.

Lindan, R. (1981, March). Urinary tract infection: A preventable disease. *The Female Patient, 6,* 36–43.

Madsen, P. O., Larsen, E. H., & Dorflinger, T. (1985, July). Infectious complications after instrumentation of urinary tract. *Supplement to Urology, 26*(1), 15–17.

Marshall, S. (1965, January). The effect of bubble bath on the urinary tract. *The Journal of Urology, 93*(1), 112.

Maskell, R., Pead, L., Pead, P. J., & Balsdon, M. J. (1984). *Chlamydia* infection and urinary symptoms. *British Journal of Venereal Disease, 60*(1), 65–67.

Messing, E. M., & Stamey, T. A. (1978, October). Interstitial cystitis: Early diagnosis, pathology, and treatment. *Urology, 12*(4), 381–392.

Neu, H. C. (1983, May). Urinary tract infections in the 1980s. *Seminars in Urology, 1*(2), 130–137.

Nichols, D. H., & Wisgirda, J. A. (1985). Gynecological urology.

In D. H. Nichols & J. R. Evrard (Eds.), *Ambulatory gynecology* (pp. 200–222). Philadelphia: Harper & Row.

Nicolle, L., Harding, G. K. M., Preiksaitis, J., & Ronald, A. R. (1982, November). The association of urinary tract infection with sexual intercourse. *The Journal of Infectious Diseases, 146*(5), 579–582.

O'Dowd, T. C. (1984, August). Frequency and dysuria in women: The tip of an iceberg. *The Practitioner, 228*(1394), 711–715.

Paavonen, J., and Vesterinen, E. (1982). *Chlamydia trachomatis* in cervicitis and urethritis in women. *Scandinavian Journal of Infectious Diseases, Supplementum, 32,* 45–54.

Parivar, F., & Bradbrook, R. A. (1986). Review: Interstitial cystitis. *British Journal of Urology, 58:*239–244.

Parsons, C. L. (1985, June). Urinary tract infections. *Clinics in Obstetrics and Gynecology, 12*(2), 487–496.

Peddie, B. A., Gorrie, S. I., & Bailey, R. R. (1986, April). Diaphragm use and urinary tract infection. *The Journal of the American Medical Association, 255*(13), 1707.

Physicians' desk reference (40th ed.). (1986). Oradell, NJ: Medical Economics Company.

Prentice, R. D., Wu, L. R., & Gehlbach, S. H., et al. (1985). Treatment of lower urinary tract infections with single-dose trimethoprim—sulfamethoxazole. *The Journal of Family Practice, 20*(6), 551–557.

A quick check for UTI. (1984, August). *Emergency Medicine, 60,* 65.

Quinlan, M. W. (1984, March). UTI: Helping your patients control it once and for all. *RN,* 39–42.

Reid, J. S. (1985, November/December). The other cystitis: Interstitial cystitis. *Journal of Nephrology Nursing,* 294–296.

Roberts, J. A. (1984, September). Urinary tract infections. *American Journal of Kidney Diseases, 4*(2), 103–117.

Ronald, A. R. (1983, May). The management of urethrocystitis in women. *Seminars in urology, 1*(2), 114–120.

Rosin, R. D., Griffiths, T., & Sofras, F., et al. (1979). Interstitial cystitis. *British Journal of Urology, 51,* 524–527.

Sabath, L. D., & Charles, D. (1980, May). Urinary tract infections in the female. *Obstetrics and Gynecology, 55*(5, Suppl.), 162S–169S.

Salmen, P., Dwyer, D. M., Vorse, H., & Kruse, W. (1983, October). Whirlpool-associated *Pseudomonas aeruginosa* urinary tract infections. *The Journal of the American Medical Association, 250*(15), 2025–2026.

Schaeffer, A. (1983, May). Bladder defense mechanisms against urinary tract infections. *Seminars in Urology, 1*(2), 106–113.

Scotti, R. J., & Ostergard, D. R. (1984, June). The urethral syndrome. *Clinical Obstetrics and Gynecology, 27*(2), 515–529.

Sheldon, C., & Gonzalez, R. (1984, March). Differentiation of upper and lower urinary tract infections: How and when? *Medical Clinics of North America, 62*(2), 321–333.

Smith, G., Brumfitt, W., & Hamilton-Miller, J. (1983, December). Diagnosis of coliform infection in acutely dysuric women. *The New England Journal of Medicine, 309*(229), 1393–1394.

Sobota, A. E. (1984, May). Inhibition of bacterial adherence by cranberry juice: Potential use for the treatment of urinary tract infection. *The Journal of Urology, 131*(5), 1013–1016.

Stamey, T. A., & Kaufman, M. T. (1975, August). Studies of introital colonization in women with recurrent urinary tract infections. II. A comparison of growth in normal vaginal fluid of common versus uncommon serogroups of *Escherichia coli. The Journal of Urology, 114*(2), 264–267.

Stamey, T. A., & Timothy, M. M. (1975, August). Studies of introital colonization in women with recurrent urinary tract infections. I. The role of vaginal pH. *The Journal of Urology, 114*(2), 261–263.

Stamey, T. A., Wehner, N., Mihara, G., & Condy, M. (1978). The immunologic basis of recurrent bacteriuria: Role of cervical vaginal antibody in enterobacterial colonization of the introital mucosa. *Medicine, 57,* 47–56.

Stamm, W. E. (1980, August). Single-dose treatment of cystitis [Editorial]. *The Journal of the American Medical Association, 244*(6), 591–592.

Stamm, W. E., Counts, G. W., Running, K. R., Turck, M., & Holmes, K. K. (1982, August). Diagnosis of coliform infection in acutely dysuric women. *The New England Journal of Medicine, 307*(8), 463–468.

Stamm, W. E., Running, K., & McKevitt, M., et al. (1981, April). Treatment of the acute urethral syndrome. *The New England Journal of Medicine, 304*(16), 956–958.

Stamm, W. E., Wagner, K. F., & Amsel, R., et al. (1980, August). Causes of the acute urethral syndrome in women. *The New England Journal of Medicine, 303*(8), 409–415.

Stanton, S. L. (1978, April). Surgery of urinary incontinence. *Clinics in Obstetrics and Gynecology, 5*(1), 83–108.

Thomas, V., Shelokov, A., & Forland, M. (1974, March). Antibody-coated bacteria in the urine and the site of urinary-tract infection. *The New England Journal of Medicine, 290*(11), 588–590.

Vosti, K. L. (1975, March). Recurrent urinary tract infections. *The Journal of the American Medical Association, 231*(9), 934–940.

Wall, E., & Baldwin-Johnson, C. (1984). Urinary tract infections among diaphragm users. *The Journal of Family Practice, 18*(5), 707–711.

Walter, S., & Olesen, K. P. (1982, May). Urinary incontinence and genital prolapse in the female: Clinical, urodynamic and radiological examinations. *British Journal of Obstetrics and Gynecology, 89*(5), 393–401.

Warwick, R. T. (1979, February). Observation on the function and dysfunction of the sphincter and detrustor mechanisms. *Urologic Clinics of North America, 6*(1), 13–30.

Warwick, R. T. & Brown, A. D. G. (1979, February). A urodynamic evaluation of urinary incontinence in the female and its treatment. *Urologic Clinics of North America, 6*(1), 203–215.

Williams, M. E., & Pannill, F. C., III (1982, December). Urinary incontinence in the elderly. *Annals of Internal Medicine, 97*(6), 895–907.

Wong, E. S., Fennell, C. L., & Stamm, W. E. (1984, January–March). Urinary tract infection among women attending a clinic for sexually transmitted diseases. *Sexually Transmitted Diseases, 11*(1), 18–23.

Wright, D., & Matsen, J. M. (1984, June). Diagnosing urinary tract infection. *Diagnostic Medicine, 44*(6), 44–53.

18

Multiorgan Disorders

Ronnie Lichtman and Suzanne M. Smith

Toxic-shock syndrome, diethylstilbestrol exposure in utero, and endometriosis are women's health problems not confined to any one organ. They are therefore discussed together in this chapter. The role of the primary care gynecologic provider in these potentially serious problems is fourfold: teaching preventive measures whenever possible and alerting women to symptomatology; screening for risk factors and signs and symptoms; co-managing or referring for emergency care or medical follow-up as necessary; and providing psychological support and recommending community resources and professional counseling when appropriate. In this chapter, each of these entities is described, and the primary care management role is discussed in detail.

TOXIC-SHOCK SYNDROME

Toxic-shock syndrome (TSS) is a multi*system* disorder, by definition involving at least three organ systems (Thomas & Withington, 1985, p. 158); however, because of its association with menstruation and particularly with tampon use, and, to a lesser extent, with certain barrier methods of birth control, as well as its increased incidence during the postpartum period, this disease is of concern to women's health care providers and their patients.

Definition

Toxic-shock syndrome was originally described by Todd, Fishaut, Kapral, and Welch in 1978 in a report of seven cases among children between 8 and 17 years old. They wrote: "During the past few years we have seen what appears to be a new and severe, acute disease characterized by hyperaemia, subcutaneous oedema, hypotension, renal failure, and liver injury, and which has been associated with the presence of toxin-producing strains of phage-group-1 *Staphylococcus aureus*" (p. 1116).

In 1980, the Centers for Disease Control (CDC) outlined criteria for diagnosing TSS (CDC, 1980b, p. 442). These appear in Table 18–1.

Incidence

After the initial description of TSS in children, the disorder was found to be associated with menstruation (Davis, Chesney, & Wand, 1980; Schrock, 1980; Shands, Schmid &

Dan, 1980). In 1982, almost 80 percent of TSS cases were menstruation related; of these, 99 percent were in women who used tampons (CDC, 1983, p. 400). As of June 1983, CDC had reported 2,204 cases of TSS. Ninety-six percent were in females, of which 90 percent were associated with menstruation. Thirty-six percent occurred in persons between 15 and 19 years of age; 97 percent of sufferers were white. In 1980, Davis and associates reported a minimum annual incidence rate of 6.2 per 100,000 menstruating women in Wisconsin, where great effort was given to TSS surveillance. Peterson (1982, p. 891) estimates a national yearly rate of 8.9 cases per 100,000 menstruating women and 0.5 per 100,000 U.S. population.

The number of known new cases of TSS increased from 1979 to 1980, but decreased progressively after 1980 (CDC, 1983, p. 398). The CDC attributes changes in the incidence rates to changes in the number of tampon users and their pattern of use; changes in available brands, composition, and absorbency of tampons; widespread publicity of a new superabsorbent tampon, Rely, in 1978, and its subsequent removal from the market; changes in the prevalence of infective strains of *S. aureus*; and early recognition and treatment of the syndrome (Reingold, Hargrelt, & Shands, 1982, p. 878).

Etiologic and Predisposing Factors

Staphylococcus aureus is associated with the development of TSS (CDC, 1980b, p. 441). This organism has been isolated in mucous membranes and infected sites of TSS patients, but not in blood, suggesting that a toxin produced by the organism is the responsible pathogenic agent (Todd et al., 1978). Named *toxic shock syndrome toxin 1* (TSST-1) at a symposium held in 1984 (Parsonnet, Hickman, Eardley, & Pier, 1985, p. 514), this substance has been demonstrated to be toxigenic in a variety of laboratory animals (Stolz, Davis, & Vergeront, 1985). Garbe and associates (1985), however, report that among 32 patients with nonmenstrual TSS, only 62.5 percent produced TSST-1, compared with 93 percent of 44 patients with menstrual TSS. They suggest that other as yet unrecognized toxins play a role in the pathogenesis of this disorder. The specific pathophysiologic action of TSST-1 and other toxins in the distinct clinical entity of TSS is not understood.

In one study of 80 patients, vomiting, mucous membrane involvement, myalgia, and abnormal urinalysis appeared to be independent of shock and have thus been

TABLE 18–1. OUTLINE CRITERIA FOR DIAGNOSING TOXIC SHOCK SYNDROME

1. Fever: temperature > 38.9°C (102°F)
2. Rash: diffuse macular erythroderma
3. Desquamation, 1 to 2 weeks after onset of illness, particularly of palms and soles
4. Hypotension: systolic blood pressure ≤ 90 mm Hg for adults or below fifth percentile by age for children under 16 years of age, or orthostatic syncope
5. Involvement of three or more of the following organ systems:
   A. Gastrointestinal: vomiting or diarrhea at onset of illness
   B. Muscular: severe myalgia or creatine phosphokinase level ≥ 2 × ULN[a]
   C. Mucous membrane: vaginal, oropharyngeal, or conjunctival hyperemia
   D. Renal: BUN or Cr ≥ 2 × ULN or ≥ 5 white blood cells per high-power field—in the absence of a urinary tract infection
   E. Hepatic: total bilirubin, SGOT, or SGPT ≥ 2 × ULN
   F. Hematologic: platelets ≤ 100,000/mm³
   G. Central nervous system: disorientation or alterations in consciousness without focal neurologic signs when fever and hypotension are absent
6. Negative results on the following tests, if obtained:
   A. Blood, throat, or cerebrospinal fluid cultures
   B. Serologic tests for Rocky Mountain spotted fever, leptospirosis, or measles

[a]ULN, upper limits of normal for laboratory; BUN, blood urea nitrogen level; Cr, creatinine level; SGOT, serum glutamic–oxaloacetic transaminase level; SGPT, serum glutamic–pyruvic transaminase level.

postulated to reflect the specific action of TSS-associated toxin (Davis et al., 1982a, p. 446), whereas other clinical features were associated with the presence of shock. Shock is due most likely to the movement of serum fluids and proteins from the intravascular compartment to the extravascular space, resulting in peripheral vasodilation, decreased blood pressure, and shock.

The Tampon Link. The role of tampon use as a predisposing factor for TSS has been actively investigated since this phenomenon was noted in 1980. In a retrospective study by CDC of 50 female victims of TSS and 50 controls, a statistically significant association between Rely tampons—both super and regular strength—and TSS was established. This study estimated the relative risk for the development of TSS with this brand of tampon to be 7.9 (CDC, 1980b, pp. 442–443).

The Tri-State Toxic Shock Syndrome Study, which was a case-control analysis of data from Iowa, Minnesota, and Wisconsin for the 1-year period 1979–1980, represents the largest TSS study to date (Osterholm, Davis, & Gibson, 1982). In this study the odds ratio (estimate of relative risk) for developing TSS while using tampons during menstruation was 18.01 for all brands, with a range of 5.29 to 27.5 for individual brands. Rely was the only brand with a statistically significantly increased odds ratio when used exclusively.

A number of possible mechanisms by which tampon use leads to TSS have been proposed. The tampon, soaked with blood in the body, may act as a medium for the growth of *S. aureus* and may enhance toxin production. Absorption of the toxin may occur through vaginal lacerations, which have been noted with continuous tampon use (Barrett, Bledsoe, Greer, & Droegemueller, 1977; Shands et al., 1980), and with the use of superabsorbent products (Friedrich & Siegesmund, 1980). Specific tampon materials may

enhance organism growth or toxin production (Shands et al., 1980). As *S. aureus* has not been found in tampons (CDC, 1980b, pp. 442–443), it is unlikely that the organism is introduced through the tampon, but it is possible that the tampon carries bacteria from the hands or perineum (Shands et al., 1980). Finally, it has been suggested that tampons, especially superabsorbent types, may remove substrates from the vaginal environment that normally allow vaginal lactobacilli to inhibit the growth of *S. aureus*. This inhibitory effect has been demonstrated in vitro by Sanders, Sanders, and Fagnant (1982).

TAMPON ABSORBENCY. The Tri-State Toxic Shock Syndrome Study found absorbency of tampons to be the most important factor in explaining increased incidence of TSS associated with tampon use. Data on absorbency *cannot* be inferred from the manufacturer's labeling because there are no standards by which to measure absorbency (National Women's Health Network, 1983, p. 3). Osterholm and associates (1982) obtained absorbency information from manufacturers based on in vitro and in vivo testing by individual companies. They evaluated Pursettes (Campana Corporation), o.b. (Johnson and Johnson Products), Playtex (International Playtex Corporation), Rely (Procter and Gamble), and Tampax (Tampax). Their data on tampon absorbency are summarized in Table 18–2. The computed odds ratios for developing TSS with the use of various brands are as follows:

Use of all tampon brand styles, with the exception of o.b. Regular, Tampax Slender/Regular, and Tampax Super, had significantly increased odds ratios when compared with no use of tampons. Tampons with the highest odds ratios were Rely Regular, Tampax Super Plus, Playtex Super Plus (deodorant/nondeodorant), Kotex Super (Security/Stick), Rely Super, and Kotex Regular (Security/Stick). All had odds ratios of >22.

Tampax Slender/Regular, o.b. Regular, and Tampax Super tampons had odds ratios between 2.60 and 4.99. When users of these three tampon brand styles were com-

TABLE 18–2. TAMPON ABSORBENCY[a]

Brand and Style	Absorbency Category[b]
Kotex Super	II[c]
Kotex Regular	III
o.b. Super-Plus	I
o.b. Super	II
o.b. Regular	III
Playtex Super-Plus	I
Playtex Super	I
Playtex Regular	II
Rely Super (no longer sold)	I
Rely Regular (no longer sold)	III
Tampax Super-Plus	I
Tampax Super	III
Tampax Slender Regular	IV
Tampax Original Regular	IV

[a]Except for Rely, data reflect tampons available approximately October 1980 to June 1981.
[b]Tampon absorbency was based on measurements made by manufacturers using the syngyna ("synthetic vagina") method and provided to Osterholm and colleagues, who summarized the data and developed the categories used here. (I) ≥ 18.4 g; (II) 15.5–18.3 g; (III) 12.1–15.4 g; (IV) ≤ 12 g.
[c]This product was in Category I before about March 1981 (see composition).

Adapted from Institute of Medicine. (1982). Toxic shock syndrome: Assessment of current information and future research needs (p. 46). Washington, DC: National Academy Press. Reprinted with permission.

bined and compared with nonusers, the odds ratio (2.98) was not significant ($P = 0.33$).

Age-adjusted odds ratios for o.b. Super and Super Plus, Pursettes Regular and Super, and Tampax Junior tampon styles could not be determined because there were too few women who used these styles. (Osterholm et al., 1982, p. 433)

This same study (Davis et al., 1982a) also found an increased risk with nighttime use of tampons. Possible reasons are increased wearing time (although this was *not* significant when evaluated separately), increased absorption of toxin, or perhaps increased vaginal blood flow during sleep. These researchers did not find an increased risk with continuous tampon use throughout the entire menstrual cycle, although Shands and associates (1980) did find this to be significant in a retrospective study of 52 women with TSS and 52 controls matched for age and sex.

TAMPON COMPONENTS. In a recent analysis, Mills and co-investigators (1985) demonstrated in laboratory medium that the production of TSST-1 is controlled by the concentration of magnesium ion (Mg^{2+}), with an increase in toxin inversely related to Mg^{2+}. They found that polyester foam fibers found in Rely tampons bind Mg^{2+} and thus lead to increased production of toxin. Tampons made of cotton, cotton and rayon, or carboxymethyl cellulose were not found to affect toxin production. These experiments were conducted in vitro, and the authors suggested that further research is needed to fully understand this effect, especially as it may be altered by the presence of blood and menstrual fluid. An analysis of 285 cases of tampon-associated TSS did not support this hypothesis (Berkley, Hightower, Broome, & Reingold, 1987). This study found that tampon absorbency, not chemical composition, was the factor related to TSS.

The consumer has little access to information regarding tampon components as manufacturers generally do not reveal this information (National Women's Health Network,

1983). Table 18–3 summarizes various tampon characteristics.

Relationship to Contraception. Firm conclusions about the relationship of TSS to contraceptive use cannot be drawn. Both Shands (1980, p. 1439) and Davis (1980, p. 1434) and their associates reported that women with TSS were less likely to use any form of contraception than controls, although the researchers admit that this finding may have been skewed because controls were selected among women attending gynecologic clinics. They speculate that oral contraceptive use may be protective as a result of the pill's effect on the endometrium and on menstrual flow or its alteration of vaginal flora. This trend was confirmed by the Tri-State Toxic Shock Syndrome Study (Lanes, Poole, Kryer, & Lanza, 1986; Osterholm et al., 1982, p. 437). Spermicides have also been suggested as protective (Shelton & Higgins, 1981, p. 632); however, cases of TSS apparently associated with certain barrier methods of contraception have been reported.

Thirteen cases of TSS associated with use of the vaginal contraceptive sponge have been reported. On the basis of data from Utah and Minnesota, the estimated relative risk of developing TSS has been calculated to be from 7.8 to 40 for sponge users compared with nonusers. The risk is highest with use during menstruation or the postpartum period, use of longer than 30 hours, difficult removal, particularly when the sponge fragments, or a combination of these factors (Faich, Pearson, Fleming, Sobel, & Anello, 1986). Nevertheless, the absolute risk is small; without predisposing factors, one case per two million sponges used has been documented.

Several cases of TSS occurring during diaphragm use have appeared in the literature. Use of the diaphragm in the postpartum weeks, for a prolonged period, and/or during adolescence may increase the risk of developing TSS (Jaffe, 1981; Lee, Dillon, & Baehler 1982; Litt, 1983; Loomis & Feder, 1981; Wilson, 1983).

In an analysis of 75 women with TSS from the Tri-state

TABLE 18–3. TAMPON COMPONENTS[a]

Brand and Style	Composition	Applicator
Kotex Super Kotex Regular	Cotton and rayon with a polypropylene or rayon cover and polyester string. Crosslinked carboxymethyl cellulose was an ingredient in samples manufactured before September 1980, and therefore it was present in shelf samples prior to about March 1981.	Wound paper stick or polyethylene tube
o.b. Super-Plus o.b. Super o.b. Regular	Cotton and rayon Cotton and rayon Cotton and rayon	None
Playtex Super-Plus Playtex Super Playtex Regular	Rayon polyacrylate fiber, cotton, and polysorbate 20. Styles come with or without deodorant. Fragrance is present in the deodorant versions.	Polyethylene tube
Rely Super (no longer sold) Rely Regular (no longer sold)	Cross-linked carboxymethyl cellulose and polyester foam	Polyethylene tube
Tampax Super-Plus Tampax Super Tampax Slender Regular	Polyacrylate rayon fiber Cotton fiber and rayon fiber Cotton fiber, rayon fiber, and high-absorbency cotton fiber (crosslinked carboxymethyl cellulose)	Tube of spirally wound strips of paper held together with water-soluble glue
Tampax Original Regular	Cotton fiber	

[a]Dimensions: Tampons are approximately between 35 and 50 mm long and 10 to 18 mm in diameter. Except for Rely, data reflect tampons available approximately October 1980 to June 1981.
Adapted from Institute of Medicine. (1982). Toxic shock syndrome: Assessment of current information and future research needs (p. 46). Washington, DC: National Academy Press. Reprinted with permission.

Study, tubal ligation was found to be positively associated with the development of TSS, but this finding was based only on three exposed cases (Lanes et al., 1986).

Other Possible Risk Factors. TSS has been reported at an increased rate among the following groups: postpartum women (and in at least one case report, it was found in a newborn as well [Green & LaPeter, 1982]); postoperative patients with *S. aureus* surgical wound infections (Bartlett, Reingold, & Graham, 1982; Dornan, Thompson, & Conn, 1982); patients with other staph infections (Reingold, Dan, Shands, 1982); adolescent women. Indeed, more than one third of TSS cases have occurred in females under 19 years of age (CDC, 1983, p. 400; Litt, 1983, p. 270).

Nonassociated Factors. Factors examined by various investigators and found to be unassociated with TSS are use of feminine deodorant sprays or douches (Osterholm et al., 1982; Shands et al., 1980); perceived amount of menstrual flow; number of tampons used daily; and methods of insertion and maximum time of use of one tampon or frequency of tampon change (Shands et al., 1980). The Tri-State Study, however, noted a trend toward significance with use of one tampon 13 hours or longer (Osterholm et al., 1982, p. 437). Other nonsignificant factors in that study included wearing of pantyhose, underwear, or tight-fitting pants; drug or alcohol use; cigarette smoking; swimming, bathing, or sauna or whirlpool use; sexual activity, including intercourse, oral sex, manual stimulation, or vibrator use; fecundity; previous illness (except in the menstrual period preceding the study period); household or family illness; recent physician visits or hospitalizations; recent pelvic examination; menstrual history, including age at menarche, length of cycle, or perceived menstrual changes in the year preceding TSS.

Clinical Presentation

The CDC offers the following description of the clinical presentation of TSS (CDC, 1980a, p. 229):

> Toxic-shock syndrome typically begins suddenly with high fever, vomiting, and profuse watery diarrhea, sometimes accompanied by sore throat, headache, and myalgias. The disease progresses to hypotensive shock within 48 hours, and the patient develops a diffuse, macular, erythematous rash with nonpurulent conjunctivitis. Urine output is often decreased, and patients may be disoriented or combative. The adult respiratory distress syndrome (ARDS) or cardiac dysfunction may also be seen.
>
> Laboratory studies reveal elevated blood urea nitrogen, serum creatinine, bilirubin, and creatine phosphokinase levels, and white blood cell counts with marked left shifts. Platelet counts are low in the first week of illness but are usually high in the second week.

Davis and co-workers (1982a, p. 442) examined 80 patients with nonfatal TSS occurring between October 1979 and September 19, 1980, all of whom presented with fever, rash or desquamation, hypotension (measured or manifested by orthostatic dizziness or, less frequently, orthostatic syncope), and multisystem involvement. Most commonly affected were the gastrointestinal system (vomiting and diarrhea at onset), the mucous membranes (conjunctival, oropharyngeal, and vaginal hyperemia), and the muscular system (myalgia or muscle pain). Central nervous system, hepatic, or renal involvement was also seen in greater than 50 percent of these patients, manifested by disorientation or combativeness, increased serum glutamic-pyruvic

transaminase or total bilirubin levels, and oliguria, abnormal urinalysis, or elevated BUN or creatinine levels. Other common clinical findings were headache; abdominal pain; pedal, hand, or facial edema; lymphadenopathy; metallic taste; dark urine; and hair thinning or loss or splitting of nails.

Less frequent complications were decreased or increased platelets and cardiopulmonary complications including ARDS, pulmonary edema, myocarditis (diagnosed by electrocardiac changes), arrhythmias, and increased cardiac silhouette. Decreased calcium and phosphate levels have also been noted. Desquamation of the skin has been reported as a late clinical occurrence, manifest 5 to 12 days after resolution of the initial rash and most commonly found on the soles of the feet, palms of the hand, and fingertips (Chow, Wong, MacFarlane, & Bartlett, 1984, p. 427).

Convalescence from TSS is usually complete by the tenth day after onset (Pope, 1981). Long-term TSS sequelae include gangrene (Chesney, Crass, & Polyak, 1982, p. 847), myopathy associated with weakness and fatigue, reported for up to 2 years, and carpal and tarsal tunnel syndromes. Cold and cyanotic extremities may persist (Chow et al., 1984). Decreased concentration and ability to retain information were noted by Rosene, Copass, Kastner, et al., (1982) in more than 50 percent of 12 patients. Loss of memory has been observed. Of course, the most serious consequence of TSS is death. CDC reported a 3 percent TSS mortality rate in 1984.

Management

Diagnosis. TSS should be ruled out in any menstruating woman who complains of fever, vomiting or diarrhea, dizziness or syncope, and erythema of the mucous membranes or a rash resembling sunburn, particularly if she is a tampon user. Indeed, it has been suggested that TSS should be considered in any woman who has used tampons during or immediately preceding the onset of fever (Smirniotopoulos, 1983). If the woman is in the postpartum period or the adolescent age group, the diagnosis is even more likely. The presence of an infection of the skin or of a postoperative wound also increases likelihood of this disease. In these instances, immediate medical referral is mandatory.

There is no specific diagnostic test for TSS, although a marker protein, the antigen defining TSS staphylococci, has been quantified in experimental TSS in animals and found in humans with the disease. Such markers, however, cannot be considered diagnostic until a definite etiologic agent is proven (Melish, Chen, & Murata 1983, p. 122a). Saadah and Andrews (1984, p. 150) point out that the diagnosis cannot be confirmed definitely at initial presentation, although a tentative diagnosis based on presenting symptoms can be made. A vaginal culture for *S. aureus* should be done, although its absence in the vaginal flora does not preclude TSS and its presence is not diagnostic. A gram stain of vaginal secretions demonstrating both polymorphonuclear leukocytes and gram-positive cocci in five or more oil immersion fields, if coupled with coagulase-positive staphylococci on culture, strongly correlates with TSS. Other initial abnormal laboratory findings are hyponatremia, abnormal urinary sediment, and altered renal and hepatic function. Leukocytosis, particularly with an elevation in immature neutrophils, thrombocytopenia, elevated creatine phosphokinase, and hypocalcemia may be seen (Shands et al., 1980, p. 1438). Table 18-1 outlines other confirmatory laboratory results.

Intervention

TREATMENT. There is no definitive treatment for TSS. Intensive care is generally warranted (CDC, 1980a, p. 229). Intravenous fluids, and possibly vasopressor agents, are necessary to counteract hypovolemic shock (Chesney et al., 1982, p. 847). Other treatments are directed at specific symptoms and organ systems involved.

Recurrences have been shown to be less likely if antistaphylococcal antibiotics are used during the initial TSS episode. These are defined as β-lactamase-resistant antibiotics and include penicillinase-resistant penicillins and cephalosporins, clindamycin, and vancomycin (Davis et al., 1982a, p. 444). Discontinuation of tampon use has also been associated with reduced recurrence rates, independently of antibiotic use (Davis et al., 1982a, 1982b).

TEACHING AND COUNSELING. Teaching and counseling are the most important functions of the nonphysician health care provider in the prevention and early detection of TSS. Teaching and counseling should be oriented to women at risk for the disease, which includes all menstruating women who use tampons and those who use—and particularly misuse—certain barrier methods of birth control. At most risk are women who have already suffered an attack of TSS; counseling of these women should be directed toward prevention of recurrence. Witzig and Ostwald (1985) recommend particular attention to prevention for adolescent females.

Teaching and counseling should also be geared toward helping women make appropriate risk–benefit assessment regarding the use of tampons and female-barrier contraceptives. Because of the publicity in the media, some women may have unrealistic fears of this disease. These often can be allayed with a discussion of absolute risks. The Institute of Medicine (1982) estimates 15 per 100,000 tampon users as the upper limit of possible annual cases. The National Women's Health Network (1983, p. 8) estimated that approximately 49,000,000 American women of menstrual age used tampons in mid-1980. There is some evidence that up to 20 percent or approximately 10,000,000 of these women are no longer using tampons, but the vast majority of menstruating women in the United States still use tampons during all or part of their menstrual cycles.

If tampon use is ascertained by history, then signs and symptoms of TSS, as previously outlined, should be discussed with the patient. The following additional recommendations are adapted from the National Women's Health Network's suggested guidelines (1983), although not all of these are based on confirmed research findings:

- The chance of contracting TSS is greatly reduced by not using tampons. Alternatives include sanitary napkins and reusable soft cloths.
- The risk of TSS can be reduced by discontinuing use of superabsorbent tampons. The least absorbent tampon capable of handling a woman's menstrual flow should be used.
- It is possible that frequent changing of tampons and use of alternatives during part of the menstrual cycle, particularly at night, may reduce TSS risk.
- Tampon package inserts should be read before using tampons, and women should be encouraged to ask any questions about their proper use if it is not clear.
- Hand washing and cleanliness should be advised when inserting tampons (Shelley, 1982).
- Adolescent women especially should not use high-absorbency tampons. Women should be advised that the risk of TSS is highest for women aged 24 or younger.
- Women who have had TSS should not use tampons.
- Postpartum women should not use tampons.
- Women should consider avoiding use of tampons if they have staph infections of the skin, such as infected pimples and parenychia.
- Women with certain heart defects should use tampons cautiously or avoid them, as bacteria could enter the bloodstream through tampon-induced vaginal lacerations.
- Women who develop any symptoms of TSS while using a tampon should remove the tampon immediately and seek medical attention as soon as possible.
- Diaphragms and contraceptive sponges should not be worn more than 24 or 30 hours and should be avoided in the first 6 to 8 weeks after childbirth.
- Local and/or state public health departments should be notified about any cases of TSS so they can be reported to CDC. Patients should do this on their own, as physicians may not.
- Any interested individuals should write to the government and to tampon manufacturers expressing concern and demanding additional research, more explicit product labeling, and premarketing testing. Reclassification of tampons as Class III Medical Devices would necessitate such testing of these products. The Food and Drug Administration, 5600 Fishers Lane, Rockville, MD 20857, can be contacted.
- Women who have suffered TSS may contact the Litigation Information Service of the National Women's Health Network, P.O. Box 5055, FDR Station, New York, NY 10150, for information and support in seeking redress through the court system.

INTRAUTERINE DIETHYLSTILBESTROL EXPOSURE

From 1948 to 1971, a synthetic, potent, nonsteroidal estrogen called diethylstilbestrol (DES) was widely prescribed to pregnant women in the United States. It was advocated as a treatment or preventive measure for a variety of complications including threatened abortion, history of spontaneous abortion, toxemia, prematurity, postmaturity, and fetal death in utero (Smith, 1948; Smith & Smith, 1949), and it was prescribed for women judged to be at high risk, such as those with diabetes (Little, 1953). Treatment often began in the first trimester and continued throughout pregnancy. It has been estimated that during those years, DES was given to four to six million pregnant women (Glaze, 1984, p. 435). The drug's use persisted despite a lack of consensus in the medical literature regarding its therapeutic value. The original study was critiqued for its lack of a placebo group. As early as 1953, a clinical trial comparing DES with a placebo in over 1,000 patients found no significant value to the administration of DES in pregnancy (Dieckmann, Davis, Rynkiewicz, & Pottinger, 1953).

In 1970, Herbst and Scully reported a surprisingly high incidence of vaginal clear cell adenocarcinoma among women under the age of 25 in New England, one of the geographic areas where DES was widely used. Prior to that, this type of cancer had been almost exclusively found in women over the age of 50. A year later, Herbst, Ulfelder, and Poskanzer (1971) reported an association between maternal stilbestrol therapy and the subsequent development of vaginal clear cell adenocarcinoma in young women who had been exposed in utero. Seven of the eight reported cases were related to first-trimester DES exposure; of four maternal controls for each case, no such exposure was found—a highly significant difference. That same year, the Food and Drug Administration (FDA) withdrew its approval for DES use in pregnancy (Adess, Brown, Hackett, & Turiel, 1984, p. 2).

Since the first report, a large volume of literature has accumulated examining cancer and other consequences of DES teratogenesis. Although it is hoped that the problems associated with DES are self-limited, because they are confined to persons born within the years 1946 and 1972, the youngest of exposed persons are still adolescents and the long-term effects of DES exposure in aging women are as yet unknown. It is important, therefore, for all gynecologic practitioners to be aware of this problem, its manifestations, and its clinical management.

Pathophysiology of Teratogenesis

It is thought that DES is a teratogen, rather than a carcinogen, and that the adenocarcinomas seen in DES-exposed women occur secondarily to changes that make the vaginal epithelium more susceptible to carcinogenic effects of endogenous estrogens (Ostergard, 1981, p. 381; Prins, Morrow, Townsend, & Disaia, 1976). This would explain why cancer in DES-exposed women appears after puberty. DES exposure in utero effects the müllerian system, which develops into the female reproductive tract. Its main teratogenic effect has been described as "the prevention of the transformation of the müllerian columnar epithelium to the stratified squamous variety" (Ostergard, 1981, p. 381). Such transformation proceeds upward, toward the cervix, explaining why vaginal changes in DES-exposed women are often found in the fornices (Prins et al., 1976, p. 249) (Fig. 18–1). Transformation begins at 10 weeks of embryonic life and is generally completed by the eighteenth week (Jefferies, Robboy, & O'Brien, 1984, p. 64). The development of the female müllerian system, however, can be traced back to the first week of embryonic existence, with the formation of the wolffian (or mesonephric) system, which precedes the müllerian system. The müllerian duct system begins to develop at 4 weeks, and the uterovaginal canal, at first divided by a septum, is formed into a single cavity at 7 weeks. In animal studies, the effects of estrogen on the development of the female müllerian system in embryos have been found to be dependent on the timing of its administration and the dose used. Estrogen generally causes rapid sexual differentiation and hypertrophy of the vagina, uterus, and tubes. With very large doses, however, the growth of the müllerian duct may be arrested (Prins et al., 1976, pp. 246–248).

Consequences of Intrauterine Exposure

Much of the data on DES exposure comes from the Diethylstilbestrol–Adenosis (DESAD) Project, a National Cancer Institute–sponsored study initiated in 1974 at Baylor College of Medicine, Massachusetts General Hospital, the University of Southern California, and the Mayo and Gundersen Clinics. To eliminate selection bias in this study,

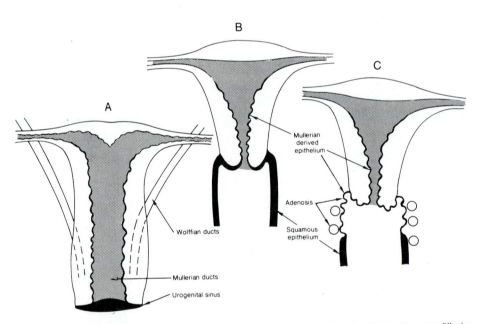

A, Cephalad progression of urogenital sinus-derived squamous epithelium (*solid black*) over müllerian duct-derived columnar mucosa (*stippled*) early in gestation. The wolffian ducts are regressing without testosterone stimulation. *B,* Vaginal canal lined by squamous epithelium up to the endocervical canal as found in late gestation in normal female fetuses. *C,* DES exposure before the nineteenth week of gestation, often causing retention of the müllerian mucosa over parts of the cervix and vagina (adenosis) by interference with the normal migration of squamous epithelium. This may also lead to structural changes in the vagina, cervix, and/or uterus.

Figure 18–1. Schematic representation of the embryologic development of the vagina in the unexposed and DES-exposed woman. *(From Stillman, R. J. [1982, April]. In utero exposure to diethylstilbestrol: Adverse effects on the male reproductive tract and reproductive performance in male and female offspring. American Journal of Obstetrics and Gynecology, 142(7), 907. Reprinted with permission.)*

four distinct groups of DES-exposed women were identified for study (Labarthe, Adam, & Noller, 1978): women traced through prenatal record review, women referred by themselves, women referred by physicians, women having gynecologic abnormalities typical of DES exposure. The last group cannot be documented specifically to have been exposed to DES. Within each group, matched controls were selected. Data for each group were analyzed separately.

Cancer has proven to be a relatively rare complication of DES exposure; other structural and functional abnormalities are more commonly encountered. These include vaginal adenosis; cervical hoods, collars, and cockscombs, as well as hypoplasia, erosion, and transverse cervical or vaginal ridges; T-shaped or hypoplastic uteri; constricting bands in the endometrial cavity; and infertility and poor reproductive outcomes. Recent evidence also suggests a possible increased risk for the development of dysplasia, a precursor of squamous cell carcinoma (Robboy et al., 1984). Abnormalities also have been reported in the male offspring of women given DES, and the possibility has been raised of increased rates of breast cancer in women who themselves took DES.

Cellular Abnormalities

ADENOSIS. Adenosis is the most common finding associated with DES exposure. This is a condition in which columnar or glandular (secretory) epithelium, resembling that of the endocervix, endometrium, or fallopian tube, is found in the vagina or on the ectocervix (Herbst, Kurman, & Scully, 1972). Most commonly, this columnar epithelium, which embryologically should have been transformed into squamous epithelium, is found in the vaginal fornices. This location is consistent with an arrest of the normally occur-ring upward growth of squamous epithelium of embryonic development.

In one study, Herbst, Poskanzer, Robboy, and associates (1975) found vaginal adenosis in 35 percent of 110 DES-exposed women aged 18 to 25 and in 1 percent of 82 control subjects. In the DESAD Project, vaginal epithelial changes (VECs) were found in 34 percent of vaginal smears of exposed women identified by prenatal record review and in 65 and 59 percent of women referred to the project and requesting examination. In this study, the findings associated with VEC were more frequently seen when DES was administered at high doses, for a long duration, or early in pregnancy.

Clinically, cervical adenosis may produce a "strawberry" appearance (Ostergard, 1981, p. 381). Vaginal adenosis may appear as red granular areas, varying from 1-mm "spots" to extensive areas, especially in the upper vagina (Herbst et al., 1972, p. 288) (Fig. 18–2). Submucosal cystlike lesions, comparable to Nabothian cysts on the cervix, may be seen, even after the adenosis regresses. The area of adenosis may be palpable as grainy and irregular. Areas of adenosis do not stain properly with acetic acid or Lugol's iodine solution.

Herbst and associates (1975, p. 339) report that both adenosis and cervical erosion have been found in cases of clear cell adenocarcinomas associated with DES exposure, yet there is no documentation of transition from adenosis to the far less common adenocarcinoma. In fact, adenosis often has been found to regress over time. This occurs by the process of squamous metaplasia (conversion), which may eventually lead to complete replacement of the adenosis with normal squamous epithelium (Burke, Antonioli, & Friedman, 1981; Robboy, Young, & Welch, 1981). This has been observed at a more rapid rate among sexually ac-

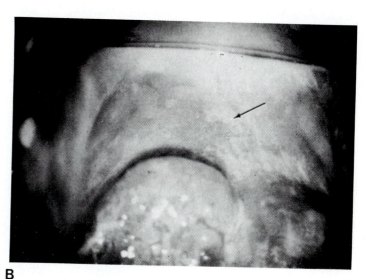

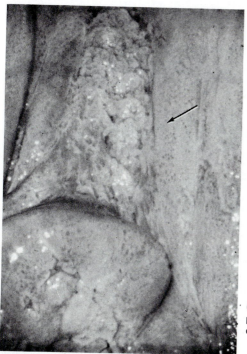

B

(A) Large triangular-shaped area of columnar epithelium in anterior vagina present at initial examination. (B) Follow-up examination at 24 months. The columnar epithelium has been replaced by grade I white epithelium.

A

Figure 18–2. Vaginal adenosis. *(From Burke, L., Antonioli, D., & Friedman, E.A. [1981, January]. Evolution of diethylstilbestrol-associated with genital tract lesions.* Obstetrics and Gynecology, *57 (1), 79–84. Reprinted with permission).*

tive than nonsexually active women (Frank, Krumholz, & Deutsch 1985). Robboy, Young, and associates (1984, p. 874) postulate that adenosis or ectropion may be a precursor of clear cell adenocarcinoma only when the vaginal or cervical columnar epithelium resembles that of the tubes or endometrium, rather than the endocervix.

CLEAR CELL ADENOCARCINOMA. The risk of developing clear cell adenocarcinoma is estimated to be .14 to 1.4 per 1,000 exposed women (Robboy, Noller, & Kaufman, 1983). As of 1980, more than 400 cases of vaginal or cervical clear cell adenocarcinoma occurring in women born after 1940 had been documented in the Registry for Research on Hormonal Transplacental Carcinogens, which is based in Chicago. About two thirds of these women are known to have suffered intrauterine exposure to nonsteroidal estrogens. They range in age from 7 to 30 years, with the peak incidence seen at approximately age 19. Whether a second peak will occur is unknown as this disease has previously been seen mostly in older women. The largest numbers of cases in the United States have been reported from California, Massachusetts, New York, and Pennsylvania. Five-year survival has been 80 percent, attributed to widespread screening and the resulting early detection (Herbst, 1981).

Women with adenocarcinoma may present with abnormal vaginal bleeding or discharge or be asymptomatic (see Fig. 18–3) or palpable as cervical or vaginal nodularities.

SQUAMOUS CELL CARCINOMA. The question of whether DES-exposed women have increased susceptibility to squamous cell carcinoma is unresolved. On colposcopy, white epithelium, mosaicism, and punctation have been noted among the DES-exposed (Ostergard, 1981, p. 388). These lesions, however, have been found to be most often associated with squamous metaplasia and not dysplasia (Welch, Robboy,

Kaufman, et al., 1985). In 1981, the DESAD Project (Robboy et al., 1981) reported no increase in squamous cell dysplasia among 1,489 study participants. In a later report, these same researchers (Robboy, et al., 1984) found a two- to fourfold increase in the incidence rates of biopsy-confirmed dysplasia among DES-exposed women over nonexposed controls. This was positively correlated with the extent of squamous metaplasia, which is often secondary to adenosis, leading to the hypothesis that this immature epithelium is more susceptible to the effects of carcinogenic factors, such as papillomavirus, often implicated in the development of dysplasia (Adam, Kaufman, Adler-Storthz, 1985; Robboy et al., 1984, pp. 2982–2983). Only further careful follow-up of DES-exposed women will answer this question.

Structural Abnormalities. Structural abnormalities among DES-exposed women involve the vagina, the cervix, the uterus, and possibly the fallopian tubes. These take a variety of forms and may or may not regress with time.

VAGINA AND CERVIX. In one study of 267 DESAD Project participants, 44 percent demonstrated structural changes of the cervix (Kaufman, Adam, Binder, & Gerthoffer, 1980, pp. 301–302). These were cervical ridges, collars, hypoplasia, and pseudopolyps (Fig. 18–4). Cervical abnormalities have been called by a number of different terms; the same finding may be called a cervical collar, hood, ridge, or cockscomb by different authors. The term *cockscomb* has also been used to encompass all these changes. In some instances it is difficult to assess whether various authors are referring to the same or different anomalies.

Jefferies and associates (1984) have analyzed structural anomalies of the vagina and cervix among participants in the DESAD project, and Table 18–4 defines and describes their classification with the synonyms often used. They found a rate of 25 to 49 percent for structural abnormalities.

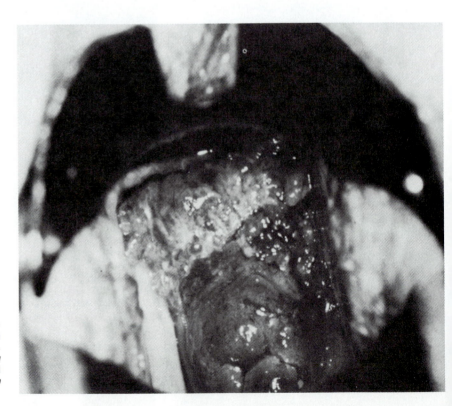

Figure 18–3. Advanced adenocarcinoma on anterior vaginal wall in a DES-exposed offspring. *(From Ostergard, D. R., [1981, June]. DES-related vaginal lesions, Clinical Obstetrics and Gynecology, 24(2), 392. Reprinted with permission).*

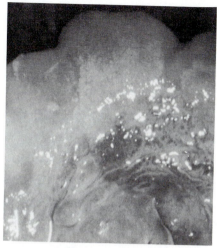

A. Cockscomb cervix.

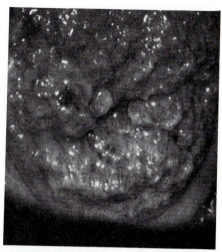

B. Portion of the cervix covered with columnar epithelium.

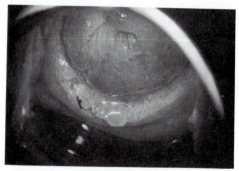

C. Posterior cervical hood or collar. Cervix covered with columnar epithelium.

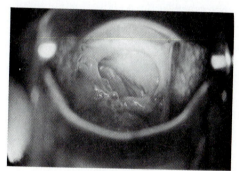

D. Circumferential.

Figure 18-4. Cervicovaginal changes following in utero DES exposure as seen on colposcopic examination. *(From Burke, L., & Mathews, B. [1977].* Colposcopy in clinical practice. *Philadelphia: F. A. Davis Co., pp. 83, 85, 86, 92. Reprinted with permission).*

TABLE 18-4. STRUCTURAL ABNORMALITIES OF THE VAGINA AND CERVIX SEEN AFTER IN UTERO DES EXPOSURE

Abnormality	Description	Synonym
Of cervix and vaginal fornix		
Cockscomb	Raised ridge, usually on anterior cervix	Hood, transverse ridge of cervix
Collar	Flat rim involving part to all of circumference of cervix	Rim, hood, transverse ridge of cervix
Pseudopolyp	Polypoid appearance of cervix results from circumferential constricting groove, thickening of stroma of anterior or posterior endocervical canal: includes endocervical stromal hyperplasia	
Hypoplastic cervix	Cervix less than 1.5 cm in diameter	Immature cervix
Altered fornix of vagina	Includes absence, complete or partial, or pars vaginalis, abnormality of fornices, fusion of cervix to vagina, partial or complete fornical obliteration	
Of vagina, exclusive of fornix		
Transverse septum, incomplete		Vaginal ridge
Longitudinal septum, incomplete		

Adapted from Jefferies, J. A. Robboy, S. J., O'Brien, P. C., et al. (1984, January 1). Structural anomalies of the cervix and vagina in women enrolled in the Diethylstilbestrol Adenosis (DESAD) Project. American Journal of Obstetrics and Gynecology, 148(1), 60. Reprinted with permission.

TABLE 18–5. RATES OF STRUCTURAL ABNORMALITIES NOTED IN DESAD STUDY GROUPS[a]

Participant Classification	Structural Changes of Cervix and Vaginal Fornix (%)								Other Vaginal Changes (%)
	Any Structural Change	Any Type	Cockscomb	Collar	Pseudopolyp	Abnormal Fornix	Hypoplastic Cervix		
Record review (N = 1,655)	25.3	24.8	9.1	13.4	3.4	3.1	3.2		0.8
Control (N = 963)	2.3[b]	2.1[b]	0.9[b]	0.8[b]	0.1[b]	0.3[b]	0.0[b]		0.2[c]
Walk-in (N = 800)	42.6	42.1	14.0	24.5	1.9	7.0	9.1		1.6
Referral (N = 1,089)	48.6	47.8	16.1	30.9	4.5	5.7	6.0		1.6

[a]Values in field are percentages of persons in each classification who had the indicated anomalies. Some participants had more than one.
[b]Significantly (P < 0.001) less than the record review group (χ^2 test).
[c]Two-sided P value = 0.059.
From Jefferies, J. A., Robboy, S. J., O'Brien, P. C., et al. (1984, January 1). Structural anomalies of the cervix and vagina in women enrolled in the Diethylstilbestrol Adenosis (DESAD) Project. American Journal of Obstetrics and Gynecology, 148(1), 60. Reprinted with permission.

Table 18–5 lists the rates for each type of cervical and vaginal change noted in three DESAD study groups and the control group. Anomalies were negatively correlated with the week of embryonic exposure to DES and positively correlated with the total DES dose, the pregnancy history of the exposed woman, and her age at menarche. Like the changes of adenosis, but unlike those of the uterus, structural changes of the cervix and vagina have been found to regress with age. Jefferies and co-workers (1984, p. 65) suggest that the presence of a vaginal or cervical structural abnormality consistent with those found among the DESAD project participants should be presumptive of a history of DES exposure and should prompt a search for maternal prenatal data.

UTERUS. The DESAD study also found a variety of uterine anomalies. Among 267 participants, 31 percent were found to have a T-shaped uterus with a small cavity, 19 percent a T-shaped uterus, 13 percent a small uterine cavity, 13 percent a T-shaped uterus with a constriction, 4 percent constriction rings, and 8 percent other abnormalities, which included uterine filling defects, synechia, diverticula, and unicornuate or bicornuate uterus (Kaufman et al., 1980, pp. 301-302). (See chapter 14, fig. 14-6).

In the DESAD study, women with cervical abnormalities were 4.5 times more likely to have abnormal uterine changes (Kaufman et al., 1980, pp. 301–302). Of women with VECs, 82 percent were found to have uterine structural abnormalities, compared with 44 percent of women without VECs. Dosage of DES did not affect the frequency of abnormal hysterosalpingograms (HSGs) but the earlier the DES was administered in pregnancy, the greater the likelihood of an abnormal HSG. Interestingly, 45 percent of women who did not receive DES until 19 weeks of pregnancy had abnormalities of the uterus. This suggests an adverse effect of DES on the development of the uterine muscle, because by the nineteenth week of embryonic life, the müllerian ducts have already fused.

FALLOPIAN TUBES. In one laparoscopic study of fallopian tubes in 16 DES-exposed women with infertility problems, DeCherney, Cholst, and Naftolin (1981, p. 741) consistently found a "foreshortened, convoluted tube, with withered fimbria and a pinpoint os."

URINARY TRACT ANOMALIES. Urinary tract anomalies were not found at a statistically significant rate in 102 DES-exposed women who underwent intravenous pyelogram (Gallup, Altaffer, & Castle 1984), although Herbst, Robboy, Scully, and Poskanzer (1974, p. 717) did find congenital urinary tract anomalies, including duplication of the ureter and unilateral renal agenesis, in 6 percent of young women with clear cell adenocarcinoma.

Functional Abnormalities: Infertility and Poor Reproductive Outcome

INCIDENCE. Although most DES-exposed women can become pregnant and carry a fetus to viability, poor reproductive outcomes are a major consequence of this exposure. Studies of DES daughters are inconclusive regarding the exact risks of infertility or poor pregnancy outcomes. Cousins, Karp, Lacey, and Lucas (1980) found no significant differences in pregnancies achieved between their DES study group and a matched control group. The numbers in this study were low, however: 71 in the study group and 69 controls. Bibbo, Gill, and Azizi, (1977) followed 229 DES-exposed women and 136 controls and found significantly lower fertility rates, as did Herbst, Hubby, Azizi, and Makii (1981) in an analysis of 338 exposed and 298 nonexposed women. Barnes and associates (1980) analyzed patient recall data from women in the DESAD Project—618 exposed and 618 controls. They found no difference in ability to conceive, but found significant differences in the numbers of women experiencing unfavorable outcomes, having a miscarriage, and never having had a full-term birth. Berger and Goldstein (1980) followed 69 DES-exposed women over an 8-year period. All were sexually active and did not use contraceptives; the overall pregnancy rate was 66.7 percent. Unfortunately, these researchers did not have a control group for comparison. Schmidt, Fowler, Talbert, and Edelman (1980), looking at a group of 276 DES-exposed women, found a "pregnancy wastage" of 43 percent for first pregnancies and 33 percent for all pregnancies. Considering only women with vaginal adenosis or cervical hoods, the pregnancy wastage was 53 percent. This study suffers from a possible selection bias, however, as all participants were self-referred, and no control group was designated.

Increased rates of spontaneous abortion, ectopic pregnancy, and premature delivery have been noted by a number of researchers (Berger & Goldstein, 1980; Herbst et al., 1981; Kaufman et al., 1980; Sandberg, Riffle, Higdon, & Getman, 1981). Mangan and associates (1982) also found a higher frequency of incompetent cervix among 98 DES-exposed women compared with 167 age-matched nonexposed women.

Overall, the percentages of women able to deliver viable infants among DES-exposed women are as high as 82 percent, among 338 patients (Herbst et al., 1981), 78 percent among 327 women with 616 pregnancies (Kaufman et al., 1984), 75.6 percent among 98 women (Mangan, Borow, & Burtnett-Rubin, 1982), 69 percent among 255 pregnancies not electively aborted (Sandberg et al., 1981), and 41 percent among 69 women (Berger & Goldstein, 1980). In studies that made distinctions between women found through prenatal chart review and self- or physician-referred women, the prenatal chart review group demonstrated better outcomes (e.g., Kaufman et al., 1984). This points to a potential bias in studies that either do not separate these groups for analysis or in which the study population is all referred because these are the patients in whom DES effects are the most obvious (e.g., Berger & Goldstein, 1980; Cousins et al., 1980; Sandberg et al., 1981).

ETIOLOGY. The causes for poor reproductive outcomes among DES-exposed women have not been clearly established. Although uterine structural abnormalities explain a large number of pregnancy complications (Berger & Goldstein, 1980; Kaufman et al., 1980), these abnormalities do not explain all the poor pregnancy outcomes seen, nor does any one structural abnormality preclude successful pregnancy (Sandberg et al., 1981) or relate specifically to a particular outcome (Kaufman et al., 1984). Barnes and associates (1980, p. 612) found no significant differences in outcome for DES-exposed women with or without structural defects. They did, however, find a dose-related relationship between exposure and premature deliveries. Herbst et al. (1981) found less frequent menses and a shorter duration of flow among the DES-exposed group. The latter finding was confirmed by Cousins and associates, (1980) and Bibbo and associates, (1977), although Schmidt and associates (1980) found an increased menstrual flow to be more common among 276 DES daughters. They also found anovulation and oligomenorrhea to be frequent menstrual irregularities.

Haney and Hammond (1983, p. 851) speculate, from their study of 33 infertile DES-exposed women, that "(1) surgical manipulation of the cervix more frequently leads to cervical stenosis and ultimately pelvic endometriosis, (2) tubal pregnancies may occur by a mechanism unrelated to salpingitis, and (3) the spectrum of problems causing infertility is similar to that in the non-DES-exposed population." Their numbers, of course, are small and their study did not have a control group.

As DES often was administered because of poor pregnancy outcomes, several investigators have examined the possibility that this occurrence in DES-exposed offspring is due not to the drug, but to hereditary factors. Kirkhope (1983) compared reproductive performance among two groups of mothers and daughters, 54 DES-exposed mother–daughter pairs and 51 in whom DES exposure could not be confirmed. The results do not support the existence of a familial tendency toward increased pregnancy loss in DES daughters. An increased ability to achieve viable pregnancies among DES daughters over their mothers was found by Mangan et al. (1982), but these same DES-exposed women achieved fewer viable pregnancies than did their non–DES-exposed sisters.

DES Mothers. An increased risk of breast cancer in women who themselves took DES in pregnancy has been noted in some studies, although these findings are not conclusive. Bibbo, Haenszel, Wied, (1978) found an increased but not statistically significant rate of breast cancer among 693 women who had taken the drug compared with 668 controls. In a reanalysis of these data, Wolfe found a significantly increased risk among women aged 50 or younger; he excluded cases in which the original slides were not available for review, and by this exclusion, the results achieved statistical significance. In addition, he reclassified six exposed women who were age 50 at diagnosis into the younger age group, and this too caused that group to reach a significantly higher level of breast cancer than the control group (Brian, Tilley, & Labarthe, 1980).

In a study of data from the Mayo Clinic center of the DESAD project, the rate of breast cancer incidence among 408 DES-treated women was not higher than that for various women in Olmsted County, Minnesota. At this clinic, however, DES doses were lower than those used at other centers where DES was frequently given, including those in Chicago, where the Bibbo study was conducted (Brian et al., 1980). In an English study conducted 27 years after treatment, 76 DES-treated women were found to have a rate of breast cancer higher than that among 76 controls. In this original treatment group, the dosages used were far greater than those administered at the Mayo Clinic and even greater than those used in Chicago (Beral & Colwell, 1980). Greenberg, Barnes, and Resseguie, (1984) compared the incidence of breast cancer in 3,033 DES-treated women with that in a control group of parous women. They found a relative risk of 1.4 in the treated group.

DES-exposed Males. Another area of controversy is whether males exposed to intrauterine DES exhibit genitourinary abnormalities. Bibbo and co-workers (1977) found epididymal cysts, hypotrophic testes, and capsular induration in 25 percent of 163 DES-exposed males compared with 6 percent of 168 controls. They also found decreased ejaculate volume and lower values for sperm density and total motile spermatozoa in exposed compared with nonexposed men, although both were in the normal range, and more cases of "severely pathologic semen." Two cases of azoospermia and one of bilateral hypotrophic testes were found in the DES-exposed group. Gill, Schumacher, and Bibbo (1976) found similar structural and functional abnormalities, although in a later study, they found fewer significant differences in semen characteristics (Leary, Resseguie, & Kurland, 1984, p. 2988). Other authors have found urethral meatal stenosis and hypospadias (Cosgrove, Benton, & Henderson, 1977; Henderson et al., 1976); varicocele and absent, hypoplastic, or undescended testes (Stenchever et al., 1981; Whitehead & Leiter, 1981); and hypoplastic penis (Gill et al., 1976). In a mailed questionnaire to which 225 exposed males and 111 nonexposed males responded, the exposed males reported more difficulty passing urine than the nonexposed and described the conditions of hypospadias and urethral stenosis at a higher rate (Henderson, Benton, & Cosgrove, 1976). Andonian and Kessler (1979), however, found no differences in semen analysis or physical or genital examination findings in a comparison of 24 DES-exposed men with 24 matched controls.

These studies vary in selection of subjects and methodology, including methods of data collection and the use of a control group; comparisons are therefore difficult to make. One group of researchers who did not find any significant abnormalities on examination of 265 males to DES compared with 274 controls (Leary, Resseguie, & Kurland, 1984) explain their conflicting findings by either a difference in selection criteria (they used only record review to identify cases) or the lower doses of DES given at the Mayo Clinic, where their study participants were recruited.

Management of DES-exposed Women

Data Collection

HISTORY. The first component in the management of DES exposure is its identification. A woman may be aware of this problem and report it to her health care provider, or she may be unaware of her exposure or of its significance. It is the practitioner's responsibility to include questions about DES exposure as part of every routine health history. If a woman is unsure of exposure, she can consult her mother, who may need to consult her physician, if still available, or request her medical records, if accessible. Women who were most likely to have received DES include those with prior pregnancy loss, miscarriage or threatened miscarriage, bleeding during pregnancy, and diabetes. History can help identify the likelihood of DES exposure where there is any doubt and alert the practitioner to the need for careful physical examination and for suggesting to the woman that she attempt to discover her history. DES-like drugs were prescribed under a variety of names, listed in Table 18–6. A patient or her mother may be aware of a specific drug taken, but may not be aware that it was DES.

Patients known to have been exposed to DES in utero should be asked about prior assessments, including Pap smears, colposcopy, and biopsy. Any treatments received should be noted (Noller, Townsend, & Kaufman 1981, p. 85).

PHYSICAL EXAMINATION AND LABORATORY TESTING. The DESAD Project has identified physical examination needs beyond the routine gynecologic assessment for DES-exposed women from which the following discussion is adapted (Robboy et al., 1983). After vulvar inspection, careful palpation of the vagina and cervix is important. The entire length of the vagina should be palpated with particular attention given to the fornices. Ridges and structural changes should be noted. Any areas of thickening, nodularity, or induration should alert the practitioner to the need for referral for possible biopsy. This palpation should precede speculum examination; therefore, only water is recommended for lubrication.

During speculum examination, all walls of the vagina should be examined; the speculum must therefore be carefully rotated as it is withdrawn. Excess mucus should be gently removed with a moist cotton swab, and a Pap smear of the cervix taken. In addition, the epithelium in the upper third of the vagina should be sampled with a wooden or plastic spatula. The spatula should be rotated along the entire circumference of the vaginal fornices. If any other area of the vaginal epithelium appears abnormal, if it is red and granular, for example, it too should be sampled. Any abnormal finding is an indication for referral. Colposcopy and iodine staining of the cervix and vagina are recommended. Ideally, these should be done by a practitioner experienced in evaluating DES-exposed women. Biopsy is indicated whenever the cervix or vagina is indurated, is granular, contains a nodule or mass, appears different in color or texture from the surrounding tissue, or is atypical on colposcopy.

Pelvic examinations of DES-exposed women should begin after menarche or by age 14 in the absence of menarche. If vaginal bleeding, spotting, or abnormal discharge occurs, then an examination is needed earlier. A narrow Pedersen speculum can be used in the young adolescent; a cystoscope has been recommended when examination is necessary in a prepubertal girl (Fuller, 1978). In the absence of abnormal changes, pelvic examinations are recommended

on a yearly basis, although some authors advocate 6-month intervals for repeat examination (Anderson et al., 1979). Interval histories should include questions about abnormal bleeding or discharge. Any abnormal symptoms or Pap smear findings necessitate repeat colposcopy.

It is advisable that DES-exposed women be managed whenever possible in conjunction with a practitioner who specializes in this area. Once an initial assessment with colposcopy has been made, repeat examination may be done by a nonphysician gynecologic practitioner if the patient chooses this type of care. Any abnormal findings on history, examination, or cytology must lead, without hesitation, to referral.

Intervention

TREATMENT. No treatment is advocated for DES exposure. Adenosis requires no therapy except continuing surveillance as outlined earlier. Specific abnormalities such as cancer or infertility are treated on an individualized basis. Treatment for clear cell adenocarcinoma may be limited to local excision and/or radiation, but this has been associated with recurrence. More commonly, radical hysterectomy with pelvic lymph node dissection is advised. Vaginectomy may be performed in cases of vaginal adenocarcinoma. Re-

TABLE 18–6. DES-TYPE DRUGS THAT MAY HAVE BEEN PRESCRIBED TO PREGNANT WOMEN

Amperone	Milestrol
Benzestrol	Monomestrol
Chlorotrianisene	Neo-Oestranol I
Comestrol	Neo-Oestranol II
Cyren A	Nulabort
Cyren B	Oestrogenine
DES	Oestromenin
DesPlex	Oestromon
Dibestil	Orestol
Dienestrol	Pabestrol D
Dienoestrol	Palestrol
Diestryl	Progravidium
Di-Erone	Restrol
Diethylstilbenediol	Stilbal
Diethylstilbestrol dipalmitate	Stilbestrol
Diethylstilbestrol diphosphate	Stilbestronate
Diethylstilbestrol dipropionate	Stilbetin
Digestil	Stilbinol
Domestrol	Stilboestroform
Estan	Stilboestrol
Estilben	Stilboestrol DP
Estrobene	Stilestrate
Estrobene DP	Stilpalmitate
Estrosyn	Stilphostrol
Fonatol	Stil-Rol
Gynben	Stilronate
Gyneben	Stilrone
Hexestrol	Stils
Hexoestrol	Synestrin
Hi-Bestrol	Synestrol
Menocrin	Synthoestrin
Meprane	Tace
Mestilbol	Teserene
Methallenestril	Tylandril
Metystil	Tylosterone
Microest	Vallestril
Mikarol	Willestrol
Mikarol forti	

From Robboy, S. J., Noller, K. L., Kaufman, R. H., & et al. (1983). Prenatal diethylstilbestrol (DES) exposure. Clinical Pediatrics, 22(2), 143. Reprinted with permission.

construction can be accomplished with grafting techniques (Fuller, 1978).

CONTRACEPTION. The choice of contraception may be influenced by DES exposure. Structural abnormalities may prevent the use of an intrauterine device or diaphragm. Many women and physicians prefer to avoid further estrogen exposure as would occur with hormonal contraceptives, although estrogen has not been demonstrated to influence either positively or negatively the development of DES-related sequelae. As most DES-exposed women, however, are not yet at the age where estrogen-related tumors are likely to be seen, current data are insufficient to draw firm conclusions regarding the use of oral contraceptives (Noller et al., 1981, p. 95).

TEACHING AND COUNSELING. All women born between 1946 and 1971 should be helped to identify whether they suffered DES exposure and, if so, counseled about appropriate follow-up. They can be reassured about the risk of clear cell adenocarcinoma, although the future incidence of this and of squamous cell cancers or their precursors remains unknown. DES-exposed women should be counseled that most can achieve viable pregnancies. Those who do face infertility or suffer untoward pregnancy outcomes need referral and counseling regarding fertility workups, treatments, and alternatives to pregnancy (see Chapter 27). Women with clear cell adenocarcinoma require intensive teaching and supportive care before, during, and after treatment (Donahue, 1978).

ENDOMETRIOSIS

Endometriosis can seriously interfere with a woman's well-being. It can lead to dysmenorrhea, dyspareunia, chronic pelvic pain, abnormal vaginal bleeding, infertility, and spontaneous abortion. Bowel symptoms, including diarrhea and pain with defecation, have been reported (Chatman & Ward, 1982). Constipation may result from an avoidance of defecation secondary to pain (dyschezia) (Luciano & Pitkin, 1984, p. 300). Endometriosis, which reportedly occurs in approximately 1 percent of women in the childbearing years (Steele, Dmowski, & Marmer, 1984, p. 34), has thus far eluded understanding. Theories abound regarding the etiology of the disease and of its consequences, but no one theory has yet provided an adequate explanation.

Definition and Pathophysiology

Endometriosis is, by definition, the presence of endometrial tissue outside of the endometrium. Such tissue has been found on the ovary, cul-de-sac of Douglas, uterine ligaments, pelvic peritoneum, rectovaginal septum, cervix, and inguinal area. About 12 percent of women with endometriosis have lesions in the gastrointestinal tract, most often in the rectosigmoid and less often in the appendix and ileum. Endometrial implants may be found in surgical scars, the vagina, vulva, perineum, urinary bladder, or umbilicus. Rarely, they are found in the fallopian tubes, lymph nodes, skin, muscle, lungs, kidneys, pleura, diaphragm, spleen, stomach, gallbladder, heart, and bone (Fox & Buckley, 1984, p. 281; Luciano & Pitkin, 1984, p. 300). Endometrial metaplasia has been suggested as the mechanism involved in the proliferation of endometrial tissue in the pelvic area (von Numers, 1965). Its widespread diffusion has been accounted for by the variety of ways this tissue may travel, via the fallopian tubes, the venous system, or the lymphatics.

Ectopic endometrial tissue consists of glands and stroma. It may respond to cyclic hormones but, if so, demonstrates only minimal proliferative or secretory activity (Fox & Buckley, 1984, p. 281). Bleeding may occur into endometrial lesions or into their surrounding tissue.

Interestingly, recent findings from electron microscopic analyses and nuclear electron binding studies of endometrial implants show differences between the appearance and hormonal receptor properties of these specimens and uterine endometrium. Additionally, differences have been noted in the ways the two types of tissue respond to treatment with progesterone and the testosterone danazol. These findings suggest an inaccuracy in the long-held belief that lesions of endometriosis duplicate endometrial tissue (Schmidt, 1985, p. 159).

Symptoms and sequelae of endometriosis result from pathophysiologic changes including bleeding from the lesions, the presence of cysts, called endometriomas, adhesions, and/or anatomic distortions or obstructions. Some specific symptoms depend on the anatomic location of the disease. In addition, the role of hormones, prostaglandins, and autoimmune factors has been examined to explain the consequences of endometriosis.

Classification

To determine and evaluate treatment for endometriosis, several authors have proposed systems of classifying the disease, from mild to severe. Classification can be made only by laparotomy or laparoscopy; symptoms themselves do not account for disease severity and are not used in classification (Ranney, 1980, p. 865). A special committee was appointed by the American Fertility Society (AFS) in 1978 to create a uniform and universally accepted classification (Buttram, 1985). Revised in 1985, this classification divides the disease into four stages—minimal, mild, moderate, and severe—on the basis of the assignment of points according to size and location of endometriomas, whether they are deep or superficial, the extent of adhesions, and associated ovarian or tubal enclosure and obliteration. Nonpelvic endometriosis is considered separately (American Fertility Society, 1985, p. 351). Reprint forms outlining the classification system are available from the American Fertility Society, 2131 Magnolia Avenue, Suite 201, Birmingham, AL 35256.

Etiology

The etiology of endometriosis remains poorly understood although a number of hypotheses have been examined. Several researchers have suspected a genetic basis for the development of endometriosis. In a comparison of 123 endometriosis patients with female relatives of their husbands, Simpson, Elias, Malinak, and Buttram (1980) found a difference in family histories. Among patients with endometriosis, 5.8 percent of sisters and 8.1 percent of mothers also had the disease, a proportion significantly higher than in the relatives of the husbands. Husband's relatives were chosen as controls on the assumption that they had socioeconomic backgrounds similar to those of study participants, thus avoiding the possible confounding of genetics with socioeconomic factors. The findings of this study are most consistent with a polygenic or multifactorial inheritance, meaning that the trait is influenced by either more than one gene or the interaction of genetics and environment, or both.

A long-debated, widely accepted hypothesis regarding

the etiology of endometriosis, first proposed in 1927, is retrograde menstruation, resulting in a reflux of endometrial tissue through the fallopian tube (Fox & Buckley, 1984, p. 280; Halme, Hammond, Hulka, 1984). A recent study based on laparoscopy of 323 women, however, demonstrated the inadequacy of retrograde menstruation as an explanation for the pathophysiology of endometriosis by showing that over 90 percent of women with patent tubes have blood in their peritoneal fluid during the perimenstrual period (Halme et al., 1984, p. 153).

Immunologic and hormonal explanations for the ectopic implantation of endometrium have been proposed more recently. Steele et al. (1984) examined a variety of parameters relating to immune function in 27 women with varying degrees of endometriosis and 26 age-matched control women. Both groups were infertile. The study found that "specific cellular mechanisms operative in limiting ectopic growth of the endometrial tissue are impaired in women with endometriosis" (pp. 35–36). The authors found this impairment to be related in degree to the extent of endometriosis present.

Sensky and Liu (1980) have proposed an "increased sensitivity to estrogen" in some women with endometriosis. Their conclusion regarding estrogen is based on an uncontrolled study of 163 women in which estrogen-related phenomena were found to be associated with endometriosis. These included menorrhagia, irregular menstrual cycles, assumed to represent anovulation, and endometrioid carcinoma. On the basis of previous studies, they could not blame elevated levels of estrogen for these occurrences because when this hormone has been measured, it has not been found to be elevated in women with endometriosis. These authors suggest that menorrhagia may be a predisposing factor to the development of endometriosis, as increased bleeding and clots might encourage retrograde menstruation (Sensky & Liu, 1980, p. 575).

Cheesman, Cheesman, Chatterton, and Cohen (1983) and Koninckx, Ide, Vandenbroucke, and Brosens (1980) found evidence in women with endometriosis for the unruptured luteinizing follicle (ULF) syndrome, in which a functioning corpus luteum exists, but the egg does not leave the follicle. Koninckx et al. postulate this as a causative factor in the development of endometriosis; they found lower than normal steroid hormone concentrations in the peritoneal fluid of women with ULF, which they believe precludes the prevention of implantation of endometrial cells by the usual steroid hormone environment of the peritoneum.

Incidence and Risk Factors

The actual incidence of endometriosis is unknown (Chatman & Ward, 1982, p. 158). Because its definitive diagnosis can be made only by laparoscopy, it is likely to be more common than believed. The condition has been reported in 15 to 25 percent of all women undergoing laparotomy and in perhaps 1 percent of women in childbearing years (Steele et al., 1984), although some authors cite its incidence as high as 7 to 40 percent of all menstruating women (Muse & Wilson, 1982, p. 145).

Endometriosis has traditionally been considered a disease of women in their thirties and forties, although in at least two series of laparoscopies performed for disabling pelvic pain or abnormal vaginal bleeding in adolescent women, a substantial percentage were found to have endometriosis (Chatman & Ward, 1982, p. 157; Goldstein, De Cholnoky, & Emans 1980). Nulliparity has also been considered a risk factor for endometriosis, although 30 to 40

percent of women with the disease are parous (Luciano & Pitkin, 1984, p. 300).

Japanese women have been found to have a high rate of the disease (Miyazawa, 1976). It has been believed that endometriosis is rare among black women; however, this does not seem to be the case. Chatman (1976) reports on 190 laparoscopies performed on black patients for a variety of symptoms including pelvic pain, dyspareunia, infertility, amenorrhea, abnormal bleeding patterns, and the presence of an adnexal mass or nodularity; 21 percent of these women had endometriosis. Lloyd (1964) also found a comparable rate of endometriosis in black and white patients undergoing gynecologic surgery. Chatman concludes (p. 988) that prejudicial attitudes may account for the belief that pelvic pain or other symptoms in black women are related to pelvic inflammatory disease rather than to endometriosis.

Consequences

Infertility

INCIDENCE. Endometriosis has been found to be strongly associated with infertility. Kistner (1975, p. 1151) reported a 30 to 40 percent rate of infertility in women with endometriosis, which is approximately two times that of the general population. Strathy, Molgaard, Coulam, and Melton (1982) estimated a 20-fold increased risk of infertility with endometriosis. Among infertility patients, approximately 6 to 15 percent are estimated to have endometriosis (Muse & Wilson, 1982, p. 145), although in an examination of 276 laparoscopies of infertile women, Peterson and Behrman (1970) found minimal endometriosis in one third of those whose infertility could not be attributed to other causes.

ETIOLOGY. In some women with endometriosis, there are obvious pathologic explanations for infertility. In extensive disease, endometriomas may leak blood and adhesions may form, possibly obscuring the fimbriated end of the fallopian tubes. Even with patent tubes, there may be interference of release, pickup, or transport of the ovum (Fox & Buckley, 1984, p. 282; Melega, Marchesini, Bellettini, et al., 1984). Fertility, however, may be impaired in less severe forms of the disease. The reason for this is unclear. Explanatory theories include changes in prostaglandin (PG) secretion, anovulation, luteal phase defect, unruptured luteinizing follicle syndrome, hyperprolactinemia, and autoimmune and genetic factors (Melega et al., 1984; Muse & Wilson, 1982).

Cheesman and colleagues (1983) found a delay in the urinary excretion of pregnanediol-3-gluconoride (PGD), the endpoint of progesterone metabolism, in 40 infertile women with varying degrees of endometriosis, possibly reflecting a shortened luteal phase in such women. Sondheimer and Flickinger (1982) did *not* find evidence of a short luteal phase in women with endometriosis, although they did not use the same criteria as the Cheesman group. They propose that alterations in ovulatory function can be a result of prostaglandins, which are known to be released by endometrial tissue and which have been found to play a role in ovulation, luteolysis, and tubal function.

A number of researchers have measured prostaglandins in the peritoneal or cul-de-sac fluid of women with endometriosis and compared their levels with those in normal women and/or infertile women without this disease. A variety of prostaglandins have been looked at, including prostaglandin $F_{2\alpha}$ ($PGF_{2\alpha}$), thromboxane B_2 (TxB_2), 6-

keto-prostaglandin $F_{1\alpha}$ (6-KF), prostaglandin E_2 (PGE$_2$), and 15-keto-13, 14-dihydroprostaglandin $F_{2\alpha}$ (PGFM) (Badaway, Marshall, Gabel, & Nusbaum, 1982; Dawood, Khan-Dawood, & Wilson, 1984; Drake, O'Brien, Ramwell, & Metz, 1981; Rock, Dubin, & Ghodgaonkar, 1982; Sond-heimer & Flickinger, 1982).

Schmidt (1985, p. 159) points out that evaluation of results of studies measuring prostaglandin levels in peritoneal fluid is problematic because of methodologic discrepancies, such as whether or not the stage of the menstrual cycle was considered in the analysis of data. Current data neither prove nor disprove the theory that prostaglandins are responsible for the infertility of endometriosis.

Weed and Arquembourg (1980) propose an autoimmune response to explain the infertility resulting from endometriosis. They demonstrated the presence of complement C3 in the uterine endometrium of women with endometriosis, but not in women without the disease, and hypothesized that endometrial proteins, released from endometriomas, may trigger an autoimmune response. This may cause the rejection of implantation or interfere with sperm passage. Mathur, Peress, and Williamson, (1982) found increased numbers of immunoglobulin G and A antibodies to endometrium and ovary in women with endometriosis, although their sample was quite small.

Muscato, Haney, and Weinberg (1982) found an increased number of macrophages in the peritoneal fluid of infertile women with endometriosis compared with the fluid of either fertile women or infertile women without endometriosis. These macrophages were found to degrade sperm at a rate double that of peritoneal macrophages from both fertile women and infertile women without endometriosis. This hypothesis was supported by the findings of Halme, Becker, Hammond, Raj, and Raj (1983).

None of the preceding theories has been supported sufficiently by research to constitute proof of its role in the etiology of infertility in endometriosis. It is also possible that a variety of mechanisms are associated with this consequence of endometriosis, working in combination or differentially affecting individual women.

Spontaneous Abortion. Naples, Batt, and Sadigh (1981) found an "inordinately high rate of spontaneous abortion" in patients with endometriosis. They based their conclusion on a retrospective study of 214 pregnancies in 100 patients with endometriosis and the rate of spontaneous abortion in a group of 65 women treated for endometriosis. Olive, Franklin, and Gratkins (1982) also found increased rates of spontaneous abortion in a retrospective study of 263 women. Forty-four percent aborted spontaneously, although the percentages were quite different in patients with prior infertility than in those without infertility: 68.7 and 17.1 percent, respectively. No control group was looked at in this study; participants were selected from private practice patients undergoing laparoscopy.

Interestingly, Wheeler, Johnston, and Malinak (1983) found a greater proportion of spontaneous abortion in patients with mild endometriosis (49 percent) than in those with moderate or severe disease (25 and 24 percent). This would preclude mechanical disruption of pregnancy as an explanation for spontaneous abortion, yet other causes have not been identified.

Other Complications. Occasionally, endometriotic tissue undergoes malignant transformation, indicated by a change in the typical pattern of pain experienced, an abrupt increase in its severity, or onset after menopause (when endometriosis usually regresses). Enlargement of a pelvic

mass or rupture of an endometrioma may be indicative of cancer (Mostoufizadeh & Scully, 1980). Reports have also appeared in the literature relating endometriosis to urinary tract obstructions with loss of kidney function (Kane & Drouin, 1985). This is a serious, though rare, consequence.

Clinical Presentation

Symptoms. The severity of symptoms of endometriosis is not always related to the extent of disease (Fox & Buckley, 1984, p. 283; Luciano & Pitkin, 1984, p. 300). Generally, women with symptomatic disease present with a history of increasing dysmenorrhea, dyspareunia, and/or pelvic pain. Green (1977, p. 337) describes the pain as "deep-seated aching or bearing down pain" in the lower abdomen, posterior pelvis, vagina, and back. It may radiate to the bowel and perineum, even the thighs. The pain generally begins a day or two before menses and may increase in intensity in the first few days of menstruation. It gradually subsides and ends just before the end of menstruation or shortly afterward, although over time it can progress in both severity and duration. Symptoms may vary, however, and include premenstrual spotting, dysfunctional uterine bleeding, dysuria, and dyschezia. Occasionally, urinary urgency, hematuria, or rectal bleeding may occur. Rarely, hemoptysis, intestinal obstruction, cutaneous nodules, or hydroureter or hydronephrosis may be present. Women with endometriosis may present with infertility, with or without other symptoms.

Physical Examination Findings. A tender nodule at the uterosacral ligament is rather specific to endometriosis (Andrews et al., 1984). Other common physical examination findings in endometriosis are general pelvic tenderness, especially at the cul-de-sac or posterior surface of the lower uterine segment or cervix, tender and/or enlarged adnexa (unilateral or bilateral), and a fixed retroflexed uterus. Ovaries affected by endometriosis may be felt as cystic. Pain on motion of pelvic structures is most apparent just before and during menses (Green, 1977, p. 338; Luciano & Pitkin, 1984, p. 300).

Differential Diagnosis. Endometriosis must be differentiated from salpingitis (or pelvic inflammatory disease), ectopic pregnancy, ovarian cysts, pelvic adhesions, uterine fibroids, ovarian cancer with peritoneal seeding, intestinal problems, and urinary tract disorders.

Endometriosis may cause generalized peritonitis if there is leakage from or rupture of a large endometrioma. This emergency situation must be distinguished from ruptured ectopic pregnancy, rupture or torsion of an ovarian cyst, acute salpingitis, or appendicitis.

Definitive diagnosis of endometriosis is made operatively. Luciano and Pitkin (1984, p. 301) recommend laparoscopy because of the "panoramic view" it provides of the pelvis and lower abdomen. The lesions of endometriosis can be identified by their characteristic appearance, and the disease is classified according to the AFS system. If there is a question about the diagnosis on laparoscopy, a transendoscopic biopsy can be taken for histologic analysis.

Management
Data Collection

HISTORY. Whenever a woman in the childbearing years has complaints characteristic of this disease, the practitioner should suspect endometriosis. A careful history, including a family history, will help support this suspicion. A concrete current and historical description of any symptoms should be elicited. A woman may need to be guided to remember and describe explicitly details such as the onset of the problem, when in her cycle pain occurs, and how it has changed over time. Parity and gravidy are important pieces of data, as endometriosis is more common in, although certainly not limited to, nulliparas.

PHYSICAL EXAMINATION. A complete abdominal and pelvic assessment is crucial in confirming a suspicion of endometriosis and ruling out other conditions whose symptoms may be similar (see Chapter 3). A rectal examination must be included, because the uterus may be fixed in a retroverted position, and nodularity of the uterosacral ligaments, cul-de-sac, and posterior uterine wall may be better appreciated rectally.

LABORATORY TESTING. There are no specific laboratory tests to assess for endometriosis, although tests to rule out other conditions may be appropriate. A sonogram may be useful if masses are felt (Dawood, 1983, p. 458). Definitive diagnosis is made by laparoscopy.

Intervention

TREATMENT. Many authors advise early treatment of endometriosis because of the progressive nature of the disease (Luciano & Pitkin, 1984, p. 300). For this reason, any woman in whom endometriosis is suspected deserves the option of a prompt referral to a gynecologist for possible laparoscopic diagnosis and treatment. The nonphysician health care provider, however, should be familiar with treatment options so that anticipatory guidance can be offered and questions answered.

The goals of treatment for endometriosis include prevention of disease progression, alleviation of pain, and establishment or restoration of fertility. A variety of treatment approaches have been advocated. In women not desiring to maintain their reproductive capacity, hysterectomy and bilateral salpingo-oophorectomy constitute the only definitive cure, although more conservative medical and surgical approaches may control symptoms and cause disease regression. Surgery may be performed, with conventional or laser techniques, to remove endometrial implants while conserving the reproductive organs. A variety of medical therapies have been used. These include the induction of pseudopregnancy with oral contraceptives, the use of androgens, and, most recently, creation of a pseudomenopause with danazol, a testosterone derivative, and suppression of ovarian function with gonadotropin-releasing hormone (GnRH) agonists, a so-called medical oophorectomy (Yen, 1983). As a treatment for infertility secondary to endometriosis, danazol is used for 3 to 6 months, then discontinued to allow for conception.

Some gynecologists have suggested pregnancy as a treatment for endometriosis for women in whom infertility is not a consequence of the disease, or possibly as a preventive measure in women at risk for endometriosis, that is, those with a family history (Dawood, 1983, p. 459, 465; Green, 1977, pp. 341–342). One study that considered this factor, however, found that pregnancy delayed, but did not prevent, reoccurrence of the disease (Wheeler & Malinak, 1983). Similarly, some authors have advocated the use of oral contraceptives as a method of family planning for women at risk, although its value is purely speculative

(Sensky & Liu, 1980, p. 575). For mild endometriosis, in the absence of disabling symptoms, some advocate expectant management, even with infertility. In a comprehensive and careful review of the treatment literature for infertility, Schmidt (1985) points to the lack of prospective controlled studies to show the value of treatment over expectancy for mild forms of the disease.

Many researchers have attempted to evaluate the efficacy of surgical and medical treatment in endometriosis. Most have looked at correction of infertility, assessing the number of pregnancies achieved after surgery, medical treatment, or a combination of surgery and medicine. In a limited number of studies, treatment has been compared with no treatment. Conclusions are varied and, given the methodologic problems that characterize this body of literature, must be considered tentative. Table 18–7 summarizes this literature, dividing various studies into those that evaluate treatment of infertility, spontaneous abortion, and disease recurrence or pain relief.

DANAZOL. Because of the widespread use of danazol as a treatment for endometriosis, this drug deserves further discussion. Danazol, a synthetic steroid, is a derivative of α-ethinyl testosterone with antigonadotropic properties that has been shown to suppress serum follicle-stimulating hormone and luteinizing hormone levels. Amenorrhea is seen in the majority of danazol users after 6 to 8 weeks of treatment, and some women experience other menopausal symptoms. Side effects are related to anabolic and androgenic properties of the drug. These include weight gain, acne, and oily skin. Vaginal spotting has been observed (Dmowski & Cohen, 1975). Arthralgia, rash, hemoptysis, muscle cramps, hirsutism, vaginitis, hand tremors, depression, fatigue, decreased libido, headache, nausea, voice changes, and decreased breast size have all been noted (Buttram, Reiter, & Ward, 1985, p. 354). In one study, which compared side effects of 800- and 400-mg regimens of danazol, therapy was discontinued secondary to side effects in 10 of 190 patients receiving the higher dose and in 5 of 119 receiving the lower dose (Buttram, et al., 1985).

An additional problem is danazol's cost, which, in 1983, was reported to be about $150 per month (Menaker, 1984, p. 268). Guzick and Rock (1983, pp. 582–583) conclude, on the basis of a lack of clearly demonstrated benefit to either medical or surgical treatment, "the recommendation of danazol or surgery should be individualized on the basis of the patient's particular clinical situation, also taking into account the risks of surgery versus the side effects of danazol." Combination therapy has also been recommended, especially for women with severe endometriosis and significant pelvic adhesions (Moore, Harger, Rock, & Archer, 1981, p. 19).

TEACHING AND COUNSELING. Patients in whom there is a high suspicion of endometriosis need to be counseled regarding diagnosis and possible treatments. This, of course, requires referral to a gynecologist. Once diagnosed, women deserve a frank discussion of treatment options with potential risks and benefits. Each woman, depending on the particular effects suffered from endometriosis, must make an individualized and informed decision. Any woman participating in a clinical trial of a treatment modality must be provided with all components of informed consent.

Psychological support may be needed for women experiencing severe, disabling pain, sexual difficulties secondary to dyspareunia, and infertility (see Chapter 27). Appro-

TABLE 18-7. TREATMENT OF ENDOMETRIOSIS

Studies of Infertility							
Study	*Year*	*Number of Patients*	*Therapy Used*	*Control Group (Y/N)*	*Randomization (Y/N)*	*% Conceptions*	*Comments*
Garcia and David	1977	119	1. Expectant 2. Surgery	Y	N	Expectant: 32.4% (minimal disease) Surgery: 32.4% Surgery with minimal disease: 66.7% Surgery recommended but refused: 6.7% Surgery not done (secondary to male involvement): 0% Surgery not recommended but done secondary to patient's request: 0%	F/U[a]: 2 years
Dmowski and Cohen	1978	99 (84 infertile)	Danazol	N	N	46.4% Corrected[b]: 72.2%	F/U: 37 months
Daniell and Christianson	1981	66 35 Mild 25 Moderate 6 Severe	Combined: surgery and postop or preop danazol	N	N	54% Corrected[b]: 68%	
Moore et al.	1981	38 28 attempted, pregnancy	Danazol, four dose schedules: 100, 200, 400, 600 mg/day/6 months	N	Y	Overall: 28% 100 mg: (2/7) 29% 200 mg: (4/8) 50% 400 mg: (0/5) 0% 600 mg: (2/10) 20%	F/U: 6-24 months after Rx discontinued
Seibel et al.	1982	65 Minimal disease only	1. Danazol 2. No Rx after laparoscopic D&C and tubal lavage	Y	Y	Danazol: 30% No Rx: 50%	F/U: 6 months
Schenken and Malinak	1982	90 Mild	1. Expectant 2. Surgery	Y	N	Expectant: 72-75% Surgery: 72.4-76.2%	F/U: 1 year
Rantala et al.	1983	129	Surgery	N	N	51.2%	F/U: 1 year
Portuondo et al.	1983	31	Expectant	N	N	61.2%	F/U: 36 months Not adjusted for male factor
Guzick and Rock	1983	313 Mild or moderate	1. Danazol 2. Surgery	N	N	Danazol: 68.3% Surgery: 74%	
Puleo and Hammond	1983	39 (29 infertile)	Danazol	N	N	33% Corrected[b]: 56%	F/U: 16.5 months
Butler et al.	1984	75 Mild	Danazol	N	N	28%	
Bellina et al.	1984	108 (84 "at-risk" for pregnancy)	CO_2 laser	N	N	Mild-moderate: 55% Severe-Extensive: 88% Ectopic: 3% Abortion rate: 17%	F/U: 12 months 26 months

Buttram et al.	1985	157	1. Danazol
			2. Surgery
			3. Preop danazol, then surgery
			4. Surgery, then postop danazol
				N	N	1. Danazol
						  Minimal: 58%
						  Mild: 39%
						  Moderate or severe: 67%
						2. Surgery
						  Mild: 73%
						  Moderate: 56%
						  Severe: 40%
							7% discontinued medications secondary to side effects

TABLE 18–7. TREATMENT OF ENDOMETRIOSIS (CONTINUED)

Studies of Infertility

Study	Year	Number of Patients	Therapy Used	Control Group (Y/N)	Randomiza-tion (Y/N)	% Conceptions	Comments

						3. Danazol, surgery
						  Mild: 83%
						  Moderate: 67%
						  Severe: 50%
						4. Surgery, Danazol
						  (severity not speci-
						  fied)	

Starks and Grimes	1985	105 minimal disease	1. Danazol 2. No Rx	Y	N	Danazol: 71% Untreated: 30%	Patients selected Rx
Martin	1985	50	1. CO_2 laser at laparoscopy 2. CO_2 laser with postop laparoscopy (severe only)	N	N	11% Other reasons for not becoming pregnant: 59%	F/U: 7–19 months

Feste	1985	112
		  92 Mild
		  17 Moderate
		  3 Severe
			Laser	N	N	72%
						Other conditions present: 31%
							F/U: 1 year

Studies of Spontaneous Abortion

Study	Year	Number of Patients	Therapy Used	Control Group (Y/N)	Randomiza-tion (Y/N)	Rate of Spontaneous Abortion

Naples et al.	1981	Group 1: 100
		Group 2: 65
			1. Various medical treatments
			2. Surgery
				Y[c]	N	Medical Rx
						  Before dx:
						    <2 years: 63%
						    2–4 years: 43%
						  After Rx: 25%
						Surgical Rx
						  Before surgery: 46%
						  After surgery: 8%

Wheeler et al.	1983	226 pregnancies	1. Expectant
			2. Surgery
				Y	N	Before surgery: 35%
						  Mild: 49%
						  Moderate: 25%
						  Severe: 24%
						After surgery
						  9% with secondary infertility
						  13% with primary infertility

Groll	1984	80	1. Expectant 2. Surgery 3. Danazol	Y	N	Expectant: 52% Surgery: 12% Danazol: 7%

Studies of Disease Recurrence or Pain Relief

Study	Year	Number of Patients	Therapy Used	Control Group (Y/N)	Randomiza-tion (Y/N)	Findings

Dmowski & Cohen	1975	39	Danazol	N	N	On repeat laparoscopy
						  No disease: 59%
						  Adhesions, no active disease: 26%
						  Residual disease: 15%

Moore et al.	1981	38	Danazol: four dosage schedules	N	Y	Improvement at laparoscopy: 71% Symptomatic relief after 6 months: 89% Recurrent symptom within 1 year of Rx discontinued: 51%
Puleo & Hammond	1983	39	Danazol	N	N	Complete pain relief: 47% Pain recurrence at 6.9 months: 38%
Wheeler & Malinak	1983	423	Surgery	Y	N	Cumulative 3- and 5-year recurrence rates: 13.5 and 40.3%
Feste	1985	37	1. Laser 2. No laser	Y	N	Pain relief: 72% (no results non-Rx group)
Kauppila & Ronnberg	1985	20	1. Naproxen sodium 2. Placebo	Y	Y	Treated: 83% complete or partial relief Placebo: 41% relief

[a]F/U = time of follow-up (where specified).
[b]Corrected rate excludes those women or couples for whom there is another reason for infertility.
[c]Control group is pregnancies among same women before treatment.

priate referrals for individual or group therapy should be offered as necessary.

REFERENCES

Adam, E., Kaufman, R. H., Adler-Storthz, K., et al., (1985, January 15). A prospective study of association of herpes simplex virus and human papillomavirus infection with cervical neoplasia in women exposed to diethylstilbestrol in utero. *International Journal of Cancer, 35*(1), 19–26.

Adess, N., Brown, K., Hackett, S., & Turiel, J. (1984). *Fertility and pregnancy guide for DES daughters & sons.* Long Island, NY: DES Action National.

American Fertility Society. (1985, March). Revised American Fertility Society classification of endometriosis. *Fertility and Sterility, 43*(3), 351–352.

Anderson, B., Watring, W. G., Edinger, D. D., et al., (1979, March). Development of DES-associated clear-cell carcinoma: The importance of regular screening. *Obstetrics and Gynecology, 53*(3), 293–299.

Andonian, R. W., & Kessler, R. (1979). Transplacental exposure to diethylstilbestrol in men. *Urology, 13*(3), 276–279.

Andrews, W. C., Buttram, V., & Cohen, M., et al., (1984). Open Forum. *International Journal of Fertility, 29*(1), 1–12.

Badaway, S. A. Z., Marshall, L., Gabel, A. A., & Nusbaum, M. L. (1982, August). The concentration of 13,14-dihydro-15-keto prostaglandin $F_{2\alpha}$ with and without endometriosis. *Fertility and Sterility, 38*(2), 166–169.

Barnes, A. B., Colton, T., & Gundersen, J., et al., (1980, March 13). Fertility and outcome of pregnancy in women exposed in utero to diethylstilbestrol. *The New England Journal of Medicine, 302*(11), 609–613.

Barrett, K., Bledsoe, S., Greer, B. E., & Droegemueller, W. (1977, February 1). Tampon-induced vaginal or cervical ulceration. *American Journal of Obstetrics and Gynecology, 127*(3), 332–333.

Bartlett, P., Reingold, A. L., & Graham, D. R., et al., (1982, March). Toxic Shock Syndrome associated with surgical wound infections. *Journal of the American Medical Association, 242*(10), 1448-1450.

Bellina, J. H., Voros, J. I., Fick, A. C., & Jackson, J. D. (1984). Surgical management of endometriosis with the carbon dioxide laser. *Microsurgery, 5*(4), 197–201.

Beral, V., & Colwell, L. (1980, October 25). Randomised trial of high doses of stilboestrol and ethisterone in pregnancy: Long-term follow-up of mothers. *British Medical Journal, 281*(6248), 1098-1101.

Berger, M., & Goldstein, D. P. (1980, January). Impaired reproductive performace in DES-exposed women. *Obstetrics and Gynecology, 55*(1), 25–27.

Berkley, S. F., Hightower, A. W., Broome, C. V., & Reingold, A. L. (1987, August 21). The relationship of tampon characteristics to menstrual toxic shock syndrome. *Journal of the American Medical Association, 258*(7), 917–920.

Bibbo, M., Gill, W. B., & Azizi, F., et al., (1977, January). Follow-up study of male and female offspring of DES-exposed mothers. *Obstetrics and Gynecology, 49*(1), 1–8.

Bibbo, M., Haenszel, W. M., & Wied, G. L., et al., (1978, April 6). A twenty-five-year follow-up study of women exposed to diethylstilbestrol during pregnancy. *The New England Journal of Medicine, 298*(14), 763–767.

Brian, D. D., Tilley, B. C., & Labarthe, D. R., et al., (1980, February). Breast cancer in DES-exposed mothers: Absence of association. *Mayo Clinic Proceedings, 55*(2), 81–93.

Burke, L., Antonioli, D., & Friedman, E. A. (1981, January). Evolution of diethylstilbestrol-associated genital tract lesions. *Obstetrics and Gynecology, 57*(1), 79–84.

Burke, L., & Mathews, B. E. (1977). Evaluation of the diethylstilbestrol exposed offspring. In *Colposcopy in clinical practice.* Philadelphia: F. A. Davis.

Butler, L., Wilson, E., Belisle, S., et al., (1984, March). Collaborative study of pregnancy rates following danazol therapy of stage I endometriosis. *Fertility and Sterility, 41*(3), 373–376.

Buttram, V. C. (1985, March). Evolution of the revised American Fertility Society classification of endometriosis. *Fertility and Sterility, 43*(3), 347–350.

Buttram, V. C., Reiter, R. C., & Ward, S. (1985, March). Treatment of endometriosis with danazol: Report of a 6-year prospective study. *Fertility and Sterility, 43*(3), 353–360.

Centers for Disease Control. (1980a, May). Toxic-shock syndrome—United States. *Morbidity and Mortality Weekly Report, 29*(20), 229–230.

Centers for Disease Control. (1980b, September 19). Follow-up on toxic-shock syndrome. *Morbidity and Mortality Weekly Reports. 29*(37), 441–443.

Centers for Disease Control. (1983, August 5). Update toxic-shock syndrome—United States. *Morbidity and Mortality Weekly Reports, 32*(30), 398–400.

Centers for Disease Control. (1984, February). Toxic-shock syndrome and the vaginal contraceptive sponge. *Morbidity and Mortality Weekly Reports, 33*(4), 43–49.

Chatman, D. L. (1976, August). Endometriosis in the black woman. *American Journal of Obstetrics and Gynecology, 125*(7), 987–989.

Chatman, D. L., & Ward, A. B. (1982, March). Endometriosis in adolescents. *The Journal of Reproductive Medicine, 27*(3), 156–160.

Cheesman, K. L., Cheesman, S. D., Chatterton, R. T., & Cohen, M. R. (1983, November). Alteration in progesterone metabolism and luteal function in infertile women with endometriosis. *Fertility and Sterility, 40*(5), 590–594.

Chesney, P. J., Crass, B. A., & Polyak, M. B., et al., (1982, June). Toxic shock syndrome: Management and long-term sequelae. *Annals of Internal Medicine, 96*(6, Part 2): 847–851.

Chow, A. W., Wong, C. K., MacFarlane, A. M. G., & Bartlett, K. H. (1984, February 15). Toxic shock syndrome: Clinical and laboratory findings in 30 patients. *Canadian Medical Association Journal, 130*(4), 425–430.

Cosgrove, M., Benton, B., & Henderson, B. E. (1977, February). Male genitourinary abnormalities and maternal diethylstilbestrol. *The Journal of Urology, 117*(2), 220–222.

Cousins, L., Karp, W., Lacey, C., & Lucas, W. E. (1980, July) Reproductive outcome of women exposed to diethylstilbestrol in utero. *Obstetrics and Gynecology, 56*(1), 70–76.

Daniell, J. F., & Christianson, C. (1981, May). Combined laparoscopic surgery and Danazol therapy for pelvic endometriosis. *Fertility and Sterility, 35*(5), 521–525.

Davis, J. P., Chesney, P. J., Wand, P. J., et al., (1980, December 18). Toxic-shock syndrome: Epidemiologic features, recurrence, risk factors, and prevention. *The New England Journal of Medicine, 303*(25), 1429–1435.

Davis, J. P., Osterholm, M. T., Helms, C. M., et al. (1982a, April). Tri-state toxic-shock syndrome study. II. Clinical and laboratory findings. *The Journal of Infectious Disease, 145*(4), 441–447.

Davis, J. P., Osterholm, M. T., & Helms, C. M., et al. (1982b, June). Tristate toxic shock syndrome study: Evaluation of case definition and prevention of recurrence. *Annals of Internal Medicine, 96*(6, Part 2), 903–905.

Dawood, M. Y. (1983). Endometriosis and adenomyosis. In J. W. Ellis & C. R. B. Beckman (Eds.), *A clinical manual of gynecology.* Norwalk, CT: Appleton–Century–Crofts.

Dawood, M. Y., Khan-Dawood, F. S., & Wilson, L., Jr. (1984, February 15). Peritoneal fluid prostaglandins and prostanoids in women with endometriosis, chronic pelvic inflammatory disease, and pelvic pain. *American Journal of Obstetrics and Gynecology, 148*(4), 391–395.

DeCherney, A. H., Cholst, I., & Naftolin, F. (1981, December). Structure and function of the Fallopian tubes following exposure to diethylstilbestrol (DES) during gestation. *Fertility and Sterility, 36*(6), 741–744.

Dieckmann, W. J., Davis, M. E., Rynkiewicz, L. M., & Pottinger, R. E. (1953, November). Does the administration of diethylstilbestrol during pregnancy have therapeutic value? *American Journal of Obstetrics and Gynecology, 66*(5), 1062–1078.

Dmowski, W. P., & Cohen, M. R. (1975, August). Treatment of endometriosis with an antigonadotropin, danazol: A laparoscopic and histologic evaluation. *Obstetrics and Gynecology, 46*(2), 147–154.

Dmowski, W. P., & Cohen, M. R. (1978, January 1).Antigonadtropin (Danazol) in the treatment of endometriosis: Evaluation of posttreatment fertility and three-year follow-up data, *American Journal of Obstetrics and Gynecology, 130*(1), 41–48.

Donahue, D. (1978, June). DES: A case study. *Cancer Nursing, 1*(3), 207–210.

Dornan, K. J., Thompson, D. M., & Conn, A. R., et al. (1982, January). Toxic shock syndrome in the postoperative patient. *Surgery, Gynecology and Obstetrics, 154*(1), 65–68.

Drake, T. S., O'Brien, W. F., Ramwell, P. W., & Metz, S. A. (1981, June 15). Peritoneal fluid thromboxane B$_2$ and 6-ketoprostaglandin F$_{1\alpha}$ in endometriosis. *American Journal of Obstetrics and Gynecology, 140*(4), 401–404.

Faich, G., Pearson, K., & Fleming, D., et al. (1986, January 10). Toxic shock syndrome and the vaginal contraceptive sponge. *Journal of the American Medical Association, 255*(2), 216–218.

Feste, J. R. (1985, May). Laser laparoscopy: A new modality. *The Journal of Reproductive Medicine, 30*(5), 413–417.

Fox, H., & Buckley, C. H. (1984, April). Current concepts of endometriosis. *Clinics in Obstetrics and Gynecology, 11*(1), 279–287.

Frank, A. R., Krumholz, B. A., & Deutsch, S. (1985, May). Regression of cervicovaginal abnormalities in DES-exposed women. *The Journal of Reproductive Medicine, 30*(5), 400–403.

Friedrich, E., & Siegesmund, K. A. (1980, February). Tampon-associated vaginal ulcerations. *Obstetrics and Gynecology, 55*(2), 149–156.

Fuller, A. F. (1978, June). The DES syndrome and clear cell adenocarcinoma in young women. *Cancer Nursing, 1*(3), 201–205.

Gallup, D. G., Altaffer, L. F., & Castle, C. A. (1984, October). Urinary tract evaluation of diethylstilbestrol-exposed female progeny followed in a colposcopy clinic. *The Journal of Reproductive Medicine, 29*(10), 717–721.

Garbe, P. L., Arko, R. J., & Reingold, A. L., et al. (1985, May 3). *Staphylococcus aureus* isolates from patients with nonmenstrual toxic shock syndrome. *Journal of the American Medical Association, 253*(7), 2538–2542.

Garcia, C. -R., & David, S. S. (1977, December). Pelvic endometriosis: Infertility and pelvic pain. *American Journal of Obstetrics and Gynecology, 129*(7), 740–747.

Gill, W. B., Schumacher, G. F. B., & Bibbo, M. (1976, April). Structural and functional abnormalities in the sex organs of male offspring of mothers treated with diethylstilbestrol (DES). *The Journal of Reproductive Medicine, 16*(4), 147–153.

Glaze, G. M. (1984, February). Diethylstilbestrol exposure in utero: Review of literature. *Journal of the American Osteopathic Association, 83*(6), 435–438.

Goldstein, D. P., De Cholnoky, C., & Emans, S. J. (1980, September). Adolescent endometriosis. *Journal of Adolescent Health Care, 1*(1), 37–41.

Green, S. L., & LaPeter, K. S. (1982, January). Evidence for post-partum toxic-shock syndrome in a mother–infant pair. *The American Journal of Medicine, 72*(1), 169–172.

Green, T. H. (1977). *Gynecology: Essentials of clinical practice* (3rd ed.). Boston: Little, Brown, 1977.

Greenberg, E. R., Barnes, A. B., & Resseguie, L., et al. (1984, November 29). Breast cancer in mothers given diethylstilbestrol in pregnancy. *The New England Journal of Medicine, 311*(22), 1393–1398.

Groll, M. (1984, June). Endometriosis and spontaneous abortion. *Fertility and Sterility, 41*(6), 933–935.

Guzick, D. S., & Rock, J. A. (1983, November). A comparison of danazol and conservative surgery for the treatment of infertility due to mild or moderate endometriosis. *Fertility and Sterility, 40*(5), 580–584.

Halme, J., Becker, S., & Hammond, M. G., et al. (1983, February 1). Increased activation of pelvic macrophages in infertile women with mild endometriosis. *American Journal of Obstetrics and Gynecology, 145*(3), 333–337.

Halme, J., Hammond, M. G., Hulka, J. F., et al. (1984, August). Retrograde menstruation in healthy women and in patients with endometriosis. *Obstetrics and Gynecology, 64*(2), 151–154.

Haney, A. F., & Hammond, M. G. (1983, December). Infertility in women exposed to diethylstilbestrol in utero. *The Journal of Reproductive Medicine, 28*(12), 851–856.

Henderson, B. E., Benton, B., & Cosgrove, M., et al. (1976, October 4). Urogenital Tract Abnormalities in sons of women treated with diethylstilbestrol. *Pediatrics, 58*(4), 505–507.

Herbst, A. L. (1981, July 15). Clear cell adenocarcinoma and the current status of DES-exposed females. *Cancer, 48*(2, Suppl.), 484–488.

Herbst, A. L., Hubby, M. M., Azizi, F., & Makii, M. M. (1981, December 15). Reproductive and gynecologic surgical experience in diethylstilbestrol-exposed daughters. *American Journal of Obstetrics and Gynecology, 141*(8), 1019–1028.

Herbst, A. L., Kurman, R. J., & Scully, R. E. (1972, September). Vaginal and cervical abnormalities after exposure to stilbestrol in utero. *Obstetrics and Gynecology, 40*(3), 287–298.

Herbst, A. L., Poskanzer, D. C., & Robboy, S. J., et al. (1975, February 13). Prenatal exposure to stilbestrol: A prospective comparison of exposed female offspring with unexposed controls. *The New England Journal of Medicine, 292*(7), 334–339.

Herbst, A. L., Robboy, S. J., Scully, R. E., & Poskanzer, D. C. (1974, July 1). Clear-cell adenocarcinoma of the vagina and cervix in girls: An analysis of 170 registry cases. *American Journal of Obstetrics and Gynecology, 119*(5), 713–724.

Herbst, A. L., & Scully, R. E. (1970, April). Adenocarcinoma of the vagina in adolescence: A report of 7 cases including 6 clear-cell carcinomas (so-called mesonephromas). *Cancer, 25*(4), 745–757.

Herbst, A. L., Ulfelder, H. & Poskanzer, D. C. (1971, April 22). Adenocarcinoma of the vagina: Association of maternal stilbestrol therapy with tumor appearance in young women. *The New England Journal of Medicine, 284*(16), 878–881.

Institute of Medicine. (1982). *Toxic shock syndrome: Assessment of current information and future research needs.* Washington, DC: National Academy Press.

Jaffe, R. (1981, December 24). Toxic-shock syndrome associated with diaphragm use [letter]. *The New England Journal of Medicine, 305*(26), 1585–1586.

Jefferies, J. A., Robboy, S. J., & O'Brien, P. C., et al. (1984, January 1). Structural anomalies of the cervix and vagina in women enrolled in the Diethylstilbestrol Adenosis (DESAD) Project. *American Journal of Obstetrics and Gynecology, 148*(1), 59–66.

Kane, C., & Drouin, P. (1985, January 15). Obstructive uropathy associated with endometriosis. *American Journal of Obstetrics and Gynecology, 151*(2), 207–211.

Kaufman, R., Adam, E., Binder, G. L., & Gerthoffer, E. (1980, June 1). Upper genital tract changes and pregnancy outcome in offspring exposed in utero to diethylstilbestrol. *American Journal of Obstetrics and Gynecology, 137*(3), 299–308.

Kaufman, R., Noller, K., & Adam, E., et al. (1984, April 1). Upper genital tract abnormalities and pregnancy outcome in diethylstilbestrol-exposed progeny. *American Journal of Obstetrics and Gynecology, 148*(7), 973–984.

Kauppila, A., & Ronnberg, L. (1985, March). Naproxen sodium in dysmenorrhea secondary to endometriosis. *Obstetrics and Gynecology, 65*(3), 379–383.

Kirkhope, T. G. (1983, November). Reproductive performance among DES exposed daughters compared with that of their mothers. *The Ohio State Medical Journal, 79*(11), 867–869.

Kistner, R. W. (1975, December). Management of endometriosis in the infertile patient. *Fertility and Sterility, 26*(12), 1151–1166.

Koninckx, P. R., Ide, P., Vandenbroucke, W., & Brosens, I. A. (1980, June). New aspects of the pathophysiology of endometriosis and associated infertility. *The Journal of Reproductive Medicine, 24*(6), 257–260.

Labarthe, D., Adam, E., Noller, K. L., et al. (1978, April). Design and preliminary observations of National Cooperative Diethylstilbestrol Adenosis (DESAD) Project. *Obstetrics and Gynecology, 51*(4), 453–458.

Lanes, S., Poole, C., Kreyer, N. A., & Lanza, L. L. (1986, May). Toxic shock syndrome, contraceptive methods, and vaginitis. *American Journal of Obstetrics and Gynecology, 154*(5), 989–991.

Leary, F. J., Resseguie, L. J., & Kurland, L. T., et al. (1984, December 7). Males exposed in utero to diethylstilbestrol. *Journal of the American Medical Association, 252*(21), 2984–2989.

Lee, R. V., Dillon, W. P., & Baehler, E. (1982, January 23). Barrier contraceptives and toxic shock syndrome [Letter]. *Lancet, 1*(8265), 221–222.

Litt, I. F., (1983, December). Toxic shock syndrome. *Journal of Adolescent Health Care, 4*(4), 270–274.

Little, B. (1953, November). Discussion. *American Journal of Obstetrics and Gynecology, 66*(5), 1079–1080.

Lloyd, F. P. (1964). Endometriosis in the Negro woman: A five year study. *American Journal of Obstetrics and Gynecology, 89*(4), 468–469.

Loomis, L., & Feder, H. M., Jr. (1981, December 24). Toxic-shock syndrome associated with diaphragm use [Letter]. *The New England Journal of Medicine, 305*(26), 1585.

Luciano, A. A., & Pitkin, R. M. (1984). Endometriosis: Approaches to diagnosis and treatment. *Surgery Annual, 16,* 297–312.

Mangan, C. E., Borow, L., & Burtnett-Rubin, M. M., et al. (1982, March). Pregnancy outcome in 98 women exposed to diethylstilbestrol in utero, their mothers, and unexposed siblings. *Obstetrics and Gynecology, 59*(3), 315–319.

Martin, D. C. (1985, May). CO_2 laser laparoscopy for the treatment of endometriosis associated with infertility. *The Journal of Reproductive Medicine, 30*(5), 409–412.

Mathur, S., Peress, M. R., & Williamson, H. O., et al. (1982, November). Autoimmunity to endometrium and ovary in endometriosis. *Clinical and Experimental Immunology, 50*(2). 259–266.

Melega, C., Marchesini, F. P., & Bellettini, L., et al. (1984, August). Diagnostic value of laparoscopy in endometriosis and infertility. *The Journal of Reproductive Medicine, 29*(8), 597–600.

Melish, M. E., Chen, F. S., & Murata, S. M. (1983). Quantitative detection of toxic shock syndrome marker protein in human and experimental toxic shock syndrome (TSS). *Clinical Research, 31*(1), 122A.

Menaker, J. S. (1984, October). Diagnosis and management of endometriosis. *The Journal of the Kansas Medical Society, 85*(10), 267–268, 277.

Mills, J., Parsonnet, J., & Tsai, Y. C., et al. (1985, June). Control of production of toxic-shock syndrome toxin-1 (TSST-1) magnesium ion. *The Journal of Infectious Diseases, 151*(6), 1158–1161.

Miyazawa, K. (1976, October). Incidence of endometriosis among Japanese women. *Obstetrics and Gynecology, 48*(4), 407–408.

Moore, E. Harger, J. H., Rock, J. A., & Archer, D. F. (1981, July). Management of pelvic endometriosis with low-dose danazol. *Fertility and Sterility, 36*(1), 15–19.

Mostoufizadeh, G. H. M., & Scully, R. E. (1980, September). Malignant tumors arising in endometriosis. *Clinical Obstetrics and Gynecology, 23*(3), 951–963.

Muscato, J. J., Haney, A. F., & Weinberg, J. B. (1982, November 1). Sperm phagocytosis by human peritoneal macrophages: A possible cause of infertility in endometriosis. *American Journal of Obstetrics and Gynecology, 144*(5), 503–509.

Muse, K. N., & Wilson, E. A. (1982, August). How does mild endometriosis cause infertility? *Fertility and Sterility, 38*(2), 145–152.

Naples, J. D., Batt, R. E., & Sadigh, H. (1981, April). Spontaneous abortion rate in patients with endometriosis. *Obstetrics and Gynecology, 587*(4), 509–512.

National Women's Health Network. (1983). *Tampons and toxic shock syndrome.* Washington, DC: National Women's Health Network.

Noller, K. L., Townsend, D. E., & Kaufman, R. H. (1981). Genital findings, colposcopic evaluation, and current management of the diethylstilbestrol-exposed female. In A. Herbst & H. A. Bern (Eds.), *Developmental effects of diethylstilbestrol (DES) in pregnancy.* New York: Thieme–Stratton.

Olive, D. L., Franklin, R. R., & Gratkins, L. V. (1982, June). The association between endometriosis and spontaneous abortion: A retrospective clinical study. *The Journal of Reproductive Medicine, 27*(6), 333–338.

Ostergard, D. R. (1981, June). DES-related vaginal lesions. *Clinical Obstetrics and Gynecology, 24*(2), 379–394.

Osterholm, M. T., Davis, J. P., & Gibson, R. W., et al., (1982, April). Tri-state toxic shock syndrome study. I. Epidemiologic findings. *The Journal of Infectious Diseases, 145*(4), 431–440.

Parsonnet, J., Hickman, R. K., Eardley, D. D., & Pier, G. B. (1985, March). Induction of human interleukin-1 by toxic-shock-syndrome toxin-1. *The Journal of Infectious Diseases, 151*(3), 514–522.

Peterson, D. R. (1982, June) Epidemiologic comparisons of incidence of toxic shock syndrome. *Annals of Internal Medicine, 96*(6, Part 2), 891.

Peterson, E. P., & Behrman, S. J. (1970, September). Laparoscopy of the infertile patient. *Obstetrics and Gynecology, 36*(3), 363–367.

Pope, T. L. (1981, September/October). Toxic shock syndrome. *Nurse Practitioner, 6*(5), 31–32.

Portuondo, J. A., Echanojauregui, A. D., Herran, C., & Alijarte, I. (1983, January). Early conception in patients with untreated mild endometriosis. *Fertility and Sterility, 39*(1), 22–25.

Prins, R., Morrow, C. P., Townsend, D. E., & Disaia, P. J. (1976, August). Vaginal embryogenesis, estrogens, and adenosis. *Obstetrics and Gynecology, 48*(2), 246–250.

Puleo, J. G., & Hammond, C. B. (1983, August). Conservative treatment of endometriosis externa: The effects of danazol therapy. *Fertility and Sterility, 40*(2), 164–169.

Ranney, B. (1980, September). Endometriosis, pathogenesis, symptoms, and findings. *Clinical Obstetrics and Gynecology, 23*(3), 865–873.

Rantala, M. L., Kahanpaa, K. V., Koskimies, A. I., & Widholm, O. (1983). Fertility prognosis after surgical treatment of pelvic endometriosis. *Acta Obstetricia et Gynecologica Scandinavica, 62*(1), 11–14.

Reingold, A. L., Dan, B. B., Shands, K. N., & Broome, C. V. (1982, January 2). Toxic-shock syndrome not associated with menstruation: A review of 54 cases. *Lancet, 1*(8262), 1–4.

Reingold, A. L., Hargrelt, N. T., & Shands, K. N., et al. (1982, June). Toxic shock syndrome surveillance in the United States, 1980–1981. *Annals of Internal Medicine, 96*(6, Part 2), 875–880.

Robboy, S. J., Noller, K. L., & Kaufman, R. H., et al. (1983, February). Prenatal Diethylstilbestrol (DES) exposure: Recommendations of the Diethylstilbestrol–Adenosis (DESAD) Project for the Identification and Management of Exposed Individuals. *Clinical Pediatrics, 22*(2), 139–143.

Robboy, S., Noller, K. L., & O'Brien, P., et al. (1984, December 7). Increased incidence of cervical and vaginal dysplasia in 3,980 diethylstilbestrol-exposed young women: Experience of the National Collaborative Diethylstilbestrol Adenosis Project. *Journal of the American Medical Association, 252*(21), 2979–2983.

Robboy, S., Young, R. H., & Welch, W. R., et al. (1984, September 1). Atypical vaginal adenosis and cervical ectropion: Association with clear cell adenocarcinoma in diethylstilbestrol-exposed offspring. *Cancer, 54*(5), 869–875.

Robboy, S. J., Szyfelbein, W. M., & Goellner, J. R., et al. (1981, July 1). Dysplasia and cytologic findings in 4,589 young women enrolled in Diethylstilbestrol–Adenosis (DESAD) Project. *American Journal of Obstetrics and Gynecology, 140*(5), 579–586.

Rock, J. A., Dubin, N. H., & Ghodgaonkar, R. B., et al. (1982, June). Cul-de-sac fluid in women with endometriosis: Fluid volume and prostanoid concentration during the proliferative phase of the cycle—days 8 to 12. *Fertility and Sterility, 37*(6), 747–750.

Rosene, K. A., Copass, M. K., & Kastner, L. S., et al. (1982, June). Persistent neuropsychological sequelae of toxic shock syndrome. *Annals of Internal Medicine, 96*(6, Part 2), 865–870.

Saadah, H. A., & Andrews, Z. M. (1984, May). The gram stain and culture of vaginal secretions in toxic shock syndrome. *Oklahoma State Medical Association, 77*(5), 150–151.

Sandberg, E. C., Riffle, N. L., Higdon, J. V., & Getman, C. E. (1981, May 15). Pregnancy outcome in women exposed to diethylstilbestrol in utero. *American Journal of Obstetrics and Gynecology, 140*(2), 194–205.

Sanders, C., Sanders, W. E., Jr., & Fagnant, J. E. (1982, April 15). Toxic shock syndrome: An ecologic imbalance within the genital microflora of women? *American Journal of Obstetrics and Gynecology, 142*(8), 977–982.

Schenken, R. S., & Malinak, L. R. (1982, February). Conservative surgery versus expectant management for the infertile patient with mild endometriosis. *Fertility and Sterility, 37*(2), 183–186.

Schmidt, C. L. (1985, August). Endometriosis: A reappraisal of pathogenesis and treatment. *Fertility and Sterility, 44*(2), 157–173.

Schmidt, G., Fowler, W. C., Talbert, L. M., & Edelman, D. A. (1980, January). Reproductive history of women exposed to diethylstilbestrol in utero. *Fertility and Sterility, 33*(1), 21–24.

Schrock, C. (1980). Disease alert [Letter]. *Journal of the American Medical Association, 243*(12), 1231.

Seibel, M. Berger, M.J., Weinstein, F. G., & Taymor, M.L. (1982, November). The effectiveness of danazol on subsequent fertility in minimal endometriosis. *Fertility and Sterility, 38*(5), 534–537.

Sensky, T. E., & Liu, D. T. (1980, May/June). Endometriosis: Association with menorrhagia, infertility and oral contraceptives. *International Journal of Gynecology and Obstetrics, 17*(6), 573–576.

Shands, K., Schmid, G. P., & Dan, B. B., et al. (1980, December 18). Toxic-shock syndrome in menstruating women: Association with tampon use and *Staphylococcus aureus* and clinical features in 52 cases. *The New England Journal of Medicine, 303*(25), 1436–1442.

Shelley, W. B. (1982, January 23). Preventing tampon-associated toxic shock [Letter]. *Lancet, 1*(8265), 221.

Shelton, J., & Higgins, J. E. (1981, December). Contraception and toxic-shock syndrome: A reanalysis. *Contraception, 24*(6), 631–634.

Simpson, J. L., Elias, S., Malinak, L. R., & Buttram, V. C. (1980, June 1). Heritable aspects of endometriosis. I. Genetic studies. *American Journal of Obstetrics and Gynecology, 137*(3), 327–331.

Smirniotopoulos, T. T. (1983, October). Update on toxic shock syndrome: Recognizing and treating the mild case. *Postgraduate Medicine, 74*(4), 369, 372.

Smith, O. W. (1948, November). Diethylstilbestrol in the prevention and treatment of complications of pregnancy. *American Journal of Obstetrics and Gynecology, 56*(5), 821–833.

Smith, O. W., & Smith, G. V. S. (1949, November). The influence of diethylstilbestrol on the progress and outcome of pregnancy as based on a comparison of treated with untreated primigravidas. *American Journal of Obstetrics and Gynecology, 58*(5), 994–1009.

Sondheimer, S. J., & Flickinger, G. (1982). Prostaglandin $F_{2\alpha}$ in the peritoneal fluid of patients with endometriosis. *International Journal of Fertility, 27*(2), 73–75.

Starks, G., & Grimes, E. M. (1985, June). Clinical significance of focal pelvic endometriosis. *The Journal of Reproductive Medicine, 30*(6), 481–484.

Steele, R. W., Dmowski, W. P., & Marmer, D. J. (1984, July/August). Immunologic aspects of human endometriosis. *American Journal of Reproductive Immunology, 6*(1), 33–36.

Stenchever, M. A., Williamson, R. A., & Leonard, J., et al. (1981, May 15). Possible relationship between in utero diethylstilbestrol exposure and male fertility. *American Journal of Obstetrics and Gynecology, 140*(2), 186–193.

Stillman, R. J. (1982, April 1). In utero exposure to diethylstilbestrol: Adverse effects on the male reproductive tract and reproductive performance in male and female offspring. *American Journal of Obstetrics and Gynecology, 142*(7), 905–921.

Stolz, S. J., Davis, J. P., & Vergeront, J. M., et al. (1985, May). Development of serum antibody to toxic shock syndrome among individuals with toxic shock syndrome in Wisconsin. *The Journal of Infectious Diseases, 151*(15), 883–889.

Strathy, J., Molgaard, C. A., Coulam, C. B., & Melton, L. J. (1982, December). Endometriosis and infertility: A laparoscopic study of endometriosis among fertile and infertile women. *Fertility and Sterility, 38*(6), 667–672.

Thomas, D., & Withington, P. S. (1985, May). Toxic shock syndrome: A review of the literature. *Annals of the Royal College of Surgeons of England, 67*(3), 156–158.

Todd, J., Fishaut, M., Kapral, F., & Welch, T. (1978, November). Toxic-shock syndrome associated with phage-group-1 staphylococci. *Lancet, 2*(8100), 1116–1118.

von Numers, C. (1965). Observations on metaplastic changes in the germinal epithelium of the ovary and on the aetiology of ovarian endometriosis. *Acta Obstetricia et Gynecologica Scandinavica, 44*, 107–116.

Weed, J. C., & Arquembourg, P. C. (1980, September). Endometriosis: Can it produce an autoimmune response resulting in infertility? *Clinical Obstetrics and Gynecology, 23*(3), 885–893.

Welch, W. R., Robboy, S. J., & Kaufman, R. H., et al. (1985, July). Pathology of colposcopic findings in 2635 diethylstilbestrol-exposed young women. *Gynecologic Oncology, 21*(3), 227–286.

Wheeler, J. M., Johnston, B. M., & Malinak, L. R. (1983, May). The relationship of endometriosis to spontaneous abortion. *Fertility and Sterility, 39*(5), 656–660.

Wheeler, J. M., & Malinak, L. R. (1983, June 1). Recurrent endometriosis: Incidence, management, and prognosis. *American Journal of Obstetrics and Gynecology, 146*(3), 247–253.

Whitehead, E. D., & Leiter, E. (1981, January). Genital abnormalities and abnormal semen analyses in male patients exposed to diethylstilbestrol in utero. *The Journal of Urology, 125*(1), 47–50.

Wilson, C. (1983, December). Toxic shock syndrome and diaphragm use. *Journal of Adolescent Health Care, 4*(4), 290–291.

Witzig, D. K., & Ostwald, S. K. (1985, January). Knowledge of toxic shock syndrome among adolescent females: A need for education. *Journal of School Health, 55*(1), 17–20.

Yen, S. S. C. (1983, March). Clinical applications of gonadotropin-releasing hormones and gonadotropin-releasing hormone analogs. *Fertility and Sterility, 39*(3), 1257–1266.

SECTION IV
Menstrual Issues

The Significance of Menstruation

Perhaps more than any other body process, menstruation throughout history has been cloaked in a veil of mystery, myth, and taboo. It has been called by a variety of names, many with a connotation of ill-health. It has been the source for mythologies of female power and of female evil. It has been used, even through modern times, to deny economic, political, and social opportunity to women. All this, despite the fact that half of society menstruates with some regularity for approximately one third to one half of their lives.

Menstruation is a normal, expected, physiologic process. Indeed, the absence of regular menses, not its presence, is a cause for medical concern. It is, in fact, a process that allows for the continuation of life. We have, therefore, chosen to separate menstrual disorders from the section on pathophysiology. Some problems relating to this physiologic function certainly qualify as pathology; others are less clear. Is dysmenorrhea that does not incapacitate a woman a disease? Is premenstrual syndrome (PMS) that a woman understands and controls with diet, exercise, and stress management really a pathology? We think not.

We have devoted separate chapters to the entities of PMS and dysmenorrhea, although some research focuses on "perimenopausal" issues. We believe that current knowledge points to distinct etiologies for these problems and therefore the need for different management approaches. Although we are aware that definitive discussion of these issues cannot be achieved at this time, the extent to which women are concerned with dysmenorrhea and PMS warrants attention worthy of entire chapters.

We hope this section, although based on incomplete and evolving knowledge, will help remove menstruation from the realm of myth into the realm of scientific understanding.

19

Premenstrual Syndrome

Dayle Peck

Premenstrual syndrome (PMS) is a relatively new term. The concept entered the medical literature in 1931 when Dr. Robert Frank, an American gynecologist, coined the phrase *premenstrual tension* to describe a variety of emotional and physical symptoms occurring prior to each menstrual period. The cyclic recurrence of such symptoms is by no means new, however, and to understand the attitudes and the confusion involved in PMS today, we need to look at some of the social and cultural conditioning surrounding the phenomenon of menstruation.

This chapter provides a brief historical and social look at attitudes toward menstruation and PMS. It then defines PMS and discusses its prevalence and symptomatology. Suggested etiologies are reviewed along with proposed treatments specific to each particular theory of causality, although readers are cautioned to remember that much of this information remains speculative. A proposed classification for PMS is outlined. A framework for primary care management of PMS is offered. This includes diagnosis, teaching and counseling, patient self-assessment and self-help, and nonpharmacologic remedies such as exercise, nutrition, nutritional supplementation, and a variety of relaxation techniques.

HISTORICAL AND SOCIAL PERSPECTIVE

Since earliest recorded history, menstruation and childbearing have been at once a threat and a source of envy to men. A commonly held belief was that the unseen and mysterious forces that controlled the regular flow of blood possessed the power to create life, a power made obvious during childbearing. If these forces could create life, then they could also destroy life; hence the source of fear.

Menstrual blood has been endowed over time with both positive and negative powers. In ancient Rome, Pliny wrote in his *Natural History:* "Contact with it [menstrual blood] turns new wine sour; crops touched by it become barren, grafts die, seeds in gardens are dried up, the fruit of trees falls off, the edge of steel and the gleam of ivory are dulled, hives of bees die, even bronze and iron are at once seized by rust and a horrible smell fills the air; to taste it drives dogs mad and infects their bites with an incurable poison" (Delaney, Lupton, & Toth, 1976, p. 28).

Conversely, menstrual blood has been reputed to cure leprosy, warts, birth marks, gout, goiter, hemorrhoids, epi-

lepsy, worms, headache, and plague. It has been said to be effective as a love charm, has been claimed to ward off river demons and evil spirits, and was occasionally seen as fit to be an offering to a god (Delaney et al., 1976).

Many such myths and taboos have persisted into recent times; these ingrained social attitudes still retain significant influence. The literature regarding PMS is replete with unproven assumptions, and to this day relatively little scientific research into the syndrome has been conducted. On one extreme, the very existence of PMS as a biologic entity has been questioned, whereas, on the other, PMS has been blamed for female incompetence and, indeed, antisocial behavior.

In 1895, Dr. Mary Putnam Jacobi pinpointed the reason behind an increased medical awareness of menstrual disorders: "[I]t is in the increased attention paid to women and especially in their new function as lucrative patients . . . that we find explanation for much of the ill health among women freshly discovered today" (Jacobi, 1895, p. 175).

Many psychiatrists have claimed that PMS symptoms are nervous disorders and reflect a failure to adjust to a woman's role. Karen Horney, who authored a pioneer psychoanalytic essay on PMS, suggested that tension preceding menses is caused by the unconscious denial of a desire for a child and that the premenstruum is a burden only for those women who have conflicts about mothering (Horney, 1967).

A differing view is provided by Karen Paige who believes that premenstrual and menstrual distress is the result of cultural conditioning, that it is a social response rather than a reaction to shifts in hormone balance. Paige (1973) found that women most distressed premenstrually are those most tied to home, children, and traditional female roles.

Psychologist May Brown Parlee (1973) maintains that there is no scientific proof that PMS even exists. She points out that correlational studies fail to include control groups and that questionnaires bias responses by focusing on negative symptoms and on experiences just before and during menses. Many research tools have been designed more to assess women's incompetence than to emphasize their strengths (d'Orban, 1981; Press & Clausen, 1982).

Conversely, Katharina Dalton, a British gynecologist who pioneered research into PMS, largely from the 1950s to the 1970s, has compiled a collection of behavioral changes of women who are premenstrual. These include home, factory, and road accidents (Dalton, 1960b), misbehavior and lowered grades among schoolgirls (Dalton, 1960a, 1960c), and criminal activity (Dalton, 1961, 1980a).

An effort has also been made to implicate the premenstrual syndrome as a mitigating factor in various crimes. Some forensic psychiatrists believe that severe and ascertainable premenstrual disorders should be considered grounds for a plea of insanity.

Two unusual cases in Britain forced the legal profession to give more attention to PMS. In one, a woman was convicted of stabbing a barmaid to death, but was put on probation possibly because of her plea of PMS as an extenuating circumstance. The second case involved a woman who killed her lover. She was allowed to plead guilty to manslaughter rather than face murder charges on the grounds of ''diminished responsibility'' resulting from PMS (Dalton, 1980a).

A 1981 case in Brooklyn, New York, involved a mother of six who was arrested for beating her 4-year-old daughter. Her lawyer wanted to take the plea of PMS beyond that of a mitigating circumstance and use it as a complete defense. The lawyer claimed that the defendant's attack of PMS was so severe that she blacked out and did not know what she was doing. The lawyer's motion was denied (Holtzman, 1988).

Feminists and legal experts are concerned that such attention to PMS may cause a revival of old myths about raging hormones and female instability. They advocate treating the syndrome as a health issue, but do not support using it as a legal defense. They fear that it could be used to further discriminate against women (Holtzman, 1988; Press & Clausen, 1982).

This historical and social look toward menstruation and PMS reveals that medical, psychologic, and legal formulations are influenced by social attitudes. It highlights the many questions that remain concerning PMS. Researchers and practitioners today must consider PMS seriously, but without prejudice, seek its causes, and investigate treatments and preventive measures.

DEFINITIONS

A cohesive pathophysiologic formulation for PMS has yet to be established; however, physiologists, gynecologists, nurses, and psychiatrists agree on certain fundamental facts:

1. Premenstrual syndrome is a clinical entity that is somatic, not psychic, in origin.
2. PMS is a complex mechanism. It may have its origin in the disturbance of the ovarian cycle and the balance of hormones, but it reaches out to involve other endocrine gland functions and both the autonomic and central nervous systems.
3. Disturbances of endocrine control with repercussions on the nervous system lead to marked changes in the physiochemical equilibrium of the body. A predominant alteration is retention of body fluids.

Although there is no universally accepted definition of PMS, some researchers have defined criteria for inclusion of women into studies of PMS. Walton and Youngkin (1987, p. 175) accepted women into their study as PMS sufferers only if their symptoms occurred cyclically 1 to 14 days before menses or during the first days of menses; were relieved by menses; were absent for at least 7 days after menstruation; and caused difficulty in coping with daily activities and interpersonal relationships during the symptomatic period. Haskett, Steiner, Osmun, and Carroll (1980) used the following criteria for inclusion into their study: premenstrual dysphoric symptoms for at least six menstrual cycles; moderate to severe physical and psychological symptoms; symptoms only during the premenstrual period with relief at the onset of menses; age between 18 and 45 years; not pregnant; not using hormonal contraception; regular menses for six previous cycles; no psychiatric disorder; normal physical examination and laboratory profile; no drugs for 4 weeks preceding the study and no use during the study of antianxiety medications, diuretics, hormones, or neuroleptics. With such rigid criteria, five out of six volunteers for this study did not qualify.

PREVALENCE

Although bias in studies of PMS leads to overestimation of its prevalence, most authors believe it to occur in 20 to 60 percent of women of menstrual age (Hargrove & Abraham, 1982; Reid & Yen, 1981; Woods, Most, & Dery, 1982). Up to 20 to 40 percent of women suffer some degree of incapacitation (Reid & Yen, 1981). Golub (1988) reports higher rates of PMS among women in their thirties and forties than among younger women.

SYMPTOMS

PMS encompasses a wide variety of symptoms and a spectrum of severity ranging from mild to severe. Reported manifestations of PMS include the following (Greene & Dalton, 1953; Reid & Yen, 1981; Woods et al., 1982):

Somatic

- Headache/migraine
- Breast swelling/tenderness
- Abdominal bloating
- Nausea
- Edema of extremities
- Joint pain
- Backache
- Pelvic/low abdominal pain
- Increased thirst or appetite
- Hay fever/asthma/coryza (allergic rhinitis)
- Cravings for sweets or salty foods
- Cold sweats
- Feeling not quite well
- Palpitations
- Ulcerative stomatitis
- Herpes
- Dermatosis/acneiform eruptions
- Hives
- Pinkeye/sties
- Glaucoma
- Increase in refractive errors in vision
- Hot flashes
- Epileptiform seizures
- Spot bruising
- Constipation
- Lack of coordination

Psychogenic

- Fatigue
- Depression
- Irritability and tension
- Lack of concentration/distractibility

- Insomnia
- Aggressiveness
- Moodiness/mood swings
- Indecision, inefficiency
- Psychotic episodes precipitated by PMS
- Forgetfulness
- Crying easily
- Confusion
- Loneliness

Among the symptoms attributed to PMS, those affecting motor and cognitive function are the most controversial (Coyne, Woods, & Mitchell, 1985). In a critical review of the literature, Sommer (1983) concluded that the aggregate evidence does not support menstrual cycle effect on cognitive ability or work or academic performance. Even investigators whose studies have shown cyclic differences in cognitive task performance have pointed out that such changes "should not be taken as evidence of a functionally significant impairment or enhancement of abilities at different stages of the cycle" and have noted that males also experience cyclicity in cognitive performance (Broverman et al., 1981, p. 653).

CLASSIFICATION

As interest in PMS has grown and analysis has become more detailed, symptoms have been grouped and classified

TABLE 19-1. CLASSIFICATION OF PREMENSTRUAL SYNDROME (PREMENSTRUAL TENSION)

PMT-A

Most common

Symptoms: anxiety, irritability, nervous tension (Sufferers may report increased consumption of dairy products and refined sugar.)

Physiology: high serum estrogen, low serum progesterone

Treatment: vitamin B_6 200 to 800 mg daily, to reduce serum estrogen; magnesium 340 mg daily; progesterone

PMT-B

Symptoms: edema, adbominal bloating, mastalgia, weight gain

Physiology: high sodium and water retention; high serum aldosterone

Treatment: vitamin B_6, 100 to 200 mg daily, to suppress aldosterone and cause diuresis; reduction of sodium intake to 3 g per day; increase in vitamin E up to 600 units daily to improve breast symptoms; increase in intake of natural diuretics

PMT-C

Symptoms: increased appetite, craving for sweets; increased intake of refined sugar followed by palpitations, fatigue, fainting spells, headache, tremors

Physiology: increased carbohydrate tolerance, low red cell magnesium

Treatment: magnesium 340 mg daily.

PMT-D

Least common, most serious

Symptoms: depression, withdrawal, insomnia, forgetfulness, confusion

Physiology: low serum estrogen, high progesterone, elevated adrenal androgens

Treatment: complete medical evaluation and prescription medication as indicated

From Hargrove, J. T., and Abraham, G. E. (1982). The incidence of premenstrual tension in a gynecologic clinic. Journal of Reproductive Medicine, 27(12), 721–724.

and causes and treatments for each group have been explored, although not proven. A proposed classification of PMS is outlined in Table 19-1. In this classification system, premenstrual syndrome is referred to as premenstrual tension (PMT). This terminology has the potential for confusion, however, as tension symptoms are only one manifestation of premenstrual symptomatology. Some authors use the terminology *premenstrual tension syndrome* (PTS).

SUGGESTED CAUSES AND TREATMENTS

To date, there is no proven cause of PMS or universally accepted treatment for the syndrome. A variety of treatments have been proposed over the years, based on theorized etiologic agents. Because the body organs and systems involved in PMS are often multiple and the symptoms not well defined, it is difficult to demonstrate a single etiologic agent. The methodologies used in studies examining treatment efficacy have varied. Not all researchers have used clinical trials with control groups; it is difficult to compare the therapies. Although impressive results have been demonstrated, many studies lack adequate controls and/or large sample sizes and must, therefore, be regarded as dubious. Uncontrolled studies often result in a favorable outcome for the product in question.

The suggested etiologies and treatments discussed in this section are progesterone deficiency/progesterone replacement; endogenous hormonal changes/exogenous hormonal therapy; endogenous hormone allergy/desensitization therapy; prolactin/bromocriptine therapy; aldosterone/aldactone therapy; electrolyte changes/diuretic therapy; psychogenic causes/lithium carbonate, antidepressant therapy; and prostaglandin/prostaglandin inhibitors.

Self-help measures, including exercise, nutrition and nutritional supplementation, and relaxation techniques are considered under Primary Care Management.

Progesterone Deficiency/Progesterone Replacement

Progesterone deficiency is a popular etiologic theory for PMS. As early as 1931, Frank proposed that PMS was due to excessive blood levels of the female sex hormone—estrogen. In 1938, Israel maintained that excess estrogen was not the cause of PMS; deficient progesterone production, leading to unopposed estrogen, actually was responsible for PMS. Unopposed estrogen was believed to cause fluid retention, hyperplasia of breast tissue, abnormal carbohydrate metabolism—an increased tolerance to sugar—and central nervous system manifestations secondary to accumulation of estrogen within the limbic system (Reid & Yen, 1981).

Dalton (1980b) maintains the following:

1. Progesterone is formed in the adrenals from simpler compounds. It is present throughout the entire menstrual cycle and is the essential basis for all corticosteroids.
2. Progesterone is produced by the ovary only during the luteal phase of the menstrual cycle.

Dalton suggests that if production of progesterone by the ovary is insufficient in the premenstruum to meet the requirements of the uterus, some is taken from the adrenals, leaving them deficient for the production of corticosteroids. This may result in water retention; imbalance of sodium and potassium, both intra- and extracellularly; and failure to control allergic reactions.

Dalton also contends that it is not the estrogen or progesterone that is significant, but the ratio between the two, and that PMS results from an imbalance in this ratio.

Dalton began experimenting with the administration of natural progesterone, extracted from yam and soybean plants, in the early 1950s. This progesterone cannot be administered orally because it is rapidly metabolized by the portal system of the liver and has a half-life of 15 minutes. Unlike medroxyprogesterone acetate (Depo-Provera) or the hormones in oral contraceptives, this compound is identical to the body's own. It must be given by the rectal, vaginal, or parenteral route (Gonzalez, 1981a).

An intramuscular dose of 100 mg results in midpregnancy levels of progesterone that are maintained for about 48 hours. When it is given vaginally and rectally, normal luteal phase levels are reached in 4 and 8 hours, respectively, and then gradually decline to follicular phase levels after 24 hours.

Dalton has used progesterone with apparent success for over 30 years. She recommends rectal or vaginal dosages ranging from 100 to 400 mg three times a day or intramuscular dosages from 50 mg on alternate days to 100 mg daily. Treatment should begin approximately 5 days before symptoms are expected. Dalton believes that these dosages cannot be dangerous, because in pregnancy progesterone levels reach 15 times the normal. She reports an 83 to 95 percent success rate with this regimen with no significant alteration of menstrual cycles (Dalton, 1980b; Gonzalez, 1981b; Greene & Dalton, 1953; Sampson, 1979; Swaffield, 1980).

Not all studies have reflected the high success rate achieved by Dalton, and her research has been widely criticized for its lack of controls. In 1979, Sampson conducted a double-blind, controlled study using progesterone in both 200- and 400-mg doses against a placebo. Thirty-one percent of the women receiving 200 mg per day reported progesterone to be more effective than placebo in relieving their symptoms. Forty-three percent, however, reported placebo more effective than progesterone. When the dose was increased to 400 mg per day, only 27 percent reported progesterone more effective and 35 percent gave the placebo the higher rating. Fifteen percent reported both equally helpful. There was never a statistically significant difference between the two.

Maddocks, Hahn, Moller, and Reid (1986) conducted a double-blind, placebo-controlled crossover clinical trial of progesterone. Twenty women used a 200-mg vaginal suppository twice a day for 12 days before menses for 3 months, followed by a placebo for 3 months. The researchers found only marginal effectiveness of progesterone compared with placebo.

There are few side effects proven to be caused by progesterone, but patients have reported nausea, breast discomfort, increased edema, and alterations in the menstrual cycle including irregular bleeding, dysmenorrhea, excessive bleeding, and complete suppression of menstruation (Kerr et al., 1980; Sampson, 1979).

Because of the inconvenience, discomfort, and expense of natural progesterone therapy, some research has examined the efficacy of synthetic compounds. The most prominent among these is dydrogesterone, a stereoisomer of progesterone. It has similar effects but does not inhibit the gonadotropins, so it does not prevent ovulation or disrupt the menstrual cycle. It serves to balance existing progesterone in relation to 17β-estradiol during the second half of the cycle.

Dydrogesterone is given orally, 10 mg twice a day. Good results have been reported especially in relief of depression, headache, and edema, and poor results in alleviation of breast tenderness (Kerr et al., 1980; Taylor, 1977).

Endogenous Hormonal Changes/Exogenous Hormonal Therapy

One of the earliest causal theories for PMS suggested an imbalance in the premenstrual phase between the ovarian steroids estradiol and progesterone (Israel, 1938). Exogenous hormonal therapy in the treatment of PMS includes various oral contraceptives and danazol, an androgenic steroid.

Studies in this area are relatively inconclusive. Many methodologic concerns exist that create problems in drawing accurate conclusions regarding the effectiveness of oral contraceptives in treating PMS. These include selection bias, poor choice of experimental design, and lack of adequate controls (Goldzieher, Moses, Averkin, Scheel, & Taber, 1971). The birth control pills used in many studies are of high dose compared with pills used today.

One study of 398 subjects involving Oracon, Ovulen, and Norinyl (see Chapter 7) yielded no statistically significant success in alleviation of PMS sysmptoms (Goldzieher et al., 1971). Another study of 152 oral contraceptive users showed improvement in premenstrual depression and irritability but not in premenstrual headache or swelling (Herzberg & Coppen, 1970); however, 6 percent of the pill group complained of depression, compared with 2 percent of the control group of 40. A study of more than 5,000 women revealed that those taking combination pills had significantly less severe premenstrual depression than sequential users (Kutner & Brown, 1972).

Some experimentation also has been done with Enovid, a high-dose oral contraceptive containing 0.15 percent of the 3-methyl ether of ethinyl estradiol (mestranol). As a treatment for PMS it is given orally, 10 mg per day, beginning on day 5 of the cycle and continuing for 20 days. Enovid seems to afford good relief of some symptoms including irritability, acne, and cramping, but is associated with a high incidence of side effects. Almost 90 percent of 25 users studied reported mild to marked nausea, 44 percent demonstrated delayed menses, 32 percent reported increased bloating, and 88 percent complained of excessive breast engorgement. It would appear that in this case the treatment is as bad or worse than the disease (Hood & Bond, 1959). Such high-dose oral contraceptives are no longer used for contraception.

Minimal experimentation has been done with danazol, a weakly androgenic, anabolic steroid that is a powerful antigonadotropin. Its exact mechanism of action is unclear but it decreases the formation of the endometrium and renders the patient amenorrheic. Taken throughout the cycle, in daily doses of 200 to 800 mg, with a mean of 400 mg, danazol suppresses plasma estradiol to levels comparable to those found in the early follicular phase and decreases amounts of plasma estrone, progesterone, and prolactin. Sarno, Miller, and Lundblad (1987) found significant results in a double-blind, crossover clinical trial of 14 women taking 200 mg of danazol or placebo daily. Although this study demonstrated good results with minimal side effects, danazol can cause increased serum sodium, potassium, and albumin; weight gain from 3 to 5 kg; decreased libido; breast reduction; deepening of the voice; and menopausal symptomatology. A large number of women give up its use for these reasons (Day, 1979; Hood & Bond, 1959). This drug is also very expensive. Chapter 18 discusses danazol more extensively in the section on Endometriosis.

ENDOGENOUS HORMONE ALLERGY/ DESENSITIZATION THERAPY

Gerber (1921) and Urbach (1939) were among the first to demonstrate experimentally that premenstrual urticaria resulted from hypersensitivity to some specific substance that appeared in the serum during the premenstruum. Symptoms could be produced in sensitive individuals, but not in normal subjects, by injection of serum collected premenstrually. Patients could be desensitized by intradermal injection with serum from affected women (Reid & Yen, 1981; Rogers, 1962).

It has been demonstrated that symptoms of PMS in selected cases can be attributed to a similar hypersensitivity to endogenous hormones or their metabolites. Intracutaneous injection of estradiol/estrone has yielded a positive reaction in women with severe PMS but not in women without the disease (Reid & Yen, 1981). In 1945, in a series of women with disorders related to the menstrual cycle, 80 percent of 79 women were found, on skin testing, to be allergic to pregnanediol, a metabolite of progesterone. One study found that if pregnanediol were given orally in small doses, patients decreased their sensitivity to it. Good results were obtained in the relief of depression, irritability, nervousness, bloating, mastalgia, and weight gain (Reid & Yen, 1981; Rogers, 1962).

A study of 138 women revealed a high incidence of personal or familial history of allergy, positive skin test reactions to conventional allergens, eosinophilia, low titers on histamine latex test, and high levels of immunoglobulin E in the PMS patients compared with normal controls. Another study tested the results of a course of treatment using a γ-globulin/histamine complex in a group of 40 women known to suffer from PMS. Subcutaneous injection of the complex on days 6, 13, and 20 of the first cycle, days 13 and 20 of the second cycle, and day 20 of the third cycle, with a booster 6 months after the last injection, yielded a 70 percent satisfactory response. After 2 years the success rate remained at 60 percent. This was especially effective in patients with premenstrual migraine headaches (Atton-Chamla et al., 1980).

Prolactin/Bromocriptine Therapy

Prolactin affects water and electrolyte balance and influences cerebral function. Because of these properties it has been implicated in PMS.

Normal plasma prolactin levels are reported to show a circadian-type rhythm, with higher levels occurring during sleep and marked individual fluctuation from day to day, peaking about the time of ovulation. Prolactin levels are higher in the luteal phase than in the follicular phase. The hypothalamus plays an essential role in controlling prolactin levels, exerting primarily an inhibiting effect on its production. Prolactin can inhibit luteinizing hormone-releasing factor (LHRF), which in turn suppresses formation of the gonadotropic hormones (luteninizing hormone follicle-stimulating hormone). It thus alters the amounts of estrogen and progesterone secreted (Andersch & Hahn, 1982; Andersch, Abrahamsson, Wendestam, Ohman, & Hahn, 1979; Elsner, Buster, Schlinder, Nessim, & Abraham, 1980).

Bromocriptine (Parlodel) is an ergot alkaloid that acts at the dopamine receptor sites in the hypothalamus to enhance prolactin inhibitory factor activity. It also causes the prolactin secretory cells in the anterior pituitary gland to suppress prolactin production (Graham, Harding, Wise, & Berriman, 1978).

It is possible that the fluid retention, mood changes, and altered prolactin secretion found in PMS patients are all secondary to changes in the neurotransmitter function of the central nervous system and that the effect of bromocriptine is directly related to its dopaminergic action at one or more sites. The drug does not alter levels of estrogen or progesterone and does not affect menstrual cycle length (Andersch et al., 1979).

The most significant improvements with bromocriptine therapy have been found in the symptoms of breast tenderness, bloating, and depression. These symptoms have also responded well to placebo, however, which may emphasize the psychological component of PMS as well as the need for caution in the interpretation of any uncontrolled trials of therapy (Elsner et al., 1980).

Aldosterone/Aldactone Therapy

Estrogen possibly causes increased synthesis of plasma renin substrate in the liver. This causes elevation of plasma renin activity and plasma angiotensin II, which in turn results in elevated secretion and excretion of aldosterone.

Aldosterone is probably the most potent naturally occurring sodium hormone known. Its most important effect is to increase the rate of tubular reabsorption of sodium, which in turn increases water retention.

Progesterone, conversely, is sodium depleting and appears to be a partial antagonist to aldosterone by blocking its action at the renal tubules. Changes in progesterone levels usually are followed by parallel changes in aldosterone levels.

Because spironolactone or aldactone is a specific aldosterone antagonist, a few studies have tested its effectiveness in relieving PMS symptoms. Aldactone acts primarily by competing with aldosterone for receptor sites at the aldosterone-dependent sodium–potassium exchange site in the distal convoluted tubule. It causes excretion of water and sodium while sparing potassium. It has been found useful in relieving the edema and ascites found in congestive heart failure, hepatic cirrhosis, and nephrotic syndrome and in treating hypertension.

Aldactone dosages range from 25 to 200 mg. orally per day. Peak serum levels are attained 2 to 4 hours after administration. The few studies investigating its effect have been inconclusive at best. Treatment with aldactone has resulted in decreased weight gain and improvement of psychological symptoms in 80 percent of 28 treated patients. Aldosterone levels have not been significantly altered, however, and in some instances have been raised. It is generally believed that whatever positive effects aldactone may have are due to its action as a diuretic. Its side effects include gastrointestinal symptoms and palpitations, and it is known to be a carcinogen in higher doses. Its routine use in the treatment of PMS is therefore questionable (O'Brien, Craven, & Selby, 1979).

Electrolyte Changes/Diuretic Therapy

Another school of thought proposes that PMS is a result of the electrolyte changes brought about by the hormonal shifts toward the end of the menstrual cycle. Specifically, this involves retention of the sodium ion, which directly influences the accumulation of extracellular fluid in body tissues. According to this theory, neurologic symptoms result from edema of the nervous system, particularly the brain. Nausea and bloating are due to fluid buildup in the intestine, and other symptoms stem from edema of individual organs (Greenhill & Freed, 1940; Reeves, Garvin, & McElin, 1971).

Several authors have recommended the use of exogenous diuretics to alleviate PMS symptoms. Because potassium deficiency correlates with edema and its replacement has been effective in treating cyclic edema, potassium chloride has been investigated as a possible therapy for PMS. Studies, however, have not proven it to be any more effective than a placebo for symptomatic relief in cases of PMS (Reeves et al., 1971).

Investigators also have tested the efficacy of ammonium chloride or ammonium nitrate—salts often used to eliminate retained fluid in cardiac and renal disturbances. In the few studies conducted, patient groups have been small, and, although researchers claim almost 100 percent success, no controls have been used; findings are therefore unreliable (Greenhill & Freed, 1940).

One study tested the effectiveness of a drug called Tenavoid, which is a combination of bendrofluazide, a diuretic, and 200 mg of meprobamate (Miltown), a tranquilizer. Tenavoid was compared in a crossover study with placebo, bendrofluazide alone, and meprobamate alone. One tablet was taken by 105 subjects three times a day on the days when symptoms occurred, up to a maximum of 7 days before the expected onset of menstruation. The study reported a higher success rate with Tenavoid than with each of its separate ingredients or placebo. Side effects included palpitations, dyspnea, weakness, nocturia and urinary frequency, vertigo, indigestion, and headache (Carstairs & Talbot, 1981). Tranquilizers also have the potential for addiction.

Psychogenic Causes/Lithium Carbonate, Antidepressant Therapy

Researchers have postulated that because lithium carbonate has been proven beneficial in the control of manic states and schizophrenia and because PMS seems to be clinically similar to these excitement conditions, this drug could be beneficial in treating PMS. Lithium has the capacity to affect enzymes, alter nerve excitability, influence hormonal behavior, and favorably influence clinical states resembling PMS. It is possible that lithium competes with sodium ions for enzyme sites and regularly causes a considerable diuresis of sodium and water. Of the several studies investigating lithium, most are skewed because the groups used were already under psychiatric care for other disorders and were on other medications including oral contraceptives (Glick & Stewart, 1980).

To maintain serum concentrations at an optimal level, daily oral dosages of lithium ranging from 750 to 2,400 mg in divided doses are used. In some instances, lithium has served to stabilize mood swings and decrease episodic aggressive and hyperactive behavior (Glick & Stewart, 1980). Most findings, however, are that lithium is ineffective against somatic PMS symptoms and has little influence on behavioral symptoms in most women (Steiner, Haskett, Osmun, & Carroll, 1980). When lithium has been compared with placebo, minimal, if any, difference has been demonstrated (Singer, Cheung, & Schou, 1974; Steiner & Carroll, 1977). In addition, lithium has significant side effects including tremors, weakness, nausea, vomiting, abdominal cramping, confusion, blurred vision, and water retention. For these reasons it is not generally recommended for use unless the woman has other concomitant psychological dis-

orders for which it is effective. Such patients should receive ongoing psychiatric care.

In a double-blind, placebo-controlled crossover study, oral alprazolam was prescribed in low doses (25 mg three times a day) for PMS (Smith, Rinehart, Ruddock, & Schiff, 1987). This drug has antianxiety, antidepressant, and smooth muscle relaxant effects. Significant reductions in severity of nervous tension, mood swings, irritability, anxiety, depression, fatigue, forgetfulness, crying, cravings for sweets, abdominal bloating, abdominal cramps, and headache were found. The only side effect demonstrated was daytime sedation.

Prostaglandin/Prostaglandin Inhibitors

Some work has been done recently on the use of prostaglandin inhibitors for relief of premenstrual symptoms. Forms of prostaglandins are found throughout the body. Varying levels in the reproductive tract affect the cyclic regression of the corpus luteum and the decidual reaction and menstrual endometrial shedding. Prostaglandins play a significant role in dysmenorrhea (see Chapter 20).

Prostaglandins in the breast tissue may cause premenstrual vasodilation and pain. Prostaglandins are also formed at multiple sites in the central nervous system and may play a part in regulation of body water content, appetite, and body temperature, and stimulate release of antidiuretic hormone. Produced in both the medulla and cortex of the kidney, prostaglandins participate in the control of renal blood flow and renin release, as well as mediate the action of loop diuretics, modulate the water permeability response of the kidney to vasopressin, and maintain the glomerular filtration rate at normal levels. They may play a part in certain affective disorders.

Antiprostaglandins such as mefanamic acid (Ponstel) may relieve such symptoms as breast tenderness, abdominal bloating, and ankle swelling, but no improvement has been found in decreasing tension, lethargy, or depression. No studies yet have produced reliable conclusions and further research is required in this area (Budoff, 1983; Wood & Jakubowicz, 1980).

PRIMARY CARE MANAGEMENT

Diagnosis

Data Collection

HISTORY TAKING. The diagnosis of PMS is made through careful history taking. No physical findings or laboratory tests have proven useful although some chemical alterations have been found. PMS must be distinguished from dysmenorrhea; PMS is not primarily a pain response (Shangold, 1983).

Some women present to care providers because of PMS. Others, believing it is woman's lot to suffer, or simply unaware of the existence of treatment modalities, do not consider it valuable to seek help for their symptoms. It is up to the practitioner to take a thorough menstrual history (see Chapter 2) and assist each woman in recognizing and reporting her symptoms and assessing their severity. This assessment is necessarily subjective and can be made only in terms of each woman's life-style, activities, expectations, and goals for herself. A diagnosis based on the classification of PMS presented in Table 19–1 can then be made.

Frank (1986) describes several PMS treatment programs run by nurse-practitioners. These experts recommend conducting the initial PMS consultation during the asymptomatic follicular phase of the menstrual cycle (from menses to ovulation). History taking includes a careful delineation of symptoms, their onset, change over time, severity, degree of disability, and any treatments or self-help measures that have been tried; a nutritional history, with particular attention given to alcohol, salt, and caffeine use; a medical history to rule out symptoms or previous diagnoses of anemia, diabetes, or thyroid disorders, which may either contribute to PMS or be mistaken for it; a gynecologic history to rule out endometriosis in which symptoms also begin premenstrually (see Chapter 18); and an occupational and social history focusing on life-style, support systems, and reactions of significant others to the problem.

PHYSICAL EXAMINATION. Although physical assessment cannot diagnose PMS, it is useful in ruling out other conditions. Lauersen (1985) suggests including weight, blood pressure, heart and lung assessment, and breast and pelvic examination. A rectal examination may be useful in ruling out endometriosis. The thyroid gland should also be palpated.

LABORATORY DATA. Lauersen recommends a Pap smear, including a maturation index, taken from the upper lateral third of the vagina to indicate estrogenization of the vaginal tissues. Suggested blood tests include a CBC to rule out systemic infection and anemia, thyroid studies, and hormonal levels including follicle-stimulating hormone/luteinizing hormone, serum estradiol, serum progesterone, and serum prolactin. Hormonal levels should be drawn 1 to 7 days prior to menstruation or at the time of the woman's most severe symptoms. Hormonal levels can be correlated with the classification of PMS (Table 19–1). This type of assessment, however, has not been proven to be of value and is not widely advocated.

Intervention

It is the joint responsibility of practitioner and patient to plan the management of the patient's PMS. Counseling and education include providing information about available options. A good beginning treatment is to provide supportive teaching and counseling, to build the woman's self-esteem, and to recommend self-assessment and self-help measures including stress reduction, nutritional changes and/or a regimen of dietary supplementation, and exercise. These should be appropriate for the type of premenstrual tension experienced.

Teaching and Counseling. The first step in patient education and counseling is to assist the woman to know herself. Teach her to identify her own symptoms. Are they manifested primarily physically or psychologically? Do events in her life trigger or exacerbate any symptoms? Advise her to keep a journal or calendar, to know when symptoms occur, learn to anticipate the difficult times, and plan accordingly. Each person must examine her own life-style and determine whether or not she is doing all she can to help herself and must assess her own motivation and desire to participate in self-assessment and self-help.

Self-Assessment. A woman can be advised to keep a 3-month history of her symptoms. She can devise a check-off sheet with each of her PMS symptoms listed down the side of the page and the numbered days of the cycle across the top. She then grades the severity of symptoms on each cycle day. Grading levels are none; mild—present but not interfering with activities; moderate—present and interfering with activities but not disabling; and severe—disabling. Presence and amount of menses are also recorded. A food diary that includes all intake and cravings can also be maintained. A follow-up visit after several months of self-assessment can help a woman interpret her findings.

Self-Help. There are three cardinal rules in a self-help program for PMS:

1. Reduce stress as much as possible.
2. Build up the body's natural defenses.
3. Alleviate the symptoms.

As much as possible, affected women should reduce activities or encounters that increase stress. Tasks should be delegated when possible. Coyne, Woods, and Mitchell (1985) suggest presenting self-management strategies to women. These may include putting off important decisions or preparing ahead of time for them. These authors emphasize that this is done not because women cannot be trusted to make decisions but simply to help reduce stress that may be associated with PMS. They also urge that suggestions be offered in a positive way and women be assisted to reject premenstrual stereotyping.

A woman can be advised to discuss her problem. Partners, children, parents, or friends—the people with whom a woman lives or works—usually bear the brunt of the difficult times. In a study of the personal and family impact of PMS, Brown and Zimmer (1986) report that increased conflict, decreased family cohesion, and disrupted communication among family members may result. It is important, therefore, for PMS sufferers to be as honest as possible with family members and significant others. Their support is vital, but unless a woman communicates with them, they will have trouble understanding and helping. Family members and support persons can be welcomed to provider visits at which PMS is discussed.

Support groups or educational sessions have been advocated for PMS sufferers and their families (Heinz, 1986; Walton & Youngkin, 1987). Rome (1986) suggests that woman-run self-help groups can serve as a forum for sharing information, discussing feelings, setting up phone-support systems, and providing mutual assistance with tasks during the premenstrual period. Practitioners can certainly be instrumental in organizing such groups.

EXERCISE. A great deal is being written about the benefit of exercise; it may be as important in diminishing the symptoms of PMS as it is in promoting other aspects of health. Daily, vigorous exercise strengthens body–mind integration, promotes psychological and physical feelings of well-being, and helps the body balance itself under stress. Exercises designed to stretch and tone the muscles, performed daily or at least 3 to 4 days a week, have been found to increase oxygenation and aid in decreasing stress (Lever, Brush, & Haynes, 1982; Timonen & Procopé, 1971).

Although the effect of exercise in premenstrual syndrome has not been extensively examined, several studies have found it to be beneficial. In one, university students who were involved in competitive sports and exercised regularly reported less pain before and during menstruation and significantly less premenstrual headache, nervousness, irritability, anxiety, and depression than sedentary students, who constituted the control group (Timonen & Procopé, 1971). The active students also used less analgesia for PMS symptoms than the control group. In a prospective study, Prior, Vigna, Sciaretta, Alojado, and Schulzer (1987) found that 6 months of exercise training was associated with decreased premenstrual symptoms in 15 women compared with 6 women whose activities did not change during the study period. Particular symptoms that were affected included breast awareness and tenderness, fluid retention and bloating, and personal stress. Feelings of anxiety tended to decrease although not to a significant level. Changes in hormonal status, menstrual patterns, and weight were not noted.

Several possible mechanisms may explain positive effects of exercise on PMS. It has been suggested that a greater circulatory capacity is required premenstrually for satisfactory perfusion of the brain because of the presence of some peripheral factor, probably edema. It is reasonable to assume that exercise improves or stabilizes circulation to the brain, increases the total capacity of the circulatory system, and improves the oxygenating ability of the cardiopulmonary pump (Timonen & Procopé, 1971). Exercise has also been found to increase blood levels of β-endorphins (Colt, Wardlaw, & Frantz, 1981; Farrell, Gates, Maksud, & Morgan, 1982; Fraioli, Moretti, Paolucci, Alicicco, & Crescenzi, 1980). Although the physiologic value of this has not been definitely established, β-endorphins have been associated with analgesia and euphoria (Farrell et al., 1982). The role of these substances in PMS is the focus of ongoing research. Daily levels of β-endorphins throughout the menstrual cycle are currently being investigated to determine whether PMS patients have persistently lowered premenstrual levels (Chuong & Coulam, 1988, p. 83). A deficiency of these substances may prove to be a significant etiologic agent in PMS.

Aerobic exercise also has been shown to decrease resting muscle action potential, an effect described as tranquilizing (deVries, 1968; deVries, Wiswell, Bulbulian, & Moritani, 1981). This may be significant for PMS; in at least one study, increased muscle tension was found to be present during the premenstrual period (Coyne, 1983).

Canty (1984) suggests an exercise program for PMS consisting of 20 to 30 minutes of aerobic workouts at least four times a week with cycle modifications in intensity and type of exercise according to PMS symptoms. She acknowledges that the effects of exercise on PMS need further testing before it can be scientifically considered beneficial.

NUTRITION. Few researchers have actually looked at the relationship of PMS to diet. One study, however, of 295 college sophomores showed a positive correlation between consumption of caffeine-containing beverages and PMS, although this does not prove causality (Rossignol, 1985). In addition, many women have an altered glucose tolerance during the premenstrual phase that results in an actual or at least relative hypoglycemia; this can add to the fatigue, depression, and irritability of PMS (Lever et al., 1982).

Many women with PMS symptoms have poor eating habits. They may be deficient in many nutrients. A woman should eat sensibly even if on a diet. She should be aware of the cycles of her body. There may be food cravings and a small weight gain during the few days before menses. A balanced, nutritious diet is most important for the prevention and/or relief of PMS during this time, though it may be harder to stick to a diet during premenstrual days.

Dietary revisions should include the following:

1. Limiting consumption of refined sugar (up to 5 tablespoons/day), salt (up to 3 g/day), red meat (up to 3 oz/day), alcohol (no more than 1 oz/day), and substances with caffeine—coffee, tea, and chocolate
2. Limiting tobacco use
3. Limiting intake of protein to 1 g/kg body weight per day
4. Relying more on fish, poultry, whole grains, and legumes as sources of protein and less on red meat and dairy products
5. Limiting dairy products to two servings per day. Using low-fat or no-fat dairy products (Calcium supplementation may be necessary; see Chapter 24.)
6. Limiting intake of fats, mainly saturated and cooked, to less than 20 percent of total calories
7. Increasing intake of complex carbohydrates to between 60 and 70 percent of calories
8. Increasing intake of green leafy vegetables, legumes, whole grains, and cereals
9. Eating smaller, more frequent meals to maintain blood sugar levels
10. Using natural diuretics to reduce fluid retention (These include water, celery juice, cucumber, watermelon, and many herbal teas such as parsley tea.)

Instruct patients to read food labels carefully. Be sure it is understood that dietary adjustments must be adhered to daily and for several months for effects to be noticeable. Referral to a nutritionist may be beneficial.

NUTRITIONAL SUPPLEMENTS. Certain minerals and vitamins can be supplemented. Calcium, magnesium, vitamins A, B6, and E, and evening primrose oil all have been suggested for relief of PMS.

Although Dalton believes that there is no scientific basis for the addition of calcium, it may help to ease stomach cramps and muscle pain. Begin with 800 to 1,000 mg in tablet form. (See Chapter 24 for additional discussion of calcium supplementation.) Magnesium may be beneficial in view of the fact that many women with PMS symptoms have demonstrated low serum magnesium levels (Abraham & Lubran, 1981; Kumar, Zourlas, & Barnes, 1963). Good results have been obtained with the administration of magnesium 340 mg daily in the form of magnesium sulfate for at least 6 weeks (Abraham, 1983).

Some research has been done into the use of vitamin A for PMS. The underlying mechanism of its action is not entirely clear. Carotene inactivates thyroxine and reduces thyroid hyperactivity, as well as the accompanying increased tone of the sympathetic nervous system that often exists premenstrually. Carotene also is believed to participate in the inactivation of estrogen in the liver, thus helping to counteract premenstrual hyperestrogenism. Still another theory is that it acts purely as a diuretic, although this has not been substantiated.

In one study, 218 patients were given vitamin A 200,000 to 300,000 units a day on the days symptoms were usually experienced. Ninety percent of the patients reported moderate to good improvement of symptoms, especially tension and headache. Unfortunately, the evaluation was subjective and no controls were used (Block, 1960). Overdosage with vitamin A is possible; women must be cautioned against megadoses.

Pyridoxine (vitamin B6) has recently gained much popularity for the treatment of PMS symptoms. Vitamin B_6 exists in the cells in the form of pyridoxal phosphate. Its most important role is that of coenzyme for the synthesis of amino acids. It is also believed to act in the transport of some amino acids across cell membranes.

In the 1940s, vitamin B_6 was thought to play some part in correcting aberrant estrogen metabolism, but, more recently, attention has turned to its role in the regulation of brain monoamine production. It is now known that vitamin B_6 in the form of pyridoxal phosphate acts as a coenzyme in the final step of the biosynthesis of the neurotransmitters dopamine and serotonin from tyrosine and tryptophan, respectively.

A deficiency of vitamin B_6 causes abnormal urinary excretion of tryptophan metabolites, a phenomenon observed in pregnancy and in patients treated with oral contraceptives. It may be deduced, then, that an excessive amount of unopposed estrogen may cause an actual or relative deficiency of vitamin B_6. When this happens, the vitamin's function as a coenzyme is impaired and a deficiency of dopamine and serotonin results. This, in turn, can cause depression, irritability, and a decrease in mental alertness. Vitamin B_6 in high doses suppresses aldosterone and results in diuresis.

Good results have been reported with administration of vitamin B_6 50 to 200 mg daily for 10 days prior to the onset of menses. More than 200 mg a day may cause some gastric disturbances, but is otherwise not contraindicated if required for relief of symptoms (Abraham, 1983).

Other research indicates that the best success can be obtained with administration of vitamin B_6 up to 100 mg/20 kg body weight per day in three divided doses throughout the menstrual cycle. After 3 to 6 months of therapy, B_6 is beneficial in its impact on prolactin levels, estrogen metabolism in the liver, and glucose utilization in the brain (Abraham, 1983; Rose, 1978; Wilhelm-Haas, 1984).

Some work is currently being done to determine the effectiveness of vitamin E on certain PMS symptoms. It is possible that vitamin E enhances production of prostaglandin E, which has an inhibitory effect on prolactin (although prolactin's role in PMS is still questionable). Vitamin E has shown some success in alleviating fibrocystic breast changes (see Chapter 10); because symptoms of fibrocystic breasts increase during the luteal phase, vitamin E is being studied for use in PMS at 150, 300, and 600 units per day in divided doses (Abraham, 1983; London, Sundaram, Murphy, & Goldstein, 1983; Simmons, 1983).

Some studies using evening primrose oil have found a favorable response rate of about 50 percent, but the studies are not well controlled. Evening primrose oil contains γ-linoleic acid and vitamin E. Symptoms most improved include headache, craving for sweets, increased appetite, heart pounding, fatigue, dizziness, fainting, depression, forgetfulness, crying, confusion, and insomnia (Abraham, 1983; London et al., 1983; Simmons, 1983).

OTHER SELF-HELP MEASURES.   Success has been attained in alleviating the symptoms of PMS through the use of several natural means. Techniques that are relatively easy to learn and implement without professional help include progressive relaxation and imaging. Reports indicate a 75 to 80 percent effectiveness for biofeedback. The primary focus of this technique is to increase blood flow to the uterine muscle. Patients are taught the method in four steps. First, they are instructed in general relaxation techniques. Second, they learn to warm their hands by opening the arteries and increasing blood flow. Third, they are taught to increase blood flow to the feet in the same way. Skin thermometers monitor success. The fourth step is to increase blood flow to the pelvic region. The process takes 10 to 15 sessions over about 3 months to learn. For detailed information, contact the Biofeedback Society of America, 3201 Owen Street, Wheat Ridge, CO 80033 (Perlmutter, 1983).

Self-hypnosis is also increasing in popularity. The initial phase takes from 1 to 3 hours to learn and the patient is taught how to totally relax. Discomfort is not diminished, but awareness of it is blocked. The patient learns to dissociate from the unpleasant feelings. A list of qualified hypnotherapists in the United States can be obtained from the Institute for Research in Hypnosis and Psychotherapy, 10 West 66 Street, New York, NY 10023 (Perlmutter, 1983).

Evaluation and Referral. Success at alleviating PMS requires active patient participation; the chosen regimen must therefore be acceptable to the woman. After implementation for an adequate time period, the treatment should be evaluated. If self-help measures have not afforded sufficient relief, as measured by the patient, referrals can be made for other natural therapies or more interventionist treatment with prescribed medications. The latter is especially appropriate for women with PMT—D (see Table 19–1). Practitioners should develop a list of health professionals offering various treatments in their area. It is the responsibility of the practitioner to assess their training and integrity and make sure, for example, that those prescribing medications such as progesterone do so within the confines of a scientific study with all the provisions of informed consent provided to the patient.

REFERENCES

Abraham, G. E. (1983, July). Nutritional factors in the etiology of the premenstrual tension syndromes. *Journal of Reproductive Medicine, 28*(7), 446–464.

Abraham, G. E., & Lubran, M. M. (1981, November). Serum and red cell magnesium levels in patients with premenstrual tension. *American Journal of Clinical Nutrition, 34*(11), 2364–2366.

Andersch, B., & Hahn, L. (1982). Bromocriptine, and premenstrual tension: A clinical and hormonal study. *Pharmatherapeutica, 3*(2), 107–113.

Andersch, B., Abrahamsson, L., & Wendestam, C, et al. (1979, December). Hormonal profile in premenstrual tension: Effects of bromocriptine and diuretics. *Clinical Endocrinology, 11*(6), 657–664.

Atton-Chamla, A., Favre, G., Goudard, J. -R., Miller, G., Rocca-Serra, J. P., Teitelbaum, M., Vallette, C., & Charpin, J. (1980). Premenstrual syndrome and atopy: A double blind clinical evaluation of treatment with a gamma-globulin/histamine complex. *Pharmatherapeutica, 2*(7), 481–486.

Block, E. (1960). Use of vitamin A in PMS. *Acta Obstetricia et Gynecologica Scandinavica, 39*(4), 586–592.

Broverman, D. M., Vogel, W., Klaiber, E. L., Majcher, D., Shea, D., & Paul, V. (1981, August). Changes in cognitive task performance across the menstrual cycle. *Journal of Comparative and Physiological Psychology, 95*(4), 646–654.

Brown, M. A., & Zimmer, P. A. (1986, January/February). Personal and family impact of premenstrual symptoms. *Journal of Obstetric, Gynecologic, and Neonatal Nursing, 15*(1), 31–38.

Budoff, P. W. (1983, July). The use of prostagladin inhibitors for the premenstrual syndrome. *Journal of Reproductive Medicine, 28*(7), 469–478.

Canty, A. P. (1984, November). Can aerobic exercise relieve the symptoms of premenstrual syndrome (PMS)? *Journal of School Health, 54*(10), 410–411.

Carstairs, M. W., & Talbot, D. J. (1981, November/December). A placebo controlled trial of Tenavoid in the management of the premenstrual syndrome. *British Journal of Clinical Practice, 35*(11/12), 403–409.

Chuong, C. J., & Coulam, C. B. (1988). Current views and the beta-endorphin hypothesis. In L. H. Gise (Ed.), *The premenstrual syndromes.* New York: Churchill Livingstone.

Colt, E. W. D., Wardlaw, S. L., & Frantz, A. G. (1981, April). The effect of running on plasma β-endorphin. *Life Sciences, 28*(14), 1637–1640.

Coyne, C. (1983, December). Muscle tension and its relation to symptoms in the premenstruum. *Research in Nursing and Health, 6*(4), 199–205.

Coyne, C. M., Woods, N. F., & Mitchell, E. S. (1985, November/December). Premenstrual tension syndrome. *Journal of Obstetric, Gynecologic, and Neonatal Nursing, 14*(6), 446–453.

Dalton, K. (1960a, January). Effect of menstruation on schoolgirls' weekly work. *British Medical Journal, 1*(5169), 326–328.

Dalton, K. (1960b, November). Menstruation and accidents. *British Medical Journal, 2*(5210), 1425–1426.

Dalton, K. (1960c, November). Schoolgirls' behavior and menstruation. *British Medical Journal, 2*(5210), 1647–1659.

Dalton, K. (1961, December). Menstruation and crime. *British Medical Journal, 2*(5269), 1752–1753.

Dalton, K., (1980a, November). Cyclic criminal acts in premenstrual syndrome. *Lancet, 2*(8203), 1070–1071.

Dalton, K. (1980b, July). Progesterone, fluid and electrolytes in premenstrual syndrome [Letter]. *British Medical Journal, 281*(6232), 61.

Day, J. (1979). Danazol and the premenstrual syndrome, *Postgraduate Medical Journal, 55*(5 Suppl.), 87–89.

Delaney, J., Lupton, M. J., & Toth, E. (1976). *The curse: A cultural history of menstruation.* New York: E. P. Dutton.

deVries, H. (1968, March). Immediate and long term effects of exercise upon resting muscle action potential level. *The Journal of Sports Medicine and Physical Fitness, 8*(1), 1–11.

deVries, H., Wiswell, R. A., Bulbulian, R., & Moritani, T. (1981, April). Tranquilizer effect of exercise: Acute effects of moderate aerobic exercise on spinal reflex activation level. *American Journal of Physical Medicine, 60*(2), 57–66.

d'Orban, P. T. (1981). PMS—A disease of the mind? [Letter]. *Lancet, 2*(8260/8261), 1413.

Elsner, C. W., Buster, J. E., & Schlinder, R. A., et al. (1980, December). Bromocriptine in the treatment of premenstrual tension syndrome. *Obstetrics and Gynecology, 56*(6), 723–726.

Farrell, P. A., Gates, W. K., Maksud, M. G., & Morgan, W. P. (1982, May). Increases in plasma β-endorphin/β-lipotropin immunoreactivity after treadmill running in humans. *Journal of Applied Physiology, 52*(5), 1245–1249.

Fraioli, F., Moretti, C., Paolucci, D., Alicicco, E., Crescenzi, F., & Fortunio, G. (1980). Physical exercise stimulates marked concomitant release of β-endorphin and adrenocorticotropic hormone (ACTH) in peripheral blood in man. *Experientia, 36*(8), 987–989.

Frank, E. P. (1986, February). What are nurses doing to help PMS patients? *American Journal of Nursing, 86*(2), 137–140.

Frank, R.H.T. (1931, November). The hormonal causes of premenstrual tension. *Archives of Neurology and Psychiatry, 26*(5), 1053–1057.

Gerber, H. (1921). Einige Daten zur Pathologie der Urticaria Menstruationalis. *Dermatologische Zeitschrift, 32*(1), 143–150.

Glick, I. D., & Stewart, D. (1980, July/August). A new drug treatment for premenstrual exacerbation of schizophrenia. *Comprehensive Psychiatry, 21*(4), 281–287.

Goldzieher, J. W., Moses, L., Averkin, E., & Taber, B. (1971). Nervousness and depression attributed to oral contraceptives. *American Journal of Obstetrics and Gynecology, 111*(8), 1013–1020.

Golub, S. (1988). A developmental perspective. In L. H. Gise (Ed.), *The premenstrual syndromes.* New York: Churchill Livingstone.

Gonzalez, E. R. (1981a). Even oral progesterone may be effective. *Journal of the American Medical Association, 245*(14), 1394 (inset).

Gonzalez, E. (1981b). Premenstrual syndrome: An ancient woe deserving of modern scrutiny. *Journal of the American Medical Association, 245*(14), 1393–1396.

Graham, J. J., Harding, P. E., Wise, P. H. & Berriman, H. (1978). Prolactin suppression in the treatment of premenstrual syndrome. *Medical Journal of Australia, 2*(3, Suppl.), 18–20.

Greene, R., & Dalton, K. (1953). The premenstrual syndrome. *British Medical Journal, 1*(4818), 1007–1014.

Greenhill, J. P., & Freed, S. C. (1940). The mechanism and treatment of premenstrual distress with ammonium chloride. *Endocrinology, 26*(3), 529–531.

Hargrove, J. T. & Abraham, G. E. (1982). The incidence of premenstrual tension in a gynecologic clinic. *Journal of Reproductive Medicine, 27*(12), 721–724.

Haskett, R. F., Steiner, M., Osmun, J. N., & Carroll, B. J. (1980). Severe premenstrual tension: Delineation of the syndrome. *Biological Psychiatry, 15*(1), 121–139.

Heinz, S. A. (1986). Premenstrual syndrome: An assessment, education, and treatment model. In V. L. Olesen & N. F. Woods, (Eds.), *Culture, society, and menstruation.* Washington, DC: Hemisphere.

Herzberg, B., & Coppen, A. (1970). Changes is psychological symptoms in women taking oral contraceptives. *British Journal of Psychiatry, 116*, 161–163.

Holtzman, E. (1988). Premenstrual syndrome as a legal defense. In L. H. Gise (Ed)., *The premenstrual syndromes.* New York: Churchill Livingstone.

Hood, W. E., & Bond, W. L. (1959). Enovid therapy for premenstrual tension. *Obstetrics and Gynecology, 14*(2), 239–240.

Horney, K. (1967). *Feminine psychology.* New York: W. W. Norton.

Israel, S. L. (1938). Premenstrual tension. *Journal of the American Medical Association, 110*(21), 1721–1723.

Jacobi, M. P. (1895). Modern female invalidism. *Boston Medical and Surgical Journal, 137*(7), 174–175.

Kerr, G. D., Day, J. B., Munday, M. R., Brush, M. G., Watson, M., & Taylor, R. W. (1980). Dydrogesterone in the treatment of the premenstrual syndrome. *The Practitioner, 224*(1346), 852–855.

Kumar, D., Zourlas, P., & Barnes, A. (1963). In vitro and in vivo effects of magnesium sulfate on human contractility. *American Journal of Obstetrics and Gynecology, 86*(8), 1036–1040.

Kutner, S. J., & Brown, W. L. (1972). Types of oral contraceptives, depression and premenstrual symptoms. *Journal of Nervous and Mental Diseases, 155*(3), 153–162.

Lauersen, N. (1985). Recognition and treatment of premenstrual syndrome. *Nurse Practitioner, 10*(3), 11–12, 15, 18–22.

Lever, J., Brush, M., & Haynes, B. (1982). *Premenstrual tension.* New York: Bantam Books.

London, R. S, Sundaram, G. S., Murphy, L., & Goldstein, P. J. (1983). Evaluation and treatment of breast symptoms in patients with the premenstrual syndrome. *Journal of Reproductive Medicine, 28*(8), 503–508.

Maddocks, S., Hahn, P., Moller, F., & Reid, R. L. (1986). A double-blind placebo-controlled trial of progesterone vaginal suppositories in the treatment of premenstrual syndrome. *American Journal of Obstetrics and Gynecology, 154*(3), 573–581.

O'Brien, P. M., Craven, D., & Selby, C. (1979). Treatment of premenstrual syndrome by spironolactone. *British Journal of Obstetrics and Gynaecology, 87*(2), 142–147.

Paige, K. E. (1973). Women learn to sing the menstrual blues. *Psychology Today, 7*(4), 41–46.

Parlee, M. B. (1973). The premenstrual syndrome. *Psychological Bulletin, 80*(6), 454–465.

Perlmutter, C. (1983, January–February). PMS. *McCalls,* 17.

Press, A., & Clausen, P. (1982, November). Not guilty because of PMS? *Newsweek,* 111.

Prior, J. C., Vigna, Y., Sciaretta, D., Alojado, N., & Schulzer, M. (1987). Conditioning exercise decreases premenstrual symptoms: A prospective, controlled 6-month trial. *Fertility and Sterility, 47*(3), 402–408.

Reeves, B. D., Garvin, J. E., & McElin, T. W. (1971). Premenstrual tension: Symptoms and weight changes related to potassium therapy. *American Journal of Obstetrics and Gynecology, 109*(7), 1036–1040.

Reid, R. L., & Yen, S. S. C. (1981). Premenstrual syndrome. *American Journal of Obstetrics and Gynecology, 139*(1), 85–104.

Rogers, W. D. (1962). The role of endocrine allergy in the production of premenstrual tension. *Western Journal of Surgery, Obstetrics and Gynecology, 70*(2), 100–102.

Rome, E. (1986). Premenstrual syndrome (PMS) examined through a feminist lens. In V. L. Olesen & N. F. Woods (Eds.), *Culture, Society, and Menstruation.* Washington, DC: Hemisphere.

Rose, D. P. (1978). The interactions between vitamin B_6 and hormones. *Vitamins and Hormones, 36,* 53–79.

Rossignol, A. M. (1985). Caffeine-containing beverages and premenstrual syndrome in young women. *American Journal of Public Health, 75*(11), 1335–1336.

Sampson, G. (1979). Premenstrual syndrome: A double blind controlled trial of progesterone and placebo. *British Journal of Psychiatry, 135,* 209–215.

Sarno, A. P., Miller, E. J., & Lundblad, E. G. (1987). Premenstrual Syndrome: Beneficial effects of periodic low-dose danazol. *Obstetrics and Gynecology, 70*(1), 33–36.

Shangold, M. H. (1983). Drug therapy for the premenstrual syndrome. *Journal of Reproductive Medicine, 28*(8), 525–526.

Simmons, M. K. (1983). Possible new relief for premenstrual syndrome. *Journal of the American Medical Association, 250*(11), 1371–1375.

Singer, K., Cheung, R., & Schou, M. (1974). A controlled evaluation of lithium in the premenstrual tension syndrome. *British Journal of Psychiatry, 124,* 50–51.

Smith, S., Rinehart, J. S., Ruddock, V. E., & Schiff, I. (1987). Treatment of premenstrual syndrome with alprazolam: Results of a double-blind, placebo-controlled, randomized crossover clinical trial. *Obstetrics and Gynecology, 70*(1), 37–43.

Sommer, B. (1983). How does menstruation affect cognitive competence and psychophysiological response? *Women and Health, 8*(2/3), 53–90.

Steiner, M., & Carroll, B. J. (1977). The psychobiology of premenstrual dysphoria: Review of theories and treatments. *Psychoneuroendocrinology, 2*(4), 321–335.

Steiner, M., Haskett, R. F., Osmun, J. N., & Carroll, B. J. (1980). The treatment of premenstrual tension with lithium carbonate: A pilot study. *Acta Psychiatrica Scandinavica, 61*(2), 96–102.

Swaffield, L. (1980). Menstruation: Pre-menstrual syndrome. *Nursing Times, 76*(10), 412–413.

Taylor, R. W. (1977). Treatment of premenstrual tension with dydrogesterone. *Current Medical Research and Opinion, 4*(Suppl. 4), 35.

Timonen, S., & Procopé, B. J. (1971). Premenstrual syndrome and physical exercise. *Acta Obstetricia et Gynecologica Scandinavica, 50*(4), 331–337.

Urbach, E. (1939). Menstruation allergy or menstruation toxicosis. *The New International Clinics, 2*(New Series 2), 160–168.

Walton, J., & Youngkin, E. (1987). The effect of a support group on self-esteem of women with premenstrual syndrome. *Journal of Obstetric, Gynecologic, and Neonatal Nursing, 16*(3), 174–178.

Wilhelm-Haas, E. (1984). Premenstrual syndrome: Its nature, evaluation and management. *Journal of Obstetric, Gynecologic, and Neonatal Nursing, 13*(4), 223–229.

Wood, C., & Jakubowicz, D. (1980). The treatment of premenstrual symptoms with mefanamic acid. *British Journal of Obstetrics and Gynaecology, 87*(7), 627–630.

Woods, N. F., Most, A., & Dery, G. K. (1982). Prevalence of perimenstrual symptoms. *American Journal of Public Health, 72*(11), 1257–1264.

20

Dysmenorrhea

Nancy Sullivan

The past two decades have seen a revolutionary change in perspective on dysmenorrhea. From the 1930s to the early 1970s, dysmenorrhea was believed by many health professionals and the lay public alike to be mainly a psychosomatic illness. An afflicted woman was offered little hope for relief and often was made to feel that the pain she suffered was due to some inability on her part to adapt to her feminine role or was "all in her head." Medical textbooks and research studies reinforced the psychogenic basis for dysmenorrhea, despite certain data that belied its validity. Although, beginning in the early part of the century, some work was done on evaluating exercise for the relief of dysmenorrhea, most medical practitioners provided little in the way of treatment. Women, therefore, tended not to seek medical care for this problem, preferring to cope as best they could.

Today, dysmenorrhea is considered seriously as a health problem. Research into its prevalence, causes, and treatments has been carried out in many disciplines including nursing, biochemistry, physiology, epidemiology, social science, gynecology, and pharmacology. Women with dysmenorrhea are no longer blamed for their discomfort, and health practitioners give serious attention to helping women find relief from the disorder. Nevertheless, there remain many questions about the etiology of dysmenorrhea.

This chapter reviews past and current perspectives on dysmenorrhea and outlines for the primary women's health care provider what is known about its causality and treatments. Both pharmacologic and nonpharmacologic remedies are discussed.

DEFINITION

Dysmenorrhea is a term of Greek origin meaning "difficult and painful menstruation" (*Stedman's Medical Dictionary* 1976, p. 432). Dysmenorrhea usually is designated as primary or secondary. Primary dysmenorrhea, also referred to as intrinsic, idiopathic, essential, or functional dysmenorrhea, is dysmenorrhea unexplained by anatomic factors or pathophysiology. The majority of cases fall into this category. In the light of present knowledge, this designation is somewhat incorrect. As most primary dysmenorrhea has as its basis an endogenous and identifiable substance—prostaglandin—it can no longer be considered to be of unknown etiology (Seegar-Jones, 1980). The exact mechanism

by which prostaglandins cause dysmenorrhea is still not understood, however, and what causes some women to have either an excess of this substance or an increased sensitivity to it remains a question. Nevertheless, the discovery of prostaglandins and extensive studies on their effect on the female reproductive organs have dramatically changed the understanding of dysmenorrhea. It is scientifically demonstrable that prostaglandins are implicated in dysmenorrhea and that prostaglandin synthesis (or synthetase) inhibitors (PGSIs) can eliminate or substantially reduce symptoms in a great majority of women.

Secondary dysmenorrhea, also referred to as extrinsic or acquired dysmenorrhea, is dysmenorrhea caused by known anatomic factors or pelvic pathology (other than prostaglandins). Some entities related to this condition are endometrial polyps, endometriosis, submucous or interstitial myomas, endometrial cancer, pelvic inflammatory disease, use of an intrauterine contraceptive device (IUD), and, rarely, a uterine or vaginal anomaly with outflow obstruction (Rosenwaks & Seegar-Jones, 1980). See Section III, Gynecologic Pathophysiology, for discussion of these various disorders.

There remains a small but significant minority of women with dysmenorrhea unexplained by anatomic factors and for whom prostaglandin synthesis inhibitors fail to provide relief. These women continue to represent a challenge to medical researchers and to health professionals.

Dysmenorrhea should not be confused with premenstrual syndrome, although many researchers and practitioners do not differentiate these syndromes. Because many women do have symptoms of both entities, it often has been assumed that they were one and the same. Some observers have noted a difference between "congestive dysmenorrhea" and "spasmodic dysmenorrhea" (Dalton, 1977) but treated them as different manifestations of the same problem. Recently, several researchers have developed the concept of "perimenstrual distress." A body of literature is accumulating around this concept based on retrospective survey data among women showing no significant distinctions between symptoms experienced premenstrually and during menses (Woods, Most, & Dery 1982).

Nevertheless, the discovery of prostaglandins and the ability of exogenous prostaglandins, when administered to symptom-free women, to produce certain symptoms but not others point to a clear distinction between dysmenorrhea and premenstrual syndrome. The fact that premenstrual symptoms are not alleviated by PGSIs appears to substantiate that this symptom complex is unrelated etiologically to dysmenorrhea (Jay, Durant, Shoffitt, & Linder, 1986; Rosenwaks & Seegar-Jones, 1980).

As early as 1964, researchers using personality tests concluded that the two syndromes were separate (Kessel & Coppen, 1964). Several questionnaires have been developed to differentiate between premenstrual syndrome and dysmenorrhea (Chesney & Tasto, 1975; Cox & Santirocco, 1981). Differentiation of the two syndromes will improve diagnosis and treatment of both, and also will improve the reliability and validity of research studies in these areas.

At the present time there is no objective definition of dysmenorrhea, and the criteria for inclusion in studies are vague. Several authors suggest, as a practical matter, making a diagnosis of dysmenorrhea if the woman seeks relief for her pain, either from a physician or by self-medication (Lamb, 1981; Ylikorkala & Dawood, 1978).

SYMPTOMS

Primary dysmenorrhea is not a disease in itself. It has been accurately described as a symptom complex (Dingfelder, 1981) or a syndrome (Sobczyk, 1980). The pain itself is located in the lower abdomen and may be described as sharp, spasmodic, crampy, or colicky, similar to the pain of angina pectoris. It may radiate to the lower back or upper thighs. Over 50 percent of dysmenorrheic women have systemic symptoms accompanying the pelvic pain. These include nausea and vomiting, headache, dizziness or fainting, fatigue, nervousness, lower backache, and diarrhea (Ylikorkala & Dawood, 1978).

Monthly symptoms usually begin at the onset of menstruation or several hours before the onset, and may continue from several hours to several days. The range and severity of symptoms vary enormously from woman to woman, and from month to month in the same woman. Some dysmenorrheic women who have experienced childbirth have described their menstrual cramps as more severe than labor pain. Told to come to the hospital when labor began to feel like cramps, they arrived fully dilated or never made it to the hospital (Weidiger, 1976).

Dysmenorrhea usually is associated with ovulatory cycles, although it has been noted in anovulatory cycles (Morrison & Nicolls, 1981). It is usually absent at menarche, making its first appearance quite abruptly 6 to 12 months later, when ovulatory cycles begin. It may become progressively more severe over time (Sobczyk, 1980). It occurs in some women on oral contraceptives, although most women experience lesser or no symptoms while on the pill.

The pain of secondary dysmenorrhea can be differentiated from that of primary dysmenorrhea. It frequently occurs several days before the onset of menses, during ovulation (mittelschmerz), or during intercourse. It can be present at any point in the menstrual cycle. The pain may begin with or even precede menarche or it may not appear until age 20 or later. One recent literature review noted that secondary dysmenorrhea should be suspected in that group of women—from 9 to 22 percent in various studies—who do not benefit from treatment with PGSIs (Owen, 1984).

EPIDEMIOLOGY

Israel (1967) reviewed the literature and found that the prevalence of primary dysmenorrhea in gynecologic patients varied from 3 to 37 percent. He surveyed his own patient records and found that dysmenorrhea as the chief complaint accounted for 8 percent of 4,000 patient visits; he cited this as twice the prevalence among a similar number of office patients analyzed by Bickers in 1954. After a more recent literature review, Dingfelder (1981, p. 874) contented himself with the statement that dysmenorrhea ''is an extremely common problem of everyday practice.''

The occurrence of dysmenorrhea has been studied in association with a number of variables. Margaret Mead (1955) noted that it is common in some cultures and seemingly absent in others. Age has been studied extensively as a factor in dysmenorrhea. Fifty to seventy-five percent of all dysmenorrheic women experience symptoms during adolescence, within 24 months of menarche, which itself varies from culture to culture (Morrison & Nicolls, 1981). There is some evidence that the prevalence and severity of symptoms decrease when women reach their twenties (Sobczyk, 1980). Dysmenorrhea is the primary cause of recurrent, short-term absence from school among adolescent females (Klein & Litt, 1981). In 1958, Golub, Lang, and Menduke found that frequent dysmenorrhea occurred in one third of public high school girls in Philadelphia, occasional dysmenorrhea occurred in another third, and the rest were free from the disorder. Klein and Litt (1981) examined data from the National Health Examination survey collected between 1966 and 1970 by the National Center for Health Statistics. They found that 59.7 percent of postmenarcheal adolescent girls reported dysmenorrhea. In a random sample of urban 19-year-olds in Sweden, 72 percent reported dysmenorrhea and 15 percent reported limitation of daily activity secondary to the disorder. In this latter group, dysmenorrhea was unrelieved by analgesics. More than 50 percent of these young women had at least one episode of school or work absence because of dysmenorrhea (Andersch & Milsom, 1982).

Other factors have been studied with varied results. Parity may be a relevant factor, with several studies showing nulliparous women to have both greater prevalence and severity of symptoms than parous ones (Andersch & Milsom, 1982; Sobczyk, 1980; Sobczyk, Braunstein, Solbert, & Schuman, 1978). Studies concerning the relation of weight, socioeconomic status, marital status, menstrual irregularity, family history, race, and body type to dysmenorrhea have been less conclusive (Morrison & Nicolls, 1981; Sobczyk, 1980). Smoking was found in one study to be related to menstrual disorders, including dysmenorrhea (Sloss & Frerichs, 1983), and in another to be negatively related to dysmenorrhea (Andersch & Milsom, 1982). This deserves further investigation.

Morrison and Nicolls (1981, p. 96) note that ''consideration of menstrual pain as 'normal' by many health care providers, patients, and parents has led to hesitation on the part of affected individuals to seek medical consultation,'' leading to underreporting of both prevalence and severity of the problem. Morrison and Nicolls also point out that dysmenorrhea has an enormous social and economic impact, which also is difficult to assess statistically.

ETIOLOGY

Currently, any discussion of the etiology of dysmenorrhea begins with prostaglandins, although as recently as 1975 a noted textbook on gynecologic disorders acknowledged that the real cause was unknown (Willson, Beecham, & Carrington, 1975, p. 104). A number of theories had been propounded for centuries. The physiologic theories included an imbalance in the normal estrogen–progesterone equilibrium, incomplete disintegration of the endometrium, hypoplasia of the uterus, acute uterine anteflexion, obstruction of the cervical canal, an allergic or altered reactivity of certain tissues to substances that do not affect non-sensitized individuals, and poor posture. The posture theory led to a number of studies on the effects of exercise on dysmenorrhea, which are reviewed under Intervention.

Psychogenic Theories

Psychogenic theories concerning the etiology of dysmenorrhea were widely held from the 1930s to the 1970s, despite evidence that physiologic factors were involved. All pain has a psychological component, as modern researchers have demonstrated. Dysmenorrhea, however, "seems to have attracted a disproportionate amount of psychological speculation when compared with other medical conditions" (Cox & Santirocco, 1981, p. 77). Lennane and Lennane (1973) argue that the conceptualization of dysmenorrhea as a result of psychological factors is a manifestation of sexual prejudice rather than a product of sound scientific thinking. Lennane (1980) has noted that in the light of present knowledge, such psychogenic theories seem "incredible" and are being abandoned. The most common psychogenic explanation was rejection or resentment of the feminine role or feminine role conflicts (Menninger, 1939; Willson et al., 1975). One author even suggested that marriage could either cure dysmenorrhea by "providing happy security" or cause the problem if the marriage proved to be "disharmonious" (Jeffcoate, 1975, p. 538).

Psychiatrists described women with dysmenorrhea as experiencing "hate-laden fantasies and dreams" and having a "tendency to pugnacity and violence as well as self-destruction" (Israel, 1967). A number of authors believed that suggestion or "psychological seeding" during adolescence was significant (Green, 1977; Jeffcoate, 1975; Schauffler, 1967). This idea was promulgated especially in literature for the lay audience. Even Benjamin Spock, in twenty million copies of *Baby and Child Care*, wrote, "It's the girl who has developed a worried attitude about health and menstruation who is more apt to have severe cramps" (Spock, 1968, p. 342).

Perhaps the most extreme position for the psychogenic theory was that of Margaret Chadwick in 1938. Chadwick described the menstruating woman as temporarily unstable, with impaired memory and unreliable actions, exhibiting strange longings for meat, feeling impaired by her condition, and wishing to seek revenge (Morrison & Nicolls, 1981).

Specific personality components attributed to dysmenorrhea have included anxiety, neurosis, overconformity, insecurity, instability, immaturity, dependency, identity problems, shyness, underachievement, and perfectionism (Frisk, Widholm, & Hortling, 1965; Green, 1977; Jeffcoate, 1975; Robbins, 1953; Willson et al., 1975). Recently, several scientifically conducted, controlled studies examining personality and its relationship to primary dysmenorrhea found no demonstrable relationship (Iacono & Roberts, 1983; Lawlor & Davis, 1981). In one study, items associated with "traditional" versus "feminist" dimensions such as work in female-dominant jobs, sex-role orientation, and attitudes toward women, as well as personal characteristics, were found to be unrelated to dysmenorrhea (Brown & Woods, 1984, p. 263).

In an analysis of life changes and dysmenorrhea, Jordan and Meckler (1982) found a small, but significant, correlation between life changes and dysmenorrhea. Woods, Most, and Longenecker (1985) similarly found a small rela-

tionship between a group of perimenstrual symptoms and both major stressful life events and daily stressors. In their definition of perimenstrual symptomatology, they include symptoms usually associated with both premenstrual syndrome and dysmenorrhea. Daily stressors were more important influences on symptoms than major life events. Stress related to children was particularly correlated with symptoms experienced during menses.

Biochemical Theories

Recent studies show that dysmenorrhea has a biochemical basis that is relatively easy to conceptualize and explain although the mechanism is not understood fully. Dysmenorrhea is associated with increased activity of the uterine myometrium—increased baseline tone as well as greater frequency and intensity of contractions. Increased uterine pressure results in decreased blood flow, tissue ischemia, and pain (Rosenwaks & Seegar-Jones, 1980).

Pickles, in 1957, was the first to suggest that the cause of increased myometrial activity and its resulting ischemia and pain might be some chemical produced by the menstruating uterus itself. Pickles termed this substance *menstrual stimulant*; subsequently, it was shown to be a group of substances containing prostaglandins E and F. In 1965, Pickles, Hall, Best, and associates noted that menstrual fluid of women with primary dysmenorrhea had a prostaglandin $F_{2\alpha}$ concentration higher than that of normal women, leading eventually to an interest in prostaglandins as an etiologic agent in primary dysmenorrhea.

Prostaglandin synthesis, the role that prostaglandins play in uterine activity, and the effects that PGSIs have are as yet poorly understood phenomena. Rosenwaks and Seegar-Jones (1980, p. 211) outlined the following theory for the role of prostaglandins in the etiology of menstrual bleeding and dysmenorrhea:

> Prostaglandin synthesis appears to be initiated by lysosomal enzyme release at menstruation. These hydrolytic enzymes trigger phospholipases, which allow the release of phospholipids—basic units for the formation of prostaglandin precursors (such as arachidonic acid). Prostaglandins increase myometrial contractions and cause constriction of small endometrial blood vessels, with consequent tissue ischemia, and endometrial disintegration, bleeding, and pain. Dysmenorrhea may be due to tissue ischemia resulting from increased intrauterine pressure, vessel constriction, and decreased uterine blood flow. Prostaglandins may also sensitize the nerve endings to other pain-producing substances.

Several researchers believe it is the high resting or baseline tone of the myometrium, rather than the frequency or intensity of uterine contractions, that is responsible for the pain of dysmenorrhea (Csapo, 1980). Interestingly, a trial utilizing a β stimulator to cause uterine relaxation was found not to relieve dysmenorrhea any more than a placebo (Hansen & Secher, 1975).

The extragenital effects of prostaglandins probably result from leakage or penetration of prostaglandins from their origin in the uterus to the general circulation (Csapo, 1980). The ability of exogenous prostaglandins to cause these symptoms when administered either locally or intravenously and the ability of PGSIs to relieve these symptoms as well as uterine pain support such a theory.

It is not clear whether women with dysmenorrhea synthesize more prostaglandins than other women or are more sensitive to a normal level. Pickles and associates (1965) found the level of prostaglandin $F_{2\alpha}$ in the menstrual fluid of dysmenorrheic women to be elevated compared with that of nondysmenorrheic women. This was corroborated by Rees, Anderson, Demers, and Turnbull (1984). Conversely, Wilks, Wentz, and Jones (1973) assayed the blood levels of normal and dysmenorrheic subjects immediately prior to and during menstruation and found no difference in prostaglandin levels.

The role of other hormones in prostaglandin regulation (and dysmenorrhea) is unclear. In vitro evidence indicates that prostaglandin synthesis and release in the endometrium may be caused by estrogen, but women with dysmenorrhea have not demonstrated increased estrogen concentrations through the menstrual cycle (Wenzloff & Shimp, 1984). Vasopressin and/or oxytocin have been proposed as possible mediators of myometrial response to prostaglandins (Strömberg, Forsling, & Åkerlund 1981). Studies in animals have shown that the uterine response to prostaglandins may be controlled by progesterone. Even before the discovery of prostaglandins, progesterone was suspected to play a role in the etiology of dysmenorrhea. In a study of the effect of exogenous intrauterine progesterone (administered via a Progestasert IUD) on the prostaglandin content of menstrual blood in dysmenorrheic women, Trobough and associates (1978) found lower levels of prostaglandin and improvement in dysmenorrhea in women using these devices compared with a control group. Future research may substantiate the role of progesterone in dysmenorrhea.

MANAGEMENT

Data Collection

History. The practitioner who takes a thorough history and listens carefully to a woman's description of her pain should be able to assess with some accuracy the severity of the woman's problem and the possibility of concomitant pathology and, consequently, to prescribe or suggest an appropriate treatment or referral. Remedies the woman has already utilized and their effects should be assessed. A history of management strategies may indicate a woman's attitude toward her discomfort, her willingness and desire to attempt various treatments, and her value system regarding pharmacologic versus nonpharmacologic remedies (Brown, 1982).

Physical Examination. A complete physical assessment is necessary to rule out pathologic causes of dysmenorrhea such as endometriosis and uterine myoma (see Chapters 18 and 14).

Laboratory Testing. No specific laboratory tests exist to demonstrate dysmenorrhea. If secondary dysmenorrhea with an underlying pathology is suspected, then appropriate laboratory tests should be utilized as necessary.

Treatment

General Approach. For women with mild symptoms who want to avoid medication if possible, nondrug remedies might be effective. For the woman with severe symptoms, prostaglandin synthesis inhibitors are available, although if she prefers, therapy with acupuncture or biofeedback may lead to relief of all or some distress. Every woman, of course, deserves a comprehensive review of possible remedies.

For women with IUDs, the alleviation of dysmenorrhea may be as simple as removal of the device. If a woman wishes to continue using this method of birth control, PGSIs may be helpful. If these medications fail to provide relief, the IUD may have to be removed. Ultimately, this is the woman's choice.

Pharmacologic Treatments. Current therapy for primary dysmenorrhea centers on the prostaglandin synthesis inhibitors. These compounds have been used as analgesic treatment for dysmenorrhea since the early 1970s. The PGSIs are nonsteroidal, anti-inflammatory analgesics that can be divided into two groups: the aryl carboxylic acids, including the salicylic acids (aspirin) and the fenamates, and the aryl alkanoic acids, including the aryl propionic acids (ibuprofen, ketoprofen, and naproxen) and the indole acetic acids (indomethacin) (Owen, 1984).

The mechanism of action of the PGSIs in the treatment of dysmenorrhea is unknown, although evidence suggests that their inhibitory effect on prostaglandin synthesis causes a concomitant reduction of intrauterine pressure and reduction of pain (Henzl & Izu, 1979). One known positive effect of PGSIs is a decrease in loss of menstrual blood, which may contribute to pain relief (Ylikorkala & Dawood, 1978). Anderson, Guillebaud, Haynes, and Turnbull (1976) showed a significant reduction of menstrual blood from an average of 119 mL to an average of 60 mL during treatment with fenamate PGSIs.

Numerous clinical trials have been conducted to evaluate the effectiveness of various PGSIs in the treatment of dysmenorrhea. Table 20–1 summarizes PGSI trials through 1983. For a majority of women, each of the PGSIs studied afforded significant pain relief. When only double-blind studies were assessed, however, the percentage of pain relief declined; still, 56 to 87 percent of women experienced significant results.

Owen (1984) enumerates numerous drawbacks to the clinical trials she evaluated, detracting from the validity and reliability of these studies. First, a number of studies permitted the use of confounding factors including IUDs, oral contraceptives, and other analgesics during the trial and did not control for such use. A number of the studies were not double blind, were open trials (with no placebo or other drug control), or were parallel rather than crossover in design. In parallel studies each drug tested is administered to a different group of women, rather than each drug being given sequentially to each participant, allowing each participant to act as her own control. Dysmenorrhea was rarely defined, nor were selection criteria included. The criteria and methods used to assess and analyze drug response were often imprecise and inadequate. Nevertheless, the accumulated body of research makes conclusions possible.

All PGSIs, including aspirin, share potential side effects. Women should be advised to note and report changes indicative of possible serious side effects, and practitioners should provide adequate follow-up for women regularly taking these medications. Side effects and the changes to be noted, as well as contraindications, include the following (Long, 1985; Modell, 1984):

1. Gastrointestinal disturbances ranging from indigestion, nausea and vomiting, diarrhea, and constipation, to gastrointestinal bleeding secondary to gastritis or peptic ulcer disease: Dark-colored stools might be indicative of gastrointestinal bleeding.
2. Salt and water retention ranging from mild weight gain and edema to exacerbation of hypertension and

TABLE 20-1. SUMMARY OF PGSI TRIALS IN THE TREATMENT OF DYSMENORRHEA

PGSI	Number of Trials	Number of Patients/cycles[a]	Number DB[b]	Number yes or NR[b] Adjunctive Treatment	Pain Relief (Overall Average)		Pain Relief, DB Only	Pain Relief to Placebo (Average)
					Excellent	*Poor*		
Fenamate (flufenamic acid/mefenamic acid; Ponstel)	9	279/1353	5(56%)	7(78%)	90%	9%	87%	9%
Ibuprofen (Motrin)	12	325/1146	7(58%)	6(50%)	66%	22%	58%	17%
Indomethacin (Indocin)	11	345/1052	7(64%)	9(82%)	68%	19%	68%	16%
Naproxen (Anaprox)	18	712/1785	13(72%)	12(66%)	62%	21%	56%	16%

[a]Number of cycles is obtained by multiplying number of patients/study by number of cycles for which they were followed in that study and adding all studies together.
[b]DB, double blind; NR, no report.
Adapted from Owen, P. (1984). Prostaglandin synthetase inhibitors in the treatment of primary dysmenorrhea: Outcome trials reviewed. American Journal of Obstetrics and Gynecology, 148*(1), 96–103. Reprinted with permission.*

congestive heart failure: Weight and blood pressure should be monitored periodically.

3. Hepatic toxicity: Hepatitis can occur with any of these drugs. Clinical symptoms of hepatitis or jaundice should be reported. These symptoms necessitate discontinuation of the drug as does elevation of transaminase levels to three times normal.
4. Renal toxicity, mild to severe, and reversible to irreversible renal insufficiency: Women should report any signs of renal damage.
5. Potentiation of oral anticoagulants and inhibition of platelet aggregation: All PGSIs should be avoided by persons taking anticoagulants. Abnormal brusing or bleeding should be noted.
6. Skin rashes, itching, hives, tinnitus, neurologic symptoms such as headaches, blurred vision, retinal changes, and dizziness, and bone marrow toxicity: Tinnitus is the earliest and most reliable symptom of aspirin toxicity or salicylism.
7. Allergic reactions: Persons with a history of aspirin sensitivity or allergy, including anaphylactic reactions, should avoid other PGSIs as cross-reactivity can occur.

It must be remembered that persons being treated with PGSIs for long-term, intransigent problems such as arthritis and rheumatism take many times the dosage, and on a continual basis, as women using the medications for dysmenorrhea. For the latter, most side effects are relatively infrequent and mild and are usually reported to be tolerable (Ylikorkala & Dawood 1978, p. 843). The side effects most frequently mentioned by dysmenorrheic patients are gastrointestinal. Budoff (1980) states that these effects can be prevented or minimized by taking the medication with milk or food. It may be difficult to tell whether such symptoms are drug related or are part of the dysmenorrhea syndrome itself. Certainly, exacerbation after use of a PGSI indicates that a symptom may be medication induced.

One PGSI drug, indomethacin, is responsible for frequent and serious adverse reactions. Twenty-five percent or more of all patients receiving indomethacin have adverse or toxic reactions; most of these are central nervous system or gastrointestinal reactions. Hematologic changes have been noted (Andersson, 1979). Central nervous system re-

actions include headache, dizziness, depression, mental confusion, and other psychic reactions such as detachment and depersonalization, often severe enough to force discontinuation of the drug. Adverse gastrointestinal effects include anorexia, epigastric distress, and abdominal pain. Peptic ulcers and perforation or hemorrhage of the stomach or duodenum have been reported (Modell, 1984). Boehm and Sarrat (1975) reported that 17 of 30 patients complained of side effects while using indomethacin for dysmenorrhea and 8 of these stopped taking the medication because of these effects.

Although a perusal of Table 20–1 shows the fenamates to provide pain relief to the greatest percentage of women, direct comparisons among the types of PGSIs cannot be considered valid from a review of the literature because of inconsistencies in study methodologies and variation in the number of women studied among the different medications. A study directly comparing PGSIs found ibuprofen, administered either before or at the onset of menses, to provide the best results (Chan, Dawood, & Fuchs, 1979). Accordingly, this drug is frequently the first choice when a woman begins a regimen of PGSI therapy. Delaying administration of this or any PGSI to onset of menses has the advantage of safeguarding against possible teratogenic effects.

Ibuprofen is currently available as a nonprescription, over-the-counter drug in 200-mg tablet form (Advil), which makes it convenient for health care providers to recommend and for women to obtain. Articles and advertisements in the lay media are touting the benefits of this medication, so more women will become aware of its existence. Certainly, as with any easily available drug, there are problems associated with inappropriate self-medication.

Aspirin is a satisfactory drug for many women complaining of mild to moderate dysmenorrhea (Klein, Litt, Rosenberg, & Udall, 1981). It, too, should be administered either before or at the onset of menses for maximum results. The low cost and universal availability of aspirin make it an attractive choice.

It is sometimes necessary to try several of the PGSIs until the one with the maximum efficacy for a particular woman is found. This requires patience on the part of the patient as well as the practitioner. Table 20–2 outlines the dosages for the various forms of available PGSIs.

TABLE 20–2. PROSTAGLANDIN SYNTHETASE INHIBITORS: DOSAGE INFORMATION

Generic Name	Trade Name	Strength/Dosage	Available Dosage Forms and Strengths
Aspirin	Many brands	600–1,200 mg qid to 5 g[a]	150-, 300-, 600-mg tablets; 300-mg coated tablets; 600-mg prolonged-action capsules
Fenoprofen	Nalfon (Dista)	300–600 mg qid to 2,400 mg[a]	600-mg tablets; 200-, 300-mg capsules
Ibuprofen	Motrin (Upjohn) Advil (Whitehall) Rufen (Boots) Nuprin (Upjohn)	400–600 mg qid to 2,400 mg[a]	200-, 300-, 400-, 600-mg tablets
Indomethacin	Indocin (Merck, Sharp, & Dohme) Indocin SR (Merck, Sharp, & Dohme)	25–50 mg tid to 200 mg[a]	25-, 50-mg capsules; 75-mg prolonged-action capsules
Mefenamic acid	Ponstel (Parke–Davis)	500 mg initially, then 250 mg qid[a]	250-mg capsules
Naproxen	Anaprox (Syntex) Naprosyn (Syntex)	250–500 mg bid to 1 g[a]	250-, 275-, 375-, 500-mg tablets

Compare to alleve

[a]Dosage should be limited to smallest amount that produces relief.
Adapted from Modell, W. (Ed.) (1984). Drugs of choice: 1984–1985. *St. Louis, MO: C. V. Mosby. Reprinted with permission.*

As mentioned previously, from 9 to 22 percent of women treated with PGSIs do not obtain significant relief from the medication. These women should be suspected of having some underlying pelvic pathology (secondary dysmenorrhea); referral for further diagnostic studies should be considered. Surgery is frequently necessary both to diagnose and to treat such problems.

Finally, there is that group of women, fortunately small, who do not obtain pain relief from PGSIs or other medication, and in whom no pelvic pathology is found on laparotomy or through other diagnostic techniques. Perhaps it is to this group of women that the designation of idiopathic or essential dysmenorrhea belongs at the present time. The challenge for medical researchers and gynecologic practitioners is to find an etiology and a treatment for the symptoms these women present.

NON-PGSI MEDICATIONS. Before the introduction of PGSIs, numerous drugs were given in an attempt to alleviate the pain of dysmenorrhea. Narcotics, estrogen, antispasmodics, and minor tranquilizers were tried according to the mode of the times (Schauffler, 1967, p. 797), rarely with good results. Since the 1960s, oral contraceptives have been utilized in the treatment of dysmenorrhea. It has been proposed that their effectiveness in relieving dysmenorrhea is related to their ability to decrease prostaglandin levels (Chan, Dawood, & Fuchs, 1981) although this remains speculative. Oral contraceptives, of course, have many side effects (see Chapter 7), and women not needing or desiring to use them for contraceptive purposes may object to their use for dysmenorrhea. They also are contraindicated for many women.

Over-the-counter preparations designed specifically for dysmenorrhea, such as Femcaps and Midol, are principally aspirin with other ingredients and are probably less effective than plain aspirin (Chan et al., 1979). Other products for menstrual pain, such as Pamprin, Femicin, Femeze, and Her-Caps, which contain acetaminophen rather than aspirin, are even less useful, as acetaminophen does not have the antiprostaglandin properties of aspirin.

NONPHARMACOLOGIC REMEDIES. A number of nondrug remedies for dysmenorrhea have been tried and can be effective, principally for mild to moderate cases. They also can be used to reduce the medication dosages necessary to relieve severe dysmenorrhea. In a small, but well-designed, controlled study, acupuncture was found to be highly effective in relieving primary dysmenorrhea and in reducing the amount of medication taken for this problem (Helms, 1987). Biofeedback also has been shown to bring relief, after about 2 months of feedback treatment (Balick, Elfner, May, & Moore, 1982).

The New Our Bodies, Ourselves (Boston Women's Health Collective, 1984) suggests relaxation, massage, biofeedback techniques, raspberry leaf tea, calcium supplements, heat, orgasm, yoga, aspirin, marijuana, and, for difficult cases, antiprostaglandins. Certainly alcohol and caffeine have been used for many years, although neither can actually be considered a "nondrug" remedy (Israel, 1967). A list of remedies in a book for lay readers in 1976, obtained from reader questionnaires, included "marijuana, sex, yoga, having a nice friend put his warm hands on my ovaries, peppermint tea . . . raspberry tea, a stiff drink, curling up with a heating pad, bone meal tablets, Alka-Seltzer, Premarin, aspirin, a good shot of gin, seeing my lover smile" (Weidiger, 1976, p. 175). Budoff (1980), however, tells her readers that most of these methods are no more effective than placebo. Some may have other effects: bone meal tablets, for example, may contain lead, and marijuana and alcohol are certainly not benign.

Exercise. Exercise also has been used as a remedy for dysmenorrhea. A number of studies have found exercise to increase blood levels of β-endorphins—the body's endogenous opiates—making its use in pain relief plausible (Colt, Wardlaw, & Frantz, 1981; Farrell, Gates, Maksud, & Morgan, 1982; Fraioli, Moretti, & Paolucci et al., 1980). Research, however, is not yet conclusive on the physiologic role of these substances or on the relationship between blood and central nervous system levels of endorphins (Farrell et al., 1982).

In a study of Philadelphia high school girls, Golub and associates (1958) found an inverse relationship between severity of pain and participation in sports during menses. No attempt was made, however, to quantify participation in sports. In another study of female students enrolled in the national gymnastics school of a Scandinavian country, there was no difference in the frequency of dysmenorrhea between gymnastic students and nongymnastic students, nor between students enrolled in the gymnastics program for 1 year and those enrolled by 2 years (Morrison & Nicolls, 1981). Nevertheless, the paucity of recent literature in this area speaks to the need for more research examining the effects of exercise on menstrual pain.

Specific exercises for the relief of dysmenorrhea were proposed by Mosher in 1914, by Billig in 1943, and by Golub in 1959. The purpose of the Mosher and Billig exercises was to correct a postural defect presumed to cause dysmenorrhea.

Mosher's exercise is done on a flat surface in the horizontal position, with knees flexed and a hand placed on the abdomen. The woman is instructed to raise her hand as far as possible by lifting the abdominal wall, and then to lower it by contracting the abdominal muscles. Mosher advised ten repetitions of this exercise each morning and night in a well-ventilated room while wearing no restrictive clothing. She reported several case studies documenting improvement.

Billig's exercises involved a sideward stretch of the hips done with the legs 18 inches apart while standing at a right

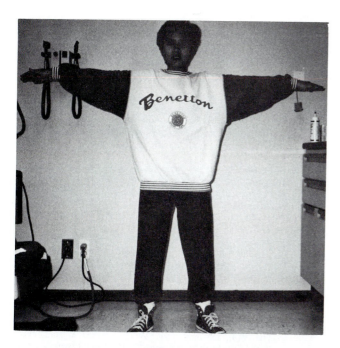
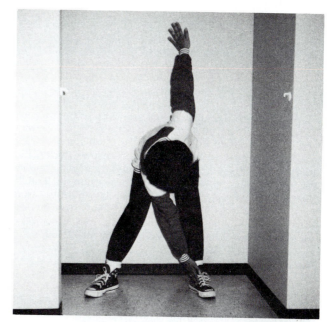
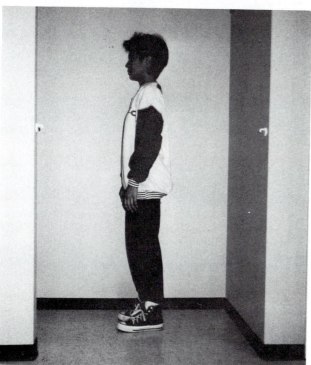
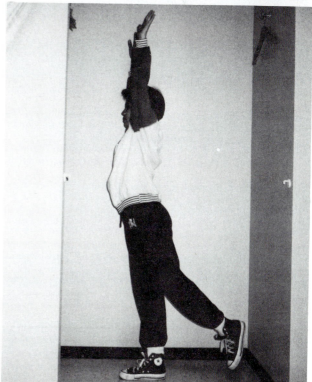

Figure 20–1. Proposed exercises for dysmenorrhea.

angle to a wall. Abdominal and gluteal muscles are contracted during the stretch. He advised doing three stretches on each side, three times a day. This exercise has been criticized as requiring supervision for proper performance (Golub, 1959).

Golub suggests two types of trunk twisting, bending, and stretching exercises, each done ten times on each side every morning and repeated later in the day. Figure 20-1 illustrates these exercises. Instructions are as follows (Golub, 1987):

1. Keep legs apart and arms stretched out to each side at shoulder height. Twist the trunk as far to the left as possible with knees straight. Touch the right hand to the left foot, the outer part if possible. Keep heels on the floor.
2. Start in a standing position, with arms straight at the sides. Swing the arms forward and upward while simultaneously swinging one leg backward. Repeat ten times with each leg.

In a study of 141 high school girls with dysmenorrhea, 92 percent were improved or cured with the Golub exercise and 91 percent with the Billig exercise (Golub et al., 1958). Cure was defined as three pain-free menstrual cycles. In a study of junior high school girls, results were less dramatic, but improvement was shown with these exercises (Golub, Menduke, & Lang, 1968). It is impossible to judge, from these studies, whether the specific exercises were helpful in reducing dysmenorrhea or whether any exercise or relaxation technique would show similar beneficial results.

Teaching and Counseling. For any woman seeking relief from dysmenorrhea, sympathetic understanding is always therapeutic. An explanation that there is a biochemical cause for the problem, and that treatment is available and effective, can be reassuring. The gynecologic practitioner today is finally able to offer a woman that reassurance.

REFERENCES

Andersch, B., & Milsom I. (1982, November 15). An epidemiologic study of young women with dysmenorrhea. *American Journal of Obstetrics and Gynecology, 144*(4), 655–660.

Anderson, A., Guillebaud, J., Haynes, P., & Turnbull, A. (1976, April 10). Reduction of menstrual blood loss by prostaglandin-synthesis inhibitors. *Lancet, 1*(7963), 774–776.

Andersson, K.-E. (1979). Side-effects of prostaglandin synthetase inhibitors. *Acta Obstetricia et Gynecologica Scandinavica,* Suppl. 87, 101–104.

Balick, L., Elfner, L., May, J., & Moore, J. D. (1982, December). Biofeedback treatment of dysmenorrhea. *Biofeedback and Self-Regulation, 7*((4), 499–520.

Billig, H. E. (1943, May). Dysmenorrhea: The result of a postural defect. *Archives of Surgery, 46*(5), 611–613.

Boehm, F. E., & Sarrat, H. (1975, August). Indomethacin for the teatment of dysmenorrhea. *Journal of Reproductive Medicine, 15*(2), 84–86.

Boston Women's Health Collective. (1984). *The new our bodies, ourselves.* New York: Random House.

Brown, M. A. (1982, March). Primary dysmenorrhea. *Nursing Clinics of North America, 17*(1), 145–152.

Brown, M. A., & Woods, N.F. (1984, July/August). Correlates of dysmenorrhea: Challenge to past stereotypes. *Journal of Obstetric, Gynecologic, and Neonatal Nursing, 13*(4), 259–266.

Budoff, P. (1980). *No more menstrual cramps and other good news.* New York: Penguin Books.

Chan, W., Dawood, M. Y., & Fuchs, F. (1979, September). Relief of dysmenorrhea with the prostaglandin synthetase inhibitor ibuprofen: Effect on prostaglandin levels in menstrual fluid. *American Journal of Obstetrics and Gynecology, 135*(1), 102–108.

Chan, W., Dawood, M. Y., & Fuchs, F. (1981, March). Prostaglandins in primary dysmenorrhea: Comparison of prophylactic and nonprophylactic treatment with ibuprofen and use of oral contraceptives. *The American Journal of Medicine, 70*(3), 535–541.

Chesney, M., & Tasto, D. (1975, October). The development of the menstrual symptom questionnaire. *Behaviour Research and Therapy, 13*(4), 237–244.

Colt, E.W.D., Wardlaw, S. L., & Frantz, A. G. (1981). The effect of running on plasma β-endorphin. *Life Sciences, 28*(14), 1637–1640.

Cox, D., & Santirocco, L. (1981). Psychological and behavioral factors in dysmenorrhea. In M.Y. Dawood (Ed.), *Dysmenorrhea.* Baltimore: Williams & Wilkins.

Csapo, A. (1980, October). A rationale for the treatment of dysmenorrhea. *Journal of Reproductive Medicine, 25*(4, Suppl.), 213–221.

Dalton, K. (1977). *The premenstrual syndrome and progesterone therapy.* Chicago: Year Book Medical Publishers.

Dingfelder, J. (1981, August 15). Primary dysmenorrhea treatment with prostaglandin inhibitors: A review. *American Journal of Obstetrics and Gynecology, 140*(8), 874–877.

Farrell, P. A., Gates, W. K., Maksud, M. G., & Morgan, W. P. (1982, May). Increases in plasma β-endorphin/β-lipotropin immunoreactivity after treadmill running in humans. *Journal of Applied Physiology, 52*(5), 1245–1249.

Fraioli, F., Moretti, C., & Paolucci, D., et al., (1980, August). Physical exercise stimulates marked concomitant release of β-endorphin and adrenocorticotropic hormone (ACTH) in peripheral blood in man. *Experientia, 36*(8), 987–989.

Frisk, M., Widholm, O., & Hortling, M. (1965). Dysmenorrhoea—Psyche and soma in teenagers. *Acta Obstetricia et Gynecologica Scandinavica, 44,* 339–347.

Golub, L. J. (1959, July). A new exercise for dysmenorrhea. *American Journal of Obstetrics and Gynecology, 78*(1), 152–155.

Golub, L. J. (1987, May). Exercise that alleviates primary dysmenorrhea. *Contemporary Ob/Gyn, 29*(5), 51–59.

Golub, L. J., Lang, W. R., & Menduke, H. (1958, May/June). Dysmenorrhea in high school and college girls: Relationship to sports participation. *Western Journal of Surgery, Obstetrics and Gynecology, 66*(3), 163–165.

Golub, L. J., Menduke, H., & Lang, W. R. (1968, October). Exercise and dysmenorrhea in young teenagers: A 3-year study. *Obstetrics and Gynecology, 32*(4), 508–511.

Green, T. H. (1977). *Gynecology: Essentials of clinical practice* (3rd ed.). Boston: Little, Brown.

Hansen, M. K., & Secher, N. J. (1975, February 15). Beta-receptor stimulation in essential dysmenorrhea. *American Journal of Obstetrics and Gynecology, 121*(4), 566–567.

Helms, J. M. (1987, January). Acupuncture for the management of primary dysmenorrhea. *Obstetrics and Gynecology, 69*(1), 51–55.

Henzl, M., & Izu, A. (1979). Naproxen and naproxen sodium in dysmenorrhea: Development from in vitro inhibition of prostaglandin synthesis to suppression of uterine contractions in women and development of clinical efficacy. *Acta Obstetricia et Gynecologica Scandinavica, 877*(Suppl.), 105–117.

Iacono, C. U., & Roberts, S. J. (1983). The dysmenorrhea personality: Actuality or statistical artifact? *Social Science and Medicine, 17*(21), 1653–1655.

Israel, S. (1967). *Diagnosis and treatment of menstrual disorders and sterility* (5th ed.). New York: Hoeber Medical Division, Harper and Row.

Jay, M. S., Durant, R.H., Shoffitt, T., & Linder, C. W. (1986, November). Differential response by adolescents to naproxen sodium therapy for spasmodic and congestive dysmenorrhea. *Journal of Adolescent Health Care, 7*(6), 395–400.

Jeffcoate, T.N.A. (1975). *Principles of gynecology* (4th ed.). Boston: Butterworths.

Jordan, J., & Meckler, J. R. (1982, June). The relationship between life change events, social supports, and dysmenorrhea. *Research in Nursing and Health, 5*(2), 73–79.

Kessel, H., & Coppen, A. (1964). The prevalence of common menstrual symptoms. *Obstetrical and Gynecological Survey, 19,* 146–149.

Klein, J. R., & Litt, I. F. (1981, November). Epidemiology of adolescent dysmenorrhea. *Pediatrics, 68*(5), 661–664.

Klein, J. R, Litt, I. F., Rosenberg, A., & Udall, L. (1981, June). The effect of aspirin on dysmenorrhea in adolescents. *The Journal of Pediatrics, 98*(6), 987–990.

Lamb, E. (1981). Clinical features of primary dysmenorrhea. In M. Y. Dawood, (Ed.), *Dysmenorrhea.* Baltimore: Williams & Wilkins.

Lawlor, C. L., & Davis, A. M. (1981, March). Primary dysmenorrhea: Relationship to personality and attitudes in adolescent females. *Journal of Adolescent Health Care, 1*(3), 208–212.

Lennane, K. (1980, October). Social and medical attitudes toward dysmenorrhea. *The Journal of Reproductive Medicine, 25*(4, Suppl.), 202–206.

Lennane, K., & Lennane, R. (1973, February) Alleged psychogenic disorders in women: A possible manifestation of sexual prejudice. *New England Journal of Medicine, 288*(6), 288–292.

Long, J. W. (1985). *The essential guide to prescription drugs* (4th ed.). New York: Harper & Row.

Mead, M. (1955). *Male and female.* New York: Mentor Books.

Menninger, K. (1939, April). Somatic correlations with the unconscious repudiation of femininity in women. *Journal of Nervous and Mental Disease, 89*(4), 514–527.

Modell, W. (Ed.) (1984). *Drugs of choice: 1984–1985.* St. Louis, MO: C.V. Mosby.

Morrison, J., & Nicolls, C. (1981). Epidemiologic, social, and economic aspects of dysmenorrhea. In M. Y. Dawood (Ed.), *Dysmenorrhea.* Baltimore: Williams & Wilkins.

Mosher, C. D. (1914, April 25). A physiologic treatment of congestive dysmenorrhea and kindred disorders associated with the menstrual function. *Journal of the American Medical Association, 62*(18), 1297–1301.

Owen, P. (1984, January 1). Prostaglandin synthetase inhibitors in the treatment of primary dysmenorrhea: Outcome trials reviewed. *American Journal of Obstetrics and Gynecology, 148*(1), 96–103.

Pickles, V. (1957, November 30). A plain muscle stimulant in the menstruum. *Nature, 180*(4596), 1198–1199.

Pickles, V., Hall, W., & Best, F., et al. (1965, April). Prostaglandins in endometrium and menstrual fluid from normal and dysmenorrheic subjects. *British Journal of Obstetrics and Gynecology, 72,* 185–192.

Rees, M. C. P., Anderson, A. B. M., Demers, L. M., & Turnbull, A. C. (1984, July). Prostaglandins in menstrual fluid in menorrhagia and dysmenorrhoea. *British Journal of Obstetrics and Gynecology, 91*(7), 673–680.

Robbins, F. P. (1953, October). Psychosomatic aspects of dysmenorrhea. *American Journal of Obstetrics and Gynecology, 66*(4), 808–815.

Rosenwaks, Z., & Seegar-Jones, G. (1980, October). Menstrual pain: Its origin and pathogenesis. *The Journal of Reproductive Medicine, 25*(4, Suppl.), 194–212.

Schauffler, G. C. (1967, May 10). Dysmenorrhea in and near puberty. *Annals of the New York Academy of Sciences, 142*(3), 794–800.

Seegar-Jones, G. (1980, October). A new perspective on dysmenorrhea [Foreword]. *The Journal of Reproductive Medicine, 25*(4, Suppl.), 193–194.

Sloss, B. M., & Frerichs, R. R. (1983, March). Smoking and menstrual disorders. *International Journal of Epidemiology, 12*(1), 107–109.

Sobczyk, R. (1980, October). Dysmenorrhea: The neglected syndrome. *The Journal of Reproductive Medicine, 25*(4, Suppl.), 198–201.

Sobczyk, R., Braunstein, M., Solberg, L., & Schuman, S. (1978, August). A case control survey and dysmenorrhea in a family practice population: A proposed disability index. *Journal of Family Practice, 7*(2), 285–290.

Spock, B. (1968). *Baby and child care.* London: New English Library.

Stedman's medical dictionary (23rd ed.). (1976). Baltimore: Williams & Wilkins.

Strömberg, P., Forsling, M. L., & Åkerlund, M. (1981, August). Effects of prostaglandin inhibition on vasopressin levels in women with primary dysmenorrhea. *Obstetrics and Gynecology, 58*(2), 206–208.

Trobough, G., Guderian, A. M., & Erickson, R. R., et al., (1978, September). The effect of exogenous intrauterine progesterone on the amount and prostaglandin $F_{2\alpha}$ content of menstrual blood in dysmenorrheic women. *The Journal of Reproductive Medicine, 21*(3), 153–157.

Weidiger, P. (1976). *Menstruation and menopause: The physiology and psychology, the myth and the reality.* New York: Alfred A. Knopf.

Wenzloff, N. J., & Shimp, L. (1984, January). Therapeutic management of primary dysmenorrhea. *Drug Intelligence and Clinical Pharmacy, 18*(1), 22–26.

Wilks, J. W., Wentz, A. C., & Jones, G. S. (1973, September). Prostaglandin $F_{2\alpha}$ concetrations in the blood of women during normal menstrual cycles and dysmenorrhea. *The Journal of Clinical Endocrinology and Metabolism, 37*(3), 469–471.

Willson, J. R., Beecham, C. T., & Carrington, E. R. (1975). *Obstetrics and gynecology* (8th ed.), St. Louis, MO: C. V. Mosby.

Woods, N. F., Most, A., & Dery, G. K. (1982, September). Toward a construct of perimenstrual distress. *Research in Nursing and Health, 5*(2), 123–136.

Woods, N. F., Most, A., & Longenecker, G. D. (1985, September-October). Major life events, daily stressors, and perimenstrual symptoms. *Nursing Research, 34*(5), 263–267.

Ylikorkala, O., & Dawood, M. Y. (1978, April 1). New concepts in dysmenorrhea. *American Journal of Obstetrics and Gynecology, 130*(7), 833–847.

21

Bleeding Disorders

Joanna Ferber Shulman

As the average age of menarche in the United States is 12.8 years and the average age of menopause is approximately 50, the average woman has *menses* (Latin for "months") for about 40 years (Treloar, 1981; Zacharias, Rand, & Wurtman, 1976). Once the pattern of her monthly bleeding becomes established, a woman becomes concerned about any deviation from that pattern. She may also become troubled if her menstrual pattern differs from those of her peers or from the publicized norms for the entire menstruating population. Thus, "abnormal" vaginal bleeding—too much or too little, too soon or too late, too often or too seldom—is one of the most common complaints that the woman of menstruating age brings to the gynecologic office or clinic. Frequently, such concerns require only reassurance from the caregiver, but reassurance that is founded on knowledge of both physiologic variation and pathologic causes of vaginal or uterine bleeding and thorough evaluation of the individual situation. The primary care practitioner must be able to recognize disorders that need more extensive study and/or therapy, initiate such studies, and seek consultation or referral as necessary.

Many abnormalities of menstruation require diagnostic steps and therapeutic modes that lie outside the province of the nonphysician practitioner; however, some bleeding phenomena that are physiologic or related to a clearly identifiable cause such as contraception, a known chronic disease that is under medical care, or stress and life-style may be handled most effectively by the practitioner of well-woman gynecology. In addition, even the woman with a severe problem will benefit from the caring explanation and listening that she can receive from her informed primary caregiver. Furthermore, knowledge about the causes and diagnosis of bleeding disorders enables the primary care provider to make preliminary assessments and perform certain screening tests, in the absence of emergency situations, and thus choose the most appropriate specialist for referral. For these reasons, some detail about various problems is provided in this chapter, even though thorough management frequently requires referral.

This chapter outlines the differential diagnosis of bleeding disorders, describes the data collection necessary when a woman presents with a problem relating to abnormal bleeding, and discusses several specific entities: amenorrhea, oligomenorrhea/hypomenorrhea, intermenstrual bleeding (metrorrhagia), and hypermenorrhea (menorrhagia).

ASSESSMENT

Differential Diagnosis

A host of possible diagnoses fall under the general heading of bleeding disorders. These are listed, in broad categories, in Table 21-1. Some of these entities are discussed in Section III, Gynecologic Pathophysiology. Table 21-1 is not intended to provide an exhaustive compilation of causes of bleeding abnormalities. Rather, it is an attempt to subdivide a complex subject into some clinically useful categories, as an initial approach to diagnosis.

The ability to evaluate a bleeding pattern as normal or abnormal depends on an understanding of physiologic variations in several age groups. The adolescent girl is usually anovulatory for more than half of her first postmenarcheal year (Altchek, 1977; Spellacy, 1983). It takes approximately 15 months for completion of the first 10 cycles and an average of 20 cycles before ovulation occurs regularly (Altchek, 1977). Therefore, irregular bleeding, both in timing and in amount, is the rule in early adolescence, rather than the exception. Similarly, the vast majority of older women experience an increased variation in menstrual interval and quantity during the 5 years preceding the menopause (Spellacy, 1983; Treloar, Boynton, Behn, & Brown, 1967).

Normal menstrual patterns are described as averages derived from observations of large groups of healthy women:

1. Cycle length (first day of menses to *next* first day of menses): 29.5 days, range 21–40 (Reindollar & McDonough, 1983) *or* 26–28 days, range 22–38 (Treloar et al., 1967), depending on age,
2. Duration of menses: 3–8 days (Reindollar & McDonough, 1983) *or* 4–6 ± 2 days (Speroff, Glass, & Kase 1983, p. 233)
3. Blood loss: 40–100 mL (Reindollar & McDonough, 1983) *or* 30–40 mL, upper limit 80 mL (Hallberg, Hogdahl, Nilsson, & Rybo, 1966)
4. Ovulatory bleeding: spotting around the time of ovulation, generally 14 days before the next menses
5. Age-related changes: gradual decrease in cycle length with increasing age (Treloar et al., 1967)

TABLE 21–1. CAUSES OF BLEEDING DISORDERS

A. Amenorrhea

Pregnant
Not pregnant
  Adolescent
    Eugonadal
      Anovulation
        Physiologic
        Polycystic ovarian syndrome
        Hypothalamic
        Hyperprolactinemia
        Other endocrine diseases
      Outflow tract abnormality
        Transverse septum
        Absent uterus and vagina
        Androgen insensitivity syndrome
    Hypogonadal
      Hypergonadotropic
        Ovarian failure
      Hypogonadotropic
        Physiologic delay
        Hypothalamic
        Hyperprolactinemia
        Other endocrine diseases
        Central nervous system tumor
        Chronic disease
  Mature
    Hypothalamic
    Pituitary
      Hyperprolactinemic
      Not hyperprolactinemic
    Ovarian
      Polycystic ovarian syndrome
      Premature ovarian failure
    Uterine scarring
  Menopausal

B. Oligomenorrhea

  Hypothalamic
    Stress, weight loss, exercise
    Drugs that affect neuroendocrine functions, for example,
      some antipsychotic medications, narcotics,
      some antihypertensive agents
  Pituitary
    Hyperprolactinemia
    Other pituitary disorders, such as Cushing's syndrome
    Some drugs
  Ovarian
    Polycystic ovarian syndrome
    Premature ovarian failure
  Other
    Disorders of thyroid or adrenal function, including mild
      forms of congenital adrenal hyperplasia
    Chronic disease

C. Single Episode of Heavy or Unexpected Bleeding

Pregnant
  Abortion
    Threatened
    Incomplete
    Complete
  Trophoblastic disease
  Placental accident
    Placenta previa
    Abruptio placentae
  Cervical change (labor)

Not pregnant
  Adolescent
    Dysfunctional uterine bleeding (anovulation)
      Physiologic
      Stress
        Emotional
        Physical
      Coagulation disorders
    Trauma
    Anatomic/organic
      Malignancy
      Arteriovenous malformations
      Infection
  Mature
    Dysfunctional uterine bleeding (anovulation)
      Stress
    Trauma
    Anatomic/organic
      Leiomyomata
      Polyps
      Retained products of conception
      Subinvolution (postpartum)
      Infection
      Malignancy
  Menopausal
    Dysfunctional uterine bleeding (anovulation)
      Physiologic
    Trauma
    Anatomic/organic
      Leiomyomata
      Polyps
      Infection
      Malignancy

D. Chronic Episodes of Abnormal Bleeding

Pregnant
    Threatened abortion
    Ectopic pregnancy
    Cervical disease
Not pregnant
  Adolescent
    Physiologic
    Anatomic/organic
      Genital tract malformations
      Infection
      Benign neoplasia
      Cervical dysplasia
      Malignancy
      Endocrine disorders
      Chronic disease
    Other
      Drugs
      Stress
      Contraceptive related
  Mature
    Anatomic/organic
      As for Adolescent
      Leiomyomata
      Polyps
      Adenomyosis
    Other
      As for adolescent
  Menopausal
    Physiologic (perimenopausal)
    Pathologic (postmenopausal)
      Malignancy
      Polyps
      Atrophic tissues

Despite the fact that many patients' descriptions of bleeding problems may fall within the range of normalcy just described, the practitioner must search for any pathologic cause for a perceived problem before offering reassurance. Because the causes of bleeding disorders are manifold, the diagnostic and therapeutic procedures range from simple, noninvasive steps that can be managed by the patient and her care provider in the home and office to extensive medical or surgical interventions that require highly specialized medical care.

Data Collection

History. It should be apparent that the first step in diagnosis of abnormal bleeding is the taking of a very detailed history, of which the most important initial piece of information is the patient's age. The incidence of various causes of bleeding problems changes dramatically, depending on whether a woman is peripubertal, reproductively mature, or perimenopausal. Particular attention also must be paid to the description of the vaginal bleeding itself—timing, amount, color, character, onset, and duration of the problem. This information is of crucial importance, yet may be very difficult to obtain accurately. Indeed, an important element of well-woman care is to encourage every woman to record on a calendar the days, amount, and character of her bleeding as a menstrual-life–long habit.

The history taking must proceed to a discussion of associated symptoms, including foul odor; pain, its location, type, duration, and what relieves or worsens it; fever; shaking chills; nausea and vomiting; diarrhea, constipation or rectal straining; urinary frequency, urgency, and dysuria; recent sexual activity; dyspareunia; known pregnancy (current or recent); trauma; and method and use of contraception. After this, the woman's complete gynecologic history must be reviewed. Significant clues to diagnosis may be obtained from knowledge of the woman's age at menarche and, if relevant, menopause, prior menstrual pattern, and any previous treatment for infection or for abnormal bleeding and its results. In addition, obstetric, contraceptive, and sexual histories are important as are observations made at the time of previous gynecologic examinations and surgical procedures. Unfortunately, patients are not always told clearly the indications for and results of such procedures; "my doctor did a scraping and told me everything was fine" is useless. If necessary, previous practitioners or institutions may have to be contacted; once the information is obtained, it should be shared fully with the patient, in writing if necessary.

A thorough history of the woman's general medical status, as well as a review of systems that might point to a hitherto overlooked medical problem, must be obtained. For example, a woman with diarrhea, weight loss, palpitations, and a tremor might be suspected of having hyperthyroidism, which is a well-known cause of menstrual problems, especially oligomenorrhea. Changes in hair pattern or in visual or auditory acuity may be symptoms of hormone-secreting or pituitary tumors. Chronic illness, recent acute illness, changes in weight, appetite, or activity, particularly strenuous exercise, and intake of medications or other substances may all affect the menstrual cycle. Symptoms of systemic bleeding, such as petechiae, bruising, or other bleeding, also must be investigated. Exposure to radiation or toxic chemicals that could damage the ovaries, endometrium, or hypothalamus should be considered (Gaines, 1981a). A nutritional history is valuable, and symptoms of such eating disorders as anorexia nervosa

should be explored. The practitioner must inquire about the patient's social situation, support systems, and psychological status, with attention to any recent changes or increased stress. Finally, a family history may be helpful, as some entities that cause bleeding problems may have a familial association, for example, endometriosis and endometrial or ovarian cancer.

As is generally the case in clinical practice, a well-taken history will lead the practitioner almost to the end of the diagnostic path, even before the patient has been examined formally and without a single laboratory test or diagnostic procedure performed.

Physical Examination. In assessment of abnormal vaginal bleeding, the physical examination should be just as thorough as the history, encompassing far more than the pelvic examination. The woman's general condition and vital signs provide an immediate estimate of the severity of the problem. A patient whose skin is pale and clammy and who has a rapid pulse and a low blood pressure may be in hypovolemic shock from a ruptured ectopic pregnancy, despite her mild complaints of irregular spotting and vague, crampy lower abdominal pain. Conversely, a woman who appears vigorous, with pink mucous membranes and nail beds and a normal pulse and blood pressure, has most likely not had the hemorrhagic quantity of bleeding that she has been describing. She needs reassurance that her problem will be taken seriously but that it is not life threatening. If there is some doubt as to the degree of blood loss, or hypovolemia, the patient can be tested for orthostatic changes in pulse and blood pressure.

The complete physical examination may reveal disorders of nutrition, endocrine function, or coagulation, in addition to or instead of specific abnormalities of the reproductive organs. Relevant findings include obesity or anorexia; delayed or precocious sexual maturation; galactorrhea; hirsutism; signs of thyroid disease such as thyroid enlargement, excessively dry or moist skin, palmar erythema, and exophthalmia; signs of Cushing's syndrome such as facial plethora, moon face, buffalo hump, and excessive acne; and petechiae and ecchymoses.

The speculum examination should include assessment of the source, amount, color, character, and odor of any observed bleeding and the performance of Pap smears, wet preps for diagnosis of vaginitis, cervical cultures for gonorrhea and chlamydia, and an analysis of the cervical mucus. Ferning of cervical mucus, viewed microscopically, implies adequate estrogenization and also constitutes a negative pregnancy test. The bimanual examination, of course, aims to discover any abnormal enlargements, masses, tenderness, or fixation of organs in the pelvis, including the rectum.

Laboratory Tests. Although the history and physical examination will have narrowed the diagnostic pathway, additional studies may be necessary to reach a firm diagnosis. Any woman who complains of heavy bleeding or who might have internal bleeding must have a spun hematocrit measured on capillary or venous blood before leaving the office or clinic. A rapid urine pregnancy test may also be helpful, especially if positive. Other blood tests may be considered, including a complete blood count (CBC) to check for infection, anemia, or thrombocytopenia; coagulation studies; β subunit of human chorionic gonadotropin (hCG) for early pregnancy; and various endocrine parameters such as prolactin (PRL), thyroid-stimulating hormone (TSH), follicle-stimulating hormone (FSH), and luteinizing hormone (LH). In addition, a variety of diagnostic procedures may be necessary, most of which will need to be performed by a gynecologist or other specialist. These may include culdocentesis, uterine sounding, endometrial biopsy, biopsy of a visible lesion, and colposcopy with cervical biopsy. Ultrasound and x-ray studies, such as hysterosalpingogram, intravenous urogram, and barium enema, may be indicated, and diagnosis by surgery may finally be required, such as a fractional dilation and curettage (D&C), hysteroscopy, or laparoscopy.

If a bleeding problem is chronic and the diagnosis unclear, the most useful information may be obtained not by laboratory studies but rather by the patient's keeping a bleeding chart and a basal body temperature (BBT) and cervical mucus chart and returning with it in 1 to 3 months. A biphasic temperature chart with ovulatory mucus patterns (see Chapter 5) ensures normal hypothalamic–pituitary–ovarian function and may save the patient part of a lengthy and costly diagnostic workup (Gaines, 1981b).

AMENORRHEA

Definition and Description

The normal menstrual cycle depends on the integrated functioning of the hypothalamus; the pituitary; the ovary, including the follicle, ovum, cumulus, and corpus luteum; the uterus, particularly the endometrium; and the cervix and vagina or outflow tract. Amenorrhea may result from abnormalities of function or structure of any of these organs. Functional disorders may affect levels of hypothalamic gonadotropin-releasing hormone (GnRH); pituitary follicle-stimulating hormone and luteinizing hormone; and/or ovarian estrogens, progesterone, and androgens.

Speroff and associates (1983, p. 142) established three criteria for the clinical problem of amenorrhea:

1. No period by age 14 in the absence of growth or development of secondary sexual characteristics
2. No period by age 16, regardless of the presence of normal growth and development, and appearance of secondary sexual characteristics
3. Absence of periods in a woman who has been menstruating for a length of time equivalent to a total of at least three of the previous cycle intervals or for 6 months

Of course, any woman who is suspected or known to have a hormonal or anatomic abnormality that could cause amenorrhea should not have her workup delayed until she satisfies the preceding criteria.

Differential Diagnosis and Evaluation

The initial evaluation of the amenorrheic woman can be done in a simple and logical fashion to identify the source of the problem. Note that Speroff and associates do not retain the traditional distinction between primary (criteria 1 and 2) and secondary (criterion 3) amenorrhea; the investigative scheme that is needed "applies comprehensively to all amenorrheas" (Speroff et al., 1983, p. 142). The very first step, sometimes overlooked, with most unfortunate consequences, is to be certain the woman is not pregnant. Table 21-1 (part A) broadly outlines the kinds of disorders that may be responsible for amenorrhea.

Data Collection

THE ADOLESCENT. In the adolescent, combined historical, physical, and laboratory data reveal whether and when the patient has passed the normal pubertal developmental milestones. If there is breast development and if superficial cells are present in a cytologic (Pap) smear of the vaginal epithelium, then the patient is eugonadal. Once pregnancy is definitively excluded, confirmation can be obtained by giving a progestational challenge, consisting of parenteral progesterone-in-oil 200 mg IM or medroxyprogesterone acetate 10 mg orally for 5 to 10 days. A positive withdrawal bleed, which generally occurs within 2 to 7 days of the injection or the last tablet, ensures eugonadal status by demonstrating that the patient is adequately estrogenized. It also confirms a normal outflow tract. The cause of her amenorrhea then is anovulation, which may be physiologic or may result from polycystic ovarian syndrome (a misnomer for a complex set of hormonal abnormalities leading to persistent anovulation) or from hypothalamic causes such as weight loss and strenuous exercise. Hyperprolactinemia and a pituitary tumor should, however, be ruled out by means of a serum prolactin assay and a coned-down (specially focused, limited field) x-ray of the sella turcica before this diagnosis is made.

In a eugonadal adolescent, failure to have withdrawal bleeding after a progesterone challenge suggests a defect of the uterus or vagina. Such a defect may have already been found on physical examination, for example, an imperforate hymen or transverse vaginal septum with associated hematocolpos or hematometra (blood accumulated in the vagina or uterus, respectively), or an absent vagina and perhaps uterus, indicative of Mayer–Rokitansky–Kuster–Hauser syndrome or of the androgen insensitivity syndrome (testicular feminization). In the case of the androgen insensitivity syndrome, there would be absent or only meager pubic and axillary hair. At the identification of a lower tract defect, the woman should be referred to a specialist in gynecologic endocrinology for possible further studies and treatment. See Chapters 11, 13, and 14 for further discussion of congenital anomalies.

A hypogonadal patient lacks breast development or superficial epithelial cells in her vaginal smear, or both. She does not have a withdrawal bleed after a progesterone challenge. In this case, the status of the outflow tract can be tested by administering orally active estrogen to stimulate endometrial proliferation (for example, 2.5 mg conjugated estrogens orally daily for 21 days) followed by the progestational agent during the last 5 to 10 days. If bleeding does not occur, especially after a second course of estrogen and progestin, a uterine or vaginal abnormality can be assumed. If bleeding does occur, then the problem is due to the failure to produce estrogen.

The next step is to determine whether this failure originates in the ovary or at the hypothalamic–pituitary level. Measuring serum gonadotropins (FSH, LH) will make this distinction; if these levels are high, the patient has ovarian failure, with some rare exceptions, and further studies by a gynecologic endocrinologist are in order.

If the gonadotropin levels are low or normal, then a pituitary tumor must be considered; a coned-down roentgenographic view of the sella turcica in the lateral projection may demonstrate its presence or absence. Alternatively, computerized tomography (CT) or magnetic resonance imaging (MRI) may be employed to search for a pituitary tumor or other intracranial abnormality. Serum prolactin, thyroid-stimulating hormone, and other hormones, such as adrenocorticotropin (ACTH), cortisol, and growth hormone, may be at abnormal levels in the presence of a pituitary tumor. Other lesions of the central nervous system, for example, craniopharyngioma, infection, trauma, and hydrocephalus, may cause hypogonadotropism, as may certain genetic disorders, such as Kallman's syndrome, which is hypogonadotropic hypogonadism associated with anosmia (absence of the sense of smell) (Tagatz, Fialkow, Smith, & Spadoni, 1970).

In the absence of any of the preceding pituitary lesions, the hypogonadotropism must result from hypothalamic problems. With this in mind, it is important once again to review the history for recent stress, weight loss, strenuous exercise, and chronic systemic disorders. The relationships between stress, weight loss, exercise, and amenorrhea are discussed under Intervention in some detail, because the primary care provider can offer valuable advice to the woman whose problem seems to result from these causes. A number of chronic diseases, however, have been implicated in causing pubertal and menstrual delay by interfering with hypothalamic–pituitary maturation. These include malabsorption syndromes, renal, pulmonary, and cardiovascular diseases, hemoglobinopathies, and neoplasia (Reindollar & McDonough, 1983). Correct management of these disorders requires referral to the appropriate medical or surgical specialist. The practitioner should be aware that the most common cause of reversible hypogonadotropism is physiologic or constitutional delay for which teaching, reassurance, and follow-up are the only necessary treatments.

THE MATURE WOMAN. If the patient is a postpubertal woman who has had menses for some time, but becomes amenorrheic, a similar search for the responsible reproductive organ or ''compartment'' (Speroff et al., 1983, p. 143) must be undertaken, although the list of underlying causes is altered a bit from that pertaining to the adolescent. For example, a woman who has menstruated in the past cannot have congenital obstruction or absence of the uterus or vagina. But she may subsequently develop uterine synechiae (Asherman's syndrome) during an abortion or postpartum curettage, or endometrial fibrosis as a result of tuberculous endometritis or other granulomatous disease, and will not have withdrawal bleeding to progestin, nor estrogen plus progestin, challenge.

The role of contraception should be considered. Amenorrhea may occur with progestin-only oral contraceptives or with progesterone-containing injectable contraceptives. Amenorrhea may follow discontinuation of oral contraceptives; this temporary condition is known as postpill amenorrhea. If it persists more than 6 months, a thorough investigation is needed.

In the evaluation of the amenorrheic patient, the scheme proposed by Speroff and associates (1983, pp. 145–145) is both simple and complete in leading to identification of the responsible compartment of the reproductive system. It is presented here in modified outline form, as most of the problems uncovered require referral for detailed diagnosis and therapy (Table 21–2).

THE PERIMENOPAUSAL WOMAN. Amenorrhea may signal the menopause; this usually follows a period of menstrual disturbances of both flow and frequency. The diagnosis of menopause on clinical grounds alone requires 6 to 12 months of amenorrhea in a woman over the age of 45. The diagnosis can be confirmed by finding of elevated LH and FSH levels (hypergonadotropic hypogonadism). Serious confusion may occasionally result when a woman in her mid forties has a short period of amenorrhea and then a

TABLE 21–2. LABORATORY STUDIES

1. Pregnant?	Yes	Stop.
	No	Proceed to 2.
2. Galactorrhea?	Yes	Add sella turcica film to steps in 3, regardless of PRL level (see 5).
	No	Proceed to 3.
3. a. TSH level	High	Diagnosis—*primary hypothyroidism.*
	Normal	Proceed to 3b.
b. PRL level	High ($\geq$ 100 ng/mL)	Sella turcica film (see 5).
	Normal	Proceed to 3c.
c. Progestin challenge	Positive (with normal TSH, Negative PRL)	Diagnosis—*anovulation.*
		Proceed to 3d.
d. Estrogen and progestin challenge	Positive	Diagnosis—*hypogonadism.* Proceed to 4.
	Negative	Diagnosis—*uterine or vaginal problem.*
4. FSH and LH levels	High	Diagnosis—*ovarian failure.*
	Normal or low	Sella turcica film (see 5).
5. Sella turcica film (coned-down view)	Abnormal	CT scan.
	Normal	PRL elevated: Diagnosis—*pituitary microadenoma.* PRL normal: Diagnosis—*hypothalamic amenorrhea.*

positive pregnancy test. Tests for pregnancy which measure hCG, not just the β chain of hCG, also measure FSH and LH, because these three polypeptide hormones have a common α chain. Therefore, pregnancy testing in a woman in this age group should be done by means of a specific assay for the β subunit of hCG. See Chapter 4 for more discussion of pregnancy testing.

Role of the Primary Care Provider. The extent to which the primary care provider pursues diagnostic screening for a woman of any age depends on clinic or practice protocols and consultation agreements. Certainly, blood work can be obtained by the primary care provider but special X-rays, like sella turcica views, CT, or MRI, are done after consultation or referral. Administration of a progestin or estrogen-progestin challenge generally requires consultation.

Intervention

Once the compartment responsible for amenorrhea is identified, the detailed pathology and treatment generally are pursued by specialists (Marut & Dawood, 1983; Rebar, Coulam, Little, & Schnatz, 1984; Speroff et al., 1983, pp. 141–184; Yen, 1986a, 1986b). In some practice settings, hormonal therapy may be co-managed with care provided by the primary practitioner in consultation with a gynecologist. Only hypothalamic amenorrhea, which is diagnosed by excluding pituitary lesions in the context of hypogonadotropism, may not require extensive medical therapy. Indeed, a caregiver other than a physician may, at times, be better equipped to manage the potentially reversible causes of hypothalamic dysfunction such as stress, weight loss for nonorganic reasons, and strenuous exercise programs.

In the not-too-distant past, many so-called female problems, either of menstruation or of fertility, were treated with the general advice to relax—advice that reflected either well-intentioned ignorance or disinterest on the part of the practitioner. Today, however, research on the interaction between nervous system or neurotransmitter functions and hormonal regulation throughout the body is revealing a biologic basis for the relation of stress to physiologic phenomena.

The hypothalamus is a major arena for this interaction as it receives neurotransmitter signals from various parts of the brain and responds with the release of a wide variety of hormones, including GnRH (Yen, 1986c). Any disruption of the normal pulsatile pattern of GnRH release leads ultimately to amenorrhea; the release of GnRH from the hypothalamus is regulated or affected by a number of neurotransmitters and brain hormones. Dopamine inhibits and norepinephrine stimulates a variety of hypothalamic functions; these two neurotransmitters may provide the control of GnRH production (Kase, 1983a). Serotonin, another major neurotransmitter in the hypothalamus, does not seem to have a direct role, but may influence GnRH secretion by way of its conversion to melatonin in the pineal gland (for which organ a role in human reproduction has long been sought) (Cardinali, 1981; Kase, 1983b). Additionally, β-endorphins, which are produced from "big ACTH" or pro-opiomelanocortin (POMC) in response to stress, have been shown to decrease gonadotropin production, presumably by affecting GnRH secretion (Blankstein, Reyes, Winter, & Faiman, 1981; Quigley, Sheehan, Casper, & Yen, 1980); they also stimulate prolactin secretion (Reid, Hoff, Yen, & Li, 1981; Stubbs et al., 1978).

As the interaction between nervous system functions and hormonal regulation is better understood, the biochemical basis for hypothalamic amenorrhea is becoming clearer; what is needed is further knowledge of the effects of stress, both physical and mental, on neurotransmitter function and thus on endocrine activities. Meanwhile, the job of the primary caregiver is to help the amenorrheic patient to identify, cope with, and perhaps ultimately resolve the sources of stress in her life. The principles of the psychosomatic approach to diagnosis and treatment may be most helpful (Youngs & Reame, 1983). Referrals for psychological therapy or for stress reduction therapies such as biofeedback may be indicated. The source of stress in a woman's life, however, may be self-chosen and presumably enjoyable, that is, strenuous exercise, and therefore her amenorrhea must be managed within the context of continuation of this activity, if that is her choice.

That strenuous exercise causes amenorrhea is well-documented (Feicht et al. 1978; Frisch et al., 1981; Hale, 1983; Malina, Harper, Avent, & Campbell 1973; Shangold & Levine, 1982; Speroff, 1984; Warren, 1980). What is less clear is whether the amenorrhea results from exercise alone (Abraham, Beumont, Fraser, & Llewellyn-Jones, 1982; Bullen et al., 1985) or from the associated weight loss (Frisch, 1977; Frisch & McArthur, 1974; Vigersky, Andersen, Thompson, & Loriaux, 1977), decrease in body fat even without a change in weight (Boyden et al., 1982), or emotional stress associated with maintaining a rigorous training schedule. It has been suggested that there is a critical weight that must be achieved by a woman of a given height for her to establish menarche and regular menses. Even more important is the percentage of body weight that is fat (Frisch, 1977); a loss of body weight of 10 to 15 percent may include a loss of body fat sufficient to cause amenorrhea. This theory, however, has been seriously questioned (Billewicz, Fellowes, & Hytten, 1976; Ellison, 1981; Johnston,

Malina, & Galbraith 1971; Johnston, Roche, Schell, & Wettenhall, 1975). Several studies of young ballet dancers with menarcheal delay show that sexual development and onset of menarche correlate with periods of forced rest without change in body weight or composition (Abraham et al., 1982; Warren, 1980). The incidence of exercise-induced amenorrhea varies with the nature of the activity (dancing > running > swimming and cycling), the amount of training (in runners and dancers), and the age of onset of training: girls who begin training before menarche have menarcheal delay and also experience more subsequent menstrual disorders than do those who start training after menarche (Frisch et al., 1981).

If, after careful study according to the scheme outlined earlier, the cause of amenorrhea in a given woman is determined to be her exercise program, there are several options for treatment. She may choose to reduce the intensity or duration of exercise or to gain some weight and see whether her problem resolves. If she remains amenorrheic, she requires hormonal therapy to prevent subsequent problems. If a progestin challenge induces withdrawal bleeding, she is producing sufficient estrogen to be at risk for endometrial hyperplasia or carcinoma, and therefore should be treated with medroxyprogesterone acetate 10 mg daily for 10 days each month. If a progestin challenge does not induce withdrawal bleeding, then she is hypoestrogenic and at risk for osteoporosis, atrophic vaginitis, and perhaps cardiovascular diseases. She should be treated with conjugated estrogens 0.625 to 1.25 mg daily on days 1 to 25 of each month and medroxyprogesterone acetate 10 mg daily on days 16 to 25. Alternatively, low-dose oral contraceptives may be used to provide similar hormonal protection. Hormonal therapy may be co-managed or physician managed depending on the practice setting. Teaching and counseling must emphasize the preventive nature of this therapy.

Care for the perimenopausal woman requires attention to changing patterns of bleeding that result from decreasing estrogen secretion and from anovulation, as well as to attendant symptoms such as hot flushes, headaches, insomnia, and mood changes. All of these may be normal effects of declining ovarian function, but they are nonetheless real, and more or less disabling, to the woman who experiences them. Hormonal therapy with progestins, or with estrogens plus progestin, may be indicated for menstrual regulation, as well as for relief of the symptoms, and for prevention of vaginal dryness and osteoporosis. Extensive discussion of the perimenopause is found in Chapter 24.

OLIGOMENORRHEA/HYPOMENORRHEA

Definition and Description

The term *oligomenorrhea* is frequently used to describe any situation of decreased menses, in time or amount or both. Strictly, oligomenorrhea refers to too-seldom menses: normal bleeding at greater-than-usual intervals. The term *hypomenorrhea* refers to scanty (too little) bleeding at normal intervals. On the basis of these definitions, one would suspect that oligomenorrhea results from hormonal problems—hypothalamic, pituitary, or ovarian—whereas hypomenorrhea might reflect end-organ or uterine problems or hormonal influences on the endometrium itself.

Differential Diagnosis and Evaluation

Today, one of the most common causes of hypomenorrhea is the use of oral contraceptives. Recent estimates are that

8.6 million American women take OCs (Bachrach, 1984); it is therefore important to explain in advance, when prescribing OCs, that their use decreases menstrual flow by as much as two thirds. This results from the continuous action of the progestin component, which produces a decidualized endometrium with "exhausted" and atrophic glands. Indeed, OCs are often prescribed for treatment of hypermenorrhea.

Other causes of hypomenorrhea include structural abnormalities of the endometrium or of the uterus that result in either partial destruction of the endometrium itself (e.g., partial Asherman's syndrome or tuberculous endometritis) or congenitally caused partial obstruction of the outflow tract (see Chapter 14).

The clinical entities responsible for oligomenorrhea include many of those causing amenorrhea, as the difference in menstrual function may be only a matter of degree. The approach to the patient is similar to that for the patient with amenorrhea, except that tests for the intactness of the outflow tract are not necessary. The diagnostic effort focuses instead on abnormalities of ovarian, pituitary, or hypothalamic function, either as primary causes or as these organs are affected by other disorders such as thyroid, adrenal, or other endocrine diseases, chronic disease in general, or drug use or abuse.

Oligomenorrhea also may be physiologic or part of the normal pattern of events for the first few years after menarche and again for several years before the menopause (Treloar et al., 1967). These periods of oligomenorrhea may be punctuated by episodes of very heavy bleeding (dysfunctional uterine bleeding), occurring as estrogen-breakthrough bleeding.

The major pathologic causes for oligomenorrhea are listed in Table 21–1B. The diagnostic workup for these disorders has been presented under Amenorrhea. The role of the primary care provider in diagnosis is comparable.

Intervention

Treatment efforts for oligomenorrhea should be aimed at reversing the underlying cause, if possible. Alternatively, hormonal replacement therapy using progestins, with or without estrogens, should be undertaken to prevent the complications of unopposed estrogen production (endometrial hyperplasia or carcinoma) or of absent estrogen (osteoporosis, hot flushes, vaginal dryness, and other menopausal symptoms). Hormonal treatment requires consultation or referral, depending on the practice setting and protocols. The maximum time interval allowed between successive treatments with oral medroxyprogesterone is about 10 to 12 weeks (Kase, 1983a, p. 366, 1983c, p. 265), although most authors routinely suggest a monthly regimen.

Teaching and counseling should emphasize the need for women to keep careful records of vaginal bleeding. Thorough explanations of the preventive value of therapeutic regimens should be provided. See Chapters 14 and 24 for further discussion of the consequences of unopposed estrogen and decreased estrogen.

INTERMENSTRUAL BLEEDING (METRORRHAGIA)

Definition and Description

In the broadest sense, intermenstrual bleeding refers to any episode of bleeding, whether spotting or hemorrhage or "like a period," that occurs at a time other than the normal menses. This implies that the woman is indeed menstruating regularly and that the intermenstrual bleeding has a cause that is separate from the menstrual cycle itself. It may be difficult, however, to fit a given woman's bleeding disorder into just this subdivision, or any of the other categories presented in this chapter, especially in the absence of a bleeding record that has been carefully maintained over a period of months.

Differential Diagnosis and Evaluation

A small amount of bleeding at the time of ovulation, that is, 14 days before the onset of the next menses, is considered normal. The etiology of ovulatory spotting remains unclear; however, it is a common occurrence, best documented by its repetitive timing in the menstrual cycle.

Intermenstrual bleeding may be related directly to contraceptive use. Many women with an intrauterine device experience spotting between periods (as well as heavier bleeding with menses). This may be due to endometritis or salpingitis, partial expulsion of the IUD, or to any of the other causes of intermenstrual bleeding to be discussed. See Chapter 8 for more information about this contraceptive method, and Chapters 14 and 15 for further discussion of endometritis and salpingitis. If all of these entities have been ruled out, and the bleeding is not severe, the IUD may be left in place. Consideration should be given to iron supplementation by diet, pills, or both (Hatcher et al., 1984, p. 91).

Oral contraceptive use may also give rise to episodes of spotting, especially during the 3 months after initiation (Hatcher et al., 1984, p. 51). The problem may be alleviated simply by reassurance and by recommending that pills be taken at exactly the same time each day. Women can be assisted in developing a routine so that taking the pill is associated with a never-omitted daily activity. For persistent spotting, a different formulation may be tried, increasing either the estrogenic or the progestational potency of the pills. The former may be helpful for treating spotting that occurs early in the cycle, and the latter for late spotting. Chapter 7 details the management of pill-related problems.

As with diagnosis of other bleeding disorders, the practitioner must always investigate whether the patient could be, or recently was, pregnant. Perceived intermenstrual bleeding could signal such disorders as threatened abortion or actual miscarriage, ectopic pregnancy, molar pregnancy, retained products of conception (even placental polyps), subinvolution of the uterus, and postpartum or postabortal endometritis.

In the absence of any of these conditions, the practitioner must consider many other possible causes of intermenstrual bleeding; some may be obvious and/or readily treatable, whereas others may require extensive specialized workup and treatment. These include trauma, foreign objects, vaginitis, cervicitis, endocervical polyps, cervical eversion (ectopy, ectropion), cervical dysplasia, endometritis, endometrial polyps, leiomyomata, salpingitis/adnexitis, benign functional ovarian cysts, endometriosis, benign neoplasms, and malignancies of any portion of the genital tract.

Data Collection

A complete bleeding history, described earlier in this chapter under Assessment, is important, with the focus on possible association of the bleeding with any antecedent event such as coitus or douching. Although it may seem obvious, the practitioner should inquire whether the patient is certain that the bleeding is vaginal, rather than (most commonly) rectal, in origin.

The physical examination should of course concentrate on the quantity, quality, and source of any observed bleeding in addition to all of the other elements of the examination. Frequently, however, there is no visible bleeding, nor any obvious source for the bleeding, at the time the woman is present in the office. If this is the case, and if no diagnosis can be made, the patient should be asked to return at the time of the next episode of intermenstrual bleeding. This point may need special instruction and emphasis, for many women, because of a sense of modesty or of feeling unclean, are reluctant to undergo a gynecologic examination when they are bleeding. They also may have been told not to have their routine checkup and Pap smear while menstruating and therefore need to learn that the situation is different when abnormal bleeding is the complaint.

Even in the absence of active bleeding, some simple diagnostic procedures can be done, including a wet mount, in saline, of any vaginal discharge, for microscopic examination; a Pap smear; a cervical culture; and a white blood cell count and erythrocyte sedimentation rate. Any visible lesion should be biopsied, for which referral to a gynecologist is necessary. Ultrasound may reveal useful information about any palpated pelvic mass, for example, whether it is cystic or solid. Finally, a dilation and curettage (D&C) or laparoscopy or both may be indicated as diagnostic methods.

Intervention

Treatment of intermenstrual bleeding depends on the diagnosis made and ranges from reassurance for ovulatory bleeding, through observation of a presumed functional ovarian cyst for one to three menstrual cycles, adjustment of oral contraceptive regimens, removal of foreign objects and repair of trauma, to antibiotic therapy for lower and upper tract infections, removal of polyps, further evaluation of any abnormal Pap smear including colposcopy, biopsy, cautery, cryotherapy, and/or conization, and finally, to the extensive additional workup and therapy, including surgery, chemotherapy, and radiotherapy, for malignancy. The primary care practitioner must initiate timely consultation or referral. Teaching and counseling must prepare women for the diagnostic procedures necessary, to the extent the practitioner anticipates them at a given point in the evaluation. All patient concerns must be addressed and questions answered as completely as possible.

HYPERMENORRHEA (MENORRHAGIA)

Definition and Description

Profuse or prolonged bleeding occurring at normal intervals constitutes hypermenorrhea or menorrhagia. It is only one of several patterns of excessive vaginal bleeding. A precise definition of hypermenorrhea, or of excessive bleeding in general, is very difficult to establish because of the wide variations in normal. If a woman considers the amount or duration of blood flow to be excessive, however, then diagnostic and therapeutic measures are warranted. The hemoglobin concentration and hematocrit are objective guides to the actual amount of blood lost.

Polymenorrhea refers to normal bleeding at shorter-than-usual intervals. This is common in postmenarcheal girls and also in some premenopausal women. It also may be the presenting complaint of women who have intermenstrual bleeding of sufficient amount to be interpreted as a second monthly period.

Differential Diagnosis and Evaluation

The organic causes of hypermenorrhea are many and include anatomic lesions, inflammatory processes, dyscrasias, systemic diseases, and carcinoma, as well as hormonal disturbances. As with other bleeding disorders, the practitioner must not forget the possible role of contraceptive use. In particular, the IUD commonly increases the menstrual flow. Women receiving an IUD must be advised that increased bleeding is likely. For some women, an IUD may be contraindicated for this reason; however, the incorporation of progesterone into the IUD (Progestasert-T) has diminished the problem of hypermenorrhea (Hatcher et al., 1984, pp. 80, 230).

Probably the most common anatomic cause of heavy menstrual bleeding is the presence of uterine leiomyomata (myomas or fibroids). These benign tumors may be found in submucosal, intramural, or subserosal locations. The submucosal site, though the least common, causes the most problems with bleeding, apparently because of changes in the overlying endometrium and its blood supply. Submucous myomas may be felt at the time of curettage, seen by hysteroscopy, or revealed as filling defects on a hysterosalpingogram. Intramural myomas also have been cited as a cause of heavy menses; presumably they interfere with the normal contractility of the myometrium. Subserosal myomas generally are not implicated as causing hypermenorrhea. Further discussion and illustrations of uterine myomas are provided in Chapter 14.

Adenomyosis is also a fairly common cause of heavy menses, as well as of intermenstrual or premenstrual spotting, usually accompanied by dysmenorrhea. Adenomyosis is the presence of functional endometrial tissue deep within the uterine myometrium, not connected with the normal endometrium (see Chapter 14). It usually occurs in multiparous women in the fourth and fifth decades and is frequently misdiagnosed as leiomyomata, which, in fact, often accompany adenomyosis (Emge, 1962). With adenomyosis alone, the uterus becomes enlarged and may be somewhat irregular and tender; however, it is not enlarged to the extent it may be with myomas. Adenomyosis cannot be definitively diagnosed except by histopathology at the time of hysterectomy or, rarely, hysterotomy; hysterectomy is also the therapy of choice.

Even if the history and examination point clearly to the existence of leiomyomata or adenomyosis, the practitioner is not entitled to conclude that the cause of hypermenorrhea has therefore been found. Endometrial hyperplasia or carcinoma may coexist with myometrial abnormalities and must be searched for by endometrial curettage. Indeed, endometrial hyperplasia or carcinoma may frequently coexist with adenomyosis (Emge, 1962; Marcus, 1961).

Abnormalities of endometrial growth are frequent causes of heavy menstrual bleeding as well as of intermenstrual bleeding. These abnormalities range from endometrial polyps through cystic hyperplasia and adenomatous hyperplasia, to frankly malignant adenocarcinoma or other, less common, endometrial cancers. See Chapter 14 for further discussion of these disorders. Diagnosis of these entities is by endometrial curettage.

A rare anatomic cause of extremely heavy menses is an arteriovenous malformation in the uterine wall; this requires special radiographic studies (arteriography) for diagnosis, generally after all other diagnostic and therapeutic measures have failed.

Inflammatory processes such as endometritis, chronic or acute, and salpingitis may sometimes cause heavy menses. The menstrual abnormality may be the presenting complaint of a woman with only mild infection. Other clues are necessary to arrive at the diagnosis and appropriate antibiotic regimen. See Chapters 14 and 15 for more information on diagnosis and treatment of these infections.

Any woman with recurrent episodes of hypermenorrhea must be investigated for a disorder of coagulation, such as thrombocytopenia, of several possible etiologies, or von Willebrand's disease. The history may include easy bruisability, frequent nosebleeds, or bleeding from the gums. Alternatively, there may be a history suspicious for autoimmune or collagen-vascular disease. Laboratory studies should include, at least, platelet count, prothrombin time, partial thromboplastin time, and fibrinogen concentration. Referral to an internist or hematologist is indicated if the history and/or laboratory parameters suggest a coagulation defect. Hypermenorrhea may be the first clinical manifestation of a coagulopathy in an adolescent girl (Dunn & Steingold, 1985; Mishell, Fisher, & Haynes et al. 1984).

Constant or intermittent bleeding or very heavy bleeding at irregular intervals is the most common presentation of *dysfunctional uterine bleeding* (DUB). To most authors, DUB is synonymous with anovulatory bleeding; however, as with other menstrual disorders, a host of other causes must be ruled out before the diagnosis of DUB can be made. These include especially pregnancy-related events, which can be responsible for either profuse bleeding, as occurs with spontaneous abortion/miscarriage, placenta previa, or abruptio placentae; trophoblastic disease; or, for intermittent bleeding, threatened abortion and ectopic pregnancy. Additionally, the anatomic and systemic pathologies listed earlier must be sought and eliminated.

Speroff and associates (1983, p. 225) list "three major categories of dysfunctional endometrial bleeding": estrogen-breakthrough bleeding, estrogen-withdrawal bleeding, and progestin-breakthrough bleeding. Estrogen-breakthrough bleeding occurs when the endometrium is continuously stimulated by estrogen in the absence of progesterone. Similarly, progestin-breakthrough bleeding occurs when there is an abnormally high ratio of progesterone to estrogen, as in women using progestin-only hormonal contraception. Estrogen-withdrawal bleeding occurs when an estrogen source is abruptly removed, such as by bilateral oophorectomy or by discontinuation of exogenous estrogen therapy.

Of these three categories, the most important clinically is estrogen-breakthrough bleeding, which may manifest itself either by intermittent but prolonged spotting, if estrogen levels are low, or by prolonged periods of amenorrhea interrupted by episodes of profuse bleeding and attendant severe anemia, if estrogen levels are chronically high. As suggested earlier, both of these pictures are fairly common among perimenarcheal teenagers and perimenopausal women in their forties. Nevertheless, any condition that gives rise to chronic anovulation, in the context of continuing estrogen production, may lead to DUB. Such conditions include polycystic ovarian syndrome, obesity, hyper- and hypothyroidism, estrogen-secreting ovarian neoplasms, and any of the endocrine problems that have been discussed under Amenorrhea and Oligomenorrhea.

Intervention

Treatment for hypermenorrhea is dependent on the cause of the bleeding. IUDs may have to be removed or changed to the progesterone-containing type if the bleeding is se-

vere or the woman anemic. Treatment for symptomatic myomas is usually surgical: myomectomy or hysterectomy. Medical therapy may be used in conjunction with surgery. Chapter 14 discusses this in greater detail. The treatment for adenomyosis is also surgical. Hormonal manipulation does not seem to help, although minimal disease may be treated with analgesics, especially prostaglandin inhibitors. Some benign endometrial abnormalities may be treated, as well as diagnosed, by dilation and curettage. Other abnormalities require hormonal therapy; generally, progestational agents are used. In an older woman, especially with extensive or recurrent disease, hysterectomy may be a preferred method of treatment. Malignant disease, of course, requires a staging workup and extensive therapy. As a practical point, however, the practitioner should remember that some cases of endometrial hyperplasia and carcinoma arise from continuous or unopposed estrogen stimulation of the endometrium. Therefore, the practitioner must carefully ascertain whether continuous estrogen exposure could be occurring as from chronic anovulation, from a theca or granulosa cell tumor of the ovary, or from exogenous estrogen administration.

Therapy for DUB is hormonal: periodic progestin administration for the chronically anovulatory woman with adequate estrogen production or combined estrogen and progestin (as in oral contraceptive pills) for the anovulatory adolescent. This assumes that all other treatable causes of DUB have been ruled out. If this therapy fails, reevaluation is necessary.

Finally, it should be noted that for the normal woman who has heavy menses without any pathologic cause, as well as for the IUD wearer, prostaglandin synthetase inhibitors, including aspirin, ibuprofen, indomethacin, mefenamic acid, and naproxen, may be effective in decreasing the menstrual blood loss (Anderson, Haynes, Guillebaud, & Turnbull, 1976; Fraser, Pearse, & Shearman et al., 1981; Speroff et al., 1983, p. 239). The exact mechanism for this effect is not clear; however, prostaglandins, especially PGE_2 and $PGF_{2\alpha}$, are found in human endometrial tissue in increasing amounts as the menstrual cycle progresses. They are well known to have profound effects on vascular dilation or constriction and on platelet aggregation, both of which may influence the amount of menstrual blood lost.

ADDENDUM: ROLE OF THE D&C

The D (dilation of the cervix) and C (curettage, scraping of the endometrium) has recently come under suspicion as being unnecessary except as a source of income for physician and hospital. As the D&C is commonly recommended in the context of abnormal uterine bleeding, it might be useful to review both its purpose and its practice.

Curettage of the uterine cavity may at times be curative of a bleeding problem, if it removes the abnormal, causative tissue, such as products of conception, polyps, or focal endometrial hyperplasia. Its major purpose, however, is diagnostic. The tissue removed is studied in the histopathology laboratory and endometrial abnormalities are reported. Further therapy depends on the laboratory information. Additionally, the D&C provides information about the size and shape of the uterine cavity, which may be important in ruling out leiomyomata or in staging endometrial carcinoma.

The curettage procedure involves repetitive scraping of the endometrium until the entire uterine cavity is sampled. An endometrial biopsy is a single strip of endometrium, usually taken for purposes of dating the endometrium within the menstrual cycle. This might be done to confirm ovulation, or its absence, or to establish a luteal phase defect; it is not intended to find the cause of a bleeding abnormality and is certainly not sufficient to rule out the presence of a malignancy.

Most authors and clinicians agree that a D&C is a required part of the diagnostic effort for abnormal uterine bleeding, especially for heavy bleeding or intermenstrual bleeding, where endometrial abnormalities are more likely. The important exception is the adolescent woman with apparent DUB, where the likelihood of another problem is so small as not to merit the discomforts and risks of a D&C. Some authors (Grimes, 1982; Speroff et al., 1983, pp. 240–241) believe that endometrial sampling should be done only after medical therapy fails in *all* women, except those at high risk for endometrial carcinoma. Risk factors include age over 40, obesity, polycystic ovarian syndrome, and estrogen therapy without progesterone. In one retrospective study of more than 1,000 D&Cs, less than 4 percent of women under the age of 40 demonstrated malignant endometrial tissue (Smith & Schulman, 1985).

The D&C no longer has to be a hospital procedure, with a preoperative and a postoperative overnight stay and general anesthesia. The equivalent diagnostic information can be obtained from a procedure performed in the gynecologist's office, in the majority of cases (Grimes, 1982). Not only is this more convenient and less expensive, but it may also be safer. Although infrequent, possible D&C complications include infection and uterine perforation (Smith & Schulman, 1985). Complications of anesthesia are also possible.

The D&C procedure involves the following:

1. Tenaculum placement on the cervix: Local anesthesia, either topical (Rabin, Dwyer, & Kaiser, 1988) or injected, may eliminate discomfort.
2. Cervical dilation
   a. Minimal dilation is needed if the patient is of reproductive age, and if a small (4-mm-diameter), soft-suction curette is used.
   b. Paracervical block anesthesia may eliminate or reduce the pain of dilation.
   c. Topical anesthesia, inserted into the endocervical canal, may have a role here and is currently being explored (Rabin et al., 1988).
   d. Diazepam and/or a narcotic analgesic such as meperidine may rarely be needed. More often, gentle and patient explanations and techniques reduce anxiety and fear, which are well-known enhancers of pain.
3. Endometrial curettage
   a. Currently available soft curettes or endometrial samplers provide adequate tissue samples with less pain than older techniques using sharp metal curettes.
   b. Vacuum aspiration methods allow rapid sampling of the entire endometrial cavity.
   c. Prostaglandin synthetase inhibitors given 20 to 30 minutes before the procedure may significantly reduce the discomfort of curettage.
   d. Again, explanation and reassurance to the patient may provide significant psychological analgesia.
4. Postoperative cramping and bleeding
   a. Usually minimal
   b. May be controlled by prostaglandin-inhibiting agents

Hysterosalpingography and hysteroscopy also may provide useful information about the shape and contents of the uterine cavity and may be used in conjunction with the histologic sample obtained by curettage to arrive at a diagnosis and, hence, appropriate treatment for abnormal uterine bleeding.

REFERENCES

Abraham, S. F., Beumont, P. J. V., Fraser, I. S., & Llewellyn-Jones, D. (1982, July). Body weight, exercise and menstrual status among ballet dancers in training. *British Journal of Obstetrics and Gynaecology, 89*(7), 507–510.

Altchek, A. (1977, September). Dysfunctional uterine bleeding in adolescence. *Clinical Obstetrics and Gynecology, 20*(3), 633–650.

Anderson, A. B. M., Haynes, P. J., Guillebaud, J., & Turnbull, A. C. (1976, April 10). Reduction of menstrual blood loss by prostaglandin synthetase inhibitors. *Lancet, 1* (7963), 774–776.

Bachrach, C. A. (1984, November-December) Contraceptive practice among American women: 1973–1982. *Family Planning Perspectives, 16*(6), 253–259.

Billewicz, W. Z., Fellowes, H. M., & Hytten, C. A. (1976, January). Comments on the critical metabolic mass and the age of menarche. *Annals of Human Biology, 3*(1), 51–59.

Blankstein, J., Reyes, F. I., Winter, J. S. D., & Faiman, C. (1981, March). Endorphins and the regulation of the human menstrual cycle. *Clinical Endocrinology, 14*(3), 287–294.

Boyden, T. W., Pamenter, R. W., & Grosso, D., et al., (1982, April). Prolactin responses, menstrual cycles, and body composition of women runners. *Journal of Clinical Endocrinology and Metabolism, 54*(4), 711–714.

Bullen, B.A., Skrinar, G.S., & Beitins, I.Z., et al., (1985, May 23). Induction of menstrual disorders by strenuous exercise in untrained women. *New England Journal of Medicine, 312* (21), 1349–1353.

Cardinali, D.P. (1981, Summer). Melatonin: A mammalian pineal hormone. *Endocrine Review, 2*(3), 327–346.

Dunn, L. J., & Steingold, K. A. (1985). Menstrual abnormalities. In D. H. Nichols, & J. R. Evrard (Eds.), *Ambulatory gynecology.* Philadelphia: Harper & Row.

Ellison, P. T. (1981, March). Threshold hypotheses, developmental age, and menstrual function. *American Journal of Physical Anthropology, 54*(3), 337–340.

Emge, L. A. (1962, June 15). The elusive adenomyosis of the uterus: Its historical past and its present state of recognition. *American Journal of Obstetrics and Gynecology, 83*(12), 1541–1563.

Feicht, C. B., Johnson, T. S., & Martin, B. J., et al., (1978, November 25). Secondary amenorrhea in athletes. *Lancet, 2*(8100), 1145–1146.

Fraser, I.S., Pearse, C., & Shearman, R. P., et al., (1981, November). Efficacy of mefenamic acid in patients with a complaint of menorrhagia. *Obstetrics and Gynecology, 58*(5), 543–551.

Frisch, R. E. (1977). Food intake, fatness, and reproductive ability. In R. A. Vigersky (Ed.). *Anorexia nervosa.* New York: Raven Press.

Frisch, R. E., Gotz-Welbergen, A. V., & McArthur, J. W., et al., (1981, October 2). Delayed menarche and amenorrhea of college athletes in relation to age of onset of training. *Journal of the American Medical Association, 246*(14), 1559–1563.

Frisch, R. E., & McArthur, J. W. (1974, September 13). Menstrual cycles: Fatness as a determinant of minimum weight for height necessary for their maintenance or onset. *Science, 185*(4155), 949–951.

Gaines, F. (1981a, July-August). Secondary amenorrhea, Part 1: Diagnostic protocol. *Nurse Practitioner, 6*(4), 17–29.

Gaines, F. (1981b, September-October). Secondary amenorrhea, Part 2: Assessment and plans. *Nurse Practitioner, 6*(5), 14–23.

Grimes, D. A. (1982, January 1). Diagnostic dilation and curettage: A reappraisal. *American Journal of Obstetrics and Gynecology, 142*(1), 1–6.

Hale, R. W. (1983, September). Exercise, sports, and menstrual dysfunction. *Clinical Obstetrics and Gynecology, 26*(3), 728–735.

Hallberg, L., Hogdahl, A., Nilsson, L., & Rybo, G. (1966). Menstrual blood loss—A population study. *Acta Obstetrica et Gynecologica Scandinavica, 45,* 320-351.

Hatcher, R. A., Guest, F., & Stewart, F., et al., (1984) *Contraceptive technology 1984-1985* (12th rev. ed.). New York: Irvington Publishers.

Johnston, F. E., Malina, R. M., & Galbraith, M. A. (1971, December 10). Height, weight and age at menarche and the "critical weight" hypothesis. *Science, 174*(4014), 1148.

Johnston, F. E., Roche, A. F., Schell, L. M., & Wettenhall, N. B. (1975, January). Critical weight at menarche: Critique of a hypothesis. *American Journal of Diseases of Children, 129*(1), 19-23.

Kase, N. G. (1983a). Anovulation. In N. G. Kase & A. B. Weingold (Eds.), *Principles and practice of clinical gynecology.* New York: John Wiley.

Kase, N. G. (1983b, April). The neuroendocrinology of amenorrhea. *Journal of Reproductive Medicine, 28*(4), 251-255.

Kase, N. G. (1983c). Normal and abnormal menstruation. In N. G. Kase & A. B. Weingold (Eds.), *Principles and practice of clinical gynecology.* New York: John Wiley & Sons.

Malina, R. M., Harper, A. B., Avent, H. H., & Campbell, D. E. (1973, Spring). Age at menarche in athletes and non-athletes. *Medical Science and Sports Exercise, 5,* 11-13.

Marcus, C. C. (1961, August). Relationship of adenomyosis uteri to endometrial hyperplasia and endometrial carcinoma. *American Journal of Obstetrics and Gynecology, 82*(2), 408-416.

Marut, E. L., & Dawood, M. Y. (1983, September). Amenorrhea (excluding hyperprolactinemia). *Clinical Obstetrics and Gynecology, 26*(3), 749-761.

Mishell, D. R., Jr., Fisher, H. W., & Haynes, P. J., et al., (1984, October). Menorrhagia: A symposium. *Journal of Reproductive Medicine, 29*(10, Suppl.), 763-782.

Quigley, M. E., Sheehan, K. L., Casper, R. F., & Yen, S. S. C. (1980, May). Evidence for increased dopaminergic and opioid activity in patients with hypothalamic hypogonadotropic amenorrhea. *Journal of Clinical Endocrinology and Metabolism, 50*(5), 949-954.

Rabin, J. M., Dwyer, A., & Kaiser, I. (1988). A topical anesthetic for use in gynecology. Manuscript in preparation.

Rebar, R. W., Coulam, C., Little, B., & Schnatz, P. T. (1984, September). Amenorrhea: The clinical approach. *The female patient. 9,* 20-32.

Reid, R. L., Hoff, J. D., Yen, S. S. C., & Li, C. H. (1981, June). Effects of exogenous β_h-endorphin on pituitary hormone secretion and its disappearance rate in normal human subjects. *Journal of Clinical Endocrinology and Metabolism, 52*(6), 1179-1184.

Reindollar, R. H., & McDonough, P. C. (1983, September). Adolescent menstrual disorders. *Clinical Obstetrics and Gynecology, 26*(3), 690-701.

Shangold, M., & Levine, H. (1982, August 15). The effect of marathon training upon menstrual function. *American Journal of Obstetrics and Gynecology, 143*(8), 862-869.

Smith, J. J., & Schulman, H. (1985, April). Current dilatation and curettage practice: A need for revision. *Obstetrics and Gynecology, 65*(4), 516-518.

Spellacy, W. N. (1983, September). Abnormal bleeding. *Clinical Obstetrics and Gynecology, 26*(3), 702-709.

Speroff, L. (1984, February). The effect of exercise on the menstrual cycle. *Postgraduate Obstetrics and Gynecology, 4*(4), 1-5.

Speroff, L., Glass, R. H., & Kase, N. G. (1983). *Clinical gynecologic endocrinology and infertility* (3rd ed.). Baltimore: Williams & Wilkins.

Stubbs, W. A., Jones, A., Edwards, C. R. W., Delitala, G., Jeffcoate, W J., Ratter, S. J., Besser, B. M., Bloom, S. R., & Alberti, K. G. M. M. (1978, December 9). Hormonal and metabolic responses to an enkephalin analogue in normal man. *Lancet, 2*(8102), 1225-1227.

Tagatz, G., Fialkow, P. J., Smith, D., & Spadoni, L. (1970, December 10). Hypogonadotropic hypogonadism associated with anosmia in the female. *New England Journal of Medicine, 283*(24), 1326-1329.

Treloar, A. E. (1981, December). Menstrual cyclicity and the premenopause. *Maturitas, 3*(3/4), 249-264.

Treloar, A. E., Boynton, R. E., Behn, B. G., & Brown, B. W. (1967, January–March). Variation of the human menstrual cycle through reproductive life. *International Journal of Fertility, 12*(1, Part 2), 77-126.

Vigersky, R. A., Andersen, A. E., Thompson, R. H., & Loriaux, D. L. (1977, November 24). Hypothalamic dysfunction in secondary amenorrhea associated with simple weight loss. *New England Journal of Medicine, 297*(21), 1141-1145.

Warren, M. P. (1980, November). The effects of exercise on pubertal progression and reproductive function in girls. *Journal of Clinical Endocrinology and Metabolism, 51*(5), 1150-1152.

Yen, S. S. C. (1986a). Chronic anovulation caused by peripheral endocrine disorders. In S. S. C. Yen & R. B. Jaffe (Eds.), *Reproductive endocrinology: Physiology, pathophysiology and clinical management* (2nd ed.). Philadelphia: W. B. Saunders.

Yen, S. S. C. (1986b). Chronic anovulation due to CNS–hypothalamic–pituitary dysfunction. In S. S. C. Yen & R. B. Jaffe (Eds.), *Reproductive endocrinology: Physiology, pathophysiology and clinical management* (2nd ed.). Philadelphia: W. B. Saunders.

Yen, S. S. C. (1986c). Neuroendocrine control of hypophyseal function: Physiological and clinical implications. In S. S. C. Yen & R. B. Jaffe, (Eds.), *Reproductive endocrinology: Physiology, pathophysiology and clinical management* (2nd ed.). Philadelphia: W.B. Saunders.

Youngs, D. D., & Reame, N. (1983, September). Psychosomatic aspects of menstrual dysfunction. *Clinical Obstetrics and Gynecology, 26*(3), 777-784.

Zacharias, L., Rand. W. M., & Wurtman, R. J. (1976, April). A prospective study of sexual development and growth in American girls: The statistics of menarche. *Obstetrics and Gynecology Survey, 31*(4), 325-337.

SECTION V
Developmental Issues

Development and the Primary Care Practitioner

A book of this scope cannot begin to deal with human development and its significance for women. Development is a continual process. It sometimes proceeds orderly, sometimes not. It may or may not appear predictable; its stages may or may not coincide with chronological age. Our ability to develop and change keeps us alive and vital; it has been said to be the only constant in life.

Rather than provide a comprehensive view of development, we have chosen to focus on three developmental or life-cycle stages that affect the vast majority of women and directly influence gynecologic health and well-being: puberty and adolescence, the postpartum months, and the perimenopausal and aging years. These are dramatic times, times of striking change and adjustment. Whether these changes are in the direction of health depends on our physical and psychological relationship to them, determined in large part by our support systems, our general sense of self, and the way society and culture define and treat these events. The depiction of these stages as either normal or pathologic will largely determine the social and individual reactions to them. The gynecologic practitioner can assist each woman to use these life-cycle events to enhance her own growth and potential. In turn, this can help promote positive societal responses. We believe that women have much to offer throughout life and we challenge society to accept women at all life stages as the positive force we are.

22

Adolescence

Sharon Robinson

Prior to the 1950s, the adolescent was considered basically healthy and for the most part either was left out of the health care system or inadequately provided for. For the past several decades, however, the unique health care needs of the adolescent have received considerable attention from health care planners, researchers, and providers.

Three major factors account for this redirection of energy: (1) the large number of adolescents in need of health care—there are over 39 million youths aged 12 to 21 in the United States today (U.S. Department of Commerce, 1983); (2) the social upheaval that characterized the late 1960s; and (3) the legal changes that occurred in the late 1960s and early 1970s allowing increased adolescent access to health care. According to common law, any individual under the age of majority is the chattel of his or her parent and, accordingly, is not allowed to enter into a contractual relationship (including one for medical services) without parental involvement. The age of majority is now 18 years, however, and an emancipated minor (one who no longer is subject to parental control) may obtain medical care without parental consent. Laws vary by state as to interpretation of emancipation; in some states, for example, a pregnant minor or one who is a parent is considered emancipated. Under public health laws in all 50 states, a minor may receive treatment for venereal disease without parental consent (Litt, Cuskey, & Rudd, 1980).

Assuming responsibility for health and seeking appropriate health care is difficult for many adults and especially difficult for adolescents. For the inexperienced, obtaining health services without the aid of an adult can be confusing, frightening, embarrassing, and sometimes legally impossible. Once an adolescent has entered the system, adequate care still may be inaccessible for financial reasons. Consequently, even when adolescents recognize illness, they often remain outside the health care system.

In spite of the progress made toward understanding adolescent behavior and efforts made toward developing programs to address their unique needs, adolescents still remain in many ways a mystery and a challenge.

This chapter briefly reviews adolescent development, including psychosocial, cognitive, physical, and sexual; outlines health problems common to adolescents; and discusses components of adolescent health care and management of adolescent gynecologic visits. The focus is on sexually transmitted diseases and pregnancy prevention.

DEVELOPMENT

Adolescence, teenage years, and the teens are terms used interchangeably to describe the process of evolving from childhood to adulthood. The word *adolescence* is derived from the Latin *adolescere* meaning ''to grow up'' (Tyler & Woodall, 1982, p. 117). Puberty is the period during which an adolescent undergoes sexual and physical maturation. Adolescence parallels puberty but they are not synonymous. Although there is no clearly defined time frame that marks the achievement of adulthood, it is generally accepted that adolescence spans the years from 12 to 21 with the events of puberty occurring approximately over a 4-year period. Adolescence can be further subdivided into early adolescence, which usually ends at about age 16, and late adolescence (Blotcky & Looney, 1980). Some authors (Slap, 1986) divide adolescence into three periods: early adolescence (ages 12 to 14), midadolescence or adolescence proper (ages 15 to 17), and late adolescence (ages 18 to 21).

Practitioners should remember that, in spite of some general characteristics of this period, each person experiences adolescence differently. Most adolescents survive and grow into productive adults; however, for increasing numbers of teenagers, patterns developed during late childhood and early adolescence are self-destructive as reflected in teen suicide, violence, and drug and alcohol use/abuse.

The only effective way to help youth become self-sufficient adults is to build toward that goal step by step. Children need to feel that they have opportunities and options (Children's Defense Fund, 1985, pp. 7–8). Each child needs a secure family, a community that offers access to quality education and adequate recreational facilities, association with able and motivated peers, and access to adults who can serve as role models.

Psychosocial Development

Traditional societies rarely recognize a long period in which the child gradually assumes adult responsibilities. Instead, after a brief rite-of-passage ceremony the child often is expected to function as an adult. By contrast, in the United States a protracted transitional period of physical and psychosocial development is not only tolerated but is considered critical to meet the demands of a complex society. The typically depicted scenario is that the industrious, compliant, often charming school-age child becomes the outspoken rebellious teenager. Not until the adolescent matures and enters young adulthood does she become a secure, goal-directed, self-sufficient individual who is capable of making responsible decisions, accepting commitments, and contributing to her community. A classic early work on adolescence described it as a period of "storm and stress" (Hall, 1904). More recent studies, however, have shown most adolescents to be far more stable than this original description implied. Unfortunately, studies of psychological development during adolescence have concentrated on white, middle-class males. Minorities, females, and adolescents from lower socioeconomic classes have been largely neglected by psychological research (Mitchell, 1980).

The basic psychological task of adolescence is to formulate and consolidate an adult identity (Erikson, 1980). This has many components including cultural or group identity, social or class identity, career or professional identity, gender and sexual identity, and a personal identity (Tyler & Woodall, 1982, pp. 117–118).

The multiple elements involved in the establishment of identity are affected by forces from within the individual as well as from the environment. They include the growth of cognition; the establishment of independence or autonomy from one's family; the development of sexuality, peer relationships, social responsibility, a value system, and a future orientation; the selection of an occupation; and the acquisition of body image, group image, self-esteem, and competency. The extent of an adolescent's access to broad experiences, options, and resources influences identity formation. For adolescent females, however, the attempt to form an identity can lead to frustration, as women continue to be ascribed into sex roles that conflict with their developing values and beliefs.

Because of the adolescent's rapid emotional and physical changes, the period is often characterized by egocentricism. Egocentricism contributes to the adolescent's vulnerability by creating a myth of invulnerability (Tauer, 1983). The adolescent often believes that she is special, unique, and immune. This personal fable, as it has been called, leads girls, for example, to believe that they can be sexually active and not get pregnant (Elkind, 1967, p. 1025). Risk taking, often characteristic of adolescence, may also account for unprotected sexual activity (Jessor, 1984).

Cognitive Development

Formal operational thought occurs when the individual has the capacity to extrapolate from past experiences to solve problems. Piaget (1950) characterized the cognitive shift of adolescence as a movement from concrete to abstract reasoning. This process begins at age 11 or 12, but the ability to use formal operational thought is probably not achieved until age 15 or 16. The young adolescent who thinks concretely has difficulty conceptualizing or planning for the future. She may not be able to separate fantasy from fact. She is unable to think "what if" or to see that her behavior may have predictable consequences.

Adolescence is a period of experimentation. This experimentation is necessary for cognitive growth. It is through experimentation that teenagers learn their boundaries and develop inner control. Without this expansion in their range of experiences, the fewer resources they would have to draw on for problem solving (Blum & Resnick, 1982, p. 802).

Physical Development

Puberty. Puberty in the female may be defined as the stage in development when "the ovaries secrete sex hormones, primarily estradiol, in quantities sufficient to stimulate growth of genital structures and produce secondary sex characteristics" (Wallach & Bongiovanni, 1983, p. 18). Although there is great variability in the timing of the onset and duration of puberty, in females puberty usually occurs between the ages of 8 and 14.9; it generally occurs 6 to 12 months earlier for girls than for boys (Lee, 1980). A number of factors have been identified that influence the timing of puberty, including heredity, socioeconomic status, endocrine function, nutrition, physical activity, altitude, illness, stress, abuse or neglect, and geography (Moscicki & Shafer, 1986).

The onset of puberty is due to maturation of the central nervous system (Altchek, 1985, p. 40); the process involves an interplay among the hypothalamus, pituitary gland, and ovaries. During childhood, the hypothalamus is sensitive to very low levels of estrogen, which exert a negative feedback on it, reducing its activity. At puberty, the hypothalamus exhibits a decreased sensitivity to this negative feedback and increases its production of gonadotropin-releasing hormone (GnRH). This leads to increased production of gonadotropins—initially follicle-stimulating hormone (FSH)—and ovarian stimulation. Eventually, estrogen levels increase. The increased production of FSH occurs as early as 8 years of age in girls, with a rise in luteinizing hormone (LH) production several years later (Speroff, Glass, & Kase, 1983, p. 69).

The increased production of estrogens (mainly estradiol) allows for the growth and development of the uterus, fallopian tubes, vagina, labia, and breasts (particularly the ductal system). The estrogen-stimulated endometrium is eventually shed at menarche. LH stimulates maturation of the graafian follicle into the corpus luteum, which produces progesterone. Progesterone is responsible for development of a secretory endometrium and further development of the breast lobules.

The sequence of pubertal events in females is summarized in Table 22–1. The first sign of puberty generally is the appearance of the breast bud (thelarche); pubic hair usually appears right after breast development, although sometimes it may appear first (Dewhurst, 1984). Axillary hair appears about 2 years after the beginning of pubic hair growth; in a few children, however, axillary hair may be the first to appear. Tanner (1962) developed a scale for the assessment and staging of adolescent pubertal development. This scale appears as Table 22–2 and Figures 22–1 and 22–2.

TABLE 22–1. AGES OF SEXUAL DEVELOPMENT IN THE FEMALE

Characteristic	Approximate Age Range of Development	Median Age of Development
Breast bud	<8–13	9.8
Onset pubic hair	8–13	10.5
Maximal growth	10–14	11.4
Menarche	9–15+	12.8
Adult breast	12–18	14.8
Adult pubic hair	12–18	13.7

From Speroff, L., Glass, R. H., & Kase, N. G. (1983). Clinical Gynecologic endocrinology and infertility (3rd ed., p. 371). Baltimore, MD: Williams & Wilkins. Reprinted with permission.

TABLE 22–2. TANNER STAGING

Stage	Breast	Pubic Hair
I (prepubertal)	Elevation of papilla only	No pubic hair
II	Elevation of breast and papilla as small mound; areola diameter enlarged Median age: 9.8 years	Sparse, long, pigmented hair, chiefly along labia majora Median age: 10.5 years
III	Further enlargement without separation of breast and areola Median age: 11.2 years	Dark, coarse, curled hair sparsely spread over mons. Median age: 11.4 years
IV	Secondary mound of areola and papilla above the breast Median age : 12.1 year	Adult-type hair abundant but limited to the mons Median age: 12.0 years
V	Recession of areola of breast Median age: 14.6 years	Adult-type spread in quantity and distribution Median age: 13.7 years

From Speroff, L., Glass R. H., & Kase, N. G. (1983). Clinical gynecologic endocrinology and infertility (3rd ed., p. 377). Baltimore, MD: Williams & Wilkins. Reprinted with permission.

The results of the combined processes of maturation are changed proportion of limbs to torso, new hair growth, re-formed body contours, increased height and weight, voice differences, and genital development. For the young woman, these changes create a need to accept and familiarize herself with a new body (Tyler & Woodall, 1982, p. 120).

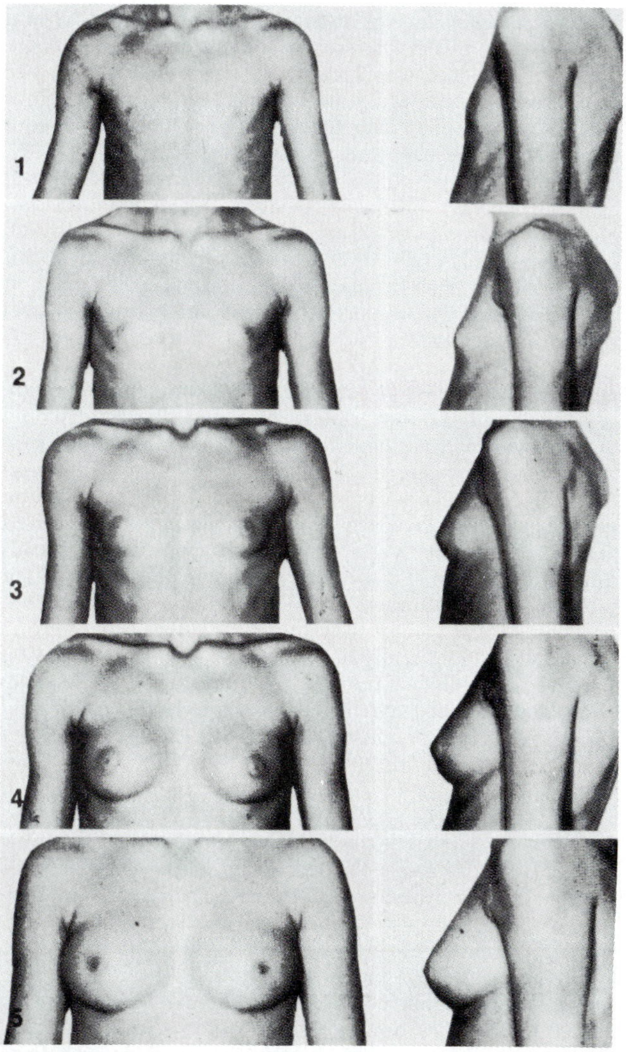

Figure 22–1. Tanner staging: breast standards. (From Tanner, J. M. [1962]. Growth at adolescence [2nd ed.]. Oxford: Blackwell Scientific. Reprinted with permission.)

Learning to appreciate and enjoy adult femininity is part of the establishment of gender identity and overall self-esteem.

Menarche. Menarche, or the onset of menstruation, is one event of puberty. Menarche is a late event, occurring after the peak of the height (or growth) spurt has been passed.

The height spurt of the typical girl occurs 2 years earlier than that of the boy, but is less marked. In the year of peak growth, a girl grows between 6 and 11 cm. The average growth in height after menarche is about 2.5 inches (Speroff et al., 1983, p. 368). Growth in height is accompanied by a peak in weight gain, accounting for over 40 percent of ideal adult weight (Slap, 1986).

The normal range of menarche in a given population is 5 years, from age 10.5 to age 15.5. The average age for menarche in the United States is now 12.8. It has been hypothesized (Frisch, 1983) that the attainment of an adequate weight for height is vital to the onset of menstruation, although this theory is not universally accepted (Billewicz, Fellowes, & Hytten 1976; Ellison 1981; Johnston, Malina, & Galbraith, 1971; Johnston, Roche, Schell, & Wettenhall, 1975). As is commonly known, early menstrual cycles are usually anovulatory, and therefore, irregular, and sometimes heavy. Anovulation typically lasts 12 to 18 months after menarche, although there are many exceptions (Speroff et al., 1983, p. 71). Menarche may be speeded or delayed by external or internal factors (Warren, 1983, p. 233). Conditions thought to speed menarche include blindness, obesity, urban residence, hypothyroidism, and the combination of retardation with being bedridden. Conditions that may delay menarche include food shortage, poor nutrition, altitude, number of children in the family, thyrotoxicosis, muscular development, and ballet dancing.

Deviations. Thus far, normal physical changes of adolescence have been described. Sometimes, however, an adolescent's growth falls outside the usually defined range of normal. This may not represent pathology. For the young woman whose physical or sexual maturation does not conform to that of her peers, there can be additional anxiety and concern; the adolescent, more than anyone else, does not like to be different. A girl may present to a health care provider complaining of being too short, too tall, or possibly less sexually developed than her friends. It becomes the responsibility of the health care practitioner to provide reas-

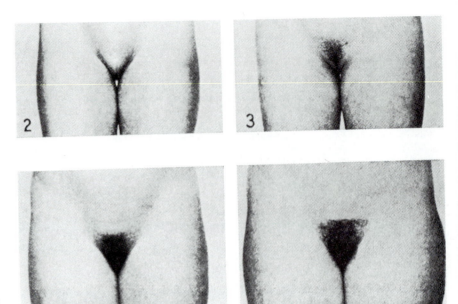

Figure 22–2. Tanner staging: Pubic hair standards. *(From Tanner, J. M. [1962]. Growth at adolescence [2nd ed.]. Oxford: Blackwell Scientific. Reprinted with permission.)*

surance and/or to make the appropriate referral for management when pathology does exist.

PRECOCIOUS PUBERTY. Puberty is considered precocious if secondary sexual development begins before age 8 or menarche before age 10 (Dewhurst, 1984, p. 91). This may be physiologic, as a result of early hypothalamic/pituitary activity, but it may be caused by a feminizing ovarian tumor or, rarely, an adrenal tumor. Young girls also have been reported to experience precocious puberty after ingestion of their mother's oral contraceptives. With an early onset, pubertal events may occur in the expected order or may vary. If vaginal bleeding is the first sign, it may signify a disorder known as the McCune/Albright syndrome. This is characterized by cafe-au-lait spots, which are light brown, irregular skin lesions, most commonly found on the shoulders, back, face, or neck (Dewhurst, 1984, p. 96). Sometimes, only one aspect of pubertal development is advanced. This is usually unexplainable. In most cases of precocious puberty, once pathology has been ruled out, reassurance can be offered. These young women function normally and do not manifest later problems. Most problems are short-lived and more psychological than physical.

DELAYED PUBERTY OR MENARCHE. Pubertal or menarcheal delay may result from pathology or may be a normal variation. The determination of whether delay is abnormal is based on an evaluation of development according to an accepted definition of delayed maturation. Speroff and associates (1984, p. 376) suggest using age 13 if no breast budding has occurred and age 18 if menarche has not occurred, because, by this age, only 1 percent of adolescent females have not menstruated. Other guidelines used by practitioners are based on the Tanner scale for adolescent physical development (Table 22–2 and Figures 22–1 and 22–2). These include (1) elapse of more than 5 years from initiation of breast growth (Tanner stage 2) to menarche or (2) elapse of more than 2.2 years from Tanner stage 3 without progression to the next stage or 1 year from Tanner stage 2 without progress to stage 3 (Litt & Cohen, 1979, p. 127). An alternative guideline is lack of menarche beyond 1 year past the mother's age of menarche, assuming hers was within normal limits (Litt & Cohen, 1979). Once delay is diagnosed, the medical assessment is then based on a determination of which patients are destined eventually to undergo spontaneous puberty and/or menarche and which have disorders that lead to sexual infantilism and require treatment.

Diagnosis of developmental disorders requires referral to a specialist in adolescent gynecology or endocrinology. Differential diagnosis includes concomitant medical disease in which delayed maturation often is secondary to malnutrition, such as with diabetes mellitus, cystic fibrosis, congenital heart disease, and uremia (Warren, 1983, p. 233); gonadal dysgenesis, often involving abnormal karyotypes, as in Turner's syndrome (see Chapter 16); structural anomalies of the female genital tract such as an absent or hypoplastic vagina or imperforate hymen (see Chapter 11) (Huppert, 1983); and male pseudohermaphroditism. A diagnostic framework for adolescent amenorrhea is presented in Chapter 21.

BLEEDING IRREGULARITIES. Irregular bleeding patterns are seen frequently among adolescents, often characterized by very heavy or prolonged bleeding. This occurs secondary to anovulatory cycles in which the endometrium is exposed to estrogen, but not to progesterone. Irregular bleeding generally resolves with time, once ovulation is established and there is cyclic formation of a functioning corpus luteum. Intervention may be advisable, however, when bleeding presents an emotional problem for the adolescent or when it causes anemia. Treatment involves progesterone (10 mg of Provera orally for 5 days) or oral contraceptives, provided pathology is ruled out (Huppert, 1983, p. 48). Occasionally, bleeding may be severe enough to warrant hospitalization. See Chapter 21 for further discussion of the management of abnormal bleeding.

Sexual Development

Sexuality, in its broadest sense, encompasses the search for identity, gender roles, sexual attitudes, behaviors and feelings, relationships, affection, caring, physical touch, recognition, and acceptance as a sexual being (Tauer, 1983, p. 275). Through sexual experimentation adolescents test their feelings and establish their sexual identity. The forms of sexual expression they experiment with include fantasy, daydreams, masturbation, petting, mutual masturbation, outercourse, homosexual experiences, and heterosexual intercourse. Although some form of physical contact with oneself and another is an important prerequisite to intimacy, the adolescent may not always experience satisfaction, but instead may feel guilt, shame, anger, fear of homosexuality, or sexual inadequacy.

Sarrel and Sarrel (1981, pp. 93–94) describe a process of ''sexual unfolding'' involving the realization of sexual capacity, recognition of sexual preferences, and development of the capacity for shared sexual pleasure within a relationship of love. These authors place sexual development within the context of other developmental processes of adolescence. The entirety of sexual unfolding consists of nine identified processes.

1. An evolving sense of the body—toward a body image that is gender specific and fairly free of distortion (particularly about the genitals)
2. The ability to overcome or modulate guilt, shame, fear, and childhood inhibitions associated with sexual thoughts and behavior
3. A gradual loosening of the primary emotional ties to parents and siblings
4. Learning to recognize what is erotically pleasing and displeasing and being able to communicate this to a partner
5. Resolution of conflict and confusion about sexual orientation
6. A sexual life, free of sexual dysfunction or compulsion
7. A growing awareness of being a sexual person and of the place and value of sex in one's life, including options such as celibacy
8. Becoming responsible about oneself, one's partner, and society (e.g., using contraception and not using sex as a means of exploitation of another)
9. A gradually increasing ability to experience eroticism as one aspect of intimacy with another person—not that *all* eroticism occurs, then, in an intimate relationship, but that this fusion of sex and love is possible

Tauer (1983, p. 275) reports that sexual activity in adolescents may serve a number of purposes that include the promotion of self-esteem, having someone to care about and caring about someone else, experimentation, accommodation of peer pressure, feeling grown up, touching and being touched, feeling good, and getting even. Using Erikson's developmental framework, Howe (1986) points out that adolescents who precede identity formation with sexual intimacy may have difficulty solving the task of establishing identity.

HEALTH NEEDS

Adolescent health presents a paradox. The adolescent commonly is believed to be at the peak of health, but the facts contradict the assumption (Marks & Fisher, 1987).

Health Problems

Mortality. Mortality figures indicate that violence in the form of traffic accidents (often associated with alcohol use), homicides, and suicides is by far the leading cause of death in this age group, with neoplasms second, and infectious or congenital conditions third (National Center for Health Statistics, 1986). For every successful suicide among adolescents, there are about 50 to 200 attempts (Marks & Fisher, 1987), and attempted suicide is two to three times more common among female adolescents.

Substance Use/Abuse. Although rates of adolescent smoking declined between 1971 and 1981, tobacco use remains a problem with no further decline since 1981 (Hansen, Ma-

lotte, & Fielding, 1987; Johnston, O'Malley, & Bachman, 1986). The greatest increase today in cigarette smoking is among teenage girls (Evans & Raines, 1982, p. 105). Problem drinking and smoking are often interrelated. Adolescent alcohol use increased after World War II until 1965, decreased between 1965 and 1975, and leveled off after 1975 (Hansen et al., 1987). In 1985, a survey of high school seniors revealed that 65.9 percent had used alcohol in the month preceding the survey, with daily drinking reported by 5 percent and binge drinking (five or more drinks in a row) reported by 37 percent (Johnston et al., 1986, pp. 20, 23). Peer use has been found to be the most important influence on adolescent drinking behavior. In 1985, this same survey showed a decline since the late 1970s in drug use, but marijuana smoking was still reported by 26 percent in the month prior to the survey and by 44 percent in the preceding year, with daily use reported by nearly 5 percent. Use of other drugs in the year preceding the survey was reported by 6 to almost 16 percent of the high school seniors. These included stimulants (15.8 percent), cocaine (13.1 percent), hallucinogens (8 percent), inhalants (7.7 percent), tranquilizers (6.1 percent), opiates (6 percent), and sedatives (5.8 percent).

Eating Disorders. Adolescence is notoriously a period of dietary excesses and deficits. Serious consequences may result including junk food addiction, adolescent obesity, or the eating disorders of anorexia nervosa and bulimia (Brockopp & Hall, 1984; Heald & Khan, 1973; Marino & King, 1980).

Gynecologic/Reproductive Problems. In an analysis of reasons for outpatient gynecologic visits among adolescents, Russo (1982) found the following to be most common: menstrual disorders; genital tract infections; postpartum, postabortion, and postoperative referrals; lower abdominal pain; routine examinations; contraception; and referrals for asymptomatic adnexal masses. Dysmenorrhea is widespread among adolescents (see Chapter 20). Sexually transmitted diseases (STDs) in adolescents have increased greatly since the 1960s (Silber & Woodward, 1982).

SEXUALLY TRANSMITTED DISEASES. STDs constitute one of the important medical and social consequences of adolescent sexual expression (see Section III, Gynecologic Pathophysiology). The actual incidence of STDs among adolescents is difficult to determine because of inadequate screening, incomplete reporting, and aggregation of reported cases into broad age categories. For most STDs, the reported rates reach a peak in the late teens or early twenties and decline with increasing age. Age-related behavioral factors affecting infection rates include the frequency, nature, and context of sexual activity (Bell & Hein, 1984, p. 77).

There is a broad spectrum of STDs; gonorrhea is the most often screened for and reported communicable disease. In the United States, the greatest increase in the rate of reported gonorrhea during the current epidemic has been seen among 15- to 19-year-old females. In 1979, 38 percent of all reported female gonorrhea, but only 17 percent of all male gonorrhea, was in adolescents (Bell & Hein, 1984, p. 77). The difference in rates between adolescent females and males may be partially explained by the tendency among adolescent females to have partners 2 to 3 years older than themselves.

Adolescent rates of gonorrhea declined slightly after 1979; however, they remain high. In 1982, 1,425 cases per 100,000 women aged 15 to 19 and 71 cases per 100,000 women aged 10 to 14 were reported (Strobino, 1987).

Syphilis is not as widespread in the United States among adolescents as gonorrhea (Bell & Hein, 1984). As with gonorrhea, there is a decreasing incidence of the disease with increasing age. In one study of syphilis among adolescents, most patients presented with signs of secondary disease, rather than with a primary chancre (Silber & Niland, 1984). A suspicion of syphilis, therefore, should be maintained when any sexually active teenager presents with skin or mucous membrane rashes or other signs of secondary syphilis (see Chapter 12).

Chlamydia trachomatis infections are estimated to be on the increase (Gump, 1984) and to exceed even gonorrhea in prevalence (Eagar, Beach, Davison, & Judson, 1985). The actual incidence of this infection is unknown because of the difficulties of in vitro cultivation of *C. trachomatis* (see Chapters 4 and 12). The prevalence rate among sexually active adolescents in various socioeconomic groups has been reported to be 8 to 25 percent or higher (Chacko & Lovchik, 1984; Fisher, Swenson, Risucci, & Kaplan, 1987; Fraser, Rettig, & Kaplan, 1983; Golden, Hammerschlag, Neuhoff, & Gleyzer, 1984; Saltz, Linneman, Brookman, & Rauh, 1981). It is believed that cervical ectropion in the adolescent female may increase the likelihood of acquisition of chlamydial infection (Bell & Hein, 1984, p. 81; Harrison, Costin & Meder, et al., 1985). Screening for chlamydia, therefore, has been advocated for adolescents with cervical ectropion (Chacko & Lovchik, 1984). Chlamydia and gonorrhea often coexist (Eagar et al., 1985); an adolescent infected with one of these organisms should be screened for the other.

Pelvic inflammatory disease (PID) or salpingitis is the most common serious complication of genital infection in adolescents, as it is in older women (see Chapter 15). PID rates are on the increase, with the highest rates among 15- to 19-year-olds (Washington, Sweet, & Shafer, 1985). The potential loss of fertility is especially devastating among this young population. There is evidence that the adolescent with anovulatory cycles is particularly susceptible to PID because of the prolonged period during each cycle when the cervical mucus is permeable to motile bacteria (Bell & Hein, 1984, p. 81).

Cervical dysplasia also is on the rise among sexually active adolescents (Spitzer & Krumholz, 1988). Routine Pap smears are recommended for all sexually active adolescents to detect this treatable condition (Jones, Russo, Dombroski, & Lentz, Russo & Jones, 1984).

The clinical manifestations and the management of STDs generally are the same for adolescents as for adults. Although adolescent compliance with therapy for STDs has not been studied, whenever possible, single-dose regimens for STDs are recommended to maximize compliance.

ADOLESCENT PREGNANCY. In 1982, 43 percent of never-married women aged 15 to 19 reported having had sexual intercourse (Hofferth, 1987a). Among these young women, 14.6 percent had never used contraception and less than one half reported consistent contraceptive use. High rates of unprotected intercourse result in more than a million adolescent pregnancies each year (Alan Guttmacher Institute, 1981). Of all U.S. teenagers, approximately 11 percent or 110 per 1,000 get pregnant each year. Most of these conceptions are unintended and unwanted, and over half of the pregnancies end in abortion. There were over 537,000 births to teens in the United States in 1981 (National Center for Health Statistics, 1984) and almost 480,000 in 1984 (Hofferth, 1987b). In each of these years, almost 10,000 births were to girls under age 15. One birth in seven today is to a teenage mother (Children's Defense Fund, 1985, p. 5).

The United States leads nearly all other developed nations of the world in rates of teenage pregnancy, abortion, and childbearing (Jones et al., 1985). Although the actual number of teen births declined during the 1970s and stabilized in the early 1980s for all adolescents except those under 15, total pregnancies, contraceptive use, abortion, and sexual activity all increased (Alan Guttmacher Institute, 1981). Twenty percent of teenagers who become pregnant do so within the first month of beginning intercourse and 50 percent within 6 months (Zabin, Schwab, Kantner, & Zelnik, 1979, p. 215).

Adolescent pregnancy is a national problem. But, like teenage unemployment and school dropout rates, it is a more serious problem in poor and minority communities. For black teens specifically, and the black community in general, the problem is quite threatening. Black teenagers account for 14 percent of the adolescent population, yet disproportionately account for 28 percent of adolescent births and 47 percent of all births to unmarried teenagers (Children's Defense Fund, 1985, p. 10).

Preventing children from having children has been a battlecry of the 1980s. Adolescent parenthood is recognized as a serious threat to individual development, family stability, and community enhancement.

Although the numbers alone are staggering, they fail to address the depth of the problem. For the pregnant teenager, there may be an increased risk of developing obstetrical complications such as preeclampsia, premature labor, and surgical delivery. For the child of teenage parents, there is an increased risk of low birth weight, prematurity, infant mortality, and child abuse (Brown, 1985). Such poor outcomes for both mother and child may result from low socioeconomic status, primiparity, and inadequate prenatal care, rather than from the biologic effects of young age (Strobino, 1987). Additionally, there is an increased risk of poverty and family instability for the mother and child (Makinson, 1985). Adolescent mothers are less likely to receive a high school diploma or equivalency degree than women whose first child is born when they are in their twenties (Mott & Marsiglio, 1985). Adolescent parents are more likely to be unemployed or have low-paying jobs (Ancrum, Andrews, & Soloway, 1987). The resultant cost to society in terms of dollars and loss of human potential is great.

According to a study done by Zelnik and Kantner (1977), the percentage of adolescent females aged 15 to 17 who have had intercourse rose dramatically during the 1970s. This declined significantly in the early 1980s, mostly accounted for by a decline in the rate of sexual activity among black adolescents, although overall rates of ever having intercourse remained higher among black adolescent females than whites (Ancrum et al., 1987, p. 21). Although there was a documented increase in use of contraceptives, data indicate that requests for contraception are initiated long after onset of sexual activity. Fifty percent of females do not use any form of birth control during their first sexual experience, and two thirds of all adolescent girls fail to use birth control routinely (Blum & Resnick, 1982, p. 800).

Reasons adolescents give for nonuse of contraception include wanting a pregnancy; wrong time of the month to get pregnant; unanticipated intercourse; dangers of or difficulty in using contraception; too young to get pregnant; and lack of contraceptive information (Zelnik & Kantner, 1979). In a study done by Zabin, Schwab, and Clark (1981, p. 205) to determine what prompted the initial family planning clinic visit, adolescents most often stated that suspicion of pregnancy was the motivating factor. Other frequently mentioned responses were that their male partner or their mother suggested that they come, they were having a closer relationship with their partner, and they just started to have sex. When asked why they did not come to the clinic earlier, the main responses were "I didn't get around to it" and "I was afraid my family would find out if I came."

There is a prevalent belief among adolescents that it is bad to plan to have sex (Kisker, 1985). If you are using contraceptives or if you start going to a family planning clinic, you are planning to have sex. Those who do prepare for sex, therefore, feel guilt and embarrassment.

Hughes and Torre (1987, p. 53) identify the following factors as related to risk of pregnancy in adolescent women: sexual inexperience; infrequent intercourse (less than or equal to one or two times a month); intercourse with an uncommitted partner; intercourse usually unplanned or "spontaneous"; perceived irregularity of menstrual cycle; contraception perceived as a shared or partner responsibility rather than the responsibility of self alone; dissatisfaction with contraceptive methods; and lower levels of maternal education. Zabin, Hirsch, Smith, and Hardy (1984), however, found that teenagers who believe contraception to be a shared responsibility are slightly more likely to use a method than those who see it as the responsibility of one or the other partner.

Effective contraceptive use is an ongoing process. The user must accept herself as sexually active, recognize that pregnancy is the likely result of her sexual activity, believe that a pregnancy would seriously interfere with her life plans, be cognizant of the techniques involved in contraception, and consistently use an effective method (Mudd, Dickens, & Garcia, et al., 1978, p. 502). In addition to barriers created by teenagers themselves, efforts to prevent unwanted pregnancies among adolescents may be further complicated by the lack of support for contraceptive use by their parents, limited access to contraceptive services, and legal and financial barriers to family planning services.

ADOLESCENT MALE CONTRACEPTIVE BEHAVIOR. National data on adolescent contraceptive behavior indicate that males have strongly regarded contraception as the female's responsibility (Blum & Resnick, 1982, p. 800). In Sorensen's (1973) National Probability Sample, nearly 60 percent of the teenage males "sometimes, usually, or always" just trusted to luck that their partner would not become pregnant; only 1 in 10 always made sure that their partner would not become pregnant, and only 1 in 10 always made sure that their partner was using some kind of contraception (Scales, 1977, p. 211). And yet, studies indicate that, although the birth control pill is the most frequently used contraceptive, the condom and withdrawal account for a significant percentage of adolescent contraceptive use (Sorensen, 1973). Consequently, a large percentage of teenage birth control depends on the male's assuming the responsibility.

Male attitudes and behavior toward contraception have been supported by institutional and sociocultural standards that have tended to discourage male participation and devalue the male role in family planning decisions (Scales, 1977, p. 212). This attitude is reflected in the common expression "boys will be boys." Scales concluded from an analysis of contraceptive behavior among males that the increased use of the pill would lead to greater alienation of the sexes by further decreasing the male's involvement with pregnancy prevention. A more recent survey of black, urban, junior high and high school males in Baltimore, however, reported a larger percentage of young men who acknowledge shared or sole responsibility for pregnancy prevention (Clark, Zabin, & Hardy, 1984). This study re-

vealed misinformation, however, about the availability and accessibility of contraception, including the condom.

The effect of male contraceptive involvement secondary to the epidemic of acquired immune deficiency syndrome (AIDS), and publicity regarding the protective role of the condom remains to be analyzed. It is interesting to note, however, that many of the media campaigns promoting condom use are directed at women. One study that assessed recent changes in perceptions and use of condoms among sexually active adolescents in San Francisco found that males had not increased use of condoms and that neither males nor females had increased intentions to use them. This was so despite a documented perception that condoms protected against STDs (Kegeles, Adler, & Irwin, 1988).

ABORTION. It is estimated that half of pregnancies to girls under age 15 and two fifths of those to adolescents aged 15 to 17 end in abortion (Alan Guttmacher Institute, 1981, p. 52). Adolescents account for a disproportionate number of abortions in the United States. Teenagers have higher abortion ratios than any other age group, except women over 40, and have higher rates of abortion at later gestational ages (Alan Guttmacher Institute, 1981, p. 55). In 1981, teenage abortions accounted for 28 percent of all induced abortions in the United States (Strobino, 1987, p. 105).

The decision to have an abortion for a woman of any age group is serious and often stressful. For the teenager who has not established her sexual identity and is struggling with dependence versus independence, the decision is even more complex. A young woman often feels helpless and at the mercy of her parents or the man or boyfriend involved (Hern, 1977, p. 266). Often, others are quick to make the decision for her and apply pressure to either carry the pregnancy or abort it. To take this responsibility away from the pregnant adolescent may provide temporary relief, but the long-term effects of a unilateral decision do not support growth or a change in behavior. Ultimately, the pregnant woman must live with her decision.

Research indicates that few adolescents experience serious psychiatric problems after an abortion (Hatcher et al., 1980, p. 189; Perez-Reyes & Falk, 1973). In fact, many teens report feeling relief. The physical risks and complications from legal abortion are similar for teens as for older women, although studies have found postabortal endometritis and cervical lacerations to be higher among women aged 17 and younger (Burkman, Atienza, & King, 1984; Schulz, Grimes, & Cates, 1983), whereas mortality has been shown to be lower (Ory, 1983). In addition, because rates of second-trimester abortion are higher in adolescents, young women face an increased number of risks from these more hazardous procedures (see Chapter 28).

In one prospective study, 77 percent of adolescents used contraception 1 year postabortion. These findings suggest that abortion is not used as a birth control method among adolescents (Abrams, 1985).

HEALTH SERVICES

Events occurring in adolescence, choices made, and habits acquired often have serious and sometimes permanent consequences. Therefore, it is critical for the primary health care worker to reach healthy children and adolescents and help them to establish and consistently practice behavior that will enhance their health and maximize their potential as productive human beings.

To provide comprehensive primary health care to adolescents, it is necessary to adapt traditional health care services to meet the unique needs of this population. In evaluating programs for adolescents, Jekel (1981, p. 139) observed that the most effective ones included a team approach with a triad of services: medical, social, and educational. Green and Horton (1982, p. 39) observed that effective programs maintained a developmental perspective gearing approaches to the cognitive and affective realities of the adolescent period; encouraged individual responsibility; involved adolescents in planning, implementation, and evaluation of programs; used peer support; encouraged staff sensitivity to confidentiality; and recruited and trained adult staff whose approach to adolescents was open, knowledgeable, supportive, flexible, and nonjudgmental.

In addition to comprehensive services, the physical setting is important. Ideally, care for adolescents should be provided in a setting separate from that used for adults and children (Adams, 1983, p. 240). There should be age-appropriate magazines and posters, an area that is conducive to group activity, and examining rooms that maximize privacy. The schedule should be flexible, providing after-school and evening sessions to accommodate teens in school or working. In considering the adolescent's need for confidentiality and independence, the service should be financially and geographically accessible for the young women it serves. Reality, however, often dictates that care must be provided in less than ideal settings. Practitioners with a basic understanding and concern for adolescents as well as a degree of creativity can offer quality personalized care anywhere.

As a word of caution, working with adolescents, although often exciting, challenging, and rewarding, can be exhausting and result in high staff turnover. To minimize this risk, the staff requires ongoing support through the use of team case management meetings, interagency collaboration and consultation, and the avoidance of unrealistic commitment to the teens. The key to making a program work lies in its overall coordination.

MANAGEMENT OF GYNECOLOGIC CARE

In 1981, the American Academy of Pediatrics' Committee on Practice and Ambulatory Medicine recommended health maintenance examinations for adolescents every 2 years. Some specialists in adolescent medicine recommend yearly examinations because of the rapid development that occurs during these years (Marks & Fisher, 1987).

Data Collection

Health Interview. The purpose of the interview is to assess the adolescent's health status and determine priorities for care based on the individual's perceived needs and those identified by the health care worker. In addition to those areas covered in Chapter 2, the components of an initial interview with an adolescent include family and peer group relationships and school performance. Immunization status and nutritional assessment are important components of the interview (Marks & Fisher, 1987). Eating disorders such as bulimia and anorexia nervosa should be asked about in a matter-of-fact, nonjudgmental manner. Adolescents should be screened for risk behaviors including smoking, alcohol and drug use, and sexual and contraceptive behavior. Questions about depression and suicidal thoughts are appropriate (Marks & Fisher, 1987).

The interview should be conducted within an atmosphere that maximizes privacy and confidentiality. The question "Am I normal?" is often foremost in the adolescent's mind. Reassurance should be given freely during the interview and physical examination, with reinforcement during the discussion after the exam. The relationship to health of all issues raised should be explained as should the need for all components of the physical examination and laboratory tests.

The interview provides an opportunity for the care provider to discuss how the teenager relates to peers and adults, to review alternatives to coitus and some of the possible consequences of intercourse, to give information about sexual anatomy and functioning, and to provide contraception. It is also a time to discuss fears and concerns related to the first pelvic examination.

Although it is important to respect the independence and confidentiality of the teenager, special care must be taken to involve the family and other significant people in the adolescent's life. In the case of the nonverbal teen, the practitioner may need to request that a family member be present for the interview. If the adolescent is alone, it may be necessary to telephone a relative for additional information or request their presence at the follow-up session. In private, the young woman should be asked about her relationship with various identified family members including their ability to communicate, knowledge of her sexual activity, and their support for contraceptive use.

Physical Examination. The routine physical examination for the adolescent should include a complete assessment as outlined in Chapter 3. Tests of vision and hearing should be included or recommended and referrals provided.

An important component of the adolescent physical examination is assessment of biologic maturity. The Tanner grading system is available to aid in this determination. Stage 1 for each criterion is the prepubertal stage; stage 5 is full maturity (see Table 22–2 and Figures 22–1 and 22–2). Using this tool, practitioners working with adolescents can accurately assess physical maturity. A teenager should be described as having, for example, stage 4 pubic hair development and stage 4 breast development, rather than with the meaningless phrase "a normal-appearing 12-year-old girl" (Rigg, 1980, p. 13).

An initial pelvic examination should be performed for any adolescent who is sexually active or has been sexually assaulted, is considering contraceptive use, or has any complaint that might be gynecologic, including vaginal discharge, abnormal vaginal bleeding, or abdominal pain (Litt & Cohen, 1979). All young women exposed to diethylstilbestrol (DES) in utero should be examined early in adolescence, although this cohort is diminishing. An initial gynecologic examination may be recommended at age 18 for all other young women, although there are no gynecologic risks for healthy, nonsexually active women at this age. Some young women request a gynecologic examination because they feel it is appropriate (Sarrel, 1981). Hein (1984) refers to the first pelvic examination as a rite of passage into American womanhood. The examination provides an opportunity for learning about the body, increasing body awareness, and developing positive health attitudes and practices.

The pelvic examination is a fundamental component of women's health care. Because of its importance and the frequency with which it must be performed, health care providers must make each pelvic examination as dignified, informative, and comfortable as possible. In a study of sources of anxiety about pelvic examinations among adolescents, fear of pain was found to be most related to anxiety, followed by fear of discovery of pathology and embarrassment about undressing and personal cleanliness (Millstein, Adler, & Irwin, 1984).

Several techniques have been developed to minimize the stress of the pelvic examination. All procedures should be explained in advance. Hein (1984) suggests using three-dimensional models showing normal anatomy to illustrate the procedure. To promote relaxation, the woman should be taught relaxation breathing to be used during the examination; this can be taught in advance with continuing verbal reinforcement provided during the examination, or explicit instructions can be presented at the time of the examination. If the young woman chooses to have a friend or family member present for the examination, the practitioner should respect this decision. The practitioner should talk her way through the examination, explaining everything she is doing and why. The patient should be alerted before her body is touched and the inner thigh gently touched before the genitalia. A hand mirror can be used to enable the woman to visualize the anatomy of the vulva, vagina, and cervix. Great care should be given to maintaining privacy and reinforcing the normalcy of the young woman's physical development whenever possible.

If the young woman's vagina will not permit insertion of a narrow or pediatric speculum, the Pap smear and cervical inspection can be deferred in most cases until the woman becomes sexually active; vaginal discharge, DES exposure in utero, or continuous vaginal bleeding, however, mandate a speculum examination to identify cervical or vaginal pathology. Referral to an adolescent specialist or practitioner with extensive experience in examining adolescents may be necessary. Chapter 18 describes in detail the components of the pelvic examination required subsequent to in utero DES exposure.

The bimanual examination can be performed using only the index or middle finger if the introitus does not permit the introduction of two fingers. Gentleness is the key word. In the adolescent who is a virgin, rectal examination may substitute for a vaginal examination if the hymen is rigid and reassurance and relaxation techniques fail to provide sufficient relaxation, or when the examination obviously creates undue emotional trauma for the adolescent.

Laboratory Testing. Laboratory tests required for adolescents are similar to those for adults. A Pap smear and appropriate STD screening should be initiated in sexually active young women. See Chapter 4 for a detailed discussion of screening and diagnostic tests used in gynecologic assessment.

Intervention

Unless pathology exists requiring treatment or referral for diagnosis and therapy, intervention at most adolescent gynecologic visits consists of the provision of contraception and teaching and counseling.

Provision of Contraception. General principles of counseling about the various forms of birth control include consideration of life-style, frequency of intercourse, number of sex partners, cultural background and beliefs, attitudes, biases, values, and motivating factors. Will this woman or couple take the time necessary before each act of intercourse to use properly a method like a diaphragm or foam or condoms? Will the woman take a pill daily in spite of sporadic intercourse? Does she possess the cognitive and emotional maturity to allow her to anticipate and plan accordingly? In addition, it is important to recognize the limitations of the practitioner role. A practitioner cannot call daily to remind someone to take her pill nor can providers prevent pregnancy in someone who wants to conceive. Nevertheless, the provision of ongoing care is vital to successful contraceptive use. Kellinger (1985) found that almost one quarter of respondents in a study of adolescents who discontinued their contraceptive method did so because of fear or side effects. This points to the need for close, personal, and frequent follow-up in this age group.

For detailed information about each contraceptive method, see Section III, Contraception. The following discussion is limited to specific considerations relating to adolescent use of the various methods.

ORAL CONTRACEPTIVES. Although the condom and withdrawal are the methods most often used at first coitus, the birth control pill is the most frequently used method of contraception among adolescents (Turetsky & Strasburger, 1983). Freeman, Rickels, Mudd, and Huggins (1982, p. 816) studied 400 girls aged 17 or younger in a teen clinic where contraceptive methods were available. Among all family planning enrollees under age 18, 75 percent used oral contraceptives, 9 percent intrauterine devices (IUDs), 9 percent foam/condoms, 2 percent diaphragms, and 6 percent no contraceptive method.

The birth control pill offers several advantages for the young woman: it is highly effective; its use need not be associated with sexual activity; it may lead to decreased menstrual flow and cramping; and it has the potential of improving acne. Taken daily, it can become a ritual (Turetsky & Strasburger, 1983).

There are a number of drawbacks to adolescent pill use. Use effectiveness for teenagers drops as a result of poor comprehension of directions and lack of motivation, especially when intercourse is infrequent. The teen may find that the need to hide pill packages from her family is a problem; she must obtain the money necessary to maintain an ongoing supply and must keep follow-up clinic appointments for refill prescriptions. An all too common response from pregnant teens who discontinued pill use prior to conception is "I ran out and did not get to the clinic for more." Planning and the ability to follow through are traits necessary to effectively use birth control pills. These may not be developed until mid- or late adolescence.

Motivation for daily pill ingestion is often clouded by infrequency of sexual activity among teenagers. Freeman and associates (1982, p. 821) found that the adolescents in their sample had intermittent or infrequent sexual activity. When sexual activity is once a month or less, daily medication may seem irrelevant, and missing or stopping pills may appear reasonable. This raises the question of whether the pill is the preferred method when sex is sporadic. To counteract this dilemma, users need extensive information about how oral contraceptives work; this may require teaching or reviewing concepts about basic reproductive anatomy and physiology. Adolescents should also learn about and practice use of alternative methods.

Although adolescents are at lower risk for complications of the pill, they can develop hypertension; thromboembolic or neurovascular disease; abnormalities in glucose tolerance with exacerbation of diabetes; exacerbation of sickle cell disease, asthma, or vascular headaches; chlamydial infections; incomplete bone epiphyseal closure; and gallbladder disease (Turetsky & Strasburger, 1983). Of importance for adolescent females is the risk of postpill amenorrhea in those with preexisting menstrual irregularities or anovulatory cycles, although it is unknown whether the amenorrhea is due to the pill or to preexisting dysfunction (Turetsky & Strasburger, 1983). Ideally, the adolescent should have well-established menstrual cycles before the introduction of oral contraceptives. The reality, however, often does not permit waiting until the young woman has had 2 years of regular menstrual cycles. Bolton (1981, p. 984) recommends a minimum of three monthly cycles at intervals of 35 days or less prior to oral contraceptive use.

INTRAUTERINE DEVICE. Although the IUD offers the teenager an effective method whose use is not directly associated with sexual activity, its association with infection and subsequent infertility make it a less desirable method than the oral contraceptive, particularly because many adolescents may have more than one sexual partner, increasing their risk of contracting a sexually transmitted disease with the possibility of ascending infection. In addition, there is greater difficulty of IUD insertion in women who have never had children, discomfort caused by increased cramping and blood flow during menses, required follow-up office visits, reluctance of adolescents to check strings, and difficulty for some adolescents in learning or recognizing danger signs (Hatcher et al., 1980, pp. 182–183). The advantages of IUD use for teens are that once inserted, few follow-up visits are required; the fear of discovery is minimal; advance planning is not required; it may remain in place for long periods; and it can be simply removed when pregnancy is wanted. Consequently, the IUD may be the method of choice for teens who are incapable of or have no motivation for using contraceptives that require planning; this advantage must be weighed carefully against the risk of infection. A sexual history revealing multiple partners can be considered a contraindication to IUD use for adolescent women.

DIAPHRAGM. Although the diaphragm has minimal dangerous or annoying side effects, the preparation and anticipation necessary for this method are often unacceptable to the adolescent. For some teenagers, however, the diaphragm is an excellent form of contraception (Fisher, Marks, & Trieller, 1987). It offers freedom from fear for those concerned about chemicals in the pill or the risk of infection associated with the IUD. It also may be appropriate for women who have sporadic intercourse. The diaphragm may be objectionable because of the fear that it will be discovered by the family, the need to touch one's body, and the need to plan prior to intercourse.

For the young woman who has chosen the diaphragm, clear instructions must be given with sufficient time allotted for practicing insertion, checking for placement, and removing the diaphragm. In addition to the instructions outlined for diaphragm use in Chapter 6, the young woman needs assistance in thinking through use of the diaphragm given various scenarios. The practitioner can explore with her patient possible safe places to store the diaphragm. For example, she may want to consider the possibilities of carrying a pouch within her pocketbook that contains the diaphragm and a small tube of spermicide, putting the diaphragm in place before going on a date, and having two diaphragms—one to keep at home and one to carry with her or to keep at her partner's home. Reinforcement should be given that the decision to use contraception is a responsible one. During this discussion the practitioner can raise with the young woman the feasibility of talking with her mother or parents about her sexual activity and contraceptive choice. With the permission of the patient, the partner can be included in the discussion of methods and encour-

aged to participate in use of the method. The woman's partner can learn how to insert the diaphragm or remind his partner to use it consistently.

CONDOMS. The condom is often the first method used when teens form sexual alliances. The condom is popular because it is available at low cost without a prescription, is easily concealable, and has a dual function: contraception and disease prevention. The condom prevents direct genital contact, which leads to both dissatisfaction and security. Some men complain of decreased sensation, whereas others laud the decreased risk of sexually transmitted infections. Young men need to be cautioned against carrying condoms for months in their pockets; the heat can lead to deterioration of the condom material with subsequent breakage during intercourse.

All sexually active teenagers should know about the availability and use of the condom. Whenever possible, supplies should be at the practitioner's disposal for ready distribution.

FOAM/SUPPOSITORIES/VAGINAL SPONGE. Spermicidal foam, vaginal suppositories, and the vaginal sponge offer sexually active teens the advantage of easy access without a prescription. Spermicides also are associated with decreased transmission of STDs. Disadvantages of these methods that may be particularly problematic for young people are relatively low effectiveness rates, the need to use them just prior to or during the sexual act, messiness, and, for the sponge, the risk of toxic-shock syndrome. Women should be encouraged to have their partners use condoms in conjunction with spermicides.

WITHDRAWAL. Withdrawal is a popular method of contraception with limited efficacy because of sperm release prior to ejaculation and the motivation required during intercourse for the male to withdraw his penis. Teenagers often have misconceptions about this method and need to have these corrected.

MALE CONTRACEPTIVE INVOLVEMENT. Practitioners can play an important role in influencing male attitudes toward contraception and contraceptive behavior among their patients. Males need to be incorporated into individual and group discussions regarding birth control. If a young woman's partner accompanies her to family planning visits, he can be welcomed to participate in part or all of the visit providing the woman agrees. This man has already demonstrated responsibility and willingness to become involved. The greater challenge is to reach out to less motivated young men. Special efforts should be made to attract males into the clinical setting; to emphasize their participation through sex education programs in schools, community agencies, and churches; to use posters, films, and magazines depicting the dual responsibility for contraception and parenting; and to employ male counselors in family planning clinics. Clinics can be expanded to include practitioners able to provide direct services to adolescent men. Most important, young men can only be expected to act responsibly as adolescents and then as adults if responsibility is taught to children within the home, school, and community.

Teaching and Counseling. Perhaps the most important task of the practitioner in dealing with adolescents is teaching and counseling. Counseling involves first listening. Specific adolescent counseling needs can relate to a variety of areas including self-image, body image, sexuality, attitude toward contraception, friendships, family relationships, communication, school, and work or career decisions. To foster a positive self-image and encourage health-promoting attitudes and behaviors, adolescents need information. The health care practitioner is in an ideal position to provide this information. Informational needs related to health include female and male development; anatomy and physiology, including the menstrual cycle; sexuality; fertility; conception and contraception; STDs; nutrition; consequences of tobacco, alcohol, and drug use; and health screening. Questions must always be encouraged and never ridiculed or dismissed.

An important component of counseling for adolescents involves the promotion of decision making. This must include decisions regarding smoking, drugs, alcohol, sex, contraception, and pregnancy. Counseling involves reinforcing the right to say no to peer pressure and helping adolescents to think through how they will react in a variety of situations. It involves providing support for rejecting unhealthy behaviors and premature sexual intercourse and working with the adolescent to prevent the unwanted or negative consequences of sexual expression.

Counseling must be oriented toward helping the adolescent assess her own values and base decisions on them (Tauer, 1983). A team approach is imperative, with consultations and referrals made as necessary for more intensive individual and group counseling.

FAMILY COUNSELING. Effective communication is key to family survival and growth during this critical period. The health care provider is in a valuable position to act as mediator when necessary. Often, adults feel a sense of helplessness with adolescents which may be based on feelings of inadequacy or a general lack of information about normal development, or both. In an attempt to establish their identity, adolescents test boundaries and challenge authority. Power struggles between adults and adolescents are inevitable.

While working with the family, the practitioner should emphasize the normalcy of certain behavior associated with adolescence. The family may need to be reminded that stress can be productive and growth producing for all members. Practitioners, however, must recognize the signs of conflict or distress that are beyond their capabilities and utilize available and appropriate resources for support, consultation, and/or referral.

PREGNANCY PREVENTION/SEX EDUCATION. With over a decade of experience in efforts established toward preventing teenage pregnancy, much has been learned although little has changed. Communication between parents and teenagers remains inadequate. In spite of studies that demonstrate no increased sexual activity after sex education, many adults are resistant to accept the reality of initiation of sexual activity at younger ages with the consequent need to provide sex education in early grades. Adolescents need to understand contraception and to have geographic, legal, and financial access to contraceptive services and methods.

Although greater accessibility to family planning services and earlier and better sex education will not solve the problem of adolescent pregnancy, they will help. Jones and co-authors (1985, p. 61) found that developed countries with the most liberal attitude toward sex, the most easily accessible contraceptive services for teenagers, and the most effective formal and informal programs for sex education have the *lowest* rate of teenage pregnancy, abortion, and childbearing. Berger and associates (1987) found increased

rates of contraceptive use after the introduction of family planning counseling in an adolescent clinic without increased rates of sexual activity. In this study, counseling included information on the establishment of sexual values, the right to say no, abstinence and alternatives to intercourse, consequences of intercourse, and contraception. Information on STD prevention has become increasingly important as well.

The approach to solving the problem of adolescent pregnancy must be multifaceted, involving a commitment from families, communities, and educational and health care systems. Model programs have been developed utilizing a variety of techniques such as teen improvisational theater, life-skills counseling programs, peer counseling, single-site multipurpose centers, comprehensive school-based programs, combination hospital-, school-, and university-based teen programs, church-based family life centers, and community-based Child Watch Programs (Dryfoos, 1985; Zabin, Hardy, Streett, & King, 1984). Assertiveness training and parent programs have been incorporated (Howard, 1985). Sensitivity to cultural variations in attitudes and practices must be developed for program effectiveness in reaching a broad spectrum of families (DeSantis & Thomas, 1987).

Some success has been reported by those involved in projects geared toward changing behavior and decreasing adolescent pregnancy rates. The St. Paul clinic, for example, is one innovative model of a successful comprehensive on-campus health clinic. The program has reduced births by more than half in five different high schools with a parallel decline in total pregnancies. The project also has been effective in keeping adolescent mothers in school (Kirby, 1984, p. 351).

Nathanson and Becker (1985) found that clinic accessibility, special attention to recruitment and follow-up of teenagers, personalized services and staff–patient rapport facilitated teenage contraceptive use. Interestingly, their study found that patients expected a more directive approach from practitioners regarding birth control method selection than did the practitioners. When the patients' and staff's role expectations were consistent, subsequent contraceptive behavior improved.

Although there is growing support for innovative programs providing sex education and contraceptive services for adolescents, there is also considerable opposition and resistance. The opposition stems from the beliefs that sex education should be taught in the home, that abstinence is the only acceptable behavior for teens, and that sex education promotes unacceptable sexual behavior. While the controversy continues, the reality confronts us and poses a growing threat to our nation.

PREABORTION COUNSELING. Preabortion counseling is vital, both for decision making and for preparation for the procedure. The practitioner should work with the ambivalent teenager and, when appropriate, her family to help them explore their options and jointly come to a decision. Questions that guide the adolescent into thinking about the reality of pregnancy and parenthood should be raised (Ruszala, 1980). Referral for more intensive crisis intervention may be necessary.

Once the abortion decision has been made, the practitioner's role is one of supporting the young woman as she works through the experience so that learning takes place and her self-image remains intact. A referral for abortion should be made and explicit information about the procedure and recovery provided. The patient should be helped to choose between local and general anesthesia. Chapter 28 gives detailed information about all components of abortion counseling.

REFERENCES

Abrams, M. (1985, May). Birth control use by teenagers. *Journal of Adolescent Health Care, 6*(3), 196–200.

Adams, B. N. (1983, June). Adolescent health care: Needs, priorities and services. *Nursing Clinics of North America, 18*(2), 237–247.

Alan Guttmacher Institute. (1981) *Teenage pregnancy: The problem that hasn't gone away,* New York: The Alan Guttmacher Institute.

Altchek, A. (1985). Pediatric and adolescent gynecology. In D. H. Nichols & J. R. Evrard (Eds.), *Ambulatory gynecology.* Philadelphia: Harper & Row.

Ancrum, L., Andrews, B., & Soloway, R. (1987, July). *Where we stand: Services for sexually active, pregnant and parenting adolescents in New York City.* New York: Center for Public Advocacy Research, Inc.

Bell, T. A., & Hein, K. (1984). Adolescents and sexually transmitted diseases. In K. K. Holmes, P. Mårdh, F. F. Sparling, & P. J. Wiesner (Eds.), *Sexually Transmitted Diseases.* New York: McGraw-Hill.

Berger, D. K., Perez, G. & Kyman, W., et al., (1987, September). Influence of family planning counseling in an adolescent clinic on sexual activity and contraceptive use. *Journal of Adolescent Health Care, 8*(5), 436–440.

Billewicz, Z. W., Fellowes, H. M., & Hytten, C. A. (1976, January). Comments on the critical metabolic mass and the age of menarche. *Annals of Human Biology, 3*(1), 51–59.

Blotcky, M. J., & Looney, J. G. (1980). Normal female and male adolescent psychological development: An overview of theory and research. *Adolescent Psychiatry, 8,* 184–199.

Blum, R. W., & Resnick, M. D. (1982, October). Adolescent sexual decision-making: Contraception, pregnancy, abortion, motherhood. *Pediatric Annals, 11*(10), 797–804.

Bolton, G. C. (1981, September). Adolescent contraception. *Clinical Obstetrics and Gynecology, 24*(3), 977–986.

Brockopp, D. Y., & Hall, S. Y. (1984, April). Eating disorders: A teen-age epidemic. *Nurse Practitioner, 9*(4), 32–35.

Brown, S. S. (1985, May/June). Can low birth weight be prevented? *Family Planning Perspectives, 17*(3), 112–118.

Burkman, R. T., Atienza, M. F., & King, T. M. (1984, August). Morbidity risk among young adolescents undergoing elective abortion. *Contraception, 30*(2), 99–105.

Chacko, M. R., & Lovchik, J. C. (1984, June). *Chlamydia trachomatis* infection in sexuality active adolescents: Prevalence and risk factors. *Pediatrics, 7*(6), 836–840.

Children's Defense Fund. (1985). *Preventing children having children.* Washington, DC: Children's Defense Fund.

Clark, S. D., Zabin, L. S., & Hardy, J. B. (1984, March/April) Sex, contraception and parenthood: Experience and attitudes among urban black young men. *Family Planning Perspectives, 16*(2), 77–82.

DeSantis, L., & Thomas, J. T. (1987, August). Parental attitudes toward adolescent sexuality. *Nurse Practitioner, 12*(8), 43–48.

Dewhurst, J. (1984). *Female puberty and its abnormalities.* New York: Churchill Livingstone.

Dryfoos, J. (1985, March/April). School-based health clinics: A new approach to preventing adolescent pregnancy? *Family Planning Perspectives, 17*(2), 70–75.

Eagar, R. M., Beach, R. K., Davison, A. J., & Judson, F. N. (1985, July). Epidemiologic and clinical factors of *Chlamydia trachomatis* in black, Hispanic and white female adolescents. *The Western Journal of Medicine, 143*(1), 37–41.

Elkind, D. (1967, December). Egocentrism in adolescents. *Child Development, 38*(4), 1025–1034.

Ellison, P. T. (1981, March). Threshold hypotheses, developmental age, and menstrual function. *American Journal of Physical Anthropology, 54*(3), 337–340.

Erikson, E. H. (1980). *Identity and the life cycle.* New York: W. W. Norton.

Evans, R. I., & Raines, B. E. (1982). Control and prevention of smoking in adolescents: A psychosocial perspective. In T. J. Coates, A. C. Peterson, & C. C. Perry (Eds.), *Promoting adolescent health.* New York: Academic Press.

Fisher, M., Marks, A., & Trieller, K. (1987, September). Comparative analysis of the effectiveness of the diaphargrm and birth control pill during the first year of use among suburban adolescents. *Journal of Adolescent Health Care, 8*(5), 393–399.

Fisher, M., Swenson, P. D., Risucci, D., & Kaplan, M. H. (1987, October). *Chlamydia trachomatis* in suburban adolescents. *The Journal of Pediatrics, 111*(4), 617–620.

Fraser, J. J., Rettig, P. J., & Kaplan, D. W. (1983, March) Prevalence of cervical *Chlamydia trachomatis* and *Neisseria gonorrhoeae* in female adolescents. *Pediatrics, 71*(3), 333–336.

Freeman, E. W., Rickels, K., Mudd, E. B. & Huggins, G. R. (1982, August). Never-pregnant adolescents and family planning programs: Contraception, continuation, and pregnancy risk. *American Journal of Public Health, 72*(8), 815–822.

Frisch, R. (1983). Fatness, menarche and fertility. In S. Golub (Ed.), *Menarche: The transition from girl to woman.* Lexington, MA: Lexington Books.

Golden, N., Hammerschlag, M., Neuhoff, S., & Gleyzer, A. (1984, June). Prevalence of *Chlamydia trachomatis* cervical infection in female adolescents. *American Journal of Diseases of Children, 138*(6), 562–564.

Green, L. W., & Horton, D. (1982). Adolescent health: Issues and challenges. In T. J. Coates, A. C. Petersen, & C. C. Perry (Eds.), *Promoting adolescent health.* New York: Academic Press.

Gump, D. W. (1984, October). A growing danger—Chlamydial infertility. *Contemporary Ob/Gyn, 24*(4), 39–43.

Hall, G. S. (1904). *Adolescence: Its psychology and its relations to physiology, sociobiology, sex, crime, religion, and education* (2 vols.). New York: Appleton.

Hansen, W. B., Malotte, C. K., & Fielding, J. E. (1987). Tobacco and alcohol prevention: Preliminary results of a four-year study. *Adolescent Psychiatry, 14,* 556–575.

Harrison, H. R., Costin, M., & Meder, J. B., et al., (1985, October) Cervical *Chlamydia trachomatis* infection in university women: Relationship to history, contraception, ectopy, and cervicitis. *American Journal of Obstetrics and Gynecology, 153*(3), 244–251.

Hatcher, R. A., Stewart, G. K., & Stewart, F., et al., (1980). *Contraceptive technology 1980–1981* (10th ed.). New York: Irvington.

Heald, F. P., & Khan, M. A. (1973, November). Teenage obesity. *Pediatric Clinics of North America, 20*(4), 807–817.

Hein, K. (1984, Summer/Fall). The first pelvic examination and common gynecological problems in adolescent girls. *Women and Health, 9*(2/3), 47–63.

Hern, W. M. (1977). *Abortion in the seventies: Proceedings of the Western Regional Conference on Abortion.* New York: National Abortion Federation.

Hofferth, S. L. (1987a). Factors affecting initiation of sexual intercourse. In S. L. Hofferth & C. D. Hayes (Eds.), *Risking the future: Adolescent sexuality, pregnancy, and childbearing* (Vol. II). Washington, DC: National Academy Press.

Hofferth, S. L. (1987b). Teenage pregnancy and its resolution. In S. L. Hofferth & C. D. Hayes (Eds.), *Risking the future: Adolescent sexuality, pregnancy, and childbearing* (Vol. II). Washington, DC: National Academy Press.

Howard, M. (1985, July). Postponing sexual involvement among adolescents: An alternative approach to prevention of sexually transmitted diseases. *Journal of Adolescent Health Care, 6*(4), 271–277.

Howe, C. L. (1986, February). Developmental theory and adolescent sexual behavior. *Nurse Practitioner, 11*(2), 65, 68, 71.

Hughes, C. B., & Torre, C. (1987, September). Predicting effective contraceptive behavior in college females. *Nurse Practitioner, 12*(9), 46-49, 53-54.

Huppert, L. (1983). Ovarian dysfunction in the adolescent. In A. M. Bongiovanni (Ed.), *Adolescent gynecology: A guide for clinicians.* New York: Plenum.

Jekel, J. F. (1981). Evaluation of programs for adolescents. *Birth Defects Original Article Series, 17*(3), 139–153.

Jessor, R. (1984). Adolescent development and behavioral health. In J. D. Matarazzo, S. M. Weiss, J. A. Herd, N. E. Miller, & S. M. Weiss (Eds.), *Behavioral health: A handbook of health enhancement and disease prevention.* New York: John Wiley & Sons.

Johnston, F. E., Malina, R. M., & Galbraith, M. A. (1971, December). Height, weight and age at menarche and the ''critical weight'' hypothesis. *Science, 174* (4014), 1148.

Johnston, F. E., Roche, A. F., Schell, L. M., & Wettenhall, N. B. (1975, January). Critical weight at menarche: Critique of a hypothesis. *American Journal of Diseases of Children, 129*(1), 19–23.

Johnston, L. D., O'Malley, P. M., & Bachman, J. G. (1986). *Drug use among American high school students, college students and other young adults: National trends through 1985.* Rockland, MD: National Institute on Drug Abuse, U.S. Department of Health and Human Services.

Jones, D. E. D., Russo, J. F., Dombroski, R. A., & Lentz, S. S. (1984, October). Cervical intraepithelial neoplasia in adolescents. *Journal of Adolescent Health Care, 5*(4), 243–247.

Jones, E. F., Forrest, J. D., & Goldman, N., et al., (1985, March/April). Teenage pregnancy in developed countries: Determinants and policy implications. *Family Planning Perspectives, 17*(2), 53–63.

Kegeles, S. M., Adler, N. E., & Irwin, C. E., Jr. (1988, April). Sexually active adolescents and condoms: Changes over one year in knowledge, attitudes and use. *American Journal of Public Health, 78*(4), 460–461.

Kellinger, K. G. (1985, September). Factors in adolescent contraceptive use. *Nurse Practitioner, 10*(9), 55, 58, 61–62.

Kirby, D. (1984). *Sexuality education: An evaluation of programs and their effects.* Santa Cruz, CA: Network Publications.

Kisker, M. E. (1985, March/April). Teenagers talk about sex, pregnancy and contraception. *Family Planning Perspectives, 17*(2), 83–90.

Lee, P. A. (1980, September). Normal ages of pubertal events among American males and females. *Journal of Adolescent Health Care, 1*(1), 26–29.

Litt, I. F., & Cohen, M. I. (1979). Adolescent sexuality. *Advances in Pediatrics, 26,* 119–136.

Litt, I. F., Cuskey, W. R., & Rudd, S. (1980). Identifying adolescents at risk for noncompliance with contraceptive therapy. *Journal of Pediatrics, 96*(4), 742–745.

Makinson, D. (1985, May/June). The health consequences of teenage fertility. *Family Planning Perspectives, 17*(3), 132–139.

Marino, D. D., & King, J. C. (1980, February). Nutritional concerns during adolescence. *Pediatric Clinics of North America, 27*(1), 125–139.

Marks, A., & Fisher, M. (1987, July). Health assessment and screening during adolescence. *Pediatrics, 80*(1, Suppl.), 135–158.

Millstein, S. G., Adler, N. E., & Irwin, C. E. (1984, April). Sources of anxiety about pelvic examinations among adolescent females. *Journal of Adolescent Health Care, 5*(2), 105–111.

Mitchell, J. R. (1980). Normality in adolescence. *Adolescent Psychiatry, 8,* 200–213.

Moscicki, A., & Shafer, M. B. (1986, November). Normal reproductive development in the adolescent female. *Journal of Adolescent Health Care, 7*(6, Suppl.), 41S–64S.

Mott, F. L., & Marsiglio, W. (1985, September/October). Early childbearing and completion of high school. *Family Planning Perspectives, 17*(5), 234–237.

Mudd, E. H., Dickens, H. O., & Garcia, C. R., et al., (1978, July). Adolescent health services and contraceptive use. *American Journal of Ortho Psychiatry, 48*(3), 485–504.

Nathanson, C. A., & Becker, M. H. (1985, January). The influence of client–provider relationships on teenage women's subsequent use of contraception. *American Journal of Public Health, 75*(1), 33–38.

National Center for Health Statistics & Ventura, S. J., (1984, September). Trends in teenage childbearing, United States 1970–1981. *Vital and Health Statistics,* Series 21, No. 41, Publication (PHS) 84-1919, Public Health Service, Washington DC: U.S. Government Printing Office.

National Center for Health Statistics. (1986). *Vital Statistics in the United States, 1982.* Vol. II: *Mortality, Part A.* DHHS Publication (PHS) 86–1122, Public Health Service, Washington, DC: U.S. Government Printing Office.

Ory, H. (1983, March/April). Mortality associated with fertility and fertility control: 1983. *Family Planning Perspective, 15*(2), 57–63.

Perez-Reyes, M. G., & Falk, R. (1973, January). Follow-up after therapeutic abortion in early adolescence. *Archives of General Psychiatry, 28*(1), 120–126.

Piaget, J. (1950). *The psychology of intelligence.* London: Routledge & Kegan Paul.

Rigg, A. C. (1980). Puberty: An introduction to adolescent medicine. In A. C. Rigg & R. B. Shearin (Eds.), *Adolescent medicine: Present and future concepts.* Chicago: Yearbook Medical Publishers.

Russo, J. F. (1982, September). The spectrum of outpatient adolescent gynecologic pathology. *Journal of Adolescent Health Care, 3*(2), 126–128.

Russo, J. F., & Jones, D. E. D. (1984, October). Abnormal cervical cytology in sexually active adolescents. *Journal of Adolescent Health Care, 5*(4), 269–271.

Ruszala, J. (1980, March/April). Adolescent pregnancy. *Nurse Practitioner, 5*(2), 22–24.

Saltz, G. R., Linneman, C. C., Brookman, R. R., & Rauh, J. L. (1981, June). *Chlamydia trachomatis* cervical infections in female adolescents. *The Journal of Pediatrics, 98*(6), 981–985.

Sarrel, L. J., & Sarrel, P. M. (1981, December). Sexual unfolding. *Journal of Adolescent Health Care, 2*(2), 93–99.

Sarrel, P. M. (1981, December). Indications for a first pelvic examination. *Journal of Adolescent Health Care, 2*(2), 145–146.

Scales, P. (1977, July). Males and morals: Teenage contraceptive behavior amid the double standard. *The Family Coordinator, 26*(3), 211–222.

Schulz, K. F., Grimes, D. A., & Cates, W., Jr. (1983, May). Measures to prevent cervical injury during suction curettage abortion. *Lancet, 1*(8335), 1182–1184.

Silber, T. J. (1986, November). Approaching the adolescent patient: Pitfalls and solutions. *Journal of Adolescent Health Care, 7*(6, Suppl.), 31S–40S.

Silber, T. J., & Niland, N. F. (1984, April). The clinical spectrum of syphilis in adolescence. *Journal of Adolescent Health Care, 5*(2), 112–116.

Silber, T. J., & Woodward, K. (1982, October). Sexually transmitted diseases in adolescence. *Pediatric Annals, 11*(10), 832–843.

Slap, G. B. (1986, November). Normal physiological and psychosocial growth in the adolescent. *Journal of Adolescent Health Care, 7*(6, Suppl.), 13S–23S.

Sorensen, R. C. (1973). *Adolescent sexuality in contemporary America.* New York: Word Publishing.

Speroff, L., Glass, R. H., & Kase, N. G. (1983). *Clinical gynecologic endocrinology and infertility* (3rd ed.). Baltimore, MD: Williams & Wilkins.

Spitzer, M., & Krumholz, B. A. (1988, January). Pap screening for teenagers: A lifesaving precaution. *Contemporary Ob/Gyn, 31*(1), 33–36, 41–42.

Strobino, D. M. (1987). The health and medical consequences of adolescent sexuality and pregnancy: A review of the literature. In S. L. Hofferth & C. D. Hayes (Eds.), *Risking the future: Adolescent sexuality, pregnancy, and childbearing.* Washington, DC: National Academy Press.

Tanner, J. M. (1962). *Growth at adolescence* (2nd ed.). Oxford: Blackwell Scientific.

Tauer, K. M. (1983, June). Promoting effective decision-making in sexually active adolescents. *Nursing Clinics of North America, 18*(2), 275–292.

Turetsky, R. A., & Strasburger, V. C. (1983, May). Adolescent contraception: Review and recommendations. *Clinical Pediatrics, 22*(5), 337–341.

Tyler, S. L., & Woodall, G. M. (1982). *Female health and gynecology: Across the lifespan.* Bowie, MD: Robert J. Brady Company.

U.S. Department of Commerce (1983). *Bureau of the Census,* Vol. 1: *Characteristics of the population,* Chap. B: *General Population Characteristics,* Part 1: *United States Summary.*

Wallach, E., & Bongiovanni, A. M. (1983). Pubertal development. In A. M. Bongiovanni (Ed.), *Adolescent gynecology: A guide for clinicians.* New York: Plenum.

Warren, M. P. (1983). Clinical aspects of menarche. In S. Golub (Ed.), *Menarche: The transition from girl to woman.* Lexington, MA: Lexington Books.

Washington, A. E., Sweet, R., & Shafer, M. A., (1985, July). Pelvic inflammatory disease and its sequelae in adolescents. *Journal of Adolescent Health Care, 6* (4):298–310.

Zabin, L. S., Hardy, J. B., Streett, R., & King, T. M. (1984, June). A school-, hospital- and university-based adolescent pregnancy prevention program: A cooperative design for service and research. *The Journal of Reproductive Medicine, 29*(6), 421–426.

Zabin, L. S., Hirsch, M. B., Smith, E. A., & Hardy, J. B. (1984, July/August). Adolescent sexual attitudes and behavior: Are they consistent? *Family Planning Perspectives, 16*(4), 181–185.

Zabin, L. S., Schwab, L., & Clark, S. D. (1981, September/October). Why they delay: A study of teenage family planning clinic patients. *Family Planning Perspectives, 13*(5), 205–217.

Zabin, L. S., Schwab, L., Kantner, J. F., & Zelnik, M. (1979, July/August). The risk of adolescent pregnancy in the first months of intercourse. *Family Planning Perspectives, 11*(4), 215–222.

Zelnik, M., & Kantner, J. F. (1977, March/April). Sexual and contraceptive experience of young unmarried women in the United States—1976 and 1971. *Family Planning Perspectives, 9*(2), 55–70.

Zelnik, M., & Kantner, J. F. (1979, September/October). Reasons for non-use of contraception by sexually active women ages 15–19. *Family Planning Perspectives, 11*(5), 289–293.

23

The Postpartum Period

Cindy Dickinson

The postpartum period has never captured the imagination of practitioners. Literature moves quickly from volumes on pregnancy and labor and delivery to child development and childrearing. Pregnancy is usually described as a period of growth and development, whereas the postpartum period is conceptualized as a backward process, an "involutionary" process. This viewpoint has resulted partially from the focus on the physical processes taking place. For the practitioner, the 6-week postpartum checkup has conventionally marked the point when the reproductive tract has returned to its normal nonpregnant state and when the nonbreastfeeding woman will soon reestablish the hormonal balance necessary for the initiation of ovulation. In many cases, from this point on, the new mother is on her own both physically and emotionally.

In fact, the postpartum period is a dynamic time, marked by intense emotional and psychological adjustments that continue much longer than 6 weeks. If its endpoint were defined by these adjustments, the postpartum period would probably be considered much longer and more variable in length.

This chapter discusses the physiologic and psychological bases for the changes experienced in the postpartum period and reviews the management of these changes—normal and abnormal. The focus is on those areas likely to be presented in an outpatient setting, after the immediate care given within the first few days of birth.

PSYCHOLOGICAL ASPECTS

That we do not have a very good understanding of the psychological development of the postpartum woman is an understatement. Most practitioners do not see postpartum women before or after the traditional 6-week appointment. Until recently, discussion of the psychological aspects of the postpartum period was restricted to postpartum depression and sexuality. Interest in how women and men adjust, develop, and change psychologically during this period has broadened somewhat in the light of the recent attention given to adaptation of working women to the transition from work to home and back to work outside the home (Majewski, 1986). Whether postpartum women undergo a common psychological process, however, remains a fascinating question that will be answered only after more research.

One way to gain an understanding of this process is to look to other cultures, many of which place greater emphasis on the postpartum period than on the antepartum period (Goldsmith, 1984; Harris, 1987). Many customs have been associated with the "lying in" period, meant to provide a concentrated time for intense nurturing for both postpartum women and infants. Traditional hallmarks of this period include rest, warmth, and care provided by the baby's father and the birth attendant, with minimal disturbance from the outside (Lang, 1984). For many cultures birth has been a time of "emptying" and the postpartum period a process of "filling." Failure to allow this might have implications throughout the rest of a woman's life.

By other cultures' standards, perhaps the end of the postpartum period would be marked by the woman's return to fullness, both physically and emotionally. This makes sense as there is a real feeling of loss after birth, with attention shifting quickly and dramatically from the woman to the infant. From this perspective, practitioners would want to emphasize ways to support nurture of the woman during the period after birth.

Andrea Eagan (1985) is one of the few researchers in the United States who has investigated the psychological process of the postpartum woman. Her nonrandom study included 58 women, most of whom were white, middle class, and college educated. She has defined the postpartum period as a developmental process lasting 9 months after birth. Eagan categorizes the first month of motherhood as "the fog" and notes that, among her study participants, women with enough help in the early weeks did not get depressed, although the experience was never easy. During the third and fourth months she describes a symbiotic relationship between mother and child and the associated loss of an independent adult identity. The fabric of this symbiotic relationship is disrupted during the fifth month as the woman begins to recall who she was before she became a mother. Husbands or significant others are mentioned more frequently at this time, as are issues related to sexuality. The central task then becomes regaining a sense of self and integrating it into the reality of motherhood.

A slightly different approach was taken by the authors of *The New Our Bodies Ourselves* (Boston Women's Health Collective, 1984) in their description of the postpartum psychological process. They focused on developmental tasks, describing three phases, without a specific time delineation. The first phase is transition from pregnancy to parenthood; the second is adjustment to life with baby; the third is handling of more long-term issues including intimacy, childcare, and work.

In their textbook on postpartum nursing, Hawkins and Gorvine (1985) characterize postpartum adaptation as a maturational crisis or potential crisis. Factors contributing to the possibility of crisis include events surrounding the birth itself, the role transition of the period, body changes, disruption in sexual relations, and the complexity of the tasks to be accomplished. Under this crisis model, the practitioner's job is to assist postpartum families in identifying and implementing coping mechanisms, thus promoting crisis resolution, growth, and wellness.

Other nursing literature has focused on the relationship between mother and infant, concentrating on the attainment of a maternal role and maternal identity (Mercer, 1985; Rubin, 1967a, 1967b, 1984; Walker, Crain, & Thompson, 1986). Mother–infant interactions and mothering behaviors have been examined extensively.

Whether the psychological process after birth is seen as the filling up of an emptiness, the reintegration of the self into a new identity, the resolution of a crisis, or the transition to parenthood, the process almost universally takes longer than 6 weeks, and the practitioner can be influential in supporting health during this time. Any practitioner who provides family planning or well-child services should always be attentive to the fact that a woman and her family may be involved with postpartum psychological adjustments for years and that ongoing assessments continue to be relevant.

Male Reactions in the Postpartum Period/Transition to Fatherhood

The postpartum period is probably as unique for men as it is for women, and there may be similarities in the way men and women experience the postpartum period. Quadagno and associates (1986) studied 21 married couples' moods prepartum, immediately postpartum, and 6 months postpartum. During the immediate postpartum period, both husbands and wives tended to rate themselves as significantly more anxious, tearful, worried, helpless, and nervous as well as significantly less angry, less energetic, and less self-confident when compared with the prepartal and 6-month postpartum periods. They also reported being significantly more happy. It is interesting to note that although wives and husbands rated themselves as more enthusiastic during the postpartum period than during the prepartum period, only the husbands indicated a decrease in enthusiasm from the immediate postpartum period to the 6-month follow-up. More research needs to be done on the psychological development of the postpartum man over time, and consideration must also be given to men who are not in traditional relationships.

Several authors have examined the phenomenon of *couvade* in postpartum fathers. Couvade is a derivative of the French verb *couver*, meaning "to brood" or "hatch" and has come to mean, in anthropologic terms, the learned, socially sanctioned behaviors and restrictions carried out by expectant fathers. In societies where ritual couvade is not practiced, it has been documented that a large number of men suffer from various health complaints during expectant fatherhood. In a study of 70 white, mostly college educated married couples in early and late pregnancy and in the sixth postpartum week, Fawcett and York (1986) found that men exhibited physical and psychological symptoms during pregnancy and in the postpartum period. Their most frequently reported physical symptoms were "feeling

tired" (22 percent) and "feeling less active than usual" (13 percent). The psychological symptoms most frequently reported by the postpartum men were "feeling anxious" (26 percent) and "feeling better than usual" (22 percent), which seem in agreement with Quadagno's findings.

In a study of 81 mainly white, married expectant fathers that included a data collection point at 6 weeks postpartum, Clinton (1986) found that men who had low incomes, had had children previously, suffered health problems, or were from ethnic minorities were at risk for the couvade syndrome postpartum. Nevertheless, because postpartum men exhibit couvadelike symptoms does not mean that explanations for these symptoms relate solely to the fatherhood experience. They may also relate to preexisting conditions, job-related stressors, or life events unrelated to pregnancy.

SEXUALITY

There is no general agreement on what to expect regarding the sexual response in the postpartum period (Reamy & White, 1985). That both physical and psychological postpartum processes affect sexuality is clear. The current research has focused on three areas of investigation:

1. Physiologic aspects of the postpartum sexual response
2. Delineation of change in libido during this period, including the direction of change, when and if libido returns to a prepregnant level, and identification of the barriers to return
3. Association between sexuality and lactation/breastfeeding

Physiologic Aspects of the Postpartum Sexual Response

Postpartum bleeding usually stops after 2 to 4 weeks. Episiotomies and lacerations are generally well healed within 10 days to 2 weeks (Brooks, 1973; Davidson, 1974), although pressure on a laceration or episiotomy during sexual intercourse may be painful much longer (Kitzinger, 1981, p. 302). From a purely physiologic point of view, coitus may be resumed when bleeding has stopped and lacerations or episiotomies are healed, well before the traditional 6-week postpartum examination. In fact, many women resume coitus before 6 weeks, despite physical and psychological deterrents and the advice of some care providers (Robson, Brant, & Kumar, 1981).

In the immediate postpartum period, the walls of the vagina are thin with fewer rugae and less lubrication. These characteristics, consistent with a steroid deprivation state, are especially true for the breastfeeding woman and contribute to a unique postpartum sexual response, as described by Masters and Johnson (1966) through observation of six postpartum women. For at least 3 months postpartum, the sexual response of the target organs (breast and external and internal genitalia) is less rapid and intense. Vasocongestion of the labia majora and minora takes longer to develop after sexual stimulation but is mature once developed. The strength of postpartum orgasmic contractions may also be less. Masters and Johnson (1966) reported that breastfeeding women may experience involuntary milk ejection during the orgasmic experience. These researchers observed, however, that by 3 months postpartum, the physiologic aspects of the sexual response return to a prepregnancy state. Normal vaginal rugae are present at this time, and vasocongestion of the labia majora and minora is no longer slow to respond to sexual stimuli. The quantity of lubrication and its development during the sexual response are also normal.

Change in Libido. There are physical, psychological, and external factors that may affect libido in the postpartum period (Hogan, 1985, p. 340). Body changes including striae gravidarum (stretch marks), a lax abdomen, and a loss of breast tone may contribute to feelings of inadequacy. Some women feel conflict between the roles of mother and lover. Some women feel more dependent on their partner in the postpartum period, whereas women working outside the home may have to deal additionally with fatigue and separation. Although it seems logical to conclude that these factors would exert a negative effect on libido, there is actually no agreement among researchers as to whether sexual desire increases, decreases, or remains the same in the postpartum period.

In interviews with 101 women early in the third postpartum month, Masters and Johnson (1966) found that 47 percent reported low or absent sexual tension. The researchers attributed this to fatigue, weakness, perineal pain, and irritative vaginal discharge. Fear of injury was a major area of concern, and breast discomfort or leakage was also a deterrent. Although no mention was made of the feelings of postpartum men, over 50 percent of the women worried about how the period of forced abstinence from coitus would affect relationship with their partners.

Fischman and associates (1986) found high, but not universal, rates of sexual discomfort among 92 women surveyed at 4 months postpartum, along with decreased sexual desire and decreased frequency of intercourse, which were often related to fatigue and dissatisfaction with bodily appearance. Robson and associates (1981) studied 113 British primiparous women, all in stable relationships, at 3 months postpartum and found that 57 percent reported sexual interest below prepregnancy levels, 33 percent reported no change, and 10 percent reported an increase. In Kenny's (1973) study of 33 postpartum women, all but one breastfeeding, about half reported an increase and 18 percent a decrease in sexual interest. Other investigations of postpartum libido further illustrate the fact that no clear pattern has emerged with respect to the postpartum sexual response (Reamy & White, 1985). It remains for the practitioner to ask questions related to libido and sexuality of both partners in the postpartum period and to investigate the ramifications of any potential problems.

Breastfeeding and Sexuality. Breastfeeding can affect sexuality, or, conversely, sexual feelings can affect a woman's or couple's comfort with breastfeeding. Studies have shown great differences among cultures concerning attitudes toward lactation and sexuality (Hinshaw, Pyeatt, & Habicht, 1972; Riordan & Rapp, 1980; Saucier, 1972). In many, abstinence during lactation is the acceptable practice (Goldsmith, 1984, p. 97) and contributes to adequate infant nutrition and to child spacing.

Research has shown both a positive effect and a negative effect, as well as no effect, of breastfeeding on sexuality. In the Masters and Johnson interviews of 101 postpartum women, the nursing group reported the highest level of postpartum sexual interest in the first 3 months, whereas three fourths of the women sampled in a study by Kenny (1973) reported little effect of lactation on their sexual life. Various interpretations can be given to these findings, providing more questions than answers. From a purely physiologic standpoint, one might expect breastfeeding to have a negative impact as it reduces vaginal lubrication (Bing & Coleman, 1977, p. 150; Hatcher, Guest, & Stewart, et al., 1986, p. 72). On the other hand, breastfeeding might be considered an erotic experience and has many physiologic responses in common with coitus, for example, nipple erection, breast warmth, uterine contractions, and milk ejection. Some women and their partners, however, may not be comfortable with the sensual responses that breastfeeding may produce (Riordan & Rapp, 1980). Possible distaste and guilt may be barriers to a woman's breastfeeding. The traditional male culture's identification of the woman's breast with her sexuality may contribute to a partner's objections to breastfeeding. Many women and men also erroneously believe that the breasts are more permanently altered by breastfeeding than by the pregnancy (Lawrence, 1985, p. 178), although, in fact, heredity and age have the most effect on breast characteristics. Practitioners should always explore the relationship of sexuality to the decision not to breastfeed or to discontinue breastfeeding early.

PHYSICAL ASPECTS

In the immediate postpartum period, women usually express concerns related to physical discomfort. Although the discomfort generally lessens after the first postpartum weeks, concerns about physiologic changes persist (Casey, 1986).

Ovulation

Postpartum women often are concerned about the return of ovulation and menstruation. Levels of progesterone and estrogen decrease rapidly after delivery in the absence of placental function. Follicular phase concentrations of estrogen and progesterone are reached at about the third postpartum week in the nonlactating woman. Likewise, levels of follicle-stimulating hormone (FSH), which are low in the initial postpartum period, rise to appropriate follicular phase levels in the third week (Martin, 1978, p. 173).

Many nonlactating women have their first menses at 6 to 8 weeks postpartum, although often, but not always, this follows an anovulatory cycle (Perez, Vela, Masneck, & Potter, 1972; Pritchard, MacDonald, & Gant, 1985, p. 376; Sharman, 1951). It has been estimated that 10 to 15 percent of nonnursing women have an ovulatory cycle by 6 weeks, 30 percent by 8 weeks, and 70 to 90 percent by 12 weeks postpartum (Martin, 1978, p. 174; Sharman, 1951).

In the nursing woman, ovulation is usually delayed. Perez and associates (1972) found that the mean day of first ovulation among women for whom lactation was artificially suspended and who never breastfed was the 49th postpartum day, with the earliest ovulation on day 36. This can be compared with a mean of postpartum day 117 for women who breastfed more than 15 days; however, there seems to be great variation in the effect of breastfeeding, depending on its frequency and whether it is full or partial. Many breastfeeding women, mistakenly trusting that breastfeeding is effective in preventing pregnancy, have become pregnant in the immediate postpartum period.

Uterus

After delivery of the placenta, the uterus contracts, and the fundus is usually found at or slightly below the level of the umbilicus. The vessels of the placental site are compressed by the contracted myometrium, which provides for hemostasis. From this point, the uterus halves its weight in the first postpartum week, not by losing cells but by decreasing the size of its cells. The uterus begins its descent into the pelvis, and, by the second postpartum week, the fundus usually cannot be felt above the symphysis. The uterus decreases from about a 20-week pregnant size to a 12-week size in this 2-week period (Pritchard et al., 1985, p. 367). At the sixth postpartum week, the uterus has returned to its nonpregnant size of a lemon, although the nonpregnant but previously gravid uterus may increase in size as the number of pregnancies increases. Afterbirth pains, the result of intermittent myometrial contraction, usually are experienced during the first postpartum days and are more painful in multiparas and during suckling of the infant. The endometrium regenerates in about 3 weeks, except for the placental site, where involution may take up to 6 weeks (Pritchard et al., 1985, p. 367).

Lochia

Lochia is the superficial layer of the uterine decidua that is sloughed off after delivery. Initially it is bright red; over the course of 1 to 2 weeks, it becomes paler and decreases in amount. The initial lochia is described as *lochia rubra*, because it contains mostly blood. Lochia rubra lasts, according to one prospective study of 261 women, about 4 days (Oppenheimer, Sherriff, Goodman, et al., 1986). The next stage is characterized by a pink *lochia serosa* containing primarily serous fluid, decidual tissue, leukocytes, and erythrocytes. The median duration of lochia serosa is about 22 days. Finally, there is *lochia alba*, a whitish discharge consisting mainly of erythrocytes and decidua (Varney, 1987, p. 478). In the study by Oppenheimer et al. (1986), the median total duration of lochia was 33 days, although it persisted to 60 days in 13 percent of women. The duration of lochia was shorter in parous women and women with smaller babies.

A lochia that remains bright red, becomes heavier, or is accompanied by excessive cramping may indicate a subinvolutionary process (incomplete obliteration of placental site vessels) or retained placental products. Lochia that is malodorous, especially if accompanied by a tender uterus and fever, may indicate endometritis and signals the need for further assessment to determine whether antibiotic treatment is required.

Cervix and Lower Uterine Segment

After delivery of the placenta, the cervix and lower uterine segment are thin, loose, soft, and malleable. The cervix is open, often with small lacerations at the lateral edges, which do not bleed and require no repair. The external os closes slowly, contracting and progressively thickening so that at the end of 1 week, the opening can admit only a fingertip; however, the external os never regains its prepregnancy appearance and remains somewhat wider at the completion of involution (Pritchard et al., 1985, p. 369). An internal cervical os that is open at the 6-week visit may indicate retained placental products and a more complete assessment should be made. The lower uterine segment, which had been large enough to contain the presenting part of the term fetus, contracts over a few weeks to its prepregnancy form.

Vagina and Perineum

After delivery, the vaginal wall is smooth and the vault is larger than before delivery because of the stretching required for the passage of the fetus. The musculature encir-

cling the vagina has also been stretched. The size of the vagina reduces slowly. This process is thought to be enhanced if the woman does the Kegel or pelvic floor exercise, a perineal muscle tightening exercise that strengthens vaginal tone (Noble, 1982) (see The 4- to 6-Week Postpartum Examination later in this chapter). Further research on the benefits of this exercise is warranted to identify the optimal postpartum exercise regime.

Vaginal rugae begin to appear at about the third postpartum week (Pritchard et al., 1985, p. 369). Abrasions, lacerations, and episiotomies heal within 7 to 14 days, usually without problems, although discomfort sometimes persists much longer, particularly with coitus. Sutures generally dissolve within the first 7 to 10 days, and pieces of suture material may be noted on the perineal pad. The vagina does not become as vasocongested or as lubricated (especially in the lactating woman) during sexual arousal in the immediate postpartum period (Bing & Coleman, 1977, p. 135; Masters & Johnson, 1966).

Abdomen

Both the peritoneum, which covers much of the uterus, and the broad and round ligaments are much more lax in the postpartum period than in the nonpregnant state as a result of their prolonged distension during pregnancy. There may be a separation or diastasis in the rectus abdominis muscles, which run longitudinally. These structures take several weeks to approximate their original shape. The abdominal wall may never resume its prepregnant appearance if the muscles remain weakened and stretched (Pritchard et al., 1985, p. 369), although some diastasis of the rectus abdominis muscles is often permanent. As the abdomen regains its prepregnancy tone, stretch marks or striae may shrink and fade, but never disappear completely.

Breasts

Although incompletely understood, the initiation of lactation seems to be a result of high prolactin levels and falling progesterone and estrogen levels after birth. During pregnancy, high levels of placental estrogen and progesterone inhibit prolactin production. When the placenta is delivered, progesterone and estrogen levels fall dramatically, decreasing prolactin-inhibiting factor (PIF) and allowing the anterior pituitary gland to produce prolactin. Prolactin is essential for milk production and is regulated by the complex interaction of pituitary, ovarian, adrenal, thyroid, and pancreatic hormones (Lawrence, 1985, p. 46). Continuation of lactation is dependent on the suckling stimulus, which continues the suppression of PIF and allows ongoing milk production (Pritchard et al., 1985, p. 372).

The letdown or secretion of milk is the second process essential to successful breastfeeding. Suckling stimulates oxytocin production by the posterior pituitary, which causes contraction of the myoepithelial cells around the alveoli of the breast. Through this process, which can be felt by many mothers, milk is expelled from the alveoli through the ducts to the lactiferous sinuses. Suckling by the infant stimulates the letdown reflex, which brings milk into the infant's mouth. The letdown process eventually may be triggered by a thought of the baby or the cry of the baby. Likewise, negative emotions can inhibit the letdown reflex, causing the breasts to empty incompletely and the infant to receive only part of the available milk. This may frustrate both the breastfeeding woman and the infant; without timely intervention on the part of a friend, family member, or practitioner, frustration may escalate to the point that breastfeeding is discontinued (Varney, 1987, p. 502).

Colostrum is the first fluid that the infant receives from the breast. It is rich in protein and contains antibodies to viral and bacterial diseases. This is of no small importance, as it has been estimated that up to 10 percent of newborns contract infections during delivery or in the first 2 months of life. Secretory immunoglobulin A is not produced in the intestinal tract until 6 weeks to 3 months of age, but is found in breast milk. Its antitoxin effect may explain why breastfed babies seem more resistant to enteric infections (Lawrence, 1985, pp. 117–118).

Breast milk may have antiallergenic properties as well. The protein in breast milk does not provoke an antibody response in the infant, whereas the protein in cow's milk may provoke a response after 18 days; the various allergic symptoms often involve the gastrointestinal tract (e.g., spitting, diarrhea, colic) (Lawrence, 1985, p. 138).

The milk produced after delivery comes in on postpartum days 3 to 5, although if a woman feeds her infant immediately after birth and nurses frequently, her milk may come in earlier.

Weaning

Weaning is the process in which the baby begins to depend on nourishment other than mother's milk. Technically, it begins when the child consumes any food besides breast milk.

Obviously, duration of breastfeeding is influenced by social and cultural norms and is not determined solely by the mother. In some countries, it is common, and indeed important for the survival of the infant, to breastfeed 2 to 3 years. In the United States and other industrialized countries, women usually wean their infants much sooner (Eiger & Olds, 1972). Social support for the nursing mother is perhaps the most significant variable determining duration of breastfeeding (Morse & Harrison, 1987). When a woman begins to consider weaning her infant, the practitioner should help her to explore her feelings about breastfeeding and clarify the circumstances prompting her decision. For example, a woman who is breastfeeding her 15-month-old infant although feeling great social pressure to stop has emotional needs very different from those of the woman who, after 3 postpartum weeks, discovers that breastfeeding is not working out for her and wants to stop even though many urge her to continue.

MANAGEMENT

The 2-Week Postcesarean Examination

A woman who has experienced a cesarean birth should be seen 2 and 6 weeks postoperatively, unless a special condition exists that requires earlier or more frequent examinations. The visit should include a careful history, appropriate components of the physical examination, and the collection of laboratory data as indicated. A major focus of assessment and management is the emotional content and impact of the cesarean birth experience.

Data Collection

HISTORY. The birth experience of the cesarean mother may leave her and her family feeling disappointed, out of control, bewildered, frightened, inadequate, and even guilty (Erb, Hill, & Houston, 1983). Because a cesarean is often unexpected and unprepared for, it may deny a woman and her family the sense of mastery and achievement often felt after birth.

Table 23–1 lists elements of the history that are specific to the cesarean experience; more general components are detailed in Chapter 2. Historical data at this visit should be gathered both by interview and by chart review whenever possible.

One of the main tasks for the practitioner at the 2-week postoperative visit is to carefully review the emotional and physical processes that preceded and followed the cesarean birth and to explore the woman's and family's understanding and interpretation of these events. One woman, for example, may feel loss because she has missed a vaginal birth experience; another woman may be most distressed by the guilt she feels from accepting epidural anesthesia for pain relief when she had planned on no medication for labor.

PHYSICAL EXAMINATION. The 2-week postoperative examination can usually be limited to those aspects listed in Table 23–1 unless a special circumstance or problem presents. The fundus is usually several fingerbreadths below the umbilicus but not as well involuted as the 2-week postpartum fundus after a vaginal birth. The fundus should not be very tender when palpated gently. The incision should be well healed and the lochia scant or absent. The pelvic exam may be deferred until the 6-week visit unless a complication is suspected.

LABORATORY DATA. The laboratory data collected at the 2-week visit relate to the findings of the history and examination. When the postoperative course is normal, no laboratory work is required. If the woman's postoperative recovery was complicated in the hospital, follow-up studies may be indicated. Appropriate tests may include, for example, a urine culture for a test-of-cure for the woman who had a urinary tract infection or a repeat complete blood count (CBC) if anemia had been present.

Screening for Complications.
As cesarean mothers generally spend at least 5 days in the hospital, most postoperative complications, such as endometritis and wound infection, manifest before discharge; however, as women who have had cesarean births are increasingly being discharged earlier than the 5 days, the practitioner must be even more aware of the full range of postoperative complications that may present in the office setting. (See Complications, later in this chapter, for a discussion of common complications.)

As all cesarean births involve indwelling catheters, all postoperative women must be screened for urinary tract infection (UTI) at 2 weeks. Routine urinalysis and culture and sensitivity are unnecessary, but the practitioner should obtain a history specific to this problem. If the woman developed a UTI while hospitalized, a test-of-cure is indicated, if the woman complains of dysuria, frequency, or urgency, urinanalysis and culture and sensitivity should be obtained. (See Chapter 17 for a more detailed discussion of this problem.)

Teaching and Counseling

EMOTIONAL RECOVERY FROM CESAREAN DELIVERY/RESOLUTION OF THE EXPERIENCE. Through a careful history, the practitioner should be able to identify specific emotional issues generated by the cesarean experience. The practitioner should find out how much information the woman has and to what extent she has reviewed the experience with those involved. Many women may not have a clear idea of the

TABLE 23–1. THE 2-WEEK POSTCESAREAN EXAMINATION

History

Birth Experience
Original plans for labor and delivery
History of events of labor and delivery and how the woman or couple feels about them
Position, size of baby, and pelvimetry
Hours of ruptured membranes
Interventions in labor including types of monitoring and medications given
Complications of labor and delivery
Indication for cesarean section/timing of the decision/participation of the woman or couple in decision making
Type of cesarean section/type of anesthesia/blood loss
Support system during labor and delivery

Hospital Experience
Number of days in hospital
Maternal and newborn complications
Interventions, for example, intravenous therapy, antibiotics
Initiation of infant feeding
Support system during hospitalization
Separation from infant/family
Laboratory data: CBCs and appropriate cultures

Home Experience
Current infant status and medical follow-up plans
Support system/family adjustment
Activity level/home responsibilities
Infant feeding
Medications
Nutritional status/diet appetite
Sleep patterns/fatigue levels
Course of physical condition: general well-being, pain, lochia, bowel and bladder function, breasts, incision, fever and chills
Emotional state

Physical Examination
Vital signs
Weight
Heart
Lungs
Breasts
Abdomen including incision
Lochia
Extremities
Pelvic (usually deferred until 6-week examination)

Laboratory Data
As indicated

indications for the cesarean section or the type of cesarean done (lower segment versus classical) and its implications for subsequent births. The hospital course should be reviewed. If no chart is available, the practitioner should speak with the people involved and/or encourage the woman to speak with the obstetrician and/or midwife to clarify the experience. This has to be a first step in the process of resolution as many women feel unnecessary guilt or focus on events that may be totally unrelated to the actual outcome.

Although it is not known whether all women have issues to resolve from the cesarean experience, there is ample evidence that the majority of cesarean women do have this need; low self-esteem, feelings of failure, and disappointment are commonly experienced (Cox & Smith, 1982; Erb et al., 1983; Lipson & Tilden, 1980). The process of resolution is important not only for a woman's postpartum adjustment, but for future pregnancy and birth. In a pilot study of 50 pregnant women, McClain (1985, p. 210) found that, after a low-segment cesarean section, the decision for a vaginal birth after cesarean (VBAC) versus elective repeat cesarean was not based on "the probabilities of particular outcomes," but rather on "constructed mental images of anticipated events based upon past childbirth experience and expected consequences of the preferred course of action."

The practitioner can refer a woman to an affordable and accessible support group like The Cesarean Prevention Movement (P.O. Box 152, Syracuse, NY 13210) or Cesarean/Support Education and Concern (22 Forest Road, Framingham, MA 01701). She can also provide or recommend appropriate literature (Cohen & Esther, 1983; Donovan, 1986).

PREPARATION FOR THE NEXT BIRTH. In recent years, it has become acceptable practice to attempt a trial of labor for women with a previous lower-segment cesarean if "there are no recurrent indications for cesarean birth" (U.S. Department of Health and Human Services, 1981). At North Central Bronx Hospital in New York, 60 to 70 percent of women who initiated a trial of labor between 1979 and 1986 delivered vaginally (Duran, 1987). Other studies show success rates between 40 and 80 percent for VBACs (Taffel, Placek, & Liss, 1987). The practitioner always should discuss this possibility, as many women are still under the impression that "once a cesarean always a cesarean."

NUTRITION AND EXERCISE. In addition to following the diet recommendations discussed under The 4- to 6-Week Postpartum Examination, the cesarean mother should continue taking prenatal vitamins and iron because of the usual blood loss experienced with this type of surgery. She should be counseled on high-iron–containing foods and on dietary measures to avoid constipation.

Exercise may begin in the hospital with breathing, foot movements, and leg and abdominal exercises (Noble, 1982). Noble believes that after leaving the hospital, most women can progress at their own pace to the normal postpartum exercises, avoiding ''lifting, straining, undue exertion, and poor body mechanics'' (see the next section).

The 4- to 6-Week Postpartum Examination

The 4- to 6-week postpartum examination is an important, although contrived, milestone in many women's lives. Although it often marks the end of the involutionary process for the practitioner, for the woman, it may mark the beginning of the postpartum experience. As this visit may be the last contact the woman has with the health care system for some time, it must be approached by the practitioner with an acute sensitivity to its importance. Specifically, the practitioner should evaluate any problems identified in the prenatal, intrapartum, or immediate postpartum period, assess the normal postpartum involutionary process, review the woman's and family's psychological adaptations to the postpartum period and parenting, and screen for postpartum complications. Appropriate consultations, referrals, interventions, and counseling and teaching should be implemented.

Data Collection

HISTORY. The history should include a review of the prenatal, intrapartum, and immediate postpartum periods to screen for problems that might still require intervention. For example, if the rubella screen was negative during pregnancy, the postpartum period is the ideal time to vaccinate, because most women do not plan to get pregnant for at least 3 months. Although congenital rubella syndrome has not been found to occur after inadvertent rubella vaccination in early pregnancy, counseling women to avoid pregnancy is wise because of the theoretical risk for congenital rubella syndrome with exposure to the live virus during pregnancy (Centers for Disease Control, 1987; Preblud, 1985). Some women require postpartum follow-up of Pap smears. If a woman had gestational diabetes, evaluation is required to ensure that she is not currently diabetic. In addition, a careful and detailed interval history of the events of the prior 4 to 6 weeks is essential, not only to identify physical problems, but to get a sense of where in the psychological continuum of the postpartum period are the woman and her family.

PHYSICAL EXAMINATION. The gynecologic examination is detailed in Chapter 3; several aspects particular to the 4- to 6-week postpartum examination are outlined in Table 23–2.

The breasts should be carefully examined. The non-breastfeeding woman will have been through her period of engorgement, and her breasts should be soft, although milk usually can still be expressed 4 to 6 weeks postpartum. The breasts of a lactating woman should be evaluated for signs of engorgement, plugged ducts, and mastitis (see Complications); nipples should be evaluated for signs of dryness, irritation, and cracking.

During the abdominal examination, special attention should be given to the rectus abdominis muscles and their separation, or diastasis, should be measured in fingerbreadths. Diastasis of these muscles is one indication of abdominal tone and should be assessed both when the muscles are relaxed and when they are contracted. To measure

the diastasis, ask the woman to lie down with her legs slightly bent. Place your fingertips below the umbilicus. Instruct the woman to tighten her abdominal muscles by raising her shoulders and head. Press your fingertips gently into the abdomen and rock them slowly from side to side until you feel the rectus abdominis muscles on either side of your fingers. Note the number of fingers needed to fill up the space between the muscles. As the woman relaxes her abdominal muscles by slowly lying back, continue to try to follow the position of the muscles as they separate further with her relaxation. Again, measure the distance of the diastasis in the relaxed position (Varney, 1987, p. 661). Varney suggests charting diastasis as number of fingerbreadths contracted/number of fingerbreadths relaxed. During the exam, have the woman feel the separation herself; this often convinces her of the need for abdominal exercises, although even with exercise some degree of separation is usually permanent.

External genitalia must be examined for their state of healing. Most episiotomies or lacerations should be well healed by 4 to 6 weeks but may still cause some discomfort, especially during coitus. Discomfort most often is felt at the posterior aspect of the hymenal ring or on the incision line. The woman should be offered the opportunity to look at the repair with a mirror.

The 4- to 6-week postpartum examination should include a complete pelvic exam as outlined in Chapter 3. The cervix should be inspected for signs of laceration. On palpation, the cervical os should be closed, and the uterus should be only slightly larger than its nonpregnant size. If the os is open and the uterus is larger than expected, the practitioner must suspect a subinvolutionary process (see Complications). A woman's pelvic tone can be evaluated by asking her to tighten her pelvic muscles around the examining fingers, although it is a rare woman who has regained her muscle tone, even with Kegel exercises, in the time since delivery. This is a good time to teach or reinforce the Kegel exercise and instruct as to its importance for good bladder control and pelvic muscle support. See Table 3–1 for a description of this exercise.

A rectovaginal examination is mandatory at the postpartum checkup after a vaginal birth. Ask the woman to tighten her sphincter around the examining finger during the rectal exam especially if a third- or fourth-degree laceration was sustained. The force of tightening should be similar to the prepregnancy force.

LABORATORY DATA. Some institutions or practices obtain routine laboratory tests at the postpartum visit. If laboratory screening was not done in pregnancy, or was done very early, some practitioners perform an annual laboratory workup at this time. Others order tests only as indicated, based on current problems.

Teaching and Counseling. What postpartum women want to know may be different from what practitioners decide to teach at the 4- to 6-week postpartum visit. In addition, what postpartum women want to know may be dependent, to some extent, on class, age, ethnicity, and time since delivery (Casey, 1986). Many researchers have found that in the immediate postpartum period, women's concerns relate most to the infant and to the physical self (Chapman, Macey, Keegan, et al., 1985; Gruis, 1977; Russell, 1974; Sumner & Fritsch, 1977). More research must be done to assist us in recognizing and assessing concerns at and beyond 4 to 6 weeks postpartum although obviously the woman herself is our best guide. Some of the common areas discussed at the 4- to 6-week postpartum visit are

TABLE 23-2. 4- TO 6-WEEK POSTPARTUM EXAM

History

Chart Review

Prenatal course, including prenatal laboratory data: Pap smear, GC and other cultures, maternal blood type and Rh factor, CBC, rubella screen and syphilis screen

Intrapartum course

Delivery and immediate postpartum period, including pre- and postdelivery vital signs and laboratory data

Interval History

Number of weeks postpartum

Concerns and questions: reaction to labor and delivery experience, postpartum concerns

General health and well being, including diet/appetite, bowel and bladder function, level of activity/exercise/fatigue, sleep patterns, pain/discomfort

Interval problems: reasons for any calls to health provider or visits to emergency room or health provider and interventions, fever, illness

Adjustments: reaction to baby, relationships with significant others, siblings, housing and financial issues

Resumption of menses: date, duration, amount, quality, associated symptoms

Resumption of coitus: when, number of times, was contraception used, if not, why not, type, discomfort if any, comfort measures used, satisfaction, sexuality issues

Family planning: plans for family, previous methods used, success, how long used, side effects, when stopped and why

Baby: any problems, feedings, problems with breastfeeding, visits for well-baby check and immunizations

Review of relevant systems

Breasts	Problems: cracked or sore nipples, mastitis, plugged ducts, engorgement
	Breastfeeding history: when initiated, frequency of feeding, enjoyment, reaction of significant others, identified support persons, when stopped and why
	Breast care practiced
Bladder function	Dysuria, urgency, flank pain, Kegel exercises, stress incontinence
Bowel function	Problems, constipation, incontinence, especially with history of a third- or fourth-degree laceration, relief measures used
Perineum	Discomfort at laceration or episiotomy site
Lochia	Duration, color sequence, odor, clots, excessive bleeding and preceding factors (e.g., exercise, heavy lifting, intercourse)
Abdomen	When and what exercises initiated
Legs	Cramps, varicosities, heat, redness, swelling, or calf tenderness

Physical Examination

Vital signs
Weight
Thyroid
Heart
Lungs
Costovertebral angle tenderness
Breasts
Abdomen
Perineum
Extremities
Speculum exam
Bimanual exam
Rectovaginal exam

Laboratory Data

As indicated

(Adapted from Varney, H. [1987]. Nurse midwifery [2nd ed., pp. 495–496]. Boston: Blackwell Scientific.)

postpartum physical and emotional changes, diet and exercise, lactation and infant feeding, sexuality and family planning, and parenting and special circumstances, such as the working mother, the single mother, the lesbian mother, and fatherhood.

POSTPARTUM CHANGES. Both physical and emotional changes of the postpartum period were discussed earlier. These should be reviewed with the woman, especially as they relate to her specific concerns.

DIET. Rest, a good diet, and exercise are essential to successful postpartum recovery. A reducing diet during the immediate postpartum period is not recommended, especially for the breastfeeding woman. The nonbreastfeeding woman should follow prepregnancy recommendations for calories and other minimum daily requirements. The literature does not give a clear idea of when the nonbreastfeed-

ing woman should begin to try to lose the weight gained during pregnancy, but common sense suggests that this can occur anytime after the sixth postpartum week and when the woman herself feels ready. For a woman who has had a heavy blood loss at delivery or a prior inadequate diet, oral iron and vitamins should be continued at least until the stores are replenished, usually 2 to 3 months (Lawrence, 1985, p. 230). It is recommended that all postpartum women continue to take 30 to 60 mg elemental iron and to increase consumption of iron-rich foods, such as green leafy vegetables, organ meats, and eggs.

Nutritional requirements for lactating women include increases in certain nutrients over prepregnant levels (Lawrence, 1985, p. 230):

Calories	+600
Protein	+20 g
Vitamin A	+400 RI

Vitamin D	$+4 \mu g$
Vitamin E	$+3$ mg d-α-tocopherol
Vitamin C	$+40$ mg
Folacin	$+100 \mu g$
Riboflavin	$+0.5$ mg
Thiamine	$+0.5$ mg

Increases in other water-soluble vitamins (e. g., other B vitamins) and minerals are also recommended. Lawrence (1985) suggests meeting postpartum dietary needs by adding to the prepregnant diet two cups of fresh milk, two ounces of meat, one-half cup of a citrus fruit, one-half cup of a dark green or yellow vegetable, one-half cup of another vegetable or fruit, and one slice of enriched or whole-grain bread. Common sense helps in ensuring that most requirements are met. For instance, varying the diet and choosing fresh rather than canned foods as much as possible help guarantee adequate nutrient intake.

Lactating women need extra fluids; a glass of liquid with each breastfeeding meets this requirement (LaLeche League International, 1983, pp. 211–213). Breastfeeding women should avoid chemical additives whose excretion in breast milk and effect on infants have not been studied (LaLeche League International, 1983, p. 202). They should avoid or limit coffee and carbonated drinks and colas that contribute to caffeine accumulation in the infant, causing caffeine stimulation (Lawrence, 1985, p. 261).

EXERCISE. The only way to restore the musculature involved in pregnancy, labor, and vaginal or cesarean birth is through exercise. Reconciling and restoring their postpartum bodies to a prepregnant body image is a major concern of women (Gruis, 1977; Russell, 1974). Some women may need guidance to accept that the return of the body to its prepregnant state is a gradual process (Strang & Sullivan, 1985). Exercises must be tailored to suit the individual woman and her birth experience. They should be begun within the first 24 hours of delivery and continued throughout a woman's lifetime to maintain strong abdominal and pelvic musculature. A number of excellent and comprehensive books on prenatal and postpartum exercises are available (Lynch-Fraser, 1983; Noble, 1982; Simkin, 1982).

Pelvic floor (Kegel) exercises aimed at restoring the tone of the pelvic floor and rectal sphincter are functionally probably even more important than abdominal exercises. Because strenuous abdominal exercises can cause an increase in pressure on the pelvic floor, pelvic floor exercises are the foundation for abdominal exercise work (Noble, 1982, p. 13). A woman can identify the pelvic muscle either by inserting two fingers into her vagina and tightening around them (or around the examiner's fingers during a vaginal exam) or by sitting on the toilet and starting and stopping the flow of urine by pulling up this muscle. Once the muscle is identified, she can do "slow Kegels," by tightening the muscle and holding it for a count of three, or "quick Kegels," by tightening and relaxing as rapidly as possible. Kegel exercises can be done during daily activities like reading, watching television, or sitting in a car, bus, or subway. They should be repeated at least five times a day (Neeson & Stockdale, 1981, p. 321).

Abdominal muscle exercises should also be started soon after birth and follow a progressive pattern from abdominal wall tightening to more demanding abdominal exercises such as curl-ups and V-sits (Noble, 1982).

BREASTFEEDING. The first-time breastfeeder is in a very vulnerable position. Today, in the United States, much discouragement exists even for a truly committed woman. These include rigid hospital schedules and regulations with extended periods of separation of mother from infant; unsupportive staff, friends, and family members; and misinformation about many aspects of breastfeeding. By the 4- to 6-week postpartum examination, initial breastfeeding problems like engorgement or sore and cracked nipples have been resolved. A woman is often ambivalent as to whether to continue breastfeeding.

Perhaps most important for the woman breastfeeding for the first time is the continued availability of support for the many ups and downs of breastfeeding. This support may come from a friend who has breastfed, a health provider, or an organization like the LaLeche League, which provides counseling by experienced women, educational materials, and advice about breastfeeding especially for difficult situations like a premature infant, twins, or a working mother (LaLeche League International, 1983). It is important for providers to be aware of all community resources available to the breastfeeding woman, particularly once she is on her own at home. At many hospitals today a special breastfeeding consultant works on the postpartum floor, providing information, devising solutions to breastfeeding problems, and working with staff in an educational capacity. She may continue her work outside the hospital by making phone calls to breastfeeding women as well as home visits after discharge. She is called a *doula*, originally a Greek word meaning "slave," but later used to describe a woman who assists the childbearing woman in any way, mainly during the postpartum period (Raphael, 1976). At North Central Bronx Hospital in New York, the *doula's* dedication, delightful presence, and extensive program was instrumental in increasing the percentage of women breastfeeding on hospital discharge, from 40 to 60 percent, since her arrival 3 years ago (personal communication with Luz Garcia, *doula* at North Central Bronx Hospital). Should a community hospital employ a *doula*, it is valuable to make her acquaintance and discuss her availability to assist women for the duration of nursing.

Breastfeeding problems encountered by women are numerous, and appropriate resources should be consulted for more specifics (Danner, 1984a,b; Eiger & Olds, 1972; La Leche League International, 1983). Many problems can be prevented by breastfeeding early (preferably at delivery), feeding frequently throughout the day and night (at least every 2 to 3 hours on demand of the infant), utilizing both breasts at each feeding, alternating the breast offered first, withholding supplementary feedings or water, and providing a good diet and a supportive relaxed environment with frequent rest periods.

Once nursing is well established, which usually occurs within a few weeks, a more flexible approach to breastfeeding can be assumed if needed. Women planning to return to work, for example, can phase out certain breastfeedings and substitute bottle feedings during working hours. Women can pump their breasts at work, provided adequate refrigeration is available, and save the milk for the next day's supply or freeze it for use up to 6 weeks later (Eiger & Olds, 1972). A manual or electric pump can be recommended for this purpose, and the practitioner should become familiar with local suppliers of such pumps or refer the woman to the LaLeche League from which they can be ordered. Formula can be introduced if pumping the breasts at work is impossible.

There are certain drugs that the breastfeeding woman should not take as they may affect milk supply or be excreted in breastmilk and have a harmful effect on the infant. Any drug that is taken during lactation should be evaluated for its effect on the infant. Such a review is beyond the scope of this chapter. There are, however, several good resources that provide the information on the effects of commonly used drugs through lactation (Lawrence, 1985, pp. 247–273). Cigarette smoking is not a contraindication to breastfeeding, but the smoking woman should be counseled not to smoke while nursing as it will affect her letdown and expose the infant to smoke in the immediate environment. Low-nicotine cigarettes should be suggested as well as reduction in the number of cigarettes per day (Lawrence, 1985, p. 389). Smoking marijuana is a different matter; some evidence from studies in animals shows that DNA and RNA formation may be affected by *cannabis,* the active ingredient in marijuana that is secreted in milk (Lawrence, 1985, p. 389; Nahas, Suciu-Foca, Armand, & Morishima, 1974). A recent study has demonstrated the presence of cocaine in breast milk with possible dangerous effects on the baby (Chasnoff, Lewis, & Squires, 1987).

Often, breastfeeding women have concerns regarding the appropriate time for weaning. The feelings of the mother and the readiness of both mother and infant should be discussed. Family attitudes and the cultural context in which a woman lives are important considerations as well. Once the decision is firmly made, weaning should be done gradually and with a lot of common sense. Anticipatory guidance should be given to the woman returning to work or school so that she plans well in advance. Several suggestions can be offered to all women (Eiger & Olds, 1972; La-Leche League International, 1983, pp. 180–181; Lawrence, 1985).

1. One nursing should be eliminated at a time, up to one per week.
2. The baby's least favorite nursing times should be omitted first.
3. The woman and her family should be encouraged to remain flexible, especially if the infant/toddler is sick or particularly upset.
4. Others can help at the time when a breastfeeding is omitted by providing extra love and attention.

SEXUALITY AND FAMILY PLANNING. The practitioner should create an environment in which a woman and her partner feel that they can discuss emotional and physiologic issues of postpartum sexuality. Often, all that is needed is for the practitioner to acknowledge that this is an important concern during the postpartum period. By the 4- to 6-week postpartum examination, many couples have resumed intercourse without much information on what to expect. Couples may need to know that the woman's sexual organs do not respond rapidly or intensely to stimulation early in the postpartum period and that the response generally returns to normal by the third postpartum month. Practitioners should also counsel that breastfeeding women experience a decrease in vaginal lubrication and that use of a water-soluble lubricating jelly like K-Y or a number of other lubricants available over-the-counter may be helpful. If a woman has had an episiotomy and/or laceration repair, she may still be experiencing some discomfort with coitus at her 4- to 6-week postpartum visit, even if the wound is essentially healed. In addition to the use of lubrication, the practitioner should suggest that any pressure be well forward on the front of the vagina and base of the clitoris (Kitzinger, 1981). Kitzinger also suggests a bedtime warm bath into which a few tablespoons of ordinary kitchen salt have been dissolved. The female-superior position for coitus helps the woman control the depth of thrusting. The couple should experiment with this and other positions as well as communicate with one another to find the best positions and techniques (Hogan, 1985, p. 342).

Some postpartum women or couples do not feel a strong desire for intercourse and should be reassured and counseled as to alternative methods of satisfying sexual needs. Couples should be reminded that the intense fatigue felt in the postpartum period, which often interferes with sexuality, will eventually subside.

Family planning is a major focus of the postpartum examination, as this often is the last contact a woman has with a practitioner for quite some time. There is evidence that in a substantial number of women, both breastfeeding and nonbreastfeeding, ovulation precedes the resumption of menstruation. This is most often true for women who have suspended breastfeeding and is sometimes true for women who are partially breastfeeding (Perez, et al., 1972; Simpson-Hebert & Huffman, 1981). A woman and her partner should be aware that the interval between delivery and the first ovulatory cycle can be short and the risk of pregnancy is inherent.

A complete discussion of contraceptive methods and decision making is contained in Section II. There are, however, special considerations for the breastfeeding woman.

Contraception and the Breastfeeding Woman. The time at which a breastfeeding woman needs to initiate contraception depends on her breastfeeding practices. A fully breastfeeding woman may not need contraception before 6 months if the infant sucks frequently and receives no supplemental feedings; however, in the United States, where infants may be fed according to a schedule or where an occasional bottle is given, ovulation should be expected sooner, requiring initiation of a contraceptive method at the 4- to 6-week postpartum examination should the woman desire (McCann, Liskin, Piotrow, et al., 1981; Simpson-Hebert & Huffman, 1981). The following discussion relates specific contraceptive methods to the breastfeeding woman.

TOTAL ABSTINENCE. Some cultures advocate a specified period of postpartum abstinence because it is believed that coitus alters breast milk (Hinshow et al., 1972; Saucier, 1972). There is no evidence that coitus has an effect on breast milk, but should a woman choose abstinence, she should be advised to develop a plan for contraception before resuming intercourse if she wishes to avoid pregnancy.

PERIODIC ABSTINENCE (SYMPTOTHERMAL METHOD OF FERTILITY AWARENESS/NATURAL FAMILY PLANNING). Lawrence (1985) reported on a Canadian study of fertility awareness during lactation using a special postpartum chart designed to record morning temperature (basal body temperature [BBT]), cervical mucus, and other signs of fertility/infertility as they relate specifically to postpartum days. The chart also provides space to note the intensity of breastfeeding. The method was apparently workable for most study participants. Special attention was given to signs of ovulation that occurred with changes in sucking patterns or with weaning or partial weaning, such as when the infant began to sleep through the night, began solid foods or partial bottle feedings, or had an illness.

Lactational infertility may be identified by the lack of mucus or by a continuous unchanging mucus flow. When ovulation resumes, irregular mucus patterns occur; these can be difficult to interpret, however. This method requires longer periods of abstinence during lactation than otherwise (Liskin, 1981, p. I50).

SPERMICIDES. It is a common assumption that spermicides have no effect on breast milk or breastfeeding and can be used safely in the postpartum period. In combination with condoms, they have usually been considered an excellent choice for the immediate postpartum period. Actually there has been little research into the relationship of spermicides to lactation or mother's milk. One study by Chvapil and associates (1980) in rats demonstrated the rapid systemic absorption of a spermicidal agent and its transfer from milk to the serum of pups. A detrimental effect on lactation per se or on the well-being of the rat pups was not investigated.

BARRIER METHODS. Condoms, cervical caps, and the diaphragm have no effect on breastfeeding and may be used in the postpartum period. Women should be advised not to use any vaginal barrier longer than 24 hours in the postpartum period because of the risk of toxic-shock syndrome (see Chapter 18). Female barrier methods should not be used for the first six postpartum weeks because of this risk. As indicated earlier, the effects of the spermicides used with these methods need more study.

INTRAUTERINE DEVICES. Because of the effect of breastfeeding on uterine contractility, there has been some concern about possible elevated intrauterine device (IUD) expulsion rates with lactation. In a study of over 3,000 women, Cole, McCann, Higgins, and Waszak (1983) found no significant difference in expulsion rates between fully breastfeeding and nonbreastfeeding women whether the IUD was inserted immediately postpartum or up to the end of a 6-month follow-up period. Expulsion rates for both breastfeeding and nonbreastfeeding women, however, were greater if the IUD was inserted immediately postpartum rather than later. The International Fertility Research Program has developed postpartum IUDs with biodegradable sutures tied to the upper arm of the IUD. This helps the IUD to stay in place while the uterus involutes and minimizes expulsions (McCann et al., 1981, p. J551).

One case-control study found that women lactating at the time of IUD insertion were ten times more likely to have a uterine perforation at the time of insertion than women with at least one live birth who were not lactating (Hartwell & Schlesselman, 1983). Caution should be used in accepting this result, as study controls were taken from other medical admissions to the hospital and there may have been a selection bias against breastfeeding women in this group.

Concern has been raised that the IUD might influence lactation by stimulating secretion of oxytocin (the hormone responsible for letdown) through uterine stimulation or by increasing prolactin levels. One study reported increased prolactin levels in women using copper IUDs compared with a control group of women using condoms or abstinence (Mehta et al., 1977), although in another study no difference was found in plasma prolactin levels before and after insertion of either inert plastic or copper IUDs (Wenof, Aubert, & Reyniak, 1979).

A study by Heikkilä, Haukkamaa, and Luukkainen (1982) demonstrated that progestin is excreted in the milk of women with progestin IUDs, thus exposing infants to synthetic progestins during the breastfeeding period. The effect on the infant was not discussed, but progestin-containing oral contraceptives do not reduce milk volume and generally are not considered to have short-term ill effects on the baby although the long-term effects are unknown (McCann et al., 1981, p. J547).

TUBAL LIGATION. If a breastfeeding woman is planning a bilateral tubal ligation after the sixth postpartum week, she should make plans for milk expression or breastfeeding in the hospital if the procedure is to be done on an in-patient basis (see Chapter 29). Regional anesthesia is the anesthesia of choice, as there is some evidence that in the initial breastfeeding period, general anesthesia and sedation may affect the establishment of breastfeeding (McCann et al., 1981, p. J552).

VASECTOMY. The postpartum period is a good time for a man to consider a vasectomy, as sperm remain in the male genital tract 2 to 3 months after this procedure. If the woman is breastfeeding, this is likely to be a period of reduced fecundity (McCann et al., 1981, p. J552).

ORAL CONTRACEPTIVES. Use of oral contraceptives while breastfeeding is an example of a situation where the needs of the woman may not be completely compatible with the needs of the infant. The authors of an extensive review of the literature on hormonal contraception during breastfeeding summarize current knowledge as follows (McCann et al., 1981, p. J544):

1. The difficulties of measuring lactation and identifying the effects of hormones make all conclusions tentative as a number of review articles have pointed out.
2. Combined estrogen–progestin oral contraceptives decrease milk volume in some cases, but pills with 0.05 mg or less estrogen do not appear to affect infant growth.
3. Progestin-only contraceptives, whether pills or injectables, either have no measurable effect on milk volume or may increase it.
4. The small doses of hormones used for contraception do not appear to prevent initiation of lactation. Limited research suggests but does not prove that, when hormonal contraceptives—combined or progestin-only—are started early, milk production may not be as great as when they are started later.
5. Minute amounts of hormones are transmitted to the infant in breast milk. Nonserious immediate effects have been observed, but long-term effects are unknown.

Given the possibility of ill effects of oral contraceptives on breastfeeding and the infant, one might ask why the discussion should continue. There are at least two reasons: First, some women consider oral contraceptives their only birth control option; given the choice of breastfeeding or using birth control pills, a woman may choose to forgo breastfeeding. The benefits of breastmilk to the infant, however, probably outweigh the risks of oral contraceptives. Second, the risks of a pregnancy may exceed the risks of oral contraceptive use during breastfeeding. Based on a review of this issue, the American Academy of Pediatrics' Committee on Drugs (1981, p. 140) concluded that practitioners should review "all the available contraceptive methods in the light of each personal situation so that an informed, individualized, and effective choice can be made." This statement was endorsed by the American College of Obstetricians and Gynecologists' Committee on Obstetrics, Maternal and Fetal Medicine.

As combination pills have been shown to have an effect on milk production, some experts suggest that progestin-only contraceptives be used by the breastfeeding woman until lactation is well established (i.e., at 6 months) or until after the first menses, when pregnancy becomes more likely. When combined estrogen-progestin pills are selected, the practitioner should offer the breastfeeding woman the following advice:

1. Use the lowest dose available.
2. Not initiate combined pills until lactation is well established—at least 2 or 3 months postpartum.
3. Take each oral contraceptive tablet daily at the beginning of the longest interval between breastfeeding.
4. Provide additional suckling time when oral contra-

ceptive use begins in order to help counteract any hormonal effect on the milk supply. If oral contraceptives are first taken at the same time that supplemental foods are added to the infant diet, a decline in milk supply should be expected, but breastfeeding can still be maintained. Breast milk will continue to benefit the child after other foods are introduced and after menses resume. (McCann et al., 1981, pp. J556–J557).

POSTPARTUM ADJUSTMENT AND TRANSITION TO PARENTHOOD. Many of a woman's early postpartum concerns relate to the infant (Bull, 1981). Often, by the second postpartum month, friends have stopped bringing in meals, partners have gone back to work, and fatigue has set in. Feelings of maternal attachment are often increasing, and the transition to parenthood is well underway. The focus seems to shift from the individual woman and the individual infant to their relationship. Therefore, it is appropriate for the practitioner to begin to raise issues about the woman's relationship with her infant and her feelings regarding her competence. Not surprisingly, excessive infant crying in the first month and additional responsibilities like other small children may work against the general trend of increasing maternal attachment in the second month (Eagan, 1985, p. 60). In many cities, parent groups are available to provide postpartum support (Dix, 1985). Referrals should be made whenever such a group might seem helpful.

Working Mothers/Single Mothers. Being both a mother and a woman who works outside the home is a fact of life for 48 percent of women with children less than a year old and for nearly 60 percent of women with children of school age ("Job Protection," 1987). Most women work because they need to; almost two thirds of working women are single, widowed, divorced, or separated or have husbands who earn less than $10,000 annually (Chavkin, 1984, p. 15). Despite the obvious reality depicted in these statistics, managing the two roles of mother and worker remains a problem, particularly because the federal government has refused to support a national maternity leave policy or national childcare program and has cut back on the little financial support previously given to these areas. The United States is the only industrialized nation in the world that does not provide a maternity leave for all its pregnant citizens. In a survey of 14 countries, the minimum paid leave was 12 weeks (Israel); the maximum leave was 9 months (Sweden) (Kammerman, 1980).

Although from a developmental point of view the timing is probably not the best, many women must consider returning to work after the sixth postpartum week, or even sooner, because disability payments, if provided, usually cover only 6 weeks. The balancing of two worlds, neither of which seems to understand the other, creates both emotional and practical problems for working mothers (Majewski, 1986; McBride, 1973; Norris & Miller, 1979). Although research supports the notion that a child can thrive in a good childcare arrangement (Vestal, 1980), guilt at leaving an infant is still perhaps nearly universal. On the one hand is the feeling that the child will somehow be shortchanged, and on the other hand is the fear that the child will love the childcare provider "more." The strictly practical issues include deciding when to return to work, how to continue breastfeeding (Van Esterik & Greiner, 1981), and finding childcare arrangements that suit a work schedule or vice versa (Shepherd & Yarrow, 1982).

The practitioner can be most helpful by raising both the emotional and the practical questions at the postpartum visit. Most women are well aware that the return to work will not be easy, but many put off serious discussion or planning until time is short. The practitioner can begin to review plans with the mother and father at this time. The practitioner should accumulate information in this area, suggest books and articles about working mothers (Boston Women's Health Collective, 1984; Norris & Miller, 1979; Shepherd & Yarrow, 1982; Vestal, 1980), and direct women to appropriate discussion groups, daycare facilities, and support organizations. Other parents can be invaluable informants on both the quality of institutional daycare in the community and alternative care arrangements such as play groups, family daycare, and parent cooperatives.

The practitioner also may want to provide counseling about pregnancy disability. Title VII of the Civil Rights Act of 1964 prohibits discrimination on the grounds of sex but it necessitated further amendment through the Pregnancy Disability Act (PDA) of 1978 to specifically prohibit discrimination against pregnant workers. The Pregnancy Discrimination Act states that "Women affected by pregnancy, childbirth, or related medical conditions shall be treated the same for all employment related purposes, including receipt of benefits under fringe benefit programs, as other persons not so affected but similar in their ability or inability to work" (Public Law 95-555; Stat. 2076; October 31, 1978).

Employers must treat pregnant women as any employee with a medical condition is treated but the law does not guarantee a minimum benefit package (Chavkin, 1984, p. 202). An employer who does not offer health care or disability coverage for other medical conditions does not have to do so for pregnancy, although the Supreme Court recently upheld a California state law giving not only equal but preferential treatment for pregnant employees ("Job Protection," 1987). "Pregnancy disability" has been interpreted widely as a physical disability lasting 6 weeks postpartum for an uncomplicated labor, delivery, and postpartum course. Extension of this period for psychological or societal reasons generally has not been accepted (Brucker & Reedy, 1983).

The practitioner should counsel women regarding their rights under federal law and any special leave and reinstatement benefits guaranteed by state law. Practitioners who want information about their own state's laws or women who feel that their employers are not complying with the law or who themselves want more information should contact the regional office of the Department of Labor.

Transition to Fatherhood. Traditionally, men have been given only an indirect role in parenting. This is changing somewhat as many fathers are seeking to be more involved parents. The postpartum period increasingly is recognized as an important time in the growth and development of men (Hangsleben, 1980).

Unfortunately, it is the rare father who comes to the 4- to 6-week postpartum visit. As the incorporation of the man into the childbirth experience continues and as his role and unique postpartum experience are recognized, his participation at this visit may become more common. For now, the practitioner may have to be aware of the man's experience from afar and counsel him through the postpartum woman. The initial step is to have both the woman and the man recognize the uniqueness of the postpartum period in their individual development.

Lesbian Mothers. There is a dearth of information on the special needs of lesbian mothers, and this section reflects that fact. Even the major studies on homosexuality have hardly focused on parenthood (Fishel, 1983), and have virtually ignored the needs of lesbian women during the postpartum period. In most respects, their needs are similar to those of all mothers.

Much of the information about gay parents has focused on the legal aspects of child custody. The authors of the chapter "Lesbian Life and Relationships" in *The New Our Bodies Ourselves* (Boston Women's Health Collective, 1984, p. 152) suggest that two lovers who have or adopt a child write a contract stating each partner's responsibilities and intentions, particularly with regard to custody and visitation rights, and that they provide in each other's will for the partner to be the child's guardian. This establishes the clear intent to parent together, although the courts do not have to honor either contract or will.

Other issues relating to the lesbian parent that have appeared in the literature reflect the heterosexual orientation of society. The gay parent's impact on the child's development has been raised as a concern, as has the forced or unconscious development of a homosexual orientation in the child (Fishel, 1983). Possible harassment from peers regarding the parent's sexual preference has been addressed. Although the lesbian mother may not have these concerns, she may be confronted with them by many elements in her life, including her health practitioners.

Many large cities have lesbian/gay parent groups that provide support and a wealth of experience on strategies for coping with a heterosexually dominated society, its myths, and its prejudices. For the child, the stress of living in a stigmatized situation is lessened when the parent is supportive. The health practitioner can foster supportive parenting by meeting the parents' needs, physically and emotionally.

COMPLICATIONS

Many postpartum complications present before the 4- to 6-week appointment. As early hospital discharge increases, however, postpartum problems may become more common in out-patient settings.

The incidence of some medical problems is increased during the postpartum period. A disease like thyroiditis (new-onset hypo- or hyperthyroidism) may present for the first time (Affonso, Andreyko, & Mills, 1987), or a preexisting condition, such as autoimmune disease, may flare or first become symptomatic in the postpartum period.

Patients taking medications for medical conditions may need dose adjustment in the postpartum period. Such medications include digoxin, insulin, and seizure medications. Failure to make appropriate changes can have life-threatening consequences.

Women also may need postpartum reevaluation of conditions discovered during pregnancy that may be altered once their bodies have returned to the nonpregnant state, for example, heart murmur. There are also certain tests that generally are delayed until the postpartum period, such as renal scans or other radiologic workups.

Discussion of these aspects of postpartum care is beyond the scope of this chapter. They are mentioned because of their relevance to the postpartum evaluation. Although their management requires medical consultation or referral, the primary care practitioner needs to be diligent in screening for such medical needs and problems during the postpartum period. This section focuses on psychological and physical complications related specifically to the childbearing process.

Postpartum Psychological Disturbances

Postpartum psychological disturbances range in expression from "baby blues" to major psychiatric illnesses.

Postpartum "blues" have been identified in anywhere from 30 to 80 percent of new mothers (Hazle, 1982; McGowan, 1977; Pitt, 1973). These blues are usually experienced within the first few postpartum weeks and involve mood swings, tiredness, irritability, and crying episodes (Ihsan, 1982; Pitt, 1973). Postpartum blues are a transitory event and resolve without the need for psychiatric intervention. Because they are so common, postpartum blues are considered a normal expression of postpartum mental health (Paykel et al., 1980; Tod, 1964). Speed of recovery is often dependent on environmental and interpersonal supports and reduction of stressors during the initial postpartum period (Hazle, 1982; McGowan, 1977). To call these blues "normal" may be reassuring to the many postpartum women who experience them, but such characterization also may trivialize the experience. Counseling should be sensitive and individualized, although all women should be given anticipatory guidance about the existence and frequency of the postpartum blues.

Paykel and associates (1980) reported on the prevalence of mild clinical depression in 20 percent of 120 women assessed at 6 weeks postpartum. This psychological expression lies between transient postpartum blues and more extreme psychiatric disturbances such as psychosis. The researchers found that the strongest factors associated with depression were occurrence of recent stressful life events and a group of factors characterized as "lack of social support." Housing problems and previous psychiatric history produced strong independent effects on the prevalence of depression both with and without stressful life events. By screening for these risks, the practitioner may be able to intervene before symptoms become disabling.

It has been estimated that major psychiatric disturbances occur in one to two of every 1,000 births (Ihsan, 1982, p. 296). Research into their etiology has taken several directions with at least three theoretical perspectives. Some researchers believe that mental illness is precipitated by childbearing and the reactivation of earlier conflicts. Others hold an organic view, maintaining that there is an effect of endocrine changes on behavior. Finally, some view postpartum disturbances as a holistic stress response resulting from psychological, physiologic, and environmental stressors (McGowan, 1977). Forms of treatment depend on the specific psychological diagnosis and the severity of symptoms and include a full range of psychological therapies including pharmacologic agents, supportive short-term psychotherapy, and institutionalization (Dix, 1985, pp. 37–55, 179–210).

At the 4- to 6-week postpartum visit, the practitioner should expect many women to report having experienced symptoms of the blues. Continuation of these symptoms after 6 weeks should not be considered a normal expression of postpartum mental health. Such psychological symptoms and their severity should be investigated in depth. Information about recent stressful life events not related to the pregnancy should be obtained as should information about the extent of family supports. In addition, any past psychiatric history should be explored.

It also is valuable to rule out postpartum thyroiditis by asking about symptoms associated with hypo- or hyperthyroid states and following up, if necessary, with thyroid function tests and antibody studies; symptoms of this transient condition often mimic those of postpartum depression. It most commonly presents between 1 to 3 months postpartum with hyperthyroidism and at 3 to 6 months postpartum with hypothyroidism (Affonso et al., 1987).

If, after intensive evaluation, the practitioner's assessment is that the presenting psychological symptoms are those of postpartum blues, the woman should be seen again in 1 to 2 weeks with telephone contact in the interim. Stressful life events should be identified and patients assisted in efforts to minimize them. Support networks should be strengthened and social services utilized if appropriate. For extended postpartum depression or more serious psychiatric disturbances, appropriate consultation and referrals should be made.

Grief or Loss

Perinatal losses include miscarriage/abortion, stillbirth, adoption, neonatal death, and loss of the anticipated "perfect" baby through congenital malformation or prematurity (Jackson, 1985). Losses of a more psychological nature are related to loss of the pregnant role or of the dyad relationship present before the entrance of the newborn (Broom, 1983). Regardless of the nature of loss, the grief process follows a definite pattern, with variations depending on the type of loss, the individual's involvement, and the particular psychological issues of pregnancy that affect the perinatal loss. Examples of such issues include motivation for pregnancy and parenthood and the relationship with the fetus during the pregnancy (Quirk, 1979). The pattern of grief work has been described as moving from the acute grief stage or initial shock, to a stage of suffering or phase of reality, and finally to a stage of resolution (Varney, 1987).

In his 1944 study of 101 bereaved patients following the disastrous Coconut Grove nightclub fire in Boston, Lindemann (1944) identified several characteristics of what he considered a normal grief reaction, including somatic distress, preoccupation with the image of the deceased, guilt, feelings of hostility and anger toward others, and breakdown of normal patterns of conduct. These responses are considered necessary for resolution of the mourning process. Although this process may take 6 months to a year, Lindemann saw a resolution to the acute grief work in 4 to 6 weeks. Therefore, the postpartum visit is an ideal time to assess the family's stage of mourning and whether or not the process seems normal (Kennell & Trause, 1978; Lindemann, 1944). Each family member—man, woman, and child—may experience the grief reaction differently and individual assessments must be made. This is yet another case in which the woman should not be the sole focus of postpartum care.

Practitioners have a particularly important role in helping grieving parents. Supports usually available to families in times of crisis are not as available after pregnancy loss (Quirk, 1979). Friends and family members often react with uncertainty and avoidance. The practitioner can provide a structure to assist the family through the crisis and provide information essential to completion of a normal grieving process.

Practitioners can support the grieving process in several ways. First, it is important to help the family accept the reality of the perinatal death (O'Donohue, 1979). Much of this work should have begun in the hospital. The practitioner should review with the family what measures were taken in the hospital. For example, did the family view and hold the infant/fetus? Were pictures, footprints, or other mementos given? Did the family choose a name? Was there a private burial or ceremony? Activities that bestow "personhood" on the infant or customs culturally appropriate to acknowledge the loss should be continued at the 4- to 6-week postpartum visit; the practitioner can specifically ask the woman and other family members about the infant's appearance and name.

The practitioner should also review with the family what happened in the interval since hospitalization and address misconceptions (O'Donohue, 1979). The practitioner may have to contact the care providers involved with the woman's hospitalization to clarify some points. These efforts are invaluable for the eventual resolution of the grief process. The postpartum visit is an appropriate time to discuss any autopsy findings, although they may not explain the cause of death.

The practitioner can encourage the family to express their emotional and physical reactions to their loss. The practitioner should discuss the couple's plans for another pregnancy. Most authorities feel that the couple should wait until the mourning reaction is completed—6 months to 1 year—before having another baby (Kennell & Trause, 1978). In addition, the practitioner should discuss any problems demonstrated by the most recent pregnancy that might necessitate particular treatments, evaluations, or referrals either before or during the next pregnancy. An example is a second-trimester loss suggestive of an incompetent cervix. Referral to a support group may be helpful for some women or couples.

Several visits may be needed during the subsequent months to help the family through this very difficult period. For the practitioner, this process is often painful. It is, however, undoubtedly instrumental in restoring a sense of well-being and health to the woman and her family.

Infection and Bleeding

Fever and heavy lochia are two of the most frequent complaints in the postpartum period. Each requires the usual thorough workup including a comprehensive history, noting predisposing factors, a complete physical examination, and the collection of laboratory data to make a diagnosis and develop an appropriate plan of management.

Infection. Low-grade temperatures are very common in the immediate postpartum period and may be nonpathologic and resolve spontaneously (Gibbs & Weinstein, 1976). Puerperal morbidity was defined in the 1930s by the Joint Committee on Maternal Welfare as "a temperature of 38.0°C (100.4°F) or higher, which occurs on any 2 of the first 10 days postpartum, exclusive of the first 24 hours; the temperature is taken by a standard technique at least four times a day" (Pritchard et al., 1985, p. 719). Because of early patient discharge, however, and rapid response to antibiotics, many postpartum infections no longer meet this criterion for morbidity.

Ledger (1986a, p. 251) describes the conditions for a clinical infection by the following "equation": "If the number or virulence of the bacteria introduced during labor or at the time of delivery plus the extent of the soft tissue damage and the amount of foreign material left in place exceed the abilities of the host's local and systemic mechanisms to eliminate the organisms, an infection will result. Any attempt to evolve methods of prevention is directed toward shifting the balance of this equation in favor of the host."

Table 23–3 lists the differential diagnosis for postpartum fever highlighting some important aspects of appropriate history taking and physical and laboratory examinations. As the diagnosis is often not straightforward or self-evident, a diagnosis is never excluded from the differential unless its irrelevance is absolutely clear. Several of the more common diagnoses presenting after the immedi-

TABLE 23–3. DIFFERENTIAL DIAGNOSIS OF POSTPARTUM FEVER

Differential Diagnosis *Fever and Infection*	History and Possible Predisposing Factors and Symptoms	Physical Examination	Laboratory Data

Endometritis	Low resistance:
	  Anemia, poor nutrition, heavy blood loss
	Cesarean section
	Long labor
	Premature rupture of membranes
	Invasive procedures or manipulations:
	  Internal monitoring, forceps, manual removal of placenta
	Size and number of lacerations and difficulty of repair
	Positive cervical culture: especially for beta strep
	Chills, severe afterbirth pains
		Vital signs:
		  Fever, tachycardia
		Fundus:
		  Tender
		Lochia:
		  May or may not have odor depending on offending organism, may be decreased in amount
		Abdomen:
		  Bowel sounds may be decreased in post-op period with mild distension
			CBC with differential:
			  Elevated or increasing WBC, with shift to left suggests infection
			Lochia/Endocervical culture (of dubious value 2° to contamination)
			Blood cultures as indicated

Wound/Laceration/Episiotomy:
  Infection, hematoma, abscess
	Type of delivery and difficulties
	Type of laceration and/or episiotomy and difficulty with repair
	History of poor tissue:
	  Vaginitis, condylomata
	Obesity
		Incision of cesarean section or laceration and/or episiotomy for signs of infection or hematoma:
		  Redness, swelling, wound separation, exudate (pus-like), induration
		Pelvic examination if hematoma or abscess is suspected to palpate for fluid collection
			Culture of exudate
			CBC and differential; pelvic sonogram if indicated to rule out hematoma or abscess

Mastitis Blocked milk duct Breast engorgement	History of missed feedings Nipple trauma Breast pain	Breast: Engorgement, localized areas of redness, warmth, tenderness, induration, nipple discharge: normal vs. pus-like	Culture of exudate from breast
Cystitis/Urinary Tract Infection (UTI) Pyelonephritis	Prior history of UTI Pyelonephritis History of bladder trauma Catherization during labor and/or delivery Sickle cell trait Urinary frequency, dysuria, urgency, oliguria, chills, suprapubic pain	Vital signs: Spiking temperatures with pyelonephritis, tachycardia Costovertebral angle tenderness (CVAT) or flank pain with pyelonephritis	Urinalysis and urine culture CBC with differential

Upper respiratory infection (URI)
Pneumonia
	History of cold, flu, or exposure to either
	History of general anesthesia
	History of asthma
	Shortness of breath, sore throat, generalized aches
		Throat:
		  Reddened with URI
		Lymph Nodes:
		  Enlarged, tender
		Lungs:
		  Rales, rhonchi, wheezing
			Throat culture
			Chest X-ray as indicated
			CBC with differential

Superficial or deep vein thrombophlebitis	History of thrombophlebitis
	Varicose veins
		Legs:
		  Redness, tenderness, swelling, positive Homan's sign, unequal pulses
		Lungs:
		  Evaluate for complication of thrombophlebitis: pulmonary embolism
			Doppler studies if deep vein thrombosis is suspected

Pelvic or femoral thrombophlebitis	History of poor response to antibiotics given for presumed infection
	History of endometritis
	History of deep vein thrombophlebitis
	Repeated severe chills
		Temperature:
		  Repeated extreme swings
		Blood pressure:
		  Hypotension with bacterial endotoxic shock
		Lungs:
		  Small pulmonary embolis can cause pleurisy and pneumonia
			Sonogram

Postpartum Bleeding Subinvolution	Endometritis Difficult delivery of placenta leading to possible retained fragments	Vital signs: If associated with endometritis, temperature and pulse may be elevated	CBC to evaluate for blood loss and possible contributing infectious process

TABLE 23-3.   (CONTINUED)

Differential Diagnosis Fever and Infection	History and Possible Predisposing Factors and Symptoms	Physical Examination	Laboratory Data

	Fibroids
	Cesearean section
		Speculum examination:
		  Lochia often profuse, reddish brown
		Bimanual examination:
		  Cervical os may remain open if there are retained placental fragments
		  Uterus is enlarged, boggy; may be tender	

Late (delayed) postpartum hemorrhage	History of endometritis Difficult delivery of placenta	Exam as above Vital signs: in extreme cases, evaluate for shock Careful inspection and bimanual for hematoma or undiagnosed laceration	As above

(Adapted from Varney, H. [1987]. Nurse midwifery [2nd ed., pp. 495–496]. Boston: Blackwell Scientific.)

ate postpartum period, including endometritis, mastitis, urinary tract infection/pyelonephritis, and episiotomy or laceration infection, are now discussed in more depth.

ENDOMETRITIS. The most common cause of puerperal morbidity, especially after cesarean section, is postpartum endometritis (ACOG, 1986). In endometritis, infection may be limited to the superficial decidua, which is shed as lochia, or, more commonly, may include the underlying myometrium. For this reason, recently some authors have referred to this infection as metritis (Pritchard et al., 1985, p. 721) or endomyometritis (Ledger, 1986b, p. 222). There is an increased risk of intrauterine infection after delivery by cesarean section (Blanco, Gibbs, & Castaneda, 1981; D'Angelo & Sokol, 1980). D'Angelo and Sokol examined five time-related risk factors—duration of labor, duration of ruptured membranes, number of vaginal exams, length of time from first vaginal exam to delivery, and duration of internal monitoring. They found that duration of labor was the most important determinant of postpartum morbidity.

Endometritis is often variable in its clinical presentation. Some women have almost no symptoms (Eschenbach & Wager, 1980, p. 1003). For example, a woman may have only mild uterine tenderness and an elevated white blood cell count possibly with a shift to the left (increased bands). In these mild cases, a healthy woman who remains afebrile may be able to get better with rest, good nutrition, and anticipatory guidance to be alert for signs of a worsening condition. In other cases, the woman might be quite sick with chills and fever to 101 to 103°F. The fundus is often markedly tender and lochia is malodorous, indicating infection by anaerobic bacteria. As infections by bacteria like β-hemolytic streptococci are not malodorous, however, the practitioner cannot be reassured by a normal-smelling lochia (Pritchard et al., 1985, p. 725).

If endometritis is suspected, consultation with a physician is indicated as the woman may need antibiotics and/or hospitalization. In the presence of a high fever, a full "fever workup" can be done as part of the office assessment. The laboratory tests may include CBC with differential, urinalysis, culture and sensitivity, blood cultures, and chest x-ray. Infections of the endometrium and myometrium are usually polymicrobial; even if one bacteria has been isolated from the cervix or placenta, other bacteria are usually involved, necessitating wide antibiotic coverage (ACOG, 1986). If intravenous antibiotics are indicated, usually several antibiotics are used, although some third- and fourth-generation cephalosporins and extended-spectrum penicillins like mezocillin are used alone. Once intravenous antibiotic therapy is begun, a woman should be counseled about the length of time that she must be afebrile before it can be discontinued—usually 24 to 48 hours. She should be helped to estimate her length of stay in the hospital. Some physicians continue oral antibiotics after initial intravenous therapy although the risks and benefits of such a practice have not been systematically studied; many specialists in infectious diseases feel this practice is unnecessary (ACOG, 1986). See Chapter 14 for more discussion of endometritis.

MASTITIS. Mastitis and its later complication, breast abscess, are the two breast infections occurring in the postpartum woman. Mastitis is an inflammation of the breast and, in the postpartum period, occurs almost exclusively in the breastfeeding woman. Since the advent of shorter hospital stays and antibiotics, it is no longer epidemic in the early postpartum period in this country (Lawrence, 1985, p. 204). Nonepidemic mastitis occurs most frequently in the second and third postpartum weeks (Devereux, 1970). Predisposing factors for mastitis include poor drainage of a breast duct and alveolus, lowered maternal resistance associated with stress and fatigue, and presence of an organism (usually *Staphylococcus aureus*, although *Escherichia coli* and rarely *Streptococcus* have been colonized).

Newbould (1974) has identified five types of lactational mastitis: subclinical (asymptomatic mastitis), acute puerperal mastitis, suppurative mastitis (breast abscess), mammary infection with uncommon organisms, and virus infection in mammary neoplasms. The first three are discussed here.

Asymptomatic mastitis usually occurs during the first 10 postpartum days, and *S. aureus* is the most common pathogen. The breast is tender and the woman may experience an occasional low-grade fever. As long as there is adequate drainage of the breast, the woman remains asymptomatic (Ezrati & Gordon, 1979).

There are two types of acute puerperal (nonepidemic) mastitis: acute puerperal mammary cellulitis and acute puerperal mammary adenitis. Marshall, Hepper, and Zirbel (1975) found acute puerperal mastitis in 2.5 percent of breastfeeding women.

Mammary cellulitis is an infection of the connective tissues between the lobes of the breast. It usually results from the introduction of bacteria through a cracked or fissured nipple and is most common in the early postpartum period. The infected area is hard, reddened, and painful. The woman is generally febrile with a temperature of at least 100.4°F (38°C) and a fast pulse. She may also have flulike symptoms, such as chills, malaise, and headache. Occasionally, the cellulitis resolves without treatment, but often, if not treated, it evolves into a breast abscess.

Mammary adenitis (or intramammary mastitis) is an infection located within the lobes and ducts of the breast. It occurs in the absence of cracked or fissured nipples. One of the theories of its causality is that staphylococci in the nasopharynx of the infant are introduced into the breast during nursing. Pus can often be expressed from the nipple of an infected breast, a finding not present in cellulitic infections. The other symptoms are similar to those of mammary cellulitis but may be less severe (Ezrati & Gordon, 1979).

High levels of sodium and chloride have been found in milk from breasts with mastitis. A woman can compare the tastes of milk from each breast to help assess whether she has an infection (Conner, 1979).

The hallmark of management of breast infection is prevention (Dilts, 1985; Eiger & Olds, 1972; Ezrati & Gordon 1979; Lawrence, 1985):

1. Prevention of engorgement by early and unrestricted nursing after delivery, with adequate rest and fluids
2. Prevention of cracked nipples by avoiding use of drying agents such as soap and alcohol directly on the nipple and by air drying and leaving milk on them after nursing
3. Wearing a supportive but not constricting bra (Constriction could lead to reduced milk flow and plugged ducts.)
4. Early identification of breastfeeding women at risk—those with cracked nipples or plugged ducts and engorgement—with a plan to eliminate the risk factors (Suggested remedies include local massage, moist heat, and rest for plugged ducts, and heat lamp therapy for cracked nipples.)
5. Antepartum and early postpartum instructions so that the breastfeeding woman can herself identify risk factors or early mastitis and initiate immediate follow-up with her practitioner
6. Scheduling of a postpartum appointment at 2 to 3 weeks postpartum for the breastfeeding woman

If mastitis is suspected, consultation with a physician is indicated as immediate antibiotic therapy may be necessary. Devereux (1970) found that abscesses were more likely if treatment or supportive measures were begun more than 24 hours after onset of symptoms.

The woman with mastitis should be counseled to continue breastfeeding (Eiger & Olds, 1972; Lawrence, 1985). Nursing decreases engorgement and congestion. Eiger and Olds note that there is no danger to the infant because his or her mouth and nose probably harbor the same organism that caused the mastitis. In two prospective studies of postpartum women with sporadic (nonepidemic) acute mastitis, no adverse effects on the mother or infant were noted when breastfeeding was continued (Devereux, 1970; Marshall et al., 1975).

Frequent nursing to reduce congestion, rest, heat to the affected breast, and analgesia should be suggested. Eiger and Olds (1972) counsel women to offer the sore breast first at each nursing so that it can be emptied more completely, but Lawrence (1985) suggests the opposite to allow the affected breast to "let down." She also advises making sure that the affected breast is emptied completely by nursing or milk expression.

Devereux (1970) found little help from cultures of the breast milk, as the attacks are usually under control by the time the identification and sensitivities were ready; in mammary cellulitis there may not be anything to culture as the infection resides in the connective tissue rather than the ductal system.

Lawrence (1985, p. 207) suggests that treatment decisions be "based on local sensitivities and length of time since delivery or exposure to resistant flora. For *staphylococcal* diseases, amoxicillin, dicloxacillin, and nafcillin may be the drugs of choice. In *streptococcal* disease, penicillin is usually preferable. In uncomplicated mastitis after 1 month postpartum, penicillin, ampicillin, or erythromycin is preferable initially." Antibiotics should be given for 10 days and must be tolerated by both the mother and the infant. Sulfa drugs, for example, should not be used if the infant is less than 1 month old.

The practitioner should consider referring the woman with mastitis to a supportive organization for what may be a difficult period of breastfeeding.

BREAST ABSCESS. Breast abscess formation is usually a result of either delayed or inadequate treatment of mastitis (Lawrence, 1985, p. 208). Most women with signs of abscess formation manifest signs of acute infection associated with mastitis. The affected breast is enlarged, painful, red, and hot. If the abscess is advanced, pointing—localized, shiny, white spots with pus just under the skin surface (Ezrati & Gordon, 1979)—may be observed. Lawrence suggests that cultures be taken of the milk and the infant's nasopharynx, although usually the milk remains clean unless the abscess has ruptured into the ductal system. With a true abscess, both surgical drainage and treatment with antibiotics are required along with rest, warm soaks, and complete emptying of the breast every few hours. If the site of drainage prohibits breastfeeding, the breast should be manually drained frequently to maintain the milk supply. Usually, an abscess heals within 4 days although antibiotics are generally continued for 2 weeks (Lawrence, 1985, p. 208).

URINARY TRACT INFECTIONS. Urinary tract infections are second only to endometritis in their contribution to puerperal infection rates. The woman catheterized during labor and delivery is at increased risk of developing a UTI (Warren, Platt, Thomas, Rosner, & Kass, 1978), particularly if the catheter had been indwelling. Signs and symptoms of urinary tract problems should be a routine topic of the 4- to 6-week postpartum history and must be given particular emphasis if a history of recent catheterization exists.

If a woman received treatment for a UTI while hospitalized a repeat urine culture should be done at the 4- to 6-week postpartum appointment. See Chapter 17 for an in-depth discussion of this problem.

EPISIOTOMY/WOUND INFECTION. Traumatized tissues are excellent culture media. Localized infection of a repaired laceration or episiotomy is most often seen after traumatic instrumental deliveries. Although not common, these infections can lead to lymphangitis, parametritis, and bacteremia (Pritchard et al., 1985, p. 721). Symptoms include localized pain, increasing rather than decreasing with time, and dysuria, possibly severe enough to cause urinary retention. Fever is uncommon but if purulent exudate cannot fully drain because of sutures, chills and fever may ensue.

Diagnosis of wound infection is made by inspection and culture of exudate. Medical consultation should always be obtained when a woman presents with an infected wound. Treatment consists of drainage and appropriate antibiotic therapy. Sutures may have to be removed to allow the wound to drain. Instruction in perineal hygiene is essential. Rest and fluids are important, and sexual activity must be avoided until healing has taken place. Analgesics may be helpful.

If a laceration or episiotomy has not healed completely by the 4- to 6-week postpartum visit, but does not show signs of infection, clean warm soaks or sitz baths and avoidance of intercourse will facilitate healing. A topical application of silver nitrate may also aid healing.

Postpartum Bleeding. Bleeding that occurs after the immediate postpartum period may be classified as secondary to subinvolution or late postpartum hemorrhage.

SUBINVOLUTION. Subinvolution of the uterus is defined as arrest or slowing of the normal involutionary process of the uterus that occurs over the 4- to 6-week postpartum period (Pritchard et al., 1985, p. 737). This process may be accompanied by excessive uterine bleeding or hemorrhage or by prolongation of the period of lochial discharge. The woman may complain of chills, fever, and/or pelvic and back pain. Predisposing factors include cesarean section, retained placental fragments, endometritis, and uterine myomas. The differential diagnosis should include ovarian cyst, pelvic adhesions, malignant uterine tumors, cystitis, and, rarely, gestational trophoblastic disease (Neeson & Stockdale, 1981, p. 119).

On bimanual examination, the subinvoluted uterus is larger and softer than expected for the particular postpartum period. The uterus may also be tender. Leukorrhea may be present.

Whenever subinvolution seems apparent, laboratory testing should include a CBC with differential. Hemoglobin and hematocrit values should be compared with previous postpartum values to assess the amount of bleeding that has taken place and the white blood cell count considered as an indicator of an infectious process. It is debatable whether lochial cultures are of value because such cultures are contaminated with normal flora and these infections are often polymicrobial. Antibiotics are generally indicated before culture results are available.

If a subinvolutionary process is suspected, physician consultation should be obtained. If bleeding is not excessive, the uterus is nontender, and the woman is afebrile, ergonovine (Ergotrate) or methyl ergonomine (Methergine), 0.2 mg po every 3 to 4 hours for 24 to 48 hours, may be the only treatment necessary (Pritchard et al., 1985, p. 737). The woman should be counseled to return immediately should she become febrile or begin to have excessive bleeding. She should be advised that ergonovine often causes painful uterine contractions.

When a woman is febrile, endometritis should be suspected. Consultation or referral should be sought immediately for antibiotic therapy. Hospitalization for intravenous antibiotic therapy may be indicated if the infection is severe.

If uterine bleeding is excessive, additional treatment may be indicated (see the next section).

DELAYED POSTPARTUM HEMORRHAGE. There are several etiologies for serious uterine hemorrhage after the immediate postpartum period (Howell, 1986; Pritchard et al., 1985, pp. 737–738):

1. Poor healing or abnormal involution of the placental site
2. Retained placental products, which necrose and deposit fibrin (Eventually, a "placental polyp" may form; when it detaches from the myometrium, hemorrhage may occur.)
3. A puerperal hematoma resulting from injury to a blood vessel beneath the skin covering the external genitalia or beneath the vaginal mucosa without a laceration to the superficial tissue (Delayed hemorrhage may occur because of sloughing of a vessel that has become necrotic from excessive pressure.)
4. Pelvic infection

With these etiologies in mind, a careful history should be taken, including a history of the bleeding and its characteristics, onset, amount, and association with other symptoms (Table 23–3).

It is easy to say that, by definition, a delayed postpartum hemorrhage means excessive vaginal bleeding, but often this is difficult to determine in all but the most extreme cases. As Oppenheimer and associates (1986, p. 755) have pointed out, lochia persists longer than is "generally appreciated." Therefore, the lochial history must be careful and detailed. In addition to a review of the presenting complaint, the practitioner should review the woman's labor and delivery with special attention to the third stage (delivery of the placenta). A problem should be suspected in any postpartum woman who reports a significant increase in lochia or continuation of lochia rubra longer than 1 week, particularly when chart review or history reveals difficulties during the third stage of labor or factors predisposing to infection.

Physical examination should include a speculum examination to assess the amount, odor, and color of the bleeding and to determine, to the extent possible, the site of bleeding. A bimanual examination should be performed to assess the size and consistency of the uterus. A degree of subinvolution may be present with retained products of conception or uterine infection. If the cervix remains open after the first postpartum week and lochia is heavy, the practitioner should suspect that some placental products have been retained. Other aspects of the physical examination are outlined in Table 23–3. A CBC with differential should be obtained for the reasons noted under Subinvolution.

If delayed postpartum hemorrhage is suspected, physician consultation should be obtained immediately as the woman may need immediate hospitalization. If the woman initially contacts the practitioner by phone, an assessment needs to be made about whether her condition dictates that she go to the nearest emergency room or be seen in an office setting.

One of the major questions facing the practitioner evaluating a woman with delayed postpartum hemorrhage is whether the woman has retained products of conception that require evacuation of the uterus by curettage or has not retained products and therefore requires more conservative management (Howell, 1986). Lee, Madrazo, and Drukker (1981) and Malvern and Campbell (1973) have demonstrated the efficacy of ultrasonic evaluation of the postpartum uterus in the management of delayed postpartum hemorrhage. Retained placental tissue or large blood clots can often be identified by sonogram. An empty uterus may spare a woman the necessity of a dilation and curettage.

REFERENCES

ACOG Technical Bulletin No. 97: Antimicrobial Therapy for Gyn Infections (1986, October). Washington, DC: American College of Obstetrics and Gynecology.

Affonso, D., Andreyko, J., & Mills, K. (1987, September/October). Postpartum thyroiditis: A new challenge in nurse midwifery. Journal of Nurse-Midwifery, 32(5), 308–316.

American Academy of Pediatrics Committee on Drugs. (1981, July). Breastfeeding and contraception. Pediatrics, 68(1), 138–140.

Bing, E., & Coleman, L. (1977). Making love during pregnancy. New York: Bantam Books.

Blanco, J., Gibbs, R., & Castaneda, Y. (1981, November). Bacteremia in obstetrics: Clinical course. Obstetrics and Gynecology, 58(5), 621–625.

Boston Women's Health Collective. (1984). The new our bodies ourselves. New York: Simon & Schuster.

Brooks, M. (1973, September). Wound healing. A review. Journal of Mississippi State Medical Association, 14, 385–390.

Broom, B. (1983, October 3). Consensus about the marital relationship during transition to parenthood. Nursing Research, 33(4), 223–228.

Brucker, M., & Reedy, N. J. (1983, September/October). Maternity leaves and the pregnancy discrimination act. Journal of Obstetrics, Gynecologic and Neonatal Nursing, 12(5), 341–343.

Bull, M. (1981, September/October). Change in concerns of first-time mothers after one week at home. Journal of Obstetrics, Gynecologic and Neonatal Nursing, 10(5), 391–394.

Casey, K. (1986). The relationship between maternal concerns and primigravidas and household membership. Unpublished master's essay, Mercy College, Department of Nursing, Masters Essay.

Centers for Disease Control. (1987, July 24). Rubella vaccination during pregnancy—United States, 1971–1986. Morbidity and Mortality Weekly Report, 36(28), 457–461.

Chapman, J. J., Macey, M. J., & Keegan, M. et al. (1985, November/December). Concerns of breast-feeding mothers from birth to 4 months. Nursing Research, 34(6), 374–377.

Chasnoff, I. J., Lewis, D. E., & Squires, L. (1987, December). Cocaine intoxication in a breast-fed infant. Pediatrics, 80(6), 836–838.

Chavkin, W. (1984). Walking a tightrope. In W. Chavkin (Ed.), Double exposure: Women's health hazards on the job and at home. New York: Monthly Review Press.

Chvapil, M., Eskelson, C., & Stiffel, V., et al. (1980, September). Studies on nonoxynol-9 intravaginal absorption, distribution, metabolism, and excretion in rats and rabbits. Contraception, 22(3), 325–338.

Clinton, J. (1986, September/October). Expectant fathers at risk for couvade. Nursing Research, 35(5), 290–295.

Cohen, N. W., & Esther, L. (1983). Silent knife: Cesarean prevention and vaginal birth after cesarean. South Hadley, MA: J. F. Bergin.

Cole, L., McCann, M., Higgins, J., & Waszak, C. (1983, April). Effects of breastfeeding on IUD performance. American Journal of Public Health, 73(4), 384–388.

Conner, A. E. (1979, June). Elevated levels of sodium and chloride in milk from mastitic breast. Pediatrics, 63(6), 910–911.

Cox, B., & Smith, E. (1982, September/October). The mother's self-esteem after a cesarean delivery. American Journal of Maternal and Child Nursing, 17(5), 309–314.

D'Angelo, L., & Sokol, R. (1980, March). Time-related peripartum determinants of postpartum morbidity. Obstetrics and Gynecology, 55(3), 319–323.

Danner, S. (1984a). Breastfeeding: Concerns and solutions. (Available from ICEA Publications, P. O. Box 20048, Minneapolis, MN 55420.)

Danner, S. (1984b). Checklist for breastfeeding. (Available from ICEA Publications, P. O. Box 20048, Minneapolis, MN 55420.)

Davidson, N. (1974, Summer). ''REEDA: Evaluating postpartum healing. Journal of Nurse-Midwifery, 19(2), 6–8.

Devereux, W. B. (1970, September). Acute puerperal mastitis—Evaluation of its management. American Journal of Obstetrics and Gynecology, 108(1), 78–81.

Dilts, C. (1985, July/August). Nursing management of mastitis due to breastfeeding. Journal of Obstetrics, Gynecologic and Neonatal Nursing, 14(4), 286–288.

Dix, C. (1985). The new mother syndrome. New York: Doubleday.

Donovan, B. (1986). The cesarean birth experience, New York: Beacon Press.

Duran, P. (1987). Vaginal birth after cesarean section: A seven year retrospective study in a large midwifery service, the North Central Bronx Experience. Unpublished manuscript.

Eagan, A. (1985). The newborn mother—Stages of her growth. Boston: Little, Brown.

Eiger, N. M., & Olds, S. (1972). The complete book of breastfeeding. New York: Bantam Books.

Erb, L., Hill, G., & Houston, Y. (1983, Summer). A survey of parent's attitudes toward their cesarean births in Manitoba hospitals. Birth 10(2), 85–92.

Eschenbach, D., & Wager, G. (1980, December). Puerperal Infections. Clinical Obstetrics and Gynecology, 23(4), 1003–1037.

Ezrati, J. B., & Gordon, H. (1979, November/December). Puerperal mastitis: Causes, prevention and management. Journal of Nurse-Midwifery, 24(6), 3–8.

Fawcett, J., & York, R. (1986, May/June). Spouses' physical and psychological symptoms during pregnancy and postpartum. Nursing Research, 35(3), 144–148.

Fischman, S., Rankin, E., Soeken, K., & Lewnz, E. (1986, January/February). Changes in sexual relationships in postpartum couples. Journal of Obstetric, Gynecologic and Neonatal Nursing, 15(1), 58–63.

Fishel, A. H. (1983). Gay parents. Issues in the Health Care of Women, 4, 139–159.

Gibbs,. R. S., & Weinstein, A. J. (1976, April 1). Puerperal infection in the antibiotic era. American Journal of Obstetrics and Gynecology, 124(7), 769–787.

Goldsmith, J. (1984). Childbirth wisdom: From the world's oldest societies. New York: Congdon Weed Inc.

Gruis, M. (1977, May/June). Beyond maternity: Postpartum concerns of mothers. American Journal of Maternal Child Nursing, 2(3), 182–188.

Hangsleben, K. (1980). Transition to fatherhood: Literature review. Issues in the Health Care of Women, 2, 81–97.

Harris, K. (1987, May/June). Beliefs and practices among Haitian American women in relation to childbearing. Journal of Nurse-Midwifery, 32(3), 149–155.

Hartwell, S., & Schlesselman, S. (1983, January). Risk of uterine perforation among users of IUD. Obstetrics and Gynecology, 61(1), 31–36.

Hatcher, R. A., Guest, F., & Stewart, F., et al. (1986). Contraceptive technology 1986–87 (13th rev. ed.). New York: Irvington.

Hawkins, J. W., & Gorvine, B. (1985). Postpartum nursing: Health care of women. New York: Springer.

Hazle, N. R. (1982, November/December). Postpartum blues—Assessment and intervention. Journal of Nurse-Midwifery, 27(6), 21–25.

Heikkilä, M., Haukkamaa, M., & Luukkainen, T., (1982, January). Levonorgestrel in milk and plasma of breast-feeding woman with a levonorgestrel-releasing IUD. Contraception, 25(1), 41–49.

Hinshaw, R., Pyeatt, P., & Habicht, J-P. (1972, April). Environmental effects on child-spacing and population increase in highland Guatemala. Current Anthropology, 13(2), 216–230.

Hogan, R. (1985). Human sexuality—A nursing perspective. East Norwalk, CT: Appleton & Lange.

Howell, R. J. S. (1986, September). Haemorrhage from the placental site. Clinics in Obstetrics and Gynaecology, 13(3), 633–658.

Ihsan, A. (1982). Gender hormones and psychopathology. In A. Ihsan (Ed.), Gender and psychopathology. New York: Academic Press.

Jackson, P. L. (1985, April). When the baby isn't perfect. American Journal of Nursing, 85(4), 396–399.

Job protection is upheld by court in pregnancy suit. (1987, January 14). New York Times, p. A1.

Kammerman, S. (1980). *Maternity and parental benefits and leaves: An international review* (Impact on Policy Series Monograph, No. 1). New York: Columbia University Center for Social Sciences.

Kennell, J., & Trause, M. (1978, July). Helping parents cope with perinatal death. *Contemporary Ob/Gyn, 12*(1), 53–68.

Kenny, J. (1973). Sexuality of pregnant and breastfeeding women. *Archives of Sexual Behavior, 2*, 215–229.

Kitzinger, S. (1981). *The experience of childbirth* (rev. ed.). New York: Penguin Books.

LaLeche League International. (1983). *The womanly art of breastfeeding* (3rd ed.). New York: New American Library.

Lang, R. (1984). Midwifery tradition: Roots and renewal. Chinese Medicine and Midwifery. [From taped speech before MANA Convention; available through Midwives Alliance of North America, (MANA).]

Lawrence, L. (1985). *Breastfeeding—A guide for the medical profession.* St. Louis: C. V. Mosby.

Ledger, W. J. (1986a). *Infection in the female.* Philadelphia: Lea & Febiger.

Ledger, W. J. (1986b). Obstetric and gynecologic infections: General considerations and antibacterial therapy. In D. N. Danforth & J. R. Scott (Eds.), *Obstetrics and gynecology* (5th ed.). Philadelphia: J. B. Lippincott.

Lee, C. Y., Madrazo, B., & Drukker, B. (1981, August). Ultrasound evaluation of the postpartum uterus in the management of postpartum bleeding. *Obstetrics and Gynecology, 58*(2), 227–232.

Lindemann, E. (1944, September). Symptomatology and management of acute grief. *American Journal of Psychiatry, 101*(2), 141–148.

Lipson, J., & Tilden, V. (1980, October). Psychological integration of the cesarean birth experience. *American Journal of Orthopsychiatry, 50*(4), 599–609.

Liskin, L. (1981, September). Periodic abstinence: How well do new approaches work? *Population Reports, I*(3), I35–I71.

Lynch-Fraser, D. (1983). *The complete postpartum guide.* New York: Ballantine Books.

Majewski, J. L. (1986, January/February). Conflicts, satisfactions, and attitudes during transition to the maternal role. *Nursing Research, 35*(1), 10–14.

Malvern, J. & Campbell, S. (1973, April). Ultrasonic scanning of the puerperal uterus following secondary postpartum haemorrhage. *Journal of Obstetrics and Gynaecology of the British Commonwealth, 80*, 320–324.

Marshall, B. R., Hepper, J. K., & Zirbel, C. (1975, September 29). Sporadic puerperal mastitis: An infection that need not interrupt lactation. *Journal of the American Medical Association, 233*(13), 1377–1379.

Martin, L. (1978). *Health care of women.* Philadelphia: J. B. Lippincott.

Masters, W., & Johnson, V. (1966). *Human sexual response.* New York: Bantam Books.

McBride, A. (1973). *The growth and development of mothers.* New York: Harper Colophan Books.

McCann, I., Liskin, L., & Piotrow, P., et al. (1981). Breastfeeding, fertility and family planning. *Population Reports, J*(24), J525–J575.

McClain, C. S. (1985, September). Why women choose trial of labor or repeat cesarean section. *Journal of Family Practice, 21*(3), 210–216.

McGowan, M. N. (1977, Summer). Postpartum disturbance—A review of the literature in terms of stress response. *Journal of Nurse-Midwifery, 22*(2), 27–34.

Mehta, S., Pawar, V., & Joshi, J., et al. (1977, March). Serum prolactin levels in women using copper IUD's. *Contraception, 15*(3), 327–333.

Mercer, R. T. (1985, July/August). The process of maternal role attainment over the first year. *Nursing Research, 34*(4), 198–204.

Morse, J., & Harrison, M. (1987, July/August). Social coercion for weaning. *Journal of Nurse-Midwifery, 32*(4), 205–210.

Nahas, G., Suciu-Foca, N., Armand, J-P, & Morishima, A. (1974, February 1). Inhibition of cellular mediated immunity in marihuana smokers. *Science, 183*(4123), 419–420.

Neeson, J. D., & Stockdale, C. R. (1981). *The practitioners' handbook of ambulatory Ob/Gyn.* New York: John Wiley & Sons.

Newbould, F. H. S. (1974). Microbial diseases of the mammary gland. In B. Larson & U. R. Smith (Eds.), *Lactation—A comprehensive treatise.* New York: Academic Press.

Noble, E. (1982). *Essential exercises for the childbearing year.* Boston: Houghton Mifflin.

Norris, G., & Miller, J. (1979). *The working mother's complete handbook.* New York: E. P. Dutton.

O'Donohue, N. (1979, September/October). The perinatal bereavement crisis, facilitating the grief process. *Journal of Nurse-Midwifery, 24*(5), 16–19.

Oppenheimer, L. W., Sherriff, E., & Goodman, J. D. S., et al. (1986, July). The duration of lochia. *British Journal of Obstetrics and Gynaecology, 93*(7), 754–757.

Paykel, E. S., Emms, E. M., Fletcher, J., & Rassaby, E. S. (1980, April). Life events and social support in puerperal depression. *British Journal of Psychiatry, 136*, 339–346.

Perez, A., Vela, P., Masneck, G., & Potter, R. (1972, December 15). First ovulation after childbirth: The effect of breastfeeding. *American Journal of Obstetrics and Gynecology, 114*(8), 1041–1047.

Pitt, B. (1973, April). Maternity blues. *Journal of Psychiatry, 122*, 431–433.

Preblud, S. (1985, July 12). Some current issues relating to rubella vaccine. *Journal of the American Medical Association, 254*(2), 253–256.

Pritchard, J. A., MacDonald, R. C., & Gant, N. T. (1985). *Williams Obstetrics* (17th ed.). East Norwalk, CT: Appleton–Century–Crofts.

Quadagno, D. M., Dixon, L., Denny, N., & Buck, H. (1986, May). Postpartum moods in men and women. *American Journal of Obstetrics and Gynecology, 154*(5), 1018–1023.

Quirk, T. (1979, September/October). The perinatal bereavement crisis theory: grief theory, and related psychosocial factors: The framework for intervention. *Journal of Nurse-Midwifery, 24*(5), 13–16.

Raphael, D. (1976). *The tender gift: Breastfeeding.* New York: Schocken Books.

Reamy, K., & White, S. E. (1985, January). Sexuality in pregnancy and the puerperium: A review. *Obstetrical and Gynecological Survey, 40*(1), 1–13.

Riordan, J. M., & Rapp, E. T. (1980, March/April). Pleasure and purpose: The sensuousness of breastfeeding. *Journal of Obstetric, Gynecologic and Neonatal Nursing, 9*(2), 109–112.

Robson, K. M., Brant, H. A., & Kumar, R. (1981, September). Maternal sexuality, during first pregnancy and after childbirth. *British Journal of Obstetrics and Gynaecology, 88*(9), 882–889.

Rubin, R. (1967a, Summer). Attainment of the maternal role. 1. Processes. *Nursing Research, 16*(3), 237–245.

Rubin, R. (1967b, Fall). Attainment of the maternal role. 2. Models and referrants. *Nursing Research, 16*(4), 342–346.

Rubin, R. (1984). *Maternal identity and the maternal experience.* New York: Springer.

Russell, C. S. (1974, May). Transition to parenthood: Problems and gratifications. *Journal of Marriage and the Family, 36*(2), 294–301.

Saucier, J. F. (1972, April). Correlates of the long postpartum taboo: A cross cultural study. *Current Anthropology, 13*(2), 238–249.

Sharman, A. (1951). Menstruation after childbirth. *Journal of Obstetrics and Gynaecology British Empire, 58*, 440–445.

Shepherd, S., & Yarrow, R. (1982, November/December). Breastfeeding and the working mother. *Journal of Nurse-Midwifery, 27*(6), 16–20.

Simkin, D. (1982). *The complete pregnancy exercise program.* New York: C. V. Mosby.

Simpson-Hebert, M., & Huffman, S. (1981, April). The contraceptive effect of breastfeeding. *Studies in Family Planning, 12*(4), 125–133.

Strang, V., & Sullivan, P. (1985, July/August). Body image attitudes during pregnancy and the postpartum period. *Journal of Obstetric, Gynecologic and Neonatal Nursing, 14*(4), 332–337.

Sumner, G., & Fritsch, J. (1977, May/June). Postnatal parental concern: The first six weeks of life. *Journal of Obstetric, Gynecologic and Neonatal Nursing, 6*(3), 27–32.

Taffel, S. M., Placek, P. J. & Liss, T. (1987, August). Trends in the United States cesarean section rate and reasons for 1980–85 rise. *American Journal of Public Health, 77*(8), 955–959.

Tod, E. (1964, December 12). Puerperal depression—A prospective epidemiological study. *Lancet, 2*(7372), 1264–1266.

U.S. Department of Health and Human Services. (1981). *Cesarean childbirth.* Bethesda, MD: National Institutes of Health.

Van Esterik, P., & Greiner, T. (1981, April). Breastfeeding and women's work: Constraints and opportunities. *Studies in Family Planning, 12*(4), 184–187.

Varney, H. (1987). *Nurse midwifery* (2nd ed.). Boston: Blackwell Scientific.

Vestal, K. (1980). The effects of day care on the child. *Issues in the Health Care of Women, 24,* 25–35.

Walker, W. O., Crain, H., & Thompson, E. (1986, March/April). Maternal role attainment and identity in the postpartum period: Stability and change. *Nursing Research, 35*(2), 68–71.

Warren, J., Platt, W. R., & Thomas, R. J., et al. (1978, September 14). Antibiotic irrigation and catheter-associated urinary tract infection. *New England Journal of Medicine, 299*(11), 570–573.

Wenof, M. Aubert, J., & Reyniak, J. (1979, January). Serum prolactin levels in short-term and long-term use of inert plastic and copper IUD's. *Contraception, 19*(1), 21–27.

24

Perimenopause and Aging

Doreen C. Harper

Past perspectives on midlife wellness for women often concentrated solely on menopausal health; however, as national awareness of the normal aging process and of women's health issues has intensified, concerns regarding well-being for midlife and older women have begun to extend beyond menopausal and reproductive health to reflect primary health care needs.

The most obvious reason for this interest in aging women and their health is increased life expectancy and its associated morbidity rates among women. It is projected that the population aged 65 and older will reach 35 million by the year 2000, of whom 20 million will be women. Women are not only living longer than men, but they are reporting a higher incidence of illness (Verbrugge, 1984).

Today, as large numbers of "baby boomers" enter the early stages of perimenopause, it becomes evident that health concerns of mature women will demand an increasing share of resources. Primary care providers, particularly nurse-midwives and nurse-practitioners, have the opportunity to deliver woman-centered care to this population, incorporating the wellness model into care for midlife and aging women, thus redefining conventional health care for women.

At what point should the primary care provider begin to *target* the special health care needs of aging? The life-cycle event most associated with the aging process in women is the menopause, which occurs during the midlife stage of development. It is this stage that determines health throughout the remainder of the life span. The health concerns of midlife women frequently become the very real health problems of elderly women. How women cope with these progressive problems in the midlife often portends their health status in old age.

An individual woman's response to growing older depends on a number of factors—the extent to which her culture values youth compared with the respect it gives to the aged; whether or not her occupation depends on physical appearance or vigor; the reactions of her significant others; her social supports and financial resources; her overall sense of self; and her past ability to cope with change. All of these factors must be considered by the practitioner providing care to women during the perimenopause and the years that follow.

This chapter begins its discussion of the health care needs of aging women with an analysis of the menopause and its surrounding years as normal parts of the aging process. The menopause and its associated physiologic changes do not constitute the entire spectrum of age-related changes in women, however. This chapter also focuses on other physical and psychosocial health concerns common to women as they age. Assessment data related to these areas are presented and followed by selected treatment and prevention interventions. A health maintenance protocol for menopausal/aging women is suggested to assist primary care providers in identifying the special health concerns of this group of women.

DEFINITION AND DESCRIPTION OF THE PERIMENOPAUSE

Although menopause is the life-cycle event most commonly associated with aging in women, there is normally a gradual transition from reproductive to nonreproductive physiologic processes. Perimenopause is the term used to describe the years during which women report the signs of this transition, years that surround the actual experience of menopause (Feldman, Voda, & Gronseth, 1985). Menopause is defined as the complete cessation of menses or the last menstrual period; it is a single physiologic event. The terms used to define the menopause and its precursors and sequelae appear interchangeably in some source books on this subject. For the purposes of this chapter, however, the perimenopause encompasses three distinct phases: the climacteric, the menopause, and the postmenopause.

The perimenopause spans a 25-year continuum from about age 35 to age 60. The average age of menopause is 49 to 51 (Cutler & Garcia 1984, p. 23; Treloar, 1981), although in a sample of 25,000 woman-years, the range was found to be 41 to 59 and to follow 2 to 8 years of menstrual changes (Treloar, 1981). Unlike menarche, the average age of menopause has remained stable since medieval times (Soules and Bremner 1982, p. 547), although it has been shown to be influenced by smoking, with increasing numbers of cigarettes smoked leading to increasingly earlier menopause (Daniell, 1976; Jick, Porter, & Morrison, 1977; Lindquist & Bengtsson, 1979), and by estrogen replacement therapy, which delays its onset by about 2 years (Treloar, 1981). As the life span for women in the United States has lengthened, the likelihood of spending more than one third of life in the postmenopausal years has increased (Utian, 1980; Woods, 1981).

Physicians have traditionally considered the perimenopause and its associated clinical phenomena as pathologic.

Prior to the midseventies, the limited research conducted about menopause was conceptualized from a disease-oriented perspective with numerous ageist and sexist overtones.

Several demographic and social trends in the late seventies and eighties have revolutionized our perspective on menopause. These have included the growth of the population of aging women, the emergence of the women's movement, the swell of research and new discoveries about menopause and its associated phenomena, the increased number of female health care providers, and the expanded utilization of midwives, nurse-practitioners, and other non-physician primary care women's health providers. The combined influence of these factors has led to a redefinition of menopause as a normal physiologic event in the medical and health care literature (MacPherson, 1981). The perimenopause, therefore, marks the beginning of the healthy aging process in women. It must be remembered, however, that perimenopause is just one element in aging. A theoretical perspective that views development as spanning the life cycle permits aging to be seen as a part of development (Reed, 1983).

PHASES OF THE PERIMENOPAUSE

The climacteric, the first phase of the perimenopause, occurs as many as 8 to 10 years prior to the onset of menopause. The term *climacteric* refers to the transitional period between the years of reproductive capability and the menopause. During the climacteric, numerous subtle changes occur as reproductive function begins to wane. These include progressive changes in the pattern of menstrual cyclicity evidenced by shortened or lengthened cycles, diminished menstrual flow, and hot flashes/flushes. The irregularities associated with the menses during the climacteric are secondary to alterations in cyclic ovarian function and may be quite variable (Soules & Bremner, 1982, p. 550). The pattern of menstrual cessation may be abrupt or may consist of irregularly spaced anovulatory cycles with profuse or scant bleeding. The ovary continues to secrete estrogen and androstenedione, even though the balance among estrogen, androstenedione, and progesterone begins to change. Associated with these changes, the gonadotropin hormones, luteinizing hormone (LH) and follicle-stimulating hormone (FSH), often fluctuate and reach excessively high levels, with the rise in FSH occurring earlier and exceeding that of LH (Cutler & Garcia, 1984, p. 20). This often leads to faster maturation of ovarian follicles and shortened follicular phases of the menstrual cycle (Upton, 1982, p. 3), although the luteal phase may also be shortened as corpus luteal activity declines.

The second phase of the perimenopause is the actual menopause itself, the last episode of menstruation, which signifies the termination of reproductive capacity in women. Menopause can be diagnosed only in retrospect. To be absolutely certain menopause has occurred, one year without spontaneous bleeding must pass.

The postmenopause is the third phase, which begins one year after the cessation of menstruation. The postmenopause is characterized by complete termination of ovarian activity and signs of estrogen decline. During this phase of the perimenopause, the majority of estrogen production occurs via the conversion of estrogen from adrenal androstenedione. The alterations in the type and source of estrogen production in the postmenopausal years lead to numerous changes in specific target organs (Fig. 24–1).

HORMONAL CHANGES OF THE PERIMENOPAUSE

The hormonal changes occurring during perimenopause are linked to the production and regulation of estrogen and to a shift in the ratio of estrogens to androgens, favoring the latter (Soules & Bremner, 1982, p. 553). Of the three types of estrogens produced in the body—estrone (E_1), estradiol (E_2), and estriol (E_3)—two types are thought to predominate during the adult female life cycle. The strongest estrogen, 17β-estradiol, is the most abundant during the premenopausal years, whereas estrone, the less potent type of estrogen, reaches its peak and predominates during the postmenopausal years. Estradiol is produced by the granulosa cells of ovarian follicles in a cyclic manner and secreted into the blood. The rate of secretion of estradiol is dependent on the stimulation and growth of ovarian follicles in response to pituitary FSH. As ovaries age, there is a gradual atresia, a decline in estradiol production, and a concomitant decline in corpus luteal activity.

The decline of ovarian function accounts for the breakdown of the negative feedback system that controls ovulation and menstruation. Because estrogen and sequential progesterone production gradually decreases throughout the normal aging process, neuroendocrine stimulation is increased. This combination of factors results in increased secretion of the pituitary hormones, FSH and LH, as the pituitary attempts to stimulate the ovaries to secrete more estrogen and progesterone (DeVane, 1983). The loss of inhibition of the gonadotropins creates a constant state of endometrial proliferation. The ovaries eventually lose their ability to respond to this hyperactive state, leading to gradual and finally permanent anovulation, known as the menopause (Fig. 24–1).

As the ovary loses its ovulatory function, becoming scarred and fibrotic, estrone becomes the major source of estrogen. The primary source of estrone production is through extraglandular aromatization of circulating androstenedione. The mechanism for estrone biosynthesis in postmenopausal women is dependent on the production of androstenedione from the adrenals and the conversion of plasma androstenedione to estrone via the aromatase enzyme in peripheral tissues, including adipose tissue, skin, hair follicles, brain, bone, muscle, and breast tissue (Fig. 24–2). The rate of extraglandular estrone formation is directly proportional to the rate of production of androstenedione and aromatase activity in the peripheral tissue sites. The most abundant source of extraglandular estrone production is adipose tissue, where androstenedione from the adrenal cortex is converted to estrone in the stromal cells. Factors known to increase the conversion of plasma androstenedione to estrone are age, liver disease, and obesity (Gambrell 1982b, p. 458). The relationships among these three factors have not been identified, however.

After menopause, levels of extraglandular estrone may be as high or even higher than they were previously. This is a significant finding, because increases in the aromatization of androstenedione to estrone have been linked to endometrial neoplasia (Casey & MacDonald, 1983).

MANIFESTATIONS OF PERIMENOPAUSAL CHANGES

The primary symptoms associated with menopause are seen in the vasomotor system, reproductive target tissues, and psychological/coping mechanisms. Vasomotor symptoms include hot flashes/flushes, perspiration, and palpita-

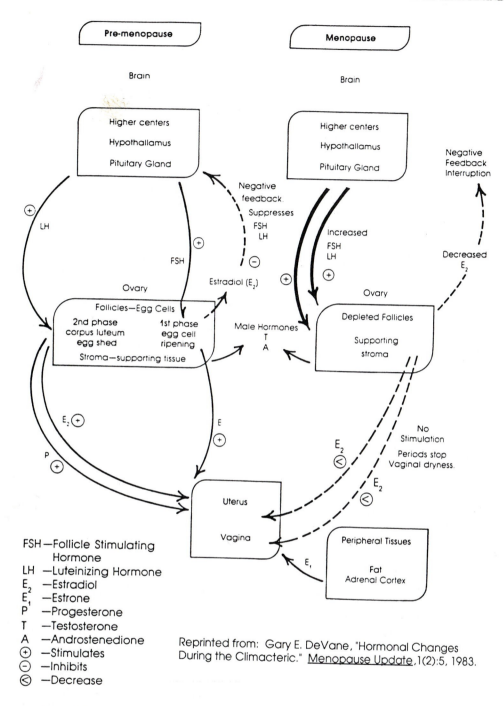

FSH —Follicle Stimulating
        Hormone
LH —Luteinizing Hormone
E_2 —Estradiol
E_1 —Estrone
P —Progesterone
T —Testosterone
A —Androstenedione
⊕ —Stimulates
⊖ —Inhibits
⊘ —Decrease

Reprinted from: Gary E. DeVane, "Hormonal Changes
During the Climacteric." Menopause Update,1(2):5, 1983.

Figure 24-1. Hormonal changes and effects on end organs. *(From DeVane, G. [1983]. Hormonal changes during the climacteric. Menopause Update, 1 [2], 2–6. Reprinted with permission.)*

tions. The target tissue symptoms include urinary urgency, frequency, and dysuria; vaginal dryness and discharge; painful intercourse; and itching and burning of the vulva. Psychological symptoms include mood swings, irritability, depression, and insomnia. This complex of symptoms, however, has been disputed by authorities, leading Notelovitz (1983) to maintain that hot flashes and vaginal atrophy are the only two reliable symptoms of the perimenopause.

Despite the supposed numerous symptoms of the perimenopause, only 25 to 30 percent of women report problems severe enough to warrant medical treatment (Notelo-

vitz 1983). Indeed, the medical and women's health literature is riddled with controversy regarding the existence and prevalence of perimenopausal signs and symptoms. The spectrum of physical and psychological changes evidenced during the menopause varies greatly from woman to woman, precluding definitive scientific explanations regarding causality. In fact, the most obvious of the vasomotor symptoms, the hot flash, does not always correlate with low blood estrogen levels (Notelovitz, 1983, p. 27; Stone, Mickal, & Rye 1975). Although alterations in estrogen levels seem to be a critical factor in triggering flushes,

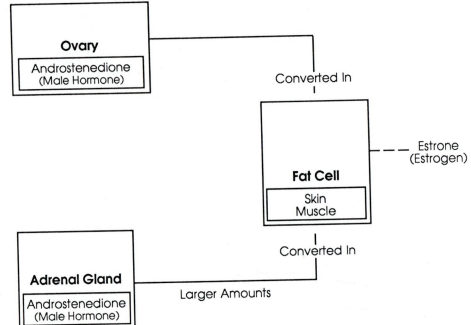

Figure 24–2. Conversion of androgen to estrogen in peripheral tissues. *(From DeVane, G. [1983]. Hormonal changes during the climacteric.* Menopause Update, 1 *(2), 2–6. Reprinted with permission.)*

it has been suggested that the hypothalamus initiates the stimulus for the hot flush and that this stimulus is related to estrogen withdrawal rather than circulating estrogen levels (Rinehart & Schiff, 1983).

Several factors may influence the development of symptoms in women including the rate of estrogen shift; genetic predisposition to aging; psychological coping responses to personal losses and crises commonly experienced in aging; social responses to aging; and individual perception of aging (Edmon, 1983). Few studies explore the complex relationship to perimenopausal symptomatology of these factors, singly or in combination. Two recent studies of 185 healthy, middle-aged women found that perimenopausal symptom severity and frequency were associated with marital role adjustment, recreation, and work role (Uphold & Sussman, 1981, 1985). Further research is needed to factor out the relationships among the physical and psychological variables associated with the perimenopause.

Vasomotor Responses

The most prevalent and obvious vasomotor symptom identified in the perimenopause is the hot flash (Feldman et al., 1985). A term often used interchangeably with hot flash is hot flush (Voda, 1983). These terms, however, describe two distinct physiologic events. *Hot flash* refers to the sudden sensation of a warm feeling in the head, neck, and chest, with a range of intensity varying from warm, to extremely warm, to hot or extremely hot. Other nonthermal body sensations may be experienced during the hot flash, including tingling, throbbing, rush of blood, lightheadedness, chills, suffocation (Voda, 1981), and a transient increase in heart rate (Edmon, 1983). *Hot flush* follows a hot flash and refers to the measurable change in skin temperature, a visible red flush in skin color, and perspiration.

The subjective symptoms of the hot flash often occur, on the average, 45 seconds prior to the hot flush. The incidence of the hot flash varies for perimenopausal women from 68 to 92 percent, depending on the age group studied. A recent study of 594 perimenopausal women reported a prevalence rate of 88 percent for women experiencing natural menopause (Feldman et al., 1985). In this study, 60 percent of the sample reported the beginning of hot flashes between ages 40 and 50, with the greatest percentage of women reporting the experience between the ages of 46 and 50.

The hot flash and its associated flush are characterized as a sudden feeling of warmth. The flash is followed by a visible redness of the face, neck, and upper thorax, which may be associated with profuse sweating in the same anatomic regions. The length of the entire experience averages 3.31 minutes (Voda, 1981). In a study of 90 women reporting hot flushes, 21 percent experienced them every few hours, and an additional 47.7 percent had them at least daily (Thompson, Hart, & Durno, 1973). The pattern of spread for the hot flash varies, but the sensation is usually located above the waist. Numerous patterns of spread have been identified including the neck to the breast area, the neck to the facial area, up the front of the body from the breast, down the front of the body from the neck, and completely above the waist.

The mechanisms responsible for the hot flash are still speculative, but it is believed that the thermoregulatory centers and the gonadotropin-releasing hormone neurons of the hypothalamus play an important role in regulating the hot flash. This configuration of vasomotor symptoms has been attributed to alterations in estrogen production and in the metabolism of catecholamines, particularly the neurotransmitters dopamine and norepinephrine. Aging decreases dopamine production and neuronal uptake of catecholamine. Decreased estrogen levels disrupt the delicate balance between norepinephrine and dopamine, creating vasomotor instability (Edmon, 1983). It is also possible that prostaglandins have a vasodilating function and are involved in the hot flash/flush (Yen, 1977, pp. 291–292).

Hot flashes generally cease approximately 4 to 6 years after the menopause, once the alterations in estrogen production have stabilized in the postmenopausal phase.

Urogenital Atrophy

The alterations in the ovarian cycle associated with the normal aging process lead to predictable changes in the vagina, vulva, uterus, ovaries, and urinary tract. With the shift in estrogen production and decline in ovarian function, the vaginal epithelium begins to atrophy. This occurs when the glycogen-rich superficial cells supporting Döderlein's bacilli and maintaining the acidic pH of the vagina begin to shrink and thin. The structure of vaginal rugae is lost, and there are concomitant decreases in vaginal fluid, glycogen production, and blood flow. Vaginal pH becomes increasingly alkaline. These normal changes increase the friability of the vaginal epithelium, leading to an increase in vaginitis among menopausal women. Other symptoms include vaginal irritation, burning, pruritis, leukorrhea, bleeding, and dyspareunia.

On physical examination, the vaginal mucosa of the postmenopausal woman may appear thin and pale. Rugae may be decreased. Petechiae, telangiectasia, ecchymoses, fissures, ulcerations, and granulation may be present. The mucosa may become thickened and hardened from irritation (called lichenification) (Rigg, 1986, p. 29).

Vaginal epithelial changes can be examined via a maturation index, which measures the relative numbers of parabasal, intermediate, and superficial cells. As estrogen decreases, parabasal cells increase, and intermediate and superficial cells decrease (Cutler & Garcia, 1984, p. 27).

Vulvar epithelium also loses its elasticity and subcutaneous fat after menopause. As the epidermal layer thins, the labia majora and minora become flattened and the introitus may lose its structural integrity. The urethra and trigone areas of the bladder may atrophy. When atrophy of the urethra occurs, symptoms of cystitis and noninflammatory urethritis are reported. Urinary stress incontinence may also occur as the pubococcygeus muscles lose their tone (Cutler & Garcia, 1984, pp. 40–41).

The uterus and ovaries shrink in size and weight. The uterine myometrium thins and the cervix becomes smaller. The external os may become almost flush with the vaginal walls. Cervical mucus decreases and the cervical canal may become stenotic (Edmon, 1983). Because of these urogenital changes, intercourse may be painful.

Skin Changes

Skin changes commonly found in aging women may relate to shifts in estradiol production during the perimenopause. Hyperpigmentation, known as senile lentigo or aging spots, occurs because of benign proliferation of melanocytes. Hypopigmentation, known as vitiligo, occurs secondary to a multifocal loss of pigmentation. Sebaceous and sweat gland activity decreases, and the epidermal skin layer begins to atrophy and thin. The skin consequently becomes less tolerant of temperature and humidity changes. Likewise, the dermal skin layer thins, reducing the integrity of the underlying collagen and, ultimately, the skin's resilience and pliability.

Breast Changes

As a target tissue for estrogen stimulation, the breasts respond to the estradiol deprivation of the perimenopause with a gradual reduction in adipose tissue and lobule size. With advanced age, the breasts eventually develop a flattened appearance.

Changes in Hair Pattern

As the sex hormonal environment of the aging woman shifts from estrogen to androgen dominance, hirsutism may occur. This may be manifest in the growth of coarse hair on the lip, chin, chest, abdomen, and back, although excess growth may indicate adrenal or ovarian pathology (Cutler & Garcia, 1984, pp. 39–40).

Changes in the Buccal Mucosa

The buccal epithelium may undergo postmenopausal atrophy similar to that of the vaginal mucosa. Changes lead to dryness, bad taste, and decreased saliva and sensation. Dryness has been associated with increased dental caries or difficulty in denture retention (Pisantry, Rafaely, & Polishuk, 1975).

Musculoskeletal Changes

Age-related bone loss is a universal phenomenon, but one that accelerates in women after the menopause. Bone is lost at an annual rate of 0.5 percent after age 40 and at an annual rate of 1.0 percent or more for at least 5 to 10 years after menopause (Ettinger 1986, p. 15; Parfitt, 1983, p. 1181; Riggs & Melton 1986, p. 1676).

Osteoporosis is the most common skeletal disorder occurring in postmenopausal women. Osteoporosis is defined as a decrease in the amount of bone minerals and matrix in a given volume of skeletal tissue (Raisz, 1982).

Bone metabolism is a complex phenomenon. Osteoblasts are the major bone-forming cells and osteoclasts are the major bone-resorbing cells. The bone remodeling sequence is responsible for the formation and resorption of bone. Normally, bone is constantly turned over via an increase in bone resorption mediated by the osteoclast which results in an increase in bone formation potentiated by the osteoblast. These processes are directly related to each other: as bone resorption increases, bone formation increases.

Bone formation is dependent on adequate circulating calcium, phosphate, and vitamin D. Numerous hormones are known to affect osteoblast and osteoclast formation either directly or indirectly. These include estrogen, progesterone, parathyroid hormone, calcitrol, prostaglandins, glucocorticoids, and calcitonin. The exact mechanisms of action of these hormones on bone formation are still unknown (Raisz, 1982).

In postmenopausal osteoporosis, data suggest that bone resorption is increased without a corresponding increase in bone formation. The net result of this accelerated bone resorption is a decrease in bone mass and a subsequent loss of bone. As osteoporotic bone mass decreases, the bone becomes more porous and predisposed to fracture (Raisz, 1982).

It has been suggested that there are two types of osteoporosis (Ettinger, 1986). Type 1 involves the trabecular bone of the spine and heads of the femur and radius, which accounts for 20 percent of the skeleton; type 2 involves dense cortical bone, which makes up most of the long bones and accounts for 80 percent of the skeleton. It is hypothesized that in type 1 osteoporosis, a dramatic demineralization takes place in trabecular bone after menopause and lasts about 10 to 15 years. With type 2 osteoporosis, cortical bone is lost more gradually without leveling off. The effects of type 2 osteoporosis, primarily hip fractures, therefore occur at a later age than do the wrist and spinal crush fractures associated with type 1 disease.

Although scientific evidence points to a relationship between lowered estrogen levels and resorption of bone, it is clear that many factors contribute to the development of postmenopausal osteoporosis. The risk factors for this disorder include low calcium intake *throughout the life cycle* (Brody, Farmer, & White, 1984; Matkovic, Kostial, Simonovic, et al., 1979; Parfitt, 1983; Riggs & Melton, 1986); inadequate exercise (Aloia, Vaswani, Yeh, et al., 1983); leanness; small stature; genetic predisposition; cigarette smoking (Williams, Weiss, Ure, et al., 1982); early menopause (Aloia et al., 1985); excessive alcohol, caffeine (Daniell, 1976) and protein intake; use of glucocorticoid and anticonvulsant drugs; and disease and surgeries, including hyperthyroidism, Cushing's syndrome, hemiplegia, rheumatoid arthritis, chronic obstructive lung disease, and gastrectomy (Cummings, Kelsey, Nevitt, & O'Dowd, 1985, p. 194; Riggs & Melton 1986, p. 1680). Osteoporosis has been found to be uncommon among blacks (Cummings et al., 1985).

The clinical features of osteoporosis may first be detected by a loss of height with kyphosis of the dorsal spine. These changes are caused by compression of the vertebrae, which in a relatively small proportion of cases develops into full compression fractures. Early stages of the disease, however, may be asymptomatic or manifest only by backache or back-muscle spasm (Whedon, 1981, p. 398). Fractures of the distal radius and femoral head resulting from minimal trauma are frequently seen as a result of osteoporosis.

Because of the significant morbidity and mortality associated particularly with hip fracture, osteoporosis is a major public health concern. It is estimated that one third of women over the age of 65 suffer fractures. Hip fractures lead to death within 4 months in 12 to 20 percent of cases (Beals, 1972; Gallagher, Melton, Riggs, & Bergstrath, 1980) and to nursing home care for half of those who survive (Cummings et al., 1985).

Diagnosis of osteoporosis is difficult, particularly in its early stages when signs and symptoms may be absent or minimal. X-ray has been criticized as inaccurate and insensitive in diagnosis of osteoporosis (Woolf & Dixon, 1984, p. 567). More sensitive techniques for its diagnosis are computerized axial tomography (CT scanning) and a radiographic technique known as dual-photon absorptiometry, which measures mineral content of trabecular and cortical bones, useful for analysis of both the spine and the proximal femur. This is considered a better technique than single-photon absorptiometry, which is less expensive, however, and more widely available. Absorptiometry involves less radiation than CT scanning (Cumming et al., 1985, p. 182). Diagnosis also includes screening to rule out endocrine abnormalities, vitamin deficiency states, or tumors that can cause bone demineralization (Upton, 1982, p. 19). Diagnosis and treatment of osteoporosis is often a multidisciplinary activity, involving women's health care providers, endocrinologists, radiologists, orthopedists, nutritionists, physical therapists, and exercise physiologists.

Sexuality

Sexuality for women has finally been recognized as more than a reproductive function. The development of the sexual self occurs throughout life and allows for expression of personality, interrelatedness, and the capacity for pleasure, intimacy, and love (Semmens, 1983). The expression of sexuality in the middle and late years may be complicated by various physical and psychosocial factors, although the perimenopausal years can begin a period of sexual renewal, particularly for women for whom this life stage affords increased time, privacy, and self-awareness.

The anatomic and physiologic changes associated with the perimenopause that have been reviewed previously may affect sexual functioning. Yet it is crucial for the provider to remember that biologic changes are just one aspect of sexual functioning for aging women. Of equal importance are psychosocial influences on motivation, interpersonal and family relationships, and comfort with self. These psychosocial factors significantly affect a woman's response to the biologic changes associated with aging (Bachmann, 1983). For example, the woman who views menopause as a relief from fear of unwanted pregnancy experiences her sexual self quite differently from the woman who views menopause as an escape from sexual demands.

The perimenopausal shift in hormone production from estradiol to estrone influences the sexual response cycle. Vaginal lubrication is slowed during the first phase of sexual excitement, requiring up to 3 to 5 minutes instead of 15 to 40 seconds. Clitoral erection and engorgement of the labia majora and minora are also diminished as a result of neurovascular changes. The orgasmic phase becomes shorter and the number of uterine contractions decreases during orgasm (Notelovitz, 1978).

These age-associated sexual changes, however, can be slowed by continued sexual activity (Masters & Johnson, 1966). Through an active sexual life, women can maintain normal vaginal pliability and function (Notelovitz, 1978), and retain their orgasmic ability. In a study of 57 women divided into a group having sexual intercourse three or more times a month and a group having intercourse fewer than ten times a year, the more sexually active were found to have less vaginal atrophy, although cause and effect were not demonstrated by this research (Leiblum, Bachmann, Kemmann, et al., 1983). Estrogen replacement also has been shown to improve neurovascular vaginal function associated with menopause, particularly vaginal congestion and lubrication (Semmens & Wagner, 1982); however, sexual activity is considered the best method of maintaining sexual response.

Concomitant medical illness in perimenopausal women, their partners, or both often interferes with sexual function. Although an illness may not have a direct effect on the neurovascular system, it may influence an individual's comfort level, body image, and physical capabilities (Semmens, 1983). Incapacitation or death of a sexual partner also mitigates against sexual activity. In addition, medications and drugs including alcohol, β blockers, antihypertensives, and anticholinergic drugs are known to inhibit sexual functioning. Stress and excessive eating may also interfere with sexual ability.

Psychosocial Changes. As a result of the longer life expectancy, personal and social perceptions about aging are being questioned. Revising expectations about advancing age means moving beyond stereotypes and overcoming ageist and sexist biases. Although the literature (Cutler, 1983) has reflected clear shifts toward more egalitarian role attitudes since the sixties, these attitudinal shifts have just recently been directed toward aging women. Yet, positive attitudes toward aging have been demonstrated among women in older age groups. In an examination of 54 women, Wernick and Manaster (1984) noted a divergence between chronological age and perception of age and attractiveness among young, middle-aged, and older women. Most notably, older participants rated pictures of old faces as younger than did young participants. This study supports the notion that perception of youthfulness and attractiveness is not synonymous with youth. In an investigation of attitudes toward menopause among several hundred women, Bowles (1986) found that positive attitude was directly associated with increasing age. Muhlenkamp, Waller, and Bourne (1983), however, found no difference in attitudes toward menopausal and nonmenopausal women among the 152 women they questioned, regardless of age of the study participant. They conclude that "women's misattribution of negative psychological characteristics to women in menopause is over" (Muhlenkamp et al., p. 23). Along with positive attitude, older women have begun to develop their mental and physical potential and to adopt health-promoting behaviors, particularly in the areas of nutrition, exercise, and risk reduction for stress and specific disease states.

During the past 40 years, women have made intense and rapid life-style changes. Many have entered the work force and have assumed increased responsibility in society. Family structures and role relationships have been altered. The impact of these changes has swept across the lives of all contemporary women, but the effect on aging women has been particularly dramatic.

Several factors have contributed to the rapid rise in the participation of women in the work force. The increased numbers of women divorced after more than 20 years of marriage (Public Health Service Task Force, 1985, p. 87), the large numbers of middle-aged women who have worked through their childbearing years, and the many older widows in the population have resulted in an increased number of working women. This trend promises to continue as younger women, motivated primarily by economics, are assuming a major responsibility for labor force participation, household management, and child care (Zajac, 1983). In 1980, however, women still earned 60 percent of a comparable male salary (Leslie & Swider, 1986). Poverty is an especially acute problem among minority women. To further complicate this picture, the crises of widowhood and divorce result in lowering the economic levels of women as they age, leading to the feminization of poverty (Estes, Gerard, & Clark, 1984, p. 57).

Recently, increased longevity and shrinking resources available for health care, reflected in changes in hospital admission and discharge policies brought about by the adoption of diagnostic-related groupings (DRGs), have increased caregiving responsibilities for women during their middle years. In addition to nurturing children, women are increasingly nurturing parents and spouses afflicted with chronic illness. These trends have thrust different sets of problems on middle-aged women, requiring them to learn new behaviors as they attempt to balance and manage multiple roles throughout the life cycle.

The most notable social change for the middle-aged woman often occurs as children leave home and she shifts from a family-centered role to a personally oriented one. Research has shown that middle-aged women are successful in adapting to multiple role changes and altering personal life-styles (Roebuck, 1983); however, specific coping strategies used need further exploration as do the stress-induced illnesses resulting from failure to adapt (Public Health Service Task Force, 1985).

The mental health hazards of aging women include alcohol and drug abuse, loneliness, depression (noted most often among women with children in the home), stress-induced illness, cigarette smoking, and violence and victimization. Women report that they are treated with less respect and dignity by the health care system and have more psychotherapeutic medications prescribed than men (Public Health Service Task Force, 1985). The significance of these factors as they relate to women's health deserves further investigation.

Psychosocial factors present the following challenges to aging women and their health care providers:

1. To recognize diversity among women as they age
2. To identify role models demonstrating successful aging
3. To identify and harness social support systems and community resources for women as they age
4. To prepare women to plan their personal finances with consideration of the likelihood of longevity and the need for eventual long-term care for family members and themselves
5. To increase public awareness about policy and health-related issues of aging women
6. To identify occupational health hazards for working women
7. To develop self-care, prevention, and health promotion practices among women as they age

EPIDEMIOLOGIC CONSIDERATIONS

The most prevalent and serious health problems among middle-aged women include cardiovascular disease, hypertension, breast cancer, lung cancer, rectal or colon cancer, reproductive cancer, arthritis, osteoporosis, diabetes, depression, alcoholism and drug dependence, obesity, endocrine disorders, and periodontal disease.

To assess the health status of middle-aged women, risk factors for these conditions must be evaluated to determine the focus of preventive care. The presence of specific problems will influence the type of therapies selected and the health team members involved in care.

MANAGEMENT OF THE PERIMENOPAUSE AND AGING

Data Collection

To make a comprehensive assessment, the provider must take into account the physiologic and psychosocial changes of menopause and aging. The specific guidelines for data collection outlined in this section are not intended as rules for practice; they merely suggest an approach to women's health care during the midlife and the aging years.

Baseline data necessary for assessing women during the perimenopause need to be repeated every 1 to 2 years, depending on the patient's age. The provider must decide which areas to emphasize. This will depend on the nature of each individual patient visit.

History. The historic data collected during the perimenopause should be specific to the risk factors associated with the perimenopause and to the breast, genitourinary, gastrointestinal, respiratory, cardiovascular, musculoskeletal, and endocrine systems (Utian, 1980). A sexual history focusing particularly on vaginal lubrication, dyspareunia, and libidinal changes is important. Table 24–1 identifies baseline data relevant to these areas.

Physical Examination. The physical changes in perimenopausal women are those common to the aging process and

TABLE 24-1. HISTORY

History of presenting symptoms
  Perspiration, night sweats
  Hot flashes/flushes
  Palpitations
  Vaginal dryness
  Vulvar itching/burning
  Dyspareunia
  Urinary stress incontinence, urgency, frequency, and dysuria
  Musculoskeletal aching
  Depression, emotional lability, irritability,
  Fatigue
  Insomnia
  Changes in mood, memory, concentration
Personal history
  Health behaviors
  Exercise
  Routine health exams
  Breast self-examination
  Medications/drugs/alcohol/tobacco/caffeine
  Nutrition and supplementation
  Stress and coping mechanisms
  Family relationships/support systems
  Work history/job satisfaction
  Financial resources
  Personal problems
  Counseling received
Menstrual history
  Past history
  Changes in menstrual cycle
  Lengthening or shortening of cycle
  Diminished flow
  Intermenstrual spotting, bleeding
Gynecologic history
  Last gynecologic examination
  Abnormal Pap smears
  Abnormal bleeding patterns
  Gynecologic disorders or surgeries
Medical history
  Hypertension
  Cardiovascular disease
  Thromboembolic disorders
  Breast disorders
  Liver/gallbladder disease
  Diabetes
  Thyroid disorders
  Allergy
  Diethylstilbestrol use
  Other health problems
  Current source(s) of medical care
Sexual history
  Libidinal changes
  Decreased lubrication
  Dyspareunia
Obstetric history
Contraceptive history
Family history
  Breast, uterine, ovarian, or cervical cancer
  Diabetes
  Hypertension
  Cardiovascular disease
  Diethylstilbestrol use by mother during pregnancy
  Osteoporosis
  Other

have been described previously in this chapter. Specific areas needing examination are identified in Table 24-2.

Laboratory Data. Laboratory data collected for the perimenopausal woman relate to the constellation of symptoms

TABLE 24-2. PHYSICAL EXAMINATION

Blood pressure, pulse, respirations
Height (compare to previous measurements)
Weight
Head and neck
Heart
Lungs
Breasts
Abdomen
Extremities
Pelvic structures
Rectum

with which she presents and to selected treatment modalities. Preliminary baseline laboratory data necessary for perimenopausal women are listed in Table 24-3.

Cytologic vaginal screening in perimenopausal women can include the maturation index, which reflects the relative number of parabasal, intermediate, and superficial cells in the vagina and indicates the state of estrogen activity in the vagina. A smear for a maturation index is taken with a spatula from the upper lateral third of the vagina and sent to the laboratory for analysis.

Preventive and Therapeutic Modalities

The most commonly prescribed treatment for menopausal symptoms is hormone replacement therapy (HRT); its use remains one of the most controversial issues in women's health care. Other, nonpharmacologic therapies used are nutrition counseling, exercise programs, and educational/support groups. In addition to therapies for specific symptomatology, menopausal women may benefit from preventive measures directed against age-related diseases including osteoporosis and cardiovascular disease.

Hormone Replacement Therapy. Although estrogens were used liberally by physicians in the treatment of menopause prior to 1975, this shotgun approach to the health care of middle-aged women came under close medical, public health, and patient scrutiny in the mid- to late seventies. A decline occurred in the use of estrogen replacement as the magnitude of the relationship between estrogen replacement therapy and endometrial hyperplasia leading to endometrial cancer became known (see, e. g., Hulka, 1980; Jelovsek, Hammond, Woodard, et al., 1980; Jick, Watkins, Hunter, et al., 1979; Shoemaker, Forney, & MacDonald, 1977; Smith et al., 1975; Ziel & Finkle, 1975).

Although the association of estrogen to endometrial cancer has been determined largely from retrospective case-control studies, most experts consider it conclusive, on the basis that more than a dozen such reports covering a

TABLE 24-3. LABORATORY DATA

Urinalysis
Complete blood count
Pap smear with hormonal maturation index
Fasting and 2-hour postprandial glucose levels
Liver function tests
Fasting plasma cholesterol and triglycerides; lipid profile
Endometrial biopsy, if HRT is considered
Progesterone challenge test, if HRT is considered
Mammography[a]
Stool for guaiac

[a]See Chapter 10 for specific recommendations.

variety of control populations have appeared in the literature (Hammond and Ory, 1982, p. 29). A prospective study reported by Gambrell, Massey, Castaneda, et al. (1980) confirmed the association.

When progesterone is added after estrogen therapy (Gambrell 1980), the risk of endometrial cancer has been shown to decrease to a rate even lower than that seen among women receiving no hormones. Flowers, Wilborn, and Hyde (1983) demonstrated that estrogen replacement alone produced hyperplasia in the cells of the endometrium, whereas progesterone and estrogen replacement prevented endometrial hyperplasia through progesterone's cellular differentiating effects.

Hormonal replacement therapy (HRT) has been advocated in the management of at least five areas associated with the perimenopause and the aging years in women: (1) physical symptomatology, including hot flashes/flushes, vaginal atrophy, and buccal mucosal and skin changes; (2) emotional symptoms including depression, sleep deprivative, and loss of libido; (3) osteoporosis prevention; (4) cardiovascular disease prevention; and (5) breast cancer prevention. It is beyond the scope of this chapter to completely review the voluminous literature on HRT. Rather, its main effects and the controversies it engenders in each of these five areas are discussed and representative studies highlighted.

Physical and Emotional Symptomatology. A number of studies have shown that HRT, including estrogen, progestin, or both, is effective in reducing menopause-associated hot flashes/flushes and atrophic vaginal changes. Reports of these benefits appeared as early as 1935 (Davis, 1935; Hammond & Ory, 1982; Mazer & Israel, 1935) and continued to be demonstrated in clinical trials. One double-blind, randomized, 3-month trial of 49 women who had undergone hysterectomy and bilateral oophorectomy found estrogen and estrogen–progesterone to be more effective than progesterone alone and found all hormonal preparations to be more effective than placebo in relieving these problems (Dennerstein, Burrows, Hyman, & Wood, 1978). Nordin, Jones, Crilly, et al. (1980) also conducted randomized prospective trials with two doses of estrogen, a progesterone, and a placebo. They followed 78 women for 3 weeks and found both doses of estrogen to be most effective. The progestin also provided relief, but to a lesser extent than the estrogen. Atrophic vaginitis has been shown to respond to estrogen replacement given locally or systemically (Gordon, Hermann, & Hunter, 1979). Semmens, Tsai, Semmens, and Loadholt (1985), however, demonstrated that it may take as long as 24 months for vaginal benefits to become evident.

Other physical and emotional benefits of hormone replacement therapy have been claimed, but, as yet, remain speculative. Although receptors for estrogen function have been identified in the skin, the benefits of exogenous estrogen on facial skin is still debatable (Utian, 1980, p. 57). Pisantry, Rafaely, and Polishuk (1975) found that the effect of gum massage on changes in the buccal mucosa was equivalent with a placebo cream and an estrogen-containing cream. Several studies have reported improvement in psychogenic depression after estrogen replacement therapy (Albrecht, Schiff, & Tulchinsky, 1981; Thomson & Oswald, 1977); however, these studies have not been prospective, limiting firm conclusions. Whether relief from insomnia or improvement of mood, libido, memory, and concentration can be achieved with HRT merits further study. The etiologies of such symptoms can be physiologic or psychologi-

cal, or combinations of both, and their variations have not been ferreted out in relation to hormonal therapy.

In at least one prospective, randomized study, estrogen replacement therapy was found to have a possible positive effect on sexual desire and enjoyment and on orgasmic frequency, although estrogen and progesterone combinations were not as beneficial (Dennerstein, Burrows, Wood, & Hyman, 1980). Evidence is not sufficient, however, to advise estrogen replacement for sexual difficulties that do not have an obvious physical cause such as debilitating hot flushes, decreased vaginal lubrication, and vaginal atrophy.

CARDIOVASCULAR DISEASE. The literature on the relationship of estrogen to cardiovascular disease is abundant, but nonetheless inconclusive. A variety of areas have been studied regarding estrogen's effect on this major cause of death in our population.

Epidemiologists have looked at cardiovascular disease risk in relation to sex, age, and hormonal environment. Studies have found risk to be lower in women than in men, but to increase in women after menopause or oophorectomy (Gordon, Kannel, Hjortland, & McNamara, 1978).

Many researchers have examined the physiologic role of estrogen in relation to specific biologic parameters determining risk for cardiovascular disease, including lipid metabolism, blood coagulation, thrombophlebitis, blood pressure, and glucose metabolism. Although estrogens in oral contraceptives have been found to adversely affect cardiovascular risk factors, there is agreement in the literature that the high-dose synthetic estrogens used in these preparations have physiologic effects different from those of the low-dose nonsynthetic estrogens used in postmenopausal treatment. Some oral contraceptives, for example, have been shown to increase low-density lipoproteins (LDLs) and to decrease high-density lipoproteins (HDLs), whereas natural or conjugated estrogens used in menopausal therapy have been shown to have the reverse—or beneficial—effect on lipids (Bush, Cowan, Barrett-Connor, et al. 1983).

Bush and Barrett-Connor (1985) carefully reviewed the literature on noncontraceptive estrogens and blood clotting mechanisms. They found "no consistent clinical evidence that noncontraceptive estrogens adversely affect coagulation factors," but also caution that "the use of these agents may predispose to a hypercoagulable state" (p. 86). Without large-scale prospective studies, detrimental effects of postmenopausal estrogens on blood coagulation cannot be ruled out, although in a study of over 5,000 postmenopausal women, those taking estrogen did not have increased rates of venous thromboembolism (Boston Collaborative Drug Surveillance Program, 1974).

Several researchers have found lowered blood pressure or protection from hypertension with postmenopausal estrogen use (Hammond, Jelovsek, Lee, et al., 1979; Lind, Cameron, Hunter, et al., 1979; Wren & Routledge, 1983), whereas others reported blood pressure increases (Coope, Thomson, & Poller, 1975; Crane, Harris, & Winsor, 1971; Pfeffer, 1978; Pfeffer, Kurosaki, & Charlton, 1979; Utian 1978; Wren & Routledge, 1981) or no change (Barrett-Connor, Brown, Turner, et al., 1979; Borglin & Staland, 1975; Christensen, Hagen, Christiansen, & Transbol, 1982; MacGillivray & Gow, 1971; Stern, Brown, Haskell, et al., 1976; Wren & Routledge, 1983).

Studies measuring cardiovascular disease among postmenopausal women have found a range of estrogen effects—protective, neutral, and detrimental. A 10-year double-blind prospective study of 168 women given either estrogen–progesterone therapy or placebo demonstrated no adverse cardiovascular changes. A possible protective role for estrogen against atherosclerotic heart disease was hypothesized but not shown conclusively (Nachtigall, Nachtigall, Nachtigall, & Beckman, 1979b). Several case-control studies have found decreased rate of cardiovascular diagnoses among women using estrogen (Hammond, Jelovsek, Lee, et al., 1979; Ross, Paganini-Hill, Mack, et al., 1981). Others have shown neither adverse nor beneficial effects of estrogen on cardiovascular health (Pfeffer, Whipple, Kurosaki, & Chapman, 1978; Rosenberg, Armstrong, & Jick, 1976). Bush and co-workers (1983) found an *overall* lower risk of death in estrogen users compared with nonusers among women aged 40 to 79 followed for 6.5 years. The greatest estrogen benefit was seen in women who had had prior oophorectomies, that is, early menopause. Estrogen's protective effect was associated with increased levels of HDL cholesterol. Most recently, Stampfer, Willett, Colditz, and co-workers (1985) surveyed over 100,000 nurses by questionnaire and found a reduced risk for coronary heart disease with estrogen therapy. Conversely, both Jick, Dinan, and Rothman (1978) and the Framingham Study (Gordon et al., 1978; Wilson, Garrison, & Castelli, 1985) found increased risk for cardiovascular disease in postmenopausal estrogen users. The Jick et al. sample, however, had a high proportion of smokers among the cases, quite possibly confounding results. The Framingham study reports failed to delineate estrogen dose or duration of its use; as the project began more than 30 years ago, it quite likely reflected higher doses than are used today.

On the basis of a complete analysis of the data, the evidence seems to support a beneficial or neutral effect of estrogen on cardiovascular disease in postmenopausal women (Bush & Barrett-Connor, 1985). Most research showing beneficial effects on cardiovascular health, however, has been done on women taking estrogens alone. Some progesterones may decrease HDL levels (Bradley, Wingerd, Petitti, et al., 1978; Gustafson & Svanborg, 1972; Hirvonen, Malkonen, & Manninen, 1981; Vilska, Punnonen, & Rauramo, 1983; Wahl, Walden, Knopp, et al., 1983). Whether estrogen–progesterone therapy has the same effect on cardiovascular health is unknown and remains controversial (Ernster & Cummings, 1986).

Because of conflicting and incomplete data, HRT is not currently recommended as a preventive measure against cardiovascular disease, although its possible value is still being researched. Estrogen–progesterone regimens, now advised because of their association with a reduced risk for endometrial cancer, particularly need to be studied. Hormonal therapy also needs to be compared with other possible protective modalities, such as nutritional change and exercise. The identification of groups for whom hormonal therapy poses risk and groups for whom it might be beneficial would be a valuable contribution.

OSTEOPOROSIS. The process of bone demineralization clearly appears to be related to estrogen, although the mechanism by which decreased estrogen causes bone change is not fully understood. Decreased levels of plasma androstenedione and estrone have been noted in women with osteoporosis symptoms (Marshall, Crilly, & Nordin, 1977). As bone cells do not contain estrogen receptors, it has been hypothesized that estrogen indirectly affects bone metabolism, probably through an effect on parathyroid hormone or calcitonin (Gallagher & Nordin, 1975).

Estrogen or estrogen–progestin replacement therapy has been demonstrated to be of clear value in preventing the progressive demineralization seen in the bones of postmenopausal women. It has been suggested that while estrogen retards bone loss, progesterone may actually build mass (Gambrell, 1982a, 1982b). Benefit has been shown in a number of prospective randomized studies, although questions still exist as to the relative value of HRT compared with the lifetime use of calcium and exercise and reduction of other risk factors such as smoking and alcohol use.

Lindsay, Hart, Aitken, and associates (1976) treated 100 women after oophorectomy with estrogen or placebo. After approximately 9 years, bone content was greater and deformity of the spine less in the estrogen group. This was a double-blind randomized trial, although it has been criticized for failing to present data on calcium intake. It has also been suggested that there may be metabolic differences between these women and women undergoing natural menopause (Albanese, Lorenze, Edelson, et al., 1981, p. 413). In another study of 258 women following oophorectomy, mestranol was found to be effective in preventing bone loss if therapy was begun within the first 6 years of surgery (Aitken, Hart, Lindsay, et al., 1976). Christiansen and co-workers (1982) studied 114 postmenopausal women for 3 years, also in a double-blind randomized study. Estrogen-treated women increased their bone mass after 2 years of therapy, whereas women in the placebo group lost 2 percent annually. Weiss, Ure, Ballard, and associates (1980) conducted a case-control study of 327 women aged 50 to 74 who had had a fracture of the hip or forearm. They found a 50 to 60 percent lowered risk of fracture in women who had used estrogens for at least 6 years. Ettinger, Genant, and Cann (1985) found a 50 percent reduction in fracture rates among nonblack estrogen users. An overall criticism of these studies is that they did not uniformly control for other associated factors such as body weight, smoking, exercise, and diet.

Nachtigall, Nachtigall, Nachtigall & Beckman (1979a) followed 84 postmenopausal women in a placebo-treated group and 84 postmenopausal women in an estrogen-progesterone-treated group for 10 years. They found that bone loss was significantly decreased in the treated group and that if estrogen-progesterone treatment was begun less than 3 years past the last menstrual period, bone mass actually increased.

Several studies have compared estrogen therapy with other preventive modalities. Recker, Saville, and Heaney (1977) randomly assigned 60 postmenopausal women to estrogen, calcium carbonate, and placebo groups. They found decreased rates of skeletal loss in both the calcium and estrogen groups, with estrogen somewhat more effective. Horsman, Nordin, Gallagher, and associates (1977) also used random assignment to test the effects in women after either menopause or oophorectomy of (1) no treatment, (2) estrogen, (3) calcium, and (4) estrogen and calcium combined. In this study, women treated with only estrogen showed greater benefit than those treated with calcium and, unlike other studies, also did better than women treated with estrogen and calcium combined. Although no significant prestudy differences were found among the four groups, the calcium and calcium–estrogen groups were 7 and 6.7 years postmenopause, respectively, compared with 5.4 and 5.2 years postmenopause for the no-treatment and estrogen-only groups, possibly biasing results.

Williams and associates (1982) identified characteristics of women most likely to benefit from estrogen prophylaxis. In a case-control study of women aged 50 to 74 with hip and forearm fractures, they found body weight and history of smoking to be the most significantly predictive factors. Obese women were found not to benefit from estrogen therapy. The National Institutes of Health (1984) point out that because most osteoporosis treatment studies have been limited to white women, beneficial effects may not apply to other racial groups.

Other preventive measures for osteoporosis are discussed under Alternative Therapies.

BREAST CANCER. Gambrell (1984) has proposed estrogen–progesterone therapy as a protection against breast cancer and its mortality. Whether such prophylaxis is indeed beneficial remains to be proven.

Gambrell bases this recommendation on retrospective data for women with breast cancer and on a prospective study that followed women on various hormonal regimens for 6 to 12 years. Retrospectively, women with cancer ($N = 256$) who had taken any hormones ($N = 63$) had a significantly higher rate of negative axillary nodes and a lower 5-year mortality than those who had not, although benefit was not demonstrated among estrogen-only users. It is possible, however, that the higher incidence of negative axillary nodes and the increased survival rates in this investigation were the result of more frequent surveillance for breast cancer for women on hormonal therapy and not the result of the therapy itself.

In Gambrell's prospective study, (1982c), a decreased incidence of breast cancer was found with estrogen use and an even lower incidence with estrogen-progesterone use, compared with an untreated group and with the incidence in the Third National Cancer Survey and the National Cancer Institute System for Electronic Evaluation and Retrieval. Other risk factors for the development of breast cancer were not mentioned in the study report. Kase (1984) points out that the rates of breast cancer in the untreated group in this study are unusually high and that the study design may have obscured the latency period for the development of breast cancer. Although Gambrell reports on large numbers of woman-years, this represents many women followed for relatively short periods. Such analysis may not yield the same data as following women for longer periods.

Several studies have found neither increased nor decreased breast cancer rates among estrogen users. The Boston Collaborative Drug Surveillance Program (1974) examined records and interviewed patients in 24 Boston hospitals in 1972. They found no association between breast cancer and estrogen use in 103 patients with either benign tumors or cancer. Kelsey, Fischer, Holford, et al. (1981) conducted a case-control study between 1977 and 1979 and found no association between breast cancer and estrogen use, comparing 332 users with 1,353 controls and analyzing other risk factors. Sartwell, Arthes, and Tonascia (1977) also carried out a case-control study of 284 breast cancer patients and similarly found no association with estrogen use.

A number of investigations, however, have shown slightly increased breast cancer rates with estrogen-only therapy. Ross, Paganini-Hill, Gerkins, and associates (1980) found a dose-related response, with the relative risk of breast cancer significantly increased once total estrogen intake exceeded 1,500 mg. These findings applied only to women with intact ovaries and were most pronounced in those with benign breast disease. Jick, Walker, Watkins, and co-workers (1980) found little association between current estrogen use and breast cancer among women with a previous hysterectomy, compared with a control group, but found a positive association between current use and breast cancer in women who had a natural menopause. These findings were stronger in women aged 45 to 54 than in older age groups. Hoover, Gray, Cole, and MacMahon (1976) followed over 1,500 women on conjugated estrogens

for 12 years and found an increasing relative risk for breast cancer associated with length of follow-up. The highest rates of breast cancer were among women who developed benign breast disease after estrogen therapy was begun. These researchers compared their cases with the expected rates of breast cancer among Southern white women, not to a specific control group, a major study flaw. Somewhat reassuringly, the increased risks found in these studies were not very high.

At best, at the time of this writing, it can be concluded that if estrogen-only therapy has an adverse effect on the development of breast cancer, it seems to be relatively small. The role of estrogen–progesterone therapy in the prevention of breast cancer deserves further long-term study.

CONTRAINDICATIONS. There is no consensus in the literature on absolute or even possible contraindications to hormonal replacement therapy during the perimenopause. Reported contraindications (Utian, 1980) to HRT include history of stroke, cardiovascular disease, cancer of the breast or endometrium, deep-vein thrombosis, liver disease, family history of breast cancer, heavy smoking, high blood pressure, diabetes, uterine bleeding, gross obesity, hyperlipidemia, superficial thrombophlebitis, and gallbladder disease (Boston Collaborative Drug Surveillance Project, 1974).

CLINICAL DECISION. Each woman should be counseled about the benefits and risks of HRT and should make an informed decision regarding its use. Assessment of risk must be individualized and based on detailed health history and physical examination of all involved body systems as noted previously in Tables 24–1 and 24–2.

The only currently valid reasons for using HRT are moderate to severe hot flashes/flushes, vaginal atrophy, and osteoporosis prevention. Although psychogenic conditions may be estrogen responsive, generally estrogen is not indicated for these conditions.

The decision to utilize hormone replacement therapy is dependent on several factors:

1. The balance between potential risks and benefits of HRT
2. The presence of valid symptoms or risk factors as indicators of the need for HRT
3. The woman's decision to choose HRT
4. The ability of the provider and patient to follow through on a plan of treatment for HRT

The provider needs to know that the risk of endometrial cancer is increased by the following factors (Utian, 1980): duration of therapy—unopposed estrogen therapy used beyond 3 years doubles the risk ratio; estrogen doses higher than 0.625 mg/day; and the type of estrogen used—for example, nonsteroidal (synthetic) estrogens and estrones, such as diethylstilbestrol, ethinyl estradiol, and mestranol, may be of greater risk than steroidal (nonsynthetic) estrogens, such as conjugated estrogens.

TREATMENT GUIDELINES. As research has shown that the major risk of estrogen replacement therapy—endometrial cancer—can be decreased by combining progesterone with estrogen (Gambrell, 1978, 1982b; Hsueh, Peck, & Clark, 1976), combination therapy is the standard recommendation. Yet even with combination therapy, the provider must consider certain guidelines for prescribing HRT and following women on the therapy (Sitruk-Ware, 1983):

1. Follow institutional or practice protocols regarding consultation and/or referral for HRT initiation and/or follow-up.
2. Prescribe the lowest possible dose of estrogen.
3. Prescribe progesterone in combination with estrogen.
4. Avoid HRT if contraindications exist or refer the woman for medical evaluation if she desires therapy and is suffering from menopausal symptoms or is at risk for osteoporosis.
5. Perform breast exam and refer for mammography and endometrial biopsy before instituting HRT.
6. Use the progesterone challenge test to evaluate the state of endogenous estrogens in the perimenopausal woman. If withdrawal bleeding occurs after 10 days of progesterone, the patient is considered to produce endogenous estrogens and to need progesterone therapy (Gambrell et al., 1980). Once withdrawal bleeding stops, prescribe estrogen.
7. Assess the patient after the first 3 months of therapy and every 6 months thereafter (Cutick, 1984; Ladewig, 1985). Assessment should include an interval history focusing on side effects, including abnormal bleeding, breast pain, cervical mucorrhea, and signs of cardiovascular problems. Physical examination should include measurement of blood pressure and weight and assessment of the breast, abdomen, pelvic organs, and rectum. Annual indicated laboratory work includes fasting blood sugar and 2-hour postprandial and cholesterol and lipid levels.
8. If breakthrough bleeding occurs during the course of treatment, refer for endometrial biopsy and gynecologic evaluation.

ADMINISTRATION.   Most estrogen, to date, is administered via the tablet form or oral route; however, parenteral forms of estrogen are available for intramuscular injection, subcutaneous implantation, transdermal application, and percutaneous administration. The main advantage of administering estrogen parenterally is that this method delivers the hormone directly to the systemic circulation, bypassing the liver. Although the oral route is still the most common method of administration, estrogen-delivering adhesive skin patches, placed on the abdomen, buttock, or thigh, recently have been made available. Studies of patches releasing 0.1 or 0.05 mg of estradiol daily have shown that this method is effective in reducing menopausal symptoms (Padwick, Endacott, & Whitehead, 1985; Place, Powers, Darley, et al., 1985); is comfortable to wear, with only minor topical reactions reported among some users (Place et al., 1985); and results in less of an increase in plasma estrone than the oral route. The last item is important because estrone has been implicated as responsible for increased endometrial stimulation (Powers, Schenkel & Darley, et al., 1985; Whitehead, Padwick, & Endacott, et al., 1985).

Estrogen is also available in cream form for vaginal application. The primary effect of intravaginal estrogen is systemic as a result of absorption through the vaginal mucosa (Rigg, Hermann, & Yen, 1978). Deutsch, Ossowki, and Benjamin (1981), however, administered varying doses of conjugated estrogen to 46 postmenopausal women and reported that daily administration of 0.3 mg did not lead to systemic absorption after 1 week. They recommend this low dosage if relief is needed only for vaginal atrophy.

Oral estrogen is prescribed in combination with progesterone to simulate the normal menstrual cycle. The usual recommended dosage is 0.625 mg of conjugated equine estrogen for 25 days with the addition of 5 mg norethindrone or 5 to 10 mg medroxyprogesterone acetate for the last 10 days of estrogen therapy (Lindsay, Hart, & Clark, 1984; Upton, 1982, p. 21). No hormones are taken for the remainder of the month.

As a treatment for menopausal symptomatology such as vaginal dryness or hot flashes/flushes, HRT is recommended for as short a time as possible. As a preventive measure against the changes associated with osteoporosis, long-term therapy has been recommended. Although a protective effect against bone loss has been shown by at least one research group even after HRT is stopped (Christiansen, Christensen, & Transbol, 1981), other investigators have found that once hormonal therapy is discontinued, the rate of bone loss accelerates greatly, offsetting the benefits of therapy (Lindsay, Hart, MacLean, et al., 1978). These different conclusions may be attributable to discrepancies in study design and methodology. Whether or not there is a rebound effect, it should be remembered that accelerated bone loss can continue 10 to 15 years after menopause.

Alternative Therapies.   Many women defer hormone replacement therapy because of contraindications or personal choice. Several other measures can be recommended as adjuncts or alternatives to hormonal treatment for relief from menopausal symptoms and prevention of disease. Therapeutic possibilities exist in the areas of nutrition, exercise, and sexual counseling.

NUTRITION.   Nutrition is a vital component of health and well-being for women as they age. Generally, caloric requirements decrease with advancing age, and dietary intake should be adjusted appropriately to maintain optimal weight. Saturated fats, nitrates, sodium, caffeine, excess sugar, alcohol, and fat aggravate menopausal symptoms. Vitamin and mineral supplementation may be helpful. Prior to initiating any supplementation, however, patients should have a thorough nutritional assessment. Food is still considered the best source of nutrients, unless deficiencies are associated with old age, chronic disease, malabsorption syndromes, or drug or alcohol abuse (Rolig, 1986).

Vitamin E in doses ranging from 100 units to greater than 2,000 units has been recommended for hot flashes since 1937, although the scientific data supporting its effectiveness are inconclusive. Excellent food sources of vitamin E are peanuts, soybeans, spinach, wheat germ, and vegetable oils. If vitamin E is taken to alleviate hot flashes, the dosage should be raised every third day to a maximum of 800 units. Patients should be advised of the serious side effects associated with vitamin E toxicity: thrombophlebitis, embolism, and breast tumors (Blair, 1986; Ladewig, 1985).

The B-complex vitamins are frequently recommended during the perimenopause, particularly B_6 (Pyridoxine) and B_{12}. As people age, vitamin B_{12} is absorbed less effectively; women, therefore, need to include good food sources of B_{12} in their diet. Foods high in B_{12} include eggs, milk, dairy products, meat, liver, and kidney. Likewise, vitamin B_6 is a nutrient that tends to be scarce in the American diet. Food sources of B_6 include pork, cereal, bran, wheat germ, milk, egg yolk, oats, and legumes. Brewer's yeast is an excellent source of B vitamins.

Vitamin C is required for the synthesis of serotonin, epinephrine, collagen, and bone tissue and for hydroxylation of adrenal hormone (Rolig, 1986). It is found in citrus fruits, peppers, tomatoes, melons, greens, raw vegetables, strawberries, pineapple, potatoes, and broccoli. Vitamin C and the B-complex vitamins are water soluble, which prevents the accumulation of toxic levels in the body; however, megadoses of vitamin C can cause rebound scurvy on withdrawal and depression of leukocyte function when consumed in quantities greater than 1 g per day (Blair, 1986, p. 31).

Dietary zinc has been found to exert a positive effect on vaginal secretion and lubrication in women. Dietary sources rich in zinc include meats, seafood, nuts, wheat germ, oats, green beans, and lima beans. The recommended daily allowance (RDA) is 15 mg per day (Tesar, 1983).

The extent to which osteoporosis can be prevented through nutritional supplementation, particularly calcium, remains controversial; yet evidence is sufficient to conclude that adequate intake of calcium throughout the life cycle is beneficial. In one evaluation of two Yugoslav populations, similar ethnically and in life-style, but with different dietary intakes of dairy products, the rate of proximal femur fractures was significantly higher in the low-intake group. Bone loss after menopause was not significantly different in the two groups, but the greater bone mass maintained throughout life was greater in the high-calcium group. It is hypothesized that this bone mass was formed in childhood. Adequate childhood calcium intake has been suggested to be the best protection against detrimental effects of later-life bone loss (Matkovic et al., 1979).

Studies examining the effect of calcium supplements in postmenopausal women show conflicting results. Nilas, Christiansen, and Rodbro (1984) provided 103 ''early'' postmenopausal women with daily calcium supplements of 500 mg for 2 years. Subsequent to providing a written dietary history, study participants were divided into three groups: those with total dietary intake of calcium less than 550 mg/day, those between 550 and 1,150 mg/day, and those above 1,150 mg/day. Bone mineral content of all participants was measured every 3 months by photon absorptiometry. The researchers found no significant differences and concluded that calcium intake has little effect on loss of bone calcium in the early menopause, which, unfortunately, they never defined. Horsman et al. (1977) also found little effect of calcium, without estrogen, in retarding bone loss.

Conversely, Lee, Lawler, and Johnson (1981) supplemented the diets of 20 elderly women with osteoporosis with calcium-rich foods and a calcium–vitamin D tablet for a total of 750 mg daily calcium for 6 months. Food intake was recorded for 1 week each month of the study and averaged 452 mg of calcium daily. An increase in mean bone density was found at the end of the experimental period, suggesting that calcium may be beneficial even in women with an average age of 70. This study suffers from the lack of a control group.

Recker, Saville, and Heaney (1977) studied three groups of women for 2 years receiving estrogen (0.625 mg/day), calcium carbonate (2,600 mg/day), or no treatment. The estrogen group had the lowest rate of decrease in skeletal mass, the control group the highest. These researchers concluded that calcium is effective in decreasing bone mass, but less so than estrogen.

In no study has calcium supplementation appeared more beneficial than HRT, although it has been suggested that it may act to increase the effectiveness of estrogen (Horsman, Jones, Francis, & Nordin, 1983). The body of literature on dietary supplementation and osteoporosis prevention suffers from a lack of prospective, randomized, controlled, long-term clinical trials with placebo groups and large numbers of study participants. Dietary evaluations are not standardized in the literature nor are methodologies for assessment of bone density. Prospective studies looking at the combined effects of calcium supplementation and exercise and controlling for smoking, body weight, and alcohol intake remain to be done. Long-term studies evaluating calcium supplementation begun early in life would also be worthwhile, although difficult to carry out.

Other dietary factors have been looked at in relation to osteoporosis. These include vitamin D, sodium fluoride, boron, phosphorus, protein, caffeine, and sodium. Vitamin D is necessary for the absorption of calcium; sodium fluoride stimulates bone formation, particularly in trabecular bone; boron, a chemical element found in fruits and vegetables, has recently been suggested as playing a role in preventing bone loss (Tufts University, 1988); excess phosphorus can adversely affect calcium balance and may accelerate bone resorption; protein, which is needed for bone growth, may, in excess, adversely affect it by increasing calcium excretion (Heaney & Recker, 1982; Margen, Chu, Kaufmann, & Calloway, 1974; Parfitt, 1983); caffeine may also adversely affect calcium balance (Heaney & Recker, 1982); excess sodium may cause bone loss (Parfitt, 1983).

Supplemental fluoride must be given in combination with calcium; otherwise defective bone mineralization may occur. Riggs, Seeman, Hodgson, et al. (1982) evaluated vertebral fracture rates in patients with prior osteoporosis. They compared women treated with calcium, estrogen-calcium, and fluoride–estrogen–calcium with a no-treatment group, two thirds of whom were given a placebo. In each treatment group, the calcium was given both with and without vitamin D. All treatment groups fared better than the control group; estrogen and fluoride were found to have effects independent of calcium alone, but the combination of calcium, fluoride, and estrogen was the most effective regimen. In this study, 38 percent of the fluoride-treated group had adverse reactions; 5 percent discontinued therapy secondary to those effects, which included joint pain or other rheumatic symptoms and gastrointestinal problems. In several patients receiving vitamin D, hypercalcemia resulted. Vitamin D was not found to improve results and is generally not recommended except in deficiency states (Woolf & Dixon, 1984, p. 571). Because of the relationship of vitamin D synthesis to sunlight, the homebound, however, may be prone to deficiency (National Institutes of Health, 1984; Parfitt, Gallagher, Heaney, et al., 1982).

Phosphorus, widely used as an additive in processed foods (Massey & Strange, 1982), has not been shown to adversely affect calcium balance in most diets (Heaney & Recker, 1982), although the effects on bone mass of very high or low phosphate intake have not been adequately studied (Parfitt, 1983).

Other hormones—calcitonin and androgens—have also been shown to have some beneficial effects on bone mass, but have additional side effects. Calcitonin, a peptide hormone secreted by the parafollicular cells of the thyroid, must be given by injection and may be associated with anorexia, nausea, and vomiting. Androgens may be virilizing and have adverse effects on HDL cholesterol (Coralli, Raisz, & Wood, 1986).

Studies have shown that the RDA for calcium of 800 mg daily is insufficient in preventing osteoporosis. In an analysis of calcium balance in 130 perimenopausal women, it was found that 1,241 mg per day was needed to maintain a zero calcium balance (Heaney, Recker, & Saville, 1977). The recommended intake of calcium for women varies from 1,000 to 1,500 mg daily (National Institutes of Health, 1984; White, 1986, p. 36; Wyman, Munier, & Spencer, 1981). Studies of the diets of postmenopausal women, however, have shown that the average daily intake of this nutrient is between 475 and 575 mg (Heaney, Recker, & Saville, 1978). Dietary sources of calcium include dairy products, sardines, and green vegetables and are listed in Table 24–4.

TABLE 24–4. CALCIUM CONTENT OF SOME COMMON FOODS

Food	Amount	Calcium (mg)
Dairy products		
Cheese		
American, processed, pasteurized	1 oz	195
Cheddar, American	1 oz	211
Cottage, creamed	1 cup	211
Edam	1 oz	225
Gruyère	1 oz	308
Mozzarella	1 oz	145
Swiss	1 oz	259
Ice cream, vanilla	1 cup	208
Ice milk, vanilla	$\frac{1}{6}$ qt	189
Milk		
Buttermilk, from skim	1 cup	296
Skim	1 cup	303
Whole, 3.5% fat	1 cup	288
Tapioca	$\frac{1}{2}$ cup	105
Vanilla pudding	$\frac{1}{2}$ cup	146
Yogurt, from skim with nonfat milk solids	1 cup	452
Grains		
All Bran (Kellogg's)	1 cup	70
Cream of Wheat, Instant, cooked	1 cup	185
Thomas protein bread	1 slice	78
Whole-wheat bread	1 slice	23
Seafood		
Flounder	3 oz	55
Lobster, boiled or broiled, 2 Tbsp butter	$\frac{3}{4}$ lb	80
Mackerel, canned	$3\frac{1}{2}$ oz	194
Sardines, canned	8 medium	354
Scallops, cooked	$3\frac{1}{2}$ oz	115
Shrimp, raw	$3\frac{1}{2}$ oz	63
Eggs		
Boiled	1 medium	26
Scrambled, milk and fat added	1 medium	52
Fruit		
Dried figs	5 medium	126
Orange, California navel	1 medium	56
Orange, Florida	1 medium	65
Prunes, dehydrated, uncooked	8 large	90
Seeds and nuts		
Almonds, unshelled	1 cup	102
Sunflower seeds	$3\frac{1}{2}$ oz	120
Vegetables		
Artichoke, cooked	1, edible part— base and soft end of leaves	51
Beans		
Lima, green, cooked	6 tbsp	47
Snap, green, cooked	1 cup	62
Wax, yellow, cooked	1 cup	50
Beets, cooked, pickled	1 cup	41
Beet greens, cooked	$\frac{1}{2}$ cup	99
Broccoli		
Raw	1 stalk (5 in.)	103
Cooked	$\frac{2}{3}$ cup	88
Cabbage, savoy, raw shredded	2 cups	67
Chicory	30–40 inner leaves	86
Collard greens, cooked	$\frac{1}{2}$ cup	152
Endive	20 leaves, long	81
Escarole	4 leaves, large	81
Fennel, raw	$3\frac{1}{2}$ oz	100
Lettuce, romaine	$3\frac{1}{2}$ oz	68
Mustard greens, cooked	$\frac{1}{2}$ cup	138
Parsley, raw	$3\frac{1}{2}$ oz	203
Parsnips, raw	$\frac{1}{2}$ large	50
Rutabagas, cooked	$\frac{1}{2}$ cup	59
Soybean curd (tofu)	$3\frac{1}{2}$ oz	128

TABLE 24–4. (CONTINUED)

Food	Amount	Calcium (mg)
Sweet potato, baked in skin	1 large	72
Squash, acorn, baked	$\frac{1}{2}$	61
Watercress, raw	$3\frac{1}{2}$ oz	151
Other		
Blackstrap molasses	1 Tbsp	116

From Pennington, J., & Church, H. N. (1980). Bowes & Church's food values of portions commonly used (13th ed.). Philadelphia: J. B. Lippincott.

Women who consume a large amount of processed foods, including soft drinks, may need increased dietary calcium to maintain the appropriate calcium:phosphorus ratio (Massey & Strange, 1982). Moderate protein and sodium intake should also be advised, and caffeine cautioned against.

Few side effects have been noted with calcium supplementation. Constipation can be alleviated with dietary measures. Some authors warn against the use of calcium in renal stone formers (Woolf & Dixon, 1984), although others believe this risk can be offset by adequate fluid intake (Whedon, 1981). The National Institutes of Health (1984) recommend that anyone with a history of kidney stones take calcium only under the guidance of a physician.

Supplemental calcium is available in a number of forms with 40 percent elemental calcium available from calcium carbonate, 13 percent available from lactate, and 9 percent from gluconate (White, 1986, p. 38). Microcrystalline hydroxyapatite compound, made from bone with physiologic amounts of calcium, phosphates, and fluoride, is well absorbed and well tolerated, although more expensive than other compounds. It has been shown to be more effective in some studies (Woolf & Dixon, 1984, p. 570). Dolomite or bone-meal preparations should be avoided because they may contain lead (White, 1986, p. 36).

EXERCISE. A regular vigorous exercise program, 15 to 60 minutes at least three to five times a week, is recommended for older women (Shangold, 1982). Walking, aerobics, tennis, and biking all prevent bone loss, burn calories, improve muscle tone, and have positive effects on cardiovascular health.

In one study of 18 women, half of whom exercised for 1 hour three to four times a week, total body calcium was found to increase after 1 year (Aloia, Cohn, Ostuni, et al., 1978). In another study (Aloia, Cohn, Vaswani, et al., 1985), lumbar spine mineral content increased in women between the ages of 50 and 73 randomly assigned to a twice-weekly 1-hour exercise group, whereas it decreased in a nonexercise control group. The optimal exercise program for osteoporosis prevention has not been firmly established, although weight-bearing exercises are considered best. Swimming is not a weight-bearing exercise; however, it is an excellent method for increasing muscle tone and flexibility, improving cardiovascular function, and burning calories.

Before prescribing exercise programs for perimenopausal women, it is incumbent on the provider to assess for contraindications and the need for referral to an exercise physiologist or sports medicine program for graded exercise evaluation. Certainly if the patient has a history of cardiovascular disorders and/or a risk profile that is positive for heart disease, referral for stress testing should be made prior to recommending an exercise program. A physical therapist should be involved for patients in whom a diagnosis of osteoporosis has been made to provide exercise

therapy and instruction in proper body mechanics (Coralli et al., 1986).

The National Institutes of Health (1984) also recommends implementing strategies to prevent falls in elderly women. Medication dosages may need to be adjusted and the home environment made safe.

SEXUAL COUNSELING. The perimenopausal woman and her partner need information regarding the normal age-related changes in sexual functioning during the midlife and aging years. The provider should alert the patient to sexual behaviors that may need modification. Specific recommendations may include more time for foreplay to achieve sexual orgasm; lubrication with an over-the-counter water-soluble lubricant; more gentle stimulation of sensitive genital tissue; frequent communication between partners about bodily changes and new sexual rhythms; and variation of sexual positions. Continuation of sexual activity throughout the midlife and into old age should be discussed in a positive manner. The use of estrogen therapy may be advisable if symptoms warrant it. From clinical observations, the Kegel exercise seems to be an excellent measure for improving sexual functioning for women, promoting perineal muscle tone, relieving hemorrhoids, and preventing or correcting urinary stress incontinence. The provider should advise all women in the perimenopause to perform at least 50 to 100 Kegels each day.

Although either partner may experience sexual discomfort as a result of chronic illness and the pharmacologic effects of medications, these preclude neither sexuality nor sensuality in the midlife or later years. On the contrary, chronically ill women and men need to continue to express themselves sensually. Recommendations based on specific conditions can be made to help partners achieve sexual pleasure and satisfaction. Consultation with a patient's medical or rehabilitation providers can clarify sexual limitations should any exist.

Midlife couples may have acquired set patterns of behavior that are monotonous and boring. As a provider, you can jog your patient's memory, reminding her to modify usual sexual patterns. In turn, sexuality in the later years of life can be as rewarding as earlier, or even more so.

Contraception. Women maintain their ability to conceive until the menopause, and must be considered fertile until free from menstruation for 1 year. As a woman ages, the medical risks associated with hormonal contraceptive methods increase (see Section II). Therefore, the provider must perform a thorough and complete health evaluation prior to recommending specific contraceptive methods. Lifestyle, frequency of intercourse, and attitudes toward contraception must also be assessed.

Sterilization, of the woman or man, is the leading method of contraception among middle-aged couples married 10 years or more. This permanent form of birth control is relatively safe with a less than 2 percent risk of complications and appropriate for individuals or couples who want no more children (see Chapter 29). The intrauterine device (IUD) is a viable option for women during the perimenopause, provided they have no bleeding disorders or structural anomalies and no history of pelvic infections or autoimmune system disorders; a monogamous sexual relationship also decreases the risks associated with this method. The barrier methods, when used properly, are highly effective in perimenopausal women. Barrier methods cause little iatrogenesis and can be used only when necessary, eliminating long-term effects. Oral contraceptives, however, have serious cardiovascular side effects that are potentiated by age and smoking. Women over 35 or 40 are usually advised to select another form of birth control, although in recent years, some practitioners have advocated low-dose triphasic pills for nonsmoking women over age 40 (Upton, 1986). Surveillance of women using oral contraceptives after this age requires consultation and comanagement.

New technologies continue to be developed and evaluated. It is certain, with the increasing number of women who maintain midlife sexual functioning, that contraception for women in this age group will emerge as a significant area in women's health care.

Teaching and Counseling. Educating women about normal and abnormal menopausal changes is a vital function of the primary care provider. Knowledge equips each woman to assume an active part in her care and make informed decisions about therapeutic and preventive modalities. In one study of women aged 40 to 60, participants responded correctly to an average of 59 percent of questions asked about menopause (LaRocco & Polit, 1980). This research suggests that myths about menopause persist and underscores the need for teaching. Nolan (1986) suggests individualization of health care planning for the midlife woman based on multiple factors including developmental and physiologic changes and environmental stresses. Counseling should be geared toward the woman's life situation and needs.

Self-help Measures. Women's health and well-being during the middle and aging years have improved during the last decade. These improvements have been related to changes in social and environmental conditions, changes in life-style and health behaviors, and the participation of women in their own health care. Nevertheless, women report more health problems and utilize health services more often than men. Through interactions with their health care providers, aging women can be educated and motivated to become more deeply involved in their own health care and that of their families (Verbrugge, 1984).

The self-help measures that enable women to participate in their health care have been identified throughout this chapter:

1. Maintaining a life-style throughout the life cycle that encourages the development of self-worth, social support systems, and economic independence
2. Avoiding smoking and excess alcohol
3. Revising eating habits to reduce caloric intake as necessary; increase calcium intake; increase fiber; avoid excess fat, salt, caffeine, and sugar intake; and include sufficient vitamin B complex and vitamin C and E foods
4. Practicing cancer screening regularly through breast self-examination, annual gynecologic checkups, Pap smears, and mammograms

5. Exercising aerobically at least three to five times a week for a total of 15 to 60 minutes with an accompanying warmup before the exercise and a cool down after it (Weight-bearing exercises are recommended to prevent osteoporosis.)
6. Maintaining regular sexual activity by using water-soluble lubricants, performing Kegel or pelvic floor exercises, communicating expectations to partners, and altering sexual practices to incorporate the deceleration of the sexual response cycle and biologic changes associated with aging
7. Monitoring hormonal replacement therapy, if selected by the woman and her provider, through regularly scheduled follow-up visits with additional follow-up should side effects be noted

MacPherson (1985) recommends the formation of self-help groups among menopausal women. Primary care practitioners can be instrumental in forming such groups among their patients.

The transition to the menopause and aging has become a vital area in well-woman gynecology as one third to one half of the life of the American woman is spent beyond the menstruating years. Projections have been made that by the next century, 30 percent of the women in this country will be postmenopausal. This phenomenon will undoubtedly influence the delivery of health care to aging women. Primary care practitioners, in particular, have an opportunity to provide leadership in the delivery of holistic woman-centered health care to this population and to influence society to accept more responsibility for the humane care of its aging population.

REFERENCES

Aitken, J. M., Hart, D. M., & Lindsay, R., et al. (1976, July). Prevention of bone loss following oophorectomy in premenopausal women. *Israel Journal of Medical Sciences, 12*(7), 608–614.

Albanese, A. A., Lorenze, E. J., & Edelson, A. H., et al. (1981, August). Effects of calcium supplements and estrogen replacement therapy on bone loss of postmenopausal women. *Nutrition Reports International, 24*(2), 403–414.

Albrecht, B. H., Schiff, I., & Tulchinsky, D. (1981, March 15). Objective evidence that placebo and oral medroxyprogesterone acetate diminish menopausal vasomotor flushes. *American Journal of Obstetrics and Gynecology, 139*(6), 631–635.

Aloia, J. F., Cohn, S. H., & Ostumi, J. A., et al., (1978, September). Prevention of involutional bone loss by exercise. *Annals of Internal Medicine, 89*(3), 356–358.

Aloia, J. F., Cohn, S. H., & Vaswani, A., et al. (1985, January). Risk factors for postmenopausal osteoporosis. *The American Journal of Medicine, 78*(1), 95–100.

Aloia, J. F., Vaswani, A. N., & Yeh, J. K., et al. (1983, September). Determinants of bone mass in postmenopausal women. *Archives of Internal Medicine, 143*(9), 1700–1704.

Bachmann, G. (1983). Sexual response and hormone therapy. *Menopause Update, 1*(2), 23–26.

Barrett-Connor, E., Brown, V., & Turner, J., et al. (1979, May 18). Heart disease risk factors and hormone use in postmenopausal women. *Journal of the American Medical Association, 241*(20), 2167–2169.

Beals, R. K. (1972, April). Survival following hip fracture. *Journal of Chronic Disease, 25*(4), 235–244.

Blair, K. (1986, July). Vitamin supplementation and megadoses. *Nurse Practitioner, 11*(7), 19–34.

Borglin, N.E., & Staland, B. (1975). Oral treatment of menopausal symptoms with natural oestrogens. *Acta Obstetricia et Gynecologica Scandinavica, 43* (Suppl.), 1–11.

Boston Collaborative Drug Surveillance Program. (1974, January

3). Surgically confirmed gallbladder disease, venous thromboembolism, and breast tumors in relation to postmenopausal estrogen therapy. *New England Journal of Medicine, 290*(1), 15–18.

Bowles, C. (1986, March/April). Measure of attitude toward menopause using the semantic differential model. *Nursing Research, 35*(2), 81–85.

Bradley, D. D., Wingerd, J., & Petitti, D. B., et al (1978, July 6). Serum high-density-lipoprotein cholesterol in women using oral contraceptives, estrogens and progestins. *New England Journal of Medicine, 299*(1), 17–20.

Brody, J., Farmer, M., & White, L. (1984, December). Absence of menopausal effect on hip fracture occurrence. *American Journal of Public Health, 72*(12), 1397–1398.

Bush, T. L., & Barrett-Connor, E. (1985). Noncontraceptive estrogen use and cardiovascular disease. *Epidemiologic Reviews, 7,* 80–104.

Bush, T. L., Cowan, L. D., & Barrett-Connor, E., et al. (1983, February 18). Estrogen use and all-cause mortality. *Journal of the American Medical Association, 249*(7), 903–906.

Casey, M. L., & MacDonald, P. C. (1983). Origin of estrogen and regulation of its formation in postmenopausal women. In H. Buchsbaum (Ed.), *The Menopause.* New York: Springer-Verlag.

Christiansen, C., Christensen, M. S., & Transbol, I. (1981, February 28). Bone mass in postmenopausal women after withdrawal of oestrogen/gestagen replacement therapy. *Lancet, 1*(8218), 459–461.

Christensen, M. S., Hagen, C., Christiansen, C., & Transbol, I. (1982, December 15). Dose–response evaluation of cyclic estrogen/gestagen in postmenopausal women: Placebo-controlled trial of its gynecologic and metabolic actions. *American Journal of Obstetrics and Gynecology, 144*(8), 873–878.

Coope, J., Thomson, J. M., & Poller, L. (1975, October 18). Effects of "natural estrogen" replacement therapy on menopausal symptoms and blood clotting. *British Medical Journal, 4*(5989), 139–142.

Coralli, C. H., Raisz, L. G., & Wood, C. L. (1986, September). Osteoporosis: Significance, risk factors and treatment. *Nurse Practitioner, 11*(9), 16–35.

Crane, M. G., Harris, J. J., & Winsor, W. (1971, January). Hypertension, oral contraceptive agents, and conjugated estrogens. *Annals of Internal Medicine, 74*(1), 13–21.

Cummings, S. R., Kelsey, J. L., Nevitt, M. C., & O'Dowd, K. J. (1985). Epidemiology of osteoporosis and osteoporotic fractures. *Epidemiologic Reviews, 7,* 178–208.

Cutick, R. (1984, March-April). Special need of perimenopausal women and menopausal women. *Journal of Obstetric, Gynecologic, and Neonatal Nursing, 13*(2, Suppl.), 685–735.

Cutler, S. (1983). Aging and changes in attitudes about the women's liberation movement. *International Journal of Aging and Human Development, 16*(1), 43–51.

Cutler, W. B., & Garcia, C. R. (1984). *The medical management of menopause and premenopause: Their endocrinologic basis.* Philadelphia: J. B. Lippincott.

Daniell, H. W. (1976, March). Osteoporosis of the slender smoker. *Archives of Internal Medicine, 136*(3), 298–304.

Davis, M. E. (1935, November). The treatment of senile vaginitis with ovarian follicular hormone. *Surgery, Gynecology and Obstetrics, 61*(5), 680–686.

Dennerstein, L., Burrows, G. D., Hyman, G., & Wood, C. (1978, November). Menopausal hot flushes: A double blind comparison of placebo, ethinyl oestradiol and norgestrel. *British Journal of Obstetrics and Gynaecology, 85*(11), 852–856.

Dennerstein, L., Burrows, G. D., Wood, C., & Hyman, G. (1980, September). Hormones and sexuality: Effect of estrogen and progestogen. *Obstetrics and Gynecology, 56*(3), 316–322.

Deutsch, S., Ossowski, R., & Benjamin, I. (1981, April 15). Comparison between degree of systemic absorption of vaginally and orally administered estrogens at different dose levels in postmenopausal women. *American Journal of Obstetrics and Gynecology, 139*(8), 967–968.

DeVane, G. (1983). Hormonal changes during the climacteric. *Menopause Update, 1*(2), 2–6.

Edmon, C. D. (1983). The climacteric. In H. Buchsbaum (Ed.), *The Menopause.* New York: Springer-Verlag.

Ernster, V., & Cummings, S. (1986, November). Progesterone and breast cancer. *Obstetrics and Gynecology, 68*(5), 715–717.

Estes, C., Gerard, L., & Clark, A. (1984). Women and the economics of aging. *International Journal of Health Services, 14*(1), 55–68.

Ettinger, B. (1986). Preventing postmenopausal osteoporosis with estrogen replacement therapy. *International Journal of Fertility, 31* (Suppl.), 15–20.

Ettinger, B., Genant, H. K., & Cann, C. E. (1985, March). Long-term estrogen replacement therapy prevents bone loss and fractures. *Annals of Internal Medicine, 102*(3), 319–324.

Feldman, B., Voda, A., & Gronseth, E. (1985, September). The prevalence of hot flash and associated variables among perimenopausal women. *Research in Nursing and Health, 8*(3), 261–268.

Flowers, C. E., Wilborn, W. H., & Hyde, B. M. (1983, February). Mechanisms of uterine bleeding in postmenopausal patients receiving estrogen alone or with a progestin. *Obstetrics and Gynecology, 61*(2), 135–143.

Gallagher, J. C., Melton, L. J., Riggs, B. L., & Bergstrath, E. (1980, July-August). Epidemiology of fractures of the proximal femur in Rochester, Minnesota. *Clinical Orthopaedics and Related Research, 150,* 163–170.

Gallagher, J. C., & Nordin, B. E. C. (1975). Effects of oestrogen and progestogen therapy on calcium metabolism in postmenopausal women. *Frontiers of Hormone Research, 3,* 150–176.

Gambrell, R. D. (1978, September). The prevention of endometrial cancer in postmenopausal women with progestogens. *Maturitas, 1*(2), 107–108.

Gambrell, R. D. (1982a, August). Clinical use of progestins in the menopausal patient. *The Journal of Reproductive Medicine, 27*(8, Suppl.), 531–538.

Gambrell, R. D. (1982b, April). The menopause: Benefits and risks of estrogen–progestogen replacement therapy. *Fertility and Sterility, 37*(4), 457–474.

Gambrell, R. D. (1982c). Role of hormones in the etiology and prevention of endometrial and breast cancer. *Acta Obstetricia et Gynecologica Scandinavica, 106* (Suppl.), 37–46.

Gambrell, R. D. (1984, September 15). Proposal to decrease the risk and improve the prognosis of breast cancer. *American Journal of Obstetrics and Gynecology, 150*(2), 119–128.

Gambrell, R. D., Massey, F. M., & Castaneda, T. A., et al. (1980, June). Use of the progestogen challenge test to reduce the risk of endometrial cancer. *Obstetrics and Gynecology, 55*(6), 732–738.

Gordon, T., Kannel, W. B., Hjortland, M. C., & McNamara, P. M. (1978, August). Menopause and coronary heart disease: The Framingham Study. *Annals of Internal Medicine, 89*(2), 157–161.

Gordon, W. E., Hermann, H. W., & Hunter, D. C. (1979, July). Treatment of atrophic vaginitis in postmenopausal women with micronized estradiol cream—A follow-up study. *Journal of the Kentucky Medical Association, 77*(7), 337–339.

Gustafson, L., & Svanborg, A. (1972, August). Gonadal steroid effects on plasma lipoproteins and individual phospholipids. *Journal of Clinical Endocrinology and Metabolism, 35*(2), 203–207.

Hammond, C. B., Jelovsek, F. R., & Lee, K. L., et al. (1979, March 1). Effects of long-term estrogen replacement therapy. I. Metabolic effects. *American Journal of Obstetrics and Gynecology, 133*(5), 525–536.

Hammond, C. B., & Ory, S. (1982, March). Endocrine problems in the menopause. *Clinical Obstetrics and Gynecology, 25*(1), 19–38.

Heaney, R. P., & Recker, R. R. (1982, January). Effects of nitrogen, phosphorus, and caffeine on calcium balance in women. *Journal of Laboratory and Clinical Medicine, 99*(1), 46–55.

Heaney, R. P., Recker, R. R., & Saville, P. D. (1977, October). Calcium balance and calcium requirements in middle-aged women. *American Journal of Clinical Nutrition, 30*(10), 1603–1611.

Heaney, R. P., Recker, R. R., & Saville, P. D. (1978, December). Menopausal changes in calcium balance performance. *Journal of Laboratory and Clinical Medicine, 92*(6), 953–963.

Hirvonen, E., Malkonen, M., & Manninen, V. (1981, March). Effects of different progestogens on lipoproteins during postmenopausal replacement therapy. *New England Journal of Medicine, 304*(10), 560–562.

Hoover, R., Gray, L. A., Cole, P., & MacMahon, B. (1976, August 19). Menopausal estrogens and breast cancer. *New England Journal of Medicine, 295*(B), 401–405.

Horsman, A., Jones, M., Francis, R., & Nordin, C. (1983, December 8). The effect of estrogen dose on postmenopausal bone loss. *New England Journal of Medicine, 309*(23), 1405–1407.

Horsman, A., Nordin, B. E. C., & Gallagher, J. C., et al. (1977, May). Observations of sequential changes in bone mass in postmenopausal women in a controlled trial of oestrogen and calcium therapy. *Calcified Tissue Research, 22*(Suppl.), 217–224.

Hsueh, A., Peck, E. J., & Clark, J. H. (1976, February). Control of uterine estrogen receptor levels by progesterone. *Endocrinology, 98*(2), 438–444.

Hulka, B. (1980, June). Effect of exogenous estrogen on postmenopausal women: The epidemiological evidence. *Obstetrical and Gynecological Surgery, 35*(6), 389–399.

Jelovsek, F. R., Hammond, C. B., & Woodard, B. H., et al. (1980, May 1). Risk of exogenous estrogen therapy and endometrial cancer. *American Journal of Obstetrics and Gynecology, 137*(1), 85–91.

Jick, H., Dinan, B., & Rothman, K. J. (1978, April 3). Noncontraceptive Estrogens and nonfatal myocardial infarction. *Journal of the American Medical Association, 239*(4), 1407–1408.

Jick, H., Porter, J., & Morrison, A. S., (1977, June 15). Relation between smoking and age of natural menopause. *Lancet, 1*(8026), 1353–1355.

Jick, H., Walker, A. M., & Watkins, R. N., et al. (1980). Replacement estrogens and breast cancer. *American Journal of Epidemiology, 112*(5), 586–591.

Jick, H., Watkins, R. N., & Hunter, J. R., et al. (1979, February). Replacement estrogens and endometrial cancer. *New England Journal of Medicine, 300*(5), 218–222.

Kase, N. (1984, May). Does steroid replacement reduce breast cancer risk? *Contemporary Ob/Gyn, 23*(5), 71–82.

Kelsey, J. L., Fischer, D. B., & Holford, T. R., et al. (1981, August). Exogenous estrogens and other factors in the epidemiology of breast cancer. *Journal of the National Cancer Institute, 67*(2), 327–333.

Ladewig, P. A. (1985, October). Protocol for estrogen replacement therapy in menopausal women. *Nurse Practitioner, 10*(10), 44–47.

LaRocco, S. A., & Polit, D. F. (1980, January-February). Women's knowledge about the menopause. *Nursing Research, 29*(1), 10–13.

Lee, C. J., Lawler, G. S., & Johnson, G. H. (1981, May). Effects of supplementation of the diets with calcium and calcium-rich foods on bone density of elderly females with osteoporosis. *American Journal of Clinical Nutrition, 34*(5), 819–823.

Leiblum, S., Bachmann, G., & Kemmann, E., et al. (1983, April 22/29). Vaginal atrophy in the postmenopausal woman. *Journal of the American Medical Association, 249*(16), 2195–2198.

Leslie, L. A., & Swider, S. M. (1986, March). Changing factors and changing needs in women's health care. *Nursing Clinics of North America, 21*(1), 111–123.

Lind, T., Cameron, E. C., & Hunter, W. M., et al. (1979). A prospective, controlled trial of six forms of hormone replacement therapy given to postmenopausal women. *British Journal of Obstetrics and Gynaecology, 86*(Suppl. 3), 1–29.

Lindquist, O., & Bengtsson, C. (1979, February). The effect of smoking on menopausal age. *Maturitas, 1*(3), 171–173.

Lindsay, R., Hart, D., & Aitken, J., et al. (1976, May 15). Long term prevention of postmenopausal osteoporosis by oestrogen. *Lancet, 1*(7968), 1038–1041.

Lindsay, R., Hart, D. M., & Clark, D. M. (1984, June). The minimum effective dose of estrogen for prevention of postmenopausal bone loss. *Obstetrics and Gynecology, 63*(6), 759–763.

Lindsay, R., Hart, D. M., & MacLean, A., et al. (1978, June 24). Bone response to termination of oestrogen treatment. *Lancet, 1*(8078), 1325–1327.

MacGillivray, I., & Gow, S. (1971, April 10). Metabolic, hormonal, and vascular changes after synthetic oestrogen therapy in oophorectomized women. *British Medical Journal, 2*, 73–77.

MacPherson, K. I. (1981, January). Menopause as disease: The social construction of a metaphor. *Advances in Nursing Science, 3*(2), 95–113.

MacPherson, K. I. (1985, July). Osteoporosis and menopause: A feminist analysis of the social construction of a syndrome. *Advances in Nursing Science, 7*(4), 11–22.

Margen, S., Chu, J.-Y., Kaufmann, N. A., & Calloway, D. H. (1974, June). Studies in calcium metabolism. I. The calciuretic effect of dietary protein. *American Journal of Clinical Nutrition, 27*(6), 584–589.

Marshall, D. H., Crilly, R. G., & Nordin, B. E. C. (1977, November 5). Plasma androstenedione and oestrone levels in normal and osteoporotic postmenopausal women. *British Medical Journal, 2*(6096), 1177–1198.

Massey, L. K., & Strange, M. M. (1982, June). Soft drink consumption, phosphorus intake, and osteoporosis. *Journal of the American Dietetic Association, 80*(6), 581–583.

Masters, W., & Johnson, V. (1966). *Human sexual response.* Boston: Little, Brown.

Matkovic, V., Kostial, K., & Simonovic, I., et al. (1979, March). Bone status and fracture rates in two regions of Yugoslavia. *The American Journal of Clinical Nutrition, 32*(3), 540–549.

Mazer, C., & Israel, S. L. (1935, July). The symptoms and treatment of the menopause. *Medical Clinics of North America, 19*(1), 205–226.

Muhlenkamp, A. F., Waller, M. W., & Bourne, A. E. (1983, January/February). Attitudes toward women in menopause: A vignette approach. *Nursing Research, 32*(1), 20–23.

Nachtigall, L. E., Nachtigall, R. H., Nachtigall, R. D., & Beckman, E. M. (1979a, March). Estrogen replacement therapy. I. A ten-year prospective study in the relationship to osteoporosis. *Obstetrics and Gynecology, 53*(3), 277–281.

Nachtigall, L. E., Nachtigall, R. H., Nachtigall, R. D., & Beckman, E. M. (1979b, July). Estrogen replacement therapy, II. A prospective study in the relationship to carcinoma and cardiovascular and metabolic problems. *Obstetrics and Gynecology, 54*(1), 74–79.

National Institutes of Health. (1984). Consensus Development Conference Statement. *Osteoporosis, 5*(3).

Nilas, L., Christiansen, C., & Rodbro, P. (1984). Calcium supplementation and postmenopausal bone loss. *British Medical Journal, 289*(6452), 1103–1106.

Nolan, J. W. (1986, March). Developmental concerns and the health of midlife women. *Nursing Clinics of North America, 21*(1), 151–159.

Nordin, B. E. C., Jones, M. M., & Crilly, R. G., et al. (1980, October). A placebo-controlled trial of ethinyl oestradiol and norethisterone in climacteric women. *Maturitas, 2*(3), 247–251.

Notelovitz, M. (1978, October). Gynecologic problems of menopausal women. Part 3. Changes in extra genital tissues and sexuality. *Geriatrics, 33*(10), 51–58.

Notelovitz, M. (1983). Menopause: When to treat. *Menopause Update, 1*(1), 27–31.

Padwick, M. L. Endacott, J, & Whitehead, M. I. (1985, August 15). Efficacy, acceptability, and metabolic effects of transdermal estradiol in the management of postmenopausal women. *American Journal of Obstetrics and Gynecology, 152*(8), 1985–1991.

Parfitt, A. M. (1983, November 19). Dietary risk factors for age-related bone loss and fractures. *Lancet, 2*(8360), 1181–1185.

Parfitt, A. M., Gallagher, J. C., & Heaney, R. P., et al. (1982, November). Vitamin D and bone health in the elderly. *American Journal of Clinical Nutrition, 36*(5), 1014–1031.

Pennington, J., & Church, H. N. (1980). *Bowes & Church's food values of portions commonly used* (13th ed.). Philadelphia: J. B. Lippincott.

Pfeffer, R. I. (1978, July). Estrogen use, hypertension and stroke in postmenopausal women. *Journal of Chronic Diseases, 31*(6/7), 389–398.

Pfeffer, R. I., Kurosaki, T. T., & Charlton, S. K. (1979, October). Estrogen use and blood pressure in later life. *American Journal of Epidemiology, 110*(4), 469–478.

Pfeffer, R. I., Whipple, G. H., Kurosaki, T. T., & Chapman, J. M. (1978, June). Coronary risk and estrogen use in postmenopausal women. *American Journal of Epidemiology, 107*(6), 479–487.

Pisantry, S., Rafaely, B., & Polishuk, W. Z. (1975, September). The effect of steroid hormones on buccal mucosa of menopausal women. *Oral Surgery, Oral Medicine, Oral Pathology, 40*(3), 346–353.

Place, V. A., Powers, M., & Darley, P. E., et al. (1985, August 15). A double-blind comparative study of Estraderm and Premarin in the amelioration of postmenopausal symptoms. *American Journal of Obstetrics and Gynecology, 152*(8), 1092–1099.

Powers, M. S., Schenkel, L., & Darley, P. E., et al. (1985, August 15). Pharmacokinetics and pharmacodynamics of transdermal dosage forms of 17β-estradiol: Comparison with conventional oral estrogens used for hormone replacement. *American Journal of Obstetrics and Gynecology, 152*(8), 1099–1104.

Public Health Service Task Force. (1985, January–February). Report of the Public Health Service Task Force on Issues in Women's Health, Volume I. *Public Health* Reports, 10(1), 73–106.

Raisz, L. L. (1982, February). Osteoporosis. *Journal of the American Geriatric Society, 30*(2), 127–137.

Recker, R. R., Saville, P. D., & Heaney, R. P. (1977, December). Effect of estrogens and calcium carbonate on bone loss in postmenopausal women. *Annals of Internal Medicine, 87*(6), 649–655.

Reed, P. G. (1983, October). Implication of the life-span developmental framework for well-being in adulthood and aging. *Advances in Nursing Science, 6*(10), 18–25.

Rigg, L. A. (1986). Estrogen replacement therapy for atrophic vaginitis. *International Journal of Fertility, 31*(Suppl.), 29–34.

Rigg, L. A., Hermann, H., & Yen, S. S. C. (1978, January 26). Absorption of estrogens from vaginal creams. *New England Journal of Medicine, 298*(4), 195–197.

Riggs, B. L., & Melton, L. J. (1986, June 26). Involutional osteoporosis. *New England Journal of Medicine, 314*(26), 1676–1684.

Riggs, B. L., Seeman, E., & Hodgson, S. F., et al. (1982, February 25). Effect of the fluoride/calcium regimen on vertebral fracture occurrence in postmenopausal osteoporosis. *New England Journal of Medicine, 306*(8), 446–450.

Rinehart, J. S., & Schiff, I. (1983). Hormonal imbalance: Hormonal treatment. *Menopause Update, 1*(2), 13–16.

Roebuck, J. (1983). Grandma as revolutionary: Elderly women and some modern patterns of social change. *International Journal of Aging and Human Development, 17*(4), 249–266.

Rolig, E. (1986, July). Vitamins: Physiology and deficiency states. *Nurse Practitioner, 11*(7), 19–34.

Rosenberg, L., Armstrong, B., & Jick, H. (1976, June 3). Myocardial infarction and estrogen therapy in post-menopausal women. *New England Journal of Medicine, 294*(23), 1256–1259.

Ross, R. K., Paganini-Hill, A., & Gerkins, V. R., et al., (1980, April 25). A case-control study of menopausal estrogen therapy and breast cancer. *Journal of the American Medical Association, 243*(16), 1635–1639.

Ross, R. K., Paganini-Hill, A., Mack, T. M., et al. (1981, April 18). Menopausal oestrogen therapy and protection from death from ischaemic heart disease. *Lancet, 1*(8225), 858–860.

Sartwell, P. E., Arthes, F. G., & Tonascia, J. A. (1977, December). Exogenous hormones, reproductive history, and breast cancer. *Journal of the National Cancer Institute, 59*(6), 1589–1592.

Semmens, J. (1983). Sexuality. In H. Buchsbaum (Ed.), *The Menopause.* New York: Springer-Verlag.

Semmens, J., Tsai, C. C., Semmens, E. C., & Loadholt, C. B. (1985, July). Effects of estrogen therapy on vaginal physiology during menopause. *Obstetrics and Gynecology, 66*(1), 15–18.

Semmens, J., & Wagner, G. (1982, July 23/30). Estrogen deprivation and vaginal function in postmenopausal women. *Journal of the American Medical Association, 248*(4), 445–448.

Shangold, M. M. (1982, March). How exercise benefits older women. *Contemporary Ob/Gyn. 19*(3), 81–86.

Shoemaker, E. S., Forney, J. P., & MacDonald, P. C. (1977, October 3). Estrogen treatment of postmenopausal women: Benefits and risks. *Journal of the American Medical Association, 238*(14), 1524–1530.

Sitruk-Ware, R. (1983). Newer and alternative methods of hormone administration. *Midlife Wellness, 1*(3), 13–17.

Smith, D., Prentice, R., Thompson, D. J., & Herrmann, W. L. (1975, December 4). Association of exogenous estrogen and endometrial carcinoma. *New England Journal of Medicine, 293*(23), 1164–1166.

Soules, M. R., & Bremner, W. J. (1982, September). The menopause and climacteric: Endocrinologic basis and associated symptomatology. *Journal of the American Geriatrics Society, 30*(9), 547–559.

Stampfer, M. J., Willett, W. C., & Colditz, G. A., et al. (1985, Octo-

ber 24). A prospective study of postmenopausal estrogen therapy and coronary heart disease. *New England Journal of Medicine, 313*(17), 1044–1049.

Stern, M. P., Brown, B. W., & Haskell, W. L., et al. (1976, February 23). Cardiovascular risk and use of estrogens or estrogen-progestagen combinations. *Journal of the American Medical Association, 235*(8), 811–815.

Stone, S. C., Mickal, S., & Rye, P. (1975, June). Postmenopausal symptomatology, maturation index and plasma estrogen levels. *Obstetrics and Gynecology, 45*(6), 625–627.

Tesar, R. (1983). Zinc: And all important trace elements. *Midlife Wellness, 1*(2), 38–40.

Thompson, B., Hart, S. A., & Durno, D. (1973, January). Menopausal age and symptomatology in a general practice. *Journal of Biosocial Science, 5*(1), 71–82.

Thomson, J., & Oswald, I. (1977, November). Effect of estrogens on the sleep, mood, and anxiety of menopausal women. *British Medical Journal, 2*(6098), 1317–1319.

Treloar, A. E. (1981, December). Menstrual cyclicity and the premenopause. *Maturitas, 3*(3/4), 249–264.

Tufts University. (1988, March). Fruits and vegetables for your bones. *Diet & Nutrition Letter, 6*(1), 1.

Uphold, C., & Sussman, E. (1981, March-April). Self-reported climacteric symptoms as a function of the relationship between marital adjustment and childrearing stage. *Nursing Research, 30*(2), 84–88.

Uphold, C., & Sussman, E. (1985, March). Childrearing, marital, recreational and work role integration and climacteric symptoms in midlife women. *Research in Nursing and Health, 8*(1), 73–81.

Upton, G. V. (1982, January). The perimenopause: Physiologic correlates and clinical management. *The Journal of Reproductive Medicine, 27*(1), 1–27.

Upton, G. V. (1986). The contraceptive and hormonal requirements of the premenopausal woman: The years from forty to fifty. *International Journal of Fertility, 30*(4), 44–52.

Utian, W. H. (1978, June). Effect of postmenopausal estrogen therapy on diastolic blood pressure and bodyweight. *Maturitas, 1*(1), 3–8.

Utian, W. H. (1980). *Menopause in modern perspective: A guide to clinical practice.* New York: Appleton–Century–Crofts.

Verbrugge, L. M. (1984, Summer). Longer life but worsening health? Trends in health and mortality of middle-aged and older persons. *Milbank Memorial Fund Quarterly, 62*(3), 475–519.

Vilska, S., Punnonen, R., & Rauramo, L. (1983, August). Long-term post-menopausal hormone therapy and serum HDL-C, total cholesterol and triglycerides. *Maturitas, 5*(2), 97–104.

Voda, A. (1981, March). Climacteric hot flash. *Maturitas, 3*(1), 73–90.

Voda, A. (1983). A descriptive analysis. *Menopause Update, 1*(2), 17–20.

Wahl, P., Walden, C., & Knopp, R., et al. (1983, April 14). Effect of estrogen/progestin potency on lipid/lipoprotein cholesterol. *New England Journal of Medicine, 308*(15), 862–867.

Weiss, N., Ure, C., & Ballard, J. H., et al. (1980, November 20). Decreased risk of fractures of the hip and lower forearm with postmenopausal use of estrogens. *New England Journal of Medicine, 303*(21), 1195–1198.

Wernick, M., & Manaster, G. (1984, August). Age and the perception of age and attractiveness. *The Gerontologist, 24*(4), 408–414.

Whedon, G. D., (1981, August 13). Osteoporosis, (Editorial). *The New England Journal of Medicine, 305*(7), 397–399.

White, J. E. (1986, September). Osteoporosis: Strategies for prevention. *Nurse Practitioner, 11*(9), 36–50.

Whitehead, M. I., Padwick, M. L., Endacott, J., & Pryse-Davies, J. (1985, August 15). Endometrial responses to transdermal estradiol in postmenopausal women. *American Journal of Obstetrics and Gynecology, 152*(8), 1079–1084.

Williams, A. R., Weiss, N. S., & Ure, C. L., et al. (1982, December). Effect of weight, smoking, and estrogen use on the risk of hip and forearm fractures in postmenopausal women. *Obstetrics and Gynecology, 60*(6), 695–699.

Wilson, P. W. F., Garrison, R. J., & Castelli, W. P. (1985, October

24). Postmenopausal estrogen use, cigarette smoking, and cardiovascular morbidity in women over 50: The Framingham study. *New England Journal of Medicine, 313*(17), 1038–1043.

Woods, N. F. (1981). Health promotion and maintenance for women. In C. I. Fogel & N. F. Woods (Eds.), *Health care of women*. St. Louis: C. V. Mosby.

Woolf, A. D., & Dixon, A. St. J. (1984, December). Osteoporosis: An update on management. *Drugs, 28*(6), 565–576.

Wren, B. G., & Routledge, A. D. (1981, November 14). Blood pressure changes: Oestrogens in climacteric women. *Medical Journal of Australia, 2*(10), 528–531.

Wren, B. G., & Routledge, A. D. (1983, August). The effect of type and dose of oestrogen on the blood pressure of post-menopausal women. *Maturitas, 5*(2), 135–142.

Wyman, S. M., Munier, W. B., & Spencer, E. R., Jr. (1981, August 13). Osteoporosis. *New England Journal of Medicine. 305*(7), 397–399.

Yen, S. S. C. (1977, June). The biology of menopause. *The Journal of Reproductive Medicine, 18*(6), 287–295.

Zajac, D. L. (1983). Women's health: Problems and options. An overview. *Issues in Health Care of Women, 6*, 287–310.

Ziel, H. K., & Finkle, W. D. (1975, December 4). Increased risk of endometrial carcinoma among users of conjugated estrogens. *New England Journal of Medicine, 293*(23), 1167–1170.

SECTION VI

The Supportive Role

The Supportive and Extended Roles

The involvement of most primary women's health care providers in the areas of sexuality, sexual abuse, infertility, abortion, and sterilization is fourfold: screening, teaching and counseling, referral, and, at times, post-procedure care. Screening involves identifying problems or needs and, when possible, their causes. Teaching and counseling includes preventive measures, self-help, and, where appropriate, as for a woman seeking an abortion or sterilization, all components of informed consent (see the introduction to Section II for a complete discussion of informed consent). Referral involves collaborating with the patient to find an appropriate source of care for a particular problem. A variety of referrals may be made, or several diagnostic or treatment options may be given. Referral systems must be developed that include gynecologists and gynecologic endocrinologists, urologists, and specialists in such areas as infertility, and sexual counselors and other therapists, who may include social workers, psychologists, and psychiatrists. Practitioners should also become familiar with self-help, support, or special interest groups, such as Resolve for patients with infertility. Management may be assumed by the nonphysician for post-abortion care and ongoing gynecologic assessment following sterilization.

Some primary care practitioners may provide services that go beyond these four-fold functions. Some practitioners, for example, insert laminaria before abortion, others perform semen analysis and may actively participate in treatments for infertility such as artificial insemination. Some perform diagnostic ultrasounds. Practitioners may be competent to provide in-depth sexual counseling.

The extent to which a given practitioner becomes involved in direct care in these areas depends upon her personal interest, patient needs, and availability of other services in her geographic region. Generally, expertise is developed through continuing education and ongoing performance of a particular function. References provided in the bibliographies of these chapters can be consulted for additional information as can gynecology or specialized textbooks. The American College of Nurse-Midwives provides guidelines for the incorporation of a new function into practice and these appear as Appendix II.

25

Sexual Health

Marian E. Dunn*

Sexuality is an important aspect of many women's lives. It adds greatly to feeling intimate and loving, is a form of adult play, helps enhance a woman's sense of femaleness, and often is life affirming. Practitioners concerned about total health care ought not to neglect this area. Women often turn to their care providers for information, reassurance, guidance, and support.

What interferes with professional availability to address sexual concerns? Many times practitioners feel uncomfortable discussing sexual matters, worrying about a lack of knowledge or inexperience. The practitioner may not be sure of her own sexual responses and may wonder whether those responses are unusual or idiosyncratic. She may believe that it would be voyeuristic to ask sexual questions and may fear offending patients. Practitioners are not always used to speaking openly, yet professionally, about an intimate area like sexuality. All of these feelings may collude to keep the practitioner silent or cause her to deflect patients' questions. Feeling comfortable talking about sexuality develops with practice.

In this chapter, we review the female and male sexual response cycles, discuss the components of a sexual history and offer methods for asking questions about sexuality, outline a simple model for helping patients with sexual concerns, and provide strategies for the practitioner to use in the brief counseling setting. Through these discussions, some of the commonly encountered sexual problems of women are addressed. Aspects of sexuality that relate specifically to sexually transmitted diseases are covered in Chapters 2, 4, 11, and 12.

Although the clinical illustrations used in this chapter are of heterosexual women, homosexual patients often have similar questions and concerns. It is often bias and apprehension that make it difficult for lesbian patients to receive the same quality of counseling all women deserve.

Adolescent and aging women may have specific sexual needs (Bernhard & Dan, 1986). See Section V for discussion of some of their particular sexual concerns.

THE SEXUAL RESPONSE CYCLE

Although a discussion of all facets of sexuality is beyond the scope of a single chapter, familiarity with current understanding of sexual response is important for the practitioner interested in providing some sexual counseling to patients. Two models of the sexual response cycle have been proposed: the Masters and Johnson model and the Kaplan model. It is important to remember that Masters and Johnson's data are based on observations of healthy volunteers in their laboratory. These volunteers had to be both coitally and manually orgasmic while being wired, observed, and monitored. The extent to which these observations can be generalized to the population at large is not known.

Masters and Johnson (1966) have divided both the female and male sexual response cycles into four separate phases: excitement, plateau, orgasm, resolution. Although acknowledging variations in sexual reactions, Masters and Johnson propose one major pattern of sexual response for men (Fig. 25–1) and three for women (Fig. 25–2). In the male, rearousal is impossible during the refractory period of the cycle. The three female patterns reflect the woman's ability to achieve single orgasm, multiple orgasm, or a return to resolution from the plateau phase without orgasm.

Each of the four phases of the sexual response cycle involves distinct physiologic reactions, genitally and extragenitally. Briefly, in the female, body responses to the four phases are as follows (adapted from Hogan, 1985, and Masters & Johnson, 1966):

Excitement

Genital response (Fig. 25–3): vaginal lubrication, resulting from vasocongestion around and in the vagina, referred to as a sweating reaction; vaginal lengthening and distension; thinning and flattening of the labia majora with separation and elevation away from the vaginal outlet in nulliparous women; venous distension of the labia majora in parous women; engorgement and protrusion of the labia minora; increase in the size of the clitoral glans; uterine elevation away from the vagina and bladder.

Extragenital response: nipple erection; venous engorgement of the breasts; increase in breast size.

Plateau

Genital response (Fig. 25–4): vasocongestion of the anterior third of the vagina, called the orgasmic platform; slight increase in width and depth of the vagina; elevation of the cervix creating a tenting effect in the midvagina and increasing the vaginal transcervical depth (except when the

Much of the structure and content of this chapter was developed during years of cooperative and pleasurable team teaching with Leonore Tiefer, PhD.

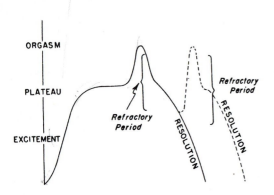

Figure 25-1. The male sexual response cycle. *(From Masters, W. H. & Johnson, V. E. [1966].* Human sexual response. *New York: Little, Brown, p. 5. Reprinted with permission.)*

uterus is markedly retroverted); increase in labial diameter with vivid color changes—pink to bright red in nulliparous women and bright red to deep wine in parous women; elevation and retraction of the clitoral body (shaft and glans).

Extragenital response: areolar engorgement; increased breast size in the woman who has never breastfed; mottling of the breast skin; engorgement of the tissues around the nipple, which decreases the evidence of nipple erection; sex flush of the breasts and chest wall; perspiration; myotonia; hyperventilation; tachycardia; increased blood pressure.

Orgasm

Genital response (Fig. 25-5): lengthening of the vaginal cul-de-sac; vaginal and uterine contractions; contraction of the external rectal sphincter and pelvic floor muscles. Controversy exists as to whether some women experience ejaculation during orgasm. Some researchers (Ladas, Whipple, & Perry, 1982) have demonstrated the existence of an ejaculate after orgasmic stimulation of the G spot (see Chapter 1), but this finding has not been widely accepted.

Extragenital response: hyperventilation, tachycardia, increased blood pressure; muscular tension throughout the body with rhythmic contractions; involuntary distension of the external urinary meatus.

Resolution

Genital response (Fig. 25-6): return of the labia to their usual color within seconds and their unstimulated thickness and position within minutes, although they may remain edematous if orgasm has not occurred; descent of the clitoris to its unstimulated position within seconds, although venous engorgement may persist if orgasm has not occurred; return of the vagina to its unstimulated size within minutes; return of the cervix and uterus to its usual position; minimal dilation of the external cervical os for up to 20 or 30 minutes if orgasm has occurred.

Extragenital response: disappearance of the mottling of the breast and sex flush; return of normal muscle tone, heart and respiratory rate, and blood pressure within minutes.

In the postmenopausal woman, all of these responses occur, but less dramatically. Chapter 24 describes menopausal changes that affect genital reactions.

The Kaplan Model

In contrast to the preceding four-phase model, Kaplan (1979, p. 9) believes that the sexual response cycle in both females and males is actually triphasic. Phase 1 is desire, which is "an appetite or drive . . . produced by the activation of a specific neural system in the brain." The physiology of this phase is not entirely understood but an interaction between the sex hormone testosterone and possibly luteinizing hormone–releasing factor (LH-RF) and neurotransmitters in the brain may be involved. Serotonin and dopamine may respectively inhibit and stimulate desire. Phases 2 and 3 of Kaplan's model involve the genital organs. Phase 2 consists of excitement or the genital vasocongestive reaction, which leads to penile erection in men and vaginal lubrication and swelling in women. The third phase comprises the reflex clonic muscular contractions that constitute orgasm in both genders. The functions of vasocongestion and orgasm differ in their nervous system innervation (parasympathetic and sympathetic, respectively); their vulnerability to the effects of physical trauma, drugs, and aging; and the clinical syndromes produced by dysfunction (Kaplan, 1974).

Because of the differences in the physiology of the three phases, the triphasic model is useful in providing a framework for sexual therapy. Most sexual dysfunction can be classified as disturbances of desire, excitement, or orgasm. Identifying whether a problem relates to desire, vasocongestion, or orgasm can help the practitioner assess its cause and determine treatment. Disorder of desire include hypo-

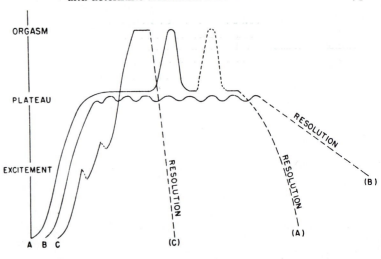

Figure 25-2. The female sexual response cycle. *(From Masters, W. H. & Johnson, V. E. [1966].* Human sexual response. *New York: Little, Brown, p. 5. Reprinted with permission.)*

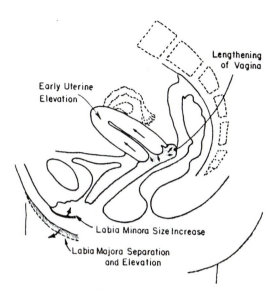

Figure 25-3. Female genital response: Excitement phase. *(From Masters, W. H. & Johnson, V. E. [1966]. Human sexual response. New York: Little, Brown, p. 72. Reprinted with permission.)*

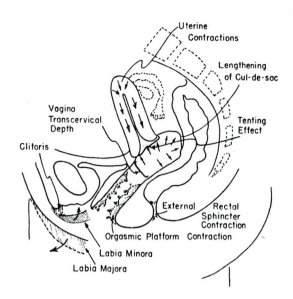

Figure 25-5. Female genital response: Orgasmic phase. *(From Masters, W. H. & Johnson, V. E. [1966]. Human sexual response. New York: Little, Brown, p. 77. Reprinted with permission.)*

active sexual desire and inhibition of desire. Disorders of excitement include difficulty with lubrication in the female and, in the male, erectile dysfunction (difficulty in attaining or maintaining an erection). Disturbances of orgasm vary in both males and females from mild situational difficulties to total anorgasmia. According to Kaplan, only vaginismus, the involuntary painful spasm of the vaginal muscles, certain types of male ejaculatory pain, and sexual phobias do not relate to a particular sexual phase (1979, pp. 21–22).

The practitioner must, of course, always bear in mind that the physiologic manifestations of sexual response form but one small part of the sexual experience. Sexuality must be seen within the context of a woman's entire life (Kitzinger, 1983); it relates to her emotions, relationships, and life choices. It is a way of communicating and an expression of trust (Bernhard & Dan, 1986).

MANAGEMENT OF SEXUAL CONCERNS

Setting the Stage—Creating an Atmosphere

Availability to discuss sexual matters is signaled in many ways: by the questions asked, but perhaps even more important, by the practitioner's manner, both verbal and non-verbal. Interest is communicated by maintaining eye contact and projecting a relaxed yet attentive body language—all the subtle physical signs that encourage discussion and openness. When the practitioner nods, leans forward, or shows that she is following the patient's story with other cues, it is easier for the patient to continue talking. People often feel most open when there is an atmosphere of privacy. In some clinic settings, true privacy is difficult to achieve. Taking the patient aside to arrange for quiet, pri-

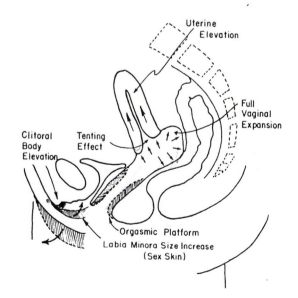

Figure 25-4. Female genital response: Plateau phase. *(From Masters, W. H. & Johnson, V. E. [1966]. Human sexual response. New York: Little, Brown, p. 76. Reprinted with permission.)*

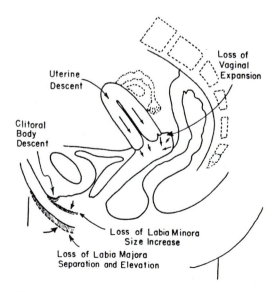

Figure 25-6. Female genital response: Resolution phase. *(From Masters, W. H. & Johnson, V. E. [1966]. Human sexual response. New York: Little, Brown, p. 78. Reprinted with permission.)*

vate space communicates sensitivity. In more difficult physical settings, practitioners can create an atmosphere of privacy by the intensity of their interest and the quality of their attention. Patients respond best when the practitioner seems not to be rushed. A clearer sexual history can be taken in a shorter time when the practitioner gives the impression of not being pressured for time.

Language

Practitioners are sometimes concerned about what language to use when asking or talking about sexuality. Both highly technical/medical terms for genitals or sexual activities and slang terms that often have pejorative connotations may seem inappropriate. Using lots of synonyms can help. To a technical term like "vaginal lubrication," the practitioner can add "when you get wet." The practitioner can speak of "intercourse," "penetration," "having sex," "orgasm," "coming," "climaxing," and so forth. The use of several descriptive words can ensure the practitioner that the patient understands her meaning and that she understands the patient's meaning. Simple, clear language is best. If the patient uses a pet term, check out the meaning. Adopting the patient's language can sometimes foster communication. If a woman speaks, for example, of "not wanting to be bothered" when she means she is not interested in having sex, using her phrase may help her feel understood.

Repeating back to the patient the essence of what you have understood her to say provides immediate feedback. "If I hear you correctly, you do desire your husband but when he starts making love to you, he seems to rush the foreplay and you do not get excited enough. Do I have it right?" The patient is then free to clarify or expand or correct what you believe you have heard. Never be afraid to check out what you believe you have heard. Patients are often vague, or a bit confused. Messages are not always clearly sent or received. By periodically checking out what you have heard, you can ensure greater understanding.

It is best not to interrupt when the patient is speaking, unless she is drifting in all directions. In that case, help the woman to focus on the central issue that concerns her. "It looks like many things are bothering you. What is the most important thing you would like my help with? What troubles you the most?"

The time-honored technique of asking "Can you tell me more about that?" is preferable to asking specific questions again and again. This allows the woman to choose the direction in which she would like to go. When we ask the patient to clarify, to give us a fuller picture, she leads and becomes more focused and better organized. If the patient seems genuinely stuck or unable to put her feelings or questions into words, it is sometimes useful to offer some possible choices. For example, a woman may be struggling to describe a lack of interest in sex. If she is unable to point to what is troubling her, the practitioner should think through a variety of possibilities. "Is it that she never has sexual thoughts or feelings, or occasionally has desire, but when an opportunity exists rejects it, or is it that she feels desire and is aroused but gets turned off in the middle of activity?" Suggesting these possibilities to the patient may give her a chance to consider her own situation and express her particular feelings and concerns.

Data Collection

Introducing Sexual Topics. Three excellent techniques can be used to introduce the topic of sexuality into clinical practice: asking questions as a routine part of the review of systems or gynecologic history; using permission-giving questions; and incorporating discussion of sexuality into the physical examination.

REVIEW OF SYSTEMS/HISTORY TAKING. In a setting where the practitioner is reviewing systems or taking a comprehensive history, it is appropriate to routinely include some trigger questions during the genitourinary review or gynecologic history. Three questions are useful and address three common dysfunctions in women: problems of lubrication, orgasmic difficulties, and dyspareunia.

1. "Any trouble with lubrication, 'getting wet,' during sex?"
2. "Any trouble with orgasm, coming, climaxing?"
3. "Any pain during sex?"

If the woman has a sexual concern that is different from these, she will usually volunteer it. She may say no to all questions but tell you she has not felt any desire lately. She may say no to all questions on this occasion, but on her next visit spontaneously bring up a problem. The stage has been set with these trigger questions. The patient can use the opportunity or choose to use it in a later visit.

Often the trigger questions serve to make women conscious of subtle physical changes that have been disturbing them. Women often equate, for example, how much desire they have for how aroused they are by how well they lubricate. Lubrication may be diminished in the estrogen-deprived woman, postmenopausal woman, breastfeeding woman, or woman on certain medications, such as antihypertensives, antihistamines, anticholinergic drugs, or psychotropics (Kaufman, 1983b). Sometimes a woman may describe herself as having less desire when she has noticed less copious lubrication, is alarmed by it, and sees it as a sign of diminished arousal. Her worry about inadequate lubrication may further inhibit her from becoming aroused, setting up a vicious cycle. This demonstrates the importance of considering all components of a woman's health history in evaluating sexual problems, particularly her age and menstrual status, chronic illnesses, and current medications.

Some women accept a level of pain during sex without bringing it to a professional's attention. This might be pain experienced during penetration, deep thrusting, or orgasm. Often a vicious cycle develops. The woman has the experience of pain and anticipates it when she is going to have sex. Her apprehension may cause her to tighten up, to become less aroused, to lubricate less, all increasing her discomfort. Sex becomes repeatedly and increasingly uncomfortable. Although the origin of the difficulty might have been mild pain or an organic or treatable cause, the pain ends up causing apprehension and inhibition of arousal. The woman then ends up with a psychological sexual problem too.

If a woman has pain, ask her to describe exactly where and when she feels the pain. It is then possible to look for organic causes during the gynecologic examination. If the cause of the dyspareunia is a minor irritation or infection or something more pronounced, such as a Bartholin's cyst or abscess, endometriosis, or pelvic inflammatory disease, treatment can be initiated (Kaufman, 1983a). If treatment is inadvisable, such as in mild obstetric scarring or a small fibroid causing pain during deep thrusting, the patient can be informed and given suggestions for greater comfort. Shallower penetration that avoids vigorous pressure on the uterus may help if the uterus or cervix is sensitive. The woman can control the depth of the thrusts by communicating with her partner or by keeping her hands at the base of her partner's penis. If there is a sensitive area in the vagina, the woman can angle her body so that the thrusting is not against that area. The woman can thus avoid discomfort and have more pleasure.

PERMISSION-GIVING QUESTION. When a review of systems is not done, an alternative way of initiating a discussion of sexual concerns is to begin with a permission-giving statement, that is, a phrase that makes having a sexual question or concern acceptable. "Most pregnant women have questions about sex and pregnancy; what questions do you have?" The first half of the statement gives the woman permission to have a question, as "most women" do. The second half is a query phrased on the assumption that the woman has a question. This encourages her more than when the practitioner asks, "Do you have any questions?" She can more easily say "no" in the latter context. For almost any clinical situation, a permission-giving question exists. "Many women I see have questions or concerns about sex; what questions do you have?" is a broadly applicable example.

GYNECOLOGIC EXAMINATION. The gynecologic examination presents an appropriate situation for attending to sexual issues. An area of tenderness, a pale and dry vagina mucosa, an atrophic vagina—all can affect sexual response. If such conditions are found, ask the patient if she experiences pain or vaginal dryness or has some difficulty with penetration. This can be very useful for the woman who may never have connected her discomfort with any organic cause, and who may be shy talking about what are to her seemingly minor sexual concerns. An involuntary muscle spasm or constriction of the musculature surrounding the outer portion of the vagina is indicative of a more serious, involuntary problem—vaginismus.

Brief Sexual History. A useful sexual history can be gathered in about 10 minutes. The technique presented here is a modification of Annon's (1975). It is suitable for the clinician in practice because of its brevity yet thoroughness.

1. *What is the problem?* Clarify, focus, get a clear picture.
2. *Problem's onset and course.* Ascertain when and how the problem began, when it is better or worse, and what events precipitate it. Does it occur in all situations, during all acts, with all partners?
3. *Why the patient thinks she has the problem?* Learn about her myths and misconceptions, significant life events, any sexual traumas.
4. *Patient's attempts at solution.* Ask the patient what she has tried, how often, with what success?

When these questions are answered, the practitioner is in a good position to help the patient. The picture is fairly complete. Each case situation, of course, is different. In some circumstances all this information is not needed. In others, it is necessary to have a sense of the answers to most of these questions.

WHAT IS THE PROBLEM? Helping the woman organize her thoughts and present her sexual difficulties in a clear manner is among the most useful functions of the practitioner. Problems are more solvable when someone can point to what is causing specific difficulties. Therefore, the first intervention of the sexual history, asking the woman to describe exactly what is bothering her, in itself is beneficial. People often couch complaints in vague terms, for example, "not in the mood lately," "not feeling turned on." By helping the patient clarify and focus in on what is disturbing,

both practitioner and patient become clearer about the source of the difficulty and more capable of providing solutions.

Patient: Oh, I'm not feeling turned on lately.

Practitioner: Can you tell me more? What do you mean "not turned on"?

Patient: I feel like having sex, but when we start making love, I lose it.

Practitioner: You "lose it"? Can you tell me what you and your partner are doing together and what you are feeling before you "lose it" and what you mean by "losing it"?

Patient: Well, we are petting, I feel excited, I get very excited and then we go to have intercourse and I feel less excited.

Practitioner: So, if I understand you right, you feel excited during the petting, but when your partner penetrates, the excitement goes down?

Patient: Yes.

Practitioner: Why do you think that happens? What are you feeling? What are you thinking at the time?

Patient: Well, when he is touching me, I feel very excited but the intercourse is not as exciting. I think I wish he would touch me more, because I know I will lose it during intercourse.

Practitioner: So, you really enjoy being touched (on your genitals or on your breasts?) but you feel less during intercourse and you expect to lose excitement once it begins? Is that right?

Patient: Yes, that is it.

PROBLEM'S ONSET AND COURSE. Health care practitioners are used to inquiring about symptoms and trying to find their causes. A sexual symptom is not very different. When did the woman's problem begin? Has she always had this problem? With all her partners? In all sexual situations, on vacations, when children are away, when feeling romantic? During all kinds of sexual stimulation? Does she have difficulty during petting, during oral sex, during intercourse? Are there times when her problem has been better, or worse? What else was going on in the patient's life when her problem began? All these questions need not be asked or answered in every case, but they suggest the kind of information that may be important to have.

Practitioner: When did you begin to feel that you were losing excitement? Has this always been true for you with your partner?

Patient: Well, before we were married, we used to pet for hours. Usually I would feel very excited and I even came before we had intercourse. I guess the trouble began after we got married.

Practitioner: What seemed different? Why do you think this happened?

Patient: Well, I have not thought about it before, but I think the petting is much shorter. We are together more. We get down to business faster.

Practitioner: So, before marriage, foreplay was much longer; now it is more rushed?

Patient: Yes.

Practitioner: Why do you think?

Patient: I think my husband rushes more to get to intercourse.

Practitioner: You used to enjoy longer petting. Now you feel a little rushed. Have you ever let your husband know that?

Patient: No, I did not realize it myself until now.

WHY THE PATIENT THINKS SHE HAS THE PROBLEM. People often have ideas about why a sexual problem has developed. It is a good idea to find out what the patient believes caused the problem or why the problem is continuing. People are often strongly influenced by myths, fears, and misinformation.

Practitioner: When you have thought about it, why do you think you have this problem?

Patient: Well, I don't know, but I used to masturbate when I was in college. Maybe I've gotten too used to being touched to have an orgasm and I've ruined myself for having intercourse. Can that happen?

PATIENT'S ATTEMPTS AT SOLUTION. People sometimes feel helpless in being able to change a situation, but most often they have attempted to solve a problem themselves. Sometimes the approach was misguided or based on misinformation ("If I avoid sex for a while, maybe I'll feel more turned on"). Occasionally, patients are overaggressive or say some things that hurt or offend their partners ("You have always been a lousy lover," "You are selfish"). Sometimes they have used the right approach to solve the problem, but have used it sporadically or incorrectly, for example, the patient who reads about self-stimulation as a means to learn orgasm, tries the technique once for a few seconds, and then gives up. It is good to ascertain the solutions the patient has tried and how these have worked out for her.

Practitioner: What have you tried to do to feel more turned on?

Patient: I thought if I had less sex, it might help, but it didn't. I tried telling myself to concentrate more. That didn't work. I wonder if you might find something physical; perhaps my clitoris is too small. Nothing I've done so far has worked.

WHAT THE PATIENT WOULD LIKE FROM YOU. The practitioner can get a good sense of what the patient wants from her as the history unfolds. Some patients seem to want reassurance and information. They may believe that their problem is organic in origin, and sometimes may want referral to a specialist. In the case presented here, the patient seems to need information, reassurance, and some simple suggestions. She wonders whether there is an anatomic problem (too small a clitoris). She worries that masturbation might have harmed her. She imagined that sexual abstinence might make her more easily aroused.

In using the brief sexual history technique with this patient, the practitioner gathered valuable information within a short period. The question now is what is a useful way for the practitioner to intervene.

Intervention: The P-LI-SS-IT Model

The PLISSIT model for sexual counseling provides four different levels of approach to sexual difficulties (Annon, 1975): *Permission, Limited Information, Specific Sugges-* tions, and *Intensive Therapy;* hence the acronym PLISSIT. The model moves from the simplest level of intervention, permission, to the most complex and highly skilled level of intervention, intensive therapy. The first three intervention levels can be implemented by any health care practitioner who is interested. Intensive therapy requires special training in sexual therapy.

Permission. Permission giving is meant to help the patient feel more comfortable about thoughts, feelings, and reactions. Many persons wonder whether their sexual responses, fantasies, and past or present behaviors are "normal." Because sexuality is not discussed openly, many are often concerned about whether their own activities or thoughts are odd or unusual.

Permission giving is aimed at making patients feel more relaxed and comfortable with what they are describing; examples are the statements "many women feel . . ." "some women enjoy . . ." and "other women are uncomfortable with. . . ." These statements help patients put their behavior in an appropriate perspective. They no longer need to feel different for having a range of feelings or reactions. When permission-giving statements reflect diversity, as in "many persons do . . ." and "many persons do not . . ." patients are in the position of deciding for themselves which group they prefer to belong to.

Permission-giving statements are often an excellent means of encouraging sexual questions or drawing out sexual concerns. For example, the practitioner who asks a patient "Most women have some concern about sex after giving birth. What concerns do you have?" is using a permission-giving technique that gives the woman greater freedom to ask questions and voice concerns. When, in the course of taking the sexual history, the practitioner notes that "most of us feel a little uncomfortable talking about sex," it often helps facilitate the patient's ability to open up and talk.

Permission giving may be all that the patient needs from the practitioner. Young or inexperienced women often simply wish to be reassured that what they feel or think falls into the normal range. When issued by the professional, a person in a position of authority, permission-giving statements are believable. Sometimes, all the practitioner does is reassure a woman and give her permission to continue doing exactly what she has been doing. The importance of this technique, however, should not be minimized.

The permission-giving statement also can be helpful when a patient asks what the practitioner would do in a particular sexual situation or what the practitioner does in her own sex life. A professional and sensitive response might be, "It doesn't matter what I do in my own life but I think it is important that you know that many women do enjoy that activity and there are many women who do not. What do you think you might feel comfortable doing? What do you think you might enjoy?" In this way, the practitioner has removed herself from direct personal questioning and yet has been of use to the patient; she has helped the patient to understand that although there is nothing abnormal about what she is describing, it is up to her to decide whether a particular behavior suits her needs.

Limited Information. A practitioner provides limited information usually in conjunction with permission giving. This factual information about sexual concerns, sexual practices, and sexual response is geared specifically to the problem or question presented by the patient. Correcting myths and misinformaton and teaching the woman about her body and how her body works are part of the limited information level. At this level the practitioner serves as sex educator, passing on to the patient corrective information, as shown in these examples: "Most women need to feel relaxed to become aroused and to lubricate." "After menopause, women may find that it takes longer for them to become more lubricated." "During the last trimester of pregnancy, many women feel somewhat uncomfortable about having sexual intercourse." All of these statements aim at providing a particular patient with information about something that is bothering her.

In the case discussed earlier, for example, permission giving and limited information might be combined as follows:

Practitioner: From what you have told me, it might be that you are more aroused by manual stimulation than you are by intercourse. There are many women who seem to be more sensitive to touch than to coitus. When you and your husband had long periods of petting, you became aroused and were orgasmic. Now, as you described it, when the foreplay is much shorter, you have difficulty becoming as aroused and reaching a climax.

Patient: But wouldn't a normal woman be aroused and excited by intercourse and able to come just from intercourse?

Practitioner: Some women are orgasmic from intercourse alone, but many seem to need the extra stimulation of direct clitoral stimulation to reach an orgasm. You can find both reactions among normal, healthy, passionate women. We believe this to be a natural and healthy response, not a problem.

In this exchange, the practitioner has provided the patient with some limited information—corrective information to clear up misunderstandings and to educate about sexual functioning. The permission-giving statements are woven in to give the woman a sense of her own normality. For example, this patient seems to be a woman who is more easily orgasmic through manual stimulation. She may be able, now, to feel a little more comfortable with her own sexual response. The practitioner could go on to correct the misunderstandings about masturbation and the belief that perhaps there is something anatomically wrong. She could discuss more fully the role and responses of the clitoris in orgasm and give the woman the opportunity to view her external and internal genitalia with a mirror during the pelvic examination (see Chapter 3).

Specific Suggestions. At the third level of intervention, the practitioner offers the patient specific suggestions for improving sexual technique, achieving greater response, enhancing communication with a partner, or selecting positions and sexual activities in specific types of situations. To provide helpful suggestions, the practitioner needs to have some knowledge of sexual response and some knowledge of how sexual response is interfered with or affected by a variety of health, illness, and disability states (see, for example, Kolodny, Masters, & Johnson, 1979). A specific suggestion, for example, for a postpartum woman might be to suggest extending foreplay to allow for the increased time needed for vaginal lubrication or to use a topical lubricant; many over-the-counter water-based, lubricants are available today that are designed to feel like natural lubrication. A specific suggestion with regard to enhancing overall sex-

ual response might be to encourage a particular patient to read a book on developing orgasmic potential and increasing sexual pleasure, such as those by Barbach (1975) and Heiman, LoPiccolo, and LoPiccolo (1976). Very often, the practitioner may suggest that the patient talk to her partner about what is bothering her or read a book, such as that by Zilbergeld (1978), on male sexuality to sensitize herself to the psychological and social sexual conditioning of the male.

These specific suggestions might be used in the case presented in this chapter:

Practitioner: I guess if we understand what has been happening for you, it sounds like you need the longer foreplay that you and you husband used to enjoy?

Patient: Yes, I guess that's true. I suppose I have been feeling a bit rushed.

Practitioner: Have you ever spoken to your husband about this and let him know how you feel?

Patient: No, I haven't . . . ah . . . I didn't realize it myself. Do you think I should?

Practitioner: Well, it might be a good idea. What do you think you might say to him to let him know how you feel?

Patient: Well, I guess I could tell him that I used to really like it when we took longer petting and that I miss that and could we do that more.

Practitioner: That sounds like a good idea. How do you think he would respond?

Patient: Oh, John's a real sweetie. I think if he knew that I needed it, he'd be happy to go along with me.

Several things occurred during this encounter. The practitioner encouraged the woman to talk to her partner, checked out how the woman would talk to her partner and what she might say, and affirmed her right to do so. When encouraging patients to speak to partners, it is often beneficial to find out what they plan to say. Sometimes, the patient may be planning to say something that is overaggressive or might be hurtful or cause discord. Helping the patient to rephrase her remarks in a constructive, more positively communicative manner can be useful.

In a difficult situation, the practitioner might choose to role play with the patient how she might express herself to her partner. For example, if the woman is planning to tell her partner that his touch is "too rough," the practitioner can encourage her to rephrase her statement more positively. "It would really feel wonderful if you touched me with light strokes." Most partners respond favorably when told what would feel good or exciting, but recoil from criticism. Verbal and nonverbal cues that indicate pleasure are erotic and tend to invite repetition.

It is generally easier for health care practitioners to offer suggestions than to listen and encourage the patient to formulate her own solutions. It is more therapeutic, however, to serve primarily as facilitator, to help the patient brainstorm and figure out her own solutions whenever possible. This leaves the woman with a greater sense of self-esteem and with enhanced problem-solving ability. The suggestions that are provided should not overwhelm the patient. It is better to offer one or two suggestions that can be followed up with the woman. When patients are given too many possibilities, they often feel confused and are unable to implement any of them.

Intensive Therapy. Intensive therapy, the final and deepest level of intervention, should not be attempted by a practitioner who has not had advanced training in sexual therapy, marital therapy, or psychotherapy. In general, appropriate referral for intensive therapy may be indicated if a patient seems overwhelmed by anxiety, has great difficulty in listening and talking, and/or has been given permission, limited information, and specific suggestions and has been unable to utilize any of them. Referral for sexual therapy should be made with care, as in most states, a person does not require a license to call her- or himself a sexual therapist. Usually, the best way to find a qualified therapist is to contact a major teaching hospital's sexual therapy unit and ask for a referral. The American Association of Sex Educators, Counselors, and Therapists (AASECT), based in Washington, DC, provides a directory of fully trained, qualified sexual therapists.

The practitioner of well-woman gynecology has the opportunity to help women feel more comfortable with the sexual part of their lives. Often, simple, educative counseling can alleviate tremendous pain and anxiety. Sexual health is a vital component of well-woman gynecology.

REFERENCES

Annon, J. S. (1975). *Behavioral treatment of sexual problems.* Vol. I. *Brief Therapy.* New York: Harper & Row.

Barbach, L. G. (1975). *For yourself: The fulfillment of female sexuality.* Garden City, NY: Doubleday.

Bernhard, L. A., & Dan, A. J. (1986, March). Redefining sexuality from women's own experiences. *Nursing Clinics of North America, 21*(1), 125–136.

Heiman, J., LoPiccolo, J., & LoPiccolo, L. (1976). *Becoming orgasmic: A sexual growth program for women.* Englewood Cliffs, NJ: Prentice–Hall.

Hogan, R. (1985). *Human sexuality: A nursing perspective.* East Norwalk, CT: Appleton–Century–Crofts.

Kaplan, H. S. (1974). *The new sex therapy.* New York: Brunner/Mazel.

Kaplan, H. S. (1979). *Disorders of sexual desire and other new concepts and techniques in sex therapy.* New York: Simon & Schuster.

Kaufman, S. A. (1983a). The gynecologic evaluation of female dyspareunia and unconsummated marriage. In H. S. Singer (Ed.), *The evaluation of sexual disorders: Psychological and medical aspects.* New York: Brunner/Mazel.

Kaufman, S. A. (1983b). The gynecologic evaluation of female excitement disorders. In H. S. Singer (Ed.), *The evaluation of sexual disorders: Psychological and medical aspects.* New York: Brunner/Mazel.

Kitzinger, S. (1983). *Woman's experience of sex: The facts and feelings of female sexuality at every stage of life.* New York: Penguin Books.

Kolodny, R. B., Masters, W. H., & Johnson, V. E. (1979). *Textbook of sexual medicine.* Boston: Little, Brown.

Ladas, A. K., Whipple, B., & Perry, J. D. (1982). *The G spot and other recent discoveries about human sexuality.* New York: Holt, Rinehart & Winston.

Masters, W. H., & Johnson, V. E. (1966). *Human sexual response.* Boston: Little, Brown.

Zilbergeld, B. (1978). *Male sexuality.* Boston: Little, Brown.

26

Sexual Abuse

Judith V. Becker and Emily Coleman

Sexual abuse is a major concern for the majority of women in our society: those who have been sexually victimized, those who will be victimized, and those who will, fortunately, somehow avoid sexual abuse are all affected to various degrees by this threat. Sexual abuse can have long-lasting traumatic effects. Additionally, fear of sexual abuse seriously restricts women's life-styles, job opportunities, and general freedom of movement. Women rank rape second only to murder in listing crimes that generate fear (Heath, Rigen, Gordon, & LeBailly, 1979).

In this chapter, sexual abuse is defined and its incidence is discussed. The myths generated around the subject of sexual abuse are addressed, as is management of the acute case of abuse. Short- and long-term sequelae and treatment are outlined and prevention is reviewed.

DEFINITION

Definitions of sexual abuse or rape vary both in the legal system and in the attitudes of the general population. Traditionally, sexual abuse or rape has been defined as intercourse physically forced on a woman by a man. This is a very limited definition excluding marital rape, date rape, sexual abuse of men, and nonintercourse sexual abuse. For the purpose of this chapter, any nonconsensual sexual act is considered sexual abuse. Practitioners should be knowledgeable regarding their state sexual abuse laws.

INCIDENCE

There are several methods of assessing the incidence of sexual abuse in our society. Whether the data are gained through crime statistics, reports through victim agencies, retrospective studies, or studies of the offenders themselves, the numbers are staggering.

The reliability of information obtained through crime reports is hampered by more than differences across jurisdictions and over time. Variations in local legal codes, crime enforcement, accuracy, and completeness of record keeping contribute to underreporting of sexual abuse (Rabkin, 1979). In addition, the victim of sexual abuse has often been reluctant to come forward, fearing a second victimization by the police or legal system. Too frequently, significant others, crucial sources of support at this time, have accused the victim of complicity and withdraw from them. All of these factors lead to further underreporting of sexual abuse. Data indicate that minimally 2.2 rapes are actually committed for every one reported (Curtis, 1975). The Law Enforcement Assistance Administration (LEAA) (1975a, 1975b) has noted that 40 to 50 percent of forcible rapes are reported.

In 1980, the FBI statistics reported the rate of rape to be 71 per 100,000 women (U.S. Department of Justice, 1980). This statistic becomes more impressive when the data on underreporting are considered. In the last 40 years, rape has had the greatest increase among crimes (Bowker, 1979). Nevertheless, conviction rates for rape are among the lowest for any crime. According to FBI figures, of every 100 reported cases of rape, there are 51 arrests. Sixteen of these arrests are convictions for forcible rape, and four are convictions for lesser charges (Rabkin, 1979).

Studies of both victim populations and offender populations also point to the severity of this problem. A retrospective study of 1,200 college-aged women indicated that 26 percent of these women had been sexually abused before age 13 (Gagnon, 1965).

Usually, the offender is not a reliable or valid source of information; yet, most of the data regarding incidence rates are from incarcerated offenders whose self-reports are questionable. When Abel, Becker, Blanchard, and Flanagan (1981) offered confidentiality to rapists participating in an outpatient treatment clinic, the rapists reported an average of six victims.

RAPE MYTHS

Myths about rape are believed by both men and women, victim and offender, young and old. False beliefs regarding sexual abuse tend to exonerate the offender, shift blame to the victim, and lead to the victim's feelings of guilt. It is important that everyone in our society be educated regarding sexual abuse. One common rape myth is that women provoke rape, or ask for it, through various means; for example, (1) by wearing provocative clothes (tight jeans, no bra, etc.), (2) by going to dangerous places (to a bar alone, to a man's apartment, on the street alone at night), (3) by behaving in a suspect manner (flirting, talking to strangers). Believing the preceding serves two functions: the victim population can feel safe by thinking that only certain women get abused sexually, and offenders can feel that the victims deserved what they got.

The reality is that anyone can be abused sexually any-where, anytime. Not only young women are raped; babies and the aged are also victims. One study notes that victims range in age from 15 months to 81 years (Hayman & Lanza, 1971). Correspondingly, anyone can be the perpetrator of sexual abuse: doctors, lawyers, priests, husbands, fathers, welfare recipients, young girls, and young boys. Sexual abuse is a crime of opportunity (Amir, 1971), and victims are selected on the basis of their availability, not their physical characteristics.

Sexual abuse is also not recognized in certain circumstances. Rape is often not perceived as rape if (1) the perpetrator is the victim's spouse, (2) the victim has previously been sexual with the perpetrator, (3) the victim is a prostitute, (4) the victim is drunk, and (5) the sexual abuse occurs during war (''All is fair in love and war''). Yet, in each of these circumstances, coercion can be employed for sexual purposes and the victim cannot consent. Other misconceptions regarding sexual abuse are exemplified by such comments as ''her lips said 'no' but her eyes said 'yes''' and ''all that woman needs is a good——.''

The media often bolster these attitudes in scenes such as that from the classic film *Gone With the Wind*. Vivian Leigh as Scarlett O'Hara smiles contentedly in the morning after being raped the night before by Clark Gable as Rhett Butler. Sexual abuse can be used to keep all women in a subservient position (Brownmiller, 1975). There are too many myths about sexual abuse to list them all here, but women and men need to be aware of these attitudes within themselves and others.

Fortunately, many states are revising their antiquated rape laws so that women who are raped by their husbands can be defined as rape victims. States are also modifying laws to make the woman's past sexual history inadmissible. Through legal reform, we will be able to ensure on at least one level that women receive justice. Society must continue, however, to confront the myths held by most people. Otherwise, even though the laws exist, jury members who hold the attitudes of society might be lax in convicting offenders.

MANAGEMENT OF CARE OF RAPE VICTIMS

Victims of sexual abuse may present at hospital emergency rooms, rape crisis centers, women's resource centers, or private clinics. Women respond to this personal crisis in different ways. Burgess and Holstrom (1973) have noted ''an expressed style'' in which the sexually abused victim openly ventilates her fear, anger, or anxiety. In such cases, crying, trembling, and restlessness may be evident. Other victims may react in a calm, subdued, and controlled manner. Some women may laugh or smile, defending against or psychologically avoiding the trauma.

Whether the woman is controlling, ventilating, or avoiding her feelings, she requires nonjudgmental support from the health care team. The task of medical personnel should not be to determine whether the rape occurred or whether the woman was at all culpable. Rather, their initial concern should be to provide the woman with needed physical and psychological care. Physical evidence should be collected in the event that the woman elects to prosecute.

Immediate Concerns

The sexual abuse victim should not be left alone. She may be accompanied by family or friends or may wish family or friends to be contacted. If available, victim advocates who are knowledgeable about medical and legal procedures can provide support throughout. The medical procedures take approximately 2 hours, excluding any waiting period. Sexual abuse victims should have a high priority in the emergency room or clinic. If a more immediate emergency takes priority, the delay should be explained to the victim. The victim should not be referred to by her first name or by such terms as ''honey.'' Treating the victim with respect and preserving her dignity are crucial. Privacy should be provided as soon as possible.

Many hospitals and clinics have written guidelines in sexual abuse cases. Several direct and comprehensive protocols are available in the literature (Bay Area Women Against Rape, 1975; Foley & Davies, 1983). Rape kits, containing instructions to the examining practitioner, specially labeled test tubes, microscopic slides, plastic bags, and combs, are available commercially or from the police. Some states require that sexual abuse cases be reported to the police, and the results of the medical examination may be used as legal evidence. The victim should be informed of this, although she does not necessarily need to make a decision on prosecuting at this time.

It is important to remember throughout the medical procedure that control and power were taken away from the woman during the sexual assault. Therefore, every effort should be made to return control to her by explaining fully the rationale and protocol involved and obtaining her written and informed consent, if she should decide to participate.

Data Collection

HISTORY. A medical and gynecologic history (see Chapter 2), as well as a description of the assault must be obtained before the physical examination to alert the practitioner to relevant information, including allergies and current medications. Again, the need for this information should be made as clear as possible. For example, it is necessary to know the day and time of last intercourse to appropriately collect evidence during the pelvic exam. Although sperm can remain in the cervix several days, they remain in the vagina only 6 to 12 hours. Therefore, if the victim had intercourse several days before the assault, the practitioner should obtain a swab from the vagina and avoid the cervix (Braen, 1980). Foley and Davies (1983) suggest recording the medical and gynecologic history on a form separate from the sexual assault history to avoid potentially biasing a jury against the victim by the use of information unrelated to the crime. Questions regarding the assault should be limited to information absolutely necessary for the location of possible evidence and trauma.

PHYSICAL ASSESSMENT. The physical assessment begins with external examination of the body to collect evidence of the sexual assault and to assess the injuries of the victim. The pubic hair is combed to collect any foreign pubic hair that may have been transferred during the assault. Whole-blood samples, saliva samples, and fingernail clippings or scrapings are also obtained. Clothing may be retained, as semen or blood stains may be present.

Careful inspection for trauma should be performed. The mouth, particularly the inside of the lips, the buttocks, the breasts, the back, and the neck are common sites of injury (Cabaniss, Scott, & Copeland, 1985). Often, this part of the physical examination is performed by a nurse (DiNitto, Martin, Norton, & Maxwell, 1986).

Pelvic Examination. Women who have not been sexually victimized often dread, fear, or avoid pelvic examinations and perceive the exam as an invasion of privacy. The lithotomy position is a particularly vulnerable one for any woman. It is important then to be sensitive to the feelings of the sexually abused woman. Meeting her when she is sitting on the examining table or on a chair in the room is preferable to meeting her in the lithotomy position. In most areas, physicians perform genital and pelvic examinations of rape victims. A model program in Florida, however, has demonstrated that nurses can perform these examinations and serve as credible witnesses in court (DiNitto et al., 1986).

The woman should be asked if she has had a pelvic exam before. Each procedure should be explained beforehand. She should be shown the speculum, which should be warmed with water (other lubricants can affect the results of the acid phosphatase test) before its use.

Lights in the examining room are then turned off. An ultraviolet light, for example, a Woods Light, is used to find semen on the body. The practitioner should look for specimens from the oral and vaginal areas, even though the victim may report only forced intercourse. Some victims are too embarrassed to admit being forced to perform fellatio or anal intercourse. Any pertinent areas showing evidence of sexual abuse are swabbed for the presence of semen. In some areas of the country, practitioners also perform an aspiration of the vaginal contents. Prostatic secretions, confirming the presence of semen, can be identified by a significant prostatic acid phosphate level, which may remain positive up to 18 hours. Examination of specimens for acid phosphate is done in the laboratory; when it is not performed quickly, the specimen should be frozen immediately (Root, Ogden, & Scott, 1974).

Careful inspection should also be made of the genital area for signs of trauma. A 1 percent solution of toluidine blue can be applied to the vaginal fourchette with a cotton-tip applicator; this chemical is easily wiped away from intact skin with lubricating jelly on a cotton swab, but when it stains blue, it indicates parakeratosis, signifying laceration (Cabaniss et al., 1985).

Routine procedures including Pap smear, gonorrhea and chlamydia cultures, and assessment of uterine or rectal tenderness and masses are completed at the end of the examination. All specimens must be dated, timed, labeled, and initialed by the examiner. Meticulous documentation, including diagrams and photographs, if the woman consents, are important (Cabaniss et al., 1985).

INFORMATION ON SEXUALLY TRANSMITTED DISEASES. It is estimated that one in 30 rape victims develops gonorrhea and one in 1,000 rape victims develops syphilis as a result of the assault (Warner, 1980). Testing at the time of the physical examination indicates only whether the victim had sexually transmitted diseases prior to the sexual assault. Therefore, it is important to emphasize the need to return for tests for gonorrhea and chlamydia in 2 weeks and for syphilis in 4 to 6 weeks. Preventive doses of penicillin may not be sufficient to cure gonorrhea or syphilis and may give the victim the mistaken impression that there is no cause for further intervention. The practitioner should present this information in a matter-of-fact way, without unduly disturbing the rape victim. Rape victims do have concerns about whether or not they will develop gonorrhea; consequently, the practitioner should stress the importance of returning for a follow-up visit. If at all possible, permission should be obtained from the victim to call in 2 weeks to remind her to return for the appointment.

Pregnancy. It has been estimated that 1 to 5 percent (Foley & Davies, 1983) of sexual assault victims become pregnant.

If the victim thinks she may already be pregnant, a urine test should be done. The sexual assault victim should be fully informed regarding the advantages and disadvantages of all the options, including postcoital oral contraception (see Chapter 7), menstrual extraction, and abortion (see Chapter 28). Again, decisions regarding treatment are made by the victim. This information should be reported to her in a nonjudgmental fashion; the practitioner should make herself available or offer the victim the services of a rape advocate to help the victim in making these decisions.

Follow-up Care. After the physical examination, the woman usually wishes to shower. Other personal needs such as clothes, mouthwash, and makeup may be needed. Medication (tranquilizers may be considered) and safe transportation home need to be arranged. Families or friends can be called to bring clothes and escort the woman home if she chooses.

Written aftercare instructions are helpful as recall is difficult under stress. An appointment schedule, copies of consent forms, and names and phone numbers of resource agencies and community services should also be provided.

Emotional Sequelae. The majority of women who are sexually assaulted experience posttraumatic stress disorder in which the woman experiences all or some of the following behaviors; the extent of debilitation varies with the individual. Sexual assault victims frequently have recurring thoughts about the assault. It is not unusual for a woman to feel as if the assault were happening again. One woman who was raped in the parking lot of the university she attended found it difficult to return to the university; as she approached the university, she recalled the rape and felt as if the event were recurring.

Frequently, sexual assault victims have difficulty falling asleep or experience early-morning awakenings. They might have recurrent dreams about the rape. These dreams can take different forms. Some women feel that they are being attacked either sexually or nonsexually. Other women report dreams in which they are extremely angry and attempting to harm someone else.

Sexual assault victims have also reported feeling numb. Frequently, events do not seem real to them, and they report a lack of interest in life and daily activities. A sexual assault can be so traumatic that it affects thought processes, such as the ability to concentrate. Other women have reported feeling quite jumpy and easily startled. These women frequently avoid situations or activities that arouse memories of the rape. When they are exposed to such situations, there appears to be an intensification of symptoms.

One symptom observed in the majority of sexual assault victims is guilt. Usually, the woman feels that she should have or could have done something to ward off the attacker or that she may somehow have been responsible for the assault. One woman treated by the first author was raped in her home while she was sleeping and while her infant son was sleeping in another room. This woman felt guilty because she did not have more secure locks on the door. Even though she had felt that she was living in a secure environment, after the assault she believed that the security was insufficient. Paradoxically, this guilt may help the woman make sense out of a basically irrational situation. Someone breaking into a woman's home and assaulting her is a frightening and unjust phenomenon. Feeling that she could have done something might help the victim psychologically deal with the irrationality and injustice of the situation.

One model used by individuals who counsel sexual assault victims is the crisis model. The major goal when seeing a woman immediately after an assault is to aid the victim in regaining control of her life. The health practitioner's role is to listen to the victim and to help her express her feelings. As with any type of crisis counseling, empathy is expressed toward the victim. Again, it is crucial that the practitioner be aware of her own feelings and prejudices regarding rape. It is not unusual for a health care professional to feel uncomfortable in providing treatment to a sexual assault victim because it brings the practitioner in touch with her own feelings of vulnerability, that is, "if it happened to this woman, it could happen to me." If the practitioner has such feelings, she may emotionally withdraw from the victim and not provide her with the needed empathy and services.

It is helpful to let the victim know that at some point, over the next couple of days, weeks, or months, she may experience the signs and symptoms of posttraumatic stress disorder. The woman should have this information so that if she starts having a sleep disturbance or if specific fears develop—fear of being alone, fear of strangers, fear of new situations, fear of going to sleep at night—she knows that these are expected sequelae to sexual assault. When victims are not informed of the expected course of posttraumatic stress disorder, they can, on occasion, feel they are "going crazy" because of their increased fear level, and this serves to upset them even further.

Over the past 15 years, numerous rape crisis centers have been established in this country and have served the needs of sexual assault victims in providing escort services, information, and counseling. The practitioner should be aware of the crisis centers in the neighborhood so that she can make an appropriate referral. Rape crisis centers are usually listed in the telephone book under victim services.

Another issue the victim faces is whether to report the crime and prosecute. In doing an acute examination and interview, the practitioner should be systematic in collecting both the medical evidence and the victim's statement in the event she elects to prosecute. There are advantages and disadvantages for the victim in deciding to prosecute. Some women have been unsuccessful in their prosecution of cases and this has served to traumatize them further. Other women have reported that they were clearly unable to resolve the traumatic experience while they were involved in criminal justice proceedings because they were constantly reminded of the rape whenever they were contacted by the prosecution or had to appear in court. It is helpful to inform the victim of the pros and cons of prosecution and to ensure that she will have a support system through the prosecutorial system if she elects to engage in criminal procedures.

Victims resolve the rape trauma and posttraumatic stress disorder at different rates. If, at 6 months, a woman is still experiencing some of the effects of the rape, she may have chronic posttraumatic stress disorder, necessitating further treatment. Various clinical researchers have investigated the long-term reactions to sexual assault. Atkeson, Calhoun, Resick, and Ellis (1982) found that depression in sexual assault survivors may persist months after the assault. Depression levels of a group of victims and a matched control group of nonassaulted women were significantly different up to 4 months after the assault. In addition, a number of the victims continued to exhibit depressive symptoms 12 months after the assault. Becker, Skinner, and Abel (1983) interviewed 181 women with sexual assault histories. Depression was measured using the Beck Depression Inventory. Fifty percent of the victims were at least mildly depressed as compared with less than 12 percent of the nonassaulted women. The mean number of years since the most recent assault was more than 12 and ranged from 3 to 40 years. Increased levels of fear are common in sexual assault victims (Becker et al., 1982; Burgess & Holmstrom, 1974; Kilpatrick, Veronen, & Resick, 1979). Becker et al. assessed fear levels in 181 sexual assault victims using the modified fear survey developed by Veronen and Kilpatrick. The group was compared with 79 women with no history of sexual assault. The mean time since the assault was 3 years. Assaulted and nonassaulted women differed significantly not only in overall fear level but on other subscales of this instrument. These results indicate that the victims had higher levels of rape-related fears as well as non–rape-related, generalized fears than did the women with no history of sexual assault. Women who reported experiencing emotional and/or psychiatric problems prior to their first sexual assault experienced greater levels of fear.

Sexual dysfunctions have also been reported in victim populations (Becker, Skinner, Abel, & Cichon, 1986; Feldman-Summers, Gordon, & Meagher, 1979). Becker et al., in a study of 371 sexual assault victims and 99 women with no history of sexual assault, found that 58.6 percent of the sexual assault survivors were experiencing sexual dysfunctions. Seventy-one percent of the victims reported that their sexual assaults were related to their development of sexual problems. In contrast, only 17.2 percent of the nonassaulted women reported experiencing any sexual problems. Differences were also found in the type of sexual problems experienced. Of the victims, 88.2 percent experienced early response cycle–inhibiting problems, such as desire dysfunctions and arousal dysfunctions, compared with 47.1 percent of the nonassaulted women. The time elapsed since the most recent assault ranged from 2 months to 40 years in this population.

These studies indicate that a significant number of sexual assault victims continue to experience depression, anxiety, and sexual problems for months, if not years, after the assault. Several studies have looked at those factors associated with recovery from an assault. Frank, Turner, and Stuart (1980) and Norris and Feldman-Summers (1981) examined factors surrounding the rape and found that familiarity with the rapist, use of a weapon, and degree of threat were not systematically related to rape recovery. Another factor that has been investigated is prerape psychological functioning and postrape symptoms (Becker, et al., 1983; Frank, Turner, Stuart, et al., 1981). Frank et al. found that a history of psychotherapy or psychiatric treatment prior to the assault was predictive of poor adjustment to the sexual assault.

Treatment. Very few studies evaluating the effectiveness of specific treatment strategies with sexual assault victims have been conducted to date. The model used by most crisis centers is the crisis intervention model, which generally provides empathy to the woman, encourages her to talk about her feelings and the assault at her own pace, and basically helps her regain control of her life. Several case studies have been done with sexual assault victims. Blanchard and Abel (1976) used biofeedback in the treatment of a woman with a 15-year history of sinus tachycardia that began shortly after she was raped at age 14. Becker and Abel (1981) report on three single-case studies. Two involve victims who developed specific fears related to stimuli present during the assault, and were then successfully treated with systematic desensitization. In the third case, the woman developed a sexual dysfunction secondary to the assault. Becker and associates (1984) reported on the use of a time-limited, behaviorally oriented sex dysfunction treatment package with 68 sexually assaulted women. Treatment gains were greatest when the treatment was exercised in a group therapy format rather than in an individual format. Therapeutic progress was found to be maintained at 3 months posttreatment.

In the area of depression, Turner and Frank (1981) used cognitive behavior therapy with 25 sexual assault victims. They report that victims made a significant improvement. The study indicates that such procedures as negative practice, systematic desensitization, cognitive behavior therapy, biofeedback, and sex dysfunction treatment have proved effective in treating specific problems of sexual assault victims.

What is lacking in the literature are well-controlled studies, in which some groups of victims receive treatment while others do not, to determine if, indeed, the untreated victims do not recover at the same rate as the other victims.

IMPLICATIONS FOR GYNECOLOGIC PRACTICE

Whenever a health practitioner takes a history from a patient, as part of a review of systems, the practitioner should ask the patient whether, as a child, adolescent, or adult, she engaged in sexual behavior that was nonconsensual. The interviewer should avoid use of the words *raped* and *molested,* as these words are emotionally charged and the patient might not acknowledge having been a victim of such experiences. If the patient acknowledges that she participated in sexual acts against her will, the practitioner should then determine how old she was at the time, the relationship of the perpetrator to the victim, the age of the perpetrator, whether the incident was disclosed, and how she feels the incident has affected her life. The practitioner should offer the patient the opportunity to talk openly about the experience, if she so desires.

PREVENTION

If our society is to deal with the problem of rape, then prevention must be focused in a number of areas. First, we must determine exactly why our society has such a high rape rate. What is it about our culture that facilitates the development of sexually aggressive arousal patterns in men? The second area of research involves identification of those persons at risk for becoming sexual aggressives and then providing treatment to them.

Prevention efforts for women and children should focus on safety training and provide treatment to all victims of sexual assault.

REFERENCES

Abel, G., Becker, J. V., Blanchard, E., & Flanagan, B. (1981). The behavioral assessment of rapists. In J. R. Hays, T. K. Roberts, & K. S. Solway, *Violence and the Violent Individual.* New York: Medical and Scientific Books.

Amir, M. (1971). *Patterns of Forcible Rape.* Chicago: University of Chicago Press.

Atkeson, B., Calhoun, K., Resick, P. & Ellis, E. (1982, February). Victims of rape: Repeated assessment of depression symptoms. *Journal of Consulting and Clinical Psychology, 50*(1), 96–102.

Bay Area Women Against Rape. (1975). Medical protocol for emergency room treatment of rape victims. Oakland, CA: Bay Area Women Against Rape.

Becker, J. V., & Abel, G. (1981). Behavioral treatment of victims of sexual assault. In S. Turner, K. Calhoun, & H. Adams, (Eds.), *Handbook of clinical behavior therapy.* New York: John Wiley & Sons.

Becker, J. V., Skinner, L., Abel, G., et al. (1983). Sequelae of sexual assault: The survivor's perspective. In J. Greer & I. Stuart (Eds.), *The sexual aggressor,* New York: Van Nostrand

Becker, J. V., Skinner, L., Abel, G., & Cichon, J. (1984, Fall). Time limited therapy with sexually dysfunctional sexually assaulted women. *Journal of Social Work and Human Sexuality, 3*(1), 97–115.

Becker, J. V., Skinner, L., Abel, G., & Chichon, J. (1986, February). Level of post assault sexual functioning in rape and incest victims. *Archives of Sexual Behavior, 15*(1), 37–49.

Becker, J. V., Skinner, L., Abel, G., & Treacy, E. (1982, Spring). Incidence and types of sexual dysfunctions in rape and incest victims. *Journal of Sex and Marital Therapy, 8*(1), 65–74.

Becker, J. V., Skinner, L., & Abel, G., et al. (1984, Fall). Depressive symptoms associated with sexual assault. *Journal of Sex and Marital Therapy, 10*(3), 185–192.

Blanchard, E., & Abel, G. G. (1976, January). An experimental case study of the biofeedback treatment of rape-induced psychophysiological cardiovascular disorder. *Behavior Therapy, 7*(1), 113–119.

Bowker, L. H. (1979). The criminal victimization of women. *Victimology: An International Journal, 4,* 371–384.

Braen, G. R. (1980). Physical assessment and emergency medical management for adult victims of sexual assault. In G. C. Warner (Ed.), *Rape and sexual assault.* London: An Aspen Publication.

Brownmiller, S. (1975). *Against our will: Men, women and rape.* New York: Simon & Schuster.

Burgess, A. W., & Holstrom, L. L. (1973, October). Rape victims in the emergency ward. *American Journal of Nursing, 73*(10), 1741–1745.

Burgess, A., & Holstrom, L. (1974). *Rape: Victims of crisis.* Bowie, MD: Robert J. Brady.

Cabaniss, M., Scott, S., & Copeland, L. (1985, March). Gathering evidence for rape cases. *Contemporary Ob/Gyn, 25*(3), 160–174.

Curtis, L. (1975). Victimization: Present and future measures of victimization in forcible rape. In *Research, action, prevention: Proceedings of the Sixth Symposium on Justice and the Behavioral Sciences.* University of Alabama, Report 29.

DiNitto, D., Martin, P., Norton, D., & Maxwell, M. (1986, May). After rape: Who should examine rape survivors? *American Journal of Nursing, 86*(5), 538–540.

Feldman-Summers, S., Gordon, P., & Meagher, J. (1979, February). The impact of rape on sexual satisfaction. *Journal of Abnormal Psychology, 88*(1), 101–105.

Foley, T. S., & Davies, M. R. (1983). *Rape—Nursing care of victims.* St. Louis, MO: C. V. Mosby.

Frank, E., Turner, S., & Stuart, B. (1980, March). Initial response to rape: The impact of factors within the rape situation. *Journal of Behavioral Assessment, 2*(1), 39–52.

Frank, E., Turner, S., & Stuart, B., et al. (1981, September-October). Past psychiatric symptoms and response to sexual assault. *Comprehensive Psychiatry, 22*(5), 479–487.

Gagon, J. (1965, Fall). Female child victims of sex offenses. *Social Problems, 13*(2), 176–192.

Hayman, C., & Lanza, C. (1971, February). Sexual assault on women and girls. *American Journal of Obstetrics and Gynecology, 109*(3), 480–486.

Heath, L., Rigen, S., Gordon, M., & LeBailly, R. (1979, September). *Rape stereotypes and fear: A control paradox.* Paper presented at American Psychological Association Meeting, New York.

Kilpatrick, D., Veronen, L., & Resick, P. (1979, June). Assessment of the aftermath of rape: Changing patterns of fear. *Journal of Behavioral Assessment, 1*(2), 133–148.

Law Enforcement Assistance Administration (1975a). *Criminal victimization surveys in the nation's five largest cities.* Washington, DC: U.S. Government Printing Office.

Law Enforcement Assistance Administration. (1975b). *Criminal victimization surveys in 13 American cities.* Washington, DC: U.S. Government Printing Office.

Norris, J., & Feldman-Summers, S. (1981, December). Factors related to the psychological impacts of rape on the victim. *Journal of Abnormal Psychology, 90*(6), 562–567.

Rabkin, J. C. (1979, October). The epidemiology of forcible rape. *American Journal of Orthopsychiatry, 49*(4), 634–647.

Root, I., Ogden, W., & Scott, W. (1974, April). The medical investigation of rape. *Western Journal of Medicine, 120* (4), 329–333.

Turner, S., & Frank, E. (1981). Behavior therapy in the treatment of rape victims. In L. Michalson, M. Herson, & S. Turner (Eds.), *Future perspectives in behavior therapy*. New York: Plenum Press.

U.S. Department of Justice. (1980). *Rape: Guidelines for a community response. An executive summary*. Washington, DC: U.S. Government Printing Office.

Warner, C. G. (1980). *Rape and sexual assault: Management and intervention*. London: An Aspen Publication, 1980.

27

Infertility

Sarah G. Potter

Consider the circumstances that prompt infertile women or couples to seek an infertility evaluation. They have been trying to conceive for as many months or years as it has taken them to become frustrated, or admit "failure," and hence seek outside help. The initial patient may be either the woman alone, with or without her partner's knowledge, or the couple. The patients' knowledge of the facts of human reproduction and fertility may be scant or sufficient. The solution to their problem, if there is one, may range from "simple" reeducation to complex hormonal manipulation or surgery. The essential screening tests, therefore, are only the beginning of a complete assessment of the infertile patient-couple. In dealing with infertility the health care provider must consider many other factors, including the patients' motivation for having a child, their ability to comprehend the diagnosis and to follow through with the plan of treatment, and their evolving emotional response to the difficulties encountered in the course of their struggle to achieve a pregnancy.

Infertility is defined as the inability of a couple to conceive after 1 year of unprotected intercourse, or the inability of the female to carry a pregnancy to term. Estimates of the incidence of infertility in the United States vary from 10 to 15 percent of all couples (Menning, 1982, p. 155; Speroff, Glass, & Kase, 1983, p. 469); of these, as many as 60 percent, depending on the underlying etiology, ultimately conceive, whereas 40 percent suffer absolute infertility, or sterility.

The changing role of women in American society has contributed toward the trend for couples to delay starting a family. Many couples opting to postpone childbearing past the early thirties may face declining female fertility (Federation CECOS, Schwartz, & Hayaux, 1982). Moreover, change in sociosexual mores during the past two decades has resulted in increased exposure of the childbearing population to infections that compromise both male and female fertility. In fact, a study by the National Center for Health Statistics found that infertility in women 20 to 24 years of age increased from 4 percent in 1965 to 11 percent in 1982 (Brooks, 1986, p. B12). Today, in part because of the legalization of abortion and the increased acceptability of single parenting, relatively few children are available for adoption by those unable to conceive. For these and other reasons, infertility, once a hidden health problem, is currently the object of rising public concern. This concern is clearly documented by the proliferation of articles in the lay literature that describe both the growing magnitude of the problem and some of the sensational high-technology solutions that are being developed (e.g., Clark, 1982, pp. 102–110; Wallis, 1984).

In this chapter, the causes of infertility are reviewed, and the management of the infertile woman or couple, including evaluation and possible treatments, is discussed. Also addressed are the emotional needs of women and men facing infertility.

CAUSES

An understanding of the multiple causes of infertility requires familiarity with the process of conception. (See Chapter 1 for a more detailed description of this process.) A simplified scheme for comprehending the process of conception starts with the monthly development of an ovarian follicle, which, after appropriate hormonal stimulation by the pituitary gland and the hypothalamus, releases a matured oocyte at midcycle. This process is called ovulation. The oocyte is propelled into the fimbriated (fringed) ends of the fallopian tube, where it remains receptive to sperm only 12 to 24 hours. Meanwhile, ejaculate is deposited into the vagina. There the sperm begin the long journey up the female reproductive tract where physiologic barriers, including cervical mucus and internal environmental conditions such as temperature and pH, select out unhealthy sperm. Only some 200 sperm from any given ejaculate of perhaps 200,000,000 reach the oocyte. As a single sperm penetrates the outer protective layers of the oocyte, it undergoes a complex and incompletely understood process called capacitation. This process enhances the sperm's ability to fertilize the oocyte by piercing the zona pellucida and the vitelline layer of the egg and then releasing its haploid chromosomal matter into the haploid oocyte. After fertilization in the ampullary part of the tube, the cleaving embryo must be propelled into the uterus, which takes 60 to 70 hours. Here the embryo must implant and, given the appropriate endometrial and hormonal support, develop into a trophoblast and then into a healthy pregnancy.

The panel of screening tests for infertility must therefore evaluate a wide variety of factors: adequacy of coital timing and technique; the production of healthy gametes by the male and the female; anatomy and function of the conduit system for spermatozoa and oocytes; presence of an interactional dysfunction such as an immune incompatibility that may interfere with transport or fertilization; and mechanisms of fertilization, implantation, and endometrial support that initiate and sustain gestation. These tests also assess the integrity of the female hypothalamic-pituitary-ovarian axis, which consists of a number of organs working in synchrony to create the cyclic hormonal environment necessary for reproductive capability.

Some of these factors cannot be directly tested or evaluated. For example, patency of the fallopian tubes can be demonstrated by hysterosalpingogram, but this test cannot measure the normal function of intraluminal cilia and tubal micromusculature. After tubal reconstruction, with demonstrated patency of the fallopian tubes, a normal semen analysis, and an adequate postcoital test, dysfunction of the tubes can be inferred only from the patient's failure to become pregnant. In addition, some of the mechanisms of human fertilization and implantation have only very recently become accessible to study through the advent of such techniques as in vitro fertilization and embryo transfer.

MANAGEMENT OF THE INFERTILE PATIENT-COUPLE

Goals of Evaluation

Many commonly held myths about infertility exist (Table 27–1). One goal of evaluation should be to dispel such mistaken beliefs and to teach the woman or couple accurately and completely what they need to know about infertility and about their case in particular. This goal is second only to the diagnosis and treatment plan. The patients must understand the long-term ramifications of their situation and, if treatment is not successful, must be guided toward future acceptance of either the absence of a diagnosis, which unfortunately occurs in 10 to 15 percent of all cases (Wallach, 1980, pp. 405–406), or failure. Thus, it is important for the care provider to address the subject of the woman or couple's attitudes toward adoption as a feasible alternative to pregnancy well before a failure to diagnose or to treat their infertility makes it inevitable (Speroff et al., 1983, p. 468).

TABLE 27–1. ONE DOZEN MISCONCEPTIONS ABOUT INFERTILITY AND ITS TREATMENT

1. Infertility is not that common.
2. Infertility is a female problem.
3a. Infertility is all in the patient's head.
3b. Infertility is all related to anxiety and nervousness.
4. Adoption increases fertility; those who adopt will conceive shortly thereafter.
5. Infertility can be the result of a small uterus.
6. Infertility can be related to a retroverted uterus.
7. A uterine suspension can improve fertility in a woman with a retroverted uterus.
8. Routine dilation of the cervix may be useful in case the cervix is stenotic.
9. Dilation and curettage ("D&C") can enhance fertility.
10. Screening tests should routinely include skull x-ray, serum levels of 17-ketosteroids, and radioimmunoassay of gonadotropins.
11. Administration of thyroid hormones can increase fertility, even in a euthyroid woman.
12. Therapy with "fertility drugs" without prior workup is worth a try.

Compiled from Resolve (1982) and Speroff et al. (1983).

When a couple presents to a health professional who does not specialize in infertility, that provider can and should perform a basic set of screening and evaluation tests before referring them to a specialist. The solution may lie in reeducation alone. The referral, if necessary, should be well supported and appropriate. For example, a physician skilled in tubal reconstruction may not be the proper infertility specialist to perform a complex immunologic evaluation of a couple.

The Initial Assessment

An initial assessment, including interview, physical examination, and laboratory tests, is within the scope of function of a primary care provider. Indeed, this investigation can sometimes negate the need for a more intensive workup or, more commonly, can help in identifying an appropriate source of referral for further evaluation and treatment.

History. The first step in the workup is, of course, to compile a complete data base on the woman or couple, starting with a complete health history. The following data should be obtained: ages of the couple; their general health; complete pregnancy history of the female and paternity history of the male; length of infertility including prior workup, if any; the coital history including frequency, timing and adequacy, use of lubricants (some of which may be spermicidal), and postcoital habits such as douching or voiding. For fertility purposes, the adequacy of sexual intercourse depends on penetration of the vagina and ejaculation by the male.

Relevant past history of the female should encompass the menstrual history including age at menarche, regularity of and discomfort during menses, and date of the last menstrual period; the complete gynecologic history covering contraceptive use and all conditions requiring medical or surgical investigation or intervention; and questioning about any nongynecologic abdominal surgery or episodes of abdominal pain that may indicate undiagnosed pelvic inflammatory disease. Detailed nutrition and exercise histories are very important. This must include discussion of the eating disorders anorexia nervosa and bulimia (Andersen, 1985; van der Spuy, 1985) (see Chapters 2 and 21). The most significant data for the interviewer to elicit from the male are history of reproductive tract infections or treatment for such received by both his present and past partners and himself; other genitourinary problems requiring surgery or other treatment; and the results of any previous infertility evaluation.

Long-term and occasional use of medications, cigarettes, alcohol, and other drugs by either the male or female can also be significant. The number of cigarettes smoked per day should be asked of all women who smoke, as a recent prospective study of over 4,000 women showed an increase in reduction of fertility with increasing number of cigarettes smoked daily. Marked differences were noted among women who smoked more than 15 cigarettes daily (Howe, Westhoff, Vessey, & Yeates, 1985). Previous cigarette smoking, however, was not found to be significantly related to fertility. The biologic effect of smoking on fertility is not entirely clear; it may induce hormonal changes or cause oocyte destruction (Hatch, 1984, p. 165). An increased percentage of morphologic sperm abnormalities were also found in a study of 43 male cigarette smokers compared with 43 nonsmokers attending an infertility clinic. Further study is needed to determine the relationship of such changes to the number of cigarettes smoked (Evans, Fletcher, Torrance, & Hargreave, 1981).

Exposure of either partner to toxic chemicals or radiation during military service, or at present or previous places of employment or residence, should be ascertained. The following exposures specifically have been shown to affect the concentration, shape, or mobility of sperm: the pesticide dibromochloropropane (DBCP), lead, radiation, antineoplastic drugs, and toluene diamine (Glass, Lyness, Mengle, et al., 1979; Lancranjan, Popescu, Gavanescu, et al., 1975b; Rowley, Leach, Warner, & Heller, 1974; Sieber & Adamson, 1975). Daily high doses of marijuana, alcohol, diethylstilbestrol (DES) exposure in utero, carbon disulfide, nonionizing radiation, long-term exposure to microwaves, and the pesticides kepone and carbaryl have possible effects on sperm or other aspects of male sexual function (Hatch, 1984, p. 166; Hembree, Nahas, Zeidenberg, & Huang, 1979; Whitehead & Leiter, 1981; Lancranjan, Maicanescu, Rafaila, et al., 1975a; Wyrobek, Watchmaker, Gordon, et al., 1981). Further investigation is required before definitive conclusions can be drawn. Many of these effects are reversible (Glass et al., 1979; Hembree et al., 1979).

As part of a complete review of systems of the female, special attention should be paid to the endocrine system. This may yield clues to an underlying medical problem, such as thyroid dysfunction, that could interfere with fertility. Specific questions regarding change of bowel habits, weight gain or loss, appetite changes, and intolerance to heat or cold should be asked. The woman should also be queried as to existing conditions, such as a cardiac problem or collagen vascular disease, which could either affect or be affected by pregnancy. In gathering the family history, the interviewer should ask about possible in utero exposure of either partner to DES. Other relevant family data would include a history of recurrent miscarriages or other fertility problems, hereditary diseases such as diabetes that could affect the woman's ability to conceive or to carry a healthy pregnancy, and prior medical treatments such as chemotherapy or radiation.

Assessment of the psychosocial context within which the couple presents for management should be ongoing. The initial interview, however, should include specific questions regarding vocation, leisure time and activities, and financial status. Eliciting information concerning the personal, emotional, and financial resources that the couple have earmarked for this effort may help assess their readiness to begin an infertility investigation (Draye, 1985). Questions about the size and makeup of the couple's families may yield insight into family pressures and expectations that may be affecting the patients' own attitudes about infertility. Every such interview should include a brief psychiatric evaluation designed to reveal how the couple, both as individuals and as a unit, may handle the stress of the workup and the chance that they may fail. Not all couples cope well with such intense scrutiny into what is usually such an intimate and private part of relationships.

Physical Examination. The physical examination performed at the initial interview often involves only the female. Complete physical assessment of the male, usually by a urologist, is generally done only if his semen analysis is abnormal. Thorough examination of the female is necessary to determine overall health. The examiner should be alert for signs of endocrine abnormalities, such as the stigmata of a thyroid disease, hirsutism, or a deviation of more than 20 percent from standard weight. Abdominal scars should be noted.

The pelvic exam can be very informative. Externally, the patient should be checked for discharge or clitoromegaly. The cervix should be assessed for discharge and signs of chronic inflammation or tenderness. Pap smear and cervical cultures for gonorrhea, chlamydia, and mycoplasma are standard procedures. On bimanual exam, any decrease in the normal mobility of the pelvic organs may indicate the presence of binding adhesion from previous infections. Fibroids and cystic ovaries should be ruled out. Any unusual tenderness may be significant. On rectovaginal exam, the skilled examiner can occasionally palpate endometrial implants. A careful and thorough pelvic exam is essential for proper diagnosis and treatment.

Laboratory Tests. After the intake interview and examination, the practitioner should confer with the couple and explain his or her evaluation and treatment plan for their problem. Both partners will be subjected to a battery of basic laboratory tests: for the woman, along with the aforementioned Pap smear and cervical cultures, a complete blood count (CBC), an erythrocyte sedimentation rate (ESR), blood chemistries, thyroid function tests, liver function tests (if therapy with clomiphene citrate is anticipated), and a urinalysis; for the man, blood chemistries, a urinalysis and urine culture, and a urethral culture. In women with an apparent ovulatory dysfunction, evaluation should include serum levels of prolactin (PRL), follicle-stimulating hormone (FSH), and luteinizing hormone (LH).

Recently, more attention has been paid to the impact on infertility of sexually transmitted diseases other than gonorrhea. Chlamydia and mycoplasma have been increasingly implicated in asymptomatic pelvic inflammatory disease, but treatment can halt the process and perhaps enhance fertility (Toth, Lesser, Brooks, & Labriola, 1983, pp. 505–507). (See Chapter 12 for further discussion of treatment for this problem.) Treatment for mycoplasma in the male can involve a course of antibiotics as long as 3 months to span the life cycle of the spermatozoa. Pregnancies sometimes result after such treatments, thereby supporting the theory that the mycoplasma interferes with the fertilization capacity of the spermatozoa (Friberg, 1980, pp. 351–359).

Battery of Infertility Screening Tests

A battery of screening tests is administered to evaluate the function of the essential steps in the conception process. Infertility screening tests for the previously unevaluated woman or couple begin with several months of careful recording of the woman's basal body temperature (BBT) and analysis of one or two semen specimens from the male. These tests can be performed while four other procedures are being scheduled: postcoital test (PCT), endometrial biopsy, hysterosalpingogram (HSG), and laparoscopy. As the male infertility factor accounts for between 25 and 40 percent of infertility cases with currently diagnosable etiologies, the semen analysis is an essential part of the infertility workup (incidence of infertility of different etiologies compiled from Collins, Wrixon, James, & Wilson, 1983, 1201–1206; Shane, Schiff, & Wilson, 1976; Speroff, et al., 1983, pp. 468–469; Warren, 1981, pp. 547–578). Semen analysis must be performed before a woman is exposed to more invasive tests.

Prior to each test, patients should be educated as to why and when in the menstrual cycle the test is being performed, as well as the necessary preparation, possible discomfort, and anticipated recovery time. Whoever arranges the evaluation schedule for the couple should do so with the convenience of the patients in mind. No scheduling consideration is more important, for example, than the relaxation benefit to the patients of a long-awaited vacation.

In general, the biopsy, PCT, and HSG can be performed during the first two menstrual cycles, and the laparoscopy later during the workup.

Basal Body Temperature and Endometrial Biopsy: Testing for Ovarian and Hormonal Function. Screening for hormonally mediated or ovarian factor infertility begins with BBT charting and includes the endometrial biopsy. Approximately 15 to 25 percent of infertility cases can be attributed to failure to ovulate. During the follicular phase of the normal menstrual cycle (the first 2 weeks), one follicle and the oocyte it contains mature. The normal body temperature during this phase ranges from 97.2 to 97.6°F. The endometrial lining of the uterus proliferates and thickens as a result of hormonal stimulation. At midcycle the ovum is extruded, may be fertilized any time from 12 to 24 hours later, and passes into the uterus. During the luteal phase (the third and fourth weeks of the typical menstrual cycle), the residual follicle becomes a corpus luteum. The corpus luteum secretes progesterone, which in turn converts the lining of the uterus to a secretory endometrium in preparation for the implantation of a potential pregnancy. Ovulation and the development of the corpus luteum manifest as an increase in BBT to 98°F and above. This level is sustained throughout the luteal phase. Some patients' temperatures dip just before the day of ovulation and then rise. This change from lower to higher ranges produces the classic biphasic pattern characteristic of normal BBT (Figure 27–1).

Daily BBT recording is an inconvenient yet informative test required of all women undergoing infertility evaluation. For the test to be successful, the patient needs careful instruction and counseling, which are appropriate functions of a primary care provider. The woman must take her temperature before arising at approximately the same time every morning. She may use a standard oral or rectal thermometer, or a special ovulation thermometer the gauge of which ranges only from 97 to 99°F, calibrated in tenths of degrees and therefore easier to read. The patient should also record days of menstrual flow; other discharge, especially mucus; concomitant illnesses; and nights on which she stayed up late or slept less than 6 hours; and days on which the couple have intercourse. This record should be kept for 2 to 6 months, depending on the age of the patient and the length of the infertility problem, while other tests are being done.

BBT provides presumptive evidence of normal oocyte production and related hormonal change. The charting method also reveals whether the couple's frequency and timing of coitus are optimal. The standard recommendation is that coitus occur 2 days before ovulation is expected and every 2 days thereafter until 2 to 4 days have passed following the rise in body temperature. Interpretation of BBT charts is not always simple, because the common biphasic pattern may not always be clear. See Chapter 5 for an in-depth discussion of these changes. Initially, many women find it difficult to comply with temperature charting; eventually, however, it becomes a part of the patient's life—a daily reminder of the problem. Some women maintain BBT records for years and become dependent on the ritual; stopping BBT charting would mean admitting failure.

The endometrial biopsy is a sampling of the uterine lining late in the luteal phase. This test is scheduled 10 days

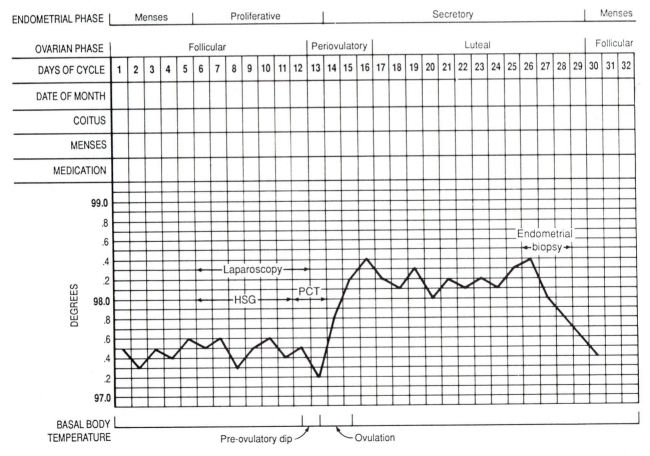

Figure 27–1. The menstrual cycle and the scheduling of infertility tests.

after the woman's BBT increase, or 2 to 3 days before the onset of her next menses. The test carries a small risk of disrupting a pregnancy (Buxton & Olson, 1969, p. 702) or of perforating the uterus. The biopsy is performed as a sterile office procedure, usually without any anesthesia. Some nonphysician health care workers receive on-the-job training to perform endometrial biopsies. Detailed discussion of the technique is beyond the scope of this text, but, in brief, a curette is introduced through the cervix into the uterus and a strip of endometrial tissue is removed under light suction. The specimen is placed in a preservative and sent for analysis in which the endometrial sample is dated within the menstrual cycle according to the types of cells present. The patient should be counseled prior to the procedure that a mild to moderate cramp may be experienced. It is important to talk her through each step of the procedure as it is performed. Infrequently, a patient may experience a vasovagal response; if this occurs, she should rise slowly and be given time to regain her equilibrium.

The biopsy is a valuable tool for infertility evaluation. It provides useful anatomic data about the cervix and the uterus. Performance of this procedure requires a patent cervix. Often, a measurement of the depth of the uterus, called a "sounding," is made, and the examiner can quickly assess the uterine cavity. A normal secretory endometrium and the absence of inflammation indicate that implantation is feasible. Finally, the biopsy yields information about normal gamete production and ovulation in the female by providing histologic evidence of ovulation. If testing at this stage determines that there is an ovulatory dysfunction, the provider should request further studies, such as prolactin, FSH, and LH assays, to determine the underlying cause of the dysfunction (Table 27–2). A normal BBT and biopsy provide evidence that the hypothalamic-pituitary-ovarian axis in the female is intact and functions normally.

Semen Analysis: Screening for Male Factor Infertility. Unlike the periodicity that characterizes oocyte maturation, normal spermatogenesis is a continuous process in the male; the germ cell takes $2\frac{1}{2}$ to 3 months to become a mature sperm. To assess the functioning of this process, a semen sample is collected by masturbation in a clean glass jar after 2 or 3 days of abstinence, or whatever is the normal interval between acts of intercourse for the particular couple. It is important, especially in winter, that the sample not be chilled during transport to the laboratory. The sample is

assessed for count, volume, motility, progression, morphology, and liquefaction (Table 27–3). Semen analysis can be performed by a primary care provider, but it is extremely important that the provider have adequate training and experience.

The variation in the values for a healthy male is so great that the first step after an abnormal result is to repeat the test. If the results obtained for the second sample are similarly abnormal, then a further workup of the male by a specialist is necessary. This workup should include physical examination and semen culture (if not already done), further endocrine evaluation, and perhaps testicular biopsy if the count is extremely low. Occasionally, a carefully taken history reveals simple causes for the poor results such as frequent hot baths, saunas, or the wearing of tight-fitting pants or underwear. Nevertheless, only a small percentage of the infertility cases resulting from the male factor are so easy to remedy (Speroff et al., 1983, p. 510).

Postcoital Test: Assessing Cervical Mucus and Male–Female Incompatibility. Probably the most crucial aspect of the PCT, also called the Sims–Huhner test after its developers, is its careful timing within the immediate preovulatory stage. The BBT should not yet show the ovulatory rise. The couple are instructed to have sexual intercourse at home either the night before or the morning of the examination. For a discussion of the optimal interval between coitus and this examination, and of the merits of the so-called "fractional postcoital tests" see Davajan and Kunitake (1969, 197) and Speroff et al. (1983, 469–473). Information about temperature, cycle day, and hours since intercourse should be elicited before the examination and recorded in the chart. During the examination, observations about the character, quality, and *spinnbarkheit* of the mucus should be made initially (Table 27–4). *Spinnbarkheit* is the elasticity of the cervical mucus. Just prior to ovulation, when the mucus is thinnest, mucus threads of 6 to 10 cm can be stretched out from the cervix. Samples of the cervical mucus should be extracted first from the exocervix and then from the endocervix. A small nasal septum forceps or a needleless tuberculin syringe is used for this purpose. Specimens are placed on a glass slide, covered with a coverslip, and examined under low and high magnification. This examination can be made by any experienced practitioner.

The presence of at least five to ten motile sperm per high-powered field is normal. For this to occur, mucus conducive to sperm survival must be present in the cervical canal. During the periovulatory stage, when the mucus in the cervix becomes copious and thin, the mucous glycoproteins line up so as to create a pathway for sperm to travel up the cervical canal. Some women never manufacture conducive mucous because of infection or other injury to the endocervical mucous glands or because of congenital or hor-

TABLE 27–2. CAUSES OF OVULATORY DYSFUNCTION

Dysfunction	Cause
Hypothalamic	Stress
	Exercise
	Weight loss
	Medications
	Destructive lesions
Pituitary	Destructive lesions
	Infarcts
	Tumor
Ovarian	Resistance
	Failure
Adrenal	Enzyme defects
Prolactin disorders	Drug related
	Idiopathic
Chronic anovulatory syndrome	Polycystic ovarian syndrome

From Zacur, H. A. (1985). Ovulation induction with gondaotropin-releasing hormone. Fertility and Sterility, 44(4), 436. Reprinted with permission.

TABLE 27–3. NORMAL VALUES FOR SEMEN ANALYSIS

Concentration	At least 20 to 40 × 10⁶ sperm/mL
Volume	2–5 mL per ejaculate; normal range, 1–7 mL
Motility	50–60 percent, with good forward progression, within 2 hours of collection
Morphology	60 percent normal
Liquefaction	Within 15–30 minutes of collection; normal range, 5–45 minutes

Compiled from Schoenfeld (1982), Speroff et al. (1983), and Warren (1981).

TABLE 27–4. THE POSTCOITAL TEST

Timing within menstrual cycle	1–2 days prior to ovulation
Time after coitus	Opinion as to optimal time after coitus varies among practitioners from less than 2 hours, to 2–4 hours, to 4–12 hours
Quality of optimal periovulatory cervical mucus	
Spinnbarkheit	>6–7 cm
Ferning	Present on slide allowed to dry without coverslip
Amount	Copious
Character	Clear, watery, acellular, thin
Sperm as counted on slide with coverslip	≥5–10 motile sperm per high-power field

Compiled from Davajan and Kunitake (1969) and Speroff et al. (1983).

monal factors. Poor timing of the PCT is the other cause of suboptimal mucus. In either case, a finding of poor mucus on initial PCT is an indication to repeat the test, either later in the current cycle as long as the BBT is still down or in a subsequent cycle. Given favorable mucus and a normal semen analysis, a poor PCT indicates a likely incompatibility between mucus and sperm. This merits further investigation by a specialist, as there exist procedures and treatments that can circumvent this problem in some cases.

Hysterosalpingogram: Indirect Visualization of the Female Reproductive Tract. Under fluoroscopic visualization during a hysterosalpingogram a radiopaque iodine-based dye is injected through the cervix, from which it follows the normal anatomic pathway into the uterus, the fallopian tubes, and finally the abdominal cavity. Performed on an outpatient basis by a radiologist, usually assisted by a gynecologist, this study reveals abnormalities of the internal configuration of the uterine cavity, such as submucous fibroids and synechiae, or congenital abnormalities such as a bicornuate uterus (see Chapter 14). It also allows the physician to determine the patency of the tubes. The configuration of the spillage from the distal ends of the tubes may show signs of loculation, that is, some restriction to free flow caused by adhesions. Remember that even given free "filling and spilling" on HSG, there is no way to ensure normal function of the fallopian tubes. The HSG is an indirect study at best.

The hysterosalpingogram should be scheduled for the interval between cessation of menstrual flow and ovulation to avoid retrograde flow of menstrual tissue into the tubes and the abdominal cavity. It can be a very uncomfortable procedure, especially if the patient's tubes are blocked, and the patient should be given anticipatory guidelines. Some patients may experience a transient vasovagal reaction after injection of the dye. A supportive attitude on the part of the examiner, along with careful step-by-step explanations of the procedure, can enhance patient relaxation. The patient should be told that the dye used in this study is nontoxic and, indeed, that forcing dye through the tubes may have a beneficial effect. If one or both tubes are found to be open, there is a slight increase in conception after HSG (Gillespie, 1965, p. 301).

Diagnostic Laparoscopy: Direct Visualization of Uterus, Tubes, and Ovaries. The diagnostic laparoscopy is the final screening examination for infertility. Performed by a gynecologist who specializes in laparoscopy, the procedure is usually done in the first 2 weeks of the menstrual cycle to ensure that the patient is not pregnant, and to prevent retrograde displacement of endometrial tissue if a dye study of the fallopian tubes is included. With the patient under general anesthesia, the abdomen is insufflated with carbon dioxide and the laparoscope is inserted through the umbilicus. Direct visualization of the pelvic organs provides data about degree of adhesion formation, presence of endometriosis or fibroids, and possibility of surgical repair of damaged tubes. By means of chromopertubation (injection of dye through the cervix to the uterus), the laparoscopist can observe whether the tubes fill and spill with dye. It is not entirely uncommon to discover that tubes seen as obstructed on HSG may fill during laparoscopy; it is presumed that a spasm may have occluded the tube during the radiographic study, and that this is eliminated by the relaxation obtained through general anesthesia.

In addition to routine preanesthesia and preoperative counseling, the patient should be forewarned that residual insufflated carbon dioxide may be trapped in the abdominal cavity and cause pain for the first few postoperative days, especially in the shoulders. This pain resolves as the gas is absorbed. Laparoscopy is more and more frequently performed in day-surgery units from which the patient is discharged home within 3 to 5 hours.

Treatment

Counseling. The treatment of each couple must be tailored to the etiology of their infertility problem. The first step in therapy, which can be initiated by the primary care provider, is counseling geared to specific findings revealed by history or physical examination. Reeducation can remedy inadequacies in coital pattern. The provider should establish that adequate coitus includes vaginal penetration and ejaculation into the vagina. For conception to occur, intercourse should take place every other day around ovulation. Less frequent intercourse may cause the couple to miss ovulation; more frequent intercourse may result in a decrease in the number of sperm ejaculated at ovulation. Occasionally, the couple may need referral for more intensive sexual counseling.

Counseling can also alter some habitual behaviors such as diet or exercise, an imbalance of which can contribute to amenorrhea (Andersen, 1985; Goldin, Adlercreutz, Dwyer, et al., 1981; van der Spuy, 1985, pp. 588, 595). Extremely underweight or overweight anovulatory women have been shown to resume normal ovulatory function after ideal weight has been achieved (Padilla & Craft, 1985). Informing the couple of the possible deleterious effects on fertility of cigarettes, marijuana, or certain chemicals, if relevant, may be the first step in eliminating these exposures; however, referral for further therapy, as appropriate, may also be necessary.

Psychological counseling also may be necessary to help women and couples deal with both the reality of infertility and the demands of infertility diagnosis and treatment. Although basic counseling can be undertaken by the primary care provider, referral for more intensive therapy may be warranted. The practitioner should develop a network of appropriate local referrals for individual or group counseling or for educational, informational, and other supportive services. She can also organize a support group among her patients (Christianson, 1986). Practitioners are advised to locate and contact organizations and providers, find out what services they offer, and assess the extent to which they will be helpful to patients.

The Male Factor. As mentioned previously, most of the workup for disorders of male gamete production is done by a urologist or male reproductive endocrinologist. Causes of male infertility include azoospermia and oligospermia. The former may result from neurogenic damage or testicular failure caused by hormonal disturbances. Infection, sperm autoimmunity, or a varicocele may lead to oligospermia (Daly, 1985, p. 61). Treatments for male factor infertility range from hormonal and antibiotic treatment, to surgery (specifically varicocele repair), to artificial insemination using the partner's sperm. Unfortunately, none of these treatments is remarkably successful (deKretser, 1974, p. 409). Recent studies have called into question the value of varicocele repair (Baker, Burger, deKretser, et al., 1985; DeFazio, 1986b).

For those couples for whom it is acceptable, donor sperm may be utilized in artificial insemination. For those couples whose only identifiable problem is oligospermia, in vitro fertilization provides an additional therapeutic option in which fewer sperm are required to fertilize the oocytes. It must be noted, however, that, as of this writing, the number of pregnancies that have resulted from in vitro fertilization is small (DeFazio, 1986a). Furthermore, an evaluation of 244 such pregnancies among eight in vitro fertilization centers in Australia showed an increase in ectopic pregnancy, spontaneous abortion, premature birth, and low birth weight after this procedure (Australian in Vitro Fertilisation Collaborative Group, 1985).

Sperm antibodies, which may be present in either the male, representing autoimmunity, or the female, defy easy treatment. Use of condoms over an extended period may decrease the female's sensitivity to sperm. Corticosteroids may be effective; in vitro manipulation of semen is currently under investigation (Bronson, Cooper, & Rosenfeld, 1984).

The Female Factor. Treatment of female infertility also depends on its etiology. The treatment for ovarian dysfunction is mostly hormonal, involving a number of drugs used either singly or in combination. The most common "fertility drugs" are the antiestrogen clomiphene citrate [or tamoxifen, which is a similar agent (Pepperell, 1983, p. 7)], human menopausal gonadotropin (hMG), human chorionic gonadotropin (hCG), and gonadotropin-releasing hormone (GnRH). Through different mechanisms these drugs stimulate the development of multiple ovarian follicles. Clomiphene citrate is the easiest of these to administer and therefore the first choice for induction of ovulation (Pepperell, 1983, p. 7).

Side effects of clomiphene citrate are hot flashes (the most common), gastrointestinal symptoms such as nausea and vomiting, and abdominal or pelvic tenderness, which may indicate hyperstimulation (Pepperell, 1983, p. 7).

Gonadotropin therapy is initiated if clomiphene citrate fails to work. Because it is more powerful, however, it should be administered only under the direction of an experienced specialist and only to patients in whom other sources of infertility have been ruled out or treated (Schwartz & Jewelewicz, 1981, p. 5). It is administered intramuscularly, and treatment regimens must be individualized to the woman's particular hormonal profile and response to the medication.

During the course of drug treatment, intercourse is

carefully timed around ovulation, as determined by BBT, serum estrogen levels, cervical mucus, and sometimes ultrasound studies. The ovaries must also be monitored for signs of cyst formation or hyperstimulation which, in the case of gonadotropin therapy, may occasionally be severe. Abdominal heaviness, tension, swelling, and pain may signify ovarian hyperstimulation, and patients should be advised to report such changes (Schenker & Weinstein, 1978, p. 256). Multiple cysts as large as 5×5 cm may be felt with mild hyperstimulation, and cysts 12 cm or larger may be present with a severe case. Severe hyperstimulation, occurring rarely, causes multiple systemic problems including ascites, pleural effusion, electrolyte imbalance, hypovolemia, oliguria, and hypovolemic shock. Hemocentration, increased blood viscosity, and thromboembolism may be observed (Schenker & Weinstein, 1978, p. 257). Judicious dosage regimens and careful follow-up of serum estradiol levels should help prevent the occurrence of this syndrome (Schenker & Weinstein, 1978, p. 265).

Infertility drugs increase the likelihood of multiple gestation, with this occurring twice as often in gonadotropin therapy. Patients should be informed of this possibility. Pepperell (1983, p. 7) reports a 10 percent rate of twin pregnancies after clomiphene citrate therapy; the incidence of multiple gestation with gonadotropin therapy is reported to be 21 to 34 percent (Schwartz & Jewelewicz, 1981, p. 10). Multiple pregnancies with more than two fetuses have been reported more often with gonadotropin therapy (Pepperell, 1983, p. 7).

GnRH therapy is a new modality for treating women with ovulatory dysfunction who have failed to conceive with other medications (Molloy, Hancock, & Glass, 1985; Phansey, Toffle, Curtin, et al., 1985; Zacur, 1985). This treatment became more effective after it was discovered that it needed to be given in a pulsatile manner. Administration is via a mechanical pump or "mechanical hypothalamus" ("A Mechanical 'Hypothalamus,'" 1984).

Hormonal therapy may also be implemented to correct a luteal phase defect detected on repeated endometrial biopsies. Clomiphene citrate and hMG have been used with some success to correct luteal phase inadequacy (Hammond & Talbert, 1982). A more common regimen is the administration of hCG or progesterone during the luteal phase of the cycle (Soules, Wiebe, Askel, & Hammond, 1977; Wentz, Herbert, Maxson, & Garner, 1984). This probably does raise serum progesterone levels, but no one has yet demonstrated clearly that higher serum levels correlate with an improved endometrium. For specific information regarding dosage regimens, side effects, and necessary counseling and follow-up for women receiving these treatments, see Murthy, Arronet, and Parekh (1970, p. 758).

Bromocriptine, a prolactin antagonist, has been used to treat infertility in women with increased blood levels of prolactin, with or without a pituitary tumor. This drug is given orally, in increasing doses, until ovulation occurs. Gastrointestinal side effects are minimized by starting the patient on a low dose (1.25 mg or half a tablet) twice a day for 1 week, with meals. The dose is doubled after 1 week. Mild nausea and postural hypotension are the only reported side effects. Serum prolactin levels are monitored to further determine dosage elevations (Lenton, Sobowale, & Coke, 1977; Pepperell, 1983, p. 3-5).

Occasionally, estrogen therapy can improve the quality and quantity of the cervical mucus at midcycle. This treatment may improve the postcoital test and enhance the migration of sperm through the cervical canal. Treatment of cervical infection can also improve mucus production; however, there are some recalcitrant cases in which the mucus never improves.

Fibroids theoretically can result in a failure in implantation by creating a chronic inflammatory response. A myectomy could be performed to treat infertility in which fibroids are the only identifiable pathology. In a recent study of 17 infertile patients with at least one 5-cm or larger submucosal leiomyoma, 61.5 percent of women with adequate sexual exposure achieved a pregnancy after surgery (Garcia & Tureck, 1984).

Dysfunction of the conduit system, more commonly termed tubal infertility, is usually treated by surgery. The approach, ranging from conservative lysis of adhesions to tubular reconstruction, is tailored to the pathology. The risk of infertility for women with endometriosis has been reported to be twice that of the general population, and a variety of theoretical mechanisms have been proposed (Muse & Wilson, 1982). Medical induction of pseudomenopause by administration of danazol for 6 to 12 months is now considered the treatment of choice, although in cases of mild endometriosis, this remains controversial (Schmidt, 1985). In a prospective study of 65 women with minimal disease who, after diagnostic laparoscopy, dilation and curettage (D&C), and tubal lavage, were randomly assigned to a danazol treatment group and a nontreatment control group, pregnancy rates of both groups were similar (Siebel, Berger, Weinstein, & Taymor, 1982). When medical treatment fails, or is inadequate, surgical excision may be necessary. (See Chapter 18 for extensive discussion of this disorder.)

If all of these procedures fail, in vitro fertilization (IVF) provides, in essence, an artificial fallopian tube—the culture dish in the incubator. After surgery to remove oocytes from the woman, fertilization and early cleavage occur in the laboratory; the embryos are then replaced in the uterus as if they had been propelled there from the tube. A newer technique, gamete intrafallopian transfer (GIFT), involves placement of both sperm and oocytes directly into the fallopian tubes, where fertilization takes place as it would naturally. This technique promises to result in success rates greater than those achieved with IVF (DiMattina & Liu, 1987). The addition of IVF and GIFT to the therapeutic armamentarium has also begun to provide insights into hitherto poorly understood processes in fertility: human fertilization and implantation. This technologic advance and other developments in the science of fertility, such as surrogate mothering, however, raise many as yet unsolved ethical and legal questions (Arditti, Klein, & Minden, 1984; Strickland, 1981).

EMOTIONAL RESPONSES OF THE PATIENT-COUPLE

It is understandable that obstacles to the realization of the need to reproduce will evoke complex emotional responses. In dealing with an infertile couple, consideration must be given to both the extrinsic and the intrinsic forces acting on them. Some inferences about the motivation of the patient-couple can be drawn from their ages, which determine the amount of pressure they may feel from the "biological clock." The magnitude, cause, and significance of age-related reductions in female fertility are a source of controversy (Bongaarts, 1982; Federation CECOS, Schwartz, & Hayaux, 1982; Howe et al., 1985; James, 1979). Nevertheless, as many women pass their midthirties, their desperation level rises with the onset of each menses.

Many couples in this age group present for evaluation long before one full year of attempting to conceive. In these instances, the initial interview should be geared toward reassurance, patient education, and counseling, unless the history points to a particular diagnosis. As first steps, the woman should begin a temperature charting and the man should supply a semen sample for analysis.

Many other aspects of a couple's life can affect their desire for children. Previous marriage and/or parenthood of one spouse may result in uneven dedication to the present search for fertility. This may or may not be problematic for the couple or for the progress of their infertility evaluation. Pressures from the extended family may come to bear: an only son may feel driven to continue the family name, or the youngest of several daughters may feel left out in family gatherings involving numerous young grandchildren. On the other hand, the families may provide unquestioning support to the couple or may not care at all. Membership in an organized religion may have some influence, either in shaping the couple's attitudes toward children or their difficulty in conceiving, or in providing fundamental support during the quest for fertility. The financial resources of the couple certainly affect how far they are willing and able to go in evaluation and treatment. For example, gonadotropin therapy can cost upward of $500 per month and insurance may not always cover this expense.

Finally, the other interests in each partner's life must be considered. The degree of satisfaction or frustration each may have found in a career can affect the vigor with which parenthood is pursued. Some working women may find it difficult to schedule all the tests and office visits the workup may require. Interests outside of work may influence a couple's overall satisfaction with the life they have built together. These and many other external factors affect a couple's response to their infertility and to the process of evaluation and treatment that they undergo.

Even more complex, however, are the intrinsic psychological drives and responses that are inextricably linked to the preceding. The motives behind the desire for a child are too fundamental and complex for discussion here, but the couple may be forced at some point to probe these by themselves. Frustration, disappointment, or grief may be experienced by either or both partners (Davis, 1987; Wedell, Billings, & Fayez, 1985). Loss of fertility can represent loss of control over an essential part of the male–female relationship, namely, the couple's sexual life. The workup demands disclosures of intimacies that may prove very uncomfortable for many couples. One danger in focusing so much attention on the timing and "success" of sexual relations is that it may result in a mechanistic approach to love making, loss of pleasure, and even sexual dysfunction.

Blame and guilt may arise within either or both partners and affect the couple's relationship, as well as the course of infertility treatment. Such feelings commonly result from the circumstances surrounding contraction of previous infections, use of contraception, and abortions. Underlying personality disorders may be brought to the fore and aggravate stresses on the couple to the extent that counseling is required. Finally, the effect of stress itself on fertility has been much studied, but no definitive medical conclusions have been drawn. The example of couples who conceive soon after adopting, despite years of infertility, is proposed as evidence that stress may negatively affect fertility. Certainly, the attitude of and support from the health care provider to whom the couple presents initially for help with their infertility can in some small measure minimize this added pressure and, perhaps, contribute to the occasional non–treatment-related spontaneous pregnancy.

Role of the Primary Care Provider

Throughout the evaluation of a woman or couple presenting with an inability to conceive, the role of the primary care provider is multifaceted. Gathering an accurate, comprehensive, and insightful history is crucial. Given the sensitive nature of some of the questions and the broad spectrum of data that are relevant, this process presents quite a challenge. Moreover, it is during this interview that the groundwork for the patient–provider relationship is laid. The primary care provider plays the role of teacher, counselor, and patient supporter as appropriate.

This therapeutic interaction becomes more important as the workup proceeds. At the outset, the provider must assess the adequacy of frequency and timing of coitus and teach as needed to correct any deficiency in this area. Before each subsequent step, the patient or couple must be counseled as to why and how each test is being performed. The primary provider orders the semen analysis and starts the patient on basal body temperature charting. If qualified, the primary provider also performs the postcoital test and endometrial biopsy. Otherwise, the patient may be referred to an infertility specialist for these tests, the hysterosalpingogram, and the diagnostic laparoscopy.

Depending on the needs and desires of the patient-couple, the relationship with the primary provider may or may not continue after the patient is referred to the infertility specialist. After this testing, it is possible that the primary care provider will be the one to explain the findings to the patients and work with them to determine the next step. If all attempts fail, it may fall to the primary care provider, as the professional best acquainted with the patients, to help them deal with that failure. Whatever the outcome, in each case, the vicissitudes of dealing with infertile women and couples present unique rewards as well as unique frustrations for the primary care provider.

REFERENCES

A mechanical "hypothalamus" for ovulation induction therapy (1984, March 16). *Journal of the American Medical Association, 251*(11), 1477.

Andersen, A. E. (1985). *Practical comprehensive treatment of anorexia nervosa and bulimia.* Baltimore, MD: Johns Hopkins University Press.

Arditti, R., Klein, R. D., & Minden, S. (Eds.) (1984). *Test-tube women.* Boston: Pandora Press.

Australian in Vitro Fertilisation Collaborative Group. (1985, October 26). High incidence of preterm births and early losses in pregnancy after in vitro fertilisation. *British Medical Journal, 291*(6503), 1160–1163.

Baker, H. W. G., Burger, H. G., & deKretser, D. M., et al. (1985, December 14). Testicular vein ligation and fertility in men with varicoceles. *British Medical Journal, 291*(6510), 1678–1680.

Bongaarts, J. (1982, March/April). Infertility after age 30: A false alarm. *Family Planning Perspectives, 14*(2), 75–78.

Bronson, R., Cooper, G., & Rosenfeld, D. (1984, August). Sperm antibodies: Their role in infertility. *Fertility and Sterility, 42*(2), 171–183.

Brooks, A. (1986, February 10). Insurers refusing to pay some costs in infertility cases. *The New York Times,* p. B12.

Buxton, C. L., & Olson, L. E. (1969, November 1). Endometrial biopsy inadvertently taken during conception cycle. *American Journal of Obstetrics and Gynecology, 105*(5), 702–706.

Christianson, C. (1986, July/August). Support groups for infertile patients. *Journal of Obstetric, Gynecologic, and Neonatal Nursing, 14*(4), 293–296.

Clark, M. (1982). Infertility: New cures, new hopes. *Newsweek, C*(23), 102–110.

Collins, J. A., Wrixon, W., James, L. B., & Wilson, E. H. (1983, November 17). Treatment-independent pregnancy among infertile couples. *New England Journal of Medicine, 309*(20), 1201–1206.

Daly, D. C. (1985, May). Advances in infertility therapy. *Comprehensive Therapy, 11*(5), 60–65.

Davajan, V., & Kunitake, G. M. (1969, March-April). Fractional in-vivo and in-vitro examination of postcoital cervical mucus in the human. *Fertility and Sterility, 20*(2), 197–210.

Davis, D. C. (1987, January/February). A conceptual framework for infertility. *Journal of Obstetric, Gynecologic, and Neonatal Nursing, 15*(1), 30–35.

DeFazio, J. (1986a, January). Clinical comment. *Ob/Gyn Clinical Alert, 2*(9), 34.

DeFazio, J. (1986b, February). Clinical comment. *Ob/Gyn Clinical Alert, 2*(10), 37.

deKretser, D. M. (1974, August). The management of the infertile male. *Clinics in Obstetrics and Gynecology, 1*(2), 409–427.

DiMattina, M., & Liu, J. (1987, October). Benefits of GIFT for treating infertility. *Contemporary Ob/Gyn, 30*(4), 145–146, 148–150.

Draye, M. A. (1985, February). An approach to infertility investigation. *Nurse Practitioner, 10*(2), 13–14, 16, 21–22.

Evans, H. J., Fletcher, J., Torrance, M., & Hargreave, T. B. (1981, March 21). Sperm abnormalities and cigarette smoking. *Lancet, 1*(8221), 627–629.

Federation CECOS, Schwartz, D., & Hayaux, M. J. (1982, February 18). Female fecundity as a function of age. *New England Journal of Medicine, 306*(7), 404–406.

Friberg, J. (1980, April). Mycoplasmas and ureaplasmas in infertility and abortion. *Fertility and Sterility, 33*(4), 351–359.

Garcia, C.-R., & Tureck, R. W. (1984, July). Submucosal leiomyomas and infertility. *Fertility and Sterility, 42*(1), 16–19.

Gillespie, H. W. (1965, April). The therapeutic aspect of hysterosalpingography. *British Journal of Radiology, 38*(448), 301–302.

Glass, R. I., Lyness, R. A. N., Mengle, D. C., et al. (1979, March). Sperm count depression in pesticide applicators exposed to dibromochloropropane. *American Journal of Epidemiology, 109*(3), 346–351.

Goldin, B. R., Adlercreutz, H., & Dwyer, J. T., et al. (1981, September). Effect of diet on excretion of estrogens in pre- and postmenopausal women. *Cancer Research, 41*(9, Part 2), 3771–3773.

Hammond, M. G., & Talbert, L. M. (1982, March). Clomiphene citrate therapy of infertile women with low luteal phase, progesterone levels. *Obstetrics and Gynecology, 59*(3), 275–279.

Hatch, M. (1984). Mother, father, worker: Men and women and the reproduction risks of work. In W. Chavkin (Ed.), *Double exposure: Women's health hazards on the job and at home.* New York: Monthly Review Press.

Hembree, W. C., Nahas, G. G., Zeidenberg, P., & Huang, H. F. S. (1979). Changes in human spermatozoa associated with high dose marihuana smoking. In G. C. Nahas & W. D. M. Paton (Eds.), *Marihuana: Biological effects.* New York: Pergamon Press.

Howe, G., Westhoff, C., Vessey, M., & Yeates, D. (1985). Effects of age, cigarette smoking, and other factors on fertility: Findings in a large prospective study. *British Medical Journal, 290*(6483), 1697–1700.

James, W. H. (1979, Winter). The causes of the decline in fecundability with age. *Social Biology, 26*(4), 330–334.

Lancranjan, I., Maicanescu, M., Rafaila, E., et al. (1975a, September). Gonadic function in workmen with long-term exposure to microwaves. *Health Physics, 29*(3), 381–383.

Lancranjan, I., Popescu, H. I., Gavanescu, O., et al. (1975b, August). Reproductive ability of workmen occupationally exposed to lead. *Archives of Environmental Health, 30*(8), 396–401.

Lenton, E., Sobowale, O. S., & Coke, I. D. (1977, November 5). Prolactin concentrations in ovulatory but infertile women: Treatment with bromocriptine. *British Medical Journal, 2*(6096), 1179–1181.

Menning, B. E. (1982, March). The psychosocial impact of infertility. *Nursing Clinics of North America, 17*(1), 155–163.

Molloy, B. G., Hancock, K. W., & Glass, M. R. (1985, January). Ovulation induction in clomiphene nonresponsive patients: The place of pulsatile gonadotropin-release hormone in clinical practice. *Fertility and Sterility, 43*(1), 26–32.

Murthy, Y. W., Arronet, G. H., & Parekh, M. C. (1970, November).

Luteal phase inadequacy. *Obstetrics and Gynecology, 36*(5), 758–761.

Muse, K. N., & Wilson, E. A. (1982, August). How does mild endometriosis cause infertility? *Fertility and Sterility, 38*(2), 145–152.

Padilla, S. L., & Craft, K. S. (1985, December). Anovulation: Etiology, evaluation and management. *Nurse Practitioner, 10*(12), 28–30, 33–34, 43–44.

Pepperell, R. J. (1983, July). A rational approach to ovulation induction. *Fertility and Sterility, 40*(1), 1–13.

Phansey, S. A., Toffle, R., & Curtin, J., et al. (1985, November). Alternative indications for pulsatile gonadotropin-releasing hormone therapy in infertile women. *Fertility and Sterility, 44*(5), 589–594.

Resolve. (1982). Resolve Information Brochure. Belmont, MA: RESOLVE (a self-help group providing medical information, referral, and emotional support to infertile women and couples).

Rowley, M., Leach, D. R., Warner, G. A., & Heller, C. G. (1974, September). Effect of graded doses of ionizing radiation on the human testis. *Radiation Research, 59*(3), 665–678.

Schenker, J. G., & Weinstein, D. (1978, September). Ovarian hyperstimulation syndrome: A current survey. *Fertility and Sterility, 30*(3), 255–268.

Schmidt, C. L. (1985, August). Endometriosis: A reappraisal of pathogenesis and treatment. *Fertility and Sterility, 44*(2), 157–173.

Schoenfeld, C. (1982). Semen analysis. In C.-R. Garcia, L. Mastroianni, Jr., R. D. Amelar, & L. Dubin (Eds.), *Current therapy of infertility 1982–1983*. Trenton, NJ: B. C. Decker.

Schwartz, M. & Jewelewicz, R. (1981, January). The use of gonadotropins for induction of ovulation. *Fertility and Sterility, 35*(1), 3–12.

Shane, J., Schiff, I., & Wilson, E. A. (1976). The infertile couple: Evaluation and treatment. *Clinical Symposia, 28*(5).

Siebel, M. M., Berger, M. J., Weinstein, F. G., & Taymor, M. L. (1982, November). The effectiveness of danazol on subsequent fertility in minimal endometriosis. *Fertility and Sterility, 38*(5), 534–537.

Sieber, S. M., & Adamson, R. H. (1975). Toxicity of antineoplastic agents in man: Chromosomal aberrations , antifertility effects, congenital malformations, and carcinogenic potential. *Advances in Cancer Research, 22*, 57–93.

Soules, M. R., Wiebe, R. H., Aksel, S., & Hammond, C. B. (1977, October). The diagnosis and therapy of luteal phase deficiency. *Fertility and Sterility, 28*(19), 1033–1037.

Speroff, L., Glass, R., & Kase, N. (1983). *Clinical gynecologic endocrinology and infertility* (3rd ed.). Baltimore, MD: Williams & Wilkins.

Strickland, O. L. (1981, March). In vitro fertilization: Dilemma or opportunity. *Advances in Nursing Science, 3*(2), 41–51.

Toth, A., Lesser, J. L., Brooks, C., & Labriola, D. (1983, March 3). Subsequent pregnancies among 161 couples treated for T-mycoplasma genital-tract infections. *New England Journal of Medicine, 308*(9), 505–507.

van der Spuy, Z. (1985, September). Nutrition and reproduction. *Clinical Obstetrics and Gynecology, 12*(3), 579–604.

Wallach, E. (1980, October). The frustrations of being "normal" yet infertile. *Fertility and Sterility, 34*(4), 405–406.

Wallis, C. (1984). The new origins of life. *Time, 124*(11), 46–53.

Warren, J. C. (1981). Reproductive failure. In S. Romney et al. (Eds.), *Gynecology and obstetrics—The health care of women* (2nd ed.). New York: McGraw-Hill.

Wedell, M. A., Billings, P., & Fayez, J. A. (1985 July/August). Endometriosis and the infertile patient. *Journal of Obstetric, Gynecologic, and Neonatal Nursing, 13*(4), 280–283.

Wentz, A. C., Herbert, C. M., Maxson, W. S., & Garner, C. H. (1984, June). Outcome of progesterone treatment of luteal phase inadequacy. *Fertility and Sterility, 41*(6), 856–862.

Whitehead, E. D., & Leiter, E. (1981, January). Genital abnormalities and abnormal semen analyses in male patients exposed to diethylstilbestrol in utero. *The Journal of Urology, 125*(1), 47–50.

Wyrobek, A. J., Watchmaker, G., & Gordon, L., et al. (1981, August). Sperm shape abnormalities in carbaryl-exposed employees. *Environmental Health Perspectives, 40*, 255–265.

Zacur, H. A. (1985, October). Ovulation induction with gonadotropin-releasing hormone. *Fertility and Sterility, 44*(4), 435–448.

28

Abortion

Phyllis Turk

Throughout the ages women have used abortion as a solution to unwanted pregnancy. Abortions have been induced by swallowing various potions, douching with curious and often dangerous solutions, and injuring various body parts, with varying degrees of success. Prior to the nineteenth century these practices, often described as unblocking the obstruction to menstrual flow, were not addressed in U. S. law if they were performed before *quickening*, the time when fetal existence was recognized (Mohr, 1978, p. 3). Legal restraints began to be applied as authorities in religion, medicine, and industry decreed that abortion was immoral, unsafe, or wasteful, and by 1880 every state had passed some kind of antiabortion law (Mohr, 1978, p. 229). Over the next decade, just as the advantages of antiseptic technique were being accepted by physicians, leading to safer abortion procedures, the practice was driven underground (Mohr, 1978, p. 239).

During the hundred or so years during which pregnancy termination was proscribed, legal "therapeutic abortion" remained an option for economically privileged women. A therapeutic abortion, one deemed necessary by the medical establishment for the woman's physical or psychological health, was socially acceptable because the decision to terminate the pregnancy was made by authority figures, not the woman herself (Smith, 1982, p. 3). Accurate data on the women who had illegal abortions in the United States during these years are unavailable, and estimates inferred from the morbidity and mortality statistics vary so much as to render the numbers useless.

Abortion law reform came gradually state by state until the 1973 *Roe* v.*Wade* Supreme Court ruling that during the first 3 months of pregnancy, the decision to abort can be made by a woman and her physician without interference from the state. After the first trimester, the state can impose safeguarding regulations. One immediate result of legalization was a decrease in mortality from illegal abortion, from 39.3 per year during the 5-year period 1972 to 1976 to zero in 1979 (Hatcher, Guest, Stewart, et al., 1984, p. 187). Abortion-related morbidity rates have also decreased significantly.

In this chapter, preabortion care, including counseling, screening, and diagnosis of pregnancy, is reviewed. The various abortion procedures available and their benefits and risks are described. Components of follow-up care, including physical assessment, intervention for complications, provision of contraception, and emotional support, are also discussed.

PREABORTION CARE

Abortion Counseling

The woman who is seeking an abortion must be helped to deal with her feelings about the abortion, assisted in the decision-making process if necessary, prepared for the abortion itself, and given anticipatory guidance concerning the outcome. One hundred years of criminality and the continuing vociferous arguments about the morality of abortion only add to the ambivalent feelings that many women must work through when they are considering terminating a pregnancy.

The woman may have come to the practitioner for pregnancy confirmation or for another reason, either suspecting that she is pregnant or surprised to be so. If she has come to have her suspicions confirmed, she may still be shocked by the news. She may be reacting to a medical problem or a positive genetic screening test in an otherwise much wanted pregnancy. Throughout the examination, the practitioner gathers clues to her thoughts and her decision-making process. Such statements as "I want an abortion," "I need an abortion," and "I have to have an abortion," as well as body language, can indicate very different feelings about the same situation and require different responses.

Along with confirmation of her pregnancy, the woman needs a supportive, nonjudgmental person with whom to explore her feelings about this pregnancy. The practitioner needs to provide information to help the woman understand and cope with her feelings, to facilitate decision making, and to help prevent future unplanned pregnancies. The information needed depends on the requests, needs, and wishes of the individual woman (and her partner or other involved person if she wishes), but the provider should not assume that a woman has knowledge in an area that has not been discussed. Some women desire and need extensive discussion concerning pregnancy versus abortion options, reproductive physiology, emotional responses, and contraception; others require minimal time on these topics.

Ambivalence is often the response to an accidental pregnancy. Unplanned pregnancy can force a woman to reassess everything from her immediate relationships to her life goals, as all these can be affected by her decision to continue or terminate this pregnancy. She may feel overwhelmed by the unexpected difficulty in making a decision that she had thought would be easier. Hern (1984, p. 78) notes that an essential component of counseling is providing support for the woman (and partner) through active listening. The counselor may help her to identify areas of conflict by acting as a sounding board. The woman may have an antichoice background or religious considerations that require exploration; she may be involved in a destructive relationship that is only now being questioned; she may be unaccustomed to making her own decisions. There are numerous reasons for ambivalence in this situation. According to Widdicombe (1981), "responses to this basic question are based more upon the woman's situation at that point in time than upon a basic attitude for or against abortion." Ultimately, the decision must be hers and for her own reasons.

Decision making means recognizing that there are only two alternatives in any pregnancy—termination or continuation to term (whether ultimately keeping the baby or giving it up)—and choosing between these. The undecided woman must sometimes be reminded that the pregnancy will progress while she is thinking about it and that by not making a decision to terminate the pregnancy she is making a decision to continue it. The type of abortion procedure to be considered depends on the length of gestation. To make an informed decision the woman must understand how the abortion will be done, the discomforts, safety, and risks that go with each choice, and the degree to which the risks increase as the decision is delayed. Midtrimester patients tend to have more ambivalence about having an abortion, and this ambivalence is frequently a chief factor in delaying the decision (Hern, 1984, p. 77). The midtrimester abortion candidate is often a teenager whose pregnancy progressed while she denied it or a woman who is having an abortion for medical reasons. In one study, couples who had undergone therapeutic abortions because of fetal defects (Jones, Penn, Schuchter, et al., 1984) expressed more anger, depression, guilt, and sadness than those who terminated pregnancies for "social" reasons. Forty-three percent of the women felt that they were to blame for having an abnormal fetus, which added to their guilt. Effective counseling, including offering the couples an opportunity to express their grief and loss, is likely to relieve preoperative anxiety and improve ability to cope with these feelings later (Hern, 1984, p. 78). Research over the last 20 years shows few long-term psychiatric sequelae to abortion. Widdicombe (1981) suggests that "as a health care community, we should foster the understanding that everybody does not feel good about everything at all times and that human responses, including grieving, are normal."

No counseling about an unplanned pregnancy is complete unless it includes consideration of prevention of future unplanned pregnancies. Basic reproductive physiology and effective contraception must be considered with the woman's specific needs in mind. As information is collected during the history and physical examination, the contraceptive methods that the woman considers appropriate must be assessed. She may have been using a reliable contraceptive method when she conceived and may have reasonable doubts about using any method. Initiation of contraception immediately after termination of a pregnancy is an option only if the patient is aware of this possibility. Ultimately, this too is her decision.

Some women delay seeking pregnancy confirmation because of a history of irregular menses, denial, lack of access to abortion services, their age and lack of experience, lack of knowledge about available options, or the cost of abortion and counseling services (Schneider, 1984). Anger and depression may contribute to the woman's delay in making a decision and acting on it. Delay may also be based on a mistaken idea of the length of the pregnancy. A significant number of women have some bleeding at or shortly after implantation that is interpreted as a menstrual period, confusing the gestational age assessment.

An unwanted pregnancy is not an isolated problem, and an abortion is generally a last resort, chosen when no other alternative is possible for the pregnant woman and her family. The decision is never taken lightly, regardless of the final choice.

Screening

Preabortion screening consists of a history and physical examination with emphasis on confirming the presence and duration of the pregnancy (see Chapters 2 and 3 for discussion of a complete history and physical examination). This is necessary to ensure the safest abortion procedure and choice of facility for each woman's needs. The aims of the screening exams are to confirm the pregnancy and determine the length of gestation, to determine if there are any medical or surgical conditions that may limit options or require medical consultation before abortion referral, and to initiate or continue counseling as needed.

History. The history should include a menstrual and contraceptive history, obstetric, medical, and surgical information, and a review of the systems. The menstrual history includes the date of onset of the last *normal* menstrual period and the previous menstrual period and any history of irregular or missed menses. What (if any) contraceptive method was she using? Was she using it correctly with a good understanding of how it works? Lack of confidence in a contraceptive method certainly affects decisions regarding postabortion contraception. The obstetric history includes number of pregnancies and their outcome. Has she had a cesarean delivery, excessive postpartum bleeding, or any other problem that the abortionist ought to be aware of? Has she ever had any surgery, particularly uterine, cervical, and other pelvic procedures? Does she have or have a history of any medical problems (especially hematologic, endocrine, or cardiac disorders)? Is she currently taking *any* medication? Does she have any allergies, specifically to local anesthetics, analgesic agents, or antibiotics?

Physical Examination. The physical examination should include vital signs, heart, lungs, breasts, abdomen, and pelvic assessment. The size of the uterus palpated on bimanual examination should confirm the length of the pregnancy, estimated by calculating from the onset of the last menstrual period. The very early pregnancy is the most challenging to diagnose, and it is crucial for accuracy as well as her comfort that the woman have an empty bladder for this exam. The woman who is "a few days late" and "feels pregnant" is probably correct especially if she has been pregnant before (Derman, 1981). The onset of nipple tingling, the first subjective indication of pregnancy, occurs 3 to 4 weeks from the last menses (Myles, 1985, p. 67). Breast engorgement, usually present prior to any uterine change, has been called the most accurate early physical change (Derman, 1981). The signs of early pregnancy are considered either presumptive or probable. Because each sign can have other causes, no one sign is diagnostic.

By 6 to 8 weeks from the onset of the last menstrual period, the uterine isthmus is considerably softer and more compressible on palpation (Hegar's sign) than in the nonpregnant woman. On speculum examination, portions of the cervix, vaginal mucosa, and vulva can be observed to have a blush or purplish coloration (Chadwick's sign). Cervical softening (Goodell's sign) is quite pronounced before any uterine enlargement is palpated.

At 8 weeks from the last menses, the uterus is the size of a tennis ball (Myles, 1985, p. 67) but more ovoid in shape. Early uterine enlargement is not always symmetric, and the area of implantation may be detected at about 8 to 10 weeks by its irregular contour (Piskacek's sign).

The uterus is described as filling the pelvic cavity at 12 weeks. Feeling like a medium-sized cantaloupe (or large grapefruit) (Nichols, 1987), it can be palpated abdominally at the level of the symphysis pubis. The fetal heart can be auscultated with a doppler device, which may be convenient for diagnosis as long as the woman's feelings are considered.

At 16 weeks from the last menstrual period, the uterus, again ovoid in shape, reaches halfway between the symphysis pubis and the umbilicus, and at 20 weeks, it is approximately one fingerbreadth below the umbilicus. It is important to remember that these descriptions are generalities. The uterus of the shorter (or taller)-than-average woman reaches these landmarks at an earlier (or later) time than stated here. Differences can also be observed throughout pregnancy with grand multiparas and, obviously, with a multiple gestation. Ultrasound becomes a reliable tool for precise dating of the pregnancy about 4 weeks after ovulation, when the gestational sac can be seen (Derman, 1981).

When assessing for gestational age, the provider must be alert to any unexpected findings. The woman with a urine slide test positive for pregnancy and a firm, walnut-sized uterus is probably not pregnant but should be rechecked in 2 weeks to be sure (Hern, 1984, p. 68). If the woman conceived with an intrauterine device in place or while taking oral contraceptives, the possibility of an ectopic pregnancy must be considered. The presence of any uterine or other pelvic anomalies should be noted. *Any discrepancy between physical findings and expected findings must be settled by an ultrasound examination before the method of pregnancy termination can be determined.*

Laboratory Tests. The minimum laboratory tests to be done before any abortion procedure are blood count (hemoglobin/hematocrit), blood type and Rh determination, and urine or serum test for pregnancy. The necessity of receiving Rh$_0$ (D) immune globulin [e.g., RhoGAM or MICRho-GAM, Gamulin Rh, Resonativ, HypRho-D, or Mini-Dose Rh$_0$ (D)] after the abortion should be explained to all women with Rh-negative blood. Pap smear, gonorrhea screening culture, and urinalysis are recommended. Chlamydia screening, although relatively expensive and not always available, is also recommended, especially for women at risk (see Chapters 4 and 12). The practitioner should be aware of which laboratory tests are performed routinely at each abortion facility so that tests that may otherwise be missed are included but replication is avoided.

PREGNANCY TESTS. Until a few years ago it was impossible to diagnose pregnancy with certainty until at least one menstrual period had been missed. Now, more sensitive pregnancy tests provide conclusive results at or before the first missed period. When a pregnancy test is performed or ordered, it is essential that the provider be familiar with the type of test and its sensitivity, and relate that information to the patient's history to interpret the test results accurately.

All of the currently used pregnancy tests are based on detecting human chorionic gonadotropin in either urine or blood. Human chorionic gonadotropin (hCG) is secreted by the syncytiotrophoblast by gestational day 8 (Derman,

1981) and is estimated to double in amount every 36 to 48 hours (Brucker, 1985) during the first month after conception. In normal pregnancy, hCG levels rise predictably, peak during the first 10 weeks, then decrease to about 5,000 mIU/mL during the remaining weeks of the pregnancy (Batzer, 1985) (Table 28–1). hCG consists of α and β subunits; the α component is chemically identical to the β subunit of luteinizing hormone (LH). This explains the LH cross-reaction observed in many pregnancy tests resulting in a false-positive reading, especially in the perimenopausal woman with higher LH levels. Pregnancy tests are classified in five general categories according to the method used to detect hCG: latex agglutination inhibition, hemagglutination inhibition, radioreceptor assay, radioimmunoassay, and enzyme-linked immunoabsorbent assay tests.

Latex agglutination inhibition (LAI) tests are widely available and inexpensive and provide rapid results. These 2-minute slide tests are the least sensitive of the current tests. They are able to detect 1.0 to 3.5 IU hCG/mL so they are accurate 1 to 2 weeks after a missed menstrual period. LAI tube tests require $1\frac{1}{2}$ to 2 hours to perform but may detect as little as 0.25 IU hCG/mL, the amount secreted at the time of the missed menses or within that week. The accuracy of the agglutination inhibition tests can be altered by several factors including proteinuria and storage. Derman (1981) urges that every urine specimen be tested for protein content and that those with significant amounts of protein be interpreted cautiously if positive for hCG. The benefit of testing a first morning urine specimen is commonly noted, but although refrigeration of the specimen appears to have no effect on accuracy, freezing it greatly increases the likelihood of a false-positive test (Derman, 1981). Drugs such as methadone and phenothiazine tranquilizers can also produce a false-positive result.

Hemagglutination inhibition (HAI) tests are the most commonly used tube tests. They are similar to LAI tube tests in sensitivity, reaction time, and confounding factors including possible LH cross-reaction. This category includes many of the home pregnancy tests, which tend to be less accurate and more expensive than laboratory-performed HAI tests (Brucker & Macmullen, 1985).

The radioreceptor assay (RRA) can be performed on urine or serum and is accurate at the time of, or a few days before, the missed menses by detecting hCG levels as low as 0.2 IU/mL. Researchers initially believed serum testing to be the method of choice but have since found hCG to be more concentrated in urine than in serum (Derman, 1981).

TABLE 28–1. APPROXIMATE URINARY HUMAN CHORIONIC GONADOTROPIN LEVELS IN PREGNANCY

Interval from Conception (wk)	hCG Level (mIU/mL)
2	12
3	50– 200
4	500–1,000
5	10,000
6	50,000
7–10[a]	100,000
11	50,000
12	20,000
13	15,000
14	10,000

[a]Peak.

From Batzer, F. (1985). Guidelines for choosing a pregnancy test. Contemporary Obstetrics and Gynecology Technology 1986, 26 (Special Issue), 37–52. Reprinted with permission.

Because hCG is not surrounded by as many other proteins in urine as it is in serum, urinary hCG may be detected more easily and earlier than serum hCG. RRA testing requires only an hour to perform, but the expense and short shelf life of the reagents mean that the laboratory must hold specimens to run in a batch once or twice a week. Cross-reaction with LH can occur.

Radioimmunoassay (RIA) tests use radioactively labeled markers that bind only to the β subunit of hCG, eliminating the possibility of an LH cross-reaction. Because of their enhanced sensitivity (0.005 to 0.04 IU hCG/mL), these "β-subunit tests" can be used to confirm a pregnancy 8 days after conception. Qualitative test results can be available from the laboratory in 1 hour; if greater sensitivity is required, a quantitative report can be obtained within 24 hours.

In an enzyme-linked immunoabsorbent assay (ELISA), an enzyme rather than a radioactive compound is used to identify the antigen of the hCG β subunit (Batzer, 1985). Because ELISA tests use a specific monoclonal antibody, they now have the advantage in sensitivity (able to detect hCG 8 days after conception), specificity (no cross-reactions), and reaction time. Available in a less sensitive version as home test kits as well as the laboratory kits, ELISAs are beginning to replace agglutination tests in popularity (Table 28–2).

ABORTION PROCEDURES

First Trimester

The method employed to terminate a pregnancy depends on the length of the pregnancy and the existence of contraindications to a particular method. The risks, complications, and cost of the abortion vary, contingent on the length of gestation, experience of the practitioner, type of procedure performed, and availability of the procedure in a given geographic area. The abortion may be performed under general anesthesia, local anesthesia, sedation, or without any of these. Anesthesia (especially general anesthesia) adds risks of its own to whatever termination method is used. The abortion performed earlier in pregnancy (first trimester) is an easier procedure, more readily available, safer, and less costly. As pregnancy progresses,

abortion procedures take longer to perform, expose the patient to greater risk of complications, are more physically and emotionally trying, and are more expensive. The woman who chooses to terminate her pregnancy because of positive findings on genetic screening by amniocentesis has no choice but to undergo a second-trimester abortion procedure. Amniocentesis (removal of amniotic fluid from the uterine cavity) for genetic studies cannot be performed before 15 to 16 weeks gestation; cell culture and study require another 3 to 4 weeks. If first-trimester chorionic villus sampling becomes widely available as an effective method of genetic testing, we should see fewer second-trimester abortion procedures performed for this reason.

In 1983, 91 percent of all abortions were done at or before 12 weeks gestation (Henshaw, 1987). First-trimester abortion procedures include menstrual extraction, vacuum curettage, laminaria insertion, and a combination of these. Not all these procedures are available everywhere, and the preferred method varies with the experience of the individual abortionist.

First-trimester abortions may be performed in a physician's office, a clinic, or a hospital; morbidity and mortality statistics show no difference with setting except to suggest that outpatient facilities may offer greater counseling and emotional support. The abortion may be done under general or local anesthesia, and here there is a difference. Local (paracervical block) anesthesia offers the advantages of simplicity and convenience (Van Lith, Wittman, & Keith, 1984). Local anesthesia costs less, has fewer side effects, and requires a shorter administration and recovery time than general anesthesia. Most important is the safety factor; there is less risk of a uterine perforation during the abortion procedure under local anesthesia, and any intraoperative complication that does occur is detected immediately. General anesthesia brings risks of its own depending on the agent selected, costs more because an anesthetist must be present, and results in a higher incidence of uterine perforation and heavy blood loss (Henshaw, 1982; Van Lith, et al., 1984).

Menstrual Extraction. Menstrual extraction, also known as menstrual regulation, endometrial aspiration, or "mini-abortion," may be performed up to 6 weeks from the last menstrual period. Originally, the term designated a procedure done before the diagnosis of pregnancy could be con-

TABLE 28–2. SUMMARY OF PREGNANCY TESTS

Type	Sensitivity (mIU hCG /mL)	Days from Conception[a]	Reaction Time	Comments
Latex (LAI) and hemagglutination (HAI) inhibition tests (urine)				Simple to perform False negative: too early, too dilute, or old specimen
Slide	1,500–3000	21–24	2 min	False positive: LH cross-reaction,
Tube	200–1,000	14–21	1–2 hr	drug use, recent pregnancy
Radioreceptor assay (RRA) (serum)	200	10	1 hr	LH cross-reaction requires sophisticated equipment
Radioimmunoassay (RIA) (serum)	1.5–40	8	20 min–1 hr 1–24 hr	Qualitative Quantitative β-subunit specificity Sophisticated equipment, required, expensive
Enzyme-linked immunoabsorbent assay (ELISA)				β-subunit specificity Simple to perform
Serum (lab)	20–50	8	5–30 min	
Urine (home)	50–300	14–17	20–30 min	

[a]Earliest detection

firmed and thus may or may not be an abortion. Opponents of the menstrual extraction procedure note that without accurate early pregnancy testing, as many as 40 to 45 percent of the women having this procedure were not pregnant (Derman, 1981). Menstrual extraction proponents questioned the alternative of asking the woman with a very early pregnancy to wait a few weeks longer for a positive diagnosis and observed that there has never been a case of menstrual regulation anywhere in the world where death was attributed to the procedure (Derman, 1981). With the increasing availability of more sensitive pregnancy tests, the number of unnecessary procedures should be limited.

Menstrual extraction is a relatively simple outpatient procedure. In some states this procedure may be performed by trained nonphysician health care providers; in most states this would be illegal (Boston Women's Health Collective, 1984, p. 294). Only a hand suction device (bulb or syringe) and a small flexible polyethylene cannula are required. Discomfort during the procedure can be minimized by mild analgesia or a paracervical block. After the cervix and vagina are cleansed with an antiseptic solution, a sterile cannula is introduced into the uterus through the cervix; then, as the suction is applied, the uterine contents are aspirated.

The advantages of menstrual extraction are its simplicity, minimal cost, and early resolution once the abortion decision is made. Some physicians feel that the procedure is technically more difficult, particularly in the young nullipara, because the cervix is not yet soft (risking a possible uterine perforation), nor is the uterus enlarged (Derman, 1981). The major disadvantage of this procedure is the failure rate, which ranges from 2.5 continued pregnancies per 1,000 abortions performed at 7 weeks or earlier (Fielding 1984) to as high as 6 percent (Derman, 1981). This is not due to the technique per se, but because this early in pregnancy the small amount of tissue can be missed. If a woman understands that the longer the interval after a missed menses (up to 6 weeks from the last menstrual period) the greater the likelihood of a positive pregnancy test and the greater the chance of a positive histologic diagnosis after the menstrual extraction (Hern, 1984, p. 121), she is better able to make an informed decision about this procedure. She should also know that cramping, nausea, diaphoresis, and syncope are possible side effects, and that some women find this procedure much more painful than they expected.

After a menstrual extraction the patient can expect bleeding, not heavier than her menstrual period, which lasts from a few days to a week, though she may not have more than spotting. She ought to avoid strenuous exercise for a few days, and avoid douching, tampons, and coitus until the bleeding stops. She should be aware of the signs of possible complication—abdominal pain, elevated temperature, and heavy bleeding—and know who to contact should any of these occur. The necessity of a 2- to 3-week postoperative examination (especially with the possibility of continued pregnancy) should not be overlooked; the practitioner should arrange with the woman in advance where she will return for her postabortion checkup: to her usual practitioner or to the physician who performs the procedure.

Suction Curettage. Suction curettage, also called vacuum aspiration, is the most commonly performed abortion procedure, representing 85 percent of all abortions in the United States in 1981 (Henshaw, Binkin, Blaine, & Smith, 1985). It may be utilized from the time a pregnancy is diagnosed until 12 weeks from the last menstrual period in any setting that is appropriate to the individual woman's needs

(physician's office, outpatient clinic, or hospital). The procedure, which takes about 15 minutes, is similar to the menstrual extraction technique except that the cervix must be dilated to allow for a wider-diameter suction cannula, and an electrically powered suction machine is employed. The cervix may be mechanically dilated with metal dilators, or laminaria may be inserted in the cervix for a slower, less traumatic dilation. The extent to which the cervix needs to be dilated depends on the cannula diameter required (generally 6 to 10 mm), which is determined by the length of the pregnancy. When the suction tubing is connected to the cannula and the suction is applied, the woman feels cramping, which lasts from a few minutes to half an hour. Some physicians curette the uterus if there is any question that it is not completely evacuated; others curette routinely after suction abortions.

After the abortion, the woman is observed in a recovery area for 1 to 2 hours. Vital signs, bleeding, and signs of any untoward reaction are checked at frequent intervals, and light refreshment is usually available. Most physicians prescribe an oxytocic drug for this time. Before discharge from the facility, the patient should be given instructions on what to do if she has any signs of infection or hemorrhage, and where to go for her 2-week checkup.

Most women say that a vacuum aspiration abortion hurts but the pain is tolerable. The factors that correlate with increased pain perception include younger age, increasing pregnancy duration, need for greater cervical dilation, and higher preoperative fear–anxiety levels (Schneider, 1984). Some women naturally express a preference for general anesthesia, which is available in many first-trimester facilities. With general anesthesia, an intravenous infusion must be started preoperatively, and the patient is exposed to possible anesthetic complications. Postabortion, the woman is at greater risk for heavy bleeding, requires a longer recovery time until the anesthesia wears off, and wakes up to uterine cramps and possibly nausea. Postprocedure instructions are the same as for a menstrual extraction.

Second Trimester

When first-trimester vacuum aspiration is possible, it is clearly the pregnancy termination method of choice. Second-trimester abortion presents additional problems. As Grimes and Cates (1981, pp. 119–120) explain, "The uterus has evolved to retain its contents tenaciously in the second trimester of pregnancy, while reserving the capacity to expel defective pregnancies in the first trimester and viable fetuses later in the third trimester. Thus, the second trimester is the least physiologic time during pregnancy for the uterus to empty itself." The uterus does not respond well to oxytocic drugs, the cervix is not readily dilated, and the fetus is larger and more difficult to get through the cervix with induction or with instruments. Early in the second trimester the uterus is too small and there is not enough amniotic fluid for consistently successful amnioinfusion terminations; later, too much fluid may dilute the infused solution and the larger fetus is less affected by it (Hern, 1984, p. 123).

There is no second-trimester abortion method of choice; rather, what has evolved is a combination of pharmacologic and surgical methods in an effort to add comfort and safety to what has been a slow, unpredictable, and painful procedure. The ideal second-trimester procedure would be safe, simple to perform, inexpensive, and readily available. Dilation and evacuation (D&E) is the predominant method of termination during the 13- to 15- week interval and appears to be the safest method through 20 weeks (Grimes & Cates, 1981; Grimes & Schulz, 1985). Pre-

TABLE 28–3. SUMMARY OF ABORTION PROCEDURES

Procedure	Weeks from LMP[a]	Facility	Average cost[b]	Time Required for Procedure	Comments
Menstrual extraction	Up to 6	Office, clinic, hospital		15 min	Fees generally same as for vacuum aspiration
Vacuum aspiration	Up to 12	Office, clinic, hospital	$190 $735	15 min (add 4 + hr for laminaria)	Hospital range is $275–1,300, including physician's fee
Dilation and evacuation	13–20	Clinic, hospital	At 16 wk, $358 At 16 wk, $740	30 min (add 4–12 hr for laminaria)	
Amnioinfusion	16–20 (to 24 in some states)	Hospital	$940		Fee scales for outpatient procedures not available

[a]Last, menstrual period.
[b]Nationwide averages; does not include RhoGAM. First trimester (clinic), add average $45 for general anesthesia. Fees vary significantly by geographic area and number of procedures performed at facility.
From Henshaw, S. (1982). Freestanding abortion clinics: Services, structure, fees. Family Planning Perspectives, 14 *(5), 248–256. Reprinted with permission.*

dilation with laminaria makes this procedure technically less difficult and less traumatic, as does performing an amnioinfusion prior to a D&E at 18 to 20 weeks. Laminaria insertion prior to amnioinfusion also shortens the time necessary for that procedure (Table 28–3).

Laminaria. Laminaria tents are small sticks of dried, compressed seaweed that readily absorb moisture. When laminaria are inserted into the cervical canal they absorb secretions and swell to four times their original diameter or more, depending on the length of time they are left in place (Fig. 28–1). The laminaria softens the cervix and initiates slow, gentle cervical dilation, decreasing the need for manual dilation in late first-trimester and in second-trimester terminations.

The procedure for laminaria insertion may be somewhat uncomfortable but should not be painful. After a routine pelvic examination, the cervix and vagina are cleansed with antiseptic and the uterus may be sounded. The laminaria tent may be soaked in sterile water (to speed swelling) (*Dilateria*, 1982) or in a bacteriostatic lubricant (*Dilateria*, 1984), before it is inserted in the cervical canal. Moistened gauze is then placed in the vagina over the ends of the lami-

naria to prevent outward migration. Insertion of the laminaria tent produces minimal discomfort but insertion of three or four tents (if needed for greater cervical dilation) usually produces pain that resolves in a few minutes. The patient is kept recumbent several minutes after insertion to avoid vasovagal syncope (Stubblefield, 1981). She should be warned that if several laminaria are inserted, she will feel cramps or pain in several hours as the laminaria swell. Oral analgesics are routinely prescribed for this. Depending on the length of gestation, the laminaria tent(s) is removed in 1 to 12 hours. The woman should be instructed to report any bleeding greater than her menstrual flow, any unusual pain, and fever greater than 100°F. She may be given a bacteriostatic or bacteriocidal cream to apply intravaginally (*Dilateria*, 1984), and is told when to return for removal of the laminaria and the evacuation procedure.

The obvious disadvantage of using laminaria tents for cervical dilation is the increased time required over mechanical dilation. If the tent is to be left overnight, the outpatient abortion candidate will be left unmonitored during most of the waiting period (though she may be with supportive friends, which may not be possible in the hospital). Theoretically, the risk of infection is greater, but this has

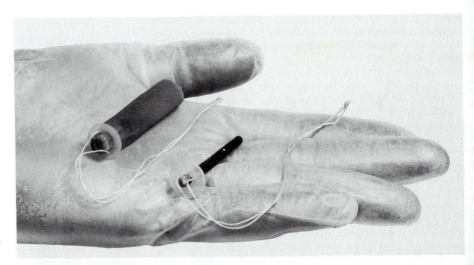

Figure 28–1. Laminaria. *(Courtesy of Milex Products Incorporated.)*

not occurred in practice (Altman, Stubblefield, Schlam, et al., 1985; Stubblefield, 1981). The advantage of using laminaria is safety. Use of laminaria alone for cervical dilation significantly decreases the risk of uterine perforation (Grimes, 1984), increases uterine contractility, and decreases any potential for cervical incompetence in subsequent pregnancies (Grimes & Cates, 1981).

Dilation and Evacuation. Dilation and evacuation may be done as a single procedure or in combination with other second-trimester methods, depending on the length of gestation and the preference of the provider. When it is done as a single procedure, the cervix is mechanically dilated and the uterine contents are crushed and evacuated with a large-bore vacuum curette. This single-procedure method is most frequently used at 13 to 15 weeks of gestation and may be done under local (paracervical block) or general anesthesia. Laminaria are frequently used because the products of conception are larger, and the cervix requires greater dilation than with a first-trimester vacuum aspiration abortion. Although use of laminaria requires at least two visits and therefore a greater time investment, the gentler cervical dilation may mean better long-term results.

The patient should be prepared to fast 6 hours prior to the evacuation. Most clinicians provide intravenous hydration during the abortion procedure, adding oxytocin during or immediately afterward to encourage uterine contractions and limit blood loss. The dilation and evacuation procedure takes approximately one-half hour; the length of the immediate recovery period depends on whether local or general anesthesia is used. Analgesia may be necessary postabortion if cramping is severe, and the woman should be advised of relief measures for engorged breasts should this present a problem (Smith, 1982, p. 64).

The advantages of dilation and evacuation compared with other techniques for second-trimester pregnancy termination are relative safety, lower cost, predictable procedure time, lack of need for hospitalization, and availability of anesthesia options. Unlike the amnioinfusion procedure, also performed in the second trimester, the patient does not experience prolonged labor or fetal expulsion, and there are no medical contraindications (Hern, 1984, p. 132; Smith, 1982, p. 64). The disadvantage is the limited availability of the procedure because more physician time is required than for amnioinfusion methods and because many providers object to performing the procedure (Hern, 1984, p. 132; Smith, 1982, p. 64).

Amnioinfusion. Amnioinfusion, for many years the second-trimester termination technique of choice, is still more widely available than dilation and evacuation. The pregnancy must be at least 16 weeks so that the uterus is an accessible abdominal organ and a pocket of amniotic fluid can be located easily. This is why women presenting themselves for vacuum aspiration abortions at 13 to 14 weeks of gestation (before D&E was an acceptable procedure) were told that they would have to wait a few weeks before terminating the pregnancy. The best time for amnioinfusion is at 16 to 18 weeks of gestation. It may also be used as an adjunctive method prior to dilation and evacuation in a later pregnancy (20 weeks or greater). Laminaria may or may not be employed. The effect of the amnioinfusion is to create uterine contractions that dilate the cervix and expel the fetus and placenta. This procedure is best done by admitting the patient to the hospital for a 2- to 3-day stay; however, some facilities offer amnioinfusion as an outpatient procedure, with the woman returning in labor. The woman is instructed to fast 6 hours prior to amni-

oinfusion. If laminaria tents are to be used, they are inserted prior to or immediately after the amnioinfusion. Necessary blood specimens are obtained and an intravenous infusion is started. The woman assumes a supine position, and the site is prepped and draped. After the skin over the site is infiltrated with a local anesthetic, an 18-gauge spinal needle is inserted into the uterine cavity, a small amount of amniotic fluid is aspirated to verify placement, and the prostaglandin solution is infused. When hypertonic (20%) saline or urea is used, approximately 200 mL of amniotic fluid is aspirated before the solution is infused by gravity drainage or through a syringe (Hatcher, Guest, Stewart, et al., 1984, p. 194; Smith, 1982, p. 67). (Figs. 28–2 to 28–5). The patient is instructed to report any unusual sensations during the instillation (dizziness and anxiety are common; other possible effects depend on the solution used), and her vital signs are monitored throughout. The procedure is frightening to many women but not painful; some feel bloated after the instillation. When it is done in an ambulatory setting, the woman is instructed to go to the hospital when labor begins. Although this arrangement leaves her more "vulnerable to physical and psychological complications without professional support or monitoring" (Smith 1982), some women choose to await labor with a close friend and pay lower hospital costs. Obviously the ambulatory procedure would be a poor option for the woman whom the provider knows will be alone or away from home.

Clinicians have different preferences regarding the amnioinfusion solution based on the advantages and disadvantages of each (Table 28–4). Increasingly, amnioinfusions are combinations of solutions intended to increase effectiveness while reducing side effects (Hatcher et al., 1984, p. 193). Prostaglandins have the shortest injection-to-abortion time but are not always fetocidal; thus, a relatively large number (estimated at up to 7 percent) of fetuses show signs of life (Hern, 1984, p. 125). Prostaglandins present no danger of coagulopathies or hypernatremia and can be used satisfactorily in clients with cardiac disease or if the clinician obtains a bloody amniotic fluid sample (Hern, 1984, p. 125). As about one third of the patients experience no effect from this drug, some clinicians advocate routine repeated amnioinfusion 6 hours after the first. Other disadvantages of prostaglandin infusion include higher incidence of nausea, vomiting, diarrhea, cervical trauma, retained placenta, and hemorrhage and relatively high cost. Prostaglandins are contraindicated in patients with a history of asthma, pulmonary hypertension, glaucoma, epilepsy, and hypertensive disease (Schneider, 1984).

Hypertonic (20%) saline offers a predictable infusion-to-expulsion time, which can be considerably shortened by the addition of oxytocin to the intravenous infusion after amnioinstillation. Its advantages are effectiveness, relatively low rate of retained tissue, and inexpense. The disadvantages lie in the potentially fatal complications of hypernatremia and disseminated intravascular coagulation (DIC) syndrome (if the saline solution is extravasated), complications that can be minimized through the use of preventive procedures (Hern, 1984, p. 124). Hypertonic saline amnioinfusion is contraindicated in patients with a bloody tap (unless the clinician chooses to wait and attempt the procedure again after a few hours) and those with cardiac disease.

Hyperosmolar urea offers the advantages of no absolute contraindications (Hern, 1984, p. 125) and a short instillation-to-contraction time, but these are balanced by a high failure rate and a high (30 to 40 percent) retained placenta rate. Urea is frequently the solution chosen when the

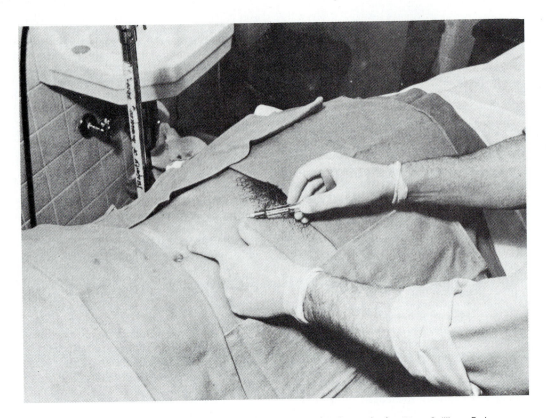

Figure 28–2. Amnioinstallation procedure. Injection of local anesthetic. *(From Quilligan, E. J., Zuspan, F. P. [1982]. Douglas-Stromme operative obstetrics [4th ed.]. New York: Appleton–Century–Crofts.)*

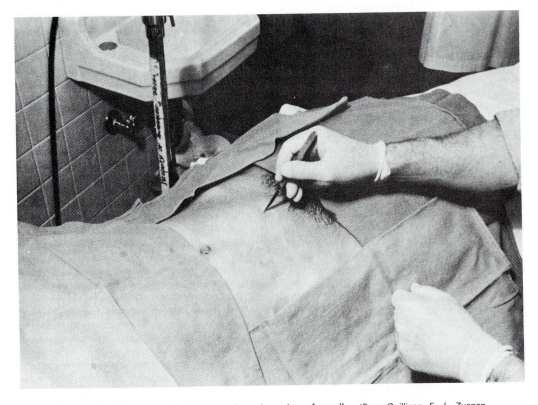

Figure 28–3. Amnioinstillation procedure. Insertion of needle. *(From Quilligan, E. J., Zuspan, F. P. [1982]. Douglas-Stromme operative obstetrics [4th ed.]. New York: Appleton–Century–Crofts.)*

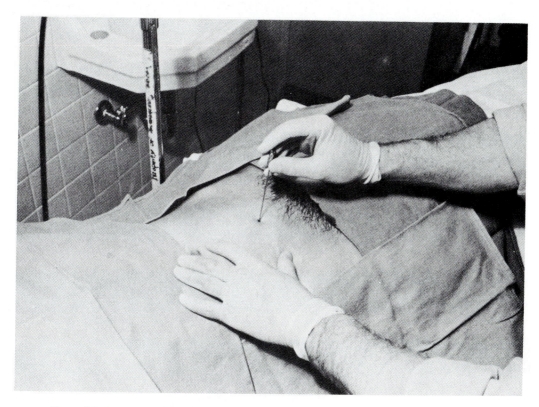

Figure 28–4. Amnioinstillation procedure. Aspiration of amniotic fluid. *(From Quilligan, E. J., Zuspan, F. P. [1982]. Douglas-Stromme operative obstetrics [4th ed.]. New York: Appleton–Century–Crofts.)*

abortion is to be a combination of techniques, such as an amnioinfusion to induce uterine contractions prior to dilation and evacuation at 20 (or more) weeks of gestation.

After the amnioinfusion, the patient is offered a fluid diet until regular active contractions are established. In some facilities she may ambulate (with or without an intravenous infusion); in others, bedrest is required. She may receive analgesics when her labor is established, but she should be aware that she will be awake when the fetus is expelled. The actual abortion occurs in bed with a nurse (generally not a physician) in attendance. If the products of conception are not complete, the nurse clamps and cuts the cord and monitors the patient closely until the placenta is delivered (or a dilation and curettage performed). The patient should remain in the hospital for observation for 12

hours after expulsion. Most women do not have extensive discomfort from cramps after the abortion, but instruction on comfort measures to relieve engorged breasts should be offered (Smith, 1982, p. 104).

Hysterotomy. Hysterotomy, a surgical incision into the uterus to remove the fetus and placenta, requires the same preparation and recovery as any major surgery. Hysterotomy may be done after a failed second-trimester abortion or when another need to enter the pelvic cavity exists (Hatcher et al., 1984, p. 192), although current investigators feel that there is no place in contemporary abortion practice for this procedure. The overall morbidity and mortality rates are several times higher than those resulting from combined abortion–sterilization procedures (Grimes, 1984).

TABLE 28–4. AMNIOINFUSION SOLUTIONS

	Advantage	Disadvantage
Prostaglandins	Contractions start within 4 hours Oxytocin augmentation not necessary No risk of coagulopathy or hypernatremia	May need repeat infusion High incidence of gastrointestinal side effects Higher risk of hemorrhage Medical contraindications Possible live fetus Expensive
Hypertonic sodium chloride	Predictable infusion-to-abortion time Effective, low retained tissue rate Inexpensive	Potential hypernatremia (0.01/100 abortions) Potential coagulopathy (0.3/100 abortions) Medical contraindications
Hyperosmolar urea	No absolute contraindications Short instillation-to-contraction time Low cost	High failure rate when used alone High retained placenta rate

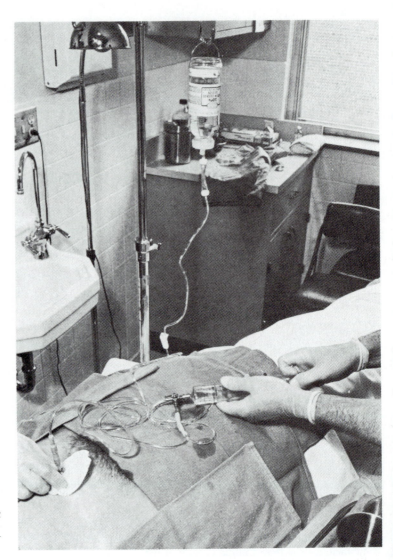

Figure 28-5. Amnioinstillation procedure. Hypertonic saline is infused. *(From Quilligan, E. J., Zuspan, F. P. [1982]. Douglas-Stromme operative obstetrics [4th ed.]. New York: Appleton–Century–Crofts.)*

The surgery may be performed under regional (usually spinal) or general anesthesia. The patient should also be aware that this major abdominal surgery leaves a permanent vertical scar on the uterus, necessitating that any future deliveries be by cesarean section.

FUTURE TECHNIQUES

Investigators looking for simple, safe pregnancy termination techniques are focusing on noninvasive methods that can be used very early in pregnancy. With the availability of more specific, sensitive pregnancy tests, these methods may soon provide a prompt resolution to an unwanted pregnancy.

Prostaglandins in the form of vaginal suppositories offer a noninvasive early termination option that may be self-administered at home (Rosen, von Knorring, Bygdeman, & Christiensen, 1984); however, the frequency and severity of gastrointestinal side effects may limit the use of these suppositories (Borten & Friedman, 1985; Foster, Smith, McGruder, et al., 1985), just as these side effects have limited the use of prostaglandins for termination later in preg-

nancy. Use of prostaglandin suppositories for cervical dilation prior to abortion has been studied with favorable results (Kajanoja, Mandelin, Makila, et al., 1984).

RU 486 is an antiprogestational compound under investigation in Europe. As progesterone is essential during implantation and early pregnancy, blocking its action would theoretically result in an early abortion (Kovacs, Sas, Resch, et al., 1984). In one study of 100 pregnant women treated within 10 days of a missed menstrual period, 85 had complete abortions. Eighteen percent of these women had prolonged bleeding, but transfusion or curettage was not required (Couzinet, Le Strat, Ulmann, et al., 1986). Investigators are also looking to RU 486 as a possible once-a-month contraceptive pill to be taken at the expected menstrual time without knowing whether fertilization has occurred (Spitz & Barden, 1985). Because it is available in oral form for self-administration, RU 486 has great potential for patient acceptance.

Less invasive procedures with fewer complications for cervical dilation are under investigation. In one small but controlled trial, Ying, Lin, and Robins (1985) found acupuncture to be an effective method for achieving cervical dilation in first-trimester abortions. This deserves further research.

POSTABORTION CARE

Immediate postabortion care consists of frequent monitoring of vital signs and bleeding, administration of Rh_0 (D) immune globulin, and education. All unsensitized Rh-negative women should receive Rh_0 (D) immune globulin regardless of the length of gestation to avoid the risk of Rh sensitization. A lower dose of Rh_0 (D) immune globulin, available as MICRhoGAM or Mini-Dose Rho_0 (D), which contains approximately 50 μg of anti-Rho_0 (D) (compared with 300 μg), has been recommended for abortions of fetuses less than 13 weeks (*Physicians' desk reference*, 1988, pp. 1439, 1494–1495). In many facilities, Rh_0 (D) immune globulin involves an extra charge.

The postoperative monitoring varies from an hour or two after a first-trimester procedure under local anesthesia to 12 hours or longer after a second-trimester amnioinfusion or a complicated termination. If oxytocic drugs (usually methergine) or antibiotics are ordered, they are initiated during this time.

Postabortion teaching focuses on instructions for self-care, the follow-up appointment, contraception, and any other concerns of the patient. The woman may eat and drink anything she desires. Although it is advisable to avoid strenuous exercise for a few days, it is usually safe for her to resume normal activities, guided by how she feels.

Bleeding and cramping vary, with a few women having none at all (particularly after an early pregnancy termination). Most women have cramps and bleeding during the first 2 weeks after an abortion. If the bleeding is heavier than the heaviest day of a menstrual period or if the cramping is severe, a woman should call or see her provider. Normal cramping should be relieved by any over-the-counter analgesic. A regular menstrual period should begin in 4 to 6 weeks, sooner if oral contraceptives are started immediately after the abortion.

For 2 weeks after an abortion, the woman should put nothing into her vagina: no tampons, no douching, and no sexual intercourse. After a second-trimester termination, which requires greater cervical dilation, a longer wait of 4 weeks is advised. The patient should be told to take her temperature twice a day for the first week and to call if it is 100°F or higher or if the bleeding develops a foul odor. Some practitioners order prophylactic antibiotics after abortion procedures; the patient taking antibiotics must also be instructed to call if she has any untoward effects, such as a rash or hives. Before her discharge from the abortion facility, the patient must know where she should call or go if she has any complications (at any hour), and must be given an appointment for a follow-up checkup in 2 weeks (some practitioners suggest 4 weeks after an amnioinfusion).

Immediate postabortion complications include uterine perforation, hemorrhage, trauma to abdominal or pelvic organs, and postabortion syndrome. The incidence of complications immediately after an abortion procedure depends on the length of gestation (increasing with increasing gestation), the technique used, the operator's skill, and the patient's general state of health (Van Lith et al., 1984). The most feared complication is uterine perforation, which, though infrequent at a rate of 0.9 per 1,000 abortions (Grimes, Schulz, & Cates, 1984a), greatly increases the morbidity and mortality rates if it results in infection, hemorrhage, trauma to abdominal organs, or hysterectomy. Perforation usually is detected easily during the procedure by the abortionist when the instrument responsible is not obstructed in its passage by the uterine wall (Pritchard, MacDonald, & Gant, 1985, p. 481). The severity of the perforation determines how it is treated, from simple observation to hysterectomy. Reliable gestational age assessment prior to the abortion procedure, use of laminaria for cervical dilation, use of local anesthesia, and performance of the abortion by an experienced physician lessen the chance of perforation.

Hemorrhage may result from uterine perforation, cervical laceration, or postabortion syndrome, and all of these are more likely to occur when the abortion is performed under general anesthesia. Postabortion syndrome is the name given to the uterine atony that may inexplicably occur after an uncomplicated abortion. The patient complains of excruciating pain a few hours after the abortion and the exam reveals a tender, larger-than-preabortion-size uterus (Van Lith et al., 1984) filled with blood and no bleeding from the cervical os. Prompt reaspiration or curettage followed by oxytocin cures this syndrome.

Complications that may manifest after the immediate postabortion period are infection, retained tissue, subinvolution, continuing pregnancy, and Asherman's syndrome. The potential for infection can be minimized by preabortion gonorrhea and chlamydia screening and treatment, treatment of severe cervicitis, complete emptying of the uterus, and prophylactic antibiotics after the procedure (Grimes, Schulz, & Cates, 1984b; Hatcher et al., 1984). Although few clinical trials have evaluated the advantages and disadvantages of routine postabortion antibiotics, several studies show their effectiveness in decreasing postabortion infection. A broad-spectrum antibiotic like tetracycline, or the longer-acting doxycycline, is advised, with prophylaxis continuing only 24 hours to minimize alterations of fecal or vaginal flora.

The patient who complains of continuing, worsening, or severe cramping or pelvic discomfort, fever, or discharge needs immediate attention. Pelvic infections are associated with subsequent infertility, so early treatment should be stressed. Whether the patient needs to be hospitalized for administration of parenteral antibiotics or can be treated as an outpatient depends on the extent of the infection.

Retained tissue can also present as severe, cramping pain, with or without signs of infection, usually within the first 5 days of abortion (Hatcher et al., 1984, p. 199). This complication is treated by evacuating the uterus and providing antibiotics as indicated.

The possibility of continued pregnancy is greater after attempted termination of a very early pregnancy or of a multiple or ectopic gestation. The continuation rate may be as high as 2.47 per 1,000 abortions at 7 weeks of gestation or earlier (Fielding, Lee, Borten, & Friedman, 1984). Careful examination of the tissue obtained at the time of the procedure reduces the likelihood of this complication, and, of course, continuing pregnancy symptoms and an enlarged uterus are indications of it.

Although all abortion patients should be monitored for these complications, the overwhelming majority of women suffer none of these effects. The safety of abortion, especially relative to the risks of term pregnancy and delivery, has been amply documented (Digest, 1982). Changes in the legal status of abortion, in its social acceptability, and in the increased availability of this service have resulted in women seeking terminations earlier in pregnancy when the risks are lowest. Legalization has spurred technologic innovations and hence provided more, and less traumatic, techniques. The skill and experience of the operating physician constitute variables to be considered when assessing abortion risks (Altman et al., 1985; Hern, 1984, p. 278).

Studies of the long-term effects of legal induced abortion

demonstrate no loss of fertility (Stubblefield, 1981; World Health Organization Task Force on Sequelae of Abortion, 1984) and no adverse psychological effects in women who aborted compared with women who carried their pregnancies to term (Bradley, 1984). The concern that induced abortion leads to cervical incompetence has not been demonstrated in women who have one abortion (Schneider, 1984), although this may be a problem after several abortions.

Adolescents (aged 17 and younger) have been shown to have a greater risk of postabortion endometritis than women aged 20 to 29 (Burkman, Atienza, & King, 1984), even when they were treated for their (higher rates of) preexisting gonorrhea and urinary tract infections. There are no studies available comparing morbidity in adolescents who have had elective abortions with adolescents who have delivered babies. Routine prophylactic antibiotics may be of benefit in this group.

FOLLOW-UP VISIT

A 2-week postabortion visit is recommended. The purposes of this visit are to assess the body's return to its prepregnant state, to screen for complications, to provide contraception if it wasn't initiated at the time of the procedure, and to offer emotional support and counseling.

Data Collection

History. A careful interval history should include how the woman is feeling, duration and amount of bleeding and cramping, and signs or symptoms of infection or continuing pregnancy (Table 28–5). Also significant are the resumption of sexual relations, use of contraception, and passage of a menstrual period (expected 4 to 6 weeks after an abortion). If any complications did occur during or after the abortion, the practitioner should have knowledge of how the patient was treated and whether the problem was resolved. The practitioner should also ascertain what, if any, medications were prescribed after the abortion and whether they were taken. Laboratory reports from the abortion procedure should be reviewed to see if any follow-up is warranted. It is particularly important to review the pathology report to make sure that products of conception were removed. If the woman is Rh negative, administration of Rh_0 (D) immune globulin should be confirmed.

Physical Examination. Depending on the type of procedure and the specific interval history, the patient is assessed for cervical lacerations, infection, and uterine involution. By this time, the uterus should be of normal size and nontender. Other components of the physical examination should be performed as indicated. A regular annual screening physical can be done at this time if necessary (see Chapter 3).

Laboratory Data. No routine laboratory tests are necessary at a normal postabortion follow-up visit; however, if abnormalities were apparent on the laboratory tests performed at the time of the procedure, repeat examinations may be appropriate.

If the history and pelvic examination suggest continued pregnancy, a sensitive pregnancy test will ordinarily pick up hCG 2 weeks after a pregnancy has terminated. A quantitative β subunit should be obtained to help differentiate between an ectopic pregnancy, a multiple gestation, and an incomplete abortion. If more than 3 or 4 weeks has elapsed since the termination, the possibility of a new pregnancy exists. The quantitative β-hCG will help differentiate the latter from other possible diagnoses.

If infection is suspected, a complete blood count with differential is warranted. Cervical and urine cultures are ordered depending on the symptomatology. Blood culture may be valuable if the woman presents with a high fever, and consultation, of course, is necessary.

Intervention

Generally, after an abortion procedure, women need contraceptive initiation, teaching and counseling, and emotional support. In the presence of suspected or confirmed complications, however, consultation is also required.

Complications. The following complications require medical intervention: continued pregnancy, whether intrauterine or ectopic, infection, and Asherman's syndrome. Asherman's syndrome, characterized by uterine adhesions and associated with dilation and curettage postabortion (see Chapter 14), may not be detected at this visit. It is suspected if the nonpregnant woman does not resume menstruation at the expected time or if the subsequent menses is unusually scanty. Patients should be advised to call if menses is not resumed by 8 weeks postabortion. Referral is necessary; treatment consists of dilation and curettage or hysteroscopic examination with cutting of adhesions (DeCherney & Friedman, 1985, p. 288; Nichols & McGoldrick, 1985, p. 441).

In the absence of pregnancy, if the uterus is still large and soft, uterine subinvolution may be diagnosed, especially after a second-trimester procedure. If this is accompanied by prolonged, excessive, or irregular bleeding, an ergot preparation can be prescribed, provided the patient's blood pressure is within normal limits. Ergotrate maleate

---

TABLE 28–5. WHAT TO EXPECT AFTER AN ABORTION

	Expected Effect	Warning Signs
Vaginal bleeding	Bleeding lasting up to 2 weeks Spotting up to 4 weeks No bleeding	Bleeding heavier than menses Bleeding more than 2 weeks Foul odor
Cramps	Menstrual-like Mild to moderate, relieved by mild analgesia	Severe, persistent un-cramplike abdominal pain
Temperature (oral)	Less than 100.0°F	100.0°F or higher
Menses	Resume within 4 weeks or after first package of oral contraceptives completed	No menses within 8 weeks Continued symptoms of pregnancy
Other	Fatigue	Appearance of rash or hives if antibiotics were given

(or methergine) 0.2 mg every 6 hours for six doses should alleviate this problem. Repeat follow-up should be scheduled for approximately 1 week. If there is no bleeding, the patient can be counseled regarding rest and seen again before treatment is instituted. Depending on practice or institutional protocols, consultation may be necessary.

Subinvolution may be associated with infection of the uterus. Symptoms of infection include abdominal pain, chills and fever, foul lochia, and general malaise. Physical examination reveals a tender uterus and possibly adnexae. Consultation is essential whenever infection is suspected.

Contraception. An ideal time to start oral contraceptives is on the day (or within a week) of a first-trimester abortion. If the woman is an appropriate candidate but for any reason has not yet started the pill, she can begin with her next period. What cannot be overstressed is the need for contraceptive measures and the possibility of another pregnancy soon after an abortion. Diaphragms can be fitted at this visit, or arrangements can be made for the woman to return during her menses for insertion of an intrauterine device if this is an appropriate method for her. An interim method must be provided. If she avoids selecting a contraceptive method or chooses abstinence, explore her reasons with her. The reasons may be unrealistic or quite appropriate. It is only by understanding the options available to her that she can make an informed decision.

Emotional Support. Many factors affect emotional reactions after an abortion. Most common are relief, mixed with some sadness or regret, and depression. Some women are alarmed at feeling depressed, especially when there were no reservations beforehand about the decision to abort. The woman who is recovering from the end of an unsatisfactory relationship (or one she thought was good) may feel doubly burdened. Other women find they are closer to their partners or have gained personal insight. Ambivalence before the abortion may make resolution of these feelings more difficult. The single most important factor affecting a woman's reaction to her abortion is the level of support provided by those who are important to her (Schneider, 1984). Recognition of her feelings and assurance that these feelings are common and short-lived are usually all that is necessary. The provider may offer a referral for individual or group counseling if the woman is interested. Some abortion facilities themselves offer support groups where feelings and issues related to the abortion can be explored before or after the procedure. The attitude of the provider can also contribute to the woman's feelings about herself and her experience. The practitioner whose manner expresses concern for the woman and support for her decision can be an important factor in the patient's coming to terms with a significant event in her life.

REFERENCES

Altman, A., Stubblefield, P., & Schlam, J., et al. (1985, August). Midtrimester abortion with laminaria and vacuum evacuation on a teaching service. *Journal of Reproductive Medicine, 30*(8), 601–607.

Batzer, F. (1985, October). Guidelines for choosing a pregnancy test. *Contemporary Obstetrics and Gynecology Technology 1986, 26*(Special Issue), 37–52.

Borten, M., & Friedman, E. (1985, October). Early pregnancy interruption with a single PGF2α 15-methyl-analogue vaginal suppository. *The Journal of Reproductive Medicine, 30*(10), 741–744.

Boston Women's Health Collective. (1984). *The new our bodies ourselves.* New York: Simon & Schuster.

Bradley, C. (1984, October). Abortion and subsequent pregnancy. *Canadian Journal of Psychiatry, 29*(6), 494–498.

Brucker, M., & Macmullen, N. (1985, September–October). What's new in pregnancy tests? *Journal of Obstetric, Gynecologic, and Neonatal Nursing, 14*(5), 353–359.

Burkman, R., Atienza, M., & King, T. (1984, August). Morbidity risk among young adolescents undergoing elective abortion. *Contraception, 30*(2), 99–105.

Couzinet, B., Le Strat, N., & Ulmann, A., et al. (1986, December 18). Termination of early pregnancy by the progesterone antagonist RU 486 (Mifepristone). *New England Journal of Medicine, 315*(25), 1565–1570.

DeCherney, A., & Friedman, A. (1985). Endoscopy. In D. Nichols & H. Evrard (Eds.), *Ambulatory gynecology.* Philadelphia: Harper & Row.

Derman, R. (1981, April). Early diagnosis of pregnancy. *The Journal of Reproductive Medicine, 26*(4s), 149–178.

Digest. (1982, September–October). Researchers confirm induced abortion to be safer for women than childbirth: Refute claims of critics. *Family Planning Perspectives, 14*(5), 271–272.

Dilateria: Laminaria japonica. (1982, June). Chicago: Milex Products, Inc.

Dilateria: A cervical dilator with more than a century of use. (1984, November). Chicago: Milex Products, Inc.

Fielding, W., Lee, S., Borten, M., & Friedman, E. (1984, March). Continued pregnancy after failed first-trimester abortion. *Obstetrics and Gynecology, 63*(3), 421–424.

Foster, H., Jr., Smith, M., McGruder, C., et al. (1985, May). Postconception menses induction using prostaglandin vaginal suppositories. *Obstetrics and Gynecology, 65*(5), 682–685.

Grimes, D. (1984, November–December). Second-trimester abortions in the United States. *Family Planning Perspectives, 16*(6), 260–266.

Grimes, D., & Cates, W. (1981). Dilatation and evacuation. In G. S. Berger, W. E. Brenner, & L. Keith (Eds.), *Second trimester abortion.* Boston: John Wright.

Grimes, D., & Schulz, K. (1985, July). Morbidity and mortality from second-trimester abortions. *The Journal of Reproductive Medicine, 30*(7), 505–514.

Grimes, D., Schulz, D., & Cates, W., Jr. (1984a, April 27). Prevention of uterine perforation during curettage abortion. *Journal of the American Medical Association, 251*(16), 2108–2111.

Grimes, D., Schulz, K., & Cates, W., Jr. (1984b, November 15). Prophylactic antibiotics for curettage abortion. *American Journal of Obstetrics and Gynecology, 150*(6), 689–694.

Hatcher, R., Guest, F., & Stewart, F., et al. (1984). *Contraceptive Technology 1984–1985* (12th rev. ed.), New York: Irvington.

Henshaw, S. (1982, September–October). Freestanding abortion clinics: Services, structure, fees. *Family Planning Perspectives, 14*(5), 248–256.

Henshaw, S. (1987, January–February). Characteristics of U.S. women having abortions, 1982–1983. *Family Planning Perspectives, 19*(1), 5–9.

Henshaw, S., Binkin, N.J., Blaine, E., & Smith, J. C. (1985, March–April). A portrait of American women who obtain abortions. *17*(2), 90–96.

Hern, W. (1984). *Abortion practice.* Philadelphia: J. B. Lippincott.

Jones, O., Penn, N., & Schuchter, S., et al. (1984, July–August). Parental response to mid-trimester therapeutic abortion following amniocentesis. *Prenatal Diagnosis, 4*(4), 249–256.

Kajanoja, P., Mandelin, M., & Makila, U., et al. (1984, March). A Gemeprost vaginal suppository for cervical priming prior to termination of first trimester pregnancy. *Contraception, 29*(3), 251–260.

Kovacs, L., Sas, M. & Resch, B., et al. (1984, May). Termination of very early pregnancy by RU 486—An anti-progestational compound. *Contraception, 29*(5), 399–410.

Mohr, J. (1978). *Abortion in America.* New York: Oxford University Press.

Myles, M. (1985). *Textbook for midwives* (10th ed.), Edinburgh: Churchill Livingstone.

Nichols, C. (1987, July–August). Dating pregnancy: Gathering and using a reliable data base. *Journal of Nurse-Midwifery, 32*(4), 195–204.

Nichols, D., & McGoldrick, E. (1985). Minor and ambulatory surgery. In D. Nichols & J. Evrard (Eds.), *Ambulatory gynecology*. Philadelphia: Harper & Row.

Physicians' desk reference (42nd ed.) (1988). Oradell, NJ: Medical Economics Co.

Pritchard, J., MacDonald, P., & Gant, N. (1985) *Williams obstetrics* (17th ed.). Norwalk, CT: Appleton–Century–Crofts.

Quilligan, E. J., & Zuspan, F. P. (1982). *Douglas-Stromme operative obstetrics* (4th ed.). New York: Appleton–Century–Crofts.

Rosen, A., von Knorring, K., Bygdeman, M., & Christensen, N. (1984, May). Randomized comparison of prostaglandin treatment in hospital or at home with vacuum aspiration for termination of early pregnancy. *Contraception, 29*(5), 423–435.

Schneider, T. (1984, March–April). Voluntary termination of pregnancy. *Journal of Obstetric, Gynecologic, and Neonatal Nursing, 13*(2, Suppl.), 77s–84s.

Smith, E. (1982). *Abortion: Health care perspective*. New York: Appleton–Century–Crofts.

Spitz, I., & Barden, C. (1985, November–December). Antiproges-

tins: Prospects for a once-a-month pill. *Family Planning Perspectives, 17*(6), 260–262.

Stubblefield, P. (1981). Laminaria and other adjunctive methods. In G. S. Berger, W. E. Brenner, & L. Keith (Eds.), *Second trimester abortion*. Boston: John Wright.

Van Lith, D., Wittman, R., & Keith, L. (1984, December). Early and late abortion methods. *Clinics in Obstetrics and Gynaecology, 11*(3), 585–601.

Widdicombe, J. (1981). Counseling issues. In G. S. Berger, W. E. Brenner, & L. Keith (Eds.), *Second trimester abortion*. Boston: John Wright.

World Health Organization Task Force on Sequelae of Abortion. (1984, November–December). Secondary infertility following induced abortion. *Studies in Family Planning, 15*(6), 291–295.

Ying, Y.-K., Lin, J.-T., & Robins, J. (1985, July). Acupuncture for the induction of cervical dilation in preparation for first-trimester abortion and its influence on HCG. *The Journal of Reproductive Medicine, 30*(7), 530–534.

29

Sterilization

Susan Papera

Voluntary sterilization is the elective termination of reproductive capacity. Although advances in surgical techniques have now made reversal of sterilization procedures possible, because reversal cannot be guaranteed, sterilization should be considered permanent.

While sterilization is the single most popular method of family planning for couples whose family is complete (Huggins & Sondheimer, 1984, p. 337), the decision to become sterile is not made easily. The ability to procreate is strongly embedded in self-perception and may contribute to a positive self-image. The choice may be seen as a last resort, because of financial and social constraints or an inability to use any available method of reversible contraception. For whatever reasons it is made, the decision evokes strong feelings and may not always be satisfying, as evidenced by the reversals sought.

Persons considering sterilization may need help in placing the decision into the context of their whole life, both current and future. They need truthful and adequate information and time to come to an appropriate decision.

In this chapter, the types of sterilization procedures available, their risks, benefits, and complications, and the role of the nonphysician health care practitioner in providing services to persons seeking sterilization are discussed. The issues of sterilization abuse, informed consent, and dissatisfaction and reversal also are addressed.

FEMALE STERILIZATION

"Voluntary female sterilization is the most widely used contraceptive method in the world" (Liskin & Rinehart, 1985, p. C125). Many reasons for the current popularity of female sterilization have been proposed, including advances in surgical techniques that have made the procedures safer; changes in cultural attitudes, especially in recognizing equal rights for women (Droegmuller, Weinstein, & Morell, 1983); economic shifts increasing the number of female-headed households and the participation of women in the workforce combined with cutbacks in social services (Petchesky, 1979); complications attributed to oral contraceptives and intrauterine devices and the publicity surrounding these; and a relaxation of barriers that had once hampered women from obtaining sterilizations.

Surgical Procedures

All female sterilization procedures involve blocking the fallopian tubes so that the ovum and sperm cannot meet. The tubes can be reached through the abdomen, the cervix, or the vagina and can be blocked by ligation and excision, electrical methods, or mechanical devices (Liskin & Rinehart, 1985). A common term for female sterilization is *tubal ligation* regardless of the blocking method used. A tubal ligation can be performed during cesarean section, after vaginal delivery or abortion, or as an interval procedure (not related to a pregnancy or its termination). This section first describes the surgical approaches to the tubes and then discusses some of the ways of effecting tubal occlusion.

Abdominal Approaches

LAPAROTOMY. Laparotomy involves a 5- to 10-cm transverse incision into the abdomen, through which instruments are introduced to reach the tubes. Because the incision is large, general or spinal anesthesia is necessary. Laparotomy requires the longest operating and recovery times among the sterilization procedures. It always requires an inpatient hospital stay. Any of the blocking techniques to be described can be used with laparotomy.

Prior to the development of other techniques in the 1960s, laparotomy was the only method of sterilization available. Today, gynecologists are reluctant to use laparotomy solely for tubal ligation. This method is more appropriate in conjunction with cesarean section or another major gynecologic or surgical procedure (Rioux & Soderstrom, 1987); however, laparotomy may be the only procedure to use if other approaches fail or if complications arise during another procedure that require more extensive surgery.

MINILAPAROTOMY. Developed in the 1970s, minilaparotomy requires a smaller incision than laparotomy, usually less than 5 cm. The transverse incision is made just above the pubic hairline. A uterine sound inserted through the cervix is used to move the uterus and bring the tubes up through the incision. Each tube is then grasped by a finger or an appropriate instrument, ligated or blocked by a mechanical device, and replaced into the abdomen (Liskin & Rinehart, 1985).

Minilaparotomy appears to be an ideal sterilization method for most women as it is simple to perform, safe, and effective. Women have fewer complications than with laparotomy because there is a smaller incision and less operating time and exposure to anesthesia. The procedure can be performed on an outpatient basis but is usually done in hospital with at least an overnight stay. It is the procedure of choice for postpartum sterilizations with the incision made periumbilically because of upward displacement of the tubes.

Contraindications to minilaparotomy are obesity, fixed uterine retroversion (Rioux & Soderstrom, 1987), and current peritoneal infection (Liskin & Rinehart, 1985). Difficulty can be encountered during the minilaparotomy if the tubes had been damaged previously by infection and/or surgery and are immobilized by pelvic adhesions.

LAPAROSCOPY. Laparoscopy involves the use of a laparoscope—a tube containing a fiberoptic light source. Inserted through a trocar into the abdomen, the laparoscope allows visualization of the internal organs. The abdomen is first punctured with a needle and inflated with 1 to 3.5 L of gas, through a special insufflation apparatus that controls pressure and volume (Wheeless & Katayama, 1985). Carbon dioxide, nitrous oxide, or room air can be used. Insufflation is done to separate the abdominal organs from the abdominal wall, allow a clear view of the pelvic organs, and provide space for insertion of the trocar (Liskin & Rinehart, 1985).

After insufflation, a small incision (1.0 to 1.5 cm) is made in the lower edge of the umbilicus or just below it, and the trocar, which guides the laparoscope, is inserted. The tubes can then be occluded by electrocoagulation or placement of a mechanical device. The incision is closed after the gas leaves the abdomen. The one-puncture or one-incision technique has been called "band-aid" surgery. In the hands of a skilled physician it can be performed with local anesthetics (Rioux & Soderstrom, 1987). Laparoscopy is often an outpatient procedure.

The two-puncture or two-incision technique, however, is easier to learn and perform. With this procedure, a second 1.0- to 1.5-cm incision is made midway between the umbilicus and the pubic bone. The first incision is for the light source, the second to insert the instruments to block the tubes. The two-incision technique can also be done under local anesthesia on an outpatient basis.

Contraindications to laparoscopy include those for minilaparotomy. Severe chronic heart or lung disease is an additional contraindication because of the Trendelenberg position and gas insufflation required by laparoscopy (Liskin & Rinehart, 1985). Laparoscopy is not appropriate for postpartum sterilization.

Vaginal Approaches: Colpotomy/Culdoscopy. In a colpotomy procedure, access to the tubes is gained through an incision in the posterior vagina while the woman is in the knee–chest position. Once found, the tubes are ligated or blocked by mechanical devices. Culdoscopy is similar to colpotomy except that a culdoscope is used to help locate the tubes.

Both colpotomy and culdoscopy have been found to have higher complication rates and slightly higher pregnancy rates than laparotomy, minilaparotomy, or laparoscopy. Common complications include pelvic infection, hemorrhage, or inadvertent proctotomy or cystotomy (Rioux & Soderstrom, 1987). These procedures are therefore performed infrequently.

Contraindications to vaginal procedures include being in the immediate postpartum period and an inability to assume the knee–chest position (Liskin & Rinehart, 1985).

Methods of Tubal Occlusion

The fallopian tubes can be occluded by surgical ligation and excision, electrocoagulation, or mechanical devices. The choice of method depends on the skill of the operator and the desire of the woman for potential reversal. The current trend is to choose methods that are highly effective yet least destructive to increase the possibility of subsequent tubal reconstruction.

Surgical Ligation and Excision. Many surgeons have developed and given their names to different methods of ligating and excising varying portions of the fallopian tubes to effect sterilization. A few of the common techniques are briefly described here.

POMEROY. In the Pomeroy procedure of ligation and excision, the fallopian tube is held up in the middle creating a loop. This loop is ligated in the midportion (ampulla) of the tube with an absorbable suture and then cut off. The two ends retract away from each other (Liskin & Rinehart, 1985; Rioux & Soderstrom, 1987). Using absorbable suture and taking care not to crush the tubes decrease the postoperative incidence of inflammation and fistula formation.

IRVING. The Irving procedure was developed in 1924 to be used in conjunction with a cesarean section. In this procedure the tube is ligated and cut in two places. The cut portion nearest the uterus (proximal or isthmus) is buried within the uterine myometrium. The distal portion (infundibulum) is fixed in the broad ligament. In a modified version often performed today, the distal portion is not fixed into the broad ligament (Wheeless & Katayama, 1985, p. 423). The Irving procedure is more difficult to perform than other techniques of surgical ligation but is extremely effective.

KROENER. The Kroener technique involves removal of the fimbriated end of the fallopian tube and a small section of the ampulla (mid- or lateral portion). The Kroener technique has been associated with a high failure rate and the development of hydrosalpinx (Rioux & Soderstrom, 1987). It is not amenable to reversal.

Electrocoagulation (Cautery). Electrocoagulation (cautery) uses high-frequency electrical energy to heat the tubal cells causing coagulation. This method is used primarily with the laparoscope.

Both unipolar and bipolar means are used for electrocoagulation. In the unipolar method, the electrical current passes through the operating forceps, the tube, and the woman's body to a ground or return plate, completing the electrical circuit (Rioux & Soderstrom, 1987). This method, however, has been found to be associated with an unacceptable number of bowel burns not related to faulty technique of the surgeon but to the electrical delivery system itself.

The bipolar method was developed in response to this complication and is increasingly popular (Huggins & Sondheimer, 1984, p. 338). With this system, the electrical current is delivered to the tubes and returns through the same instrument (Wheeless & Katayama, 1985, p. 421). The only tissue involved is that of the tube held within the instrument, unless bowel or other tissue is inadvertently grasped. Because a smaller area of the tube is destroyed with bipolar coagulation than unipolar coagulation, some operators burn the tube in three or four places to ensure blockage (Liskin & Rinehart, 1985, p. C133). Thermal burns may still occur. The complication rate is related to the operator's experience and attention to safety guidelines (Rioux & Soderstrom, 1987, p. 90).

Mechanical Devices. Mechanical devices were developed to eliminate the problems of electrocoagulation. The use of mechanical devices is associated with high rates of sterilization reversal (Owen, 1984).

TUBAL RING. The tubal ring, also known as the Falop ring, is designed to be applied with a special applicator and can be used with laparotomy, minilaparotomy, laparoscopy, or a vaginal procedure. A loop of each tube is drawn into the applicator and a ring placed over each tube. The loop portion of the tube gradually atrophies (Rioux & Soderstrom, 1987, p. 97). Spraying 2 mL of 4 percent lidocaine on the tubes before placing the rings decreases immediate postoperative pain (Wheeless & Katayama, 1985, p. 422).

CLIPS. The Hulka clip is made of two serrated elastic pins that are held in place on the tubes by a stainless-steel spring (Wheeless & Katayama, 1985, p. 423). The clips are applied to the isthmus (proximal portion) of the tubes. The closures of the clips leave no space for tubal recanalization. Because crushing of the tube occurs over time, fistulas, which are associated with acute crushing, do not form.

Nonsurgical Methods. Nonsurgical methods of tubal occlusion are under investigation although not currently approved for use by The Food and Drug Administration (FDA). Chemical blocking agents can be delivered through a hysteroscope or directly through the cervix. These include formed-in-place plugs, preformed plugs, and various chemicals. Electrocoagulation can be accomplished from inside the uterus without an abdominal incision.

FORMED-IN-PLACE PLUGS. Promising results have been achieved with a formed-in-place silicone plug, delivered through a hysteroscope as liquid silicone mixed with radiopaque silver powder. The plug can be inserted on an outpatient basis under local anesthesia. In a study of 206 women having this procedure, Loffer (1984) found that 91.3 percent or 188 women were effectively sterilized, which meant that the plugs were in place after 3 months as demonstrated on x-ray. Only 166 women were sterilized by one procedure however; 20 required two procedures and 2 women required three. These 188 women were followed for 2,910 patient months without contraception and there were no pregnancies. Plugs are removable but data on reversibility are not available.

Reported complications with silicone plugs include uterine perforation, changes in menstrual pattern, intramenstrual spotting, and foreign-body reactions including pain, cramping, and low-grade fever (Sterilization by Silicone Plug, 1984).

PREFORMED PLUGS. Preformed plugs made of a variety of materials can be placed into varying portions of the tube through the cervix and uterus. One plug, for example, blocks the uterotubal junction; another, called the Hamov intratubal device, has an intrauterine loop for later retrieval, which, theoretically, would enhance reversibility (Rioux & Soderstrom, 1987, p. 103).

OTHER CHEMICAL AGENTS. Other chemical agents under investigation include methyl cyanoacrylate (MCA) and quinacrine hydrochloride. MCA is a tissue adhesive and blocks the tubes by causing an inflammatory response, tissue necrosis, and fibrosis (Laufe & Cole, 1980). Quinacrine is a cytoxic agent used originally as an antimalarial drug. When introduced into the tubes, it causes fibrosis and occlusion. Various delivery systems for quinacrine including instillation, use of pellets, and quinacrine-impregnated IUDs are being studied. Side effects with the different placement

systems range from vaginal discharge to toxic psychosis manifested by auditory and visual hallucinations, increased psychomotor activity, anorexia, and delusions (Laufe & Cole, 1980).

Complications

Complications may arise with any method of female sterilization. They range from mild abdominal pain and infections to life-threatening hemorrhage and anesthesia accidents. Fortunately, major complications have been reported in less than 2 percent of all procedures (DeStefano, Greenspan, Dicker, et al., 1983a). Table 29–1 (Hatcher, Guest, Stewart, et al., 1984, pp. 220–221) presents the various sterilization methods, advantages, disadvantages, and failure rates.

Mortality. The Centers for Disease Control (CDC) estimate the death rate from all sterilization techniques to be 3.6/100,000 women sterilized (Huggins & Sondheimer, 1984, p. 342). The risk of death or serious morbidity from a tubal ligation is less than that associated with term pregnancy or oral contraceptive use in women older than 35 years (Hatcher et al., 1984, p. 214). It is, however, greater than the risk associated with barrier methods of contraception combined with early abortion (Tietze, Bongaarts, & Schearer, 1976).

Pain. After a laparoscopy, chest and shoulder pain may be experienced to some degree as a result of trapped gas. Among the mechanical blocking devices, the ring appears to be associated with the most postoperative pain. It also causes more pain than electrocoagulation. It has been hypothesized that this initial pain occurs because the ring cuts off the blood supply to a loop of the tube while nerve endings take several days to die (Liskin & Rinehart, 1985). Mild analgesia is usually sufficient to control postprocedure pain.

Infection/Hemorrhage. Wound infections and hematomas have been associated with the minilaparotomy. Pelvic infections and hemorrhage are associated with vaginal approaches.

Anesthesia Complications. General anesthesia is associated with more serious complications than local anesthesia. Peterson, DeStefano, Rubin, and associates (1983) reported on 29 deaths attributed to sterilization between 1977 and 1981. Eleven of these were attributable to anesthesia complications.

Failure of Sterilization. Another major complication is the failure to effect sterilization. Based on an extensive review of the literature, Huggins and Sondheimer (1985, p. 342) report the first-year failure rate of sterilization to be 0.18 to 0.37 per 100 woman-years, decreasing to 0.10 to 0.12 per 100 woman-years in following years (Table 29–2).

Reasons for pregnancies after sterilization include the following (Liskin & Rinehart, 1985; Soderstrom, 1985):

1. Undetected luteal phase pregnancies at the time of the procedure
2. Surgical errors
3. Mechanical failure of rings or clips to occlude the tubes or incorrect placement of the devices
4. Spontaneous reanastomosis of the tubes
5. Incomplete tissue damage with bipolar electrocoagulation as a result of the limited range of electrical power with this method

TABLE 29-1. STERILIZATION METHODS AND FACTORS AFFECTING THEIR UTILIZATION

	Male	Female			
	Vasectomy	*Laparoscopy*	*Minilaparotomy*	*Colpotomy*	*Culdoscopy*
Advantages	Safe to slight morbidity, almost no mortality; simple—requires minimal extra training for physicians; inexpensive compared with female sterilization; brief—takes about 20 minutes	Low rate of complication; short recovery time; minimal morbidity; same equipment and skills can be used for endoscopic diagnosis procedures; leaves small scar	Can be done as outpatient procedure with local anesthesia; short recovery time; low cost; relatively easy for physicians to learn; uses simple instruments	Leaves no abdominal scar; easily performed on women of high parity; brief—takes about 20 minutes; less postoperative pain; instruments are simple, cheap, and usually available	Leaves no abdominal scar; brief—takes about 10 minutes
Disadvantages	Not effective until sperm in reproductive system are ejaculated; complications—bleeding or infection; provides indirect protection from pregnancy for women	Not recommended for immediate postpartum period; requires expensive equipment and intensive training	Difficult with obese patients; local anesthesia not suited to all patients	Not suitable in early puerperium; higher complication rate	Not suitable in early puerperium; requires greater surgical skill than laparotomy
Failure rate[a] (%)	0.15	0.2–2	0.2–0.6	0–0.55	0–0.055
Reversibility[a] (%)	5–90 (60)	About 10–90 (70)	About 10–90 (70)	About 10–60 (50)	About 10–70 (50)
Complications (%)	5	0.1–7	0–6.5	1.6–13.3	1.6–13.3
Mortality	Almost 0	Low	Low	Low	Low
Skill required	Medical	Specialist	General practitioner	General practitioner or specialist	Specialist
Anesthesia type	Local	General or local	General or local	General or local	General or local
Equipment maintenance	Easy	Difficult	Moderate	Moderate	Difficult
Recovery time (days)	1–5	0–5	0–5	1–14	1–14
Facility	Outpatient	Outpatient or operating room	Outpatient	Operating room outpatient	Operating room or outpatient

[a]Failure rates and the potential for successful reversal depend primarily on the method of tubal occlusion. Reversibility also depends on the reversal techniques used.

From Hatcher, R. A., Guest, F., Stewart, F. et al. (1984). Contraceptive technology 1984–1985 *(12th rev. ed. pp. 220–221). New York: Irvington. Reprinted with permission.*

6. Fistula formation at the occluded or coagulated end of the tube

As pregnancy can occur any time after tubal sterilization, careful follow-up of sterilized women is important. Such care is often rendered by the nonphysician practitioner.

Ectopic Pregnancy. Ectopic pregnancy is a life-threatening complication of tubal sterilization. Although a woman's absolute risk of ectopic pregnancy is lowered after tubal ligation because the incidence of pregnancy is reduced, the likelihood that a given pregnancy will be ectopic is increased. Davis (1986) reports an ectopic pregnancy rate of 10 to 20 percent among all pregnancies after sterilization. The rate can be as high as 50 percent of pregnancies after tubal cautery. Other authors report the incidence of ectopic pregnancy as ranging from 0.02 to 0.31 per 100 sterilized women (Liskin & Rinehart, 1985, p. C136).

Partial occlusion, recanalization, or formation of a tuboperitoneal fistula may account for ectopic pregnancy after tubal ligation. In these situations, a space is created

TABLE 29-2. PREGNANCY RATES AFTER STERILIZATION

Technique	Sterilizations	Failures	Intrauterine Pregnancy	Ectopic Pregnancy
Laparoscopic tubal coagulation	23,238	45 (0.19)[a]	22 (49.0)	23 (51.0)
Nonlaparoscopic tubal ligation	13,901	106 (0.76)	93 (87.7)	12 (12.3)
Laparoscopy				
Coagulation	4,309	14 (0.32)	NA[b]	NA
Silastic band	3,536	19 (0.53)	NA	NA
Spring-loaded clip (Hulka clip)	457	3 (0.65)	NA	NA
Spring-loaded clip (prototype)	1,514	66 (4.35)	NA	NA
Laparoscopy				
Coagulation and cutting	635	5 (0.80)	NA	NA
Spring-loaded clip (Hulka clip)	1,079	22 (2.30)	NA	NA
Silastic band	1,800	8 (0.78)	NA	NA

[a]Percentages given within parentheses.
[b]Not available.

From Huggins, G., and Sondheimer, S. (1984). Complications of female sterilization: Immediate and delayed. Fertility and Sterility, 41 *(3), 350. Reprinted with permission.*

that is large enough to accommodate sperm but not a fertilized ovum. Implantation, therefore, occurs outside of the uterus (Davis, 1986).

All sterilized women should be informed of the signs of an ectopic pregnancy—amenorrhea, vaginal bleeding or spotting, and abdominal pain—and advised to seek medical attention immediately if such signs occur (see Chapter 15).

Post-Tubal Ligation Syndrome. Whether the post–tubal ligation syndrome (PTLS) is a definable entity is unclear. Since tubal ligations have been performed, there have been reports of short- and long-term gynecologic consequences. Tubal ligations have been implicated in premenstrual syndrome; menstrual irregularities including increased bleeding, shortened cycle length, and dysmenorrhea; obesity; and benign breast disease. From the 1950s to 1970, some physicians advocated simple hysterectomy for sterilization to obviate these alleged complications. Much of the literature during that time, however, reported on retrospective studies, many without controls and not accounting for important variables, such as menstrual patterns prior to sterilization and length of follow-up.

Since 1975, the subjective complaints of women after sterilization have been investigated more carefully (Huggins & Sondheimer, 1984). Newer study designs take into account a woman's menstrual pattern prior to sterilization, previous contraceptive use such as pills or an IUD, and gynecologic history. Although recent data appear to refute the existence of PTLS, not all analysts consider the results definitive (Factors Seen as Possible Links, 1986).

Fortney, Cole, and Kennedy (1983) reported on a study of 1,555 women; they looked at four parameters of menstrual change: length of cycle, duration of bleeding, dysmenorrhea, and regularity. Each woman served as her own control. The researchers concluded that women under age 35 who have normal menstrual patterns continue to do so after sterilization. Some women who have abnormal patterns prior to sterilization experience a change to normal cycles but many do not.

The CDC conducted a multicenter U. S. Collaborative Review of Sterilization (CREST) in 1978. The purpose of this prospective study was to determine the safety of female sterilization and ways to make it safer. Fifteen percent of women in the CREST study reported irregular cycles before sterilization, with 7.8 percent reporting irregularity for 2 years (Liskin & Rinehart, 1985). Analysis of the CREST data by DeStefano, Huezo, Peterson, and associates (1983b) showed that among 2,500 women, the majority reported no marked change after sterilization. Vessey, Huggins, Lawless, and Yeates (1983) also concluded that there was little or no evidence of any adverse long-term consequences of tubal sterilization.

Conversely, another large prospective study analyzing earlier data (from 1968 to 1972) found that women undergoing sterilization were at a significantly increased risk for abnormal menstrual cycles, moderate to severe menstrual cramps, and adverse bleeding after 2 years (DeStefano, Perlman, Peterson, & Diamond, 1985). This research compared two groups of women: those who were sterilized and those whose husbands were sterilized. The researchers suggest that perhaps the types of procedure most commonly utilized during this period—unipolar electrocoagulation and partial salpingectomy—might cause more menstrual problems than more recently used techniques—bipolar electrocoagulation and mechanical blocking devices.

Some explanations have been offered for the cause of PTLS (Factors Seen as Possible Links, 1986; Huggins & Sondheimer, 1984; Liskin & Rinehart, 1985):

1. Disturbed ovarian blood supply secondary to tubal damage
2. Altered innervation to the tube or ovary
3. Intermittent torsion of the distal fallopian tube or ovary
4. Estrogen–progesterone imbalance caused by the sterilization

Further research is needed on PTLS.

Dissatisfaction and Reversal

The determinants of dissatisfaction with sterilization and desire for reversal are difficult to ascertain from the literature. As with the past research on PTLS, often the studies have been retrospective, poorly controlled, with small sample sizes, or have not taken into account the timing of the procedure, that is, its relation to obstetric events, either childbirth or pregnancy termination (Bledin, Cooper, MacKenzie, & Brice, 1984). Also, studies may not have provided for adequate follow-up time to account for life changes that could affect a woman's reaction to sterilization. Abraham, Jansen, Fraser, and Kwok (1986) suggest that 4 to 7 years follow-up is necessary to evaluate satisfaction.

Despite the shortcomings in the research, trends can be identified. Most women who have undergone sterilization are comfortable with their choices and are no more likely to experience serious psychiatric problems than women choosing other forms of birth control (Liskin & Rinehart, 1985). In fact, 98 percent of women having tubal ligation want the procedure to be permanent (Rioux & Soderstrom, 1987), do not feel less feminine, and do not have subsequent sexual problems. Bledin and co-workers (1984) report that among 138 women studied 6 months after sterilization, regrets and wishes for reversal were rare. Twenty-four percent reported increased sexual satisfaction, whereas 8.9 percent felt that their sex life had deteriorated.

Dissatisfaction. Although not all women who are dissatisfied with their tubal ligation seek reversal, all women who seek reversal are dissatisfied. It appears that women who seek reversals are generally younger at the time of sterilization than those who do not (Winston, 1977). A change in partners or marital status, continuing ambivalence, later gynecologic problems perceived to be caused by the procedure, and feeling that they had not made the decision themselves or that it was done for financial considerations have been implicated in dissatisfaction (Abraham et al., 1986; Huggins & Sondheimer, 1984; Liskin & Rinehart, 1985). Whether there is more dissatisfaction when sterilization is performed in conjunction with an obstetric event is unclear.

As there is no way to predict who will be dissatisfied or wish a reversal of their tubal ligation, the best approach is to fully counsel each woman/couple regarding the areas that might lead to regrets; ultimately the woman must decide for herself. See Sterilization Abuse and Informed Consent and Role of the Primary Care Practitioner for information on presterilization counseling.

Reversal. Advances in microsurgical techniques have made reversal of tubal sterilization possible in some cases. Factors affecting success include the length of remaining undamaged tube, the method and site of occlusion, the time interval since sterilization, the woman's age, and the skill of the surgeon.

Procedures that least damage the tubes and leave greater than 3 to 5 cm of undamaged tube have the highest rate of successful reversal. These include use of rings or clips and the Pomeroy and Irving methods of ligation and excision. Success rates vary from 45 to 70 percent for the Pomeroy method to 80 percent for rings and clips.

In a study of 80 previously sterilized women, 30 of 58 (52 percent) sterilized by monopolar electrocoagulation delivered a living child after reconstructive surgery compared with 19 of 22 (86 percent) sterilized by Falope ring (Rock, Guzick, Katz, et al., 1987). This investigation also found that pregnancy was least likely to occur in women whose remaining fallopian tubes were less than 4 cm in length.

Tubes that have been occluded at the isthmic portion appear to be more successfully reanastomosed than those occluded elsewhere (Owen, 1984). Hulka clips are applied to this portion of the tube and are associated with a high reversal rate.

A decrease in successful reversal over time has been attributed to gradual changes in the tubal mucosa, including loss of folds and cilia and growth of polyps (Liskin & Rinehart, 1985). Reversal procedures on women over 35 to 40 years may be less likely to succeed because of decreasing fertility.

Reversal of tubal sterilization has been associated with a 2 percent or less ectopic pregnancy rate. This increases, however, to 5 percent after reversal of an electrocoagulation procedure.

Reversing a sterilization procedure is expensive, time consuming, and requires hospitalization and general or regional anesthesia. Success cannot be guaranteed. Whenever a woman or couple seeks such a procedure, the type of sterilization she had should be reviewed and the fertility potential of both partners assessed in order for her to give fully informed consent.

The decision to seek reversal may be very emotionally charged. Counseling needs to be thorough yet sensitive.

MALE STERILIZATION: VASECTOMY

Vasectomy is the sterilization procedure for men. It blocks the vas deferens, thus preventing sperm passage. It is technically easier to perform than the female sterilization procedures, requires only local anesthesia, and is most often an outpatient procedure. It has no risk of mortality (Tietze et al., 1976, p. 13).

Surgical Procedure

Before surgery, the vas deferens is located and held in place through the scrotum. A small scrotal incision is made and the vas is occluded by tying and cutting, cautery, or mechanical means. The procedure is repeated on the other side.

In contrast to the dramatic changes that have occurred over time in surgical techniques for female sterilization, variation in vasectomy procedures has occurred primarily in the ways the vas is occluded. The "open-ended vasectomy" is said to reduce chronic orchitic pain and have a high rate of reversal success. In this method the vas deferens is brought out through the scrotum and dissected from its sheath. The abdominal (distal) end is occluded, usually with electrocoagulation. The sheath is brought over the distal end and is secured using a clip. The vas is replaced. The procedure is repeated on the opposite side. The skin is not sutured; the skin edges are pressed together and held in place with a large pressure dressing and athletic supporter (Open-Ended Vasectomy, 1986).

Complications

Complications of vasectomy include hematoma, local infection, epididymitis, granuloma, and sterilization failure. Chronic orchitic pain may occur, although this is usually mild (Factors Seen as Possible Links, 1986). Complication rates have been reported from 16 percent for hematoma up to 0.4 percent for failure (Hatcher et al., 1984).

Concern has been raised about the long-term effect of male sterilization particularly in regard to the production of antisperm antibodies and the development of atherosclerosis and immunologically mediated diseases.

One half to two thirds of vasectomized men develop sperm antibodies but there is no evidence that pathologic complications are attributable to this (Hatcher et al., 1984). Sperm antibodies have also been found in men prior to vasectomy (Fuchs & Alexander, 1983). The presence of these antibodies, however, has been implicated in reduced fertility in men with a technically successful vas deferens reanastomosis.

In 1980, Clarkson and Alexander reported that atherosclerosis was more frequent and extensive in vasectomized monkeys than in their nonvasectomized age-matched counterparts, presumably because of an immunologic response to sperm antibodies. Studies to date, however, have failed to show increased rates of cardiovascular disease in vasectomized men (Walker, Jick, Hunter, et al., 1981a, 1981b).

In a large cohort study undertaken to look at the long-term effects of vasectomy, the overall incidence of diseases in vasectomized men was similar to or lower than the incidence in paired controls. The exception was the incidence of epididymitis–orchitis (Massey, Bernstein, O'Fallon, et al., 1984). The study, which followed vasectomized men for up to 41 years postprocedure with a median of 9 years of follow-up, did not support the suggestions of immunopathologic consequences of vasectomy within the study population.

Reversal

Anatomically, the vas deferens can be reconstructed successfully 40 to 90 percent of the time; however, functional success is much lower, ranging from 18 to 60 percent. The variability is related to the surgical procedure used, the length of vas deferens removed, whether or not coagulation was used, the type of ligation material used, the time interval between the original surgery and the reversal procedure, and the presence of sperm antibodies (Fuchs & Alexander, 1983; Hatcher et al., 1984, p. 212).

STERILIZATION ABUSE AND INFORMED CONSENT

Informed consent is the crux of the 1979 federal sterilization regulations. These were developed to stop the problems of sterilization abuse.

Abusive practices such as performing sterilization without a woman's knowledge of its permanence, threatening to stop Medicaid or welfare benefits if she did not consent to sterilization, and obtaining consent under the duress of labor or at the time of birth have been documented. Many victims of sterilization abuse have been poor or from minority groups. Feminist, health activist, and other groups organized in the 1970s to fight these abuses.

In 1975, New York City became the first city in the United States to enact legislation regulating the practice of sterilization. This legislation applies to all care providers in all settings, public and private. In 1979, the federal government guidelines for sterilization went into effect (Boston Women's Health Book Collective, 1984, pp. 256–257; *Federal Register*, 42(217), November 8, 1978). These guidelines, which apply only to federally funded programs, ensure that each person electing to undergo sterilization be informed orally and in writing of the procedures involved, the risks, complications, and benefits. Consent must be obtained by someone other than the physician performing the procedure. Each person must be informed that the sterilization is to be considered irreversible. Alternate methods of birth control must be explained. All patients must always know that they are free to change their mind any time prior to the procedure without loss of welfare or Medicaid benefits or their right to future medical treatment.

An interpreter must be provided for those who do not speak or read the language and provisions must be made for those who are blind, deaf, or otherwise disabled. The person obtaining consent must offer to answer any questions the individual may have concerning the procedure. Consent may not be obtained if the woman is in labor or delivering, seeking an abortion, or under the influence of alcohol or drugs.

Only the individual seeking sterilization needs to sign the consent form along with the person obtaining the consent, the physician performing the procedure, and the interpreter if necessary. A witness chosen by the person to be sterilized may be present when consent is obtained. The regulations mandate a 30-day waiting period from the time of signing the consent to the procedure unless emergency abdominal surgery is necessary or delivery occurs prior to a woman's estimated due date. In these cases, 72 hours must have elapsed since the consent form was signed. The consent form must be re-signed just before the procedure.

The guidelines also provided for a moratorium on sterilization for persons for whom informed consent was considered unobtainable: minors (under age 21), institutionalized individuals, and those declared mentally incompetent, except, in the last category, with a special court judgment (Petchesky, 1979, p. 34).

The intent of the regulations is to provide safeguards against sterilization abuse, but a problem can arise when a newly delivered woman who desires sterilization cannot have it performed postpartally because the papers had not been signed. Sterilization may then require a subsequent hospitalization. Oftentimes a woman may not have been aware during her pregnancy of the time constraints imposed by the federal regulations. It is important for all practitioners caring for pregnant women to inform them of the postpartum sterilization option before 36 weeks gestation so that the regulations can be implemented equitably.

ROLE OF THE PRIMARY CARE PRACTITIONER

In the United States, health practitioners other than physicians do not perform sterilizations. Primary care practitioners, however, are frequently the first to initiate or receive queries concerning this method of birth control and are the care providers both prior to and after the procedure.

The practitioner's role in this area is multifaceted. It is one of listener, teacher, and counselor. The practitioner may obtain sterilization consent, explain sterilization laws and/or regulations, and dispel myths.

The care provider must be knowledgeable about all aspects of sterilization and able to impart this knowledge in a meaningful manner. The woman or couple seeking information regarding sterilization needs factual information about procedures, risks, benefits, and costs. They may also need help in putting the decision into the perspective of their present and future life and evaluating the emotional and psychological components of such a decision. All aspects of informed consent need to be understood and implemented.

In counseling a patient, the practitioner should look for clues that might identify those who are at risk for regretting their decision (Counsel for Counselors, 1986):

1. Persons who deny facts about their lifestyle, desire for sterilization, or other personal situations
2. Persons who have made the decision alone or with little thought
3. Persons who are under stress or are being pressured by others

4. Persons who remain confused about any aspect of the procedure, especially its permanence

To help women and couples make a decision about their sterilization, situations can be presented to them that may help clarify their commitment to permanent cessation of reproductive function. They can be asked, for example, whether they would be comfortable with this choice if their children died or their partner changed, particularly if a future potential partner would not enter into a relationship in which there was no possibility of childbearing. For some couples, the possibility of death of a partner may need to be discussed, as they may view their present relationship as otherwise permanent. Such questions may be difficult for the practitioner to raise, but can be valuable in helping a person realize the possible consequences of the sterilization decision.

Another useful counseling technique is to ask women or couples to consider previous patterns of decision making. Do they tend to make decisions only later to regret or reverse them or do they usually stick to decisions made? Those individuals falling into the former category may benefit from further consideration.

For the woman or man who wants no children or no more children, regardless of present or future circumstances, and who fully realizes the permanence of the surgery, sterilization can be an excellent choice of birth control. Once accomplished, it requires no additional thought, planning, or expense.

Practitioners desiring more information on counseling for sterilization can consult the Association for Voluntary Surgical Contraception (AVSC) manual, *Counseling the Sterilization Patient, the Physicians' Guide.* It can be obtained by writing to AVSC, 122 East 42nd Street, New York, NY 10168.

FOLLOW-UP

Follow-up care for a woman who has had a tubal ligation consists of a 2-week and/or 4-week postoperative visit followed by routine gynecologic care. All women should be taught the signs of an ectopic pregnancy and should be encouraged to have yearly examinations and Pap smears.

REFERENCES

Abraham, S., Jansen, R., Fraser, S., & Kwok, C. H. M. (1986, July 7). The characteristics, perceptions and personalities of women seeking a reversal of their tubal sterilization. *Medical Journal of Australia, 145*(1), 4–7.

Bledin, K. D., Cooper, J. E., MacKenzie, S., & Brice, B. (1984, May). Psychological sequelae of female sterilization: Short-term outcome in a prospective controlled study. *Psychological Medicine, 14*(2), 379–390.

Boston Women's Health Book Collective. (1984). *The new our bodies, ourselves.* New York: Simon & Schuster.

Clarkson, T. B., & Alexander, N. J. (1980, January). Long term vasectomy: Effects on the occurrence and extent of atherosclerosis in rhesus monkeys. *Journal of Clinical Investigation, 65*(1), 15–25.

Counsel for counselors: How to handle new (and old) dilemmas. (1986, May). *Contraceptive Technology Update, 7*(5), 52–54.

Davis, M. (1986, September). Recurrent ectopic pregnancy after tubal sterilization. *Obstetrics and Gynecology, 68*(3, Suppl.), 445–455.

DeStefano, F., Greenspan, J. R., & Dicker, R. C., et al. (1983a, February) Complications of internal laparoscopic tubal sterilization. *Obstetrics and Gynecology, 61*(2), 153–158.

DeStefano, F., Huezo, C., & Peterson, H. et al. (1983b, December). Menstrual changes after tubal sterilization. *Obstetrics and Gynecology, 62*(6), 673–681.

DeStefano, F., Perlman, J., Peterson, H., & Diamond, E. (1985, August 1). Long-term risks of menstrual disturbances after tubal sterilization. *American Journal of Obstetrics and Gynecology, 152*(7, Part 1), 835–841.

Droegmuller, W., Weinstein, L., & Morell, P. (1983). Surgical contraception: The optimal method. In F. P. Zuspan & C. D. Christian (Eds.), *Controversy in obstetrics and gynecology.* Philadelphia: W. B. Saunders.

Factors seen as possible links to posttubal ligation syndrome. (1986). *Contraceptive Technology Update, 7*(3), 13–15.

Fortney, J., Cole, L., & Kennedy, K. (1983, December 1). A new approach to measuring menstrual pattern change after sterilization. *American Journal of Obstetrics and Gynecology, 147*(7), 830–836.

Fuchs, E., & Alexander, N. (1983, October). Immunologic considerations before and after vasovasostomy. *Fertility and Sterility, 40*(4), 497–499.

Hatcher, R. A., Guest, F., & Stewart, F., et al. (1984). *Contraceptive technology 1984–1985* (12th rev. ed.). New York: Irvington.

Huggins, G., & Sondheimer, S. (1984, March). Complications of female sterilization: Immediate and delayed. *Fertility and Sterility, 41*(3), 337–355.

Laufe, C., & Cole, L. (1980, September and October). Nonsurgical female sterilization. *International Journal of Gynaecology and Obstetrics, 18*(5), 333–339.

Liskin, L., & Rinehart, W. (1985, May). Female sterilization. *Population Reports, Series C, No. 9, 13*(2), C125–C167.

Loffer, F. D. (1984, June 1). Hysteroscopic sterilization with the use of formed-in-place silicone plugs. *American Journal of Obstetrics and Gynecology, 149*(3), 261–270.

Massey, F., Bernstein, G., O'Fallon, W., et al. (1984, August). Vasectomy and health. *Journal of the American Medical Association, 252*(8), 1023–1029.

Open-ended vasectomy prevents pain, may enhance reversibility. (1986, May). *Contraceptive Technology Update, 7*(5), 51–52.

Owen, E. (1984, September 1). Reversal of female sterilization: Review of 252 microsurgical salpingo-salpingostomies. *Medical Journal of Australia, 141*(5), 276–280.

Petchesky, R. P. (1979, October 9). Reproduction, ethics, and public policy: The federal sterilization regulations—Protection or paternalism? *Hastings Center Report, 9*(5), 29–41.

Peterson, N. B., DeStefano, F., & Rubin, G. I., et al. (1983, May 15). Deaths attributable to tubal sterilization in the United States, 1977 to 1981. *American Journal of Obstetrics and Gynecology, 146*(2), 131–136.

Rioux, J., & Soderstrom, P. M. (1987, August). Sterilization revisited. *Contemporary Ob/Gyn, 30*(2), 80–82, 84, 87–88, 90–91, 94, 97, 101, 103–104.

Rock, J., Guzick, D., & Katz, E., et al. (1987, July). Tubal anastomosis: Pregnancy success following reversal of Falope ring or monopolar cautery sterilization. *Fertility and Sterility, 488*(1), 13–17.

Soderstrom, R. M. (1985, June 15). Sterilization failures and their causes. *American Journal of Obstetrics and Gynecology, 152*(4), 395–403.

Sterilization by cervical plug. (1984). *American Journal of Nursing, 84*(11), 1358.

Tietze, C., Bongaarts, J., & Schearer, B. (1976, January- February). Mortality associated with the control of fertility. *Family Planning Perspectives, 8*(1), 6–14.

Vessey, M., Huggins, G., Lawless, M., & Yeates, D. (1983, March). Tubal sterilization: Findings in a large prospective study. *British Journal of Obstetrics and Gynaecology, 90*(3), 203–209.

Walker, A. M., Jick, H., Hunter, J. R., et al. (1981a, June 12). Hospitalization rates in vasectomized men. *Journal of the American Medical Association, 245*(22), 2315–2317.

Walker, A. M., Jick, H., & Hunter, J. R., et al. (1981b, January 3). Vasectomy and non-fatal myocardial infarction. *Lancet, 1*(8210), 13–15.

Wheeless, C., & Katayama, K. P. (1985). Laparoscopy and tubal sterilization. In R. Mattingly & J. Thompson (Eds.), *TeLinde's operative gynecology* (6th ed.), Philadelphia: J. B. Lippincott.

Winston, R. M. L. (1977, July 30). Why 103 women asked for reversal of sterilisation. *British Medical Journal, 2*(6082), 305–307.

American College of Nurse-Midwives: Core Competencies

PART A: NURSE-MIDWIFERY MANAGEMENT

The nurse-midwifery management process has three aspects—primary management, collaborative management, and referral—as well as medical consultation. Implicit in the management process is the documentation of all its aspects.

1. Primary management
   A. Systematically obtains or updates a complete and relevant data base for assessment of the client's health status.
   B. Accurately identifies problems/diagnoses based upon correct interpretation of the data base.
   C. Formulates and communicates a complete needs/problems list with corroboration from the client.
   D. Identifies need for consultation/collaboration/referral with appropriate members of the health care team.
   E. Provides information to enable clients to make appropriate decisions and to assume appropriate responsibility for their own health.
   F. Assumes direct responsibility for the development, with the client, of a comprehensive plan of care based upon supportive rationale.
   G. Assumes direct responsibility for implementing the plan of care.
   H. Initiates emergency management of specific complications/deviations.
   I. Evaluates, with corroboration from the client, the achievement of health care goals and modifies the plan of care appropriately.
II. Collaborative management
   Collaborative management builds upon the steps of primary management; additionally the nurse-midwife:
   A. Anticipates and identifies problems and related complications.
   B. Plans and implements physician consultation and nurse-midwifery/physician management.
   C. Carries out the plan of care as appropriate.
   D. Continues nurse-midwifery care, including teaching, counseling, support, and advocacy.
III. Referral
   A. Identifies the need for management and/or care outside the scope of nurse-midwifery practice.
   B. Selectes an appropriate source of care in collaboration with the client.
   C. Transfers the care of the client to medical management as appropriate.

PART B: FAMILY PLANNING/GYNECOLOGIC CARE

A. Assumes responsibility for management of the care of women seeking family planning and/or gynecologic services, using the nurse-midwifery management process.
B. Uses a foundation for nurse-midwifery practice that includes but is not limited to the knowledge of:
   1. Anatomy and physiology of the reproductive systems through the life cycle.
   2. Anatomy and physiology of the female breast.
   3. Anatomy, physiology, and psychosocial components of human sexuality.
   4. Factors relating to steroid, mechanical, chemical, physiologic, and surgical conception control methods, including:
      a. Rationale for use
      b. Contraindications to use
      c. Effectiveness rates
      d. Mechanisms of action
      e. Advantages/disadvantages
      f. Side effects/complications
      g. Cost
      h. Client instructions/counseling
      i. Psychological factors
      j. Provision of appropriate method, including but not limited to oral contraception, vaginal diaphragms, and IUDs
      k. Discontinuation or change of method
   5. Indicators of common problems of sexuality and methods for counseling.
   6. Factors involved in decision making regarding unplanned and/or undesirable pregnancies and resources for counseling and referral.

From The American College of Nurse-Midwives. (1985). Core competencies in nurse-midwifery. *Washington, D.C. Reprinted with permission.*

From The American College of Nurse-Midwives. (1985). Core competencies in nurse-midwifery. *Washington, D.C. Reprinted with permission.*

7. Indicators of deviations from normal and appropriate interventions, including but not limited to:
   a. Vaginal pelvic infections
   b. Sexually transmitted diseases
   c. Pelvic and breast masses
   d. Abnormal Pap smears
   e. Problems related to menstrual cycle
   f. Pelvic relaxation
   g. Urinary tract infections
   h. Infertility

8. Assessment of relevant historic data about client **and** partner.

9. Assessment of general physical and emotional status of client.

10. Common screening and diagnostic tests.

Guidelines for the Incorporation of New Procedures into Nurse-Midwifery Practice

Nurse-midwifery practice will continue to evolve, depending on the needs of the client, the needs of the site, the expectations of the institution, and the nurse-midwife's desire to improve care to women and their farmilies. Procedures incorporated into the practice of nurse-midwifery should be in concert with the Philosophy of the American College of Nurse-Midwives and the Standards for the Practice of Nurse-Midwifery of the American College of Nurse-Midwives (ACNM) and should not conflict with any current clinical practice statements of the ACNM.

While the ACNM does not approve or disapprove the incorporation of new clinical procedures into nurse-midwifery practice, the following guidelines were developed by the Clinical Practice Committee and approved by the Board of Directors to assist the nurse-midwife in expanding clinical practice:

1. Identify need for the procedure, taking into consideration:
   a. Consumer demand
   b. Safety considerations
   c. Institutional request
   d. Lack of other appropriate personnel
   e. Interest of nurse-midwives

2. Cite relevant statutes/documents that would constrain or support procedure, including:
   a. Statutes and regulations
   b. Institutional by-laws
   c. Legal opinions

3. Evaluate procedure as a nurse-midwifery function, including:
   a. Relevent literature
   b. Use by other nurse-midwives
   c. Risks/benefits
   d. Management of complications

4. Develop process for educating nurse-midwives to perform this procedure, using:
   a. Bibliography
   b. Formal study
   c. Supervised practice
   d. Protocols
   e. Evaluation of learning

5. Evaluate use of procedure, documenting:
   a. Outcome statistics
   b. Satisfaction with procedure
      — consumer
      — institution
      — nurse-midwifery practice
   c. maintenance of competency

From The American College of Nurse-Midwives. (1987). Standards for the practice of nurse-midwifery. *Washington, D.C. Reprinted with permission.*

Differential Diagnosis

The following charts synopsize the management process involved when patients present with two common, but often perplexing, complaints—lower abdominal pain and vaginal discharge. More detailed information on these problems can be found in Chapters 11, 12, 13, 14, 15, 16, 19, and 20.

These tables are intended to offer a guideline for the thought process involved in diagnostic decision making. They are not comprehensive; nor do they cover all possible patient complaints.

Other common gynecologic symptoms include abnormal vaginal bleeding and vulvar pain. An entire chapter is devoted to bleeding disorders and we refer you to Chapter 21 for its discussion of differential diagnosis of vaginal bleeding. The differential diagnosis of vulvar pain is often the same as for vaginal discharge, although external skin lesions may not present with discharge. The same management process can be applied to these and other presenting complaints.

PART A: DIFFERENTIAL DIAGNOSIS OF LOWER ABDOMINAL (OR PELVIC) PAIN

Possible Diagnosis	Historic Data	Physical Exam Data	Laboratory Data	Primary Care Management

Pregnancy
  Normal intrauterine, probably round ligament pain
  Spontaneous abortion:
    Missed, threatened, incomplete, complete
  Ectopic
	LMP,[a] normalcy of; PMP
	Abnormal bleeding
	Sexual history
	Contraceptive history
	Subjective symptoms of pregnancy
	Crampy versus pressure pain, generalized or localized
	Associated bleeding
	Shoulder pain
		Breast changes
		Speculum exam: cervical changes
		Bimanual: uterine softening and enlargement
		Adnexal enlargement, tenderness
			Pregnancy test
			If suspect AB or ectopic: serial β hCG with titers, ultrasound
			For ectopic: possible culdocentesis, laparoscopy
				Normal: reassurance, teaching and counseling, refer for prenatal care or abortion
				Threatened AB: expectant management with teaching and counseling
				Inevitable or incomplete AB: expectant management versus referral for D&C
				Ectopic: immediate referral

Urinary tract infection	Urinary frequency and urgency Dysuria, hesitancy in urination Hematuria Dyspareunia Lower back pain History of UTI	CVAT; suprapubic tenderness	Urinalysis and culture and sensitivity	Antibiotics and teaching, counseling Consultation or referral as necessary
Vaginitis	See Part B: Differential Diagnosis of Vaginal Discharge.			
Uterine myoma	History of myoma Abnormal bleeding, esp. menorrhagia Pressure pain, urinary symptoms Constipation Infertility	Bimanual: uterine enlargement, firmness, irregularity	Ultrasound Possible hysteroscopy CBC if bleeding present	Follow closely Refer if very symptomatic, adnexae difficult to palpate, infertility, or rapid growth

continued

PART A: CONTINUED

Possible Diagnosis	Historic Data	Physical Exam Data	Laboratory Data	Primary Care Management
Endometriosis	Cramplike pain, pre-menstrual onset, worsening over time Family history Dyspareunia Rectal bleeding Constipation secondary to rectal pain Abdominal, pelvic, vaginal or backache Infertility	Bimanual: fixed retro-verted uterus, ad-nexal thickening with nodules, immobile, ir-regular ovarian cysts Rectovaginal: nodules in uterosacral region or on rectovaginal septum	All labs negative Ultrasound	Refer for definitive diag-nosis (laparoscopy) and medical and/or surgical treatment
Ovarian: cyst; twisted ovarian cyst; ab-scess; cancer	Unilateral adnexal pain Dyspareunia Pressure, increased girth Menstrual irregularities Flatulence, bloating, in-digestion If secondary to PID, see PID below.	Bimanual: unilateral ad-nexal tenderness, en-largement	Ultrasound—may or may not be useful	Refer for treatment: an-tibiotic or surgical, ex-pectant
Salpingitis/pelvic inflam-matory disease	Generalized abdominal pain Sexual history: multiple sexual partners, ex-posure to STDs Contraceptive history: IUD or OCs (for chla-mydia) Fever, chills, malaise	Abdominal tenderness, guarding Bimanual: cervical mo-tion tenderness, uter-ine and adnexal tenderness May have adnexal en-largement if abscess (hydro- or pyosal-pinx)	TPR, elevated CBC with differential, elevated, shift to the left ESR, elevated Ultrasound to R/O other diagnoses Gonorrhea and chlamy-dia cultures, may be positive Pregnancy test, to R/O other diagnoses	Consult or refer for an-tibiotic therapy, pos-sible hospitalization
Primary dysmenorrhea	Relationship of pain to menses Cramplike pain, may in-clude back and/or leg pain	Absence of other find-ings R/O signs of endome-triosis	None	Teaching and counsel-ing, esp. exercise, comfort measures Antiprostaglandin ther-apy Acupuncture/biofeed-back
Premenstrual syndrome	Relationship to menses Associated PMS symp-toms	Absence of other find-ings	None	Teaching and counsel-ing, especially exer-cise, nutrition, vitamin and mineral supplementation
Mittelschmerz	Occurring midcycle	Absence of other find-ings	None	Teaching and counsel-ing, reassurance
Trauma	History of trauma Obstetric history posi-tive for operative or instrumental delivery Previous pelvic surgery Dyspareunia, esp. with deep penetration	Abdominal tenderness Bimanual: cervical mo-tion tenderness, uter-ine and/or adnexal tenderness Adhesions, scar tissue may be felt	Other labs negative	Refer for evaluation May need laparoscopy, although findings may be negative May need psychological support
Postpartum or post-abortion endometritis or IUD-related endom-etritis	History of recent birth or abortion, esp. in-strumental or opera-tive Intrapartum history: PROM, long labor, long-duration internal monitoring, multiple vaginal exams, uter-ine exploration General malaise Use of IUD	Abdominal tenderness Lochia: foul-smelling, scant or profuse	TPR, elevated CBC with differential el-evated, shift to left ESR, elevated Cervical culture Labs to R/O other con-ditions: urine culture and sensitivity, wound culture, CXR, ultrasound	Consultation for anti-biotic therapy Removal of IUD
Appendicitis	Sudden onset, severe Pain generalized or lo-calized to right side or spreading from	Absence of findings Pain at McBurney's point; referred re-bound tenderness	TPR, slightly elevated CBC with differential, elevated, shift to left	Referral to internist, surgeon

PART A: CONTINUED

Possible Diagnosis	Historic Data	Physical Exam Data	Laboratory Data	Primary Care Management
	umbilical area to right lower quadrant Coughing increases pain Loss of appetite Nausea and vomiting Low-grade fever	Abdominal guarding, muscular rigidity Positive Rovsing's sign, psoas sign, obturator sign[b] Cutaneous hyper-esthesia[b]		
Other GI problem (e.g., gas, constipation, hernia, ulcer, intestinal problem)	Nausea and vomiting Diarrhea/constipation Relation to food intake Upper GI symptoms Blood in stool, dark stools, or other color change in stool	Absence of gynecologic findings	Stool for guaiac Refer for other specialized lab tests	Nutritional counseling Referral to internist
Other GU problem (e.g., kidney stones)	Vary with problem	Absence of gynecologic findings	All other labs normal	Referral as appropriate
Other nongynecologic problem (e.g., neurologic disorders, tuberculosis, sickle cell crisis, thrombophlebitis, arthritis)	Vary with problem	Absence of gynecologic findings	All other labs normal	Referral as appropriate
Psychogenic	Variable Stress or anxiety History of sexual or other abuse	Absence of gynecologic findings	All other labs normal	Pain diary Referral to internist for further diagnosis and/ or referral for psychological counseling

[a]Abbreviations used: LMP, last menstrual period; PMP, previous menstrual period; AB, abortion; D&C, dilation and curettage; β-hCG, β subunit of human chorionic gonadotropin; CVAT, costovertebral angle tenderness; UTI, urinary tract infection; CBC, complete blood count; PID, pelvic inflammatory disease; PMS, premenstrual syndrome; STD, sexually transmitted disease; IUD, intrauterine device; OC, oral contraceptive; TPR, temperature, pulse, and respiration; ESR, erythrocyte sedimentation rate; R/O, rule out; PROM, premature ruptures of membranes; CXR, chest x-ray; GI, gastrointestinal; GU, genitourinary.
[b]See Bates, B. (1987). *A guide to physical examination and history taking* (4th ed.; pp. 348–350). Philadelphia: J. B. Lippincott.

PART B: DIFFERENTIAL DIAGNOSIS OF VAGINAL DISCHARGE

Possible Diagnosis	Historic Data	Physical Exam Data	Laboratory Data	Primary Care Management
Normal vaginal discharge Leukorrhea	No associated odor, irritation, or other symptoms	Normal vaginal findings	Wet smear: normal flora Vaginal pH 3.5–4.5	Reassurance
Ovulatory mucus Pregnancy	Cyclicity of discharge Relation to LMP[a] Associated symptoms of ovulation	*Spinnbarkeit*		Teaching
	For pregnancy: See Part A: Differential Diagnosis of Lower Abdominal (Pelvic) Pain.			
Vaginitis Candidiasis (monilia or yeast)	Character of discharge: see next column Dyspareunia Mild to severe pruritus Vaginal hygiene: non-cotton underwear, pantyhose, tight clothing; frequent douching Recent antibiotic use Pregnancy/OC/steroid/ hormone use History of monilia Onset or increase of symptoms before menses Diabetes mellitus/obesity Immunosuppression	Discharge: thick or thin, white, adherent, "cottage-cheesy," musty odor Inflamed, friable cervix or vagina. Inflamed labia or perineum	Wet smear with KOH: pseudohyphae with yeast buds, WBCs Culture: Nickerson's medium Vaginal pH ≤ 4.5.	Antifungal vaginal preparations: 1–14 days Boric acid tablets Intravaginal *Lactobacillus acidophilus* as tablets or yogurt with active cultures Gentian violet Oral antifungal medications for resistance or frequent relapse Hygienic measures

continued

PART B: CONTINUED

Possible Diagnosis	Historic Data	Physical Exam Data	Laboratory Data	Primary Care Management
Trichomoniasis	Character of discharge: see next column Vaginal burning, pruritus, dyspareunia May have lower abdominal pain, cramps Sexual history: multiple partners, exposure Symptoms of UTI History of *Trichomonas* Use of hot tub, heated pools, whirlpool, shared towels Symptoms may increase during and after menses	Discharge: grayish-yellowish-green, frothy, odorous "Strawberry" cervix Inflamed, friable cervix or vagina Possible abdominal tenderness Possible lymphadenopathy	Wet smear with NaCl: motile flagellate trichomonads, WBCs Vaginal pH 5.2–6.0. Culture on simplified trypticase or Kupferberg medium (rarely necessary) Pap smear: may be unreliable	Oral metronidazole Partner(s) must be treated Abstinence or condoms during treatment Screen for other STDs
Bacterial vaginosis	May be asymptomatic May have mild pruritus or odorous discharge or just odor (partner may complain) Odor may be increased after intercourse	May have increased discharge: thin, homogeneous, milky, pooling of discharge at introitus Absence of inflammation	Wet smear with NaCl: positive clue cells; add KOH: fishy odor (positive whiff test) Culture (not useful): mixed flora, *Gardnerella* Vaginal pH > 4.5.	Oral metronidazole or ampicillin Garlic suppositories
Atrophic vaginitis	Perimenopausal Decreased vaginal lubrication	Pale, thin vaginal mucosa; few rugae; areas of punctate hemorrhage on mucosa Sparse, brittle pubic hair	Wet smear and cultures: negative Lack of lactobacilli Estrogen index on Pap smear low Maturation index: decreased superficial and intermediate cells Vaginal pH 5.5–7.0	Estrogen replacement therapy: local or systemic (with progesterone) Consultation as necessary Vaginal lubricants Psychosocial support
Gonorrhea	History of gonorrhea or other STDs Sexual history: multiple partners, exposure Symptoms in partner May have UTI symptoms	Normal findings or mucopurulent cervical or urethral discharge (with milking)	Gonorrhea culture: smears from cervix, urethra, anus and mouth as necessary on Thayer-Martin medium Gram stain: gram-negative intracellular diplococci; may not be accurate in women	Antibiotic therapy Partner(s) must be treated Screen for other STDs
Chlamydia trachomatis	History of gonorrhea or other STDs Sexual history: multiple partners, exposure Contraceptive history: OCs Nongonococcal or nonspecific urethritis in partner May have UTI symptoms History of infertility	Normal findings or mucopurulent cervical discharge May have friable, eroded cervix with ulcerations	Culture on transport medium Direct fluorescent antibody test or enzyme-linked immunoassay Gram strain: ≥ 10 WBCs per high-power field	Antibiotic therapy: generally tetracycline or doxycycline; erythromycin if allergic or pregnant Partner(s) must be treated Screen for other STDs
Herpes genitalis	Sexual history: multiple partners or exposure History of blisterlike lesions with prodrome Lesions on partner History of severe primary attack, possibly systemic Perineal pain, burning May have UTI symptoms	Normal findings if latent Reddened vesicular lesions, painful, tender Healing lesions appear as ulcerations Inguinal lymph adenopathy	Culture of lesion and its exudate on viral medium Pap smear Tzanck smear	No cure; Acyclovir ointment or oral tablets Counseling and emotional support Refer to support groups Avoid contact during attacks, from prodrome to healing Use of condoms Self-help measures Screen for other STDs

PART B: CONTINUED

Possible Diagnosis	Historic Data	Physical Exam Data	Laboratory Data	Primary Care Management
Bartholin's gland abscess	Tenderness in labial area; signs of infection: warmth, redness, swelling Possible systemic symptoms: fever, chills, malaise History of gonorrhea	Suppurating discharge in Bartholin's area Palpation of tender mass in area	TPR Culture of discharge Gonorrhea culture	Warm soaks, sitz baths, perineal hygiene Refer if febrile or abscess persists after local treatment Possible antibiotic therapy May need incision and drainage Screen for gonorrhea
Allergic reactions Dermatitis	Pruritus, burning Relation of symptoms to use of vaginal deodorants, powders, lotions, perfumes, soaps, detergents, contraceptive creams or foam, rubbers, colored or perfumed toilet paper, underwear, bubble bath, bath oils Recent change in any of above	Absence of other findings Vulvar rashes	Wet smear and cultures negative Possible positive patch test	Eliminate causative agent Possible referral to dermatologist
Foreign body	History of insertion of foreign body into vagina, including tampon Strong odor	Foreign body seen or palpated Strong foul odor Bloody, serosanguineous, or purulent discharge	Other findings absent	Removal
Trauma	History of trauma, sexual abuse, incest Bloody discharge Sexual practices reveal possible trauma	External or internal lesions Other bruises seen	Other findings absent	Local treatments Emotional support and counseling; referral as necessary Report sexual abuse if patient is minor
Salpingitis/pelvic inflammatory disease	See Part A: Differential Diagnosis of Lower Abdominal (Pelvic) Pain.			
Maligant neoplasm of lower genital tract	Associated with abnormal bleeding History of genital tract cancer Most have increased risk postmenopausally	Serous, mucoid, bloody, purulent, or thin, watery discharge May have superimposed infection with purulent, odorous discharge Lesions may be seen	Other findings absent	Referral for immediate diagnosis (including sonogram and biopsy) and appropriate treatment

[a]Abbreviations used: LMP, last menstrual period; WBCs, white blood cells; OC, oral contraceptive; UTI, urinary tract infection; STD, sexually transmitted disease; TPR, temperature, pulse, and respiration.

Index

Italicized letters following page numbers indicate tables (*t*), and figures (*f*).

Italicized letters following page numbers indicate tables (*t*), and figures (*f*).

Italicized letters following page numbers indicate tables (*t*), and figures (*f*).

Italicized letters following page numbers indicate tables (*t*), and figures (*f*).

Italicized letters following page numbers indicate tables (*t*), and figures (*f*).